Principles and Practice of Head and Neck Surgery and Oncology

Second edition

Edited by

Paul Q Montgomery BSC MB CHB FRCS (GEN. SURG.) FRCS (ORL)
Consultant Ear, Nose and Throat – Head & Neck/Thyroid Surgeon
Anglia East Head & Neck Cancer Center
Norfolk & Norwich University Teaching Hospital
Honorary Research Fellow
The School of Biological Sciences
University of East Anglia
Norwich
Norfolk
United Kingdom

Peter H Rhys Evans FRCS FACS DDC (Paris)
Consultant Otolaryngologist/Head & Neck Surgeon
Honorary Senior Lecturer, Institute of Cancer Research
Royal Marsden Hospital
London
United Kingdom

Patrick J Gullane, MB, FRCSC, FACS, FRACS (Hon)
Otolaryngologist-in-Chief, University Health Network
Wharton Chair Head and Neck Surgery
Professor and Chair, Department of Otolaryngology-Head and Neck Surgery
University of Toronto
Toronto, Ontario
Canada

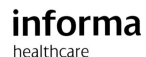

informa
healthcare

First published in the United Kingdom in 2009 by Informa Healthcare, Telephone House, 69-77 Paul Street, London EC2A 4LQ. Informa Healthcare is a trading division of Informa UK Ltd. Registered Office: 37/41 Mortimer Street, London W1T 3JH. Registered in England and Wales number 1072954.

Tel: +44 (0)20 7017 5000
Fax: +44 (0)20 7017 6699
Website: www.informahealthcare.com

A CIP record for this book is available from the British Library.
Library of Congress Cataloging-in-Publication Data

Data available on application

ISBN-10: 0 415 44412 8
ISBN-13: 978 0 415 44412 5

Distributed in North and South America by
Taylor & Francis
6000 Broken Sound Parkway, NW, (Suite 300)
Boca Raton, FL 33487, USA

Within Continental USA
Tel: 1 (800) 272 7737; Fax: 1 (800) 374 3401
Outside Continental USA
Tel: (561) 994 0555; Fax: (561) 361 6018
Email: orders@crcpress.com

Book orders in the rest of the world
Paul Abrahams
Tel: +44 (0)20 7017 4036
Email: bookorders@informa.com

Composition by Exeter Premedia Servies Private Ltd., Chennai, India
Printed and bound in India by Replika Press Pvt Ltd.

I would like to dedicate this book to my children Isabelle, Harry, and Jemima for their sacrifice of family time; to my family, friends, and colleagues for their support; and to the courage and dignity of my patients.

PQM

This book is dedicated to my wife Fran and our children Olivia, Sophie, and James who have been a source of inspiration and whose patience, encouragement, and support have been greatly appreciated. It is also dedicated to my patients whose courage and determination in the face of adversity inspire us to achieve improved chances of cure and a better quality of life.

PRE

I would like to dedicate this book to Bob and Gerardina Wharton for the generous support they provided us in establishing "The Wharton Head and Neck Centre," the endowment of three Chairs within the Princess Margaret Hospital/University of Toronto, and more recently the addition of further funds to support basic research in head and neck oncology. These contributions have helped enhance patient care, research, and education.

My thanks also to my most supportive and loving partner, Dr. Barbara Cruickshank; children, Kira and John for their patience, understanding, and sacrifice of family time' to my sister Anna and brothers Eamon and Tomas for your friendship. Finally, to my colleagues for their support of my vision and to my patients for the confidence they have placed in me.

PJG

Contents

Contributors

Nishant Agrawal MD, FACS
Fellow in Head and Neck Surgery
Department of Surgery
Head and Neck Service
Memorial Sloan-Kettering Cancer Center
1275 York Avenue
New York, New York, 10021, USA

Dr Jamil Asaria MD, BSC
Resident
Department of Otolaryngology—Head & Neck Surgery
University of Toronto
Toronto, M5S 1A1, Canada

Gideon Bachar MD
Fellow
Head and Neck Surgery
Departments of Otolaryngology/Surgical Oncology
Princess Margaret Hospital
Toronto, M5G 2M9, Canada

Alistair Balfour BSC, MBBS, FRCS(ORL-HNS)
Specialist Registrar Head and Neck Surgery
The Royal Marsden Hospital
Fulham Road
London, SW3 6JJ, United Kingdom

Emma Barker MBChB, PhD, FRCS(ORL-HNS)
Fellow
Head and Neck Surgery
Department of Otolaryngology-Head and Neck Surgery
Princess Margaret Hospital
University of Toronto
Toronto, M5G 2M9, Canada

Dr Shreerang A Bhide MRCP, FRCR
Clinical Research Fellow in Clinical Oncology
Head and Neck Unit
Royal Marsden Hospital
237 Fulham Road
London, SW3 6JJ, United Kingdom

Eric D Blom PhD
Speech Pathologist
Head and Neck Surgery Associates
Indianapolis, Indiana, 46204, USA

Dr Dominic Blunt FRCR, MRCP
Consultant Radiologist
Charing Cross Hospital
Fulham Palace Road
Imperial College Healthcare
London, W6 8RF, United Kingdom

Karen E Broadley MBBS, FRCP
Consultant in Palliative Medicine
Department of Palliative Medicine
Royal Marsden NHS Foundation Trust
Fulham Road
London, SW3 6JJ, United Kingdom

Christopher P Cottrill BSc, PhD, MRCP, FRCR
Consultant Clinical Oncologist
St Bartholomew's Hospital
West Smithfield
London, EC1A 7BE, United Kingdom

Aongus Curran MB, BCh(NUI), MD, FRCSI, FRCS(ORL-HNS)
Professor of Otolaryngology / Head & Neck Surgery
UCD School of Medicine & Medical Science
St. Vincent's University Hospital
Elm Park, Dublin 4, Éire

Pauline Doran-Williams RN, BSC, Dip HE Nursing Studies
Critical Care Unit
Royal Marsden Hospital
237 Fulham Road
London, SW3 6JJ, United Kingdom

Dr Raghav Chandra Dwivedi MBBS, MS(ORL-HNS)
Clinical Fellow
Head & Neck Unit
Royal Marsden Hospital
London, SW3 6JJ, United Kingdom

Robert L Ferris MD, PhD, FACS
Associate Professor
Vice-Chair for Clinical Operations
Chief
Division of Head and Neck Surgery
Departments of Otolaryngology and of Immunology
Co-Leader
Cancer Immunology Program
University of Pittsburgh Cancer Institute
5117 Centre Avenue
Hillman Cancer Center
Room 2.26b
Pittsburgh, Pennsylvania, 15213, USA

Dr Danny J Enepekides MD, FRCS(C)
Assistant Professor of Head and Neck Surgery
University of Toronto
Sunnybrook Health Sciences Center
Toronto, M4N 3M5, Canada

Mr Bill Fleming FRACS, FRCS
Endocrine Surgeon
Epworth Freemasons Hospital
East Melbourne, 3002, Australia

Arlene A Forastiere MD
Professor of Oncology
Sidney Kimmel Comprehensive Cancer Center
at Johns Hopkins and The Johns Hopkins
University School of Medicine
Baltimore, Maryland, 21205, USA

Ian Ganly BSC, MB, CHB, PhD FRCS(ED) FRCSORL)
Assistant Professor of Surgery
Cornell University Medical College
Assistant Attending Surgeon
Memorial Sloan-Kettering Cancer Center
1275 York Avenue
New York, New York, 10021, USA

Mr David T Gault MB, CHB, FRCS
Consultant Plastic Surgeon
London Centre for Ear Reconstruction
The Portland Hospital
London, W1W 5AH, United Kingdom

Jill Gilbert MD
Assistant Professor of Medicine
Division of Hematology/Oncology
Vanderbilt University School of Medicine
Nashville, Tennessee, 37232, USA

Ralph W Gilbert MD, FRCSC
Deputy Chief
Department of Otolaryngology-Head & Neck Surgery
University Health Network
Professor
Otolaryngology-Head & Neck Surgery
Surgical Oncology
Reconstructive Microsurgery
University of Toronto
Toronto General Hospital
200 Elizabeth Street
8N-879, Toronto, Ontario, M5G 2C4, Canada

David P Goldstein MD, FRCSC
Head and Neck Surgery/Surgical Oncology
Princess Margaret Hospital
University of Toronto
Toronto, Ontario, M5G 2M9, Canada

Patrick J Gullane MB, FRCSC, FACS, FRACS (Hon)
Otolaryngologist-in-Chief
University Health Network
Wharton Chair Head and Neck Surgery
Professor and Chair
Department of Otolaryngology-Head and Neck Surgery
University of Toronto
Toronto, Ontario, M5S 1A1, Canada

Dr Kevin J Harrington FRCP, FRCR, PhD
Senior Lecturer and Honorary Consultant in Clinical
Oncology
Head and Neck Unit
Royal Marsden Hospital
237 Fulham Road
London, SW3 6JJ, United Kingdom

Stefan OP Hofer MD, PhD, FRCS(C)
Wharton Chair in Reconstructive Plastic Surgery
Associate Professor
University of Toronto
Chief Division of Plastic Surgery
Department of Surgery and Department of Surgical
Oncology
University Health Network
200 Elizabeth Street
8N-865, Toronto, Ontario, M5G 2C4, Canada

Annabel Hooper RN Dip HE Nursing Studies
The Royal Marsden Head and Neck Unit
Royal Marsden Hospital
237 Fulham Road
London, SW3 6JJ, United Kingdom

Tihana Ibrahimpasic MD
Research Fellow in Head and Neck Surgery
Department of Surgery
Head and Neck Service
Memorial Sloan-Kettering Cancer Center
1275 York Avenue
New York, 10021, USA

Jonathan C Irish MD, MSc, FRCSC, FACS
The Kevin and Sandra Sullivan Chair in Surgical Oncology
University of Toronto
Chief
Department of Surgical Oncology
University Health Network and Mount Sinai Hospital
Professor
Department of Otolaryngology-Head and Neck Surgery
University of Toronto
610 University Av 3-954
Toronto, Ontario, M5G 2M9, Canada

Colm Irving MB, BCH, FRCA
Consultant in Anaestheria and Critical Care
Royal Marsden NHS Foundation Trust
London, United Kingdom

Dr Suzanne Kamel-Reid PhD, FACMG
Head
Laboratory Genetics and Director
Molecular Diagnostics
The University Health Network
Senior Scientist
The Ontario Cancer Institute
Professor
The University of Toronto
Dept of Pathology
The University Health Network
200 Elizabeth St
Toronto, Ontario, M5G 2C4, Canada

J John Kim MD, FRCPC
Radiation Oncology
Princess Margaret Hospital
University of Toronto
Toronto, Ontario, M5G 2M9, Canada

Jan S Lewin PhD
Associate Professor
Department of Head and Neck Surgery
Director
Section of Speech Pathology and Audiology
The University of Texas
M. D. Anderson Cancer Center
1515 Holcombe Boulevard
Department of Head and Neck Surgery Unit 1445
Houston, Texas 77030, USA

Fei-Fei Liu MD, FRCPC
Radiation Oncologist
Princess Margaret Hospital
Senior Scientist
Head of Applied Molecular Oncology Division
Ontario Cancer Institute
Dr Mariano Elia Chair in Head & Neck Oncology
Professor
Departments of Radiation Oncology
Medical Biophysics
and Otolaryngology
University of Toronto
Dept Radiation Oncology
5th Floor, 610 University Av
Toronto, Ontario, M5G 2M9, Canada

Valerie J Lund CBE
Professor of Rhinology
University College London and Honorary Consultant
ENT Surgeon
Royal National Throat
Nose & Ear Hospital (Royal Free NHS Trust)
330 Grays Inn Rd
London, WC1X 8DA, United Kingdom

John Lynn MS, FRCS
Consultant Endocrine Surgeon
Head of the Endocrine Surgical Unit
BUPA Cromwell Hospital
London, SW5 OUT, United Kingdom

Gitta Madani FRCR, MRCS, FDSRCS
Consultant Radiologist
Imperial College NHS Trust
St Mary's Hospital
Praed Street
London, WC2 INY, United Kingdom

Axel V Martin FRCR, MRCP
Specialist Registrar in Diagnostic Imaging
Royal Marsden Hospital Foundation Trust
203 Fulham Rd
London, SW3 6JJ, United Kingdom

Mr David Andrew Moffat BSc, MA(CANTAB),
MBBS, MRCS, LRCP, FRCS
Consultant in Otoneurological and Skull Base Surgery
Addenbrooke's Cambridge University Hospital NHS
Trust
Hills Road
Cambridge, CB2 0QQ, United Kingdom

Paul Q Montgomery BSc, MB, CHB, FRCS(GEN SURG) FRCS(ORL)
Consultant Ear
Nose and Throat – Head & Neck/Thyroid Surgeon
Anglia East Head & Neck Cancer Centre
Norfolk & Norwich University Teaching Hospital
Honary Reaserach Fellow
The School of Biological Sciences
University of East Anglia
Norwich, Norfolk, NR4 7T5, United Kingdom

Peter C Neligan MB, FRCS(I), FRCSC, FACS
Professor of Surgery
Director
Center for Reconstructive Surgery
University of Washington Medical Center
1959 NE Pacific St
Box 356410,
Seattle, Washington, 98195-6410, USA

Dr Kate Newbold MRCP, FRCR, MD
Consultant in Clinical Oncology
Head and Neck Unit
Royal Marsden Hospital
Downs Road
Sutton, SM2 5PT, United Kingdom

Christine B Novak PT, MSC, PhD(c)
Research Associate
Wharton Head & Neck Centre
University Health Network
200 Elizabeth Street
8N-875
Toronto, Ontario, M5G 2C4, Canada

Dr Christopher M Nutting FRCP, FRCR, MD
Consultant and Reader in Clinical Oncology
Head and Neck Unit
Royal Marsden Hospital
Fulham Road
London, SW3 6JJ, United Kingdom

Christopher J O'Brien AM, MS, MD, FRCS, FRACS
Dept of Head and Neck Surgery
Sydney Cancer Centre
Royal Prince Alfred Hospital and University of Sydney
Sydney, N5W 2050, Australia

Brian O'Sullivan MD, FRCPC, FFRRCSI(Hons)
Bartley-Smith/Wharton Chair in Radiation Oncology
Professor
University of Toronto
Head and Neck Program Leader
Radiation Oncology Sarcoma Program Leader
Princess Margaret Hospital
University of Toronto
Toronto, Ontario, M5G 2M9, Canada

Nitin A Pagedar MD
Assistant Professor
Department of Otolaryngology - Head and Neck Surgery
University of Iowa
Iowa City, Iowa, 52292, USA

Rajan S Patel MBChB, MD, FRCS(ORL-HNS)
Consultant Otolaryngologist
Head & Neck Microvascular Reconstructive Surgeon
Honorary Senior Lecturer
Auckland City Hospital
University of Auckland
Auckland, 1142, New Zealand

Snehal G Patel MD, MS, FRCS(Glas)
Associate Professor of Surgery
Cornell University Medical College
Associate Attending Surgeon
Memorial Sloan-Kettering Cancer Center
1275 York Avenue
New York, New York, 10021, USA

Caroline E Payne MBBS, MSC, FRCS(plast)
Reconstructive microsurgery fellow
Division of Plastic Surgery
University Health Network
200 Elizabeth Street
Toronto, Ontario, M5G 2C4, Canada

Frances Rhys Evans RGN ITUCERT ONCCERT MSC
106 Harley Street
London, W1N 1AF, United Kingdom

Peter H Rhys Evans FRCS, FACS, DDC(Paris)
Consultant Otolaryngologist/Head & Neck Surgeon
Honorary Senior Lecturer
Institute of Cancer Research
Royal Marsden Hospital
203 Fulham Road
London, SW3 6JJ, United Kingdom

Kevin Russell RN, BSC, DIP, HE BSC (Hons) Cancer Nursing
Critical Care Unit
Royal Marsden Hospital
237 Fulham Road
London, SW3 6JJ, United Kingdom

Andrew CH See MMed(SURG), FRCSED, FRCSGlas
Senior Consultant Head & Neck Surgeon
Gleneagles Hospital 6
Napier Road
Singapore 258500

Jatin P Shah MD MS(Surg)FACS Hon FRCS(Ed) Hon FRACS
Hon FDSRCS(Lond)
Professor of Surgery
Cornell University Medical College
Chief
Head and Neck Service
EW Strong Chair in Head and Neck Oncology
Memorial Sloan-Kettering Cancer Center
1275 York Avenue
New York, New York, 10021, USA

Ashok Shaha MD, FACS
Professor of Surgery
Cornell University Medical College
Attending Surgeon
Memorial Sloan-Kettering Cancer Center
1275 York Avenue
New York, New York, 10021, USA

Kerwin F Shannon MB, BS, FRACS
Dept of Head and Neck Surgery
Sydney Cancer Centre
Royal Prince Alfred Hospital and University of Sydney
Sydney, N5W 2050, Australia

Dr Bhuey Sharma BSC (Hons) BM, FRCR
Consultant Radiologist
The Royal Marsden Hospital NHS Trust
London and Surrey Branches
United Kingdom

Clare Shaw PhD, RD
Consultant Dietitian
The Royal Marsden NHS Foundation Trust
237 Fulham Road
London, SW3 6JJ, United Kingdom

Patrick Sheahan MB, ChB, FRCSI
Fellow in Head and Neck Surgery
Department of Surgery
Head and Neck Service
Memorial Sloan-Kettering Cancer Center
1275 York Avenue
New York, NY 10021, USA

Catherine South RN, Dip HE Nursing Studies, BA (Hons)
The Royal Marsden Head and Neck Unit
Royal Marsden Hospital
237 Fulham Road
London, SW3 6JJ, United Kingdom

Jeffrey D Spiro MD
Department of Surgery
Division of Otolaryngology/Head and Neck Surgery
University of Connecticut School of Medicine
263 Farmington Avenue
MC 6228
Farmington, Connecticut, 06030, USA

Ronald H Spiro MD
Department of Clinical Surgery
Cornell University Medical College
Head and Neck Service
Memorial Sloan-Kettering Cancer Center
1275 York Avenue
New York, New York, 10021, USA

Hin Ngan Tay MB CHB FRCS
Fellow in Head and Neck Surgery
Department of Surgery
Head and Neck Service
Memorial Sloan-Kettering Cancer Center
1275 York Avenue
New York, New York, 10021, USA

Nicola Tinne RN DIP HE Nursing Studies, BSc Cancer Nursing
The Royal Marsden Head and Neck Unit
Royal Marsden Hospital
237 Fulham Road
London, SW3 6JJ, United Kingdom

Robert M Tuttle MD, FACP
Attending Physician
Endocrinology Service
Department of Medicine
Memorial Sloan-Kettering Cancer Center
1275 York Avenue
New York, New York, 10021, USA

William Ignace Wei MS, FRCS, FRCSE, FRACS(Hon), FACS, FHKAM(ORL)(SURG)
Li Shu Pui Professor of Surgery
Chair in Otorhinolaryngology
Room 206
Professorial Block
Queen Mary Hospital
Pokfulam Road, Hong Kong

Dr John E Williams MBBS, FRCA, FFPMRCA
Consultant in Anaesthesia and Pain Medicine
Royal Marsden NHS Foundation Trust
Fulham Road
London, SW3 6JJ, United Kingdom

Ian J Witterick MD, MSc, FRCSC
Associate Professor and Vice Chair
Director of Postgraduate Education
Department of Otolaryngology-Head & Neck Surgery
University of Toronto
Ontario, M5G 2C4, Canada

Robert E Wood DDS, MDC, PhD, FRCD(C)
Associate Professor and Head
Department of Dental Oncology
Ocular and Maxillofacial prosthetics
Princess Margaret Hospital
610 University Avenue
Toronto, Ontario, M5G 2M9, Canada

Foreword

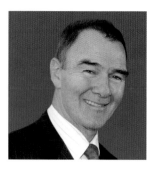

It is an honor to have been invited to contribute the Foreword to a textbook edited by colleagues whom I admire and respect and who have, in their particular ways, made an enormous contribution to the discipline of head and neck oncology. The list of contributors reads like a who's who of leaders and experts from a variety of backgrounds and many of whom I know as personal friends. It is with humility and ambivalence, therefore, that I make the following observations and comments.

A foreword should provide some context, be it historical, scientific, or philosophical, to the body of work that follows and should, moreover, induce in the reader a feeling of inquisitiveness and even excitement about the contents of the book and perhaps also a sense of satisfaction the money outlaid for the particular volume has been well spent.

I write now from a unique position, having retired from my head and neck practice prematurely following the diagnosis in November 2006 of a malignant brain tumor. It is a great gift to have been able to spend the last 20 or so years of my life treating patients with tumors and cancers of the head and neck and to now experience the vicissitudes of life as a patient.

Among the many lessons I have learned during my own cancer journey, I have been impressed with the following: first, the importance of delivering bad news to patients and their carers and families in a compassionate and gentle way. Patients these days increasingly want—and need—to know the facts about their disease, their prognosis, and the risks and benefits of the various treatment options. It is of little benefit however, to bludgeon a patient or family with statistics because it is almost impossible to apply a percentage likelihood of survival to an individual patient in a meaningful way, and to deny patients hope is utterly counterproductive.

This does not diminish in any way the importance of, and in fact the absolute necessity for, clinicians collecting their own treatment and outcome data so that information given to patients is relevant, not only to that individual's disease, but also to reflect the outcomes deliverable by the particular clinician, team, and institution.

The second point is that patients will seek their own information and additional medical opinions if their questions are not answered honestly and coherently. The ready accessibility of information on the Internet has contributed to patients being more informed than ever but this does not mean that they are necessarily able to assimilate and make effective use of the information available to them. The advice, wise counsel, and gentle guidance of experienced and compassionate clinicians are more important than ever.

Third, we are all now aware that the complimentary and alternative medicine industry is a multi-billion-dollar maze into which patients are increasingly willing to enter in the hope they will find remedies that may fill the many gaps left by conventional treatment or that may offset the complications and toxicity caused by conventional therapy. Our obligation to support our patients through their treatment has never been greater.

These comments are applicable not simply to head and neck oncology but to all cancer disciplines, particularly where rare, poor prognosis, and advanced stage cancers are concerned.

The second edition of this textbook excels once again in addressing the fundamentals of biology, epidemiology, investigation, and management of tumors and cancers of the head and neck. That patients beset with head and neck cancer require multidisciplinary evaluation and treatment is now such a truism that few currently practicing clinicians could imagine offering their patients anything but evidence-based treatment that reflected the consensus view of a multidisciplinary team that includes surgeons, radiation and medical oncologists, and allied health professionals representing nursing, speech pathology, psycho-oncology, dietetics and nutrition, and physiotherapy.

The pages of this book are filled with innumerable facts, educational pearls, treatment recommendations, and instructive diagrams. I commend the editors for their diligent efforts and the contributors for the honesty, clarity, and thoroughness of their work.

Finally, I want to recommend to the reader, whether that person is in training or practicing as a specialist, that this textbook deserves a thorough and deep reading. Armed with the knowledge and advice contained in these pages practicing clinicians should feel confident that they can offer to their patients the very best in medical care. To that I can only add my hope that all such care is given with compassion, gentleness, and humanity.

Professor Christopher J O'Brien AM MS MD FRCS FRACS
Former Director, Sydney Cancer Centre,
Royal Prince Alfred Hospital and University of Sydney
Sydney, Australia
2008-06-03

Preface

On a worldwide scale head and neck malignancy represents the 5th most common cancer and nowhere in the field of human oncology are the effects of progression of disease more readily apparent, more cosmetically deforming, and more functionally and psychologically disturbing than in this region. Unlike cancer at other sites in the body it is not a disease of one organ but it includes a wide variety of tumors affecting not only the diversity of upper aerodigestive tract organs such as the tongue, pharynx, larynx, nose, and ear, but also other related structures including the thyroid, salivary glands, skull base, skin, and lymphatics of the head and neck.

During the last 30 years progress in head and neck cancer therapy has not only benefited from an increased understanding of the molecular genetics of tumor growth and lymphatic metastatic spread, but also from a better knowledge of epidemiological and etiological factors. At the same time, cohort and accurate population-based studies have helped to identify more precisely the incidence and changing trends in head and neck cancer. Great progress has also been made in the field of diagnosis with refinement of computerized tomography (CT), magnetic resonance imaging (MRI), and positron emission tomography (PET), as well as greater use of cytology and endoscopic techniques.

A greater understanding of the clinico-pathological correlation of tumor types, tumor invasion, and patterns of spread have allowed clinicians to plan combined management for each individual patient in a more practical and objective fashion.

We have also seen a fundamental change in attitude and philosophy of patient management in the last two decades from one of prescriptive tumor treatment to a much more considered and holistic approach taking greater account of quality of life issues. This has been made possible by increased use of conservation laser and other surgical techniques as well as chemo-radiotherapeutic regimes in appropriate settings. Early patient rehabilitation following surgery has been greatly enhanced by developments in one-stage reconstructive techniques and a better understanding of the functional requirements and limitations of speech and swallowing rehabilitation.

We are indebted to the contributors to this 2nd edition which has been substantially rewritten and updated with many new authors. The combined experience and multidisciplinary philosophy is reflected in giving a broad, comprehensive and balanced view of current approaches to management of head and neck neoplasms. We hope that the book will be of value to established head & neck specialists and provide a knowledge base for trainees.

PQM
PRE
PJG

Acknowledgements

I would like to express my appreciation for the following colleagues who helped in reviewing many of the chapters and assisting in other aspects of the production of this book: Rosina Ali, Allan Bardsley, Andrew Bath, Barbara Blagnys, Tim Bradnam, Jonathan Clibbon, Erica Everitt, Jonathan Harrowven, Nichola Holton, Francesca Howe, Richard James, David Lowe, John Philips, Helena Macey, Marc Moncrieff, David Premachandra, Kate Richardson, Tom Roques, Denise Smith, Beth Southard, Michael Thomas, Paddy Wilson and Nicholas Woodhall. I would also like to thank our medical illustrator Ann Lush and medical photographer Michael Smith for their work.

PQM

We would like to express our appreciation to Informa Heathcare and in particular Kelly Cornish who has overseen the production of this book. The artists have made an invaluable contribution. We would like to express our appreciation of our secretarial support from Karen Thorp, Ann Dymond and Kathleen Nicholson.

PQM
PRE
PJG

1

Head and Neck Malignancy: An Overview

Alistair Balfour, Peter H Rhys Evans and Snehal G Patel

INTRODUCTION

On a worldwide scale head and neck malignancy represents the 5th most common cancer. However, it is not a single entity but encompasses a wide range of malignant tumors arising from many diverse and complex structures in this region of the body. The sites of origin are the upper aerodigestive tract (UADT), salivary, thyroid, and parathyroid glands and paranasal sinuses. The locally destructive effects of these tumors, or their treatment, can have a devastating effect on the lives of patients by affecting their outward appearance; the four senses of sight, smell, taste, and hearing; and the vital functions of breathing, swallowing, and talking. The complexity of the anatomical structures and functions affected present a difficult challenge to health services and require a wide variety of medical and allied specialities to ablate disease and restore function.

Primary referral of head and neck cancer may be to one of a number of specialists [ear, nose, and throat, oromaxillofacial, plastic or general surgeon, physician or medical oncologist] any of whom may take charge of management of the patient, although few are head and neck cancer specialists. This dissemination of cases, coupled with the heterogeneous nature and relative rarity of tumors at each individual site means that UADT cancer invariably forms only a small portion of the workload of these disciplines, severely restricting the experience and expertise of the individual clinician. Clinicians subspecializing in the management of head and neck cancers readily acknowledge that optimal treatment, survival, and rehabilitation can only be achieved with a detailed understanding of the anatomy, pathology, and natural history of the disease, concentrated experience in its management, and constant updating of knowledge from audit of results and published research. The management of these tumors presents a major challenge and should ideally be undertaken by an experienced multidisciplinary team with adequate resources for optimal investigation, treatment, and rehabilitation. In many countries, however, resources are very limited and the possibility of curative radiotherapy or expert surgical treatment is only available to a small minority of patients; nevertheless, great strides have been made in the last few decades to disseminate knowledge and expertise through teaching and publications as well as world health initiatives. The focus of this chapter is cancers of the UADT, but we recognize that head and neck skin cancer is a major subgroup that is discussed in separate chapters in this book.

EPIDEMIOLOGY

Incidence

The incidence of head and neck cancer varies considerably around the world from 5 to 45 per 100,000 (Figs. 1.1 and 1.2) (1). In the U.S.A., head and neck squamous cell carcinomas (HNSCC) account for 45,660 new cases: 3% of all new cancers and 11,210 deaths per year. Thyroid cancer accounts for 33,550 new cases: 2% of all new cancers, but only 1530 deaths per year (2). In England and Wales, HNSCC accounts for 6820 new cases: 3% of all new cancers and 2460 deaths per year; and thyroid cancer accounts for 1190 new cases: 0.5% of all new cancers and 260 deaths per year (3,4).

About 90% of these tumors are squamous cell carcinomas arising from the surface epithelium of the UADT, and as such they do have many common features concerning their aetiology, natural history, and classification. There are however great differences in modes of presentation and treatment depending on the individual sites within the head and neck. Worldwide, the oral cavity is the most common site of head and neck cancer (274,000 cases) and ranks as the 12th most common cancer, while cancers of the larynx, pharynx, thyroid, and nasopharynx are less common (Table 1.1) (5). However, if the HNSCCs were grouped together with thyroid cancers (784,882 cases), they would rank as the 5th most common cancer.

For HNSCCs, the male:female ratio varies from 2 to 15:1 depending on the anatomical subsite and geographical area. For thyroid cancers, the ratio is reversed with a male: female ratio of 1:3. Although head and neck cancer has higher rates in areas of deprivation within well-developed countries, it is less common in developing countries. As can be seen in Figure 1.3 (5), it is only the subsets of oral cancer in women and nasopharyngeal cancer that are more common in less developed countries.

These wide variations in the incidence of individual tumors in each country and around the world may be due to ethnic, industrial, environmental, and social influences. Oral cancer has high rates of incidence in Western Europe, India, South Africa, and Australia (Fig. 1.4) (5). There is a particularly high incidence of oral cavity cancer in males in France (Manche, Bas-Rhin, and Calvados) whereas in females the highest incidence is in India. Sharp increases in incidence of oral and pharyngeal cancer have been reported in Germany, Denmark, Scotland, Central and Eastern Europe (6). This increase is thought to be due to an increase in alcohol consumption in these groups as mean

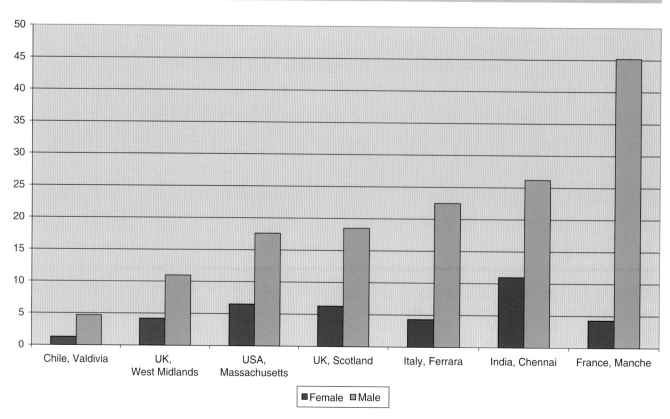

Figure 1.1   World variations in incidence of head and neck cancer (excluding thyroid) (per 100,000). *Source*: From Ref. 1.

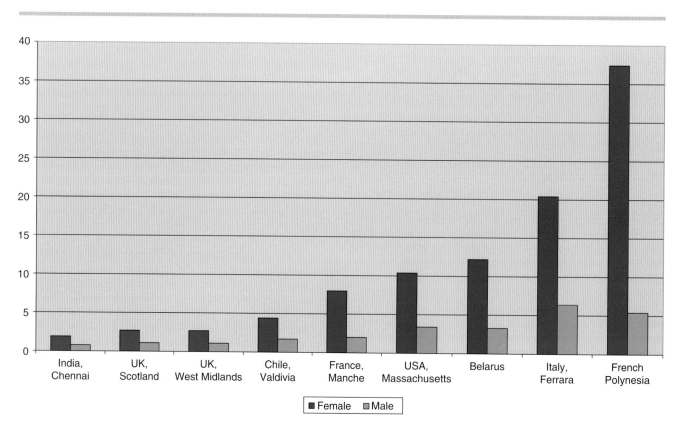

Figure 1.2   World variations in incidence of thyroid cancer (per 100,000). *Source*: From Ref. 1.

Table 1.1 Incidence and Mortality of Cancer Worldwide 2002 (5)

Rank	Cancer	Number of cases	Deaths
1	Lung	1,352,132	1,178,918
2	Breast	1,151,298	410,712
3	Colon and rectum	1,023,152	528,978
4	Stomach	933,937	700,349
5	Prostate	679,023	221,002
6	Liver	626,162	598,321
7	Cervix uteri	493,243	273,505
8	Oesophagus	462,117	385,892
9	Bladder	356,557	145,009
10	Non-Hodgkin lymphoma	300,571	171,820
11	Leukaemia	300,522	222,506
12	Oral cavity	274,289	127,459
13	Pancreas	232,306	227,023
14	Kidney etc.	208,480	101,895
15	Ovary etc.	204,499	124,860
16	Corpus uteri	198,783	50,327
17	Brain, nervous system	189,485	141,650
18	Melanoma of skin	160,177	40,781
19	Larynx	159,241	89,956
20	Thyroid	141,013	35,375
21	Other pharynx	130,296	83,993
22	Multiple myeloma	85,704	62,535
23	Nasopharynx	80,043	50,332
24	Hodgkin lymphoma	62,329	22,812
25	Testis	48,613	8,878

tar-adjusted cigarette consumption and lung cancer rates have been falling (7).

It is well recognized that nasopharyngeal cancer has especially high rates in southern China and Hong Kong with moderate rates in South East Asia, North Africa, and the Inuits of Canada and Alaska (Fig. 1.5) (5). Laryngeal cancer has higher rates in southern Europe (France, Italy, Spain), eastern Europe (Russia, Ukraine), South America, and western Asia (6). Laryngeal cancer rates have been remaining stable. Thyroid cancer has higher rates in U.S.A. and western Europe with pockets of high incidence in French Polynesia and Belarus (Fig. 1.2). The incidence of thyroid cancer has been increasing in developing countries, but the mortality rates have been decreasing.

Deprivation Effect

Significantly higher rates of UADT cancer are seen in areas of deprivation. The risk decreases by 40% in Canada and 29% in the U.S.A. as the level of average community income doubles (8). Within the U.K. there are regional variations in head and neck cancer incidence, with quite a marked increasing gradient from the relatively affluent South to the less affluent North (Fig. 1.6) (1). If the incidence of UADT cancer in all social classes was the same as the incidence in the highest affluence classes, there

would be 1430 fewer cases of UADT cancer associated with 710 fewer deaths within England and Wales alone (Table 1.2) (9,10).

AETIOLOGY

It has become increasingly apparent over recent years that the state of our health, and in particular the risks of developing cancer, depend to a large extent on our environment and our personal habits. We are being constantly reminded of the deterioration of the worldwide environment that affects us all, and our daily exposure to a number of pollutants. The majority of these pollutants are either ingested or inhaled, and initial exposure is therefore to the UADT (11). Smoking and drinking are understandably considered the most important aetiological agents (12,13) as is indicated by a great deal of clinical evidence, but less information is available on other factors such as pollutants, occupational agents, diet, viral infections and genetic influences (Table 1.3) (11,14–16).

Tobacco and alcohol are the main risk factors for UADT squamous carcinoma, and in about 90% of patients there is a history of smoking or another form of tobacco use such as chewing. Smoking tobacco is the most common aetiological factor, and the relative risks are the same for pipes and cigars as for cigarettes. The risk is increased with increased duration and intensity of smoking. Reverse smoking (in which the lit end of the cigarette is placed in the mouth so that an intense heat is experienced) is a risk factor for cancer of the hard palate (6). Alcohol is an independent risk factor but also shows significant synergy when combined with smoking in those exposed parts of the UADT (oral cavity, oropharynx, hypopharynx, and supraglottic larynx) (18,51–53). Heavy drinkers who are heavy smokers have a 35 times increased risk of oral cancer compared to those who neither drink nor smoke (54). This may be due to increased mucosal absorption of the carcinogens in tobacco from chronic inflammation and hyperaemia as well as increased solubility of the carcinogens in alcohol compared with aqueous saliva. Cessation of smoking reduces the risk of UADT cancer, and by 10 years, the risk is equal to nonsmokers (18).

Smokeless tobacco is an important risk factor for oral cancer. Chewing tobacco, oral snuff, *khaini* (oral tobacco and lime), and betel quid with tobacco are associated with a two- to sixfold increased risk of oral cancer. Betel quid with tobacco has a strong association with the development of oral leukoplakia, submucous fibrosis, and lichen planus. The role of betel quid without tobacco is not clear. Animal studies have shown that rats exposed to oral moist snuff show an increased incidence of oral, nasal, lip, and stomach cancer (55,56). Two tobacco specific nitrosamines, NNN (N-nitrosonornicotine) and NNK [4-(methylnitrosamino)-1-(3-pyridyl)-1-butanone] have been shown to independently induce oral cancers in rats (56).

A poor diet low in vegetables and fruit is a risk factor for oral cancer (57). This is supported by studies showing that a diet high in fruit and vegetables has a protective effect (20–60% reduction in risk) (6). A high intake of salted meat and fish has been shown to be an important cofactor in the development of nasopharyngeal cancer, but the mechanism is unknown (49).

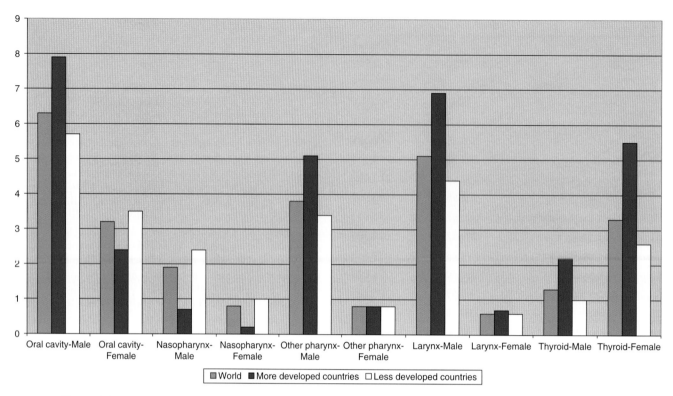

Figure 1.3 Incidence of head and neck cancers in more and less developed countries (per 100,000). *Source*: From Ref. 5.

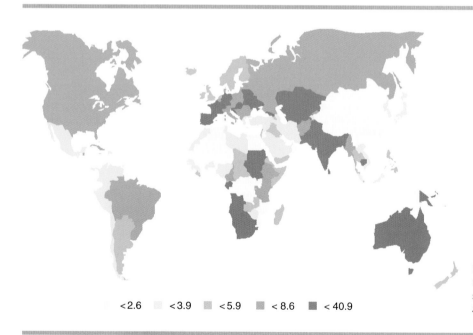

<2.6   <3.9   <5.9   <8.6   < 40.9

Figure 1.4 Worldwide variations in male incidence of oral cavity cancer (age-standardized incidence rate per 100,000). *Source*: From Ref. 5.

There is very strong evidence that Epstein Barr virus (EBV) has a major role in the development of undifferentiated nasopharyngeal carcinoma (UCNT) in high-risk populations (especially southern China). High levels of Immunoglobulin A (IgA) antibody to EBV capsid are associated with UCNT. EBV DNA and viral proteins are found in malignant cells but not in normal nasopharyngeal mucosa, and the viral DNA is present in a monoclonal form and is present in every malignant cell (49). There is also a genetic susceptibility to nasopharyngeal cancer as first- and second-generation Chinese migrants retain an elevated risk.

Human papilloma virus (HPV) 16 has been strongly implicated in UADT cancer. In a review of more than 5000 UADT cancer specimens, HPV DNA was found in 36% of

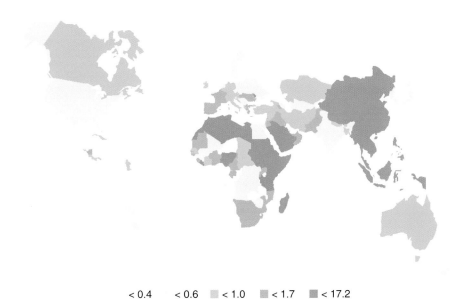

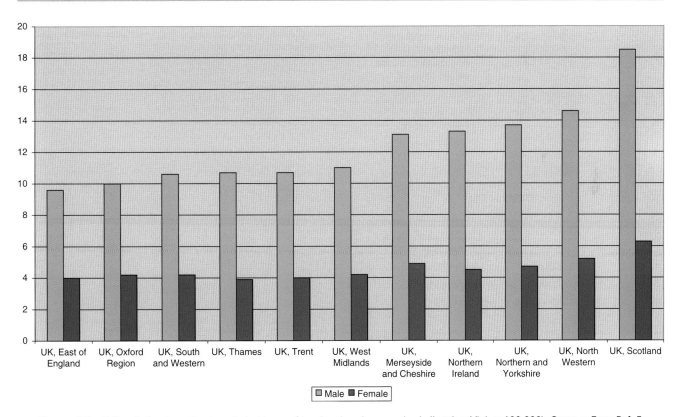

Figure 1.5 Worldwide variations in male incidence of nasopharyngeal cancer. *Source*: From Ref. 5.

< 0.4   < 0.6   < 1.0   < 1.7   < 17.2

Figure 1.6 U.K. variation by region in male incidence of head and neck cancer (excluding thyroid) (per 100,000). *Source*: From Ref. 5.

oropharyngeal tumors (of which 87% were HPV16), 24% of oral cavity tumours (68% HPV16) and 24% of laryngeal tumours (69% HPV16) (48). In comparison, HPV16 is found in only 9% of normal tonsillar tissue. HPV16 DNA integrates into the human genome at random sites and upregulates HPV oncogenes E6 and E7 (47).

There is also evidence of genetically based susceptibility and predisposition for the development of UADT cancer in patients without necessarily any history of tobacco or alcohol exposure (11). Mutagen sensitivity, which is a measure of an individual's intrinsic DNA repair capacity against free radical damage, has been demonstrated as a

Table 1.2 Number of Preventable Cases of, and Deaths from, Selected Cancers Related to Socioeconomic Deprivation in England and Wales

Site	Preventable cases			Preventable deaths		
	Male	Female	Total	Male	Female	Total
Larynx	620		620	290		290
Lip, mouth, and pharynx	710	100	810	380	40	420

The number of preventable cases/deaths is calculated as the difference between the average age-specific rate in deprivation categories 1 and 2 and the rate in each of the other deprivation categories (3 to 20), multiplied by the population in each category, summed across age groups and deprivation categories. *Source*: From Ref. 9.

Table 1.3 Aetiological Factors in Head and Neck Cancer

	Agent	Site(s)
Social	Tobacco	Oral cavity, oropharynx, hypopharynx, larynx, cervical oesophagus (12), lip, sinonasal (17,18)
	Alcohol	Oral cavity, oropharynx, hypopharynx, larynx (supraglottis), cervical oesophagus (13)
Occupational	Asbestos	Larynx (13,19–21)
	Man-made fibers	Larynx, pharynx, oral cavity (22)
	Textiles	Larynx, pharynx, oral cavity (23)
	Wood workers	Nasal cavity/sinuses (24), larynx (25), nasopharynx
	Plastics	Larynx (resins (26), rubber) (23)
		Oral cavity and pharynx (vinyl chloride) (27)
	Mustard gas	Larynx (28)
	Naphthalene	Larynx (glottic) (29)
	CME and BCME	Larynx (30)
	Pesticides	Larynx (31)
	Alcohol manufacture	Larynx (30), oral cavity and pharynx (32)
	Sulphuric acid	Larynx (32,33)
	Leatherworkers	Oral cavity, pharynx, larynx (34)
	Paint and print	Larynx (35), oral cavity (36), pharynx (35)
	Car mechanics	Larynx (25,37), oral cavity (37)
	Nickel refiners	Larynx (15,38)
	Metal workers	Larynx (35,39), Tonsil, pharynx and alveolus (36)
	Coal and stone dust	Larynx (21,30)

(Continued)

Table 1.3 Aetiological Factors in Head and Neck Cancer *(Continued)*

	Agent	Site(s)
	Cement and concrete	Larynx(39)
	Farmers	Larynx (30,39)
	Bartenders	Larynx (30,40)
Radiation	Accidental	
	Chernobyl	Paediatric thyroid (41)
	Occupational	
	Watch dial makers	Osteosarcoma of the jaw (42)
	Therapeutic	
	Acne, tinea etc.	Sarcomas (43,44)
		Thyroid (45)
	Thorotrast	Larynx, non-Hodgkin's lymphoma (46)
Genetic predisposition		UADT cancer (11)
Viral agents	HPV 16	Oral cavity, pharynx, larynx (16,47,48)
	HPV 6,11	Larynx (verrucous) (47)
	EBV	Nasopharynx (49)
Atmospheric pollution		Pharynx, larynx (50)

Abbreviations: CME, chloromethyl methyl ether; BCME, bischloro methyl ether; UADT, upper aerodigestive tract; HPV, human papilloma virus; EBV, epstein barr virus.

risk factor in the disease. A low intake of vitamins C and E was also associated with an increased risk, and when both factors were evident, patients were at greatest risk. This supports the concept that the risk of head and neck cancer is determined by a balance of factors that either enhance or protect against free radical oxygen damage, including innate capacities for DNA repair (11). Conditions carrying increased risk of head and neck cancer include DNA repair deficiency syndromes such as Bloom's syndrome, ataxia telangiectasia, Fanconi anaemia, xeroderma pigmentosum and epithelial differentiation disorders, such as dyskeraosis congenital (6).

There is good evidence that head and neck tumorigenesis proceeds through serial acquisition of genetic and phenotypic events in a stepwise manner from normal tissue to dysplasia to carcinoma in situ to invasive carcinoma to metastatic carcinoma. These events include activation of oncogenes and inactivation of tumor-suppressor genes, leading to unchecked neoplastic cell growth (58). This model helps to explain the concept of field change because cells within a mucosal area exposed to the same carcinogens and with the same mutagen sensitivity can simultaneously have advanced along one or more of these steps. The chance of developing a second primary cancer in UADT cancer is estimated at 2–3% per year and is increased by continuing exposure to carcinogens such as continued smoking.

NATURAL HISTORY

The natural history of the disease should provide the opportunity for successful intervention. The majority of head and neck cancers progress in a relatively orderly fashion, from a small primary tumor to a larger lesion and lymph node metastases. This direct size relationship generally holds true for sites such as the oral cavity and larynx; but for other sites such as the nasopharynx, oropharynx, and to a lesser extent the hypopharynx, neck metastases are seen just as frequently with T1 as with T4 lesions. Indeed the nasopharynx and oropharynx are the most commont sites of origin of the apparent "occult primary" (Table 1.4).

Distant metastases are nearly always a sequel to advanced nodal disease and remain a relatively uncommon feature, although now occurring rather more frequently as local treatment becomes more successful, as are second UADT primaries. Although distant metastases have been found at autopsy in up to 40% of fatal cases (59) progressive local disease often dominates the clinical picture during the final stages of the illness. Uncontrolled disease in the head and neck is distressing for the patient and carers, so successful elimination of the primary tumor and neck node metastases is of paramount importance. This requires early diagnosis, accurate assessment of the extent of the tumor, and radical treatment. In this respect the skill of the treating clinicians can make the difference between success and failure.

The importance of early diagnosis in UADT cancer cannot be overemphasized as survival rates rapidly diminish as the stage of tumor advances (Table 1.5) (2). Five-year survival rates fall from over 80% to approximately 50% when the disease advances from the primary site to local

Table 1.4 Relationship of Tumor Size (T) and Node Metastases (N)

Direct size relation

  Larynx

  Oral cavity

  Salivary glands

  Lip

  Nasal cavity and sinuses

No size relation

  Oropharynx

  Nasopharynx

  Hypopharynx

  Thyroid

Table 1.5 Five-Year Relative Survival Rates in U.S.A. by Extent of Disease at Diagnosis, 1996–2002 (2)

Site	All Stages %	Local %	Regional %	Distant %
Larynx	64.1	83.5	50.4	13.7
Oral cavity & pharynx	58.8	81.3	51.6	26.4
Thyroid	96.7	99.7	96.9	56.4

lymph nodes. In thyroid cancer, however, regional spread of disease generally has little effect on survival.

However, successful curative treatment of more advanced head and neck cancers may involve severe disturbance of function and/or obvious deformity. Also, many head and neck cancer patients present in poor general health because of other smoking and alcohol-related problems and may not be able to withstand very aggressive treatment. Therefore, the choice of treatment must take all these factors into account together with the wishes of the patients and their family. It is for the patients to decide whether they want the greatest possible chance of cure despite loss of an organ, for example, their larynx, or the possibility of organ preservation with a slightly lower chance of survival.

TREATMENT
Therapeutic Developments

Surgical excision of the tumor or cautery were historically the only effective methods of treatment until the early 1900s when the introduction of radium was shown to not only shrink tumors but also to eliminate some completely. The concept of combining the curative effects of surgery and radiotherapy was a logical progression introduced in the 1920s. In 1929 a report from Sweden compared the results of treatment using either radiotherapy alone or preoperatively for oral cancers and cervical metastases (60). None of the patients treated with radiotherapy alone was disease free at 5 years compared with 40% in the group treated with combined preoperative radiation and surgery. Orthovoltage irradiation dominated treatment until the 1930s curing possibly 25% of oral, pharyngeal, and laryngeal cancers (61). It became employed more commonly postoperatively, although the long-term morbidity and skin damage caused by orthovoltage was becoming apparent. As a result many oncologists reserved radiotherapy for recurrence or for palliation (62).

In the 1940s a resurgence of surgical treatment was pioneered by Hayes Martin at Memorial Hospital in New York. He introduced the concept of radical excision of the primary tumor and neck disease where feasible. This was made possible only because of improvements made in anaesthesia and blood transfusion during the Second World War and the introduction of antibiotics. Although this improved locoregional control, the complications and mutilating effects from such radical surgery were considerable. Reconstruction was usually multistaged using tubed-pedicles (Fig. 1.7), and many patients died before functional and aesthetic rehabilitation could be achieved.

By the 1950s megavoltage radiotherapy had been introduced with its skin-sparing effects, and this renewed interest in combined therapy. Other improvements in dosimetry, fractionation, and the use of electron beam therapy further reduced the limiting side effects of radiotherapy.

Head and neck surgery began to evolve as a subspecialty with the introduction of the concept of combined clinics in which the otolaryngologists became predominantly involved with the help of cosmetic surgeons. The differentiation between random and axial pattern cutaneous flaps introduced by McGregor in 1972 (63) heralded major advances in reconstructive surgery. Bakamjian's successful deltopectoral flap (1965) (64) had already gained widespread

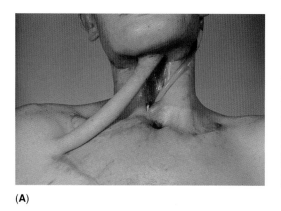

(A)

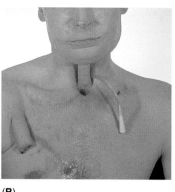

(B)

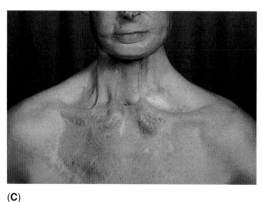

(C)

Figure 1.7   Multistage reconstruction with a tubed pedicle flap (1964). **(A)** Tubed pedicle raised from the chest. **(B)** Tube inset to reconstruct hypopharnyx. **(C)** Swallowing well 32 years later. *Source*: The Royal Marsden Hospital Head and Neck Surgery Photographic Archive.

recognition, and its axial pattern explained why it was so reliable. The ready availability and length of this and also McGregor's forehead flap permitted immediate and effective reconstruction of most defects in the head and neck. The only drawback was that most reconstructions required a second stage to divide and inset the pedicle.

The introduction in 1979 by Ariyan of myocutaneous flaps (65) allowed immediate one-stage reconstructions of large internal mucosal defects possible for the first time. Further technical and microvascular surgical advances since the 1980s have permitted widespread adoption of skin, visceral, and complex free grafts, giving the surgeon a wide variety of options for optimum reconstruction and rehabilitation. During this period there have also been significant advances in voice rehabilitation since the introduction in 1979 of the tracheo-oesophageal speech valve by Eric Blom. Transoral endoscopic minimally invasive surgery for laryngopharyngeal cancer has been practiced effectively in some parts of the world. As with most surgical operations, the technique is operator dependent and proper patient selection is crucial. More important, the scope of transoral UADT surgery is limited by the state of current instrumentation. Efforts are currently ongoing to adapt robotic instrumentation for use in the head and neck (78–80), but significant advances will be necessary for these techniques to enter common clinical use.

Single modality treatment is now well established in the management of early-stage disease, whether surgery or radiotherapy, and combined therapy gives optimal chance of cure for advanced tumors. There are exceptions, such as nasopharyngeal carcinoma that, fortunately for such a relatively inaccessible tumor, is very radiosensitive. Surgery is used for benign tumors of the head and neck, and surgical excision remains the most dependable and effective method of eliminating gross malignant disease.

Radiotherapy is most effective in eradicating microscopic disease that is less amenable to surgery; it helps reduce tumor cell dissemination by sealing lymphatics, thus confining the tumor to the primary site and decreasing the potential for metastatic spread; and it may also have an effect of enhancing the local immune reaction in irradiated tissue adjacent to the tumor (69).

Chemotherapy is playing an increasing role in the management of head and neck cancer. It was previously used primarily for palliation, but recent meta-analyses have shown that chemotherapy can improve survival when added to radiotherapy at the expense of increased acute and possibly late toxicity (66–68). Neoadjuvant chemotherapy (given prior to radiotherapy or surgery) improves local control and may allow greater organ preservation, but it does not affect overall survival. However, concurrent chemotherapy does give an 8% absolute survival benefit compared with radiotherapy alone (68). Chemotherapy with radiotherapy may improve organ preservation, but this remains under investigation. Targeted therapy using agents such as cetuximab has shown promise in combination with more standard options such as radiation (81). Biologic agents that are more specific and less toxic can be expected to play an increasing role in "organ-preserving" therapy of head and neck cancer as our understanding of the pathways and mechanisms of cancer development improves (82). It is however important to recognize that organ preservation may not equate to functional organ preservation. A retained larynx that does not protect or maintain an airway may result in less function and quality of life than a laryngectomy with voice restoration.

Multidisciplinary Presentation and Care

Head and neck cancer is primarily a mucosal disease of the UADT with 90% of tumors arising as squamous carcinomas from epithelial membranes of the oral and nasal cavities, pharynx, and larynx. Common symptomatic presentation of cancers in this region is with hoarseness, oral ulceration, sore throat, earache, bleeding, nasal obstruction, dysphagia, or cervical lymphadenopathy. Secondary symptoms may be present such as deafness due to secretory otitis media caused by eustachian tube obstruction or sinusitis due to osteomeatal obstruction. Therefore these patients commonly present to otolaryngology and oral maxillo-facial departments where the significance of these symptoms to possible underlying malignant disease is well appreciated. Management of the head and neck cancer patient should ideally be undertaken only where facilities and expertise essential for full investigation and treatment are available. The radiation and medical oncologists are essential lead clinicians in the multidisciplinary team with responsibility for radiotherapy and chemotherapy treatment.

Optimal reconstruction following ablative head and neck surgery requires a specialist head and neck reconstructive surgeon as part of the surgical team with specific training in microsurgical techniques and a broad knowledge of different free and pedicled flaps at their disposal. Also included in the multidisciplinary team are the nurse specialists, speech therapists, dieticians, dental hygienists, and physiotherapists with specialized training and expertise in head and neck cancer. Such expert teams can be developed only in units treating large numbers of patients.

IMPROVING OUTCOMES
Presentation

Patients who present with early-stage disease have better outcomes than those who present with late-stage disease (Table 1.5) (2,70). A study from Brazil showed that patients who delayed in reporting symptoms were twice as likely to present with late-stage (III and IV) disease (71). The same study also showed that the majority of delays (58%) were due to patients delaying consultations with health professionals, but health professionals were still responsible for 24% of delays. There is limited evidence that educational interventions can increase awareness among health professionals (72), and patient education on a global scale can prove very difficult and expensive.

Compliance

A significant proportion of patients with head and neck cancer are heavy users of tobacco and alcohol. Most are elderly, and many have a background of socioeconomic deprivation. Depression is common among this group. Compliance with treatment can be poor. A large meta-analysis of 2564 patients undergoing radiotherapy showed that 13% of patients did not receive the full course and 27% had their treatment protracted by more than 5 days (73). Each day of interruption equates to a 3.3% increase in the hazard rate for loco regional control and a 2.9% increase in the hazard rate for disease-free survival (74).

Timeliness of Treatment

A meta-analysis of 2427 patients receiving primary radiotherapy revealed a significant association between delaying treatment and poorer disease control and long-term survival. Five-year survival rates were 73% for those treated within 30 days of diagnosis, 62% for those treated between 31 and 40 days, and 54% for those treated more than 40 days after diagnosis (75). The same meta-analysis also reviewed 851 patients undergoing postoperative radiotherapy. Five-year survival rates were 61% for those patients whose radiotherapy started within 6 weeks of surgery, 46% for those patients treated 7 to 8 weeks after surgery, and 30% for those treated after a longer gap.

Centralization of Care

As head and neck cancer is relatively uncommon and comprises a heterogeneous group of tumors requiring complex treatment there has been a drive to centralize its management into a relatively small number of large centers to improve cure rates and functional outcomes. For example in the U.K., the National Institute for Clinical Excellence report in 2004 (76) recommended that a center treating head and neck cancer should treat at least 100 UADT cancer cases per year.

Survival

Long-term cure rates for head and neck cancer have not changed appreciably over the past 40 years because ultimate long-term survival is limited by metastatic disease, the appearance of second primaries, and other smoking-related conditions; but there is good evidence that survival rates up to 10 years have improved steadily (Fig. 1.8) (10,77).

Survival rates are heavily dependent on the stage at diagnosis, hence much poorer survival rates for hypopharyngeal cancer (20% 5-year survival) that commonly causes few symptoms until it is a T3 or T4 tumor, compared with laryngeal cancer (65% 5-year survival) that will present much earlier with dysphonia (Fig. 1.9) (10).

There is a deterioration in survival rates of head and neck cancers linked to deprivation (Fig. 1.10) (13). Possible explanations for this difference include longer delays in diagnosis, more advanced stage at diagnosis, worse general health, poorer resistance to malignancy, different histological types, poorer access to optimal health care, and lower compliance with treatment (10).

There has, however, been a definite change of emphasis in treatment of patients, not only to cure them of cancer but to rapidly restore their quality of life and functional rehabilitation. This has been made possible by tremendous improvements in reconstruction, using a variety of

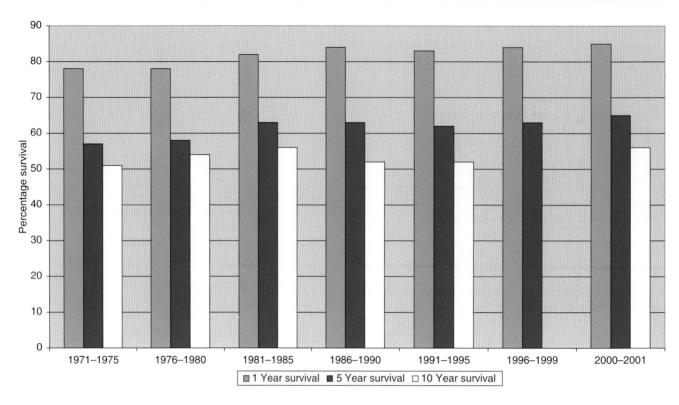

Figure 1.8   Male 1-, 5-, and 10-year survival rates for laryngeal cancer in England and Wales. *Source*: From Refs. 10, 77.

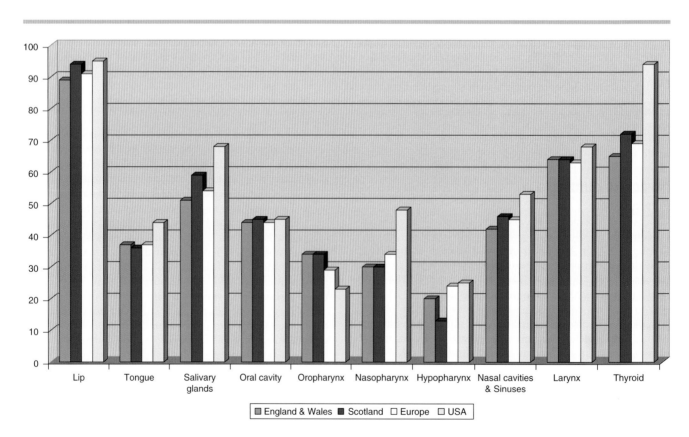

Figure 1.9   Male 5-year relative survival (%) in England and in Wales (1986–1990), Scotland (1986–1990), Europe (1985–1989), and the U.S.A. (1986–1990). *Source*: From Ref. 10.

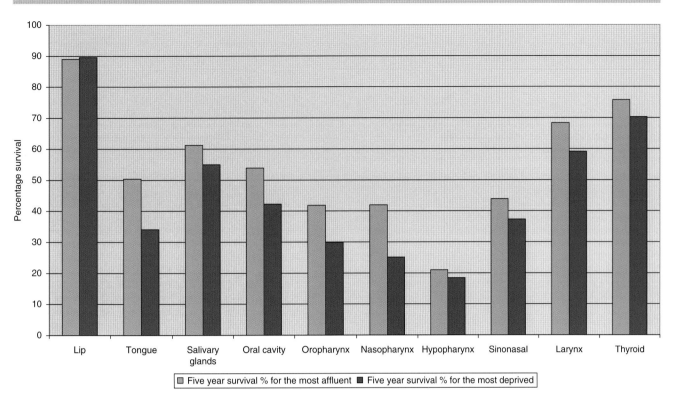

Figure 1.10 Comparison of 5-year survival in affluent and deprived patients, 1986–1990, England and Wales. *Source*: From Ref. 13.

microsurgical and pedicled reconstructions, and also rapid restoration of speech. Future advances in instrumentation and minimally invasive surgical technique will allow further improvement in outcomes. Novel targeted therapy based on individual characteristics of the tumor will become available with an increasing understanding of the genetic and molecular pathways that contribute to development of head and neck cancer. As these advances are made, the greatest challenge facing clinicians will be to select the treatment modality most likely to benefit the patient in terms of oncological and functional outcome.

SUMMARY

Although each subgroup of head and neck cancers is relative rare, collectively there are more than 780,000 new cases of head and neck cancer worldwide each year. Head and neck cancer can cause major psychological, aesthetic, and functional deficit from the disease process or the effects of treatment. Outcomes can be improved by a number of measures:

- Prevention – this requires global social measures to reduce smoking, alcohol consumption, and deprivation. HPV vaccination may have a role to play.
- Earlier detection – through increased public and healthcare awareness.
- Improved treatment – through a widely skilled multidisciplinary approach, making available the best surgical, radiotherapy, chemotherapy, and allied care available.

REFERENCES

1. Curado MP, Edwards B, Shin HR et al, eds. Cancer Incidence in Five Continents, Vol. IX (IARC Scientific Publications, No. 160). Lyon: IARC, 2007.
2. American Cancer Society. Cancer Facts and Figures 2007. Atlanta, GA: American Cancer Society, 2007.
3. Office of National Statistics (ONS). Cancer Statistics 2000: Registrations Series MB1 - No 31. London: The Stationery Office, 2003.
4. Welsh Cancer Intelligence and Surveillance Unit. Cancer incidence in Wales 1992–2001. 2002 www.wcisu.wales.nhs.uk
5. Ferlay J, Bray F, Pisani P, Parkin DM. GLOBOCAN 2002: Cancer Incidence, Mortality and Prevalence Worldwide (IARC CancerBase No. 5. version 2.0). Lyon: IARC Press, 2004. http://www-dep.iarc.fr/
6. Stewart BW, Kleihues P, eds. World Cancer Report. Lyon: IARC Press, 2003.
7. Swerdlow A, dos Santos Silva I, Doll R. Cancer incidence and mortality in England and Wales: trends and risk factors. Oxford University Press, 2001.
8. Mackillop WJ, Zhang-Salomons J, Boyd CJ, Groome PA. Associations between community income and cancer incidence in Canada and the United States. Cancer 2000; 89: 901–12.
9. Quinn MJ, Babb P, Brock A, Kirby L, Jones J. Cancer Trends in England and Wales 1950–1999. Studies on Medical and Population Subjects (Office of Population Censuses and Surveys, No. 66) London: The Stationery Office, 2001.
10. Coleman MP, Babb P, Damiecki P et al. Cancer Survival Trends in England and Wales 1971–1995: deprivation and NHS Region (Studies on Medical and Population Subjects, No. 61). London: The Stationery Office, 1999.
11. Maier H, De Vries N, Snow GB. Occupational factors in the aetiology of head and neck cancer. Clin Otolaryngol 1991; 16: 406–12.

12. Khan HA. The Dorn study of smoking and mortality among US veterans: report on 8 1/2 years of observation. J Natl Cancer Inst 1966; 19: 1896–1906.

13. Burch JD, Howe GR, Miller AB, Semenciw R. Tobacco, alcohol, asbestos and nickel in the etiology of cancer of the larynx: a case-control study. J Natl Cancer Inst 1981; 67: 1219–24.

14. Schantz SP, Zhang ZF, Spitz MS et al. Genetic susceptibility to head and neck cancer: interaction between nutrition and mutagen sensitivity. Laryngoscope 1997; 107: 765–81.

15. Jafek BW, Smith CM, Moran DT et al. Effects on the upper respiratory passages. Otolaryng Head Neck 1992; 106: 720–9.

16. Brandsma JL, Abramson AL. Association of papillomavirus with cancers of the head and neck. Arch Otolaryngol 1989; 115: 621–5.

17. IARC. Tobacco Smoking (IARC Monographs on the Evaluation of the Carcinogenic Risk of Chemicals to Humans, Vol. 38). Lyon: IARC Press, 1986.

18. IARC. Tobacco Smoke and Involuntary Smoking (IARC Monographs on the Evaluation of the Carcinogenic Risk of Chemicals to Humans, Vol. 83). Lyon: IARC Press, 2004.

19. Stell PM, McGill T. Asbestos and laryngeal carcinoma. Lancet 1973; 2: 416–17.

20. Stell PM, McGill T. Exposure to asbestos and laryngeal carcinoma. J Laryngol Otol 1975; 89: 513–17.

21. Zemla B, Wojcieszek Z. The epidemiological risk factors of the larynx cancer among the native and migrant male population. Neoplasma 1984; 31: 465–74.

22. Moulin JJ, Mur JM, Wild P et al. Oral cavity and laryngeal cancers among man-made mineral fibre production workers. Scand J Work Environ Health 1986; 12: 27–31.

23. Zagraniski RT, Kelsey JL, Walter SD. Occupational risk factors for laryngeal cancer: Connecticut, 1975–1980. Am J Epidemiol 1986; 124: 167–76.

24. Acheson ED, Cowdell H, Hadfield E, Macbeth RG. Nasal cancer in woodworkers in the furniture industry. Br Med J 1970; 2: 587–96.

25. Wynder EL, Covey LS, Mabuchi K, Mushinski M. Environmental factors in cancer of the larynx. A second look. Cancer 1976; 38: 1519–601.

26. Gerosa A, Turrini O, Bottasso F. Laryngeal cancer in a factory molding thermoplastic resins. Med Lav 1986; 77: 172–6.

27. Tabershaw IR, Gaffey WR. Mortality study of workers in the manufacture of vinyl chloride and its polymers. J Occup Med 1974; 16: 509–18.

28. Manning KP, Skegg DCG, Stell PM, Doll R. Cancer of the larynx and other occupational hazards of mustard gas workers. Clin Otolaryngol 1981; 6: 165–70.

29. Wolf O. Larynxkarzinome bei Naphtalinreinigern. Z Gesamte Hyg 1978; 24: 737–9.

30. Alderson MR, Ratten NS. Mortality of workers on an isopropyl alcohol plant and two MEK dewaxing plants. Br J Ind Med 1980; 37: 85–9.

31. Klayman MB. Exposure to insecticides. Arch Otolaryngol 1968; 88: 116–17.

32. Lynch J, Hanis NM, Bird MG et al. An association of upper respiratory cancer with exposure to diethyl sulfate. J Occup Med 1979; 211: 333–41.

33. Soskolne CL, Zeighami EA, Hanis NM et al. Laryngeal cancer and occupational exposure to sulfuric acid. Am J Epidemiol 1984; 120: 358–69.

34. Decoufle P. Cancer risk associated with employment in the leather and leather products industry. Arch Environ Health 1979; 34: 33–7.

35. Delager NA, Mason TJ, Fraumeni JF et al. Cancer mortality among workers exposed to zinc chromate paints. J Occup Med 1980; 22: 25–9.

36. Wynder EL, Bross IJ, Feldman RM. A study in etiological factors in cancer of the mouth. Cancer 1957; 10: 1300–23.

37. Schwartz E. Proportionate mortality ratio analysis of auto mechanics and gasoline service station workers in New Hampshire. Am J Ind Med 1987; 12: 91–9.

38. Pedersen E, Hogetveit AC, Andersen A. Cancer of the respiratory organs among workers at a nickel refinery in Norway. Int J Cancer 1982; 30: 681–5.

39. Flanders WD, Rothman KJ. Occupational risk of laryngeal cancer. Am J Public Health 1982; 72: 369–72.

40. Morris Brown L, Mason TJ et al. Occupational risk factors for laryngeal cancer on the Texas Gulf Coast. Cancer Res 1988; 48: 1960–4.

41. Nikiforov Y, Gnepp DR. Pediatric thyroid carcinoma after the Chernobyl disaster: pathomorphologic study of 84 cases (1991–1992) from the Republic of Belarus. Cancer 1994; 74: 748–66.

42. Martland HS. Occurrence of malignancy in radioactive persons; a general review of data gathered in the study of radium dial painters, with special reference to the occurrence of osteogenic sarcoma and the interrelationship of certain blood diseases. Am J Cancer 1931; 15: 2435–516.

43. Patel SG, See ACH, Rhys Evans PH et al. Radiation induced sarcomas of the head and neck. Head Neck 1999; 7: 346–53.

44. Mark RJ, Bailet JW, Poen J et al. Post irradiation sarcoma of the head and neck. Cancer 1993; 72: 887–93.

45. Hall P. Radiation-induced thyroid cancer. Med Oncol Tumor Pharmacother 1992; 9: 183–4.

46. van Kaick G, Wesch H, Luhrs H et al. Neoplastic diseases induced by chronic alpha-irradiation – epidemiological, biophysical and clinical results of the German Thorotrast Study. J Radiat Res (Tokyo) 1991; 32: 20–33.

47. IARC. Human Papillomaviruses (IARC Monographs on the Evaluation of Carcinogenic risks to Humans, Vol. 90), Lyon: IARC Press, 2007.

48. Kreimer AR, Clifford GM, Boyle P, Franceschi S. Human papillomavirus types in head and neck squamous cell carcinomas worldwide: a systematic review. Cancer Epidemiol Biomarkers Prev 2005; 14: 467–75.

49. IARC. Epstein-Barr Virus and Kaposi's Sarcoma Herpesvirus/ Human Herpesvirus 8 (IARC Monographs on the Evaluation of Carcinogenic Risks to Humans, Vol. 70). Lyon: IARC Press, 1997.

50. Wake M. The urban/rural divide in head and neck cancer: the effect of atmospheric pollution. Clin Otolaryngology. 1993; 18: 298–302.

51. Kabat GC, Chang CJ, Wynder EL. The role of tobacco, alcohol use, and body mass index in oral and pharyngeal cancer. Int J Epidemiol 1994; 23: 1137–44.

52. Mashberg A, Boffetta P, Winkelman R, Garfinkel L. Tobacco smoking, alcohol drinking, and cancer of the oral cavity and oropharynx among US veterans. Cancer 1993; 72: 1369–75.

53. IARC. Alcohol drinking (IARC Monographs on the Evaluation of carcinogenic risks to Humans, Vol. 44). Lyon: IARC Press, 1988.

54. Blot WJ, McLaughlin JK, Winn DM et al. Smoking and drinking in relation to oral and pharyngeal cancer. Cancer Res 1988; 48: 3282–87.

55. IARC. Tobacco habits other than smoking; betelquid and areca-nut chewing; and some related nitrosamines (IARC Monographs on the Evaluation of Carcinogenic Risks to Humans, Vol. 37). Lyon: IARCPress, 1985.

56. IARC. Smokeless Tobacco and Some Tobacco-specific N-nitrosamines (IARC Monographs on the Evaluation of Carcinogenic Risks to Humans, Vol. 89). Lyon: IARC Press, 2007.

57. Steinmetz KA, Potter JD. Vegetables, fruit, and cancer. I Epidemiology. Cancer Causes Control 1991; 2: 325–57.

58. Weinberg RA. Oncogenes, antioncogenes, and the molecular bases of multistep carcinogenesis. Cancer Res 1989; 49: 3713–21.

59. O'Brien PH, Carlson R, Steubner EA. Distant metastases in epidermoid cell carcinoma of the head and neck. Cancer 1927; 304: 1071.

60. Forssell G. Radiotherapy of malignant tumours in Sweden. Br J Radiol 1930; 3: 198–234.

61. Harrison DFN. Multimodal treatment and new approaches to therapy. In: Rhys Evans PH, Robin PE, Fielding JWL, eds. Head and Neck Cancer. Tunbridge Wells: Castle House Publications, 1983; 233–46.

62. Fletcher GH. Combination of irradiation and surgery. In: Fletcher GH, ed. Textbook of Radiotherapy, 3rd ed. Philadelphia: Lea and Febiger, 1980; 219–24.

63. McGregor IA. Fundamental Techniques of Plastic Surgery, 5th ed. Edinburgh: Churchill Livingstone, 1972.

64. Bakamjian VY. A two-stage method for pharyngoesophageal reconstruction with a primary pectoral skin flap. Plast Reconstr Surg 1965; 36: 173–84.

65. Ariyan S. The pectoralis major myocutaneous flap. A versatile flap for reconstruction in the head and neck. Plast Reconstr Surg 1979; 63: 73.

66. Munro AJ. An overview of randomised controlled trials of adjuvant chemotherapy in head and neck cancer. Br J Cancer 1995; 71: 83–91.

67. El-Sayed S, Nelson N. Adjuvant and adjunctive chemotherapy in the management of squamous cell carcinoma of the head and neck region. A meta-analysis of prospective and randomised trials. J Clin Oncol 1996; 14: 838–47.

68. Pignon JP, Bourhis J, Domenge C, Designe L. Chemotherapy added to locoregional treatment for head and neck squamous carcinoma: three meta-analyses of updated individual data. MACH-NC Collaborative Group. Lancet 2000; 355: 949–55.

69. Hewitt HB, Blake ER. The growth of transplanted murien tumours in pre-irradiated sites. Br J Cancer 1968; 22: 808–24.

70. Robertson AG, Robertson C, Soutar DS et al. Treatment of oral cancer: the need for defined protocols and specialist centres. Variations in the treatment of oral cancer. Clin Oncol 2001; 13: 409–15.

71. Kowalski LP, Franco EL, Torloni H et al. Lateness of diagnosis of oral and oropharyngeal carcinoma: factors related to the tumour, the patient and health professionals. Eur J Cancer B Oral Oncol 1994; 30B: 167–73.

72. National Institute for Clinical Excellence. Improving Outcomes in Head and Neck Cancers. The Research eVidence (Guidance on cancer services). London: NICE, 2004. www.nice.org.uk

73. Khalil AA, Bentzen SM, Bernier J et al. Compliance to the prescribed dose and overall treatment time in five randomized clinical trials of altered fractionation in radiotherapy for head-and-neck carcinomas. Int J Radiat Oncol 2003; 55: 568–75.

74. Kwong DL, Sham JS, Chua DT et al. The effect of interruptions and prolonged treatment time in radiotherapy for nasopharyngeal carcinoma. Int J Radiat Oncol 1997; 39: 703–10.

75. Huang J, Barbera L, Brouwers M et al. Does delay in starting treatment affect the outcomes of radiotherapy? A systematic review. J Clin Oncol 2003; 21: 555–63.

76. National Institute for Clinical Excellence. Improving outcomes in head and neck cancers (Guidance on cancer services). London: NICE, 2004. www.nice.org.uk

77. Coleman MP, Rachet B, Woods L et al. Trends and socioeconomic inequalities in cancer survival in England and Wales up to 2001. Br J Cancer 2004; 90: 1367–73.

78. O'Malley BW Jr, Weinstein GS, Snyder W, Hockstein NG. Transoral robotic surgery (TORS) for base of tongue neoplasms. Laryngoscope 2006; 116: 1465–72.

79. Hanna EY, Holsinger C, DeMonte F, Kupferman M. Robotic endoscopic surgery of the skull base: a novel surgical approach. Arch Otolaryngol 2007; 133: 1209–14.

80. Ozer E, Waltonen J. Transoral robotic nasopharyngectomy: a novel approach for nasopharyngeal lesions. Laryngoscope 2008; 118: 1613–6.

81. Bonner JA, Harari PM, Giralt J et al. Radiotherapy plus cetuximab for squamous-cell carcinoma of the head and neck. N Engl J Med 2006; 354: 567–78.

82. Wang LX, Agulnik M. Promising newer molecular-targeted therapies in head and neck cancer. Drugs 2008; 68: 1609–19.

2

Molecular Biology

Emma Barker, Fei-Fei Liu, Suzanne Kamel-Reid and Jonathan C Irish

INTRODUCTION

Advances in the treatment of head and neck cancer in the last 15 years have been largely limited to those that affect patient morbidity and quality of life, whereas patient survival outcomes remain relatively static. The application of new technologies however, in molecular biology and immunology, may provide the head and neck oncologist of the future with the tools to enhance patient survival.

To the clinician there appears to be an obvious qualitative "black-and-white" difference between the patient with a cancer and one without. However, at the molecular level, the mechanisms that underlie the genesis of malignant or normal tissue are so intimately related that reported molecular differences are often found to be quantitative rather than qualitative. In addition, the significance of these differences is often uncertain in the complex chain of molecular events leading to cancer.

The focus of this chapter is to provide a brief simplified description of the basic science of molecular biology for the head and neck clinician and to outline potential applications and limitations of our current knowledge. A glossary is included for the clinician who is unfamiliar with the terminology of molecular biology.

DNA, GENES, AND JARGON
DNA

The DNA molecule is a replicating chemical information system, based on a quaternary code, whose essential property is to generate more DNA in an ever-changing environment.

The information is formatted as a sequence of any of four flat nitrogen-based molecules [the nucleotide bases adenine (A), thymine (T), cytosine (C), guanine (G)] with the sequence being held on a sugar-phosphate backbone. Every strand of DNA is attached to a "complementary" DNA strand with each of the four bases being able to "bond" only with its complement: A with T and C with G. The complementary nature of these nucleic acids is critical for replication.

It is worth discussing the nature of the "bonds" between these bases, as this is very significant with respect to how DNA is studied. They are "hydrogen" bonds: the same bonds that stick water molecules to each other. When water is heated to boiling point these bonds break and the water molecules separate from each other. The same process occurs with double-stranded DNA: heating (or bathing in an alkali environment) denatures or "melts" these bonds resulting in two separate complementary single DNA strands.

The effect of cooling reverses this process allowing the separated complementary DNA strands to line up and stick to each other, a process called "annealing" or hybridization or renaturing.

The "Central Dogma"

The central dogma of molecular biology is that DNA makes RNA makes proteins and, more specifically, DNA is transcribed to messenger RNA that is then translated into protein.

Genes

A gene is a stretch of DNA that codes for a protein. In the total human genetic complement, the genome, there are approximately 25,000 genes. Less than 5% of the genome appears to code proteins and regulatory sequences with the rest having no known function. Within a gene there are some sequences that code for amino acids (exons) and some sequences that do not (introns). In gene transcription, exon and intron sequences are transcribed to mRNA but the introns are subsequently excised.

Genomic variability can be present in many forms, including single nucleotide polymorphisms (SNPs), variable number of tandem repeats (e.g., mini- and microsatellites), presence or absence of transposable elements (e.g., Alu elements) and structural alterations (e.g., deletions, duplications, and inversions). SNPs were thought to be the principal form of genomic variation and to account for much of the normal phenotypic variation (1,2). More recently, the general presence of copy number variation in normal individuals is thought to be significant in human phenotype variation (including disease resistance and susceptibility) (3,4,5,6).

GENE REGULATION

As cancer may be viewed as the deregulation of growth and death control, it is useful to review how gene expression is normally controlled.

Gene regulation has been extensively studied in bacteria, and we describe the function of a gene regulation system called an "operon" as it demonstrates important regulatory concepts. The operon model described is based on the lactose operon of the bacteria *Escherichia coli*, which is used to produce enzymes to allow the bacteria to metabolize lactose when it is in high concentrations in its environment. It is important to note there are many other regulatory models both in prokaryocytes (e.g., bacteria) and eukaryocytes (e.g., human cells), with the latter being far less well characterized.

Operons

An operon is a sequential cluster of related genes, which are needed to generate a collection of enzymes required for the metabolism or production of a substance. The purpose of this linked production is to produce functional groupings of enzymes at the correct time for the cell to react efficiently to signals in its environment. To aid the efficiency of the cell it is also designed to minimize the production of enzymes when the need for them is absent.

Operon Structure and Function

At the start of an operon is a promoter region. It is at this site where the enzyme RNA polymerase attaches to the DNA so that it can transcribe the gene-bearing area into mRNA. The next segment of the sequence is called the "operator region." This is the key controlling area as it is capable of binding a protein called the "repressor." If the repressor binds to the operator region it stops the enzyme RNA polymerase from moving onto the gene-bearing area and so stopping transcription. If the operator site is unoccupied then the RNA polymerase transcribes the genes (Fig. 2.1).

The repressor has a "signal" receptor binding site and an "operator" binding site. If the signal receptor site is occupied by the correct chemical signal then the operator binding site is distorted in such a manner as to prevent the repressor from binding to the operator, thus, transcription begins. If the signal receptor site is unoccupied then the binding site is capable of attaching to the operator so transcription is prevented.

It can be seen that an unregulated operon can occur if the repressor fails to bind to the operator. This may be due to

1. a mutation in the repressor gene code so that repressor protein does not bind to the promoter region;
2. a mutation in the promoter region so that normal repressor protein cannot bind to it;
3. mutations of the operon genes, and thus the gene products, which may affect the regulatory control of the operon by altering the signal to the repressor.

Thus, an unregulated cell growth operon could reveal qualitative and quantitative differences, for example, a mutant repressor protein and/or overexpression of normal growth enzymes.

THE CONCEPTUAL BASIS OF THE MOLECULAR BIOLOGY OF CANCER
Proto-Oncogenes and Oncogenes
Proto-Oncogenes

Proto-oncogenes are normal cellular genes that are crucially involved in normal growth regulation and cell differentiation (7). The signals for mitogenic stimulation of cells may come from different sources including growth factors, growth factor receptors, cytoplasmic signal transduction proteins, and nuclear proteins (Fig. 2.2) (8). Proto-oncogenes that function at each step of this pathway have been discovered and are thought to play an important role in a regulatory

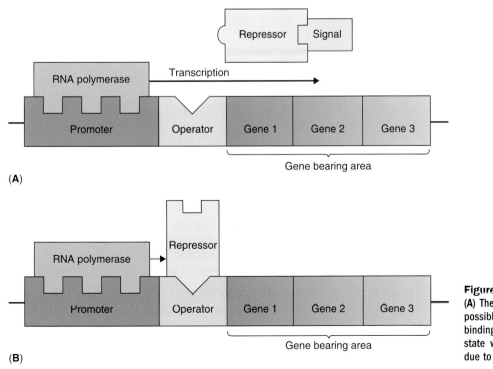

(A)

(B)

Figure 2.1 Operon structure and function. **(A)** The active state with transcription being possible due to the presence of the signal binding to the repressor. **(B)** The inactive state with transcription not being possible due to the absence of signal.

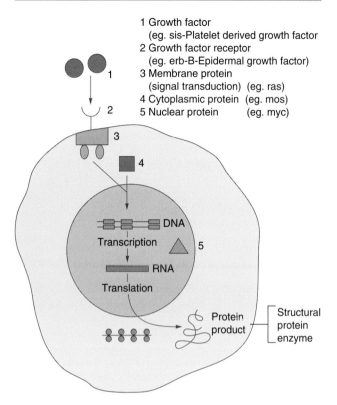

Figure 2.2 Signals of mitogenic stimulation of cells come from growth factors, with the information passed to growth factor receptors, signal transduction proteins, and nuclear proteins. Proto-oncogene products function at each step of the regulatory pathway. Dysregulation results when these genes and their protein products are altered.

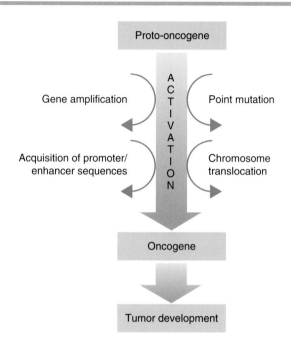

Figure 2.3 Mechanisms of proto-oncogene to oncogene activation.

network that extends from the cell surface into the cell nucleus. When mutated or deregulated these genes attain the capacity to destabilize normal cell growth and regulation and, in this state, are referred to as oncogenes (9).

Oncogenes

The resultant oncogene is a gene that can contribute to malignant transformation of cells and cause tumors in animals and humans (9). The protein product that they direct to be synthesized by the cell mediates the effect of oncogenes. The differences between the oncogene-directed protein product and that which would have been formed by the normal cellular gene can be qualitative (e.g., novel proteins secondary to mutations in the gene sequence) or quantitative (e.g., too many copies of a normal protein product) (9).

Oncogene Activation

Oncogene activation is known to occur in at least four ways (Fig. 2.3).

1. Gene acquisition of a novel transcriptional promoter. This results in gene overexpression with resultant increased gene product.
2. Chromosome translocation with resultant deregulation of a proto-oncogene close to the chromosomal breakpoints. An example of this is the Philadelphia chromosome

commonly found in chronic myelogenous leukemia (CML). In CML, the *c-abl* proto-oncogene on chromosome 9 is moved (translocated) to a region on chromosome 22 called the "breakpoint cluster region" (*bcr*) as a result of a reciprocal chromosomal movement. The resultant *bcr-abl* combination codes for a novel protein product resulting in unregulated stimulation to growth leading to chronic myelogenous leukemia.

3. Gene amplification due to increased gene copy number. This process, called "gene amplification," has been implicated in playing a causative role in a number of malignancies. For example, amplification of the 11q13 DNA sequences and overexpression of CCND1 are seen in approximately 30% of head and neck squamous cell carcinoma (HNSCC) (10).
4. Point mutation in the gene resulting in an altered protein product. An oncogene may be formed by a single nucleotide base-pair substitution in a proto-oncogene, which can result in the production of a mutant protein with loss of normal cell regulation. Analysis of a series of human papillary thyroid cancer demonstrated a 14% incidence of N-*ras* mutations (11). Other members of the *ras* gene family, such as H-*ras* and K-*ras*, have been implicated in a wide range of human malignancies. Mutagenic agents such as the components of tobacco smoke, alcohol, and radiation appear to play an important role in the etiology of some cancers.

Tumor Suppressor Genes

There is another class of genes, called "tumor suppressor genes" (TSGs), whose expression inhibits malignant transformation of cells. Mutation of such genes may lead to neoplastic transformation. TSGs were first recognized in the etiology of the inherited forms of retinoblastomas and Wilm's tumors. It is now evident that mutation in the p53 TSG occurs in a wide variety of human cancers including lung, bone, colon, mammary, and various hematological neoplasms (12). Li-Fraumeni families, who have a germ line p53 mutation, can develop cancer at any of these sites emphasizing the role of p53 as the "guardian of the genome."

The Multistage Models of Malignancy

Human cancers develop through a process involving several stages. The classical model is a successive passage of the cell through the three stages of initiation, promotion, and progression (13).

Tumor Initiation

A rapid, irreversible process that presumably results from genetic changes within the cell as a result of the cell's interaction with a carcinogenic agent. Initiated cells may be thought of as being primed for the development of malignancy although they themselves do not express this neoplastic potential unless they undergo promotion.

Tumor Promotion

Unlike initiation, the process of promotion is reversible with a prolonged latency period. Initiated cells develop into viable neoplastic lesions under the stimulus of the promoting agent. Although the generation of a tumor cell appears to be a multistep event, the activation of a single oncogene by the various mechanisms described earlier is a single discrete event. This apparent discrepancy may be explained by the fact that activation of single oncogenes may only be one facet of a complex process leading to the eventual development of a fully malignant cell.

Tumor Progression

Tumor progression is the characteristic of already established malignant tumors to successively acquire more aggressive grades of malignancy. These acquired qualities include such properties as propensity to tumor metastasis and development of radiation and chemotherapy resistance. Studies from *in vitro* models, experimental animals, and studies of human cancer have strongly supported the concept that several molecular events must occur during carcinogenesis.

The "Stem-Cell" Concept

The cancer stem cell (CSC) hypothesis suggests that there are discrete cells within a tumor that are able to direct tumorigenesis, in addition to a large population of differentiated progeny that make up the bulk of the tumor, but lack tumorigenic potential (14,15). HNSCC, consistent with other epithelial tumors, contain cellular heterogenicity. Some of this variation is attributed to genetic instability and environmental factors associated with ongoing mutations (16,17). However there is also evidence that supports the CSC hypothesis within HNSCC (18,19). Prince et al. (18) developed an immuno-deficient mouse model to test different subsets of human HNSCC cells. They found that a small subset (<10%) of cells (CD44+) were able to give rise to new tumors in vivo. This was in contrast with the CD44- cells. In addition, the CD44+ cells were able to reproduce the original tumor heterogeneity and could be serially passaged, demonstrating the two defining properties of stem cells.

INVESTIGATIONAL TECHNIQUES IN MOLECULAR BIOLOGY

Southern Blot

Southern blot technique is the analysis and comparison of the electrophoretic patterns of DNA fragments. It involves extracting DNA from a tumor sample and enzymatically digesting it into small fragments (Fig. 2.4). Electrophoresis results in a size fractionation of the DNA fragments, with the larger segments remaining close to the well of origin and the smaller segments travelling farther down the gel. The DNA is then transferred, or blotted, onto nylon or other synthetic membrane. The membrane can then be exposed ('hybridized') to radioactively labeled probes that are short DNA strands complementary to the known gene of interest. Radiolabeled probe, which has bound to homologous DNA sequence on the membrane, will result in a dark band on the X-ray film (Fig. 2.5).

Those tumors with an increased gene DNA copy number (gene amplification) will take up more radioactively labeled probe and result in a more intense signal on the radiographic film. In addition to gene amplification the Southern blot technique allows tumors to be analyzed for alterations in DNA structure. A gross deletion of a gene or point mutation at a restriction enzyme site will produce altered banding patterns [restriction fragment length polymorphisms (RFLPs)] when tumor DNA is compared with normal DNA (Fig. 2.6).

Northern Blot

The northern blot technique is the analysis and comparison of the electrophoretic patterns of RNA fragments. It involves an analogous process to the southern blot except that instead of tumor DNA being extracted and analyzed, RNA is analyzed. Whereas southern blotting can yield information about the genomic structure and the number of gene

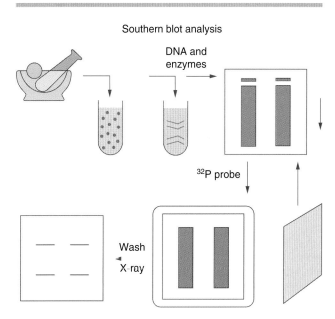

Figure 2.4 Steps involved in southern blotting.

ECORI digest

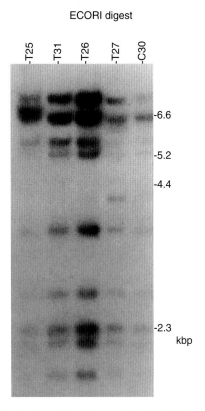

Figure 2.5 Southern blot of tumor DNA (T25, T31, T26, T27) and control DNA (C30). The DNA has been enzymatically digested resulting in characteristic DNA "fingerprints" or RFLPs. Tumor T26 showed increased uptake of the radioactive probe (*erb*-B) compared to control DNA suggesting *erb*-B amplification. *Abbreviation*: RFLP, restriction fragment length polymorphism.

HIND III digest

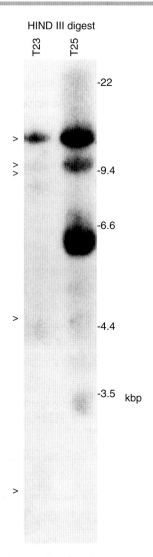

Figure 2.6 Southern blot of tumor DNA (T23, T25). In this case, the arrows mark the site of expected "fingerprints" or RFLPs. Tumor T25 demonstrates alteration of the DNA RFLP pattern (a new band at 6.6kbp) indicating gene deletion or point mutation. *Abbreviation*: RFLPs, restriction fragment length polymorphisms.

copies, northern blotting allows the expression levels of a gene to be analyzed.

Western Blot

The western blot technique is the analysis and comparison of the electrophoretic patterns of proteins. It involves the extraction of tissue protein and electrophoresis on polyacrylamide gels. Protein is then transferred onto a membrane and treated with a blocking solution. Instead of hybridization to a complementary DNA probe as in southern or northern blot techniques the western blot uses labeled antibody to detect the protein of interest.

Polymerase Chain Reaction

The polymerase chain reaction (PCR) technique creates multiple copies of a DNA segment that is amplified biochemically from a very small quantity of DNA (Fig. 2.7). The amplification involves a series of biochemical reactions consisting of three phases: denaturation, annealing and extension. The reaction consists of the DNA sample to be amplified (target), a thermostable enzyme (Taq polymerase) and two (forward and reverse) primers, which are small segments (usually 10–20 oligonucleotides long) of DNA complementary to each end of the target DNA fragment that is to be amplified. The mixture is heated to denature

the DNA double-strand and then actively cooled to allow the two primers to anneal to the now single-stranded DNA target template. The primers should only anneal to the homologous DNA sequences flanking the target template. The forward and reverse primers then act as start sites for synthesis of a new DNA strand by Taq polymerase. With each cycle of denaturation, annealing and extension the amount of target DNA between the two primers is doubled. The products of one cycle serve as templates for the next cycle so that the PCR product accumulates exponentially. Theoretically, therefore, after 30 PCR cycles 2^{30} copies of target DNA are created allowing for visualization and subsequent analysis (Fig. 2.8).

Quantitative "Real Time" PCR Analysis

The measurement of fluorescence using laser-based technology has allowed quantitation of PCR products (Fig. 2.9).

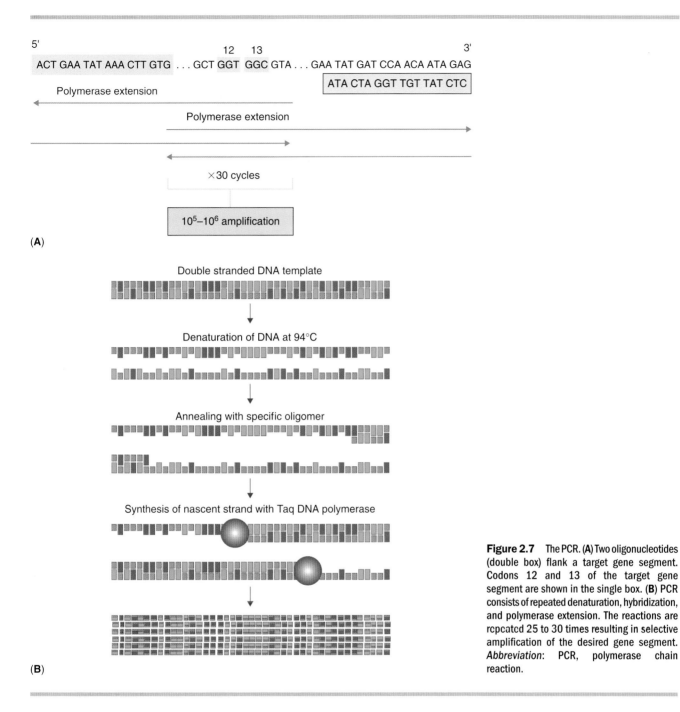

5'   12   13   3'

ACT GAA TAT AAA CTT GTG . . . GCT GGT GGC GTA . . . GAA TAT GAT CCA ACA ATA GAG

ATA CTA GGT TGT TAT CTC

Polymerase extension

Polymerase extension

×30 cycles

10^5–10^6 amplification

(A)

Double stranded DNA template

Denaturation of DNA at 94°C

Annealing with specific oligomer

Synthesis of nascent strand with Taq DNA polymerase

(B)

Figure 2.7   The PCR. **(A)** Two oligonucleotides (double box) flank a target gene segment. Codons 12 and 13 of the target gene segment are shown in the single box. **(B)** PCR consists of repeated denaturation, hybridization, and polymerase extension. The reactions are repeated 25 to 30 times resulting in selective amplification of the desired gene segment. *Abbreviation*: PCR, polymerase chain reaction.

During PCR, a fluorogenic probe, consisting of an oligonucleotide with a reporter and a quencher dye attached, anneals specifically between the forward and reverse primers in the region of interest. Owing to the 5′ to 3′ exonuclease activity of Taq polymerase, as it copies the DNA the reporter dye is cleaved from the quencher dye, allowing unquenched emission of fluorescence, which can be detected and quantified. With each cycle, additional reporter dye molecules are cleaved from their respective probes. To quantitate the amount of specific product the fluorescence intensity is measured during the PCR and compared to a standard curve that will determine absolute or relative amount of product generated. This technology has been used for many purposes, including the measurement and monitoring of disease specific transcripts (20).

DNA Sequencing

The order of bases in a DNA sequence is of great value as it is the "anatomy" of the genetic material and helps in understanding its "physiology." DNA sequencing using the Sanger and the Maxam–Gilbert sequencing techniques can determine the precise order of the nucleotide bases in a DNA strand.

The Sanger Technique

This technique is founded on the use of modified bases [dideoxynucleotides (ddN)], which terminates further base additions to a DNA sequence. A pure sample of single-stranded DNA of unknown base sequence is separated into four test tubes. Into each sample is added the ingredients

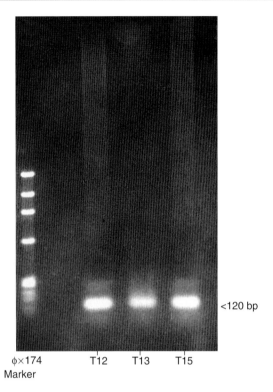

Figure 2.8 Stained gel of PCR-amplified products from three head and neck tumor specimens (T12, T13, T15). A 120-bp target of the *ras* gene from three head and neck tumors was amplified 106 times such that the product can be seen with the naked eye on this stained agarose gel. The PCR technique has allowed amplification of genetic segments of interest for further study. *Abbreviation*: PCR, polymerase chain reaction.

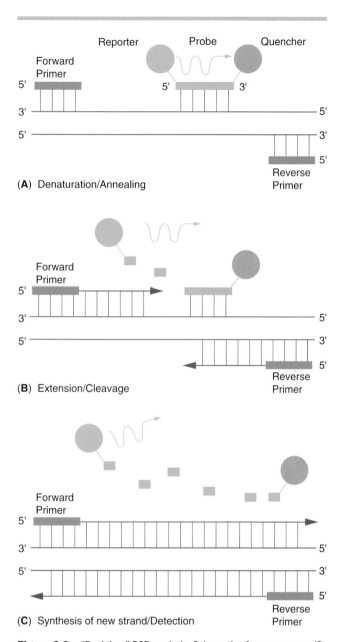

Figure 2.9 "Real time" PCR analysis. Schematic of sequence-specific annealing and 5' to 3' exonuclease-based cleavage of the fluorescent dye-labeled probe. *Abbreviation*: PCR, polymerase chain reaction.

required to generate a complementary DNA chain and small quantities of a single type of the modified bases that is incapable of allowing the polymerizing or hybridizing process to continue, thus "capping" the sequence at that complementary base point. Some of the modified bases successfully compete with the normal bases and manage to be incorporated at various complementary points on the sequence. This results in each test tube containing fragments of various lengths of complementary DNA terminated with the modified base that was added. These samples are individually electrophoresed, identified (each fragment starts with a labeled primer), and lined up next to each other; then the sequence of the original strand can be determined (Fig. 2.10). This technique can also be used to compare the bands produced from normal and tumor DNA and to allow determination of gene sequence and identification of point mutations (Fig. 2.11). More recently, sequencing is done using fluorescently labeled primers and automated technology.

Fluorescence in Situ Hybridization

Cytogenetic analysis of head and neck tumors has improved dramatically in the last 15 years due to fluorescence in situ hybridization (FISH) technology with techniques such as color karyotyping [multiplex FISH; M-FISH (21), and spectral karyotyping (SKY) (22)] and comparative genomic hybridization (CGH) (23). The traditional chromosomal banding

techniques cannot define complex karyotypes with multiple marker chromosomes as well as translocations involving regions that are cytogenetically similar by G-banding. The advent of multicolor FISH techniques, known as M-FISH and SKY, using five fluorochromes allow the detection of several targets simultaneously. Sophisticated computer analysis is required to differentiate the colors and to identify the origin of every chromosome in a hybridized metaphase cell. CGH allows screening of the whole tumor genome for DNA sequence gains or losses in a single experiment. It is based on simultaneous in situ hybridization of equal amounts of differentially labeled tumor DNA and normal DNA to a normal metaphase chromosome preparation. Differences in the fluorescence ratio between

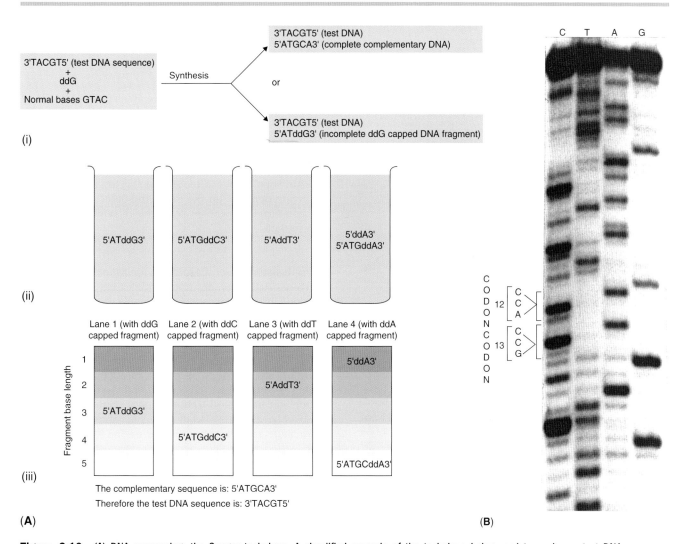

Figure 2.10 **(A)** DNA sequencing: the Sanger technique. A simplified example of the technique being used to analyze a test DNA sequence 3'TACGT5'. (i) The "capping" principle with ddG. (ii) Hybridization: one of the four modified "capping" bases is added to each of the four test tubes. The hybridization starts with a labeled primer for later identification of the fragments. (iii) Electrophoresis, identification and sequence determination. **(B)** Exposed radiograph of a sequencing gel of a head and neck cancer tumor specimen. The nucleotide sequence can be read from top to bottom. Codons 12 and 13 show sequence CCA CCG that is normal showing no evidence of point mutation (Lane 1, cysteine; lane 2, thymine; lane 3, adenine; lane 4, guanine). *Abbreviations*: ddg, dideoxy guanine; CCA CCG, cell carcinoma antigen.

the tumor and reference DNA implicate regions of abnormal DNA content in the tumor sample. Although a low-resolution technique, analysis can reveal chromosomal areas where DNA is either gained or deleted at a resolution of 2 Mbp for gains and 10 Mbp for deletions (24). Multi-color karyotyping and CGH have limitations: neither can detect chromosomal inversions or point mutations, CGH cannot detect balanced chromosomal translocations and aberrations present in low frequency, and multicolor karyotyping cannot detect subtle deletions and duplications.

Another genomic approach for the identification of chromosome changes has been developed, array-based comparative genomic hybridization, using ordered bacterial artificial chromosome (BAC) arrays, spanning the entire genome at a resolution of less than 1 Mbp (25). A BAC is a DNA construct used for transforming and cloning in bacteria. The usual insert size is 150 kbp. BACs were used

to sequence the genetic code of the human genome. In addition, BACs can be spotted onto glass slides and DNA can be hybridized to them (BAC arrays). The arrays provide improved sensitivity and resolution and can define the extent of the genomic region that is amplified or deleted and also provide an objective approach to karyotype analysis. The potential utility of these arrays for accurately quantitating chromosomal gains and losses in human tumor cell lines and tumor material derived from patients have previously been described (25). Specifically, an oral cancer genomic regional array for CGH analysis has also been described (26).

Microarray Analysis

A DNA microarray (DNA chip, gene array, or genome chip) uses a collection of co-valently attached DNA spots to a chemical matrix to qualitatively or quantitatively evaluate

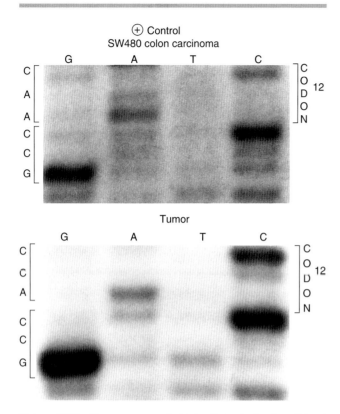

Figure 2.11 Close-up sequencing gel radiograph of codons 12 and 13 in a colon carcinoma (SW480, *Top*) known to demonstrate a CAA nucleotide sequence at codon 12 instead of the normal CCA sequence of a head and neck tumor (T15, *Below*). The SW480 cell line has a point mutation in codon 12 of the *ras* oncogene. *Abbreviation*: CCA, cell carcinoma antigen.

DNA expression. The matrix can be made up of many solid compounds including glass, plastic, or silicone. Each spot commonly represents individual genes. Using either DNA–DNA or DNA–RNA hybridization, fluorescently labeled probes allow quantification. The intensity of the fluorescence correlates with expression of the gene for which the spot codes. RNA is most commonly detected as complementary DNA (cDNA) following reverse transcription. The advantage of this system is that it can be used for expression profiling of thousands of genes simultaneously. Using either one-color or two-color fluorescent labels, an expression profile can be determined for different tissues (Fig. 2.12). This method has allowed thousands of genes to be evaluated in different normal and malignant tissues (27).

Micro-RNA

Micro-RNAs are 20 to 22 nucleotides long and bind to complementary messenger RNA (mRNA). Micro-RNAs are encoded by genes that are transcribed from DNA but not translated into protein (i.e., noncoding RNA). Their main function is to downregulate gene expression. This results in either degradation of the mRNA or inhibition of the production of protein from the mRNA. Their role in cancer formation, although not fully evaluated, appears crucial (28).

Micro-RNA expression profiles can be determined in a similar way to a DNA microarray. The micro-RNA signature of a tumor can help with tumor classification (29).

Proteomics

Proteomic studies have generated numerous data sets of potential diagnostic, prognostic, and therapeutic significance in human cancer. Two key technologies that are the foundation of these studies in cancer are two-dimensional polyacrylamide gel electrophoresis and mass spectrometry (MS). Two-dimensional polyacrylamide gel electrophoresis separates proteins in two directions at 90° to each other. The separation depends on the isoelectric point of the protein, which in turn is dependent on its charge, which is correlated with its size.

Matrix-Assisted Laser Desorption/Ionization

Matrix-assisted laser desorption/ionization (MALDI) is a technique used in mass spectrometry (30). It allows the analysis of fragile molecules (i.e., proteins and carbohydrates) that tend to fragment when ionized by more conventional ionization methods. The matrix consists of crystallized molecules. The matrix solution is mixed with the analyte (e.g., serum or saliva). It is composed of an organic solvent (dissolving hydrophobic molecules) and water (dissolving hydrophillic molecules). This solution is spotted onto a metal plate (a MALDI plate). As the solvents vaporize, the matrix and analyte are left co-crystallized on the MALDI spot. A laser is fired at the spot; and although most of the energy is absorbed by the matrix, some energy is transferred to the analyte. Thus, although protected from the disruptive energy, the analyte becomes charged. This is followed by peptide mass determination frequently using time of flight (TOF). A modification of MALDI-TOF is SELDI-TOF (surface enhanced laser desorption/ionization) (30). In SELDI the protein mixture is spotted on a modified surface. Although some samples bind to the surface, others are removed in the washing stage. Only those proteins bound will be analyzed. Again, the mass and amount of each protein is measured by irradiating the surface with a laser and measuring the TOF. Numerous uncharacterized biomarkers have been identified. Although SELDI-TOF-MS is the mainstay for serum or plasma analysis, other methods including isotope-coded affinity tag technology, reverse-phase protein arrays, and antibody microarrays are emerging as alternative proteomic technologies.

MOLECULAR BIOLOGY OF HEAD AND NECK CANCER
Genetic Susceptibility

Among genes that activate or eliminate tobacco carcinogens, the null genotypes of the carcinogen-metabolizing genes glutathione-S-transferase (GST)T1 and GSTM1, the GSTP1 (AG or GG) genotype have been shown to represent risk factors for HNSCC and markers for genetic susceptibility to tobacco-induced carcinogenesis (31). Mutagen sensitivity (a higher rate of spontaneous chromosomal aberrations in lymphoblastoid cells) induced by tobacco-associated cancer mutagen, benzo[a]pyrene diol epoxide is also associated with risk of HNSCC development (32).

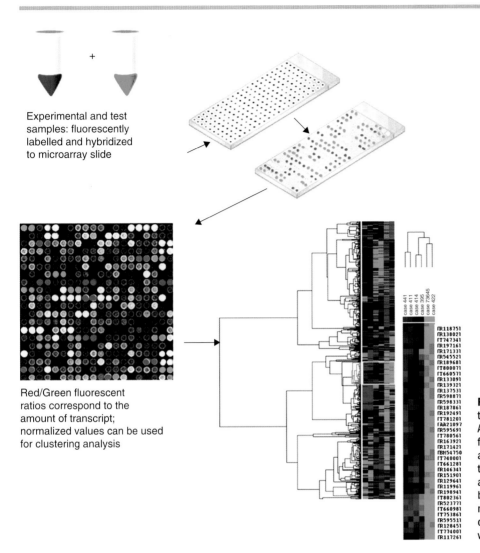

Experimental and test samples: fluorescently labelled and hybridized to microarray slide

Red/Green fluorescent ratios correspond to the amount of transcript; normalized values can be used for clustering analysis

Figure 2.12 Flow diagram to demonstrate two-color hybridization microarray method. A sample of interest is labeled with a fluorescent dye and a control is labeled with another fluorescent dye. Both samples are then hybridized onto the same spotted array and analysis carried out using the ratios between the two colors for each spot. This method minimizes potential error as a result of microarray processing. These normalized values can be used for clustering analysis.

Cytogenetic (Chromosomal) Changes

The most frequent chromosomal abnormalities in HNSCCs are unbalanced translocations leading to chromosomal deletions affecting 3p13-q24 (in >60% of tumors), 4p (43%), 5q12-q23 (30%), 8p22-p23 (65%), 9p21-p24 (43%), 10p (39%), 13q12-q24 (30%), 18q22-23 (>60%), and 21q (52%) (33). SKY analysis of seven HNSCC cell lines identified frequent structural rearrangement of the following chromosomal regions: 3q, 5p13-q11.2, 5q32-q34, 7p12-q11.2, 8p12-q12, 9p, 10p, 13p13-q12, 14q11.1-q11.2, 15p13-q11.2, 16p11.1-q11.1, 18q22-q23, and 22p13-q11.2 (34). Loss of the inactive X and loss (or rearrangement) of Y occur in 70% of tumors from female and male patients, respectively. Less common consistent changes found in 30–40% of tumors are gain affecting 3q21-qter, 5p, 7p, 8q, and 11q13-23 (35). More recently, gains were demonstrated by CGH in HHSCC lines at 3q (64%), 8q (45%), and 6q22-qter (45%) and losses at 18q22-qter (27%) (34). Allelic losses at marker loci in specific genomic regions, indicating the inactivation of critical TSGs within the regions, had also been demonstrated at 3p, 5q, 9p, 11q, 13q, 18q, and 17p (36,37). A genetic progression model for HNSCC has been postulated (38) with certain genetic events indicated as early (LOH at 3p, 9p21, and 17p13), intermediate (11q, 13q11, and 14q), and late (6p, 4q, and 8). The accumulation of genetic events is associated with histopathological progression although there may be a prolonged latency period during which clonal genetic alterations may be present before an invasive phenotype is produced (39). Some studies have correlated chromosome deletion or mutation with poor clinical outcome (LOH at 2q, 3p, 9p, 11q, 18q) (40) or biological behavior such as radiation therapy resistance (1p, 3p, 8p, 14q) (41). Using a modified CGH analysis, gains at chromosomes 10p11-12 and 11p and deletions at chromosomes 4q22-31, 9p13-24, and 14q differentiated nodal metastases from the corresponding primary tumors in human cell lines (42). In nasopharyngeal cancer, CGH has identified the most common copy number increases on chromosome arms 12p, 1q, 17q, 11q, and 12q, whereas the most frequent losses were found at 3p, 9p, 13q, 14q, and 11q (43). CGH has also demonstrated that the average number of chromosomal arms with at least one aberration was 15 in HNSCC (44). In addition, laryngeal carcinoma had significantly more aberrations than oropharyngeal carcinoma (44).

Cellular Oncogenes in Head and Neck Cancer
ErbB Receptor Proto-Oncogenes

The protein products of the *erb*B proto-oncogenes belong to the transmembrane type I receptor tyrosine kinase family (45). The *erb*B receptors have four homologous members in the family: the epidermal growth factor receptor (EGFR or *erb*B-1 or HER-1 for human EGF receptor-1), *erb*B-2 (*neu* or HER-2), *erb*B-3 (HER-3) and *erb*B-4 (HER-4). EGFR protein is expressed at low levels on the surface of the majority of normal adult cells with the exception of haematopoietic cells. Head and neck tumors analyzed for RNA expression, gene amplification, and structural alteration of the EGFR gene, *erb*B-1, showed that up to 24% displayed *erb*B-1 gene amplification and/or gene rearrangement (46,47). However, mRNA overexpression, with or without receptor protein overproduction, may be more important than gene amplification (48). Overexpression of the *erb*B-1 gene has been observed in 67% of the head and neck tumors studied whereas a stepwise increase of EGFR expression in histologically normal epithelium, premalignant, and cancerous lesions has been observed following the histologic progression (49). Those patients expressing high levels of EGFR or showing EGFR gene amplification had tumors that were clinically more advanced (50). In addition, patients with tumors with an altered EGFR copy number (particularly patients with an increased copy number) had a significantly worse outcome (47). However, gene copy number and protein expression remain controversial as accurate prognostic markers (48). Upregulation of EGFR in adjacent histologically normal tissue has been documented (51). In addition, patients with a history of alcohol and smoking have EGFR upregulation, in the absence of any mucosal abnormalities (51). Although there is no evidence for gene amplification or increased RNA transcript of *erb*B-2 in HNSCC (52–56), increased *erb*B-2 oncoprotein expression has been noted (55, 57–62). Increased HER-2 expression was associated with advanced International Union Against Cancer stage and poor prognosis (61,62). However, c-*erb*B-2 levels alone do not always correlate with the clinicopathological parameters examined, thus its value as a prognostic indicator in HNSCC remains unclear (48). Overexpression of *erb*B-3 and *erb*B-4 mRNA and protein have been found in some HNSCC lines, whereas no gene amplification was detected (54,55,63,64). In clinical settings, the roles of *erb*B-3 and *erb*B-4 in HNSCC progression are less clear (56,60,65–69). However, their ability to form heterodimers among the *erb*B family members upon stimulation by their direct ligands, that is heregulins (HRG)-b1 has been shown to enhance the signaling pathways of EGFR or *erb*B-2 and the invasive properties in HNSCC cells (70,71). Amongst the c-*erb*B family receptors studied, EGFR was the most significant factor in predicting nodal metastasis. In patients with oral squamous cell carcinoma (SCCs), the expression of all four c-*erb*B receptors was significantly associated with shortened survival and that the combination of c-*erb*B-2, c-*erb*B-3, and EGFR (but not c-*erb*B-4) significantly improved the predictive power (72).

The c-*erb*B ligand family, which are the products of distinct genes, consists of more than 30 members (73) including EGF, transforming growth factor-alpha (TGF-α), amphiregulin (AR), heparin-binding-EGFlike growth factor (HB-EGF), betacellulin (BTC), epiregulin (ER), and the several differentially-spliced variants of HRGs, also known as neuregulins. The c-*erb*B ligands can be grouped into three categories with respect to growth factor-receptor interactions (74).

The first group consists of EGF, TGF-α, and AR: These bind to and activate EGFR directly. These ligands do not induce receptor autophosphorylation or other cellular activities directly in cells expressing c-*erb*B-2, c-*erb*B-3 or c-*erb*B-4 unless EGFR is co-expressed, allowing the formation of heterodimers. The second category includes HRGs that do not interact directly with EGFR but are ligands for c-*erb*B-3 and c-*erb*B-4. They can also transactivate EGFR or c-*erb*B-2 when either c-*erb*B-3 or c-*erb*B-4 is present. The third category is classified as "bispecific" as members can bind to and activate EGFR and c-*erb*B-4 directly when either is expressed alone, and also transmodulate c-*erb*B-2 and c-*erb*B-3 when these are co-expressed. There are three established members in this group to date, including BTC, ER and HB-EGF. In HNSCC, the expression of multiple *erb*B ligands apart from EGF and TGF-α has been described (75,76). In addition, all erbB ligands can interact with each other by a mutual amplification mechanism as well as by autocrine induction (76). *Erb*B ligand receptor complex recruits a unique set of signaling proteins activating multiple distinct pathways that elicit specific biological responses associated with carcinogenesis and/or metastasis (70,71,75).

Ras Proto-Oncogene

The *ras* family of oncogenes (N-*ras*, H-*ras*, K-*ras*) encode the membrane-associated G-proteins, guanosine triphosphatases, that constitutively maintain an activated GTP-bound state and serve as signal transducers for cell surface growth factor receptors. Conflicting results have been reported regarding the importance of the *ras* family in HNSCC. NIH/3T3 transfection assay uncovered activated c-H-*ras*-1 proto-oncogenes in two squamous cell carcinoma cell lines established from human oral carcinoma patients (77). Anderson and Irish found that approximately 15% of oral and oropharyngeal malignancies demonstrate point mutations in the H-*ras* gene at codon 12 (50). K-*ras* mutations are rare (50,78,79). Yarbrough et al. (78) did not reveal point mutations of either H-*ras*, K-*ras*, and N-*ras* but did show differential protein expression. In healthy mucosa, p21 N-*ras* staining was seen in the proliferating basal layers. In dysplasia and malignancy the p21 N-*ras* staining was observed throughout the mucosa, within the cytoplasm, whereas H-*ras* and K-*ras* had variable expressions (78,79). Expression of H-*ras*, K-*ras*, and N-*ras* in HNSCC was not related to histologic differentiation or tumor, node, metastasis (TNM) staging (78).

Raf Proto-Oncogene

Raf has a serine/threonine kinase activity, functioning within the *ras-raf*-MEK-ERK mitogen activated protein kinase (MAPK) pathway (80). This signal transduction cascade is an essential mediator of a number of cellular effects including growth, proliferation, and survival. There are three known mammalian *raf* isoforms: A-, B-, and C-*raf*. There are no reports of A-*raf* mutations in HNSCC: they were observed within a leukemia cell line, but not within solid tumors (81). Activating B-*raf* missense mutations have been identified in 3/89 HNSCC (82). C-*raf* has been found overexpressed in a variety of primary human cancers including HNSCC (83). The C-*raf* oncogene has been shown to be activated from a cell line (SQ2OB) derived from a human laryngeal squamous cell carcinoma (84). Under in vitro conditions this cell line is resistant to the effects of ionizing radiation.

C-*raf* overexpression was observed in patients resistant to radiation therapy in HNSCC (83).

Cyclin D1 (CCND1: PRAD1: BCL-1)

Transition from the Gl to the S phase (the DNA synthesis phase) and from the G2 to the M phase (the mitosis phase) are critical control points in the cycle of a growing cell. A group of proteins called "cyclin-dependent kinases" (cdks) participate in the regulation of these transitions. These cdks form complexes with proteins called "cyclins," including cyclin D1. The *CCND1* gene that encodes the cyclin D1 protein is located on chromosome 11q13, and this locus is amplified in 20–52% of HNSCC. Overproduction of cyclin Dl may push a tumor cell through the G1/S transition, resulting in uncontrolled cell division and perpetuation of other genetic alterations. *CCND1* gene amplification and overexpression have been shown in HNSCC and premalignancy (85,86) and correlated with poor outcome (87–89).

EMS1 (Cortactin)

The *EMS1* oncogene is located in the same region as the *CCND1* gene on chromosome 11q13. *EMS1* encodes a cytoskeletal protein homologous to the avian F actin-binding protein (cortactin), which is involved in regulating the interactions between components in the adherens junctions. *EMS1* amplification in tumors results in overexpression of cortactin leading to a redistribution of cortactin from the cytoplasm into cell-matrix contact sites. This might affect the functioning of cytoskeleton and cell-adhesion structures and contribute to the invasive behavior of tumor cells. In HNSCC, *EMS1* amplification occurs in 20% and predicts early recurrence and reduced survival independent of other known risk factors (90). In addition, overexpression of cortactin in HNSCC cells was shown to reduce ligand-induced downregulation of EGFR (91). This resulted in continual receptor signaling to the mitogenic extracellular signal-regulated kinase MAPK pathway (91). Timpson's group recently demonstrated cortactin overexpression in a panel of HNSCC cell lines revealing enhanced serum- and EGF-stimulated proliferation under anchorage-dependent and anchorage-independent conditions and also increased resistance to anoikis (detachment-induced apoptosis) (92).

MPP11

Genetic high-copy amplification of the 7q22–31 genomic region has been recognized as an important event in the progression of HNSCC (93). A novel human candidate oncogene, *MPP11*, encoding a phosphoantigen with a regulatory role in the mitotic phase of the cell cycle, has been mapped to the critical region of 7q22–31.1 (94). *MPP11* is localized to the cytosol and associates with ribosomes (95). Increased copy number of *MPP11* and overexpression in the majority of primary HNSCC tissues and cell lines examined suggest that this gene is activated during malignant progression and may play an oncogenic role in HNSCC.

TUMOR SUPPRESSOR GENES IN HEAD AND NECK CANCER

p16

The most commonly deleted chromosome site in HNSCC is located at 9p21–p24, which is the locus for the *CDKN2/*

MTS1/INK4A TSG (37). The p16^{INK4A} gene product is an inhibitor of the cyclin/cyclin-dependent kinase complex. Loss of heterozygosity of the short arm of chromosome 9 (9p21-22) has been reported with high frequency in dysplasia, carcinoma in situ, and HNSCC (96–98), suggesting that this genetic alteration may be involved in the early developmental stages of this disease, whereas deregulation of p53 and cyclin D1 occur later (38). Although only 10–15% of HNSCCs demonstrate point mutation at the p16 gene, (99) frequent homozygous deletion in this region (100) and transcriptional silencing through promoter methylation (101) are major inactivation mechanisms in these tumors. Loss of p16 is present in 52–82% of tumors from HNSCC patients (102,103). Recently, a significant relationship between loss of p16^{INK4A} expression and adverse outcome in HNSCC was shown (88,104). Using FISH, p16 deletion was detected in 52% of patients with HNSCC and was significantly associated with development of distant metastases (105). In addition, using PCR-based techniques, a prospective study of locally advanced laryngeal SCC identified p16 mutation as an independent predictive factor for disease relapse and death (106). Despite this, there are conflicting results regarding the prognostic significance of p16 in HNSCC (107), hence the role of p16 in HNSCC carcinogenesis and progression has not been clearly established.

p53

Loss of 17p13 occurs in up to 60% of invasive SCCs and is the locus of the p53 TSG (108). Alterations of the p53 gene by allelic losses, point mutations, deletion, or inactivation disrupt its role as a guardian of the genome by impairing the cell's ability to repair and undergo apoptosis in response to DNA damage and thus leads to genomic instability. An overall p53 mutation incidence of 40–50% has been reported in a study of invasive tumors studied by direct sequencing of exons 5 through 8 (109). A higher incidence of p53 mutation has been found in the tumors of smokers and drinkers than in the tumors of patients who developed HNSCC without exposure to these agents (110). It would appear p53 mutation could be an early event in HNSCC carcinogenesis as it has been observed in premalignant lesions (109). In addition, an increasing pattern of p53 alterations has been demonstrated in premalignant lesions following histologic progression (111). Mutant p53 protein overexpression is associated with tumor recurrence, reduced disease-free and overall survival rates, and decreased rates of local control in HNSCC (112–115). In addition, p53 overexpression in regional lymph nodes was found to be an independent predictor of regional failure and poor prognosis in patients with HNSCC (115). The findings of p53 mutations in histologically negative margins of completely resected tumors and the distinct p53 genotypes in synchronous primary tumors suggest that p53 can be used as a marker for molecular staging and fingerprinting in HNSCC (110). Overexpression of p53 in tumor-distant epithelia of HNSCC patients has been reported to correlate with an increased incidence of second malignancies (116). As p53 and p16 pathways represent the two main mechanisms for cell-cycle control at the G1-S checkpoint, studies examining the prognostic role of combined alterations in these two pathways have been undertaken. Although a worse prognosis has been recognized in patients with aberrant expression of p53 and p16 in non-small-cell lung cancer (117), a prospective study of 171 patients with HNSCC demonstrated that alterations of p16 and p53 did not confer any additional information over p53 alone (104).

ING

When TSGs are inactivated, cells display neoplastic growth. Classically, both alleles need to be inactivated, such as deletion of one allele along with a mutation in the other allele. However, some TSG display haploid insufficiency, allowing hemizygous TSG to show a tumor-prone phenotype when challenged with carcinogens (118). One such family of genes is the inhibitor of growth family proteins (*ING*). *ING1*, *ING2*, *ING3*, *ING4*, and *ING5* have been described (119), although only *ING1*, *3*, and *4* have been associated with HNSCC (120–123). LOH at the chromosomal 13q33-34 region occurs in 68% of HNSCC (121), where the *ING1* TSG is located. Inhibition of *ING1* expression promotes the transformation of epithelial cells and protects the cells from apoptosis. A considerable subset of HNSCCs has been shown to harbor inactivating mutations in the *ING1* gene accompanied by selective loss of another allele (121). LOH has also been frequently detected at 7q31 in HNSCC, the location of *ING3*. Using polymorphic microsatellite markers, allelic deletion was observed in 48% of the informative cases; *ING3* was located in the proximity of D7S643. Only one missense mutation was found in HNSCC and reverse transcription polymerase chain reaction (RT-PCR) revealed decreased or absent expression of *ING3* mRNA in 50% of primary tumors compared with matched normal samples. Interestingly, 63% of tongue and larynx tumors demonstrated this reduction, with a higher mortality associated with such cases (123). *ING4* is localized to chromosome 12p13.31 (123), with LOH described in 66% of HNSCC cases. Mutation of the *ING4* gene has not been found in HNSCC; however, mRNA levels were decreased in 76% of primary HNSCC (123).

FHIT

The *FHIT* (fragile histidine triad) gene, located at 3p14, contains FRA 3B, the most common fragile site in humans, and is frequently the target of allelic loss, homozygous deletions, and genetic rearrangement in many human tumor types. Alterations of *FHIT*, such as homozygous deletions of exons at the genomic level, insertion of intronic sequences, aberrant transcripts at the mRNA level, and lack of detectable protein can be found in up to 66–68% of patients with HNSCC (124,125). Loss of *FHIT* has been shown to be an independent adverse prognostic factor for disease-free survival in HNSCC (125–127). However, high-risk tumors lacking *FHIT* expression experienced locoregional recurrence less often (18%) than high-risk patients who were *FHIT* positive (33%) suggesting that *FHIT*-negative tumors may be more sensitive to postoperative radiotherapy and therefore more susceptible to locoregional control (126). Overexpression of the *FHIT* gene has been shown to induce cell apoptosis and altered cell cycle processes although the underlying mechanism is still not well understood (128).

KLF6

The Krüppel-like transcription factor (*KLF6*) gene is a TSG dysregulated and inactivated through LOH and/or somatic mutation in 30% of HNSCC (129). *KLF6* has been shown to upregulate p21, a key regulator of cell cycle arrest, in a p53-independent manner (130). It has been associated with cancer progression, tumor recurrence, and decreased patient survival. Risk of death for patients with LOH was 8 times greater independent of tumor size, nodal status, tobacco smoking, or treatment modality. Although *KLF6* mutations were only observed in 2 of 20 samples, altered subcellular protein localization was seen in 64% of tumors (130). Targeted stable reduction of *KLF6* in HNSCC cell lines was shown to increase cellular proliferation while decreasing p21 expression. Taken together, these findings suggest that *KLF6* LOH represents a clinically relevant biomarker predicting patient survival and tumor recurrence and that dysregulation of *KLF6* function plays an important role in HNSCC progression (129).

Evidence suggests that several additional putative TSGs may reside at chromosomes 3p, 6p, 8p, 9p, 13q21, and 18q (37,38,132–135). For example, there are at least two candidate TSGs at 9p21-22 in addition to the p15/p16/p19 genes (135). and the 10q21 region (136). In addition, region 8p21.3 was shown to exhibit LOH in 87.9% of HNSCC cell lines suggesting this region harbors one or more important TSG (137). Mitochondrial TSG 1 (*MTUS1*) is a recently identified candidate TSG in this region. This gene has been shown to be consistently downregulated (RT-PCR), and a number of exon sequence variants have been noted (137). Further studies are required to identify novel markers and to discover the possible candidate genes within the consistently lost regions.

ONCOGENIC VIRUSES

There is no doubt that the main risk factor for head and neck malignancy is smoking and alcohol. Exposure to one or both accounts for more than 75% of oral cavity and pharyngeal cancers in developed countries (138). The combined effect is multiplicative rather than additive (139–141). However, viruses cause approximately 15% of all cancers, and the head and neck is no exception. DNA viruses can cause malignant transformation by inhibiting the normal function of TSG, in contrast to retroviruses (RNA viruses), which usually deregulate signal transduction pathways. Virally induced tumors can also be subdivided into acutely transforming or slowly transforming. In acutely transforming, the viral particles carry a gene that encodes for an overactive oncogene called "viral-oncogene" (v-*onc*). The infected cell is transformed as soon as v-*onc* is expressed. In contrast, slowly-transforming viruses insert their genome near a proto-oncogene in the host genome, known as transduction. The viral promoter or other transcription regulatory elements in turn cause overexpression of that proto-oncogene, resulting in uncontrolled cellular proliferation. Because viral genome insertion is not specific to proto-oncogenes and the chance of insertion near that proto-oncogene is low, slowly-transforming viruses have longer tumor latency compared to an acutely-transforming virus. With this pathogenesis it is apparent why oncogenes associated with viral transduction can also be recognized in non-virally induced malignancies. Many oncogenic viruses have been described: Epstein-Barr virus (EBV) and Human papillomavirus (HPV) are important in head and neck malignancies and are described.

Epstein-Barr Virus (EBV)

This is a double-stranded DNA virus associated with multiple diseases including Burkitt's lymphoma, nasopharyngeal carcinoma (NPC), and infectious mononucleosis. Epstein-Barr virus (EBV) infects the majority of the world's adult population, and following primary infection the individual remains a lifelong carrier of the virus. The complement regulatory protein CD21 on B cells is the principal receptor for the virus. Two types of infections can occur: either latent or lytic infection. In the former there is proliferation of the B cells, and in the latter there is generation of mature virions. Mature virion production does not inevitably lead to lysis of the host cell as EBV virions are produced by budding from the infected cell. A small viral protein set is produced during the latent cycle infection. These include Epstein-Barr nuclear antigen (EBNA)-1, EBNA-2, EBNA-3A, EBNA-3B, EBNA-3C, EBNA-leader protein (EBNA-LP) and latent membrane proteins (LMP)-1, LMP-2A, and LMP-2B and the Epstein-Barr encoded RNAs. In addition to the latent proteins, two small nonpolyadenylated (noncoding) RNAs, EBV-encoded RNA (EBERs) 1 and 2, are probably expressed in all forms of latency. Finally, EBV codes for at least 20 microRNAs that are expressed in latently infected cells. After the initial infection, it is thought that the virus stops protein production to evade the host immune system. Reactivation can occur via a number of stimuli including cross-linking of B cell receptors with antibodies.

Undifferentiated nasopharyngeal carcinoma (WHO type III; UNPC) is characterized by the presence of undifferentiated carcinoma cells together with a prominent lymphocytic infiltrate; the latter is believed to be essential for the growth of the tumor cells. A link between EBV and UNPC was suggested as early as 1966. Early studies demonstrated EBV DNA in the tumor cells of UNPCs using in situ hybridization and the anticomplement immunofluorescence assay (142). More recently, southern blot hybridization of DNA from UNPC tissues has revealed a monoclonal profile of the resident viral genome, suggesting that EBV infection had taken place before clonal expansion of the malignant cell population (143). The etiology of NPC appears to be multifactoral including EBV, geography (China and South-East Asia), and diet (nitrosamines). Serological screening identified elevated EBV-specific antibody titers in high-incidence areas; in particular, IgA antibodies to EBV viral capsid antigen (VCA) and early antigens, and these have proved useful in the diagnosis and subsequent monitoring of disease progression following treatment (144). EBNA-1 and the EBERs are expressed in all EBV-positive cases, and LMP-1 is present in up to approximately 65% of cases (145,146), although the detection of LMP-1 in a given tumor is dependent in part on the sensitivity of the method used. PCR has been shown to identify more positive cases than immunohistochemistry. PCR studies have also revealed expression of LMP-2A, though the LMP-2A protein has yet to be detected in NPCs (147). Although not validated, pretreatment circulating EBV DNA load has been shown to be an independent prognostic factor for overall survival in 376 NPC patients (148). Plasma EBV DNA using real-time PCR has been shown to be a useful marker for the disease (149) as well as predictive for recurrence in nonmetastatic NPC (149,150). In addition, it was identified as an important prognostic marker, related to tumor volume (151). Plasma EBV DNA has recently been found to be superior to serum EBV VCA antibodies in prognostic predictions for NPC in 114 paired plasma and serum samples (152). However, there are isolated reports of patients with detectable levels of EBV antibodies within their plasma, but no detectable EBV DNA (153). The association of EBV with WHO types I and II NPC remains controversial. Viral DNA is detectable in extracts from squamous cell NPCs by southern blot hybridization (154). Most in situ hybridization studies have failed to detect EBV DNA or EBERs in squamous cell NPC, and PCR only identifies EBV DNA in a small proportion of squamous cell NPCs, suggesting that EBV is present only in reactive B lymphocytes in these lesions. However, one report demonstrated the expression of the EBERs in all of 31 squamous NPCs (155). Although not all NPCs are associated with detectable EBV, the presence of the virus (detected by in situ hybridisation) was associated with a better prognosis (156). Interestingly, there is a documented association (15%) of NPC expressing viral RNA of EBV and HPV (types 6,11,16,18) (157).

Can EBV be used as a diagnostic tool in unknown primary disease? In a small study, using cellular material gained by fine needle aspiration (FNA) from metastatic lymph nodes within the cervical chain, EBV DNA was shown to be diagnostic and predictive for NPC (160). This technique was reported as 90% sensitive and 99% specific (153,158). In addition, this technique has been used to quantitate EBV DNA pre- and posttreatment using PCR (150).

Papillomaviruses

Papillomaviruses are slowly-transforming DNA viruses. The papillomavirus genome is a double-stranded circular DNA molecule approximately 8,000 base pairs in length. A single viral protein (L1) forms a capsid and self-assembled virus-like particles composed of L1 are the basis of prophylactic HPV vaccines designed to elicit virus-neutralizing antibodies to protect against initial HPV infection. The papillomavirus genome is divided into an early region (E: E1–E8), encoding various genes that are expressed immediately after initial infection of a host cell, and a late region (L) encoding the capsid genes L1 and L2. All the genes are encoded on one DNA strand. Papillomaviruses replicate exclusively in keratinocytes. Keratinocyte stem cells are the initial target of papillomavirus infections. Microtraumas (small wounds) in the skin or mucosal surface allow the virus to access the basal stem cells. Interactions between L1 and sulfated sugars on the cell surface allow initial attachment of the virus. The virus is then able to enter the cell interacting with specific receptors, including alpha-6 integrins (159) and transported to intracellular endosomes. The capsid protein L2 disrupts the membrane of the endosome, allowing the viral genome to escape and travel, with L2, to the cell nucleus (160). After successful infection of a keratinocyte, the virus expresses very low levels of the viral proteins E1 and E2, which maintain the viral DNA as a circular episome. The viral oncogenes E6 and E7, which promote cell growth by inactivating the tumor suppressor proteins p53 and pRb, respectively, may also be expressed at very low levels. Keratinocyte stem cells in the epithelial basement layer can maintain papillomavirus genomes in a dormant state for decades (161). The expression of the viral late genes, L1 and L2, is exclusively restricted to differentiating keratinocytes in the outermost layers of the skin or mucosal surface.

The increased expression of L1 and L2 is associated with a dramatic proliferation in the number of copies of the viral genome. The restriction of viral late gene expression may represent a form of immune evasion. The new infectious progeny viruses are assembled in the cell nucleus and released into the environment via desquamation, limiting any inflammatory response. Although some papillomavirus types can cause cancer in the epithelial tissues they occupy, cancer is not a typical outcome of infection. The development of papillomavirus-induced cancers typically occurs over the course of many years.

More than 118 HPVs have been described (162). Mucosal HPVs can be categorized in two major groups based on oncogenic potential. HPV 6 and 11 are "low-risk" types accounting for the majority of genital warts, while HPV 16 and 18 are the major "high-risk" types, predominating in cervical and head and neck cancers. Studies of cervical cancers have shown that the central components of HPV-induced malignant transformation are as follows: (1) inactivation of the cellular p53 gene by the E6 oncoprotein and (2) inactivation of the pRb gene by the HPV E7 oncoprotein (163). Therefore, HPV targets the same molecular pathways as the mutagens present in tobacco and alcohol (164).

A link between HPV and HNSCC was suggested 25 years ago (165). The variation in isolation of HPV DNA from tumors of the head and neck appear to be related to subsite and method of DNA detection (166,167). The strongest link was with oropharyngeal tumors (167,168) Specifically, within the oropharyngeal subsite, the association between HPV 16 and cancer was strongest for tonsil (OR: 15.1, 95% CI: 6.8–33.7). When the meta-analysis included data for the oropharynx as a whole, the OR was 4.3 (95% CI: 2.1–8.9) compared with the oral cavity (OR: 2.0, 95% CI: 1.2–3.4) and larynx (OR: 2.0, 95% CI: 1.0–4.2) (167).

Approximately 20% of head and neck cancers occur in nonsmokers and nondrinkers (169–171). There is strong epidemiologic and experimental evidence indicating that HPV accounts at least partly for this subset of cancers (172–174). It has been suggested that HPV-positive oropharyngeal cancers comprise a distinct molecular, clinical and pathologic disease entity that are likely to be causally associated with HPV infection (175) and less dependent on traditional risk factors (176). However, recently, a case-control study including newly diagnosed oropharyngeal cancer showed that oral HPV infection was strongly associated with oropharyngeal cancer among patients with or without the established risk factors of tobacco and alcohol use (177). Specifically, a high lifetime number of vaginal-sex partners was associated with oropharyngeal cancer (OR: 3.1; 95% CI: 1.5–6.5), as was a high lifetime number of oral-sex partners (OR: 3.4; 95% CI: 1.3–8.8). HPV-16 L1 seropositivity was highly associated with oropharyngeal cancer among patients with a history of heavy tobacco and alcohol use (OR: 19.4; 95% CI: 3.3–113.9) and among those without such a history (OR: 33.6; 95% CI: 13.3–84.8). The association was similarly increased among patients with oral HPV-16 infection, regardless of their tobacco and alcohol use. By contrast, tobacco and alcohol use increased the association with oropharyngeal cancer primarily among patients without exposure to HPV 16.

DIAGNOSTIC AND THERAPEUTIC APPLICATIONS OF MOLECULAR BIOLOGY

As discussed previously cellular oncogenes are cancer-causing genes that are formed when the function of a normal cellular gene is altered in some way. Like all genes the protein product that they code for mediates their effect. These proteins are usually, if not always, involved in signal transduction, which is how growth regulatory signals from outside the cell are directed to the nucleus of the cell. The differences between the oncogene-directed protein product and that which would have been formed by the normal cellular gene can be qualitative or quantitative. Activated oncogenes may differ substantively from the normal cellular gene so that its expression results in a truly novel protein specific only to the transformed cell. Alternatively, deregulation may result in a quantitative change in the levels of the gene product formed. In the second case, the protein product is not unique to the cancer cell, which limits the diagnostic and therapeutic impact of these tumor markers. The probability of curing patients with HNSCC is related to the stage of the disease. Therefore, the importance of early diagnosis cannot be overemphasized.

DIAGNOSTIC APPLICATIONS
Identification of Premalignant Lesions at Risk of Progression

Identifying patients with lesions at risk of transformation or progression is important so that exposure to risk factors can be limited and patients can be given more aggressive treatment strategies such as chemoprevention. Increased polysomies, defined as the presence of three or more copies of the chromosome, of chromosomes 7 and 17 were associated with progression from normal epithelium to dysplastic mucosae and with risk of development of oral cancer (178). Using the technique of microsatellite assay, which provides information about the frequency of allelic imbalance (AI) at polymorphic markers within chromosomal regions that harbor the TSGs, Mao et al. (179) demonstrated that the presence of AI at 3p and 9p can identify patients with dysplastic lesions at risk of progression. Further studies incorporating markers at additional chromosomal arms revealed that patients with dysplastic lesions with AI at two or more of the key chromosomal loci have a 75% chance of developing an upper aerodigestive tract tumor in 5 years (180). Identical allelic losses at 9p21, 11q13, 17p13, 3p, and 13q21 were identified in histologically benign mucosal specimens and cervical nodal metastases of patients with unknown primary HNSCC, suggesting the foci of clonal precancerous cells within these sites presumed to harbor the primary tumor (181).

Cancer Detection

Failure to diagnose HNSCC in its earliest stages is the most important factor contributing to the poor treatment outcome. Early detection is also crucial to effective surveillance after treatment of HNSCC. Although visual inspection is the most common method of detecting oral and oropharyngeal squamous carcinoma, adjunctive detection methods have been evaluated. These include use of toluidine blue to identify malignant changes in squamous mucosa

(182,183) and newer more advanced methods such as fluorescence imaging (184,185). Brush biopsies have been used to detect exfoliated cytology and DNA cytometry (186,187). Cytologic diagnosis combined with DNA-image cytometry to measure DNA aneuploidy has proven to have high specificity (>97%) and sensitivity (>98%) for malignancy in studies of patients evaluated with premalignant lesions in the oral cavity (186,188). In addition, cytology combined with DNA-image cytometry may predict malignant transformation up to 15 months before its histological confirmation (189). Head and neck cancers are among the most antigenic tumors, and several potential tumor markers for HNSCC have been suggested such as squamous cell carcinoma antigen (SCCAg) (190) and cytokeratin fragment 19 (CYFRA 21-1) (191). High urinary levels of TGF-α have been detected in patients with advanced head and neck cancer, and preliminary findings indicate that the quantity of marker detected is proportional to the clinical extent of the malignancy (192). Standard cytological methods have been shown to have potential value for the detection of second primary tumors in the esophagus of head and neck cancer patients (193). However, the lack of sensitivity and specificity remains the main problem. Using the PCR technique, Feinmeisser et al. revealed that the detection of the EBV genome in FNAs of metastatic neck nodes was highly predictive of a nasopharyngeal primary (194). These findings may carry important implications regarding the treatment of the unknown primary lesion and may result in earlier treatment of unrecognized early NPCs. Recent studies using quantitative real-time PCR have also shown that viral sequences of EBV (195) and HPV (196) may be detectable in sera of patients with advanced HNSCC and may represent novel markers for disseminated disease. Microsatellite analysis of LOH or microsatellite instability demonstrated tumor-specific DNA alterations in the serum (197) and saliva (198) of a significant percentage of patients with HNSCC. No microsatellite alterations were detected in any of the samples from healthy control patients, indicating high specificity of the assay. Soluble CD44 in saliva [solCD44 enzyme-linked immunosorbent assay (ELISA)] has recently been shown to be sensitive and specific when combined with methylation status of the CD44 gene at differentiating benign from malignant upper aerodigestive disease (199). The development of a diagnostic assay on serum reactivity to a panel of biomarkers using microarray-based serologic profiling and specialized bioinformatics has recently revealed an accuracy of 84.9% with sensitivity of 79.8% and specificity of 90.1% for HNSCC (199).

Cancer Localization

Identification of the full extent of a lesion is paramount for surgical clearance. A number of different imaging techniques, including fluorescence and spectral imaging, are currently being evaluated in HNSCC (unpublished data). Much of the literature to date is related to the upper and lower gastro-intestinal tract and the cervix (200,201).

Clinical studies have successfully used tissue autofluorescence with conventional white light endoscopy and biopsy for detecting adenomatous colonic polyps, differentiating benign hyperplastic from adenomas with acceptable sensitivity and specificity (201). It has been shown that mitochondria and lysosomes were the major intracellular fluorescent components. Normal and hyperplastic epithelial cells were weakly autofluorescent and had similar numbers of mitochondria and lysosomes, whereas adenomatous (dysplastic) epithelial cells showed much higher autofluorescence, and numerous highly autofluorescent lysosomal (lipofuscin) granules (202). Point fluorescence spectroscopy, although playing a crucial role in the pioneering mechanistic development of fluorescence endoscopic imaging, does not appear to have a predictive role due to suboptimal sensitivity and specificity. Other point spectroscopic modalities, such as Raman spectroscopy and elastic light scattering, continue to be evaluated in clinical studies but still suffer the significant disadvantages of being random and nonimaging (201). Confocal fluorescence endomicroscopy, providing real-time optical biopsy, is a recent addition to fluorescence endoscopic imaging (203). To improve detection of disease exogenous fluorescence contrast probes that specifically target a variety of disease-related cellular biomarkers using conventional fluorescent dyes and novel potent fluorescent nanocrystals (i.e., quantum dots) have been developed (204). Much of the technology can be translated into discrete anatomical areas, including the head and neck.

PROGNOSTIC APPLICATIONS
Tumor Stage Associations

As our knowledge of oncogenes increases it seems apparent that some oncogene products are necessary at the earliest stages of carcinogenesis. However, other genes are turned on late in the malignant process and seem to be required to stimulate the cancer to advanced stages of malignancy. In addition, it appears that still other genes are necessary for the development of certain tumor characteristics such as angio-/lymphangiogenesis and propensity to metastases. Overexpression of EGFR seems to be an important marker in HNSCC. Advanced clinical lesions (T4 stage) had significantly different EGFR RNA levels from those lesions of the T3 or T1/2 stages. In addition, those tumors with nodal metastases have statistically significant EGFR overexpression levels compared with those with no evidence of nodal disease (50). Another group has demonstrated in patients with oral SCCs that the expression of all four *erb*B receptors was significantly associated with shortened survival and the combination of *erb*B-2, B-3, and EGFR but not *erb*B-4 significantly improved the predicting power (60). Telomerase is a reverse transcriptase enzyme that extends telomeric repeats and is involved in cellular immortality. Like EGFR, it is overexpressed in HNSCCs and also seems to predict advanced disease (205). Telomerase activity increases with late-stage carcinoma and is present at lower levels in all earlier stages. The finding of increased telomerase activity in histologically normal tissue suggests that the enzyme may be useful as a molecular marker of disease and may play a role in the molecular assessment of tumor margins. Overexpression of p53 in initial HNSCC predicts for increased incidence of second primary tumors and recurrences of primary tumors (206).

HNSCC is characterized by its capacity to invade adjacent tissues and metastasize locoregionally. The co-operation of multiple proteolytic enzymes that are secreted by tumor cells and/or host cells and whose substrates include extracellular matrix (ECM) components is required for cancer cells to invade the ECM and penetrate the lymphatic or blood vessel wall where they may grow and metastasize to distant sites. ECM proteolysis is also involved in the angiogenesis necessary for the continued growth of solid tumors. Recent studies demonstrated that the expression of multiple key molecules involved in HNSCC invasion, angiogenesis, and metastasis including matrix metallopro-teinases (MMPs) and vascular endothelial growth factors (VEGFs) is a common feature in experimental (71,207) and clinical models of HNSCC (208–210), and the analysis of specific MMPs and VEGFs may be useful to evaluate the malignant potential in individual HNSCCs. There is convincing evidence that the invasive growth of neoplastic cells is a deregulated form of the physiological program that occurs during the formation and patterning of an embryo (211). This complex process involves many signals including hepatocyte growth factor, signaling through its receptor c-MET (212). Both molecules are mis- and over expressed in HNSCC and appear to be involved in the induction of invasive growth in HNSCC (211–213).

LOH seems to be more common than MSI in HNSCC. Although both types of microsatellite alterations have been correlated with clinico-pathological profiles, only LOH seems to have a clear prognostic value (214). The predictive value of MSI and LOH remains debatable. More research will need to be undertaken to establish LOH detection as a translational application in the HNSCC field.

Predictors of Other Aspects of Tumor Behavior

In addition to being markers for tumor staging, oncogene expression is also a predictor of tumor behavior. Activation of certain proto-oncogenes may predict radiation resistance and chemotherapy resistance. Radiation-resistant human laryngeal cancer cell lines showed evidence of altered *raf* proto-oncogenes (84). Prospective studies reveal that p53 alterations can predict tumor response to neoadjuvant chemotherapy in HNSCC (215). Increased tumor resistance to cytotoxic agents, including radiotherapy (216,217) has been associated with EGFR overexpression in HNSCC in addition to its association with more aggressive tumor behavior.

THERAPEUTIC APPLICATIONS
Anti-Oncogene Therapeutics
Anti-DNA/RNA Therapeutics

Theoretically, by preventing the flow of abnormal cellular information from the oncogene DNA to RNA to protein, one could inhibit the expression of the malignant phenotype. Specific antisense molecules could be designed to block replication or expression of oncogenic DNA (218). Similarly, blocking molecules could be directed to prevent translation of the oncogenic RNA into its abnormal oncoprotein. In vitro experiments have shown promising results. It can be difficult however, to regulate the amount of blocking that occurs due to in vivo mechanisms such as feedback regulation.

Anti-Oncoprotein Therapeutics

Immunotherapy is one particular application of this technology that may be a promising approach to cancer therapy. The created monoclonal antibody is able to recognize a specific tumor target such as an oncogene protein product. Anti-EGFR monoclonal antibody has been shown to be an effective antiproliferative agent for HNSCC via several mechanisms including induction of G1 cell cycle arrest and apoptosis (219), direct terminal differentiation (219), inhibition of production of proteolytic enzymes (207) and angiogenic factors (71), and enhancement of antitumor activity of chemotherapeutic drugs (220) and radiation therapy (221). In 2006, the U.S. Food and Drug Administration (FDA) approved cetuximab for use with radiation treatment in patients with locally advanced HNSCC (222). In this phase III trial, patients with locoregionally advanced head and neck cancer were randomly assigned to treatment with high-dose radiotherapy alone or high-dose radiotherapy plus weekly cetuximab. The results demonstrated significantly improved locoregional control and overall survival, in favor of the combination therapy. It is a human-murine chimeric monoclonal antibody (IgG) targeting the EGFR. It competitively binds to the extracellular domain of the receptor. The addition of cetuximab to cisplatin as first-line therapy in patients with recurrent or metastatic HNSCC has significantly improved the overall response rate when compared to cisplatin alone (223). Phase II data of cetuximab given as monotherapy in recurrent or metastatic HNSCC patients who had progressed on platinum-based therapy demonstrated an overall response rate of 13% with a median survival of about 6 months (224). Therefore, the FDA has also approved cetuximab monotherapy use for this indication in recurrent or metastatic HNSCC (225). Other mABs directed against different targets in HNSCC have been described, including trastuzmab and bevacizumab. Bevacizumab is an anti-angiogenic mAB directed against the VEGF. It has been demonstrated that EGFR activation can upregulate VEGF, and this phenomenon can be correlated with resistance to anti-EGFR agents (226). Some studies are ongoing, others have demonstrated encouraging results, although vascular side effects are not infrequent (227–229). Perifosine is an oral alkylphospholipid that inhibits AKT phosphorylation. Preclinical studies have demonstrated that AKT inhibition induces apoptosis and anoikis in HNSCC. The PI3K/AKT/mammalian target of rapamycin (mTOR) pathway is activated in 57–81% of patients with HNSCC, and AKT is usually upregulated (230). Perifosine does not demonstrate any anti-tumor activity in HNSCC (231). However, because AKT activation is a possible mechanism of resistance to EGFR blockade (232), the combination of AKT inhibitors with anti-EGFR agents is of potential interest. Another approach using immunotoxin is composed of an antibody or a cytokine and a conjugated molecule capable of destroying the cancer cell such as a toxin, drug, or radionucleotide. Based on the uniform expression of interleukin-4 (IL-4) receptor on HNSCC cells, a chimeric protein composed of circular permuted IL-4 and a truncated form of a bacterial toxin called *Pseudomonas* exotoxin was produced and found to be highly and specifically cytotoxic to HNSCC cells via induction of apoptosis (233).

Gene Therapy

The aim of gene therapy is to introduce new genetic material into cancer cells that will selectively kill cancer cells with no toxicity to the neighboring nonmalignant cells. Gene therapy uses a vector to deliver a DNA sequence into cells and then the DNA incorporates itself into the cellular genome and produces proteins that have a therapeutic effect. A variety of gene therapy approaches have been described as follows.

Replacing or Compensating for TSG

Active TSGs that are lost or altered through acquired genetic mutations can be reintroduced into tumor cells to control progression through the cell cycle. Transfection of human HNSCC cell lines with functional p53 temporarily arrested the growth of cells in tissue culture (234) and reduced tumor growth in nude mice (235). In addition, it has been shown that delivery of wild-type p53 can sensitize cancer cells to radiotherapy (236) and chemotherapy (237) in vitro and in vivo. A phase I study using human adenovirus/ p53 gene transfer as a surgical adjuvant in advanced head and neck cancers has been completed and revealed a survival benefit compared with that reported in chemotherapy trials (238). A number of preliminary phase II clinical trials of p53 gene therapy have been performed (239). In this trial, 18 patients with relapsed HNSCC had intratumoral injections of a viral vector expressing wild-type p53. There was a single pathological complete response, two clinical partial responses, six patients with disease stabilization, and six patients with progressive disease. In addition to the work on p53, further studies have involved other cell cycle control genes. Preclinical in vitro and in vivo studies in a number of model systems including HNSCC have demonstrated that restoration of expression of the retinoblastoma (Rb) and cyclin dependent kinase inhibitors by a variety of vectors mediated G1/S cell cycle arrest, apoptosis, and reduced tumor growth (240). Oncogene expression can lead to a significant growth advantage to the cells, or the capacity to evade normal apoptotic pathways. One approach to counteract the activating function of these mutated genes is by targeting the transcriptional/translational machinery of the cell, with the aim of preventing the cell from making functional oncogenic proteins. Two main strategies have been proposed: (1) antisense oligonucleotides (ASO) that can interfere with either transcription or translation and (2) catalytic ribozymes that interfere with translation (241). ASOs targeting several oncogene families reduced the growth of tumors in vitro and in vivo when delivered either alone and in combination with cytotoxic drugs (242). Focused experiments addressing the best mRNA to target the most effective route of administration need to be performed. In addition, it needs to be investigated whether this treatment is better in combination with other available treatments. Ribozymes are RNA molecules with catalytic activity that degrade phosphodiester bonds in mRNA molecules in a sequence specific manner. Two studies in vitro have shown activity in head and neck cancer lines (243,244); as yet, no clinical trials have been conducted in head and neck cancer patients with this modality.

Inserting Genes that Produce Cytotoxic Substances

"Suicide" gene therapy or genetic prodrug activation therapy inserts a gene into the tumor that encodes for a protein that will convert a nontoxic prodrug into a toxic substance. In HNSCC, the herpes simplex virus thymidine kinase (HSV-*tk*) gene therapy has been the most investigated (245–247).

Tumor cells are genetically modified with HSV-*tk* gene and are then treated with the prodrug ganciclovir. HSV-*tk* enzyme phosphorylates ganciclovir to ganciclovir monophosphate and then triphosphate. Ganciclovir triphosphate inhibits DNA synthesis and results in apoptosis (or programmed cell death). Nude mice were implanted with a human oral SCC cell line and treated with an adenoviral vector containing the HSV-*tk* gene and ganciclovir. The tumor cells were shown to have DNA fragmentation-positive cells (247).

Modulating the Immune System

Immunomodulation is an attractive cancer target as potentially a small immunogenic stimulus could not only trigger a primary response but also generate memory cells to prevent disease recurrence. Clinical studies to date have involved either delivering genes encoding cytokines directly into tumor cells in vivo, or using genetically modified normal or malignant cells as cancer vaccines. As an example of the former approach, intratumoral injections of cDNA encapsulated in liposomes were well tolerated in phase I and II studies and resulted in successful gene transfer. Stable disease and some partial responses were reported in patients with HNSCC (248). TNF-α, interferon-γ (IFN-γ), IL-2, and IL-4 genes have each been transfected into tumor cells in tissue culture. When these transfected cells are then introduced into humans or mice, the host immune response is amplified, thereby limiting tumor growth (249). The effect of IL-2 and IL-4 transfection has been attributed to direct stimulation and proliferation of cytotoxic T-lymphocytes by tumor cells.

Future Directions in Gene Therapy

Genes currently under investigation include suicide gene (HSV-*tk*-ganciclovir108), immune-modulatory cytokine genes (IL-2, GM-CSF, IL-12 (250)) and TSGs (p16 (251), p21 (252), p53 (253), FHIT (128), *c-myb* (254). Delivery vehicles under investigation include viral and nonviral systems (23). Viral vector systems include those based on adenoviruses, retroviruses, defective adenoviruses, adeno-associated virus, and herpes virus. Various techniques are being developed to enhance viral infection efficiency and selectivity of tumor cells such as using bispecific antibodies that recognize domains of viral vector as well as the EGFR (255) and using a modified viral vector that recognizes integrins of the a_2b_1 and a_3b_1 class frequently overexpressed in HNSCC (256). Clinical gene therapy trials using standard adenovirus 5 (Ad5)-based vectors have demonstrated limited efficacy, most likely due to low expression levels of adenoviral receptors on tumor cells. Suominen et al. (257) demonstrated in HNSCC cell lines a high CD46 expression, in contrast with the coxsackie and adenovirus receptor. In addition, Ad5/35. LacZ was more effective than Ad5.LacZ in transducing primary HNSCC cells; (257) this vector remains under further development. Nonviral gene delivery systems include liposomes and naked DNA. Another modality is "nongene gene therapy" using agents to restore the DNA binding function of key growth-regulatory elements or to target pathways that affect the ability of p53 binding protein, Mdm2, to degrade p53 (258). Targets under investigation include the inhibition of tumor angiogenesis as this will decrease vascular support required for tumor growth and support (208,259). A novel gene therapy approach uses an adenovirus called ONYX-015 that lacks the E1B region of the virus. The E1B region normally binds and inactivates p53 and is required for viral replication in normal cells. The ONYX-015 lacks E1B, thereby preferentially replicates in tumor cells lacking functional p53, leading to apoptosis (235,260). Additional mechanisms of selectivity of ONYX-015 in cancer cells also relate to viral mRNA export and processing, and its interaction with p14 (ARF) (261).

The escape of malignant cells from the local host tissues, metastasis, penetration, and then the successful acquisition of the distant host environment by sequential enzyme activation is also coded by specific proto-oncogene activation and TSG deactivation (262). Overcoming extracellular barriers to tumor spread is fundamental to the definition and spread of malignancy (262). These spreading factors are coded and can be detected at enzymatic, cytoplasmic mRNA and DNA levels. It is hoped that the "profile" of spreading factors for a tumor (208) may provide an index to later prognosis and survival, and perhaps even provide therapeutic interventions with antimetastatic factors to supplement the growing armamentarium available to the head and neck oncologist.

CONCLUSION

The understanding of how cancer cells progress has increased substantially in the last three decades. With this increased understanding, our ability to apply new technologies to control and prohibit the growth of cancer is coming closer to reality.

REFERENCES

1. International SNP Map Working Group. A map of human genome sequence variation containing 1.42 million single nucleotide polymorphisms. Nature 2001; 409: 928–33.
2. International HapMap Consortium. The International Hap-Map Project. Nature 2005; 426: 789–96. A haplotype map of the human genome. Nature 2003; 437: 1299–320.
3. Iafrate AJ, Feuk L, Rivera MN et al. Detection of large-scale variation in the human genome. Nat Genet 2004; 36: 949–51.
4. Sebat J, Lakshmi B, Troge J et al. Large-scale copy number polymorphism in the human genome. Science 2004; 305: 525–8.
5. Repping S, van Daalen SK, Brown LG et al. High mutation rates have driven extensive structural polymorphism among human Y chromosomes. Nat Genet 2006; 38: 463–7.
6. Freeman JL, Perry GH, Feuk L et al. Copy number variation: new insights in genome diversity. Genome Res 2006; 16: 949–61.
7. Weinberg R. The molecular basis of oncogenes and tumor suppressor genes. Ann NY Acad Sci 1995; 758: 331–8.
8. Hatakeyama M, Herrera R, Makela T et al. The cancer cell and the cell cycle clock. Cold Spring Harb Symp Quant Biol 1994; 59: 1–10.
9. Budillon A. Molecular genetics of cancer. Oncogenes and tumor suppressor genes. Cancer 1995; 76: 1869–73.
10. Jin C, Jin Y, Gisselsson D et al. Molecular cytogenetic characterization of the 11q13 amplicon in head and neck squamous cell carcinoma. Cytogenet Genome Res 2006; 115: 99–106.
11. Hara H, Fulton N, Yashiro T et al. N-ras mutation: an independent prognostic factor for aggressiveness of papillary thyroid carcinoma. Surgery 1994; 116: 1010–16.
12. Aurelio ON, Kong XT, Gupta S et al. p53 mutants have selective dominant-negative effects on apoptosis but not growth arrest in human cancer cell lines. Mol Cell Biol 2000; 20: 770–8.
13. Meyskens FL Jr. Strategies for prevention of cancer in humans. Oncology (Williston Park) 1992; 6(2 Suppl): 15–24.
14. Reya T, Morrison SJ, Clarke MF et al. Stem cells, cancer, and cancer stem cells. Nature 2001; 414: 105–11.
15. Pardal R, Clarke MF, Morrison SJ. Applying the principles of stem-cell biology to cancer. Nat Rev Cancer 2003; 3: 895–902.
16. Aubele M, Werner M. Heterogeneity in breast cancer and the problem of relevance of findings. Anal Cell Pathol 1999; 19: 53–8.
17. Golub TR. Genome-wide views of cancer. N Engl J Med 2001; 344: 601–2.
18. Prince ME, Sivanandan R, Kaczorowski A et al. Identification of a subpopulation of cells with cancer stem cell properties in head and neck squamous cell carcinoma. Proc Natl Acad Sci USA 2007; 104: 973–8.
19. Harper LJ, Piper K, Common J et al. Stem cell patterns in cell lines derived from head and neck squamous cell carcinoma J Oral Pathol Med 2007; 36: 594–603.
20. Pongers Willemse M, Verhagen O, Tibbe G et al. Real time quantitative PCR for the detection of minimal residual disease in acute lymphoblastic leukemia using junctional region specific TaqMan probes. Leukemia 1998; 12: 2006–14.
21. Speicher M, Ballard S, Ward D. Karyotyping human chromosomes by combinatorial multi-color FISH. Nat Genet 1996; 12: 368–75.
22. Schrock E, duManoir S, Veldman T et al. Multicolor spectral karyotyping of human chromosomes. Science 1996; 273: 494–7.
23. Bergamo N, Rogatto S, Poli-Frederico R et al. Comparative genomic hybridization analysis detects frequent over-representation of DNA sequences at 3q, 7p, and 8q in head and neck carcinomas. Cancer Genet Cytogenet 2000; 119: 48–55.
24. Jeuken J, Sprenger SH, Wesseling P. Comparative genomic hybridization: practical guidelines. Diag Mol Pathol 2002; 11: 193–203.
25. Snijders AM, Nowak N, Segraves R et al. Assembly of microarrays for genome-wide measurement of DNA copy number by CGH. Nat Genet 2001; 29: 263–4.
26. Garnis C, Campbell J, Zhang L et al. OCGR array: an oral cancer genomic regional array for comparative genomic hybridization analysis. Oral Oncol 2004; 40: 511–9.
27. Chung CH, Levy S, Yarbrough WG. Clinical applications of genomics in head and neck cancer. Head Neck 2006; 28: 360–8.
28. Tricoli JV, Jacobson JW. MicroRNA: potential for cancer detection, diagnosis, and prognosis. Cancer Res 2007 15; 67: 4553–5.
29. Lu J, Getz G, Miska EA et al. MicroRNA expression profiles classify human cancers. Nature 2005; 435: 834–8.
30. Villar-Garea A, Griese M, Imhof A. Biomarker discovery from body fluids using mass spectrometry. J Chromatogr B Analyt Technol Biomed Life Sci 2007; 849: 105–14.
31. Jourenkova-Mironova N, Voho A, Bouchardy C et al. Glutathione S-transferase GSTM1, GSTM3, GSTP1 and GSTT1 genotypes and the risk of smoking-related oral and pharyngeal cancers. Int J Cancer 1999; 81: 44–8.
32. Wang L, Sturgis E, Eicher S et al. Mutagen sensitivity to benzo (a)pyrene diol epoxide and the risk of squamous cell carcinomas of the head and neck. Clin Cancer Res 1998; 4: 1773–8.
33. Van Dyke DL, Worsham MJ, Benninger MS et al. Recurrent cytogenic abnormalities in squamous cell carcinoma of the head and neck. Gene Chromosome Cancer 1994; 9: 192–206.
34. Squire JA, Bayani J, Luk C et al. Molecular cytogenetic analysis of head and neck squamous cell carcinoma: By comparative genomic hybridization, spectral karyotyping, and expression array analysis. Head Neck 2002; 24: 874–87.

35. Carey T, Worsham M, Van Dyke D. Chromosomal biomarkers in the clonal evolution of head and neck squamous neoplasia. J Cell Biochem 1993; 17F(Suppl): 213–22.

36. Ah-See K, Cooke T, Pickford I et al. An allelotype of squamous carcinoma of the head and neck using microsatellite markers. Cancer Res 1994; 54: 1617–21.

37. Nawroz H, van der Riet P, Hruban R et al. Allelotype of head and neck squamous cell carcinoma. Cancer Res 1994; 54: 1152–5.

38. Califano J, van der Riet P, Westra W et al. Genetic progression model for head and neck cancer: implications for field cancerization. Cancer Res 1996; 56: 2488–92.

39. Califano J, Westra W, Meininger G et al. Genetic progression and clonal relationship of recurrent premalignant head and neck lesions. Clin Cancer Res 2000; 6: 347–52.

40. Partridge M. Current status of genetics for prediction, prognosis, and gene therapy. Curr Opin Otolaryngol Head Neck Surgery 2000; 8: 69–79.

41. Cowan J, Beckett M, Weichselbaum R. Chromosome changes characterising in vitro response to radiation in human squamous cell carcinoma lines. Cancer Res 1993; 53: 5542–7.

42. Wreesmann VB, Wang D, Goberdhan A et al. Genetic abnormalities associated with nodal metastasis in head and neck cancer. Head Neck 2004; 26: 10–15.

43. Chen Y-J, Ko J-Y, Chen P-J et al. Chromosomal aberrations in nasopharyngeal carcinoma analyzed by comparative genomic hybridization. Genes Chromosomes Cancer 1999; 25: 169–75.

44. Patmore HS, Ashman JN, Stafford ND et al. Genetic analysis of HNSCC using comparative genomic hybridisation identifies specific aberrations associated with laryngeal origin. Cancer Lett 2007; 258: 55–62.

45. Klapper LN, Kirschbaum MH, Sela M et al. Biochemical and clinical implications of the ErbB/HER signalling network of growth factor receptors. Adv Cancer Res 2000; 77: 25–79.

46. Irish J, Bernstein A. Oncogenes in head and neck cancer. Laryngoscope 1993; 103: 42–53.

47. Temam S, Kawaguchi H, El-Naggar AK et al. Epidermal growth factor receptor copy number alterations correlate with poor clinical outcome in patients with head and neck squamous cancer. J Clin Oncol 2007; 25: 2164–70.

48. O-charoenrat P, Rhys-Evans PH, Modjtahedi H et al. The role of c-erbB receptors and ligands in head and neck squamous cell carcinoma. Oral Oncol 2002; 38: 627–40.

49. Grandis JR, Tweardy DJ. Elevated levels of transforming growth factor alpha and epidermal growth factor receptor messenger RNA are early markers of carcinogenesis in head and neck cancer. Cancer Res 1993; 53: 3579–84.

50. Anderson J, Irish J, Ngan B-Y. Prevalence of ras oncogene mutations in head and neck carcinomas. J Otolaryngology 1992; 21: 321–6.

51. Bergler W, Bier H, Ganzer U. The expression of epidermal growth factor receptors in the oral mucosa of patients with oral cancer. Arch Otorhinolaryngol 1989; 246: 121–5.

52. Kearsley JH, Leonard JH, Walsh MD et al. A comparison of epidermal growth factor receptor (EGFR) and c-erbB-2 oncogene expression in head and neck squamous cell carcinomas. Pathology 1991; 23: 189–94.

53. Riviere A, Becker J, Loning T. Comparative investigation of c-erbB2/neu expression in head and neck tumors and mammary cancer. Cancer 1991; 67: 2142–9.

54. Rodrigo JP, Ramos S, Lazo PS et al. Amplification of ERBB oncogenes in squamous cell carcinomas of the head and neck. Eur J Cancer Part A 1996; 32A: 2004–10.

55. O-charoenrat P, Rhys-Evans P, Eccles SA. Characterization of ten newly-derived human head and neck squamous carcinoma cell lines with special reference to c-erbB proto-oncogene expression. Anticancer Res 2001; 21: 1953–63.

56. O-charoenrat P, Rhys-Evans PH, Archer DJ. C-erbB receptors in squamous cell carcinomas of the head and neck:

clinical significance and correlation with matrix metalloproteinases and vascular endothelial growth factors. Oral Oncol 2002; 38: 73–80.

57. Craven JM, Pavelic ZP, Stambrook PJ et al. Expression of c-erbB2 gene in human head and neck carcinoma. Anticancer Res 1992; 12: 2273–6.

58. Field JK, Spandidos DA, Yiagnisis M et al. c-erbB2 expression in squamous cell carcinoma of the head and neck. Anticancer Res 1992; 12: 613–20.

59. Hou L, Shi D, Tu SM et al. Oral cancer progression and c-erbB-2/neu proto-oncogene expression. Cancer Lett 1992; 65: 215–20.

60. Xia W, Lau Y-K, Zhang H-Z et al. Combination of EGFR, HER-2/neu, and HER-3 is a stronger predictor for the outcome of oral squamous cell carcinoma than any individual family members. Clin Cancer Res 1999; 5: 4164–74.

61. Cavalot A, Martone T, Roggero N et al. Prognostic impact of HER-2/neu expression on squamous head and neck carcinomas. Head Neck 2007; 29: 655–64.

62. Ma BB, Poon TC, To KF et al. Prognostic significance of tumor angiogenesis, Ki 67, p53 oncoprotein, epidermal growth factor receptor and HER2 receptor protein expression in undifferentiated nasopharyngeal carcinoma-a prospective study. Head Neck 2003; 25: 864–72.

63. Issing WJ, Heppt WJ, Kastenbauer ER. erbB-3, a third member of the erbB/epidermal growth factor receptor gene family: its expression in head and neck cancer cell lines. Eur Arch Otorhinolaryngol 1993; 250: 392–5.

64. Funayama T, Nakanishi T, Takahashi K et al. Overexpression of c-erbB-3 in various stages of human squamous cell carcinomas. Oncology 1998; 55: 161–7.

65. Shintani S, Funayama T, Yoshihama Y et al. Prognostic significance of ERBB3 overexpression in oral squamous cell carcinoma. Cancer Lett 1995; 95: 79–83.

66. Werkmeister R, Brandt B, Joos U. The erbB oncogenes as prognostic markers in oral squamous cell carcinomas. Am J Surg 1996; 172: 681–3.

67. Werkmeister R, Brandt B, Joos U. Clinical relevance of erbB-1 and -2 oncogenes in oral carcinomas. Oral Oncol 2000; 36: 100–5.

68. Ibrahim SO, Vasstrand EN, Liavaag PG et al. Expression of c-erbB proto-oncogene family members in squamous cell carcinoma of the head and neck. Anticancer Res 1997; 17: 4539–46.

69. Srinivasan R, Poulsom R, Hurst HC et al. Expression of the c-erbB-4/HER4 protein and mRNA in normal human fetal and adult tissues and in a survey of nine solid tumor types. J Pathol 1998; 185: 236–45.

70. O-charoenrat P, Rhys-Evans P, Court WJ et al. Differential modulation of proliferation, matrix metalloproteinase expression and invasion of human head and neck squamous carcinoma cells by c-erbB ligands. Clin Exp Metastasis 1999; 17: 631–9.

71. O-charoenrat P, Rhys-Evans P, Modjtahedi H et al. Vascular endothelial growth factor family members are differentially regulated by c-erbB signaling in head and neck squamous carcinoma cells. Clin Exp Metastasis 2000; 18: 155–61.

72. Xia W, Lau YK, Zhang HZ et al. Combination of EGFR, HER-2/neu, and HER-3 is a stronger predictor for the outcome of oral squamous cell carcinoma than any individual family members. Clin Cancer Res 1999; 5: 4164–74.

73. Gullick WJ. The type 1 growth factor receptors and their ligands considered as a complex system. Endocr Relat Cancer 2001; 8: 75–82.

74. Riese DJ II, Stern DF. Specificity within the EGF family/ErbB receptor family signaling network. Bioessays 1998; 20: 41–8.

75. O-charoenrat P, Modjtahedi H, Rhys-Evans P et al. Epidermal growth factor-like ligands differentially upregulate matrix metalloproteinase-9 in head and neck squamous carcinoma cells. Cancer Res 2000; 60: 1121–8.

76. O-charoenrat P, Rhys-Evans P, Eccles SA. Expression and regulation of c-erbB ligands in human head and neck squamous carcinoma cells. Int J Cancer 2000; 88: 759–65.

77. Tadokoro K, Ueda M, Ohshima T et al. Activation of oncogenes in human oral cancer cells: a novel codon 13 mutation of c-H-ras-1 and concurrent amplification of c-erb-B-1 and c-myc. Oncogene 1989; 4: 499–505.

78. Yarbrough WG, Shores C, Witsell DL et al. Ras mutations and expression in head and neck squamous cell carcinomas. Laryngoscope 1994; 104(11 Pt 1): 1337–47.

79. Ruíz-Godoy RLM, Garcia-Cuellar CM, Herrera González NE et al. Mutational analysis of K-ras and ras protein expression in larynx squamous cell carcinoma. J Exp Clin Cancer Res 2006; 25: 73–83

80. Avruch J, Zhang XF, Kyriakis, JM. Raf meets Ras: completing the framework of a signal transduction pathway. Trends Biochem Sci 1994; 19: 279–83.

81. Lee JW, Soung YH, Kim SY et al. Mutational analysis of the ARAF gene in human cancers. APMIS 2005; 113: 54–7.

82. Weber A, Langhanki L, Sommerer F et al. Mutations of the BRAF gene in squamous cell carcinoma of the head and neck. Oncogene 2003; 22: 4757–9.

83. Riva C, Lavieille JP, Reyt E et al. Differential c-myc, c-jun, c-raf and p53 expression in squamous cell carcinoma of the head and neck: implication in drug and radioresistance. Eur J Cancer B Oral Oncol 1995; 31B: 384–91.

84. Patel BK, Kasid U. Nucleotide sequence analysis of c-raf-1 cDNA and promoter from a radiation-resistant human squamous carcinoma cell line: deletion within exon 17. Mol Carcinog 1993; 8: 7–12.

85. Callender T, el-Naggar AK, Lee MS. PRAD-1 (CCND)/ cyclin D1 gene amplification in primary head and neck squamous cell carcinoma. Cancer 1994; 74: 152–8.

86. Izzo J, Papadimitrakopoulou V, Li X et al. Dysregulated cyclin D1 expression early in head and neck tumorigenesis: in vivo evidence for an association with subsequent gene amplification. Oncogene 1998; 17: 2313–22.

87. Michalides R, van Veelan N, Hart A et al. Overexpression of cyclin D1 correlates with recurrence in a group of forty-seven operable squamous cell carcinomas of the head and neck. Cancer Res 1995; 55: 975–8.

88. Bova R, Quinn D, Nankervis J et al. Cyclin D1 and p16INK4A expression predict reduced survival in carcinoma of the anterior tongue. Clin Cancer Res 1999; 5: 2810–9.

89. Higuchi E, Oridate N, Homma A et al. Prognostic significance of cyclin D1 and p16 in patients with intermediate-risk HNSCC treated with docetaxel and concurrent radiotherapy. Head Neck 2007; 29: 940–7.

90. Rodrigo J, Garcia L, Ramos S. EMS1 gene amplification correlates with poor prognosis in squamous cell carcinomas of the head and neck. Clin Cancer Res 2000; 6: 3177–82.

91. Timpson P, Lynch DK, Schramek D et al. Cortactin overexpression inhibits ligand-induced downregulation of the epidermal growth factor receptor. Cancer Res 2005; 65: 3273–80.

92. Timpson P, Wilson AS, Lehrbach GM et al. Aberrant expression of cortactin in head and neck squamous cell carcinoma cells is associated with enhanced cell proliferation and resistance to the epidermal growth factor receptor inhibitor gefitinib. Cancer Res 2007; 67: 9304–14.

93. Bockmuhl U, Schwendel A, Dietel M et al. Distinct patterns of chromosomal alterations in high- and low-grade head and neck squamous cell carcinomas. Cancer Res 1996; 56: 5325–9.

94. Resto V, Caballero O, Buta M et al. A putative oncogenic role for MPP11 in head and neck squamous cell cancer. Cancer Res 2000; 60: 5529–35.

95. Otto H, Conz C, Maier P et al. The chaperones MPP11 and Hsp70L1 form the mammalian ribosome-associated complex. Proc Natl Acad Sci USA 2005; 102: 10064–9.

96. van der Riet P, Nawroz H, Hruban R et al. Frequent loss of chromosome 9p21-22 early in head and neck cancer progression. Cancer Res 1994; 54: 1156–8.

97. Waber P, Dlugosz S, Cheng Q et al. Genetic alterations of chromosome band 9p21-22 in head and neck cancer are not restricted to p16INK4a. Oncogene 1997; 15: 1699–704.

98. Coon S, Savera A, Zarbo R et al. Prognostic implications of loss of heterozygosity at 8p21 and 9p21 in head and neck squamous cell carcinoma. Int J Cancer 2004; 111: 206–12.

99. Cairns P, Mao L, Merlo A et al. Rates of p16 (MTS1) mutations in primary tumors with 9p loss. Science 1994; 265: 415–7.

100. Wu C, Roz L, McKown S et al. DNA studies underestimate the major role of CDKN2A inactivation in oral and oropharyngeal squamous cell carcinomas. Gene Chromosome Canc 1999; 25: 16–25.

101. Reed A, Califano J, Cairns P et al. High frequency of p16 (CDKN2/MTS-1/INK4A) inactivation in head and neck squamous cell carcinoma. Cancer Res 1996; 56: 3630–3.

102. Miracca EC, Kowalski LP, Nagai MA High prevalence of P16 genetic alterations in head and neck tumors. Br J Cancer 1999; 81: 677–83.

103. Geisler S, Olshan A, Weissler M et al. p16 and p53 protein expression as prognostic indicators of survival and disease recurrence from head and neck cancer. Clin Cancer Res 2002; 8: 3445–53.

104. Ambrosch P, Schlott T, Hilmes D et al. p16 alterations and retinoblastoma protein expression in squamous cell carcinoma and neighboring dysplasia from the upper aerodigestive tract. Virchows Arch 2001; 438: 343–9.

105. Namazie A, Alavi S, Olopade OI et al. Cyclin D1 amplification and P16 (MTS1/CDK4I) deletion correlate with poor prognosis in head and neck tumors. Laryngoscope 2002; 112: 472–81.

106. Bazan V, Zanna I, Migliavacca M, Sanz-Casla M et al. Prognostic significance of p16INK4a alterations and 9p21 loss of heterozygosity in locally advanced laryngeal squamous cell carcinoma. J Cell Physiol 2002; 192: 286–93.

107. Thomas GR, Nadiminti H, Regalado J. Molecular predictors of clinical outcome in patients with head and neck squamous cell carcinoma. Int J Exp Pathol 2005; 86: 347–63.

108. Boyle J, Hakim J, Kock W et al. The incidence of p53 mutations increases with progression of head and neck cancer. Cancer Res 1993; 53: 4477–80.

109. Brennan JA, Mao L, Hruban RH et al. Molecular assessment of histopathological staging in squamous-cell carcinoma of the head and neck. N Engl J Med 1995; 332: 429–35.

110. Brennan JA, Boyle JO, Koch WM et al. Association between cigarette smoking and mutation of the p53 gene in squamous-cell carcinoma of the head and neck. N Engl J Med 1995; 332: 712–17.

111. Qin G-Z, Park J, Chen S-Y, Lazarus P. A high prevalence of p53 mutations in pre-malignant oral erythroplakia. Int J Cancer 1999; 80: 345–8.

112. Khademi B, Shirazi F, Vasei M et al. The expression of p53, c-erbB-1 and c-erbB-2 molecules and their correlation with prognostic markers in patients with head and neck tumors. Cancer Lett 2002; 184: 223–30.

113. Vielba R, Bilbao J, Ispizua A et al. p53 and cyclin D1 as prognostic factors in squamous cell carcinoma of the larynx. Laryngoscope 2003; 113: 167–72.

114. De Vicente C, Junquera Gutierrez L, Zapatero A et al. Prognostic significance of p53 expression in oral squamous cell carcinoma without neck node metastases. Head Neck 2004; 26: 22–30.

115. Cabanillas R, Rodrigo JP, Astudillo A et al. P53 expression in squamous cell carcinomas of the supraglottic larynx and its lymph node metastases: new results for an old question. Cancer 2007; 109: 1791–8.

116. Homann N, Nees M, Conradt C et al. Overexpression of p53 in tumor-distant epithelia of head and neck cancer patients is associated with an increased incidence of second primary carcinoma. Clin Cancer Res 2001; 7: 290–6.

117. Cheng YL, Lee SC, Harn HJ et al. Prognostic prediction of the immunohistochemical expression of p53 and p16 in resected non-small cell lung cancer. Eur J Cardiothorac Surg 2003; 23: 221–8.

118. Tang B, Böttinger EP, Jakowlew SB et al. Transforming growth factor-h1 is a new form of tumor suppressor with true haploid insufficiency. Nat Med 1998; 4: 802–7.

119. He GH, Helbing CC, Wagner MJ et al. Phylogenetic analysis of the ING family of PHD finger proteins. Mol Biol Evol 2005; 22: 104–6.

120. Gupta V, Schmidt A, Pashia M et al. Multiple regions of deletion on chromosome arm 13q in head-and-neck squamous cell carcinoma. Int J Cancer 1999; 84: 453–7.

121. Gunduz M, Ouchida M, Fukushima K et al. Genomic structure of the human *ING1* gene and tumor-specific mutations detected in head and neck squamous cell carcinomas. Cancer Res 2000; 60: 3143–6.

122. Gunduz M, Ouchida M, Fukushima K et al. Allelic loss and reduced expression of the ING3, a candidate tumor suppressor gene at 7q31, in human head and neck cancers. Oncogene 2002; 21: 4462–70.

123. Gunduz M, Nagatsuka H, Demircan K et al. Frequent deletion and down-regulation of ING4, a candidate tumor suppressor gene at 12p13, in head and neck squamous cell carcinomas. Gene 2005; 356: 109–17.

124. Tanimoto K, Hayashi S, Tsuchiya E et al. Abnormalities of the FHIT gene in human oral carcinogenesis. Br J Cancer 2000; 82: 838–43.

125. Lee J, Soria J-C, Hassan K et al. Loss of Fhit expression is a predictor of poor outcome in tongue cancer. Cancer Res 2001; 61: 837–41.

126. Tai SK, Lee JI, Ang KK et al. Loss of Fhit expression in head and neck squamous cell carcinoma and its potential clinical implication. Clin Cancer Res 2004; 10: 5554–7.

127. Guerin LA, Hoffman HT, Zimmerman MB, Robinson RA. Decreased fragile histidine triad gene protein expression is associated with worse prognosis in oral squamous carcinoma. Arch Pathol Lab Med 2006; 130: 158–64.

128. Ji L, Fang B, Yen N et al. Induction of apoptosis and inhibition of tumorigenicity and tumor growth by adenovirus vector-mediated fragile histidine triad (FHIT) gene overexpression. Cancer Res 1999; 59: 3333–9.

129. Teixeira MS, Camacho-Vanegas O, Fernandez Y et al. KLF6 allelic loss is associated with tumor recurrence and markedly decreased survival in head and neck squamous cell carcinoma. Int J Cancer 2007; 121: 1976–83.

130. Narla G, Heath KE, Reeves HL et al. KLF6, a candidate tumor suppressor gene mutated in prostate cancer. Science 2001; 294: 2563–6.

131. Partridge M, Emillion G, Pateromichelakis S et al. The location of candidate tumor suppressor gene loci at chromosomes 3p, 8p and 9p for oral squamous cell carcinoma. Int J Cancer 1999; 83: 318–26.

132. Ishwad C, Shuster M, Bockmuhl U et al. Frequent allelic loss and homozygous deletion in chromosome band 8p23 in oral cancer. Int J Cancer 1999; 80: 25–31.

133. Takebayashi S, Ogawa T, Jung K-Y et al. Identification of new minimally lost regions on 18q in head and neck squamous cell carcinoma. Cancer Res 2000; 60: 3397–403.

134. Toomes C, Jackson A, Maguire K et al. The presence of multiple regions of homozygous deletion at the CSMD1 locus in oral squamous cell carcinoma question the role of CSMD1 in head and neck carcinogenesis. Genes Chromosomes Cancer 2003; 37: 132–40.

135. Nakanishi H, Wang X-L, Imai F et al. Localization of a novel tumor suppressor gene loci on chromosome 9p21–22 in oral cancer. Anticancer Res 1999; 19: 29–34.

136. Beder LB, Gunduz M, Ouchida M et al. Identification of a candidate tumor suppressor gene RHOBTB1 located at a novel allelic loss region 10q21 in head and neck cancer. J Cancer Res Clin Oncol 2006; 132: 19–27.

137. Ye H, Pungpravat N, Huang BL et al. Genomic assessments of the frequent loss of heterozygosity region on 8p21.3 approximately p22 in head and neck squamous cell carcinoma. Cancer Genet Cytogenet 2007; 176: 100–6.

138. Dobrossy L. Epidemiology of head and neck cancer: magnitude of the problem. CancerMetastasis Rev 2005; 24: 9–17.

139. Blot WJ, McLaughlin JK, Winn DM et al. Smoking and drinking in relation to oral and pharyngeal cancer. Cancer Res 1988; 48: 3282–7.

140. Smith EM, Hoffman HT, Summersgill KS et al. Human papillomavirus and risk of oral cancer. Laryngoscope 1998; 108:1098–103.

141. Day GL, Blot WJ, Austin DF et al. Racial differences in risk of oral and pharyngeal cancer: alcohol, tobacco, and other determinants. J Natl Cancer Inst 1993; 85: 465–73.

142. Zur Hausen H, Schultz-Holthausen H, Klein G et al. EBV DNA in biopsies of Burkitt tumours and anaplastic carcinomas of the nasopharynx. Nature 1970; 228: 1056–8.

143. Raab-Traub N, Flynn K. The structure of the termini of the Epstein-Barr virus as a marker of clonal cellular proliferation. Cell 1986; 47: 883–9.

144. Zeng Y. Seroepidemiological studies on nasopharyngeal carcinoma in China. Adv Cancer Res 1985; 44: 121–38.

145. Young LS, Dawson CW, Clark D et al. Epstein-Barr virus gene expression in nasopharyngeal carcinoma. J Gen Virol 1988; 69: 1051–65.

146. Niedobitek G, Young LS, Sam CK et al. Expression of Epstein-Barr virus genes and of lymphocyte activation molecules in undifferentiated nasopharyngeal carcinomas. Am J Pathol 1992; 140: 879–87.

147. Brooks LA, Lear AL, Young LS et al. Epstein-Barr virus latent gene transcription in nasopharyngeal carcinoma cells: coexpression of EBNA1, LMP1, and LMP2 transcripts. J Virol 1992; 67: 3182–90.

148. Leung SF, Zee B, Ma BB et al. Plasma Epstein-Barr viral deoxyribonucleic acid quantitation complements tumor-node-metastasis staging prognostication in nasopharyngeal carcinoma. J Clin Oncol 2006; 24: 5414–18.

149. Tan EL, Looi LM, Sam CK. Evaluation of plasma Epstein-Barr virus DNA load as a prognostic marker for nasopharyngeal carcinoma. Singapore Med J 2006; 47: 803–7.

150. Makitie AA, Reis PP, Zhang T et al. Epstein-Barr virus DNA measured in nasopharyngeal brushings in patients with nasopharyngeal carcinoma: pilot study. J Otolaryngol 2004; 33: 299–303.

151. Ma BB, King A, Lo YM et al. Relationship between pretreatment level of plasma Epstein-Barr virus DNA, tumor burden, and metabolic activity in advanced nasopharyngeal carcinoma. Int J Radiat Oncol Biol Phys 2006; 66: 714–20.

152. Twu CW, Wang WY, Liang WM et al. Comparison of the prognostic impact of serum anti-EBV antibody and plasma EBV DNA assays in nasopharyngeal carcinoma. Int J Radiat Oncol Biol Phys 2007; 67: 130–7.

153. Stevens SJ, Verkuijlen SA, Hariwiyanto B et al. Noninvasive diagnosis of nasopharyngeal carcinoma: nasopharyngeal brushings reveal high Epstein-Barr virus DNA load and carcinoma-specific viral BARF1 mRNA. Int J Cancer 2006; 119: 608–14.

154. Raab-Traub N, Flynn K, Pearson G et al. The differentiated form of nasopharyngeal carcinoma contains Epstein-Barr virus DNA. Int J Cancer 1987; 39: 25–9.

155. Pathmanathan R, Prasad U, Chandrika G et al. Undifferentiated, nonkeratinizing, and squamous cell carcinoma of the nasopharynx. Variants of Epstein-Barr virus-infected neoplasia. Am J Pathol 1995; 146: 1355–67.

156. Yip KW, Shi W, Pintilie M et al. Prognostic significance of the Epstein-Barr virus, p53, Bcl-2, and survivin in nasopharyngeal cancer. Clin Cancer Res 2006; 12: 5726–32.

157. Mirzamani N, Salehian P, Farhadi M et al. Detection of EBV and HPV in nasopharyngeal carcinoma by in situ hybridization. Exp Mol Pathol 2006; 81: 231–4.

158. Tune CE, Liavaag PG, Freeman JL et al. Nasopharyngeal brush biopsies and detection of nasopharyngeal cancer in a high-risk population. J Natl Cancer Inst 1999; 91: 796–800.

159. Yoon CS, Kim KD, Park SN et al. alpha(6) Integrin is the main receptor of human papillomavirus type 16 VLP. Biochem Biophys Res Commun 2001; 283: 668–73.

160. Sun XY, Frazer I, Müller M et al. Sequences required for the nuclear targeting and accumulation of human papillomavirus type 6B L2 protein. Virology 1995; 213: 321–7.

161. Stubenrauch F, Laimins LA. Human papillomavirus life cycle: active and latent phases. Semin Cancer Biol 1999; 9: 379–86.

162. de Villiers EM, Fauquet C, Broker TR et al. Classification of papillomaviruses. Virology 2004; 324: 17–27.

163. Parker MF, Arroyo GF, Geradts J et al. Molecular characterization of adenocarcinoma of the cervix. Gynecol Oncol 1997; 64: 242–51.

164. Tran N, Rose BR, O'Brien CJ. Role of human papillomavirus in the etiology of head and neck cancer. Head Neck 2007; 29: 64–70.

165. Syrjanen K, Syrjanen S, Lamberg M et al. Morphological and immunohistochemical evidence suggesting human papillomavirus (HPV) involvement in oral squamous cell carcinogenesis. Int J Oral Surg 1983; 12: 418–24.

166. Herrero R, Castellsague X, Pawlita M et al. Human papillomavirus and oral cancer: the International Agency for Research on Cancer multicenter study. J Natl Cancer Inst 2003; 95: 1772–83.

167. Hobbs CG, Sterne JA, Bailey M et al. Human papillomavirus and head and neck cancer: a systematic review and meta-analysis. Clin Otolaryngol 2006; 31: 259–66.

168. Kreimer AR, Clifford GM, Boyle P et al. Human papillomavirus types in head and neck squamous cell carcinomas worldwide: a systematic review. Cancer Epidemiol. Biomarkers Prev 2005; 14: 467–75.

169. Wiseman SM, Swede H, Stoler DL et al. Squamous cell carcinoma of the head and neck in nonsmokers and nondrinkers: an analysis of clinicopathologic characteristics and treatment outcomes. Ann Surg Oncol 2003; 10: 551–7.

170. Lingen M, Sturgis EM, Kies MS. Squamous cell carcinoma of the head and neck in nonsmokers: clinical and biologic characteristics and implications for management. Curr Opin Oncol 2001; 13: 176–82.

171. Yamaguchi T, Shindoh M, Amemiya A et al. Identification of human papillomavirus DNA sequence in the hyperplastic epithelium of an oral denture fibroma. DisMarkers 1997; 13: 135–40.

172. Klussmann JP, Gultekin E, Weissenborn SJ et al. Expression of p16 protein identifies a distinct entity of tonsillar carcinomas associated with human papillomavirus. Am J Pathol 2003; 162: 747–53.

173. Venuti A, Badaracco G, Rizzo C et al. Presence of HPV in head and neck tumors: high prevalence in tonsillar localization. J Exp Clin Cancer Res 2004; 23: 561–6.

174. Li W, Thompson CH, Cossart YE et al. The expression of key cell cycle markers and presence of human papillomavirus in squamous cell carcinoma of the tonsil. Head Neck 2004; 26: 1–9.

175. Gillison ML, Lowy DR. A causal role for human papillomavirus in head and neck cancer. Lancet 2004; 363: 1488–9.

176. Klussmann JP, Weissenborn SJ, Wieland U et al. Human papillomavirus-positive tonsillar carcinomas: a different tumor entity? Med Microbiol Immunol (Berl) 2003; 192: 129–32.

177. D'Souza G, Kreimer AR, Viscidi R et al. Case-control study of human papillomavirus and oropharyngeal cancer. N Engl J Med 2007; 356: 1944–56.

178. Voravud N, Shin D, Ro J et al. Increased polysomies of chromosomes 7 and 17 during head and neck multistage tumorigenesis. Cancer Res 1993; 53: 2874–83.

179. Mao L, Lee J, Fan Y et al. Frequent microsatellite alterations at chromosomes 9p21 and 3p14 in oral premalignant lesions and their value in cancer risk assessment. Nat Med 1996; 2: 682–5.

180. Partridge M, Emillion G, Pateromichelakis S et al. Allelic imbalance at chromosomal loci implicated in the pathogenesis of oral precancer; cumulative loss and its relationship with progression to cancer. Oral Oncol Eur J Cancer 1997; 34: 77–83.

181. Califano J, Westra W, Koch W et al. Unknown primary head and neck squamous cell carcinoma: molecular identification of the site of origin. J Natl Cancer Inst 1999; 91: 599–604.

182. Rosenberg D, Cretin S. Use of meta-analysis to evaluate tolonium chloride in oral cancer screening. Oral Surg Oral Med Oral Pathol 1989; 67: 621–7.

183. Gray M, Elley K. Oral cancer screening. Br Dent J 2000; 189: 125.

184. Zheng W, Soo KC, Sivanandan R, Olivo M. Detection of neoplasms in the oral cavity by digitized endoscopic imaging of 5-aminolevulinic acid-induced protoporphyrin IX fluorescence. Int J Oncol 2002; 21: 763–8.

185. O'dwyer M, Day A, Padgett M et al. Detection of mucosal abnormalities in patients with oral cancer using a photodynamic technique: A pilot study. Br J Oral Maxillofac Surg 2007; 46: 6–10.

186. Maraki D, Becker J, Boecking A. Cytologic and DNA cytometric very early diagnosis of oral cancer. J Oral Pathol Med 2004; 33: 398–404.

187. Allison P. Effectiveness of screening for oral cancer not proven. Evid Based Dent 2004; 5: 40–1.

188. Remmerbach TW, Weidenbach H, Pomjanski N et al. Cytologic and DNA-cytometric early diagnosis of oral cancer. Anal Cell Pathol 2001; 22: 211–21.

189. Remmerbach TW, Weidenbach H, Hemprich A, Bocking A. Earliest detection of oral cancer using non-invasive brush biopsy including DNA-image-cytometry: report on four cases. Anal Cell Pathol 2003; 25: 159–66.

190. Snyderman C, D'Amico F, Wagner R et al. A reappraisal of the squamous cell carcinoma antigen as a tumor marker in head and neck cancer. Arch Otolaryngol Head Neck Surg 1995; 121: 1294–7.

191. Yen T, Lin W, Kao C et al. A study of a new marker, CYFRA 21–1, in squamous cell carcinoma of the head and neck, and comparison with squamous cell carcinoma antigen. Clin Otolaryngol 1998; 23: 82–6.

192. Fazekas-May M, Suen JY, Yeh YC et al. Investigation of urinary transforming growth factor alpha levels as tumor markers in patients with advanced squamous cell carcinoma of the head and neck. Head Neck 1990; 12: 411–16.

193. Pellanda A, Grosjean P, Loeni S et al. Abrasive esophageal cytology for the oncological follow-up of patients with head and neck cancer. Laryngoscope 1999; 109: 1703–8.

194. Feinmesser R, Miyazaki I, Cheung R et al. Diagnosis of nasopharyngeal carcinoma by DNA amplification of tissue obtained by fine needle aspiration. N Engl J Med 1992; 326: 17–21.

195. Lo Y, Chan L, Lo K et al. Quantitative analysis of cell-free Epstein-Barr virus DNA in plasma of patients with nasopharyngeal carcinoma. Cancer Res 1999; 59: 1188–91.

196. Capone R, Pai S, Koch W et al. Detection and quantitation of human papillomavirus (HPV) DNA in the sera of patients with HPV-associated head and neck squamous cell carcinoma. Clin Cancer Res 2000; 6: 4171–5.

197. Nawroz H, Koch W, Anker P. Microsatellite alterations in serum DNA of head and neck cancer patients. Nat Med 1996; 2: 1035–7.

198. Spafford M, Koch W, Reed A et al. Detection of head and neck squamous cell carcinoma among exfoliated oral mucosal cells by microsatellite analysis. Clin Cancer Res 2001; 7: 607–12.

199. Franzmann EJ, Reategui EP, Pedroso F et al. Soluble CD44 is a potential marker for the early detection of head and neck cancer. Cancer Epidemiol Biomarkers Prev 2007; 16: 1348–55.

200. Chang SK, Mirabal YN, Atkinson EN et al. Combined reflectance and fluorescence spectroscopy for in vivo detection of cervical pre-cancer. J Biomed Opt 2005; 10: 024031.

201. DaCosta RS, Wilson BC, Marcon NE. Fluorescence and spectral imaging. ScientificWorld Journal 2007; 21: 2046–71.

202. DaCosta RS, Andersson H, Cirocco M et al. Autofluorescence characterisation of isolated whole crypts and primary cultured human epithelial cells from normal, hyperplastic, and adenomatous colonic mucosa. J Clin Pathol 2005; 58: 766–74.

203. Tan J, Delaney P, McLaren WJ. Confocal endomicroscopy: a novel imaging technique for in vivo histology of cervical intraepithelial neoplasia. Expert Rev Med Devices 2007; 4: 863–71.

204. Karwa A, Papazoglou E, Pourrezaei K et al. Imaging biomarkers of inflammation in situ with functionalized quantum dots in the dextran sodium sulfate (DSS) model of mouse colitis. Inflamm Res 2007; 56: 502–10.

205. Mao L, El-Naggar AK, Fan YH et al. Telomerase activity in head and neck squamous cell carcinoma and adjacent tissues. Cancer Res 1996; 56: 5600–4.

206. Shin DM, Lee JS, Lippman SM et al. p53 expression: predicting recurrence and second primary tumors in head and neck squamous cell carcinoma. J Natl Cancer Inst 1996; 88: 519–29.

207. O-charoenrat P, Rhys-Evans P, Modjtahedi H et al. Overexpression of epidermal growth factor receptor in human head and neck squamous carcinoma cell lines correlates with matrix metalloproteinase-9 expression and in vitro invasion. Int J Cancer 2000; 86: 307–17.

208. O-charoenrat P, Rhys-Evans P, Eccles SA. Expression of vascular endothelial growth factor family members in head and neck squamous cell carcinoma correlates with lymph node metastases. Cancer 2001; 92: 556–68.

209. O-charoenrat P, Rhys-Evans P, Eccles SA. Expression of matrix metalloproteinases and their inhibitors correlates with invasion and metastasis in squamous cell carcinoma of the head and neck. Arch Otolaryngol Head Neck Surg 2001; 127: 813–20.

210. Shintani S, Li C, Ishikawa T et al. Expression of vascular endothelial growth factors A, B, C, and D in oral squamous cell carcinoma. Oral Oncol 2004; 40: 13–20.

211. Di Renzo MF, Olivero M, Martone T et al. Somatic mutations of the MET oncogene are selected during metastatic spread of human HNSC carcinomas. Oncogene 2000; 19: 1547–55.

212. De Herdt MJ, Baatenburg de Jong RJ. HGF and c-MET as potential orchestrators of invasive growth in head and neck squamous cell carcinoma. Front Biosci 2008; 13: 2516–26.

213. Yücel OT, Sungur A, Kaya S. c-met overexpression in supraglottic laryngeal squamous cell carcinoma and its relation to lymph node metastases. Otolaryngol Head Neck Surg 2004; 130: 698–703.

214. De Schutter H, Spaepen M, Mc Bride WH et al. The clinical relevance of microsatellite alterations in head and neck squamous cell carcinoma: a critical review. Eur J Hum Genet 2007; 15: 734–41.

215. Cabelguenne A, Blons H, de Waziers I et al. p53 alterations predict tumor response to neoadjuvant chemotherapy in head and neck squamous cell carcinoma: a prospective series. J Clin Oncol 2000; 18: 1465–73.

216. Kwok T, Sutherland R. Differences in EGF related radiosensitisation of human squamous carcinoma cells with high and low numbers of EGF receptors. Br J Cancer 1991; 64: 251–4.

217. Milas L, Fan Z, Andratschke N et al. Epidermal growth factor receptor and tumor response to radiation: in vivo preclinical studies. Int J Radiat Oncol Biol Phys 2004; 58: 966–71.

218. Yuen A, Sikic B. Clinical studies of antisense therapy in cancer. Front Biosci 2000; 5: 588–93.

219. Modjtahedi H, Affleck K, Stubberfield C et al. EGFR blockade by tyrosine kinase inhibitor or monoclonal antibody inhibits growth, directs terminal differentiation and induces apoptosis in the human squamous cell carcinoma HN5. Int J Oncol 1998; 13: 335–42.

220. Mendelsohn J, Fan Z. Epidermal growth factor receptor family and chemosensitization. J Natl Cancer Inst 1997; 89: 341–3.

221. Huang S-M, Bock J, Harari P. Epidermal growth factor receptor blockade with C225 modulates proliferation, apoptosis, and radiosensitivity in squamous cell carcinomas of the head and neck. Cancer Res 1999; 59: 1935–40.

222. Bonner JA, Harari PM, Giralt J et al. Radiotherapy plus cetuximab for squamous-cell carcinoma of the head and neck. N Engl J Med 2006; 354: 567–78.

223. Burtness B, Goldwasser MA, Flood W, Mattar B, Forastiere AA. Phase III randomized trial of cisplatin plus placebo compared with cisplatin plus cetuximab in metastatic/recurrent head and neck cancer: an Eastern Cooperative Oncology Group study. J Clin Oncol 2005; 23: 8646–54.

224. Vermorken JB, Trigo J, Hitt R et al. Open-label, uncontrolled, multicenter phase II study to evaluate the efficacy and toxicity of cetuximab as a single agent in patients with recurrent and/or metastatic squamous cell carcinoma of the head and neck who failed to respond to platinum-based therapy. J Clin Oncol 2007; 25: 2171–7.

225. Le Tourneau C, Faivre S, Siu LL. Molecular targeted therapy of head and neck cancer: Review and clinical development challenges. Eur J Cancer 2007; 43: 2457–66.

226. O-charoenrat P, Rhys-Evans P, Modjtahedi H et al. Vascular endothelial growth factor family members are differentially regulated by c-erbB signaling in head and neck squamous carcinoma cells. Clin Exp Metastasis 2000; 18: 155–61.

227. Karamouzis MV, Friedland D, Johnson R et al. Phase II trial of pemetrexed (P) and bevacizumab (B) in patients (pts) with recurrent or metastatic head and neck squamous cell carcinoma (HNSCC): An interim analysis. J Clin Oncol 2007; 25: 18s [abstr 6049].

228. Gerber HP, Ferrera N. Pharmacology and pharmacodynamics of bevacizumab as monotherapy or in combination with cytotoxic therapy in preclinical studies. Cancer Res 2005; 65: 671–80.

229. Savvides P, Greskovich J, Bokar J et al. Phase II study of bevacizumab in combination with docetaxel and radiation in locally advanced squamous cell cancer of the head and neck (SCCHN). J Clin Oncol 2007; 25: 18s [abstr 6048].

230. Mandal M, Younes M, Swan EA et al. The Akt inhibitor KP372-1 inhibits proliferation and induces apoptosis and anoikis in squamous cell carcinoma of the head and neck. Oral Oncol 2006; 42: 430–9.

231. Argiris A, Cohen E, Karrison T et al. A phase II trial of perifosine, an oral alkylphospholipid, in recurrent or metastatic head and neck cancer. Cancer Biol Ther 2006; 5: 766–70.

232. Janmaat ML, Kruyt FA, Rodriguez JA et al. Response to epidermal growth factor receptor inhibitors in non-small cell lung cancer cells: limited antiproliferative effects and absence

of apoptosis associated with persistent activity of extracellular signal regulated kinase or Akt kinase pathways. Clin Cancer Res 2003; 9: 2316–26.

233. Kawakami K, Leland P, Puri R. Structure, function, and targeting of interleukin 4 receptors on human head and neck cancer cells. Cancer Res 2000; 60: 2981–7.

234. Braun-Falco M, Doenecke A, Smola H et al. Efficient gene transfer into human keratinocytes with recombinant adeno-associated virus vectors. Gene Ther 1999; 6: 432–41.

235. Heise C, Williams A, Xue S. Intravenous administration of ONYX-015, a selectively replicating adenovirus, induces antitumoral efficacy. Cancer Res 1999; 59: 2623–8.

236. Pirollo KF, Hao Z, Rait A et al. p53 mediated sensitization of squamous cell carcinoma of the head and neck to radiotherapy. Oncogene 1997; 14: 1735–46.

237. Ogawa N, Fujiwata T, Kagawa S. Novel combination therapy for human colon cancer with adenovirus-mediated wild-type p53 gene transfer and DNA-damaging chemotherapeutic agent. Int J Cancer 1997; 73: 367–70.

238. Clayman G, Frank D, Bruso P et al. Adenovirus-mediated wild-type p53 gene transfer as a surgical adjuvant in advanced head and neck cancers. Clin Cancer Res 1999; 5: 1715–22.

239. Cayman GI, el-Naggar AK, Lippman SM et al. Adenovirus-mediated p53 gene transfer in patients with advanced recurrent head and neck squamous cell carcinoma. J Clin Oncol 1998; 16: 2221–32.

240. Rocco JW, Li D, Liggett WH Jr et al. p16INK4A adenovirus-mediated gene therapy for human head and neck squamous cell cancer. Clin Cancer Res 1998; 4: 1697–704.

241. Clark PR, Hersh EM. Cationic lipid-mediated gene transfer: current concepts. Curr Opin Molec Ther 1999; 1: 158–76.

242. Geiger T, Muller M, Monia BP et al. Antitumor activity of a C-raf antisense oligonucleotide in combination with standard chemotherapeutic agents against various human tumors transplanted subcutaneously into nude mice. Clin Cancer Res 1997; 3: 1179–85.

243. Gibson SA, Pellenz C, Hutchison RE et al. Induction of apoptosis in oral cancer cells by an anti-bcl-2 ribozyme delivered by an adenoviral vector. Clin Cancer Res 2000; 6: 213–22.

244. Wang CH, Tsai LJ, Tsao YP et al. Recombinant adenovirus encoding H-ras ribozyme induces apoptosis in laryngeal cancer cells through caspase- and mitochondria-dependent pathways. Biochem Biophys Res Commun 2002; 298: 805–14.

245. Goebel E, Davidson B, Graham S, Kem J. Tumor reduction in vivo after adenoviral mediated gene transfer of the herpes simplex virus thymidine kinase gene and ganciclovir treatment in human head and neck squamous cell carcinoma. Otolaryngol Head Neck Surg 1998; 119: 331–6.

246. Morris JC, Wildner O. Therapy of head and neck squamous cell carcinoma with an oncolytic adenovirus expressing HSV-tk. Mol Ther 2000; 1: 56–62.

247. Nishikawa M, Hayashi Y, Yamamoto N et al. Cell death of human oral squamous cell carcinoma cell line induced by herpes simplex virus thymidine kinase gene and ganciclovir. Nagoya J Med Sci 2003; 66: 129–37.

248. Gleich LL, Gluckman JL, Nemunaitis J et al. Clinical experience with HLA-B7 plasmid DNA/lipid complex in advanced squamous cell carcinoma of the head and neck. Arch Otolaryngol Head Neck Surg 2001; 127: 775–9.

249. Liu TJ, Zhang WW, Taylor DL et al. Growth suppression of human head and neck cancer cells by the introduction of a wild-type p53 gene via a recombinant adenovirus. Cancer Res 1994; 54: 3662–7.

250. Li D, Jiang W, Bishop J et al. Combination surgery and nonviral interleukin 2 gene therapy for head and neck cancer. Clin Cancer Res 1999; 5: 1551–6.

251. Rocco J, Li D, Liggett WJ et al. p16INK4A adenovirus-mediated gene therapy for human head and neck squamous cell cancer. Clin Cancer Res 1998; 4: 1697–704.

252. Mobley SR, Liu TJ, Hudson JM et al. In vitro growth suppression by adenoviral transduction of p21 and p16 in squamous cell carcinoma of the head and neck. Arch Otolaryngol Head Neck Surg 1998; 124: 88–92.

253. Clayman G, El-Naggar A, Lippman S et al. Adenovirus-mediated p53 gene transfer in patients with advanced recurrent head and neck squamous cell carcinoma. J Clin Oncol 1998; 16: 2221–32.

254. Kim SY, Yang YS, Hong KH et al. Adenovirus-mediated expression of dominant negative c-myb induces apoptosis in head and neck cancer cells and inhibits tumor growth in animal model. Oral Oncol 2008; 44: 383–92.

255. Blackwell J, Miller C, Douglas J et al. Retargeting to EGFR enhances adenovirus infection efficiency of squamous cell carcinoma. Arch Otolaryngol Head Neck Surg 1999; 125: 856–63.

256. Kasono K, Blackwell J, Douglas J et al. Selective gene delivery to head and neck cancer cells via an integrin targeted adenoviral vector. Clin Cancer Res 1999; 5: 2571–9.

257. Suominen E, Toivonen R, Grenman R et al. Head and neck cancer cells are efficiently infected by Ad5/35 hybrid virus. J Gene Med. 2006; 8: 1223–31.

258. Selivanova G, Iotsova V, Okan I et al. Restoration of the growth suppression function of mutant p53 by a synthetic peptide derived from the p53 C-terminal domain. Nat Med 1997; 3: 632–8.

259. Homer J, Greenman J, Stafford N. Angiogenesis in head and neck squamous cell carcinoma. Clin Otolaryngol 2000; 25: 169–80.

260. Heise C, Sampson-Johannes A, Williams A et al. ONYX-015, an E1B gene-attenuated adenovirus, causes cytolysis and antitumoral efficacy that can be augmented by standard chemotherapeutic agents. Nat Med 1997; 3: 639–45.

261. O'Shea CC, Johnson L, Bagus B et al. Late viral RNA export, rather than p53 inactivation, determines ONYX-015 tumor selectivity. Cancer Cell 2004; 6: 611–623.

262. Vassalli J, Pepper M. Membrane proteases in focus. Nat Med 1994; 370: 14–15.

GLOSSARY

Alleles: alternative forms of a gene at a specific chromosomal location (locus).

Allelic imbalance: a situation where one member (allele) of a gene pair is lost (loss of heterozygosity) or amplified.

Amplification: the production of many DNA copies from one or a few copies.

Aneuploidy: a chromosome profile with fewer or greater than a normal (diploid) number. This phenomenon is an index of the deregulation of the genome and is associated with carcinogenesis.

Anneal: the joining of complementary base pairs to from a double-stranded DNA molecule.

Antiparallel: the opposite orientations of the two strands of a DNA double helix; the 5" end of one strand aligns with the 3" end of the other strand.

Antisense: the complementary DNA or RNA sequence that does not code for the gene and is not transcribed. It is only important for maintaining the structure and integrity of the double helix and allows replication and transcription.

cDNA: synthetic complementary (c) DNA produced *in vitro* from an mRNA template and the initial product is double-stranded and complementary to the mRNA (it contains no introns).

Chromosome translocation: an alteration in the structure of a chromosome by movement of part or whole of a chromosome (genetic material) to another nonhomologous chromosome, that is the inter-non-homologous chromosome genetic movement. This may deregulate proto-oncogenes or tumor suppressor genes resulting in carcinogenesis.

Chromosome transposition: an alteration in the structure of a chromosome by the movement of genetic material from one site in the (homologous) chromosome to another, that is, the intra-homologous chromosome genetic movement. This may deregulate proto-oncogenes or tumor suppressor genes resulting in carcinogenesis.

Chromosomes: separate aggregates of the genome that allow cell division. The arms are classified into short arm (p) and long arm (q).

c-myc protein: a nuclear protein that activates other genes that are responsible for cell proliferation. Thus, although the protein is normal in structure it is carcinogenic due to being overexpressed.

Codon: a triplet of bases that may code for an amino acid or the end of transcription.

Cytogenetics: the study of human chromosomes, their structure and transmission.

Deletion: loss of genetic material.

Diploid: two sets of genes, one from each parent.

Disease transcripts: disease-associated mRNA sequences.

erbB proto-oncogene: this has been implicated in carcinogenesis by two mechanisms. (1) An altered version of the epidermal growth factor (EGF)-receptor gene whose mutant EGF-receptor protein product sends growth signals into the cell in the absence of bound epithelial growth factor; (2) the EGF-receptor protein product may be normal but overexpressed as seen in breast and ovarian carcinomas.

Eukaryocyte: a cell with a nucleus.

Exon: a coding fragment in a gene.

Extension: during the polymerase chain reaction (PCR) process the thermostable enzyme copies the single-stranded DNA template.

Gene amplification: an increase in the number of copies of a gene.

Gene rearrangement: the reordering of a gene sequence within a genome.

Gene: an area of DNA coding for a polypeptide.

GTL-banding or "G-banding" (giemsa/trypsin/leishman banding): chromosomes are G-banded to facilitate the identification of structural abnormalities. Slides are dehydrated, treated with the enzyme trypsin, and then stained.

Haploid: a cell (typically a gamete) with only a single copy of each chromosome.

HNSCC: head and neck squamous cell carcinoma.

Homozygous deletion: a deletion of both copies of the gene. Such deletions can be small such as a single gene or can stretch up to 10 million base pairs and delete several genes.

Hybridize: anneal.

Karyotype: the chromosome content of a cell.

Li-Fraumeni syndrome (LFS): a cancer predisposition syndrome associated with soft-tissue sarcoma, breast cancer, leukemia, osteosarcoma, melanoma, and cancer of the colon, pancreas, adrenal cortex, and brain. LFS is an autosomal dominant disorder with children of an affected individual having a 50% chance of inheriting the disease-causing mutation. About 70% of patients diagnosed clinically have an identifiable disease-causing mutation in the TP53 gene (chromosomal locus 17p13).

L-myc: a related gene to c-myc (see below) that is amplified in small-cell carcinoma.

Locus: a unique area of the chromosome where a gene or DNA sequence lies.

Loss of heterozygosity (LOH): the loss of one allele at a specific locus, caused by a deletion mutation; or loss of a chromosome from a chromosome pair. It is detected when heterozygous markers for a locus appear monomorphic because one of the alleles was deleted. When this occurs at a tumor suppressor gene locus where one of the alleles is already abnormal, it can result in neoplastic transformation.

Meiosis: the process of halving of the amount of DNA in a cell, which is seen in the generation of germ cells (gametes) with only a haploid set of chromosomes. Crossing over of homologous chromosomal elements, originally from both parents, is involved to aid gene shuffling (sexual reproduction).

Mitogenic: the promotion of mitosis.

Mitosis: the process of duplication of DNA seen in cell division producing a diploid set of chromosomes. There is no crossing over of gene sequences, and it is thus asexual: the production of identical copies.

Mutagenic: promotes malignant progression by a change in the DNA sequence.

Neu/erbB-2: a gene that specifies a cell surface mitogen receptor. It is amplified in breast and ovarian cancer. It is also termed HER-2/neu.

N-myc: a related gene to myc (see above) that is amplified in childhood neuroblastoma.

Nucleotide: the monomeric unit linked by 3″ and 5″ positions of each pentose (ribose) sugar component to form polynucleotide polymers called nucleic acids (DNA, RNA). These polynucleotide chains (DNA or RNA) have polarity (i.e., they are not the same in each direction), and are read in the 5″ to 3″ direction.

Null genotype: a mutated gene that is not transcribed into RNA and/or translated into a functional protein product.

Oncogene: an unregulated gene sequence whose product in the host presents a continuous growth stimulus by intervening in the normal growth mechanism in an unregulated manner causing carcinogenesis. (1) viral oncogenes: a parasitic viral gene sequence, denoted v-onc; (2) cellular oncogene: a cellular gene sequence, denoted c-onc, derived from the deregulation or mutated normal cellular proto-oncogene (see below).

Overexpression: the increased production by a cell of an RNA or protein product.

Paracrine: the release of a chemical substance by a cell having a local effect on adjacent cells (cf. the distant actions of hormones in the endocrine system).

Plasmids: circular double-stranded extrachromosomal DNA capable of autonomous replication. It can be used as a vector to introduce new DNA into a cell.

Point mutation: a single change in the sequence of base pairs that may result in a different amino acid or protein product.

Polymorphisms: differences in DNA sequences.

Prokaryocytes: organisms without a nucleus.

Properties of malignancy: (1) the proliferation of a cell outside the normal control mechanisms; (2) invasion of the basement membrane in epithelial tumors; (3) metastasis to aberrant sites within the body.

Proto-oncogene: a normal gene found in normal tissue, highly conserved in evolution and has central roles in signal transduction pathways that control cell growth and differentiation. If deregulated or mutated they may be carcinogenic, and thus a deregulated or mutated proto-oncogene that is carcinogenic is referred to as a cellular oncogene.

Raf proteins: growth-related proteins in the cytoplasm.

Ras protein: a cytoplasmic protein involved in signal transduction. If mutated it remains in an excited, cell growth signal-emitting mode and consequently is carcinogenic.

Recombinant DNA technology: the modification of gene sequences.

Restriction enzyme: an enzyme that breaks double-stranded DNA into fragments at sequence specific points. These enzymes work by recognizing a specific base sequence and cleave the DNA molecule at that point. This property has provided geneticists with a powerful tool for analysis and gene manipulation.

Restriction fragment length polymorphism (RFLP) analysis: this is a technique in which organisms may be differentiated by analysis of patterns derived from cleavage of their DNA. If two organisms differ in the distance between sites of cleavage of a particular restriction endonuclease, the length of the fragments produced will differ when the DNA is digested with a restriction enzyme. The similarity of the patterns generated can be used to differentiate species (and even strains) from one another.

Sense: the gene bearing DNA or RNA is called the sense strand, that is, it directly contains the genetic information.

Southern blot: the analysis and comparison of the electrophoretic patterns of DNA fragments using radioactive probes.

Telomerase: an enzyme that synthesizes the telomere, which is composed of tandem repeats of the sequence TTTAGG. This is significant as chromosome replication requires the telomere. If lost, replication ceases; if overactive then replication and cell division may continue unchecked.

Transcriptional promoter: an agent that enhances gene copying.

Transfection: the infection of a cell with isolated DNA or RNA by a viral vector.

Tumor suppressor gene: genetic elements whose loss or mutational inactivation allows cells to display one or more phenotypes of neoplastic growth.

Tyrosine kinase activity: a large number of regulatory pathways rely on enzymes that have tyrosine residues that, if phosphorylated by oncoproteins with tyrosine kinase activity, can be changed in functionality. The effect is to disrupt many regulatory pathways at the same time: a property that aids the multiplicity of effects from one change (see the section on multistage models of malignancy).

Western blot: the analysis and comparison of the electrophoretic patterns of proteins using labeled antibodies.

Wild-type genes: the normal genes found in normal tissue.

3

Imaging of Head and Neck Tumors

Axel V Martin, Bhuey Sharma, Dominic Blunt and Gitta Madani

THE ROLE OF IMAGING IN THE MANAGEMENT OF SQUAMOUS CELL CARCINOMA OF THE HEAD AND NECK

Squamous cell carcinoma (SCC) is by far the most common nonskin cancer affecting the head and neck. The clinical presentation and tendency to metastasize varies considerably, and imaging plays a vital role in the management of all such tumors. The following sections address mainly the value and limitations of diagnostic imaging at various stages in the management of patients with head and neck squamous cell carcinoma (HNSCC). Important differential diagnoses, specific clinical situations, and the rapidly emerging role of metabolic imaging are discussed.

Staging
Cross-sectional imaging has a well-defined role in the staging of patients with head and neck cancer. It is particularly useful in cases where the primary tumor is inaccessible, in defining submucosal spread, deep extension, local invasion, and in identifying synchronous primaries and distant metastases. Imaging may be utilized to answer specific questions that will affect the prognosis and further management of the patient.

Larynx
Computed tomography (CT) and magnetic resonance imaging (MRI) are equipotent in the staging of laryngeal cancers. The choice between these modalities is mainly a matter of availability and preference in the individual hospital.

All patients who clinically have glottic disease of stage T1b and higher and all patients with supraglottic or subglottic cancers should undergo a staging scan to define the deep extent and involvement of the laryngeal skeleton (Fig. 3.1).

The T staging according to the latest International Union Against Cancer (UICC) criteria from 2002 is similar for all three laryngeal levels and is dependent on the involvement/fixation of the vocal chords and local tumor spread (Fig. 3.2). Although the application of the staging is straightforward clinically and radiologically the fact that "minor thyroid cartilage erosion" alone upstages the patient to T3 in glottic and supraglottic SCC poses a problem in that no imaging modality is presently able to confidently identify this. A study correlating CT, MRI, and histopathology in 53 patients found that MRI, though superior to CT, had a reasonable sensitivity but a rather low specificity (56%) in identifying thyroid cartilage invasion (1).

In radiological terms, subtle cartilage changes, for example arytenoid cartilage sclerosis, on either CT or MRI should therefore be treated as equivocal and in terms of treatment choices, as it has been shown that minor cartilage involvement does not preclude radiotherapy with curative intent (2) in patients with T1/2 cancers (Fig. 3.1); however with clear cartilage invasion a primary surgical approach is advised (Fig. 3.3).

Early T1 cancers and tumors with a more exophytic growth pattern may be radiologically undetectable, and also subtle invasion of the anterior commissure in glottic SCC may be difficult to detect. In these cases, direct endoscopic visualization will provide diagnostic confirmation.

The prognostic significance of tumor volume and glucose avidity in laryngeal SCC is discussed later in this chapter.

Hypopharynx
Because of the growth pattern particular to the hypopharyngeal subsites, many tumors are clinically not apparent or understaged.

Often nodal disease is the first sign of malignancy with up to 75% of patients presenting with nodal involvement, often at level IV. Consequently the incidence of clinically and radiological occult nodal deposits is also very high at 30%. The overall prognosis of patients with hypopharyngeal SCC is unsurprisingly worse than those arising at other sites within the head and neck.

Posterior wall and postcricoid SCC will often spread in a submucosal fashion, masking the true extent to the clinical observer (Fig. 3.4). Depending on their origin within the piriform sinus, SCC will either spread into the lateral cervical compartments, the paraglottic space, or the glottis with early vocal cord fixation.

In either case, cross-sectional imaging is essential in defining the true disease extent, upstaging ≤90% of patients.

One important limitation of CT in the staging of posterior hypopharyngeal wall cancers is the low sensitivity in the determination of prevertebral muscle involvement—a contraindication to surgery, however, Righi et al. showed it does have a negative predictive value (NPV) of 82%, that is, preservation of the prevertebral fat plane confidently predicts the absence of infiltration in most cases (3).

The incidence of synchronous or metachronous (12%) primaries is very high, (4,5) and these should be actively excluded clinically and on staging and follow-up scans. Hypopharyngeal cancers also have a high rate of metastatic

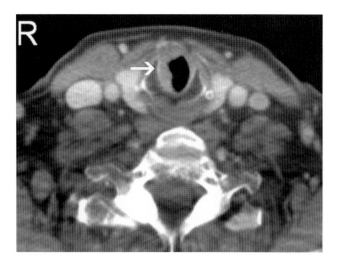

Figure 3.1 Subglottic T2 squamous cell carcinoma (arrow) in a 65-year-old male.

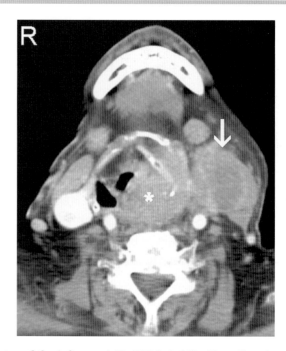

Figure 3.3 Left supraglottic SCC (asterisk) with cartilage invasion and left level 2/3 nodal involvement (arrow). T4N2. *Abbreviation*: SCC, squamous cell carcinoma.

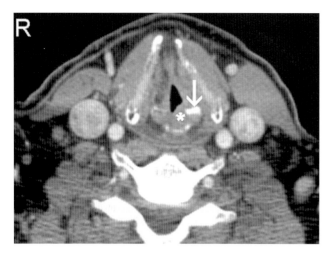

Figure 3.2 Left vocal chord SCC (asterisk) in a 51-year-old man: note arytenoid cartilage sclerosis (arrow). Due to vocal chord fixation this is a T3 tumor. *Abbreviation*: SCC, squamous cell carcinoma.

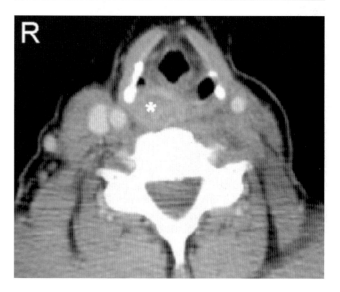

Figure 3.4 Right posterior cricoid SCC (asterisk) in a 58-year-old female with a past history of tonsillar SCC. This tumor was clinically occult. *Abbreviation*: SCC, squamous cell carcinoma.

disease (18%) at presentation compared to SCC of other head and neck regions where metastatic spread is mainly to lung, mediastinum, and bone (5).

Oropharynx

SCC in the oropharynx most frequently arises either in the anterior tonsillar pillar or the tongue base.

Early oropharyngeal tumors are often difficult to identify radiologically and clinically. Indeed, as Haas et al. found in 57 patients with carcinoma of unknown primary (CUP) referred for further investigation in a tertiary center, 10 of 15 primary sites that were subsequently identified by random biopsy of multiple sites and tonsillectomy were situated in the oropharynx (6) with 6 tumors found to arise from within the tonsil, 4 at the tongue base.

The inherent asymmetry in these structures and the physiological uptake of 18-Fluoro-deoxy-glucose (18-FDG)

in lymphoid structures reduces sensitivity in anatomical and metabolical imaging is in this situation.

In larger lesions, cross-sectional imaging is particularly useful to define the full extent of the lesion, with the size of tongue base cancers being often underestimated on clinical examination (Fig. 3.5) and the deep extent of tonsillar SCC, particularly into the parapharyngeal space (PPS), invisible to the otorhinolaryngologist (Fig. 3.6).

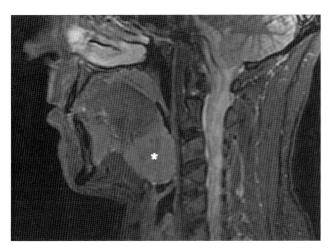

Figure 3.5 Sagittal MRI demonstrating a T2 tumor at the base of the tongue (asterisk) in a 51-year-old man. *Abbreviation*: MRI, magnetic resonance imaging.

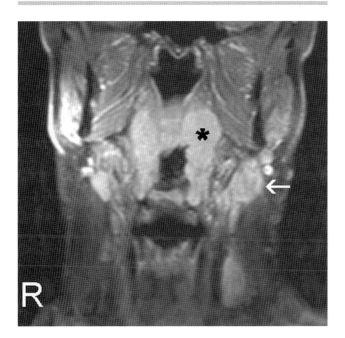

Figure 3.6 Coronal MRI showing a left tonsillar SCC (asterisk) with invasion of the parapharyngeal space and ipsilateral level-2 nodal disease (arrow). T2N1 *Abbreviations*: MRI, magnetic resonance imaging; SCC, squamous cell carcinoma.

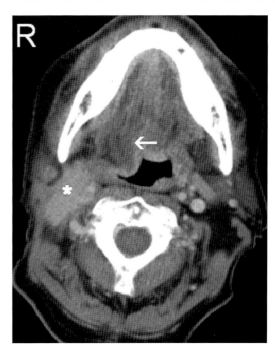

Figure 3.7 Right level-2 parapharyngeal recurrence (asterisk) with involvement of the hypoglossal nerve: Note the fatty replacement and atrophy of the ipsilateral tongue (arrow).

Retropharyngeal nodal involvement is only detectable on cross-sectional imaging.

Invasion of the prestyloid compartment of the PPS is important in the treatment planning because encasement of the internal carotid artery for more than 270° of its circumference precludes surgery. Hypoglossal nerve involvement can result in ipsilateral tongue atrophy (Fig. 3.7). Interestingly, the tumor volume is, in contrast to other subsites within the head and neck, of no prognostic relevance in the oropharynx (7).

Because of the abundance of lymphatic tissue in the oropharynx, non-Hodgkin's lymphoma is an important differential to consider, particularly in patients without risk factors for SCC. Imaging clues include a more exophytic growth pattern (Fig. 3.8) and the presence of homogenous enhancement of lymph nodes in groups other than the ones typically involved in oropharyngeal SCC (i.e., ipsilateral level II). The presence of necrosis within the primary tumor or affected lymph nodes is more typical of a squamous origin (Fig. 3.9).

Oral Cavity

The most common site of origin in the mouth is the lip, where tumors are readily identified clinically, and radiological assessment of deep invasion is rarely required in all but very advanced tumors. In the tongue, imaging is essential to allow accurate staging and determine operability. Coronal MRI sequences are preferable because they may help avoid dental artifact and produce a higher soft-tissue resolution making it easier to decide if the lesion crosses the midline—which may preclude radical surgery—and whether the lingual neurovascular bundle is involved. Nodal spread is common at presentation (up to 50%) and in the case of tongue primaries often bilateral.

Bony cortical invasion by oral cavity SCC of any size makes the tumor T4 in the UICC classification, and it is therefore essential to identify this on imaging. Imaizumi et al. documented that the specificity of MRI in this regard is inferior to CT (54 vs. 88%) (8). The authors postulated that a chemical shift artifact from bone marrow fat is responsible for the high false-positive rate. In practical

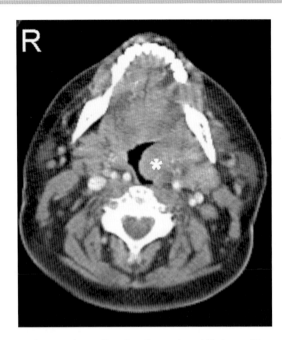

Figure 3.8 Left tonsillar lymphoma (asterisk) in a 49-year-old female.

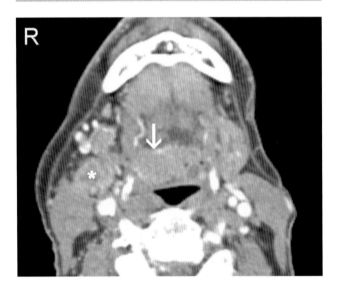

Figure 3.9 Right tongue base SCC (arrow) with ipsilateral necrotic level-2 node (asterisk) in a 77-year-old male. *Abbreviation*: SCC, squamous cell carcinoma.

terms the suspicion of bone involvement on MRI should always be confirmed on dedicated fine-slice CT acquired with a bone algorithm.

Minor salivary gland malignancies like adenoid cystic carcinoma (ACC) and muco-epidermoid carcinoma (MEC) also occur particularly in the oral cavity. They have similar imaging characteristics as SCC and cannot be differentiated radiologically (Fig. 10). Although ACC is said to have a propensity for perineural spread, this is also seen with SCC, MEC, and lymphoma. The long-term prognosis

of ACC is often dubious because it tends to be more advanced at diagnosis and distant metastases are more common (Fig. 3.11).

Nasopharynx

Nasopharyngeal carcinoma (NPC) differs significantly from other aerodigestive tract carcinomas because it has a distinctive geographical and environmental risk factor profile. It is much more common in South-East Asia where is reaches an incidence of 50/100,000 whereas in Whites it is approximately 1/100,000. There also is an association with Epstein-Barr virus infection. NPC is also distinct in its propensity for early nodal spread (up to 90% at presentation) and aggressive local behavior.

The proximity of the nasopharyngeal mucosal space to the skull base and the carotid sheath mean that these structures are often directly involved.

Cross-sectional imaging is essential for defining the local tumor extent, particularly the involvement of the parapharyngeal and masticator spaces, the carotid sheath, and skull base. Perineural and intracranial spread are also readily detected, particularly with gadolinium-enhanced MRI (Fig. 3.12).

In advanced lesions cranial nerve involvement is a common clinical symptom and can sometimes be identified on imaging either by direct visualization of the affected nerve (Fig. 3.13) or atrophic changes in neuropathic musculature.

Erosion of the skull base is well demonstrated on directly acquired coronal high-resolution bone CT. MRI is inferior in this respect because it is less suited for delineating cortical bone; however it is excellent in detecting bone marrow involvement (Fig. 3.14).

Nodal Staging and Distant Metastases

The precise nodal staging in SCC may be a clinical and radiological challenge. The classical centrally necrotic appearance of an enlarged node is only encountered in one third of cases, and size criteria have been found to be unreliable in determining involvement. A large series correlating radiological and pathological findings concluded, in the setting of head and neck SCC, 23% of nodes measuring 6–10 mm in short axis—which would be considered insignificant on cross-sectional imaging by size alone—will contain metastases (9). In consequence the reported sensitivities for CT and MRI range between 41% and 96%, with higher sensitivity always achieved at the cost of lower specificity.

18-Fluoro-deoxy-glucose-positron-emission-tomography (18-FDG-PET) is able to identify an additional 40% of metastases in affected nodes that are normal on anatomical imaging and has been reported to have a sensitivity of 90% for all nodes. It is however not able to detect micro-metastases smaller than 4 mm and may be false-negative in predominantly necrotic nodes. As the central necrosis may well be visualized on CT it is critical to assess with anatomical imaging as well (Fig. 3.15). The other inherent limitation is the relatively low specificity caused by uptake in reactive benign nodes. In clinical reality, nodal staging is still the domain of the histo-pathologist.

Extracapsular spread (ECS) in affected lymph nodes is an important prognostic factor that reduces the 5-year

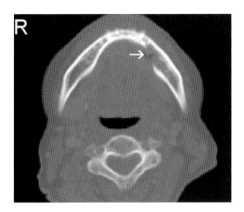
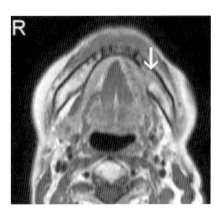

Figure 3.10 Left floor of mouth MEC with mandibular invasion on axial CT/MRI. While the CT is superior in defining the cortical erosion (arrow), the MRI delineates the marrow invasion (down arrow) better. *Abbreviations*: MEC, muco-epidermoid carcinoma; CT/MRI, computed tomography/ magnetic resonance imaging.

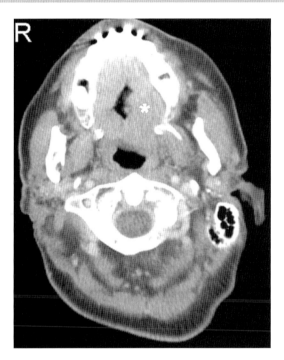

Figure 3.11 A MALT lymphoma of the hard palate (asterisk) in a 63-year-old female. *Abbreviation*: MALT, mucosa associated lymphoid tissue.

disease-free survival by 50% (1). This appears to be independent of whether ECS is macroscopic or microscopic (11). Unfortunately no imaging modality has enough diagnostic accuracy to identify particularly microscopic ECS reliably with reported sensitivities of up to 74% overall for any imaging modality.

Synchronous distant metastases and second malignancies are common particularly in patients with advanced-stage SCC and have been reported in up to 21% of patients (1). A further 9% will go on to develop metachronous distant disease with a similar incidence of second primary malignancies. It has been established that the accuracy of standard cross-sectional imaging in identifying these is insufficient, with a false-negative rate for CT of up to 50% (13). In contrast the sensitivity of positron emission tomography (PET) and PET/computed tomography (CT) in this situation has been reported as up to 100% (14) with a substantial impact on patient management. The use of PET/CT as a staging and surveillance procedure in advanced stage (III/IV) has therefore been advocated but up to this point not prospectively analyzed.

The Unknown Primary (CUP)

A common presentation of SCC of the head and neck is with nodal enlargement due to metastases but no clinical evidence of a primary tumor. The traditional work-up of this patient group included panendoscopy with multiple

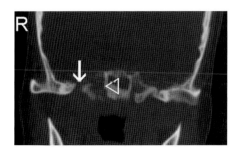
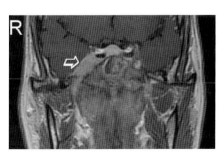

Figure 3.12 Coronal CT and MRI in a 46-year-old woman with intracranial invasion by NPC. Note widening of foramen ovale (arrow) and clivus invasion (arrowhead) on the CT. The soft-tissue disease is well demonstrated (open arrow) on the postcontrast MRI. *Abbreviations*: CT, computed tomography; MRI, magnetic resonance imaging; NPC, nasopharyngeal carcinoma.

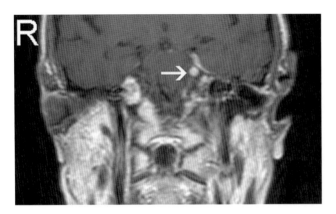

Figure 3.13 Left trigeminal nerve enhancement (arrow) on contrast-enhanced coronal MRI in a 58-year-old male with NPC and trigeminal nerve symptoms. *Abbreviations*: MRI, magnetic resonance imaging; NPC, nasopharyngeal carcinoma.

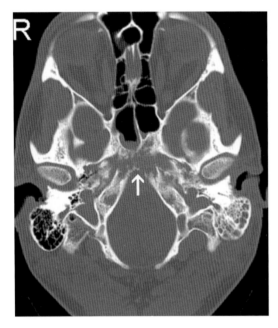

Figure 3.14 Skull base erosion (arrow) by NPC in a 40-year-old man with headache. *Abbreviation*: NPC, nasopharyngeal carcinoma.

biopsies and bilateral tonsillectomies and cross-sectional anatomical imaging.

As it has been postulated that the identification of a primary treatment target will improve outcomes, (6) the value of PET and PET/CT in this situation has been scrutinized. The reported detection rates vary widely from 30–73% (15–17). All of these studies were retrospective cohort analysis with differing inclusion criteria and diagnostic protocols.

Although it could be argued that PET/CT as the initial diagnostic modality in this clinical situation will allow a more targeted approach to a significant proportion of patients, no good quality prospective evidence for the use of PET/CT has been proffered to date.

An important point to make here is that if PET/CT is employed in the search for an unknown primary it should be performed prior to any biopsies to avoid false-positive results secondary to postsampling inflammation (Fig. 3.17).

The low sensitivity of PET for clinically occult head and neck primaries can be explained by its inability to identify lesions smaller than 5 mm and the fact that there is physiological uptake of FDG in structures like the tonsils, which may harbor the malignancy.

The Clinically Node-Negative Neck (N0 neck)

It is well established that the currently used criteria for staging neck nodal disease in patients with a known head and neck primary have a relatively low specificity and sensitivity. The commonly used size-criterion of 10 mm in short-axis diameter (SAD) on CT significantly underestimates the metastatic involvement of neck nodes as 23% of normal appearing lymph nodes with a SAD of 6–10 mm will harbor micrometastases (9).

Utilizing differential measurements depending on the nodal level has been proposed for CT and ultrasound (US) but not widely adopted.

An approach using US and fine needle aspiration has also been advocated and may indeed have a better sensitivity than other imaging modalities. However, its application is limited by the need of a skilled operator and resource requirements.

PET/CT has been investigated as a means of assessing the N0 neck, but as the size of most micro-metastases falls below the maximum spatial resolution of PET/CT (approximately 4 mm) it suffers from a relatively low sensitivity.

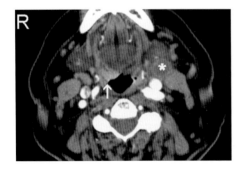
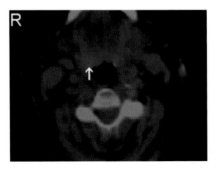

Figure 3.15 CT and PET/CT in a 66-year-old patient with a right base of tongue SCC (arrow) and contra-lateral level-2 nodal involvement (asterisk). The centrally necrotic node does not demonstrate any FDG uptake. *Abbreviation*: CT, computed tomography; PET, positron emission tomography; SCC, squamous cell carcinoma; FDG, fluoro-deoxy-glucose.

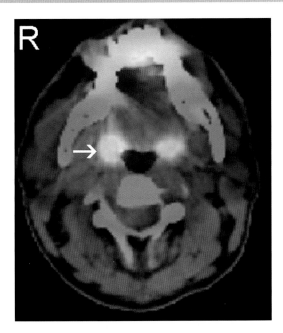

Figure 3.16 Subtle difference in uptake between right (arrow) and left tonsil on the PET/CT of a 43-year-old patient with CUP—the right tonsil was subsequently identified as the primary site. *Abbreviations*: PET, positron emission tomography; CT, computed tomography; CUP, carcinoma of unknown primary.

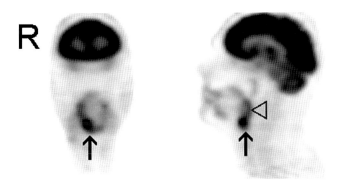

Figure 3.17 Grey-scale images of a PET scan in a patient with CUP who had undergone tonsillectomy 5 days prior to the scan. Although moderate uptake is seen in the surgical bed (arrowhead), the primary tumor at the right tongue base is also demonstrated (arrow). *Abbreviations*: PET, positron emission tomography; CUP, carcinoma of unknown primary.

However, as Ng et al. demonstrated in a study comparing anatomical imaging with PET, the detection rate for occult nodal deposits in T1–3 tumors could be doubled to 41% with PET and increased even further to 47% when correlated with a separately acquired CT or MRI (18).

The authors concluded that in patients with T1–T3 tumors the risk of failing to identify viable regional metastases after performing a PET scan can be reduced to <15%. On this basis and assuming that hybrid PET/CT will

perform even better, it appears reasonable to adopt a watch-and-wait strategy in this PET-negative patient group, thus avoiding the morbidity associated with neck dissection in at least 80% of patients. There is however no current prospective data to evaluate the long-term disease-specific outcome of this approach, and a multicenter study is warranted to validate this strategy.

A sentinel node biopsy (SNB) approach similar to the work-up of melanoma and breast cancer patients has also been proposed by Kovacs et al. in 2004 (19). After identifying truly node-negative patients with T1–3 necks by PET and SNB this group managed to avoid 59/124 hemineck dissections. During a median follow-up of 35 months none of the PET- and SNB-negative patients in their cohort recurred. This technique was recently confirmed by Tschopp et al. who in 82 sentinel nodes in 31 patients found 16 micrometastases upstaging 14 patients from cN0 to pN1. All patients subsequently underwent neck dissections. In the additional 1213 nodes from the resected specimens only one more metastasis was found, giving an overall sensitivity and NPV of 93% and 94% for SNB (20). A large multicenter trial in the United States is currently validating this method.

In summary the clinical challenge of identifying truly node-negative patients remains.

There are widely different approaches in individual centers that very much depend on local expertise and cannot be easily replicated elsewhere; however, there is promising evidence that a SNB approach has a role to play.

Prognostication

There is increasing evidence that cross-sectional imaging can offer prognostic information additional to the Tumour, Node, Metastases (TNM) classification.

Tumor volume has been shown to identify patients at risk of incomplete local control in all subsites apart from the oropharynx independently from TNM stage. For instance, a glottic T3 SCC >3.5 ml is at a risk of 50% of local failure, whereas a volume <3.5 mls predicts an 85% control rate (21,22). In hypopharyngeal cancer, the threshold volume appears to be 6.5 mls or—in the case of piriform fossa cancers—a maximum diameter of >1 cm. Exceeding those limits predicts a local failure rate of 100% (23). It has been suggested that the degree of FDG uptake on PET as expressed by the standardized uptake value (SUV) can predict local control and disease free survival. The threshold SUVs determined in different studies however vary widely from 5.5 to 10 reflecting heterogenous patient populations (24–26).

Response Assessment

Lesions that are visible on pretreatment imaging can be followed up radiologically after therapy. Hermans et al. demonstrated in laryngeal and hypopharyngeal malignancies following definitive radiotherapy a residual mass with a maximum diameter of >1 cm or an estimated volume reduction of <50% predicts local failure (27). These patients should be further investigated, ideally with metabolic imaging and targeted biopsies.

The value of FDG-PET in patients following surgery and prior to planned radiotherapy was evaluated by Shitani et al. who in 91 patients found 11 biopsy-proven

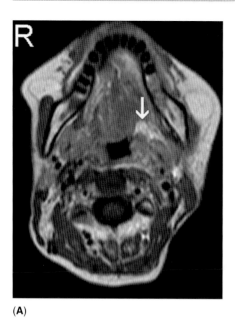
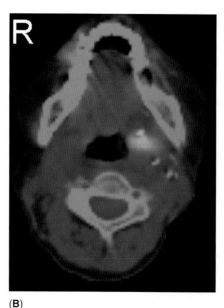

(A)   (B)

Figure 3.18   (A) Axial MRI of a patient with clinical suspicion of recurrence of a left base of tongue SCC. Appearances were stable when compared to a previous scan and were interpreted as "postsurgical changes" (arrow). (B) PET/CT at the same level demonstrates a FDG-avid SCC recurrence. *Abbreviations*: MRI, magnetic resonance imaging; SCC, squamous cell carcinoma. PET, positron emission tomography; CT, computed tomography; FDG.

PET-positive residua/relapses. Because of the early timing of the PET/CT (mean 28 days) a significant number of false-positives (n = 13) was observed (28).

Neck Dissection Following Intensity–modulated Radiotherapy (IMRT)

Because of the risk of clinically and radiologically occult viable nodal deposits the treatment paradigm for patients with node-positive SCC has been radiotherapy followed by elective neck dissection. This meant overtreating the substantial subset (up to 86%) of patients who had been cured by the radiotherapy alone. PET/CT is establishing itself as a very important tool in this setting as the reported NPV for nodal metastatic disease across all reported studies exceeds 91%, that is, the absence of FDG-avid lesions predicts the absence of viable tumor and correlates to disease-free survival (29–31). It has therefore been recommended that all patients should undergo a PET/CT following radiotherapy and before neck dissection with surgery only performed on PET positive cases. In the study by Nayak et al. this approach avoided 86% of neck dissections with an acceptable false-positive rate of 30% and no detrimental effect over a median follow-up of 18.1 months.

Timing of the PET/CT is crucial: it should be performed at least 3 months after completion of radiotherapy. Earlier scanning has been shown to be associated with a significant false-positive rate, the reason for this appears to be a combination of radiation-induced inflammation and "metabolic stunning" of viable tumor cells.

Recurrence

As surgery and/or radiotherapy will cause tissue changes that may mask or mimic tumor a baseline study 3 to 6 months following treatment is advisable in patients at risk of recurrence. Sequential morphological follow-up imaging has however been shown to have a relatively low sensitivity particularly in the postsurgical neck (Fig. 3.18). The early detection of recurrence is important to modify treatment approaches, for example, in patients undergoing multiple surgical procedures to improve cosmetic and functional outcome, some operations could be avoided if recurrence was demonstrated in the interval. The value of PET and PET/CT in identifying recurrence has been well documented in patients who have undergone surgery and those treated with chemoradiotherapy.

As Kunkel et al. demonstrated, the overall sensitivity of FDG-PET in detecting recurrence was 87%, even though in their cohort 52 of 97 patients with oral SCC had undergone major surgery. They also showed that the SUV was directly correlated to the 3-year disease-specific survival (32). Lee et al. found an overall sensitivity of 94% for detecting recurrence in 159 patients undergoing routine surveillance (33). In both studies the high NPV suggests that FDG-PET is particularly valuable in excluding recurrence.

The relatively low specificity can be improved by performing an early follow-up scan. Terhaard et al. performed a prospective study on 75 patients with laryngeal or oro-/hypopharyngeal cancer treated with radiotherapy. Of the patients who showed increased uptake but no evidence of residual disease on targeted biopsies, a reduction in SUV on an early-repeat FDG-PET correlated well with the absence of disease and increased the overall sensitivity from 63 to 82% (34).

Generally the timing of scanning is very important because many false-positives are caused by inflammatory treatment-related change. A delay of 12 weeks after the completion of treatment is now generally recommended to maximize the diagnostic accuracy of FDG-PET.

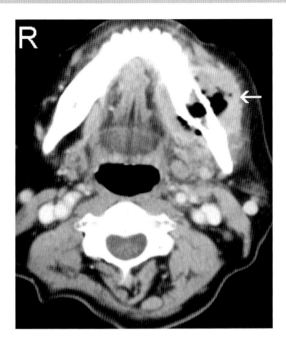

Figure 3.19 Previously irradiated left oral SCC. There is radionecrosis of the mandible associated with abnormal soft tissue on both sides of the mandible (arrow). *Abbreviation*: SCC, squamous cell carcinoma.

The value of MRI in detecting recurrence has also been scrutinized. MRI can demonstrate the cell density in a lesion by measuring the diffusion of water molecules. Pathologically inflammation correlates to extra-cellular edema, which on a molecular level leads to an increase in the mobility of water molecules. Diffusion weighted imaging (DWI) will therefore show a signal loss. Conversely the increased cell density of malignant cells will restrict diffusion, leading to an increased signal on DWI. Van de Caveye et al. have shown that this can be applied to head and neck cancer patients with clinical suspicion of recurrence. In 26 patients the apparent diffusion coefficient (a value calculated on the basis of the DWI) had a very high accuracy of 96% for differentiating recurrence from postradiotherapy change (35). This promising new technique requires further validation.

Radiotherapy Planning

Three-dimensional (3D) and, more recently four-dimensional (4D), conformal radiotherapy is used to optimize the delivery of IMRT.

CT and MRI are utilized to define the tumor volume and its local extent to maximize the delivered dose to tumor while minimizing damage to surrounding normal tissue. However, there is still controversy whether there is significant inter- and intraobserver variability when assessing gross tumor volume (GTV) (38). and reduced the time needed to delineate the target volume (39).

The same group showed that the irradiated volume and the dose to the parotid gland were significantly reduced (18% and 39%, respectively) when using PET to establish the GTV, compared to CT (40).

A current limitation of this approach is the lack of standardization of PET metabolic activity thresholds used to define the GTV.

A shortcoming of all imaging modalities is the underestimation of superficial spread. A discrepancy of clinical examination and radiological findings in this respect should be taken into account when planning RT.

Radionecrosis

Although the development and optimization of chemoradiotherapy has facilitated a more precise targeting of malignancies, short- and long-term effects on normal tissues in the irradiated field remain a considerable risk. However, long-term radiation changes may develop in a more random fashion and sometimes with considerable delay. Temporal lobe necrosis, for instance, manifests after a median interval of 5 years (41).

Osteoradionecrosis is a long-term complication that, in head and neck cancer patients, can develop particularly in oral cavity cancers and malignancies in close proximity to the skull base. Because the clinical presentation of osteoradionecrosis and local recurrence are very similar the imaging findings are often pivotal in differentiating between the two. CT has established itself as the modality of choice in this situation (42). An associated soft-tissue component is suggestive of recurrence (Fig. 3.19). Specific but infrequently observed signs of osteoradionecrosis include the appearance of intraosseus air bubbles and the formation of sequestra. Because the osteonecrosis will cause an intense inflammatory reaction, metabolic imaging has no discriminating value (43).

The inflammatory reaction in chondroradionecrosis in patients with laryngeal or hypopharyngeal SCC treated with radiotherapy may also pose a diagnostic dilemma. As Zbaeren et al. observed in 10 patients with severe chondroradionecrosis who required salvage laryngectomy, 3 harbored recurrent/residual tumor unsuspected on prelaryngectomy imaging (44). For a more general discussion of post-treatment changes please refer to the section on imaging of posttreatment changes and functional videofluoroscopic assessment.

THE ROLE OF IMAGING IN EXTRAMUCOSAL MALIGNANCIES
Malignant Sinonasal Tumors
Introduction

In contrast to inflammatory sinonasal disease, sinonasal tumors are rare. Carcinoma is the most common neoplasm but accounts for only 3% of all head and neck tumors. Due to its nonspecific and late presentation, sinonasal malignancy is generally associated with a poor prognosis (45). Early diagnosis of malignancy requires a high index of suspicion in patients who do not respond to medical treatment, suffer recurrent symptoms, or complain of unilateral symptoms. Judicious use of imaging and nasoendoscopy facilitate earlier diagnosis.

A diverse range of malignant pathology affects the sinonasal cavities. Table 3.1 demonstrates the prevalence of sinonasal tumors. Epithelial tumors are the most common, with SCC accounting for 80% of all malignant histology. Around 25–63% of sinonasal carcinomas arise in the maxillary antrum, 15–35% in the nasal cavity, 10–25% in the ethmoid complex, and 1% in the frontal and sphenoid sinuses (45,46).

The Role of Imaging

The imaging features of the majority of tumors are nonspecific. Although endoscopy is the ideal investigation for mapping the superficial extent of the tumor, the critical role of imaging is to demonstrate the deep extent.

CT is the first line of investigation in patients with persistent or recurrent sinonasal symptoms and is the best modality for the assessment of bony changes. If the CT scan is suggestive of malignancy, MRI is used to delineate the extent of tumor and to distinguish tumor from trapped secretions (Fig. 3.20). The highest diagnostic accuracy is achieved with the use of both modalities, and both modalities are routinely used in malignancy (47,48).

CT images should be reconstructed in the axial, coronal, and sagittal planes with 3-mm slice thickness. A suggested MRI protocol is as follows:

- 4 mm contiguous slices
- T1-weighted axial and coronal sequences
- T2W axial images

Table 3.1 Conditions with Intrinsic Bone Pathology but Without a Specific Site Predilection (62)

Condition	Notable facts	Radiological features
Common metastases	Most common in central SB. Perineural spread of H&N tumors or hematogenous spread of breast, bronchus, or prostate.	Lung and breast metastases are lytic, prostate lesions are usually mixed sclerotic/lytic with a soft tissue mass. Sclerotic lesions are hypointense on all sequences. Marrow replacement is best seen on T1-weighted images.
Meningioma	Maybe nodular or plaque-like. Encase vessels	Durally based hyperdense mass on CT +/− hyperostosis, strong uniform CE on CT and MRI. En-plague lesions cause slight bone expansion and extensive hyperostosis.
Uncommon myeloma and plasmacytoma	Myeloma may cause diffuse SB disease. Plasmacytoma of the skull base is unusual	Diffuse lytic lesion associated with a soft tissue mass.
Lymphoma	Leptomeningeal disease is most common CNS lymphoma and presents with cranial nerve palsies and may cause perineural spread. SB may be involves by extension of orbital or cavernous sinus lymphoma.	Lytic or mixed lytic/sclerotic lesions. Marrow replacement on MRI
Langerhans cell histiocytosis	Usually affects skull vault in children of 5–15 years. SB sometimes involved. Most often solitary.	Lytic lesion with sharp margins +/− sequestrum, sclerotic rim during healing phase.
Osteosarcoma (OS)	Rarely affect membranous bone hence SB, Paget's disease, and radiotherapy are risk factors.	Aggressive lytic lesion, soft tissue mass with ossific density foci, nonmineralized OS also occurs.
Giant cell tumor (GCT)	SB involvement is rare, sphenoid bone affected most commonly. Brown's tumors of secondary hyperparathyroidism have similar radiological appearance.	Well-defined lytic lesion +/− sclerotic rim and containing soft tissue density. Typically intermediate SI contents with low SI sclerotic rim. May be low SI throughout due to hemosiderin deposition. Strong CE.
Aneurysmal bone cysts	Most commonly in the sphenoid bone (usually body)	Multiloculated cyst with fluid-fluid levels. Solid components suggest a precursor lesion frequently a GCT
Fibro-osseous lesions	Fibrous dysplasia (FD) (children and young adults), Ossifying fibroma (OF) and Paget's disease (after the 5th decade)	FD is typically an expansile, ground glass lesion on CT but may be cystic. MRI appearances can be confusing mimicking tumor. OF has similar imaging features but a more aggressive clinical course
Osteomyelitis and pseudotumor	Extension of infection of inflammation from paranasal sinuses or external auditory canal.	Aggressive imaging features with extensive bone erosion on CT and high T2 SI on MRI which is out of proportion with the volume of soft tissue seen on CT. Endarteritis may result in vascular occlusion
Peripherally located central nervous system tumors	Slowly growing and borderline tumors cause pressure erosion of the SB (well-defined borders) whereas aggressive tumors result in permeative erosion.	

Abbreviations: SB, Skull base; H&N, head and neck; CE, contrast enhancement; SI, signal intensity; CT, computed tomography; MRI, magnetic resonance imaging; CNS, central nervous system.

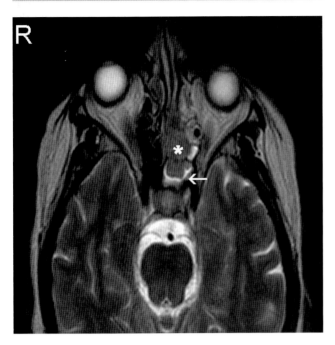

Figure 3.20 T2-weighted axial MR image showing intermediate signal intensity adenocarcinoma in the left ethmoid sinus (asterisk) as well as high signal intensity secretions (arrow). *Abbreviation*: MR, magnetic resonance.

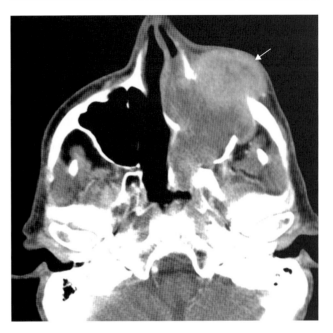

Figure 3.21 Axial CT image demonstrating squamous cell carcinoma eroding the anterior wall of the left maxillary antrum. Note invasion of the skin of the face resulting in obliteration of the subcutaneous fat. *Abbreviation*: CT, computed tomography.

- Postgadolinium T1 fat-saturation axial and coronal sequences
- Short T1 inversion recovery (STIR) coronal images of the neck.

Features Suspicious of Malignancy

The radiological features that raise the possibility of malignancy are

- unilateral sinus disease
- bony changes
- extensive soft tissue mass
- tumor necrosis
- lymphadenopathy.

Unilateral sinus disease may be due to benign or malignant tumors and should prompt the need for further investigation, even in the absence of other positive findings. In a retrospective study of 1118 CT scans of the paranasal sinuses, only 28 cases showed unilateral disease, of which 12 cases were due to neoplasia (6 malignant) (49).

The patterns of bony involvement in sinonasal disease are erosion, remodeling, sclerosis, and new bone formation. Bony erosion is suspicious of malignancy and is the typical pattern seen in SCC (Fig. 3.21); however, it may be observed in inflammatory conditions particularly in the skull base (50,51). Bony remodeling may occur in some malignancies such as olfactory neuroblastoma as well as inflammatory conditions such as mucocele. Reactive sclerosis is the hallmark of chronic inflammation. The coexistence of bony erosion and sclerosis is characteristic

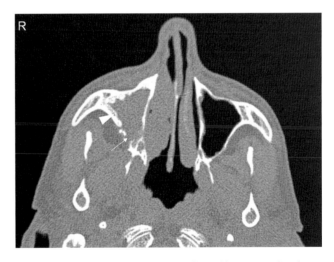

Figure 3.22 Axial CT image in a patient with recurrent lymphoma within the right maxillary antrum, resulting in bony sclerosis (arrowhead) and erosion (arrow). *Abbreviation*: CT, computed tomography.

of Wegener's granulomatosis but is occasionally seen in malignancy (Fig. 3.22).

New bone formation may be in the form of stippled "chondroid" calcification that occurs in well-differentiated chondrosarcoma; these calcified foci have low T1 and high T2 signal on MRI. A sunburst periosteal reaction is highly suspicious of osteosarcoma, but a soft tissue mass causing bony destruction and containing areas of sclerosis (due to matrix mineralization) is a more common finding (46).

The vast majority of sinonasal tumors are of low to intermediate signal intensity on all MRI sequences (Fig. 3.20) but may show areas of heterogeneous signal due to hemorrhage and necrosis. Chronic inflammation results in a variety of signal intensities on all sequences and may therefore mimic malignancy on noncontrast images. However, contrast enhancement usually allows the differentiation of moderately enhancing tumor (Fig. 3.23) from the bright peripheral enhancement of inflammation and nonenhancement of retained secretions. Furthermore, inflammatory sinonasal disease enhances more avidly than malignancy. Occasionally, tumors of salivary origin such as adenoid cystic carcinoma show high signal intensity on T2W images, potentially mimicking inflammatory disease but are usually distinguishable from inflammatory disease by their enhancement characteristics. Malignant tumors may exhibit either homogeneous or heterogeneous enhancement with failure of enhancement of areas of necrosis.

There are a few features that raise the possibility of a specific histological subtype. Peripheral areas of cystic degeneration and calcific foci are features associated with olfactory neuroblastoma (esthesioblastoma) but occur in the minority of cases (Fig. 3.24). Malignant melanoma may be hyperintense on T1W (due to hemorrhage and the paramagnetic effect of metals bound to melanin) and hypointense on T2W images and most frequently affects the nasal cavity (Fig. 3.25). The typical features of T-cell lymphoma are bony destruction in excess of the soft tissue mass (which may result in misdiagnosis as Wegener's granulomatoses on CT) and homogeneous contrast enhancement. Soft tissue sarcomas usually give rise to a large mass with rhabdomyosarcoma being the most common sinonasal

malignancy in children. Aggressive local behavior associated with regional metastases is the hallmark of sinonasal undifferentiated carcinoma and sinonasal neuroendocrine carcinomas.

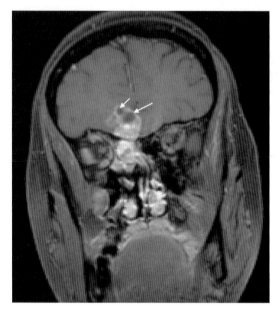

Figure 3.24 Coronal T1-weighted fat-saturated postgadolinium image demonstrating enhancing recurrent olfactory neuroblastoma in the superior nasal cavity, with intracranial extension. Note the nonenhancing peritumoral cysts.

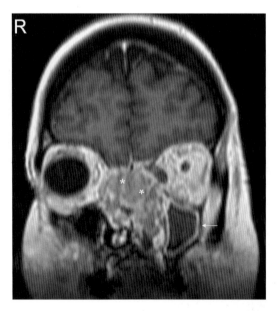

Figure 3.23 Coronal T1-weighted postgadolinium image showing moderately enhancing tumor within the nasal cavity and ethmoid sinuses (asterisks) as well as retained secretions in the left maxillary sinus and the bright peripheral enhancement of inflamed mucosa (arrow).

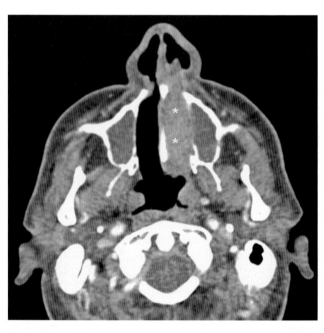

Figure 3.25 Axial CT image showing an enhancing soft tissue mass (asterisks) in this case due to melanoma, filling the left nasal cavity and vestibule. *Abbreviation*: CT, computed tomography.

Lymphadenopathy at presentation is observed in around 15% of patients and is associated with a poor prognosis, although metachronous lymph node metastases have a better outcome (45,46). The posterior nose, ethmoid, and sphenoid sinuses drain to the retropharyngeal lymph nodes as do antral tumors that invade posterior structures. This lymph node group is not clinically detectable and is only shown on cross-sectional imaging.

Patterns of Spread

Mapping the extent of tumor is essential for the planning of the surgical approach and radiotherapy fields. The major role of imaging is to demonstrate the patterns of direct, perineural, or metastatic spread.

MRI assessment of the periorbita (the continuous periosteal lining of the orbit) is essential as breach of the periosteum by tumor necessitates orbital exenteration (52). The negative predictive value of MRI is superior to the positive predictive value (53). The bony orbit and periosteum are hypointense on all MRI sequences. This low signal characteristic remains as long as the periorbita is intact, even in the presence of bony erosion. When the adjacent sinus is replaced by tumor or secretions, this sharp curvilinear hypointensity stands out against the high-signal intensity orbital fat, on T1W sequences. Infiltration of the periorbita results in loss of this well-defined low signal intensity boundary (Fig. 3.26).

Direct intracranial extension to the anterior cranial fossa (ACF) is best assessed with gadolinium-enhanced T1W sequences, allowing identification of the layers that separate the ethmoid sinus from the brain parenchyma: the hypointense cribriform plate, the dura mater (which may enhance due to inflammation), and the low signal intensity cerebrospinal fluid (CSF) (54). Progressive degrees of tumor spread to the ACF manifest initially as loss of the sharp low signal intensity bone interface, displacement of the dura mater by tumor, nodular thickening of the involved dura mater (Fig. 3.27), obliteration of the CSF within the subarachnoid space, and invasion of the brain parenchyma (Fig. 3.24) (50). Mild dural thickening (of less than 5 mm) may be inflammatory. Although intracranial tumor extension is occasionally observed in benign conditions such as mucoceles and polyps, these exhibit a smooth, rounded surface whereas malignant extension tends to be broad based and flat (55).

Perineural spread (PNS) of tumor is particularly characteristic of ACC but is also seen with SCC, lymphoma, and melanoma. Due to its higher incidence, SCC is the most likely cause of PNS from a sinonasal tumor. The presence of PNS makes curative surgery unlikely (56). Up to 40% of patients with PNS are asymptomatic whereas the remaining patients complain of various cranial neuropathies, depending on the nerve affected (57). PNS due to sinonasal malignancy usually involves branches of the maxillary nerve (V2). Extension to the pterygopalatine fossa, foramen ovale, and Meckel's cave may result in involvement of the mandibular division of the trigeminal nerve (V3) as well as facial and glossopharyngeal nerve branches traveling with V2 and V3 (57).

The imaging features of PNS are enlargement and erosion of the skull base neural foramina, abnormal enhancement within these foramina, replacement of the normally observed fat signal in the ptyerygopalatine fossa, loss of the normal CSF signal within Meckel's cave, asymmetrical enlargement of these spaces, or encasement of the internal carotid artery within the cavernous sinus (57).

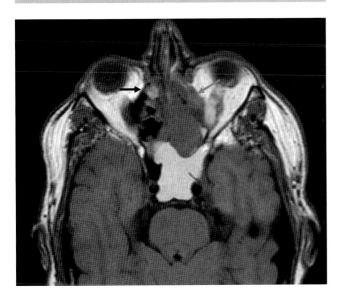

Figure 3.26 Axial T1-weighted MR image showing tumor within the superior nasal cavity and ethmoid air cells. Note the focal loss of the low-signal intensity periorbita (grey arrow) suggestive of orbital invasion and the normal linear low signal periorbita (black arrow). *Abbreviation*: MR, magnetic resonance.

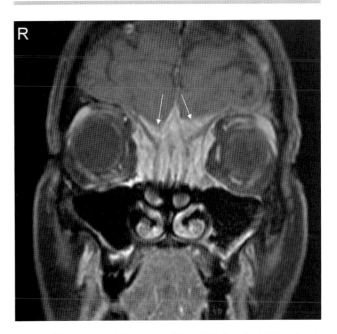

Figure 3.27 Coronal fat-saturated T1-weighted postgadolinium image demonstrating dural invasion manifesting as thick dural enhancement (arrows).

Conclusion

The majority of sinonasal malignancies are SCCs. However, a great diversity of pathologies with differing biological behavior may arise in the sinonasal cavity. The imaging features of the majority of tumors are usually nonspecific. The primary aim of imaging is to determine the tumor extent; orbital and intracranial invasion is of particular importance as this dictates the surgical approach. Close communication with the clinician and pathologist as well as knowledge of any previous treatment is essential.

Skull Base

Skull base pathology may be intrinsic to the bones of the skull, extend to the skull from below or above, metastasize to this location, or may be a part of systemic disease. Clinical assessment of the skull base is limited, and imaging is used to characterize tumors as well as to assess their extent and resectibility. Malignant tumors of the skull base are rare. Benign pathology should be considered in the differential diagnosis of imaging abnormalities of base of skull, as benign disease in this location may be locally aggressive or have aggressive imaging appearances thus mimicking malignancy. The following text summarizes malignant pathology affecting the skull base whereas a variety of benign pathology is summarized in a tabular format.

Differential Diagnosis of Skull Pathology

The skull base is divided anatomically into three regions: anterior, middle, and posterior that approximately correspond to cranial fossae of the same name. The boundary of the anterior and middle skull base is the chiasmatic sulcus, the anterior clinoid process, the posterior border of the lesser wing of the sphenoid, and the superior border of the greater sphenoid wing. The boundary between the middle and posterior skull base is the sphenooccipital synchondrosis, the petroccipital suture, and the posterior petrous ridge.

The use of these anatomical divisions aids differential diagnosis (as some tumors occur at predictable locations) and guides surgical approach.

Malignant tumors without specific site predilection include lymphoma and myeloma (Fig. 3.28). Table 3.1 summarizes this group as well as the intrinsic bony pathology affecting the base of skull. Metastases may involve any part of the skull base (Figs. 29 and 30) but most frequently occur in the middle skull base. These may result from by hematogenous spread (most commonly from breast, bronchus, and prostate) or perineural spread of head and neck malignancy. Involvement of the bones of the skull base manifests as ill-defined lytic or sclerotic foci on CT (Table 3.1). On MRI marrow replacement is best seen on T1-weighted images as replacement of the normal high fat signal, which enhances on fat-suppressed postgadolinium images. Sclerotic tumors have low signal intensity on all sequences (similar to cortical bone).

Primary osteosarcoma of the skull base is rare; osteosarcoma secondary to Paget's disease or radiotherapy occurs more frequently. CT is more specific than MRI, demonstrating an aggressive periosteal reaction and permeative bony changes (58). A variety of intrinsic lesions of

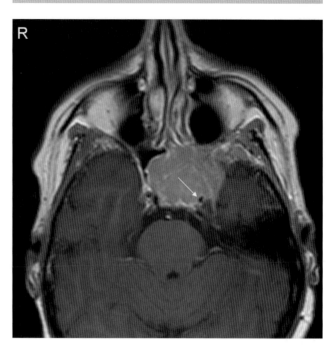

Figure 3.28 Axial T1-weighted postgadolinium MRI demonstrates a moderately enhancing myeloma deposit in the central skull base. Note encasement of the cavernous portion of the left internal carotid artery (arrow). *Abbreviation*: MRI, magnetic resonance imaging.

the skull base are included in Table 3.1 as they may mimic tumor. Fibrous dysplasia and Paget's disease have variable MRI appearances depending on the degree of sclerosis (low signal intensity on all sequences), cystic components (low T1 and high T2 signal), and marrow replacement (loss of normal high signal fatty marrow on T1 sequences). Both conditions cause bone expansion, may enhance avidly, and are easily confused with tumor on MRI but confidently diagnosed on CT.

The anterior skull base may be invaded by superior extension of sinonasal and orbital tumors. Sinonasal tumors are discussed in a separate section. Orbital tumors include lacrimal gland neoplasm, tumors of nerve sheaths, metastases, lymphoma, chloroma, and rhabdomyosarcoma. Lacrimal tumors arise in the superolateral orbit, displace the globe inferiormedially, and may erode the orbital roof and invade the anterior cranial fossa. Orbital tumor may also extend through the optic canal and orbital fissures to the middle cranial fossa. Chondrosarcoma of the chondro-vermian synchondrosis (Fig. 3.31) arises from the posterior nasal septum and may invade the anterior skull base. Table 3.2 summarizes conditions affecting the anterior skull base.

Superior extension of nasopharyngeal carcinoma (Fig. 3.32) is the most common central skull malignancy, causing bony erosion on CT and marrow replacement on MRI. Bony changes seen following treatment of NPC may be due to tumor invasion, radionecrosis, or occasionally osteomyelitis.

Juvenile angiofibroma (JAF) (Figs. 3.33 and 3.34) is locally invasive vascular lesion that occurs almost exclusively in male adolescents and probably represents hamartoma rather than a benign tumor (59). The site of origin of

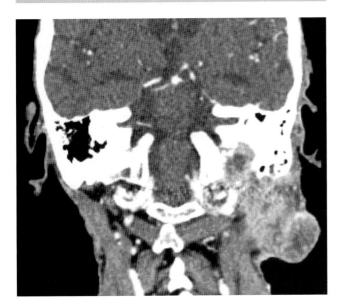

Figures 3.29 Coronal CT images demonstrating a large metastatic deposit in the left neck resulting in erosion of the temporal and occipital bones. *Abbreviation*: CT, computed tomography.

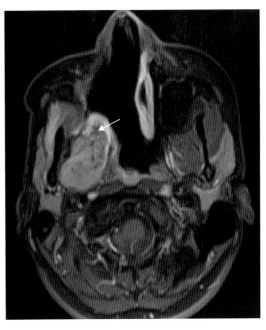

Figure 3.31 Axial fat-saturated postgadolinium T1-weighted MRI demonstrating recurrent chondrosarcoma in the right masticator space (originally arising from the chondro-vermian synchondrosis). Note the markedly heterogenous contrast enhancement (arrow). *Abbreviation*: MRI, magnetic resonance imaging.

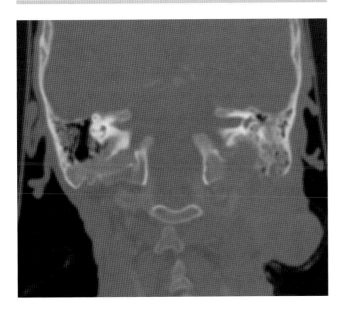

Figures 3.30 Coronal CT images, on bone windows, demonstrating the aggressive pattern of erosion of the temporal and occipital bones. *Abbreviation*: CT, computed tomography.

the tumor is believed by some to be the sphenopalatine foramen whereas others suggest it is the vidian canal aperture in the pterygopalatine fossa; regardless, there is early involvement of both of all these sites. JAF may then extend to the nasal cavity, nasopharynx (by submucosal spread), and the sphenoid, maxillary, and ethmoid sinuses (in order

of frequency) (60). Early involvement of the bone of the pterygoid root is common (60). Extension along the vidian canal or foramen rotundum may result in involvement of the basisphenoid or intracranial disease (but JAF usually remains extradural). Tumor may extend lateral to the infratemporal fossa or to the inferior orbital fissure. JAF enhances avidly on CT and MRI and exhibits flow voids on T2 and postgadolinium T1-weighted images, reflecting the vascular nature of the lesion. CT may demonstrate bony erosion or remodeling (expansion).

The most frequent malignant process affecting the cavernous sinus is metastases. Like lymphoma, cavernous sinus metastases may be unilateral or bilateral. Tables 3.3 and 3.4 summarize pathology affecting the middle skull base and the cavernous sinus.

Posterior skull base pathology may be divided into tumors of the clivus and fissures, the jugular fossa and the petrous temporal bone. Chordoma is a rare malignancy of the notocordal remnant. Skull base chordoma usually arises in the midline, most commonly from the sphenooccipital synchondrosis (Figs. 3.35 and 3.36), typically presenting with headache and ophthalmoplegia due to cranial nerve involvement. On imaging there is a large lobulated well-defined midline soft tissue mass that erodes the clivus. Around 50% of tumors contain calcific foci that represent eroded bone fragments (60). The tumor classically displays high T2 signal intensity. High signal foci on T1-weighted images reflect hemorrhage. In contrast, chondrosarcoma is a paramedian tumor that usually arises from the petro-occipital fissure (Fig. 3.37). Fifty percent of these tumors exhibit a typical "chondroid" pattern of calcification on CT

Table 3.2 Conditions Affecting the Anterior Skull Base (ASB) (58,60,62)

Condition	Notable facts	Radiology
Common malignant sinonasal tumors	Usually squamous cell carcinoma (SCC) in adults and rhabdomyosarcoma (RMS) in children.	SCC: Necrosis, bone erosion. Intermediate SI + CE RMS: Bone erosion/ expansion, homogenous mass, CE.
Uncommon orbital tumors	Lacrimal gland neoplasm, tumors of neural origin, metastases, lymphoma, chloroma, and RMS.	
Benign sinonasal pathology	A variety of conditions including mucocele, polyposis, inverted papilloma, and complicated sinusitis (bacterial, fungal or granulomatous) may involve the SB.	Benign lesions tend to cause bone expansion and remodeling, but infection and granulomatoses may have aggressive appearances with bone erosion.
Rare Cephalocele	15% of cephaloceles occur around the nose and orbit.	Mass contiguous with brain paranchyma and herniating through a bony defect
Dermoid cyst	Midline lesion; may arise in ASB, PSB, or most commonly in spinal canal. ASB cysts are associated with a bifid crista galli and large foramen caecum +/– a cutaneous sinus.	Thick-walled heterogeneous mass. May contain fat density, calcification (Ca2+) and bone. Fat-fluid levels maybe present, if cyst ruptures into ventricles + chemical meningitis, CE common. Variable SI depending on SI fat and protein content of fluid and Ca2+.
Chondroid tumors	Arising from the chondro-vermian synchondrosis (between the nasal septum and sphenoid). See posterior skull base	

Abbreviations: SB, Skull base; H&N, head and neck; CE, contrast enhancement; SI, signal intensity; Ca2+, calcification; ASB; PSB, posterior skull base.

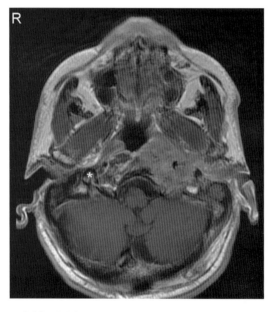

Figure 3.32 Axial postgadolinium T1-weighted MRI demonstrating a large left nasopharyngeal carcinoma that invades the central and posterior skull base. Note the normal right jugular fossa (asterisk) and replacement of the left jugular fossa with tumor. *Abbreviation*: MRI, magnetic resonance imaging.

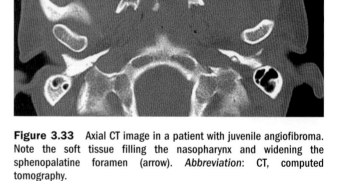

Figure 3.33 Axial CT image in a patient with juvenile angiofibroma. Note the soft tissue filling the nasopharynx and widening the sphenopalatine foramen (arrow). *Abbreviation*: CT, computed tomography.

that are low signal on T1 and high on T2-weighted imaging. The jugular fossa is generally affected by benign pathology. Tables 3.5 and 3.6 summarize tumors affecting the posterior skull base.

Endolymphatic sac tumor is a rare aggressive vascular tumor that arises from the posterior end of the endolymphatic sac. The tumor is rare but strongly associated with Von-Hippel Lindau syndrome (61). CT demonstrates bony erosion and fragments in a characteristic location at the posterior petrous ridge. On MRI areas of T1-weighted hyperintensity reflect blood products, the lesion enhances avidly and may contain flow voids.

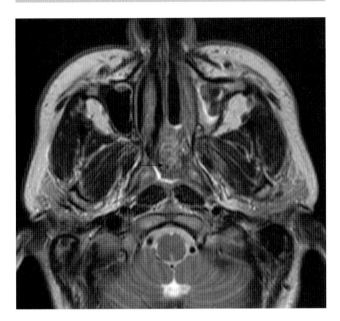

Figure 3.34 Axial T2-weighted MRI in a patient with juvenile angiofibroma. Note the heterogenous soft tissue (arrow) that fills the nasopharynx and contains occasional flow voids, reflecting its vascular nature. *Abbreviation*: MRI, magnetic resonance imaging.

Tumors arising in the jugular fossa are typically benign and include nerve sheath tumors and epidermoid. Glomus jugulare and jugulotympanicum paraganglioma are benign but locally invasive tumors that cause permeative bony erosion of the jugular fossa (Fig. 3.38). The typical salt and pepper appearance on T2-weighted and postgadolinium T1-weighted MRI is due to flow voids on a background of high signal intensity or enhancing paranchyma (Fig. 3.39).

SCC of the external auditory canal may in invade the temporal bone resulting in bony erosion. Tumor recurrence (Figs. 3.40 and 3.41) may be detectable with CT or MRI imaging, but FDG PET-CT is particularly useful for demonstrating skull base recurrence where there has been a flap reconstruction.

Salivary Imaging

The vast majority of salivary gland tumors originate in the parotid and submandibular glands; however, minor salivary gland tumors within other sites of the upper aerodigestive mucosa and sublingual gland tumors are also occasionally encountered. Lymphoma may present in a node adjacent or even within the parotid; rarities include nerve sheath tumors. Parotid tumors are usually benign; however, tumors of smaller salivary glands have a higher incidence of malignancy (64,65).

The most useful imaging modality in the initial workup of a salivary gland mass is ultrasound. The four main paired salivary glands are of smooth echo texture, slightly higher than surrounding muscle and subcutaneous fat. High-resolution, high-frequency probes give excellent

imaging except in the deep lobe of the parotid. The delineation of salivary masses from adjacent pathological lymphadenopathy is particularly useful as the most common nodal site for occult oral cavity tumors (level 2) abuts both the glands. US also is highly sensitive at differentiating acute sialadenitis or plunging ranula from a mass.

Parotid and submandibular gland tumors usually appear as hypoechoic masses relative to normal salivary tissue (Fig. 3.42). The most common tumors (pleomorphic adenomas and Warthin's tumors) are usually smooth in contour or slightly lobulated. Particularly pleomorphic adenomas may contain areas of variable echo texture and cystic change (these may be almost completely cystic). Higher grade tumors have a more varied appearance and may be less well defined giving a clue as to their nature. Intraparotid lymph nodes are common and have a highly characteristic appearance. If lymph nodes in the parotid are enlarged, however, they may cause confusion and appear much more suggestive of a tumor. Lymph nodes are not seen within the substance of the submandibular gland but may abut it. US has utility in guiding fine needle aspiration or core biopsy for preoperative planning (66).

The limitations of US are of operator variability, and limited depth resolution, nevertheless it is simple and easily available and can guide which masses require further imaging to delineate their full extent. The approximate plane of the facial nerve and the retromandibular vein posterior to the angle of the mandible can be readily appreciated and lesions infiltrating deep to this usually require CT or MRI for full delineation; however the accuracy for predicting the position of a parotid mass relative to the facial nerve is not entirely reliable, the plane of the retromandibular vein being the best marker for the position of the nerve branches on imaging (67).

CT shows the salivary glands well, the parotid usually containing a variable amount of fat and therefore being of less high attenuation than adjacent muscle. Dental artefact can obscure particularly the parotid gland although scanning with different gantry angle is an occasionally useful technique to visualize these in a different plane to that of the amalgam. Mass lesions appear denser than parotid tissue and with intravenous contrast medium tend to enhance well, but on occasions can be hard to differentiate from normal tissue. Low-density areas correspond to cystic change. The deep lobe of the parotid is usually well seen on CT as is the retromandibular vein with IV contrast.

MRI provides excellent anatomical detail of the salivary glands and tumors and is probably the modality of choice for operative planning in malignant tumors and where an infiltrating pattern is suspected. The deep lobe and relationship to the stylomandibular tunnel of any mass is generally well shown. It allows easy multiplanar imaging and assessment of difficult surrounding margins, such as the cartilage of the external auditory canal, the bone of the mandible, the carotid sheath, and other structures bordering the parapharyngeal space into which deep lobe lesions characteristically extend (64,68). With its propensity for perineural infiltration, MRI also can image cranial nerve pathways and reveal intracranial or skull base infiltration, although this may be extremely hard to appreciate. Fat-saturated T1-weighted images in multiple planes following

Table 3.3 Conditions Affecting the Middle skull base (58,62,63)

Condition	Notable facts	Radiology
Common nasopharyngeal carcinoma (NPC)	SCC of nasopharynx may be associated with Epstein-Barr Virus, most commonly centered on lateral pharyngeal recess of nasopharynx (NP).	Invasive NP mass, bone erosion (marrow replacement on MRI), 90% have nodal metastases at presentation. May invade cavernous sinus. May show only mild CE.
Uncommon juvenile angiofibroma	Posterior nasal mass, arising adjacent to spheno-palatine foramen in adolescent males; extension through vidian canal and foramen rotundum to CSB. Highly vascular and nonencapsulated	Bone remodelling +/− erosion, enlarges vidian canal, nasal cavity, pterygopalatine fossa (PPF), may invade ethmoid and maxillary sinuses. On MRI heterogenous mass with multiple flow voids, intense CE.
Cranio-pharyngioma	Tumors arise from the Rathke (pharyngo-hypophyseal) pouch remnant; majority are sellar or suprasellar. Rarely tumors arise within the sphenoid bone	Mass usually containing cystic, soft tissue and calcific foci. Surrounding inflammation may result in sclerosis of the sphenoid bone. Usually high T1 (due to proteinacious contents) and high T2 SI. Peripheral CE.
Rathke pouch cysts	Usually sellar or suprasellar. May arise within the sphenoid bone. Radiological and histological differentiation from a mucocele is difficult.	Well-defined cystic mass without a soft tissue component. Variable T1 and high T2 SI.
Pituitary adenoma (PA)	Adenoma originates in pituitary fossa and usually extends superiorly but may invade sphenoid bone. May invade cavernous sinus and encases carotid artery without narrowing it. Rarely PA is completely intraosseous.	On CT macroadenomas are isodense, contain cystic/necrotic/hemorrhagic areas and Occasional Ca2+. Bony erosion of sellar floor. Homogeneous CE of solid elements on MR. Intraosseous PA replaces fatty marrow of sphenoid, (low T1 and high T2 SI) expands the bone without erosion. Associated with empty sella, and intact sellar floor.
Chordoma	See PSB	
Neurofibroma	Most arise from trigeminal nerve (V), especially ophthalmic division (V1).	See PSB for imaging characteristics.
Schwannoma	Most arise from trigeminal nerve and ganglia. May extend to CSB, cisternal V (causing CPA mass) or be dumbell-shaped extending from the cisternal V to gasserian ganglion (constricted by Meckel's cave).	See PSB for imaging characteristics.

Abbreviations: SB, Skull base; H&N, head and neck; CE, contrast enhancement; SI, signal intensity; Ca2+, calcification; SCC, squamous cell carcinoma; PSB, posterior skull base; MRI, magnetic resonance imaging; CSB, central skull base; CT, computed tomography; PP; CPA, cerebellopontine angle.

Table 3.4 Conditions Affecting the Cavernous Sinus (62)

	Unilateral	Bilateral
Common	Schwannoma Meningioma Metastases Vascular lesions	Pituitary adenoma Meningioma Metastases
Uncommon	Lymphoma Cavernous sinus thrombosis Chordoma	Lymphoma
Rare	Lipoma Cavernous hemangioma Plexiform neurofibroma Osteo/chondrosarcoma	

intravenous gadolinium diethylene triamine pentaacetic acid (DTPA) are especially helpful in these cases, although for most operative planning in less aggressive tumors, fewer sequences usually suffice. The same is true for postoperative follow-up scans. In the evaluation of vascular malformations of the head and neck, which may present as salivary gland mass lesions, MRI is unrivalled.

Minor salivary gland tumors usually on oral cavity mucosa are best delineated with MRI. Infiltration into palate and perineural spread are assessed on postgadolinium images, but most of these tumors have a relatively nonspecific appearance and without knowledge of the histology, cannot usually be differentiated from squamous cell tumors arising at these sites. Sublingual tumors can be visualized with US, but MRI is the best modality for assessment of relationships with the muscles of the floor of the mouth and tongue.

Thyroid Imaging

Imaging of the thyroid produces considerable controversy. The management and imaging strategies of thyroid nodules will usually be agreed according to local expertise and agreement.

The incidence of thyroid nodules in postmortem studies is high, and as incidental findings on sonography of the neck these are likewise extremely common. Data on the incidence of thyroid malignancy within these is variable, with studies quoting thyroid malignancy in 10–15% (range 0–29%) (69–81). This has to be seen however in the context of uncertainty over the clinical significance of microscopic foci of papillary carcinoma that have been documented as present in a large percentage at autopsy examination (14,82). Data on "malignancy" in incidental thyroid nodules therefore needs careful interpretation. Various strategies for evaluation have been proposed by, for

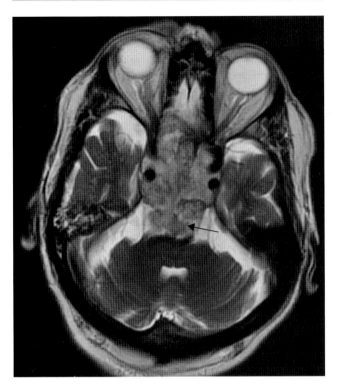

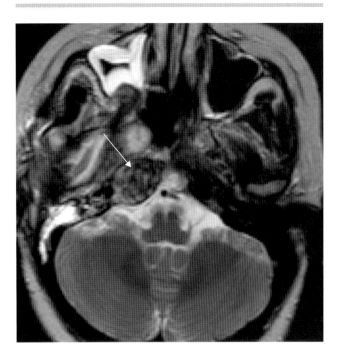

Figure 3.37 Axial T2-weighted MRI demonstrating recurrent chondrosarcoma (arrow) originating from the right petro-occipital fissure. Note the typical paramedian location. *Abbreviation*: MRI, magnetic resonance imaging.

Figure 3.35 Axial T2-weighted MRI showing the typical appearance of chordoma. Note the relatively high T2 signal intensity of the tumor and the "tumor thumb" extending into the prepontine cistern (arrow). *Abbreviation*: MRI, magnetic resonance imaging.

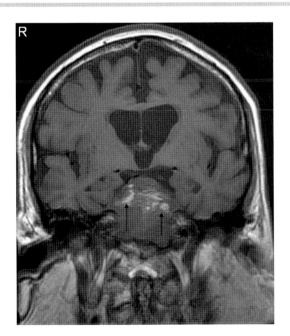

Figure 3.36 Coronal T1-weighted MRI in a patient with chordoma, demonstrating the typical midline location. The high signal foci within the tumor reflect hemorrhage. *Abbreviation*: MRI, magnetic resonance imaging.

example, the American Thyroid Association, the American Association of Clinical Endocrinologists, and the Society of Radiologists in Ultrasound (73,83). Most involve a cutoff of 10–15 mm in determining which require an fine needle aspiration (FNA), with smaller lesions requiring FNA only if there are suspicious US features. The true importance of size as a criteria for determining the utility of FNA is however not proven and is influenced in part by studies assessing the incidence of tumors on FNA of palpable lesions presenting with a mass (a different population). The approach for incidental lesions demonstrated on CT or MRI is likewise not clear. There is also a problem with a size criterion in avoiding FNA in patients with multinodular changes, in whom there may be a very large number of lesions, with several of well over 10 mm. Sonographic follow-up is not validated and has large resource implications. A consensus document from the National Cancer Institute of the United States summarizes the current evidence well, although admits to the lack of good data to support some of its recommendations (83).

Many imaging modalities are used in the assessment of thyroid masses, but US is the most useful initial assessment technique. Current scanning employs high resolution (8–14 mHz) probes, usually with a linear array footprint. With the patient's neck slightly extended over a pillow, or similar support, almost all patients can be scanned successfully. The resolution of such high-frequency probes is under a millimeter, and the detail on grey-scale scanning

Table 3.5 Tumors Arising from the Clivus and Fissures (60,62)

Tumors arising from the clivus and fissures	Notable facts	Radiology
Enchondroma	Most common osteochondral tumor in PSB	Lobulated soft tissue mass causing scalloped endosteal bone resorption. High T2 SI. "Ring and arc" pattern of CE
Chordoma	Notocord origin midline (but occasionally paramedian) aggressive malignancy, PSB is the most common location, also arise in CSB	Clival mass with bone erosion (95%) contains high density ossific fragments of destroyed bone (50%). Heterogeneous CE, with areas of cystic necrosis. On MRI heterogeneous T1 SI with high signal foci of hemorrhage and proteinacious material and hyperintense T2 SI. Tumor "thumb" typically indents the anterior surface of the pons on sagittal images.
Chondrosarcoma	Arises from petro-occipital fissure or sphenooccipital synchondrosis.	Well-differentiated tumors show stippled chondroid calcification (>50%). Low T1 SI. Markedly heterogeneous CE. High T2 SI

Abbreviations: SB, Skull base; H&N, head and neck; CE, contrast enhancement; SI, signal intensity; Ca2+, calcification; PSB, posterior skull base; CSB, central skull base.

Table 3.6 Tumors of the Jugular Fossa (JF) (60,62)

Tumor	Notable facts	Radiology
Paraganglioma	Glomus jugulare (JF), jugulotympanicum (JF and middle ear cavity), Vagale (rare)	Permeative erosive margins on CT. Strong CE on CT and MRI. "Salt-and-pepper" appearance on T2-weighted and postgadolinium T1-weighted imaging due to vascular flow voids against high SI paranchyma.
Schwannoma	JF lesion presents with sensorineural hearing loss (>90%). Encapsulated.	On CT, a well-defined fusiform or dumbbell mass; isodense to brain; enlarge JF with sclerotic rim (pressure erosion). Isointense on MRI, but large tumors may contain mural cysts, necrosis/ hemorrhage. Intense, homogeneous CE. Tend to have high T2 SI
Neurofibroma (NF)	Nonencapsulated, arising from peripheral nerves. Also arise from V and involve CSB.	Usually well-defined but may be an ill-defined infiltrating mass (diffuse NF), characteristically low density with mild CE on CT. Isointense to muscle on MRI, mild to moderate CE. Intermediate SI
Epidermoid	Midline or paramedian tumor with lobulated margins.	CSF density and SI, pressure erosion of SB, Ca2+ (25%). No CE. Exhibits restriction (bright SI) on DWI MR.

Abbreviations: SB, skull base; H&N, head and neck; CE, contrast enhancement; SI, signal intensity; Ca2+, calcification; CT, computed tomography; MRI, magnetic resonance imaging; CSB; SB, skull base; CSF, cerebrospinal fluid; DWI MR, Diffusion weighted imaging magnetic resonance.

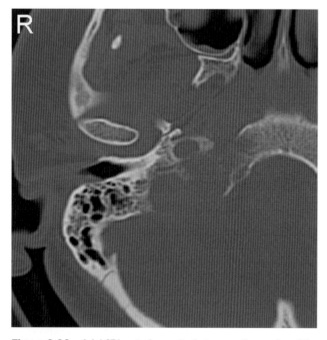

Figure 3.38 Axial CT image demonstrating permeative erosion of the right jugular fossa typical of glomus jugulare. *Abbreviation*: CT, computed tomography.

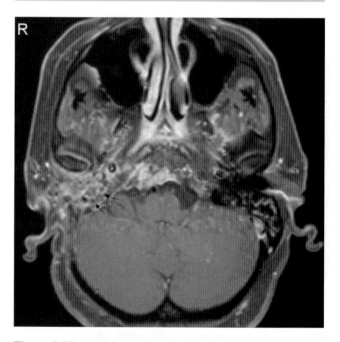

Figure 3.39 Axial image demonstrating extensive recurrence of a right glomus jugulotympanicum. Note the flow voids (arrows) resulting in a salt-and-pepper appearance).

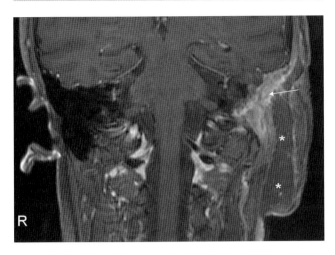

Figure 3.40 Coronal fat-saturated postgadolinium MRI demonstrating enhancing recurrent squamous cell carcinoma (arrow) of the left external auditory canal deep to the reconstruction (asterisks). *Abbreviation*: MRI, magnetic resonance imaging.

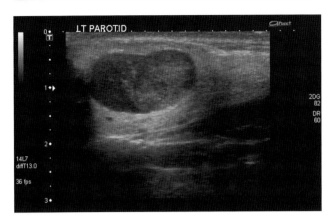

Figure 3.42 Pleomorphic adenoma of the parotid gland. Note low echogenicity relative to surrounding gland.

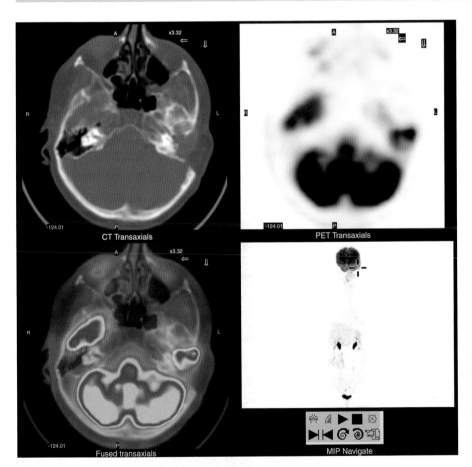

Figure 3.41 FDG PET-CT images showing recurrent squamous cell carcinoma of the left external auditory canal. Note the bony erosion on the CT image (*top left*) and the high FDG activity at the surgical site on the fused image (*bottom left*). *Abbreviations*: FDG; PET, positron emission tomography; CT, computed tomography.

allow for highly accurate delineation of normal from abnormal thyroid tissue. It has a sensitivity for thyroid masses of approaching 100%. It allows an assessment of the whole gland except in patients where there is significant retrosternal extension of a mass. It also has high utility in guiding FNA or core biopsy. In the past it has been characterized as lacking in specificity of any lesions discovered; however, there are some features of thyroid nodules that can allow for a reasonably high degree of diagnostic confidence (84) (Table 3.7) (although there is overlap between

Table 3.7 Ultrasound Findings of Benign and Malignant Thyroid Tumors

	Benign	Malignant
Margins and shape	Well circumscribed, round or ovoid, often with a "halo"	Can be smooth, or irregular with discontinuous or absent "halo," taller than wide on transverse scanning (Figs. 3.43 and 3.44)
Echogenicity	Variable. Often isoechoic. May contain very coarse calcification	Often reduced. Microcalcification common. Macrocalcification possible.
Cystic change	Common. Complex cystic content often seen following hemorrhage into cyst	Suspicious if solid component/nodule in cyst wall. Predominant cystic pattern is rare.
"Comet tail" behind echogenic foci	Characteristic of colloid in benign lesions (Fig. 3.45)	Rare
Multiple similar nodules	Frequent in the context of diffuse thyroid enlargement	Rare
Lymph nodes	Normal	Frequently involved at presentation
Blood flow pattern on Doppler	Highly vascular, usually organized pattern	Usually highly vascular, often disorganized pattern

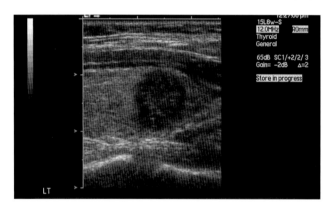

Figure 3.43 Papillary carcinoma of the thyroid. Note low echogenicity, absence of halo, and nonsmooth margin.

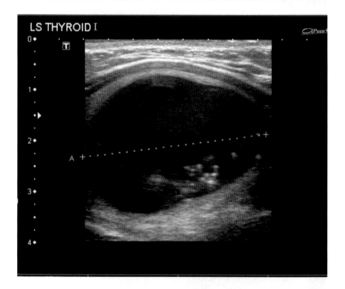

Figure 3.45 Colloid cyst containing echogenic foci.

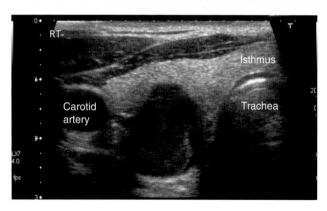

Figure 3.44 Follicular carcinoma of the thyroid.

many of these findings taken individually) which when placed in the clinical context and patient presentation can allow for avoidance of FNA in many patients. There is no evidence to support serial thyroid nodule ultrasound follow up scanning.

US is unquestionably operator dependent however, and placing it in the clinical pathway relies on good clinico-radiological liaison.

CT has limited role in evaluation of the primary lesion but is usually the mainstay of staging for local lymphadenopathy and pulmonary metastatic disease. It also has utility in defining the inferior extent of any retrosternal extension. Iodine-containing contrast media flood thyroid tissue including many thyroid malignancies and limit the use of diagnostic or therapeutic radioactive iodine for at least 6 weeks. It is important therefore to inform those responsible for scan protocolling if these are to be used.

MRI has similar efficacy in local disease and nodal evaluation to CT but currently does not allow for delineation of pulmonary disease. It is widely used for evaluation of suspicious bone lesions demonstrated on isotope bone scanning.

Isotope scanning has a particular use in evaluating functional thyroid disease, but less use in the initial evaluation of thyroid masses. Technetium 99m-pertechnetate is the most commonly used isotope for evaluating functional thyroid tissue, and the presence of photon deficient nodules requires evaluation, usually with US. The most common cause of such "cold" nodules is cystic change that is easily diagnosed on US, a solid lesion requires exclusion of malignancy. About 85–90% of solitary nodules are cold, but only 6–10% of cold nodules are malignant (85). Indeterminate nodules comprise approximately 4–7% of solitary nodules and, as with cold nodules, require biopsy. Dominant cold nodules when part of a multinodular goiter also may be malignancies and biopsy should be considered (86).

Isotope scanning has an important role in the evaluation and detection of metastatic disease or residual thyroid malignancy in the neck. This employs iodine-123 that is taken up in metabolical active lesions and can allow for planning of radioactive iodine therapy. PET is becoming more widely used in staging and follow up of thyroid malignancies.

Parathyroid Imaging

US and isotope imaging are the mainstays of parathyroid imaging. Parathyroid localization can be performed using thallium-201 and technetium-99m pertechnetate subtraction imaging; however ⁹⁹ᵐTc sestamibi offers better image quality, dosimetry, and accuracy (89). Some thyroid lesions also retain it and require subtraction techniques (90) using iodine-123 or Tc-99m pertechnetate to obtain the thyroid image.

Planar and single-photon emission tomography to give more anatomical information may be used. Sestamibi scintigraphy has the ability to detect ectopic parathyroid adenomas (Fig. 3.46) with an accuracy of more than 90%, (91–95) and sensitivities between 68–88% for solitary adenomas are quoted (89,92,93). With many of the techniques there are however false positives and negatives resulting from such difficulties as patient movement, and variable thyroid isotope uptake, as well as small size of adenomas and limited resolution (87).

On US, the typical appearance of a parathyroid adenoma is a well-circumscribed round or oval nodule, usually hypoechoic to the overlying thyroid gland (94,95) (Fig. 3.47). Larger adenomas may have more variable appearances, but on color Doppler imaging most demonstrate a hypervascular pattern.(96) In patients with multinodular thyroid disease, exophytic nodules may mask or resemble an adenoma, and it will miss ectopic adenomas (97). Sensitivity of between 72–89% for the detection of solitary adenomas with preoperative ultrasound has been reported (92,93,98). It is with concordant results with these two methods that the sensitivity and accuracy of preoperative detection and localization is probably at its highest (89,93,99,100).

IMAGING OF POST-TREATMENT CHANGES AND FUNCTIONAL VIDEOFLUOROSCOPIC ASSESSMENT

The impact of surgery and radiotherapy on the imaging appearances of the neck is profound and renders follow-up imaging one of the greatest challenges in radiology.

HERMES

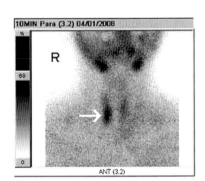

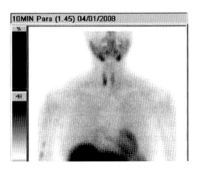

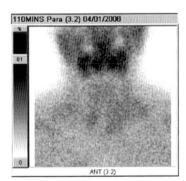

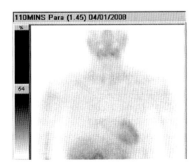

Figure 3.46 Sestamibi scintigraphy demonstrating right-sided parathyroid adenoma (arrow).

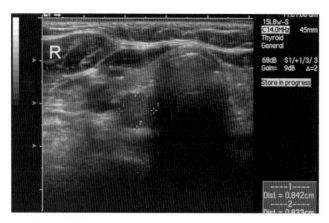

Figure 3.47 Ultrasound of the same lesion as Figure 3.46. Parathyroid adenoma.

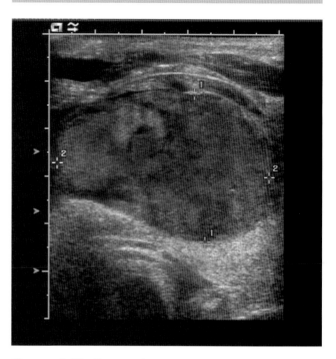

Figure 3.48 Postoperative neck collection on ultrasound. Predominantly hematoma.

Post-treatment Changes

Early Postoperative Complications

In the early postoperative stages, the most common requirements for imaging are in the assessment of collections within the neck. These include hematomas, infected collections and seromas, especially after neck dissection, and combinations of these. The presence of significant volumes of fluid deep to a flap can threaten its viability or the healing process at its margins. US is a good initial investigation and can guide percutaneous aspiration if there is a suitable collection (Fig. 3.48). CT is also a useful modality in these cases and has the advantage over US in its ability to assess collections containing gas (which cannot be visualized accurately with US) (Fig. 3.49) or in the retropharyngeal or deep tissues of the neck. Assessment of arterial flow and venous patency can be assessed by US and CT; however in the postoperative patient, it will often be a judgment based on the overall clinical picture that determines the best use of imaging.

Flaps and Grafts

The recognition of soft tissue, osseous, and fat containing flaps and grafts is key to the interpretation of the postoperative neck, following reconstructive procedures. Fat has a highly characteristic low attenuation on CT (Fig. 3.50) and similarly high signal on both T1- and T2-weighted MRI sequences. It can be rendered low signal using fat suppression or STIR, and this is particularly helpful in assessing for areas of abnormal enhancement suggesting recurrent disease. Bone flaps and grafts fixed with metallic plates produce sometimes troublesome artifact on CT and MR, although modern CT scanners produce less artifact than older generations of scanners. Common rotational flaps such as that using pectoralis major (Fig. 3.51) can be identified from the pedicle of muscle running cranially from the chest wall, but with later muscle atrophy the nature of many flaps can be less clear.

Resections and Neck Dissection

Key to the radiological interpretation of postoperative appearances is an understanding of the surgical procedure

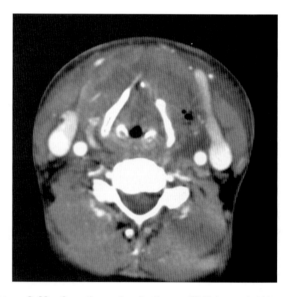

Figure 3.49 Operative neck collection on CT. Note gas bubbles and mixed attenuation. *Abbreviation*: CT, computed tomography.

undertaken. A radical neck dissection removes nodes from level I to V, the ipsilateral submandibular gland, internal jugular vein, sternocleidomastoid muscle, and the spinal accessory nerve. The appearances on CT (Fig. 3.51) or MRI show flattening of the ipsilateral neck, absence of the internal jugular vein and sternocleidomastoid muscle, loss of clear margins of local tissue planes, and the demonstration of the common carotid artery lying more superficially than normal. The trapezius muscle is recognized as atrophic.

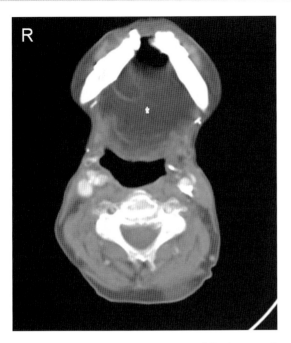

Figure 3.50 Fat containing flap (asterisk) following resection of advanced floor of mouth tumor. Note characteristic fat density on CT. *Abbreviation*: CT, computed tomography.

gland. Loss of clearly defined fat planes between adjacent structures is characteristic.

Following resections in the oral cavity and oropharynx asymmetry is the hallmark. Care is needed to not confuse absence of a structure on one side with a mass lesion on the contralateral side (most commonly when interpreting the palatine tonsils, or following partial glossectomy). The appearances after laryngectomy usually pose no radiological difficulty although following laryngopharyngectomy, with a reconstruction (e.g., using free jejunum) assessment particularly at the resection margins can be hard. Following surgery for sinonasal tumors, the resection cavity margins will characteristically demonstrate some soft tissue thickening, with recurrent tumor often appearing as more mass like and enhancing more avidly after intravenous contrast.

Radiotherapy
Tissue swelling during and after radiotherapy is recognized as diffuse usually low attenuation thickening particularly of the mucosa of the larynx. Symmetrical thickening of the epiglottis (Fig. 3.52), aryepiglottic folds and false vocal cords (Fig. 3.53), laryngeal mucosa, and subglottis occurs in the vast majority of postlaryngeal irradiation patients, and these changes may be seen for years. Elsewhere, diffuse increased attenuation of fat planes and loss of definition between adjacent structures is seen. The salivary

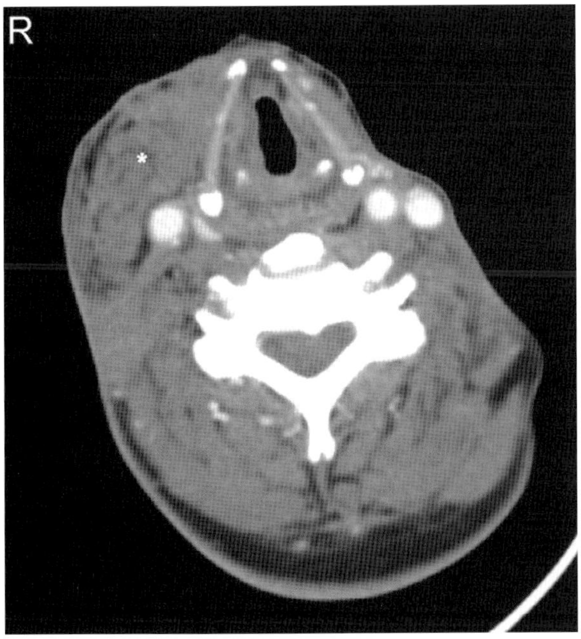

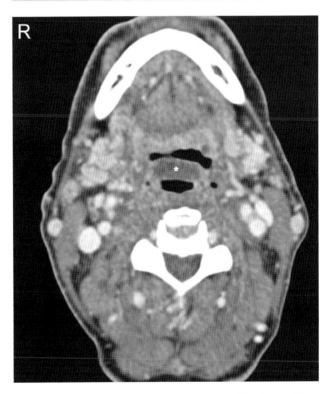

Figure 3.51 Postoperative neck CT. There has been a right radical neck dissection (absent sternocleidomastoid and internal jugular vein as well as atrophic right trapezius muscle). The soft tissue overlying the site of the resection has been covered by a pectoralis major myocutaneous flap (asterisk). *Abbreviation*: CT, computed tomography.

Figure 3.52 Postradiotherapy appearances. CT shows diffuse swelling of all mucosal surfaces, at this level seen in the epiglottis (asterisks) with increased attenuation of subcutaneous fat and loss of tissue planes. *Abbreviation*: CT, computed tomography.

Less radical approaches, with their various terminologies (functional, supra-omohyoid, selective etc.), may produce relatively little specific radiological evidence, although a level-1 dissection will usually remove the submandibular glands show diffuse swelling initially but subsequently become smaller and atrophic and generally less fatty. The arteries usually show accelerated atherosclerosis.

Videofluoroscopic Assessment

Contrast swallow after major surgical resection is most usually performed between 5 and 7 days postoperatively to identify sites of possible leak prior to reinstituting oral intake (Fig. 3.54). Water soluble contrast rather than barium should be used. If the patient has poor oral control of the bolus and laryngeal movement is likely to be impaired (e.g., following glossectomy or partial laryngectomy) then low osmolarity contrast is important as this will be harmless if aspiration occurs. If a leak is seen, the study is often repeated after a further period of time to assess healing. Positioning the postoperative patient and optimizing timing, frame rate, and projection is a very considerable challenge. A control exposure is mandatory, and usually a rapid frame rate (2–3 exposures per second) is needed to obviate difficulties with timing and ensure any leak is captured as it occurs. Once again, familiarity with the

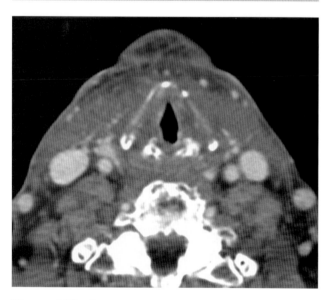

Figure 3.53 Postradiotherapy appearances. Diffuse edema of mucosal surfaces. Level of the arytenoid cartilages and false cords.

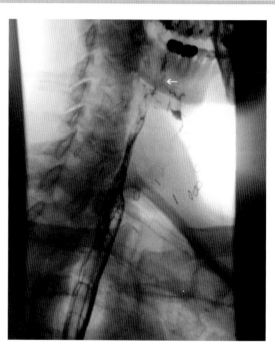

Figure 3.54 Postoperative water soluble contrast swallow. Leak from the superior margin of the laryngectomy site (arrow).

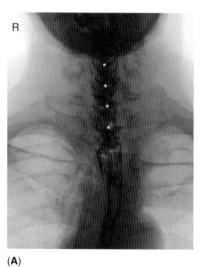

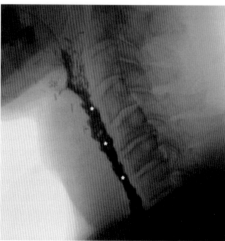

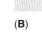

(A) (B)

Figure 3.55 Water soluble contrast swallow demonstrating a jejunal interposition (asterisks) following laryngopharyngectomy.

surgery performed greatly assists interpretation, especially if an interpositional flap has been used during a laryngo-pharyngectomy (Fig. 3.55). In later assessment of swallowing when more functional information is required, the involvement of speech and language therapists is very helpful. Continuous recording onto video or digital storage media assists assessment and analysis of swallowing or voicing pathology. Commonly different consistencies are trialed, from thin liquid to thick solids, following which various maneuvers such as chin tuck or lateral head turn are assessed for reducing risks of aspiration. In voicing assessment following laryngectomy, fluoroscopic studies during attempted phonation or after passing a tube into the esophagus and insufflating with air allow for directed therapy if the cause of dysphonia is identified. Spasm within the pharyngo-oesophageal segment is frequently seen and may respond to botulinum toxin injection.

REFERENCES

1. Becker M, Zbären P, Laeng H et al. Neoplastic invasion of the laryngeal cartilage: Comparison of MR imaging and CT with histopathologic correlation. Radiology 1995; 194: 661–9.

2. Castelijns JA, Becker M, Hermans R. Impact of cartilage invasion on treatment and prognosis of laryngeal cancer. Eur Radiol 1996; 6: 156–69.

3. Righi PD, Kelley DJ, Ernst R et al. Evaluation of prevertebral muscle invasion by squamous cell carcinoma. Can computed tomography replace open neck exploration? Arch Otolaryngol Head Neck Surg 1996; 122: 660–3.

4. Schwager K, Nebel A, Baier G et al. Second primary carcinomas in the upper aerodigestive tract in different locations and age groups. Laryngorhinootologie 2000; 79: 599–603.

5. Spector JG Sessions DG, Haughey BH et al. Delayed regional metastases, distant metastases, and second primary malignancies in squamous cell carcinomas of the larynx and hypopharynx. Laryngoscope 2001; 111: 1079–87.

6. Haas et al. Diagnostic strategies in cervical carcinoma of unknown primary (CUP). Eur Arch Otorhinolaryngol 2002; 259: 325–33.

7. Nathu RM et al. The impact of primary tumor volume on local control for oropharyngeal squamous cell carcinoma treated with radiotherapy. Head Neck 2000; 22: 1–5.

8. Imaizumi A et al. A potential pitfall of MR imaging for assessing mandibular invasion of squamous cell carcinoma in the oral cavity. Am J Neuroradiol 2006; 27: 114–22.

9. Brekel M et al. Cervical lymph node metastasis: assessment of radiologic criteria. Radiology 1990; 177: 379–84.

10. Jose J et al. Cervical node metastases in squamous cell carcinoma of the upper aerodigestive tract: the significance of extracapsular spread and soft tissue deposits. Head Neck 2003; 25: 451–6.

11. Woolgar JA et al. Cervical lymph node metastasis in oral cancer: the importance of even microscopic extracapsular spread. Oral Oncol 2003; 39: 130–7.

12. Schwartz DL et al. Staging of head and neck squamous cell cancer with extended-field FDG-PET. Arch Otolaryngol Head Neck Surg 2003; 129: 1173–8

13. Perlow A et al. High incidence of chest malignancy detected by FDG PET in patients suspected of recurrent squamous cell carcinoma of the upper aerodigestive tract. J Comput Assist Tomogr 2004; 28: 704–9.

14. Gourin CG et al. Identification of distant metastases with positron-emission tomography-computed tomography in patients with previously untreated head and neck cancer. Laryngoscope. 2008; 118: 671–5.

15. Fleming A et al. Impact of 18-F-fluorodeoxyglucose-positron-emission tomography/computed tomography on previously untreated head and neck cancer patients. Laryngoscope 2007; 117: 1173–9.

16. Waltonen J Ozer E, Schuller D, Agrawal A et al. Diagnosis of unknown primary tumors: changes in the 21ˢᵗ century. Ohio State University, Berlin, 2007.

17. Wartski M et al. In search of an unknown primary tumour presenting with cervical metastases: Performance of hybrid FDG-PET–CT. Nucl Med Commun 2007; 28: 365–71.

18. Ng S et al. Prospective study of 18-F-fluorodeoxyglucose positron emission tomography and computed tomography and magnetic resonance imaging in oral cavity squamous cell carcinoma with palpably negative neck. J Clin Onc 2006; 24: 4371–6.

19. Kovacs AF et al. Positron emission tomography with sentinel node biopsy reduces the rate of elective neck dissections in the treatment of oral and oropharyngeal cancer. J Clin Oncol 2004; 22: 3973–80.

20. Tschopp L et al. The value of frozen section analysis of the sentinel lymph node in clinically N0 squamous cell carcinoma of the oral cavity and oropharynx. Otolaryngol Head Neck Surg 2005; 132: 99–102.

21. Pameijer et al. Can pretreatment computed tomography predict local control in T3 squamous cell carcinoma of the glottic larynx treated with definitive radiotherapy? Int J Radiat Oncol Biol Phys 1997; 37: 1011–21.

22. Hermans R et al. Predicting the local outcome of glottic squamous cell carcinoma after definitive radiation therapy: value of computed tomography-determined tumour parameters. Radiother Oncol 1999; 50: 39–46.

23. Pameijer FA et al. Evaluation of pretreatment computed tomography as a predictor of local control in T1/T2 pyriform sinus carcinoma treated with definitive radiotherapy. Head Neck 1998; 20: 159–68.

24. Allal AS et al. Standardized uptake value of 2-[(18)F] fluoro-2-deoxy-D-glucose in predicting outcome in head and neck carcinomas treated by radiotherapy with or without chemotherapy. J Clin Oncol 2002; 20: 1398–404.

25. Halfpenny W et al. FDG-PET. A possible prognostic factor in head and neck cancer. Br J Cancer 2002; 86: 512–16.

26. Kitagawa Y et al. FDG-PET for prediction of tumour aggressiveness and response to intra-arterial chemotherapy and radiotherapy in head and neck cancer. Eur J Nucl Med Mol Imaging 2003; 30: 63–71.

27. Hermans R et al. Laryngeal or hypopharyngeal squamous cell carcinoma: can follow-up CT after definitive radiation therapy be used to detect local failure earlier than clinical examination alone? Radiology 2000; 214: 683–7.

28. Shintani SA et al. Utility of PET/CT imaging performed early after surgical resection in the adjuvant treatment planning for head and neck cancer. Int J Radiat Oncol Biol Phys 2008; 70: 322–9.

29. Nayak JV et al. Deferring planned neck dissection following chemoradiation for stage IV head and neck cancer: the utility of PET-CT. Laryngoscope 2007; 117: 2129–34.

30. Yao M et al. Pathology and FDG PET correlation of residual lymph nodes in head and neck cancer after radiation treatment. Am J Clin Oncol 2007; 30: 264–70.

31. Brkovich VS et al. The role of positron emission tomography scans in the management of the N-positive neck in head and neck squamous cell carcinoma after chemoradiotherapy. Laryngoscope 2006; 116: 855–8.

32. Kunkel M et al. Detection of recurrent oral squamous cell carcinoma by [18F]-2-fluorodeoxyglucose-positron emission tomography: implications for prognosis and patient management. Cancer 2003; 98: 2257–65.

33. Lee JC et al. F-18 FDG-PET as a routine surveillance tool for the detection of recurrent head and neck squamous cell carcinoma. Oral Oncol 2007; 43: 686–92.

34. Terhaard CH et al. F-18-fluoro-deoxy-glucose positron-emission tomography scanning in detection of local recurrence after radiotherapy for laryngeal/ pharyngeal cancer. Head Neck 2001; 23: 933–41.

35. Van de Caveye V et al. Detection of head and neck squamous cell carcinoma with diffusion weighted MRI after (chemo) radiotherapy: correlation between radiologic and histopathologic findings. Int J Radiat Oncol Biol Phys 2007; 67: 960–71.

36. Hermans R et al. Laryngeal tumor volume measurements determined with CT: a study on intra- and interobserver variability. Int J Radiat Oncol Biol Phys 1998; 40: 553–7.

37. Mukherji SK et al. Interobserver reliability of computed tomography-derived primary tumor volume measurement in patients with supraglottic carcinoma. Cancer 2005; 103: 2616–22.

38. Daisne JF et al. Tumor volume in pharyngolaryngeal squamous cell carcinoma: comparison at CT, MR imaging, and FDG PET and validation with surgical specimen. Radiology 2004; 233: 93–100.

39. Daisne JF et al. Tri-dimensional automatic segmentation of PET volumes based on measured source-to-background ratios: influence of reconstruction algorithms. Radiother Oncol 2003; 69: 247–50.

40. Geets X et al. Impact of the type of imaging modality on target volumes delineation and dose distribution in pharyngolaryngeal squamous cell carcinoma: comparison between pre- and per-treatment studies. Radiother Oncol 2006; 78: 291–7.

41. Lee AW et al. Retrospective analysis of nasopharyngeal carcinoma treated during 1976-1985: late complications following megavoltage irradiation. Br J Radiol 1992; 65: 918–28.

42. Hermans R. Imaging of mandibular osteoradionecrosis. Neuroimaging Clin N Am 2003; 13: 597–604.

43. Liu SH, Chang JT, Ng SH et al. False positive fluorine-18 fluorodeoxy-D-glucose positron emission tomography finding caused by osteoradionecrosis in a nasopharyngeal carcinoma patient. Br J Radiol 2004; 77: 257–60.

44. Zbären P et al. Radionecrosis or tumor recurrence after radiation of laryngeal and hypopharyngeal carcinomas. Otolaryngol Head Neck Surg 2006; 135: 838–43.

45. Barnes L, Brandwein M, Som PM. Diseases of the nose, paranasal sinuses, and nasopharynx. In: Barnes L, ed. Surgical pathology of the head and neck, 2nd ed. New York; Marcel Decker, 2001: 439–555.

46. Som PM, Brandwein MS. Tumors and tumor-like conditions. In: Som PM, Curtin DC, eds. Head and neck imaging. 4th ed. St Louis: Mosby, 2003: 261–373.

47. Lund VJ, Howard DJ, Lloyd GA et al. Magnetic resonance imaging of paranasal sinus tumors for craniofacial resection. Head Neck 1989; 11: 279–83.

48. Hahnel S, Ertl-Wagner B, Tasman AJ et al. Relative value of MR imaging as compared with CT in the diagnosis of inflammatory paranasal sinus disease. Radiology 1999; 210: 171–6.

49. Ashsan F, El-Hakim H, Kim AW. Unilateral opacification of paranasal sinus CT scans. Otolaryngology – Head and Neck Surgery 2004; 131: 53.

50. Maroldi R, Farina D, Battaglia G et al. MR of malignant nasosinusal neoplasms. Frequently asked questions. Eur J Radiol 1997; 24: 181–90.

51. Som PM, Lawson W, Lidov MW. Simulated aggressive skull base erosion in response to benign sinonasal disease. Radiology 1991; 180: 755–9.

52. Curtin HD, Rabinov JD. Extension to the orbit from paraorbital disease. The sinuses. Radiol Clin North Am 1998; 36: 1201–13, xi.

53. Maroldi R, Berlicchi M, Farina D et al. Benign Neoplasms and Tumor-like Conditions. In: Maroldi R, Nicolai P, eds. Imaging in Treatment Planning for Sinonasal Diseases. Springer Verlag, Berlin, 2005; 107–158.

54. Ahmadi J, Hinton DR, Segall HD et al. Surgical implications of magnetic resonance-enhanced dura. Neurosurgery 1994; 35: 370–7.

55. Som PM, Dillon WP, Sze G et al. Benign and malignant sinonasal lesions with intracranial extension: differentiation with MR imaging. Radiology 1989; 172: 763–6.

56. Goepfert H, Dichtel WJ, Medina JE et al. Perineural invasion in squamous cell skin carcinoma of the head and neck. Am J Surg 1984; 148: 542–7.

57. Ginsberg LE. Imaging of perineural tumor spread in head and neck cancer. Semin Ultrasound CT MR 1999; 20: 175–86.

58. Borges A. Skull base tumours part I: Imaging technique, anatomy and anterior skull base tumours. Eur J Radiol 2008; 66: 338–47.

59. Maroldi R, Lombardi D, Farina D et al. Malignant neoplasms. In: Maroldi R, Nicolai P, eds. Imaging in treatment planning for sinonasal diseases. Springer Verlag, 2005: 159–220.

60. Harnsberger HR, ed. Diagnostic imaging: Head and neck. Salt Lake City, Utah. Amirsys 2004; pp II-2-64-67.

61. Manski TJ, Heffner DK, Glenn GM et al. Endolymphatic sac tumors. A source of morbid hearing loss in von Hippel-Lindau disease. JAMA 1997; 277: 1461–6.

62. Osborn AG. Brain tumors and tumor-like masses. In: Osborn AG, ed. Diagnostic Neuroradiology. St. Louis: Mosby-Year Book, 1994: 401–528.

63. Borges A. Skull base tumours part II. Central skull base tumours and intrinsic tumours of the bony skull base. Eur J Radiol 2008; 66: 348–62.

64. Lee YY, Wong KT, King AD et al. Imaging of salivary gland tumours. Eur J Radiol 2008; 66: 419–36.

65. Madani G, Beale T. Tumours of the salivary glands. Semin Ultrasound CT MR 2006; 27: 452–64. Review.

66. Kraft M, Lang F, Mihaescu A et al. Evaluation of clinician-operated sonography and fine-needle aspiration in the assessment of salivary gland tumours. Clin Otolaryngol 2008; 33: 18–24.

67. Ragbir M, Dunaway DJ, Chippindale AJ et al. Prediction of the position of the intraparotid portion of the facial nerve on MRI and CT. Br J Plast Surg 2002; 55: 376–9.

68. Stambuk HE, Patel SG. Imaging of the parapharyngeal space. Otolaryngol Clin North Am 2008; 41: 77–101, vi.

69. Academy of Clinical Thyroidologists. Position paper on FNA for non-palpable thyroid nodules (08/2006). (www.thyroidologists.com/papers.html).

70. Brander AEE, Viikinkoski VP, Nickels JI et al. Importance of thyroid abnormalities detected in US screening: a 5-year follow-up. Radiology 2000; 215: 801–6.

71. Cooper DS, Doherty GM, Haugen BR et al. Management guidelines for patients with thyroid nodules and differentiated thyroid cancer. Thyroid 2006; 16: 109–40

72. Chung WY, Chang HS, Kim EK et al. Ultrasonographic mass screening for thyroid carcinoma: a study in women scheduled to undergo a breast examination. Surg Today 2001; 31: 763–7.

73. Frates MC, Benson CB, Charboneau JW et al. Management of thyroid nodules detected at US: Society of Radiologists in Ultrasound Consensus Conference Statement. Radiology 2005; 237: 794–800.

74. Kang HW, No JH, Chung JH et al. Prevalence, clinical and ultrasonographic characteristics of thyroid incidentalomas. Thyroid 2004; 14: 29–33

75. Kim EK, Park CS, Chung WY et al. New sonographic criteria for recommending fine-needle aspiration biopsy of nonpalpable solid nodules of the thyroid. Am J Roentgenol 2002; 178: 687–91.

76. Leenhardt L, Hejblum G, Franc B et al. Indications and limits of ultrasound-guided cytology in the management of nonpalpable thyroid nodules. J Clin Endocrinol Metab 1999; 84: 24–28.

77. Liebeskind A, Sikora AG, Komisar A et al. Rates of malignancy in incidentally discovered thyroid nodules evaluated with sonography and fine needle aspiration. J Ultrasound Med 2005; 24: 629–34.

78. Nabriski D, Ness-Abramof R, Brosh T et al. Clinical relevance of non-palpable thyroid nodules as assessed by ultrasound guided fine needle aspiration biopsy. J Endocrinol Invest 2003; 26: 61–64.

79. Nan-Goong IS, Kim HY, Gong G et al. Ultrasonography-guided fine-needle aspiration of thyroid incidentaloma: correlation with pathological findings. Clin Endocrinol 2004; 60: 21–8.

80. Papini E, Guglielmi R, Bianchini A et al. Risk of malignancy in nonpalpable thyroid nodules: predictive value of ultrasound and color-Doppler features. J Clin Endocrinol Metab 2002; 87: 1941–6.

81. Steele SR, Martin MJ, Mullenix PS et al. The significance of incidental thyroid abnormalities identified during carotid duplex ultrasonography. Arch Surg 2005; 140: 981–5.

82. Harach HR, Franssila KO, Wasenius VM. Occult papillary carcinoma of the thyroid. A "normal" finding in Finland. A systematic autopsy study. Cancer 1985; 56: 531–8.

83. US National Institutes for Health: National Cancer Institute. Final draft of the review and conclusions document; Feb 29, 2009. http://thyroidfna.cancer.gov/pages/conclusions/

84. Moon W, Jung S, Lee J et al. Benign and malignant thyroid nodules: US differentiation- multicentre retrospective study. Radiology 2008; 247: 762–70.

85. Freitas JE, Freitas AE. Thyroid and parathyroid imaging. Semin Nucl Med 1994; 24: 234–45.

86. Belfiore A, LaRose GL, LaPorta GA et al. Cancer risk in patients with cold thyroid nodules: relevance of iodine intake, sex, age and multinodularity. Am J Med 1992; 93: 363–9.

87. Palestro CJ, Tomas MB, Tronco GG. Radionuclide imaging of the parathyroid glands. Semin Nucl Med 2005; 35: 266–76.

88. Johnson NA, Tublin ME, Ogilvie JB. Parathyroid imaging: technique and role in the preoperative evaluation of primary hyperparathyroidism. AJR 2007; 188: 1706–15.

89. Merrick MV. Endocrine. In: Merrick MV, ed. Essentials of nuclear medicine, 2nd ed. Berlin: Springer-Verlag, 1998: 149–76.

90. Hindie E, Melliere D, Jeanguillaume C et al. Parathyroid imaging using simultaneous double-window recording of technetium-99m-sestamibi and iodine-123. J Nucl Med 1998; 39: 1100–5.

91. Moinuddin M, Whynott C. Ectopic parathyroid adenomas: multi-imaging modalities and its management. Clin Nucl Med 1996; 21: 27–32.

92. Ruda JM, Hollenbeak CS, Stack BC Jr. A systematic review of the diagnosis and treatment of primary hyperparathyroidism from 1995 to 2003. Otolaryngol Head Neck Surg 2005; 132: 359–72.

93. Siperstein A, Berber E, Mackey R et al. Prospective evaluation of sestamibi scan, ultrasonography, and rapid PTH to predict the success of limited exploration for sporadic primary hyperparathyroidism. Surgery 2004; 136: 872–80.

94. Gooding GAW. Sonography of the thyroid and parathyroid. Radiol Clin North Am 1993; 31: 967–89.

95. Reading CC, Charboneau JN, James EM et al. High resolution parathyroid sonography. AJR 1982; 139: 539–46.

96. Randel SB, Gooding GAW, Clark OH et al. Parathyroid variants: US evaluation. Radiology 1987; 165: 191–4.

97. Fugazzola C, Bergamo AI, Andreis I et al. Parathyroid glands. In: Solbiati L, Rizzatto G, eds. Ultrasound of Superficial Structures. London: Churchill Livingstone, 1995: 87–114.

98. Koslin DB, Adams J, Andersen P et al. Preoperative evaluation of patients with primary hyperparathyroidism: role of high resolution ultrasound. Laryngoscope 1997; 107: 1249–53.

99. Haber RS, Kim CK, Inabnet WB. Ultrasonography for preoperative localization of enlarged parathyroid glands in primary hyperparathyroidism: comparison with (99m) technetium sestamibi scintigraphy. Clin Endocrinol (Oxf) 2002; 57: 241–49.

100. Solorzano CC, Carneiro-Pla DM, Irvin GL 3rd. Surgeon-performed ultrasonography as the initial and only localizing study in sporadic and primary hyperparathyroidism. J Am Coll Surg 2006; 202: 18–24.

4

Radiation Therapy for Head and Neck Cancer

Kevin J Harrington, Christopher M Nutting, Kate Newbold and Shreerang A Bhide

INTRODUCTION

Radiotherapy (RT) is an extremely effective treatment for head and neck cancer, as a primary modality and as an adjuvant treatment following surgery. In early-stage disease, single modality radical RT can cure >90% of cancers in some tumor subsites (e.g., larynx) (1). In more advanced-stage diseases, RT is usually used in combination with cisplatin chemotherapy, either as radical chemoradiotherapy (2,3) or in an adjunctive fashion after ablative surgery (4).

Most cancers of the head and neck are squamous cell carcinomas (HNSCC) and are generally considered to be radiosensitive lesions. There is a well-established relationship between the radiation dose delivered to the tumor and the probability of tumor control (Fig. 4.1). In general terms, below a certain threshold dose, there is no chance of tumor control. Beyond this dose, for HNSCC, the tumor control probability curve plotted against radiation dose exhibits a sigmoidal relationship with a relatively steep gradient. Therefore, beyond the threshold radiation dose, the higher the radiation dose delivered to the tumor the higher the chance of cure. However, surrounding normal tissues are also contained in radiotherapy portals, and irradiation of these normal tissues limits the dose that can be delivered to the tumor safely. This phenomenon can be represented in terms of the late normal tissue complication probability curve (also shown by the dotted line in Fig. 4.1). It is the occurrence of late normal tissue complications such as fibrosis or osteoradionecrosis that limits our ability to increase cure rates simply by escalating radiation doses to tumor tissues. This limitation is exemplified by the theoretical dose escalation from 70 Gy (Gray) to 75 Gy in Figure 4.1 that leads to improved tumor control but only at the expense of an unacceptable increase in late normal tissue damage. The concept of the therapeutic index (i.e., the gap between the tumor control probability and the normal tissue complication probability curves) is a useful means of visualizing the conflict between the desire to increase the radiation dose to the tumor and concerns about normal tissue damage (Fig. 4.2). In an attempt to circumvent this limitation on radiation dose delivery, novel radiotherapy techniques and combination treatment strategies have been developed in an attempt to improve the therapeutic index (5).

THE RADIOBIOLOGICAL BASIS OF RADIOTHERAPY

Radiobiology is the study of the effect of radiation on living matter. Although a detailed account of the science of radiobiology is beyond the scope of this chapter, a brief description of five of its central themes (the five Rs of radiobiology) will serve to highlight the important areas of interest and their clinical relevance (6). The five Rs of radiobiology are repair, repopulation, reoxygenation, redistribution, and radiosensitivity.

Repair

The damage caused by radiation to the DNA of normal and malignant cells takes a number of different forms. Single- and double-strand DNA breaks are the most important phenomena, and double-stranded breaks, in particular, have been found to correlate with cell kill over a wide range of doses. However, once damage has occurred, complex cellular repair mechanisms come into effect to attempt to restore the integrity of the DNA sequence. It is thought that all reparable damage is completely repaired within 6 hours of irradiation. Although repair is a highly desirable property of normal cells, its occurrence in cancer cells will tend to reduce the efficacy of therapeutic radiation. The ability of normal and tumor cells to repair radiation-induced DNA damage varies and lies at the heart of the design of fractionated courses of radiotherapy. In general, normal tissues are said to repair damage more efficiently. Therefore, dividing a course of radiation into a number of fractions with an interval between them to allow normal tissue repair allows differential killing of normal and tumor cell populations. The *therapeutic ratio* is the term used to describe the ratio between the cell kill in the tumor compared to that in normal tissue. Changes in the pattern of fractionation alter the differential cell killing between tumors and late-responding normal tissues, in effect modifying the therapeutic ratio. Increasing the dose per fraction may be hazardous because this causes relatively more damage in normal tissues than in the tumor and reduces the therapeutic ratio. On the other hand, reducing the dose per fraction may be advantageous as there will be differential sparing of normal tissues relative to the tumor, increasing the therapeutic ratio. Balanced against this is the need to increase the total dose and the number of radiation fractions to achieve equal total tumor cell kill. If this requires undue prolongation of treatment, the beneficial effects of fractionation may be lost by the occurrence of tumor cell repopulation (see below) and a decreased chance of cure. In the case of low-dose rate interstitial brachytherapy (see below), the treatment can be viewed as a large number of very small radiation fractions given one after another. Repair occurs throughout the treatment and gives rise to differential sparing of normal tissues while allowing high curative doses to be delivered to the tumor.

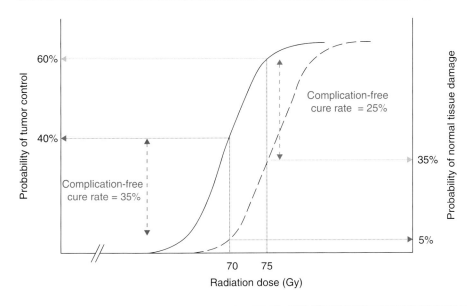

Figure 4.1 Dose-response curves for tumor (solid line) and normal (dotted line) tissues. At a radiation dose of 70 Gy, 40% of tumors are cured but at the expense of severe long-term toxicity (grade 3 or greater) in around 5% of patients. Therefore, the complication-free cure rate is 35%. If the radiation dose is increased to 75 Gy, the cure rate increases to 60% but the normal tissue damage rate also increases to 35%, for a complication-free cure rate of only 25%. In this notional example, the complication-free cure rate decreases with an increase in radiation dose. For this reason, simple radiation dose escalation is not a viable strategy to achieve improved outcomes in treating head and neck cancer.

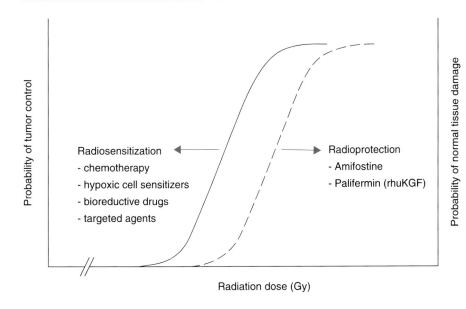

Figure 4.2 The concept of radiosensitization and radioprotection. If the tumor control probability curve (solid line) can be shifted to the left by the addition of cytotoxic chemotherapy, hypoxic cell sensitizers, bioreductive drugs, or targeted agents without also shifting the normal tissue damage probability curve (dotted line) in the same direction, the net effect is to widen the gap between the curves and to increase the therapeutic index. Similarly, if the normal tissue damage probability curve can be shifted to the right by radioprotectors without causing a similar shift in the tumor control probability curve, the net effect is to increase the therapeutic index.

Part of this advantage is lost if high-dose rate brachytherapy is used. Such treatment must be delivered in fractions with sufficient time between them to allow for repair of damage in normal tissues.

Repopulation

During a course of fractionated radiotherapy, viable tumor cells continue to divide. As some cells are destroyed by a dose of radiotherapy, new cells replace them. Some studies have suggested that after approximately 3 weeks of fractionated radiotherapy viable clonogenic tumor cells are able to enter a phase of accelerated repopulation. Therefore, to eradicate a tumor completely, the radiotherapy must destroy not only all of the original tumor cells but also any formed by repopulation during the treatment period. This has led

to the concept of "wasted" radiation dose (i.e., some of the next fraction of radiotherapy is used up in killing cells born in the interval between fractions). Therefore, prolongation of the overall treatment time would be expected to have an adverse effect on local control and patient survival. Clinical studies have confirmed this prediction for a number of different tumor types, including head and neck cancer. Changes in conventional fractionation regimens, classically 2 Gy fractions once daily for 5 days per week, are under investigation (see below).

Reoxygenation

Well-oxygenated (euoxic) cells are more susceptible to the effects of ionizing radiation than hypoxic cells. The euoxic zone around tumor blood vessels tends to contain healthy, dividing cells, whereas the areas distant from the blood vessels often show areas of necrosis thought to be due to anoxic cell death. RT is generally effective at killing the euoxic cells, and those that have already died from profound anoxia no longer pose a threat. However, in the intervening territory between the euoxic and anoxic cell populations there exists a population of hypoxic cells that is able to remain viable in a quiescent, noncycling phase. There is evidence to suggest that this group of cells is relatively radioresistant and is a major determinant of the outcome of RT. Fractionation of RT provides a mechanism to circumvent this problem. As euoxic cells are killed by radiation, they no longer absorb and metabolize oxygen allowing it to diffuse further from the blood vessels into previously hypoxic areas. This effect of tumor reoxygenation tends to reverse the relative radioresistance of the hypoxic cell population.

Redistribution

Cellular radiosensitivity varies at different phases of the cell cycle. Cells in G1, early S, and G2/M phases are highly sensitive, whereas cells in late S phase are highly resistant to the effects of ionizing radiation. Fractionated courses of RT aim to exploit the tendency for tumor cells to redistribute into different phases of the cell cycle throughout the course of treatment. Therefore, it is hoped that cells in a relatively radioresistant phase at the time of one treatment fraction will be in a more sensitive phase at the time of the next fraction.

Radiosensitivity

Different types of tumors have differing inherent sensitivities to ionizing radiation. Therefore, RT is more effective in treating some tumors than others (e.g., lymphomas and seminomas are extremely radiosensitive, and gliomas and melanomas are relatively radioresistant). However, within a given tumor type, such as head and neck cancer, it is impossible to predict in advance what the inherent radiosensitivity of any individual tumor will be. If it were possible to assay radiosensitivity on a biopsy specimen before therapeutic radiation started, it might be possible to select the most appropriate radiotherapy regimen or even to identify tumors that would be unlikely to be cured by RT. As yet, such assays have proved to be little more than a research tool and have not found their way into routine RT treatment strategies.

Knowledge of these principles of radiobiology has been used to enhance radiation treatment by guiding selection of optimal dose delivery (fractionation) schedules and informing the rational choice of agents to be combined with RT. In addition, as a parallel track of research, our technical ability to deliver RT has improved such that we are able to deliver more homogeneous doses of radiation to the tumor and reduce dose delivery to critical normal tissues. In this chapter we review how these key advances have begun to translate into improved therapeutic outcomes for patients with HNSCC.

ROLE OF RADIOTHERAPY IN HEAD AND NECK CANCERS

RT or surgery alone is effective in early stage [American Joint Committee on Cancer (AJCC) Stage I and II] HNSCC.

RT can be delivered via external beam and/or brachytherapy (see below). For stage III and IV HNSCC, surgery and postoperative (chemo)radiation (4) or definitive chemoradiation are effective (7,8). Lesions with high probabilities of cure (>70%) should ideally be treated with a single therapeutic modality (either surgical or nonsurgical). The increased morbidity of combined surgical and nonsurgical treatment is unjustified, especially when not associated with a significantly improved control rate. However, there are circumstances in which RT and surgery are used as part of a planned treatment program.

Preoperative Radiation Therapy

Preoperative RT is infrequently used and should not be considered to be a standard of care. This recommendation is based on the fact that even in the event of a complete or an excellent partial response to RT the volume of tissue that must be considered to be at risk of harboring microscopic disease is exactly the same as before the onset of RT. Therefore, preoperative RT can never be considered to represent a means of reducing the extent of a curative surgical procedure. Nonetheless, on rare occasions, preoperative RT can be considered in the following situations: (1) fixed, inoperable neck nodes; (2) in situations where the initiation of postoperative RT is likely to be delayed by more than 6–8 weeks due to the need for extensive surgical reconstruction; (3) prior to surgical approaches that will occasion the use of the gastric pull-up for reconstruction; and (4) in patients who have undergone an open, incisional biopsy of a positive neck node. In general terms, when RT is to be used in a dual modality strategy with surgery, it is best employed to treat postsurgical microscopic disease.

Postoperative Radiation Therapy

Postoperative RT is usually considered when the risk of recurrence above the clavicles exceeds 20%. The operative procedure should be one stage and should ideally allow irradiation to start no later than 6 weeks after surgery (9). An operation should be undertaken only if complete excision is anticipated. Partial removal (debulking) of irresectable gross disease should be avoided on the grounds that it may delay the start of definitive RT and may disturb the blood supply to the tumor, which may, in turn, reduce oxygenation and/or delivery of cytotoxic chemotherapy to the tumor. An exception to this would be endoscopic debulking of a laryngeal cancer obstructing the airway.

Indications for Postoperative Radiation Therapy

Absolute indications for postoperative irradiation are involved (positive) margins at the primary tumor resection site and extracapsular spread of involved lymph nodes. Near absolute indications include close (less than 5 mm) margins, two or more involved cervical lymph nodes and invasion of the soft tissues of the neck (4). The presence of lymphovascular space invasion and perineural invasion are relative indications for postoperative RT that are considered in concert with other factors. The advantages of postoperative, compared with preoperative, radiation therapy include less operative morbidity, more meaningful margin checks at the time of surgery, a knowledge of tumor spread for radiation treatment planning and no chance that RT-induced toxicity will prevent the patient from being able to undergo surgery. The potential disadvantages of postoperative RT include the delay in starting radiation therapy with the possibility of tumor growth (especially in contralateral neck nodes) and the higher radiation dose required to accomplish the same rates of locoregional control because of disturbance in vascular supply in the operative bed.

RADIATION THERAPY TECHNIQUES

The delivery of radiation to patients represents a serious undertaking with the potential for immediate and long-term consequences to the patient. The central dogma that underlies radiation treatment technique is the absolute requirement to attempt to treat all areas at high risk of harboring disease while limiting the dose delivered to uninvolved normal tissues to the minimum that is practicable. This second issue is particularly important in the head and neck region because of the close proximity of critical normal structures (spinal cord, brain stem, optic nerve and chiasm, parotid glands, and swallowing apparatus) to radiation target volumes. Therefore, in practice, radiation delivery is considered in terms of areas that contain gross macroscopic disease (the primary site and involved lymph nodes) and areas that potentially contain subclinical, microscopic disease [clinically uninvolved (elective) cervical lymph nodes]. Hence, radiation treatment planning requires a thorough understanding of the risk of microscopic lymph node involvement and the pattern of nodal failure. These variables depend on the site of the primary tumor and the disease stage at presentation. Knowledge of routes of subclinical spread at the primary site is also important.

Brachytherapy

Brachytherapy describes the situation in which radioactive sources are brought close to the tumor mass (or even implanted within it) to deliver a highly localized radiation dose. Brachytherapy approaches that are used in patients with HNSCC include (1) interstitial brachytherapy: in which radioactive sources are inserted directly in to tumor-bearing tissues (e.g., the tongue); (2) intraluminal brachytherapy: in which the radioactive source is placed within a hollow viscus (e.g., the nasopharynx); and (3) surface molds: in which the radioactive source is placed close to disease on the skin surface or lip.

Interstitial brachytherapy can yield excellent disease control and functional results in patients with tongue and floor-of-mouth tumors (Fig. 4.3). This form of treatment is particularly appropriate for thin tumors (<5 mm) in which the rates of neck relapse are <30% (10). Ten-year local control rates were reported by Yamazaki et al (1997) (11). For patients treated with either ^{226}Ra or ^{192}Ir, they obtained 10-year control rates of 79% and 83% for T1 disease and 61% and 68% for T2 disease, respectively. Interstitial brachytherapy has also been used in patients with positive local excision margins after surgery, with a 2-year local control rate of 89% (12). Intraluminal brachytherapy can be used in patients with nasopharyngeal disease—either as a tumor boost after external beam radiotherapy or as definitive treatment for relapsed disease (13).

Conventional Radiation Therapy

In recent years, the technology underlying the planning and delivery of RT has undergone something of a revolution. Historically, so-called conventional RT involved treatment planning by fluoroscopic X-ray screening and treatment delivery by one to four regular square or rectangular fields (Fig. 4.4). Blocks of lead (or of a dense alloy called Cerrobend) were positioned by hand such that they shielded parts of the radiation field encompassing normal structures. The advantage of this technique is that it is well established with known patterns of response, local control, and toxicity. However, in the head and neck region, the main disadvantage is that conventional radiation delivery offers little information on the precise doses received by normal tissues and this limits the scope for tumor dose escalation. New techniques, such as three-dimensional conformal RT (3-DCRT) and intensity-modulated radiotherapy (IMRT), have significantly changed the landscape for radiation delivery in the head and neck region and provide very real opportunities for tumor dose escalation and normal tissue sparing.

Three-Dimensional Conformal Treatment Planning

The wide availability of computed tomography (CT) scanning technology has driven the development of 3-DCRT. In this planning technique a CT scan is taken with the patient immobilized in the RT treatment position. Data from these scans provide the radiation oncologist with precise anatomical and electron density data on tumor and normal tissues. As a result, on a slice-by-slice basis, the macroscopic tumor [gross tumor volume (GTV)], the areas of probable subclinical spread [the clinical target volume (CTV)] and the margin (3–5mm) that needs to be added around the CTV to ensure accurate coverage on a day-to-day basis [the planning target volume (PTV)] can be outlined on the CT images.

The GTV should always be defined for the primary tumor and any involved nodes with the aid of the diagnostic scans, operation notes, clinical examination, and nasendoscopic assessment. It is recognized that a planning CT scan with intravenous contrast will allow better definition of this volume. The radical dose CTV (CTV1) should encompass the GTV and those areas at high risk of spread that are to be treated to a radical dose. It is obtained by adding a customised margin to the GTV. Where no obvious anatomical barrier exists, a minimum 1-cm margin should be added to the GTV. In general, barriers to tumor spread, such as bone and fasciae, can be excluded, provided they are not breached. Air is not part of the CTV1; however, the growing algorithms of some treatment planning systems are such that incorporating the air within an organ is unavoidable. Any neighboring structures involved by tumor should be included. All involved nodal levels should be included in the CTV1. Consensus guidelines on nodal outlining in the postoperative neck should be followed (14). Because of the risk of extracapsular spread, a margin around the nodal GTV of at least 1 cm should be added. This can be customized around any intact anatomical barriers (bone, fasciae, etc.) and should include any involved structures (i.e., muscle, soft tissues, bone). In a postoperative setting, CTV1 should include the preoperative GTV and surgical bed of the primary tumor and/or involved nodes with a customized

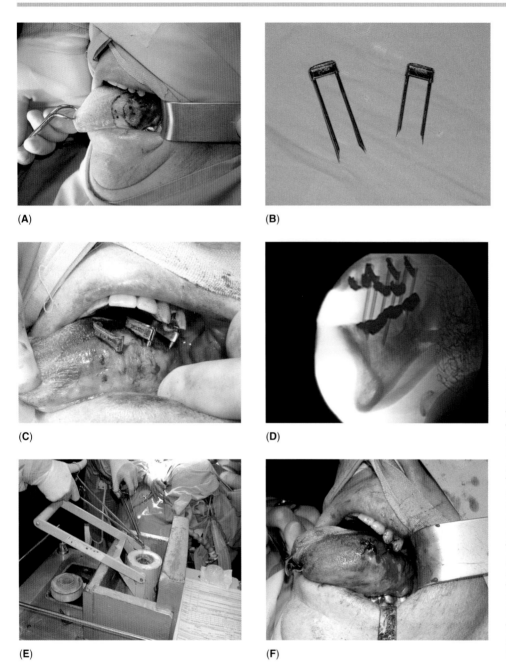

Figure 4.3 Brachytherapy for a T1 N0 carcinoma of the mobile tongue. (A) Under general anesthesia the tumor is identified and demarcated with a surrounding margin of 1 cm. (B) Rigid gutter guides of variable lengths are available. (C) The gutter guides are inserted into the area of the implant with the aim of achieving equal spacing (approx 1 cm) and a parallel distribution. (D) While the patient is still anesthetised, intraoperative fluoroscopy is used to check that the distribution of the gutter guides is acceptable (equal, parallel spacing). (E) ^{192}Ir hairpins are removed from their lead containment (using long-handled forceps) and inserted into the gutter guides. (F) Final view with hairpins sutured in place and gutter guides removed. *Abbreviation*: N0.

margin. This volume should be edited to include the entire organ where the tumor arose but to respect anatomical barriers that have not been breached (bone, fasciae, etc.). Where there is no anatomical barrier a 1-cm margin should be added. The nodal surgical bed should be included in the CTV1 if pathologically positive. For the elective CTV (CTV2), the Danish Head and Neck Cancer Study (DAHANCA), European Organisation for Research and Treatment of Cancer (EORTC), Groupe Oncologie Radiotherapie Tete Et Cou (GORTEC), National Cancer Institute of Canada (NCIC), Radiation Therapy Oncology Group (RTOG) consensus guidelines (15) are followed for target volume definition of the node-negative neck for levels I–V. In addition, a supraclavicular fossa nodal volume is defined. This level is in continuity with levels IV and V and encompasses the

fatty planes and blood vessels at the root of the neck at the level of or just below the clavicles.

The critical normal tissue structures [the organs at risk (OAR)] can also be outlined on each slice of the CT scan (Fig. 4.5). RT treatment planning computers are then used to design the optimal arrangement of radiation beams to cover the PTV and to spare the OARs. A number of different plans may be produced to allow the radiation oncologist to select the most appropriate one—usually on the basis of greatest homogeneity of coverage of the PTV for the lowest dose delivery to the most important OAR(s). For 3-DCRT shielding can be introduced using devices called multileaf collimators (MLC) consisting of multiple leaves or fingers that project into the primary beam to create any defined aperture shape to conform to the target volume.

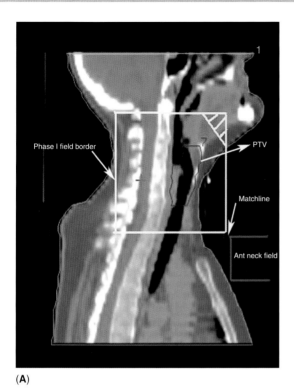
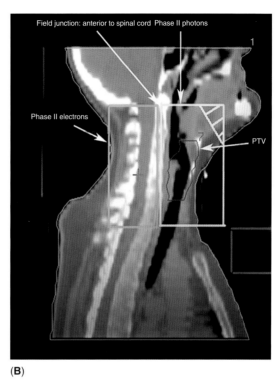

(A)   **(B)**

Figure 4.4 Two-dimensional conventional radiotherapy for a T3N0 squamous cell cancer of the supraglottic larynx. **(A)** Phase I treatment consists of two large opposed lateral photon beams (the radiograph shows the view from the right-sided beam). The PTV represents the primary tumor in the supraglottic larynx plus a margin (to include microscopic extension and technical set-up). The photon field (yellow box with hatched area representing lead shielding) encompasses the PTV and the locoregional lymph nodes that will receive elective radiotherapy. An anterior field (red line) is matched to the lateral fields to treat the low neck nodes. Note that the spinal cord receives the full radiation dose using this technique and so at about 40 Gy it is necessary to change the RT field arrangement. **(B)** Phase II field arrangement involves moving the posterior edge of the Phase I photon field forward so that it is anterior to the spinal cord. The area overlying and posterior to the spinal cord is treated using electron fields (green box) which penetrate a limited depth into tissues and do not reach the spinal cord. *Abbreviations*: N0; PTV, planning target volume.

This technique is more time-consuming than conventional RT and requires specialist technical support, but it offers the opportunity of achieving clinically important improvements in tumor control probability and reductions in normal tissue complication probability.

Intensity Modulated Radiotherapy

This is an advanced approach to three-dimensional treatment planning and conformal therapy. It optimizes the delivery of irradiation to irregularly shaped volumes and has the ability to treat concave volumes. IMRT uses sophisticated computer software and hardware to vary the shape and intensity of radiation delivered to different parts of the treatment volume. In IMRT, the physician designates specific doses of radiation (constraints) that the tumor and normal surrounding tissues should receive. The RT planning computer program then generates an individualized plan to meet these constraints. This process is called "inverse treatment planning" because the planning process starts with an ideal or target dose distribution, and through repeated trials the best approximation to this ideal is achieved. To deliver IMRT requires linear accelerators equipped with computer-controlled dynamic MLC. They use multiple movable "leaves" to conform the radiation beam to the shape

of the tumor from any angle and to shield adjacent normal structures. Dynamic MLCs allow the doses of radiation to vary within a single beam such that higher doses are delivered in some areas and lower doses in other areas (Fig. 4.6).

In the head and neck region IMRT has a number of potential advantages: (1) it allows for greater sparing of normal structures such as salivary glands, esophagus, optic nerves, brain stem, and spinal cord (16,17); (2) it allows treatment to be delivered in a single-treatment phase without the requirement for matching additional fields to provide tumor boosts and eliminates the need for electron fields to the posterior (level II, V) neck nodes (Fig. 4.4); (3) it offers the possibility of simultaneously delivering higher radiation doses to regions of gross disease and lower doses to areas of microscopic disease (the so-called simultaneous integrated boost) (18). These advantages permit the design of clinical studies aiming to escalate the doses of radiation delivered to tumor volumes. Reports on the effects of such approaches on rates of locoregional control are awaited with great interest.

As yet, no randomized trials comparing IMRT with conventional or 3-DCRT have been completed. The perceived advantage of this technique over standard RT techniques has resulted in wholesale adoption of this technique in the U.S.A. and in other countries and makes properly conducted

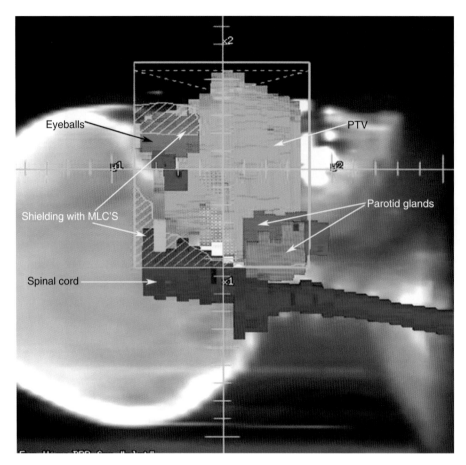

Figure 4.5 Three-dimensional conformal radiotherapy. This figure demonstrates the PTV (olive green) and a number of OARs (brain stem/spinal cord—red; right and left parotid glands—dark green and purple, respectively; right and left eyeballs—magenta and light blue, respectively; optic nerves—blue) superimposed on a digitally reconstructed radiograph. The green box represents a so-called beam's eye view of a lateral field for the treatment of a maxillary antral tumor. The PTV overlaps the parotid glands, which means that these structures can not be shielded. OARs such as the spinal cord and the eyeballs have been shielded from radiation using MLCs (hatched area in lime green) where they lie outside the PTV. *Abbreviations*: PTV, planning target volume; OARs, organs at risk; MLCs, multileaf collimators.

clinical trials virtually impossible. However, a recently completed Cancer Research UK-sponsored randomized trial of parotid-sparing IMRT versus 3-DCRT (PARSPORT) will report in 2009. A follow-on study of cochlear-sparing IMRT (COSTAR) is also open to recruitment.

Palliative Radiotherapy

RT can also be used with palliative intent in patients for whom a curative treatment option does not exist. Situations in which palliative RT may be useful include (1) as initial treatment for locally advanced tumors in patients with very poor performance status who will not be able to tolerate radical treatment; (2) for short-course treatment of local disease in patients with metastatic (M1) disease at the initial presentation; (3) for symptom relief (pain, bleeding, airway compromise) in patients with locally recurrent disease—this treatment may entail some retreatment of previously irradiated areas (reviewed in Ref. 19); (4) for symptom relief of distant metastatic disease (e.g., bone pain, spinal cord compression).

Palliative RT is usually delivered as a short course of treatment that can vary from a single fraction to 10 doses of RT over a 2-week period. A typical palliative radiation dose prescription would be 20 Gy in five fractions over 1 week. This treatment can be very effective in palliating pain, bleeding, and obstructive symptoms, but the effect is usually relatively short lived.

RADIATION-INDUCED SIDE EFFECTS

Any course of RT is associated with treatment-related adverse effects. Knowledge of the nature, extent, time course, and therapeutic interventions for these side effects is an essential part of the management of patients receiving RT. In particular, careful management of the acute side effects that occur during the course of treatment is vital to ensure that RT is not interrupted, because this can have deleterious effects on the likelihood of treatment success. The side effects of radiation are summarized in Table 4.1. The degree of radiation reaction can be influenced by treatment- and patient-related factors.

Treatment Factors

RT-induced toxicity is directly proportional to the total radiation dose delivered and the volume of tissue that is irradiated. In addition, the dose delivered per treatment fraction is important, especially for late reactions. It is this fact that underlies the use of protracted courses of small fractions of radiation over many weeks. Different types of radiation deposit their dose at different depths within tissue. Low energy (superficial) X-rays (50–200 KeV) and electrons deposit a higher proportion of their dose at the skin surface compared to high energy X- and γ-rays (1–10 MV). Therefore, skin toxicity is reduced when high energy X- and γ-rays are used. Patients with advanced HNSCC often receive

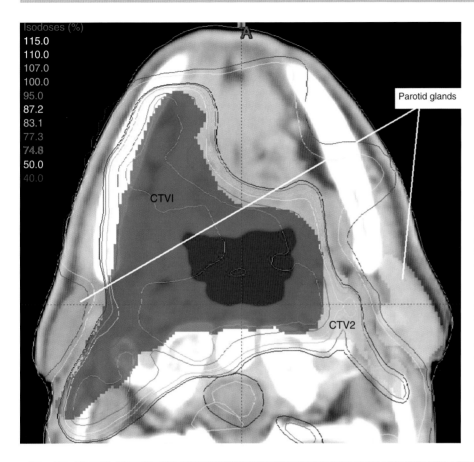

Figure 4.6 Intensity-modulated radiotherapy. This treatment technique permits the generation of concavities in the isodoses within tissues such that normal structures can be spared from excessive radiation doses. In this example, CTV1 defines an area that contains the gross tumor volume and involved lymph node disease whereas CTV2 contains clinically uninvolved nodal areas to be treated electively. The colored lines represent radiation isodoses (lines that join points of equal radiation dose) and clearly show that this technique permits a significant reduction in the dose delivered to the parotid tissue. This is in direct contrast to what would be achievable with conventional or three-dimensional conformal radiotherapy where a full radiation dose would be delivered to the parotid glands. *Abbreviations*: CTV1, Clinical target volume 1; CTV2, Clinical target volume 2.

Table 4.1 Early and Late Side Effects of Radiotherapy

Early	Late
Mucositis	Xerostomia
Desquamation	Osteoradionecrosis
Xerostomia	Fibrosis
Alopecia	Soft tissue necrosis
Loss of taste	Neurological damage
L'Hermitte's phenomenon	Second malignancy

concurrent chemotherapy and RT. This approach certainly increases acute reactions and may accentuate late reactions.

Patient Factors

Some rare genetic disorders relating to the repair of DNA damage cause increased radiation reactions (ataxia telangiectasia, Gardner's syndrome, Fanconi anaemia, xeroderma pigmentosum). Acquired disorders that can affect patients with HNSCC include conditions that affect tissue repair (e.g., poor nutritional status, high alcohol intake, smoking, and diabetes). Reduced levels of scavenger molecules (in such conditions as HIV/AIDS) may also increase reactions (20,21).

Acute Radiation Reactions

Mucositis and its Management

Mucositis occurs through death of stem cells in the basal layer of the nonkeratinized epithelium of the upper aerodigestive

tract. Because the stem cells renew the epithelium every 2 weeks or so, the acute reaction is not observed until the 3rd week of treatment when the lack of replacement epithelial cells becomes apparent. There are four recognized phases (Table 4.2) and grades (Table 4.3) for mucositis. There are no effective means of preventing the occurrence of RT-induced mucositis (22), although its extent and duration may be attenuated by therapeutic intervention. Hence, care is taken during the planning process to ensure maximal shielding of mucosa from radiation beams, without compromising tumor coverage. Once present there is no established treatment to accelerate the resolution of mucositis, although several measures are recommended to alleviate symptoms.

The main stay of therapy is the use of oral analgesics which are prescribed according to the World Health Organization (WHO) analgesic ladder—starting with nonopioid drugs, progressing to weak opioids, and finally using strong opioid medication. Although frequently prescribed, there is no convincing support for the use of mouthwashes (23,24). Normal saline and sodium bicarbonate are used, especially if there is extensive slough. Mouthwashes containing alcohol should be avoided as they may increase local inflammation and cause pain. Likewise, the patient is advised to avoid alcohol and smoking during treatment.

Cytoprotectants.
Sucralfate This agent forms ionic bonds to proteins within an ulcer and acts as a protective barrier. It may also aid healing by increasing local prostaglandin E_2 release (25).

Table 4.2   The Four Phases of Radiation-induced Mucositis

Phase1: The inflammatory phase
Cytokine release (mainly tumor necrosis factor-α, Interleukin-1,
    Interleukin-6) by the epithelium and surrounding connective tissue
    causes tissue damage.

Phase 2: The epithelial phase
Manifest by atrophy and ulceration as the damaged basal cell layer
    migrates to the surface and is exposed.

Phase 3: The ulcerative phase
Fibrinous pseudomembranes cover areas of ulceration. There is
    colonisation with gram-negative organisms with endotoxin and
    cytokine release, causing more damage to the epithelium.

Phase 4: The healing phase
The epithelium regenerates as the basal cell layer proliferates and the
    normal microflora is established.

Table 4.3   Grading of Mucositis

Grade 0: No change over baseline
Grade I: Hyperaemia
Grade II: Patchy mucositis
Grade III: Confluent mucositis
Grade IV: Ulceration, haemorrhage, necrosis

Analgesics. A large double blind, placebo-controlled trial of benzydamine reported decreased pain scores for patients on the active compound (26). Indomethacin given on the first day of treatment has also shown to decrease the severity and onset of mucositis (27).

Steroids. The role of corticosteroid mouthwashes is unclear. A few nonrandomized trials suggest they may be useful (28,29), but the risk of oral candidiasis that may accentuate mucositis must be considered.

Antimicrobials. Patients undergoing treatment may develop oropharyngeal candidal infections due to poor oral hygiene and reduced mucosal defense mechanisms. Candida is treated with nystatin mouthwash or oral fluconazole in cases of persistent infection. At present, there is no established prophylactic role for antifungal and antibacterial antimicrobials. Polymyxin E and tobramycin are active against gram-negative organisms that frequently colonize and promote mucositis by endotoxin release. There is evidence that selective depletion of gram-negative organisms by antibiotic lozenges can decrease mucositis (30).

Silver nitrate. This agent stimulates cell division in normal mucosa. There are conflicting data on its role in managing mucositis (31,32).

Xerostomia
The major salivary glands produce up to 90% of saliva. The position and size of the parotid gland means that it is frequently included in the radiation treatment field for HNSCC. The serous acini, which produce watery saliva, are more sensitive to the effects of RT than the mucous acini—resulting in the production of thick, tenacious saliva. The

decrease in the quantity and quality of saliva may lead to a change in oral flora and accelerated dental caries.

The free radical scavenger amifostine accumulates preferentially in salivary tissue. It has been shown to reduce acute and chronic xerostomia without adversely affecting the antitumor effects of RT. Amifostine is expensive and may cause nausea, vomiting, hypotension, and rarely allergic reactions (see below). More recently, there has been significant progress in the use of intensity-modulated RT as a means of sparing the parotid gland from receiving high radiation doses in patients with HNSCC. Otherwise, the management of xerostomia is palliative. Patients should sip water regularly or use artificial saliva. In severe cases, oral pilocarpine can improve symptoms (33), although unpleasant cholinergic side effects (visual, bowel, and bladder disturbance) are often limiting.

Altered Sense of Taste
Dysgeusia occurs due to RT-induced damage to the circumvallate and the fungiform papillae of the tongue. The taste buds mediating bitter/sour taste are affected more than those for sweet/salty taste. The extent of sensory disturbance is directly related to the volume of the tongue that is irradiated (34). Complete or partial recovery is usual but can be very slow and may take months to resolve. This symptom can be very distressing to the patient and is rather poorly understood.

Maintaining Nutrition
Mucositis, xerostomia, and dysgeusia all contribute to a decrease in oral intake. Many patients with HNSCC have a preexisting poor nutritional state. Management of this problem involves a multidisciplinary team including the oncologist, dietician, speech and language therapist (SALT), pain control team, and gastroenterologist. In some circumstances, a nasogastric (NG) or percutaneous endoscopic gastrostomy (PEG) tube is required to maintain nutrition while the acute reactions settle. The requirement for NG or PEG tubes is likely to increase with more widespread use of radical chemoradiotherapy. These tubes are certainly extremely important as part of the supportive care package in patients with locally advanced head and neck cancer. Rehabilitation of swallowing function often requires significant input from SALT, in terms of provision of exercises to improve oral and pharyngeal musculature and to assess the risk of aspiration using videofluoroscopy and functional endoscopic evaluation of the swallow.

Acute Skin Reactions
Normally, attempts are made to limit the acute radiation effects in the skin by using high energy X- or γ-rays that deposit their maximal dose 1–2 cm below the skin surface (the so-called skin-sparing or build-up effect). However, certain sites (e.g., back of pinna, skin over laryngeal promontory) are particularly prone to acute skin reactions because of loss of a normal skin-sparing effect. In addition, to immobilize patients and ensure day-to-day reproducibility during RT, a personalized perspex shell is used that has the effect of negating the skin-sparing effect and increasing the dose that is delivered to the skin. The perspex shell can

be cut out in areas that do not compromise the tumor dose to prevent skin soreness. Other types of radiation, such as electrons, are often used and deposit a higher percentage of their dose at the skin surface. Skin reactions can be graded as in Table 4.4 and are managed as shown in Table 4.5.

Alopecia

Alopecia occurs because the stem cells in the hair follicles are sensitive to RT. The pattern is confined within the boundaries of the radiation fields, but beam exit sites can also be affected. In treatment of HNSCC, alopecia is usually transient but it may be permanent in areas of high dose.

Neurological Side Effects

L'Hermitte's phenomenon is manifest by tingling in the arms and legs, especially when the neck is flexed. It is thought to be due to transient RT-induced demyelination and is self-limiting.

Late Radiation Reactions
Osteoradionecrosis

Osteoradionecrosis (ORN) occurs when bone cells are called upon to divide in response trauma (e.g., dental extraction) weeks, months, or even years after RT. The cells then express their DNA damage and fail to heal the wound, resulting in bone necrosis. ORN predominantly affects the mandible and maxilla (being 24 times more common in the former). The pathogenesis is one of hypocellularity, hypoxia, and hypovascularity. The incidence is related to the total dose received and the dose per fraction.

Prevention and management of ORN. To reduce the risk of ORN, patients are advised to have all preventative and restorative dental work carried out prior to RT. Good oral hygiene needs to be maintained during and after completion of RT. If dental work needs to be carried out, it must be performed by an experienced dental surgeon. Once present, ORN poses a difficult management problem. In most cases, healing will eventually take place with conservative

Table 4.4 Grading of Skin Reactions

Grade 0: No reaction
Grade I: Faint erythema
Grade II: Moderate/brisk erythema, dry desquamation
Grade III: Moist desquamation
Grade IV: Skin necrosis, full thickness ulceration

Table 4.5 Management of Acute Skin Reactions

Avoid irritants: strong soaps, sunlight
Avoid local trauma: nonabrasive towels, loose-fitting clothing
Dry desquamation
    Keep skin moisturized – aqueous cream
    1% hydrocortisone cream
Moist desquamation
    Proflavine
    Geliperm dressings
    Treat secondary infections

measures (good hygiene, adequate nutrition, and prolonged courses of antibiotics), although this can be extremely slow. Debridement of bony sequestra is sometimes required. In these situations, there has been discussion about the possible role of adjuvant hyperbaric oxygen, although there are no strong data to support its use.

Soft Tissue Fibrosis and Necrosis

Fibrosis of soft tissue is a common problem after RT for HNSCC. The tissue becomes progressively thicker and woody hard, limiting movement and causing disfigurement. There may be a role for the use of oxypentifylline that has been used to treat fibrosis at other sites. Necrosis manifests as an ulcer that fails to heal or as persisting inflammation in nonviable soft tissue. Necrosis of the laryngeal cartilages (chondronecrosis) is a particular example that represents a management dilemma. It is sometimes difficult to distinguish clinically from recurrent disease, and biopsies may be necessary. The management is conservative, keeping the area clean to prevent secondary infection. On occasions, persisting necrosis in laryngeal cartilages may necessitate laryngectomy, even in the absence of recurrent disease.

Second Malignancy

As well as treating cancer, radiation may cause second malignancies. The most common types of second malignancies are skin cancers and sarcomas. The increased risk is estimated at approximately 1–1.5% per decade.

Late Radiation-Induced Neuropathy

The tolerance of peripheral nerves for RT is higher than for the central nervous system, and acute side effects are not commonly seen. Late-onset neuropathies are caused by a combination of demyelination, fibrosis, and vascular degeneration.

OPTIMIZATION OF IMAGING FOR RADIOTHERAPY TREATMENT PLANNING

A significant cause of failure of RT to control head and neck cancer is inadequate coverage of disease by the radiation fields, a so-called geographical miss. This may happen with suboptimal staging and delineation of the extent of disease prior to treatment planning. In an attempt to improve outcomes, new anatomical and functional imaging techniques are now being assessed for integration in the radiotherapy planning process.

Cross-Sectional Imaging

Conventionally, staging of head and neck cancer has been done with anatomical imaging such as CT and magnetic resonance imaging (MRI), which give excellent morphological information. RT treatment planning is conventionally carried out using contrast enhanced CT that provides not only anatomical information but also electron density data that facilitate calculation of radiation doses in tissues. Coregistration of MRI with planning CT scans may increase the accuracy of target volume definition in some tumor types. This co-registration of anatomical imaging modalities provides superior definition of OARs. The improved certainty of the location of an OAR potentially reduces the need to compromise coverage of the target volume to a radical dose (35,36).

Functional Imaging

Imaging modalities based only on anatomy cannot provide information on disease activity if the morphology is distorted. In this respect, MRI and CT have limitations in head and neck cancer where surgery and reconstruction may alter the normal anatomy and make interpretation difficult. Functional imaging, defined as the radiological characterization of tissues in terms of their underlying biochemical pathways or physiology, has recently become more available in clinical practice. Such imaging includes the following modalities; positron emission tomography (PET), single photon emission computed tomography, magnetic resonance spectroscopy, and dynamic contrast-enhanced MRI and CT. Functional imaging may improve staging of disease by detecting subclinical (occult) carcinoma or by providing the radiation oncologist with increased information about the margins and extent of disease. As such, functional imaging may highlight the presence of disease in areas that appear structurally normal by conventional anatomical imaging. Furthermore, it can provide information on tumor characteristics such as blood flow, vascular permeability, proliferation rate, and oxygenation. Therefore, the introduction of functional imaging has a twofold benefit for RT planning in head and neck cancer. First, it may reduce the chance of a geographical miss and, second, it may delineate a biological target volume, that is, a region defined by a biochemical pathway or physiology (37).

¹⁸FDG-PET

¹⁸F-Fluoro-2-deoxy-D-glucose (¹⁸FDG) has become the most widely used tracer for PET. PET alone has been of limited value in RT planning because it only has a spatial resolution is 4–7mm and the scans lack anatomical landmarks. Integrated PET/CT scanners produce hardware fused images (Fig. 4.7) and increase accuracy compared to PET alone in head and neck cancer, 96% versus 90% in a study by Schoder et al. (38). Other studies suggest that the addition of PET/CT to treatment planning in head and neck cancer may reduce the probability of a geographical miss. Other PET tracers are being investigated and could provide information about the biology of tumors, such as proliferation rates, protein synthesis, and hypoxia (39–41).

Dynamic Contrast Enhanced Imaging

The use of dynamic contrast enhanced (DCE) or perfusion imaging has the benefit that it is a technique that can be carried out on equipment such as CT and MRI scanners already available in clinical practice. These imaging techniques permit the investigation of tumor perfusion by obtaining rapid sequences of images following the injection of a bolus of contrast agent. Contrast enhancement-time curves are produced, and these data are computed to provide parameter maps that give spatial information about perfusion and vascularity (Fig. 4.8). DCE MRI parameters have been correlated with clinical outcome following RT in head

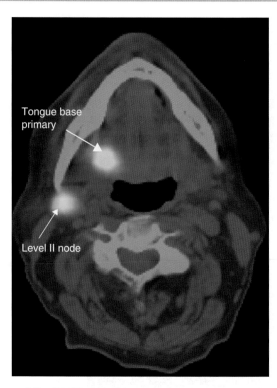

Figure 4.7 PET-CT image of a patient who presented with a right level-II neck node but no obvious primary tumor site at examination under anesthesia or standard imaging (CT and MRI). The PET-CT scan identified the primary tumor site in the right tongue base and led to a significant alteration in radiotherapy planning. *Abbreviations*: PET, positron emission tomography; CT, computed tomography; MRI, magnetic resonance imaging.

and neck cancer (42). Hermans et al. (43) found correlations between CT perfusion parameters and local control in head and neck cancer treated with radical RT.

RADIATION DOSES AND TREATMENT DELIVERY

A conventional course of RT for HNSCC is delivered over a 6–7-week course with small fractions of radiotherapy delivered 5 days a week (Monday to Friday). A standard schedule in the U.K. is 70 Gray (Gy) delivered in 35 fractions over 7 weeks. RT is delivered in multiple small fractions to allow recovery of normal tissues between doses and thus facilitate the delivery of a larger total radiation dose to the tumor. During a course of RT, tumor cells are able to repair some of the RT-induced DNA damage and continue to divide. As a result, there is an apparent repopulation of tumor cells during RT. Although this is thought to occur at a constant rate in the first few weeks of treatment, it has been suggested that after the 4th week of RT this repopulation accelerates (44,45). This is the fundamental reason for avoiding unscheduled breaks because any prolongation of the treatment course increases the total number of cancer cells to be treated. An understanding of this phenomenon is key to an appreciation of the

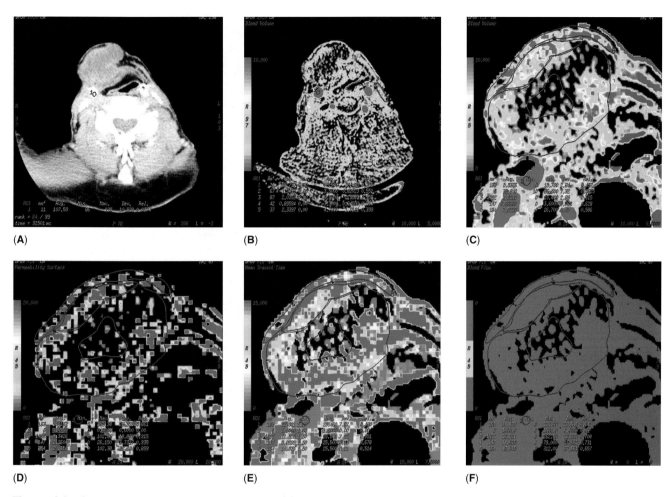

(A) **(B)** **(C)**

(D) **(E)** **(F)**

Figure 4.8   Contrast-enhanced imaging with derivation of functional parameters. (A) Baseline CT scan, (B) Perfusion map, (C) Blood volume (D) Permeability, (E) Mean transit time, and (F) Blood flow. By taking a sequence of rapid images shortly after administration of a bolus dose of intravenous contrast, detailed data can be obtained on such parameters as blood volume, blood flow, perfusion, and permeability. These data can be used in radiotherapy treatment planning to improve the therapeutic effect.

issues surrounding the selection of an optimal fractionation schedule (Fig. 4.9) (46).

Hyperfractionated Radiotherapy

Tissues that exhibit toxicity from RT many months or years following treatment, such as the spinal cord, are particularly sensitive to the radiation dose per fraction as well as the total radiation dose. For this reason, a reduction in dose per fraction to 1.1–1.2 Gy allows a larger total dose to be administered with the twin goals of better tumor control and reduced late toxicity. When more than one fraction of radiation is given per day at this lower dose, it is known as hyperfractionation. Treatment can be given in the same overall time to a larger total dose than conventional irradiation or in a shorter time to the same total dose as conventional RT (see section on accelerated radiotherapy below). In the EORTC 22791 trial, 356 patients with HNSCC were randomized to receive conventional treatment or 80.5 Gy given in twice-daily fractions of 1.15 Gy per fraction over 7 weeks. Hyperfractionation resulted in an increase in tumor control from 46% to 59% at 5 years with no increase in late normal tissue toxicity (47).

Accelerated Radiotherapy

Accelerated RT schedules have been designed to try to reduce the total treatment duration. This can be achieved in two ways: (1) more than one fraction of RT is given on each day or (2) RT must be given more than 5 days a week. If more than one fraction of RT is given in a day, the doses must be at least 4–6 hours apart to allow time for completion of DNA damage repair in normal tissues. Doses of 1.8–2.0 Gy per fraction are generally used—as in conventional fractionation.

In the EORTC 22851 trial, 512 patients were randomized to receive conventional treatment (70 Gy in 35 fractions over 7 weeks, 1 fraction per day, 5 days a week) or an accelerated spilt-course regimen of 70 Gy in 45 fractions over 5 weeks. The first course delivered 28.8 Gy in 18 fractions over 8 days (3 fractions of 1.6 Gy per fraction were delivered each day, 5 days a week, with a minimum gap of 4 hours between fractions). This was followed by a 12–14 day break, then the second course of treatment that comprised 43.2 Gy in 27 fractions over 17 days. Conventional treatment was delivered over a median of 54 days and the accelerated course treatment over a median of 33 days. Patients who received accelerated treatment showed a

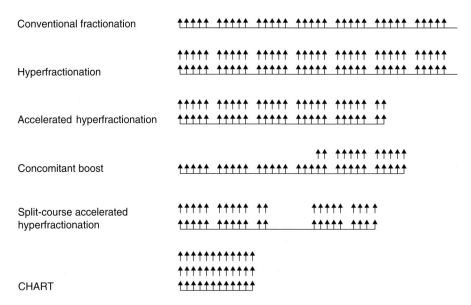

Figure 4.9 Radiation dose-fractionation schedules. Each radiation fraction is represented by an arrow. Conventional fractionation consists of 7 weeks of treatment every weekday (Monday–Friday). Hyperfractionation (without acceleration) consists of 7 weeks of treatment delivered twice a day (b.d) for 5 days a week. Accelerated hyperfractionation involves radiation delivery b.d over a shorter time scale than a conventional treatment course. In the case illustrated, treatment is delivered over 5½ weeks. Concomitant boost radiotherapy refers to the delivery of hyperfractionated treatment b.d for the last 2½ weeks. Split course hyperfractionation consists of b.d irradiation for 2½ weeks followed by a 2-week gap and then further b.d fractionated treatment over 2 weeks. CHART comprises treatment thrice daily with no breaks at the weekend. In this regimen treatment is completed in a single uninterrupted sequence of 12 days. *Abbreviation*: CHART, continuous hyperfractionated accelerated radiotherapy.

13% increase in locoregional control from 46% to 59% at 5 years. There was no increase in overall or disease-specific survival compared with conventional treatment, although a trend for disease-specific survival was noted for accelerated fractionation in longer-term survival [hazard ratio (HR) 0.78, 95% Confidence Interval 0.60–1.01, $p = 0.06$]. The incidence of early and late radiation toxicity was significantly increased in the accelerated RT group (48).

Continuous Hyperfractionated Accelerated Radiotherapy (CHART)

The continuous hyperfractionated accelerated radiotherapy (CHART) regimen was designed to test the ultimate expression of treatment acceleration through hyperfractionation. In a large randomized phase III trial, conventional RT was compared with an accelerated and hyperfractionated schedule that involved a reduction in the total dose to remain within the tolerance of acutely responding normal tissues. Nine hundred and eighteen patients with HNSCC were randomized to receive either conventional RT or the trial arm consisting of three fractions of 1.5 Gy per day on 12 consecutive days (including one weekend) to a total dose of 54 Gy. Locoregional control and overall survival rates were identical in both arms. Acute and late toxicity rates were slightly reduced in patients receiving the CHART schedule. This regimen was attractive to patients and clinicians in that it permitted a complete course of treatment to be delivered in a very short period of time. However, the need to deliver three fractions of RT a day (including the weekends) represented a significant logistical and financial burden to RT departments in the U.K. and the lack of a local control or

survival advantage meant that this regimen was not widely adopted (49).

Meta-Analysis of Altered Fractionation Regimens

Recently a meta-analysis of hyperfractionated or accelerated RT as radical treatment in HNSCC has been performed (Table 4.6). This study compared trials which randomized patients between conventional RT (66–70 Gy in 2-Gy fractions for 5 days a week) and hyperfractionated or accelerated (or both) schedules. The results showed that there was a significant survival benefit with the so-called altered fractionation that corresponded to an absolute benefit of 3.4% at 5 years. This benefit was particularly pronounced for hyperfractionated RT with an 8% benefit at 5 years (50). The benefit gained by altered fractionation is of a similar magnitude to that gained by using chemotherapy in addition to RT. The overall benefit of combining chemotherapy with RT is 5% at 5 years with an absolute benefit of 8% at 5 years for the use of chemotherapy concomitant with RT (2). Significant benefits were seen for altered fractionation in terms of overall survival and locoregional control, but not in distant metastases. It should be noted that the meta-analysis was unable to reach conclusions on rates of normal tissue toxicity due to variations in recording and reporting between trials. Future trials will have to address this issue in detail.

Despite the proven benefit of altered fractionation regimens, they have not been widely adopted in routine clinical practice in the U.K. One reason for this is that most RT departments in the U.K. are not staffed to offer treatment out of standard working hours and delivering more

Table 4.6 Summary of Data from Meta-analysis of Altered Fractionation Regimens

Fractionation schedule	Number of trials	Number of patients		HR of local control (95% CI), altered fractionated versus control RT	HR of death (95% CI), altered fractionated versus control RT	Absolute benefit at 5 years (SE)
		Altered fractionation	Control			
Hyperfractionation	4	470	507	0.75 (0.63–0.89)	0.78 (0.69–0.89)	8.2% (2.6%)
Accelerated fractionation without total dose reduction	8	1130	1128	0.74 (0.67–0.83)	0.97 (0.89–1.05)	2.0% (1.7%)
Accelerated fractionation with total dose reduction	5	713	600	0.83 (0.71–0.96)	0.94 (0.84–1.05)	1.7% (2.3%)
Total	15	2313	2235	0.77 (0.71–0.83)	0.92 (0.86–0.97)	3.4% (1.2%)

Note: A hazard ratio <1.0 with 95% confidence intervals that do not cross 1.0 is indicative of an advantage in favor of the altered fractionation regimen.
Abbreviations: HR, hazard ratio; 95% CI, 95% confidence intervals; SE, standard error.

than one fraction per day also has cost implications. In addition, all the trials analysed in the meta-analysis used RT alone—an approach that has been eclipsed by the adoption of chemoradiotherapy as the new standard of care. The next challenge is to assess the potential for developing new regimens that incorporate altered fractionation regimens and radiosensitizing chemotherapeutic agents. The necessary phase III trials are already in progress.

HYPOXIA MODIFICATION AS A MEANS OF TARGETING HNSCC

In the laboratory, the response of cells to radiation is highly dependent on the amount of oxygen they contain at the time of irradiation. This is due to the fact that the damage which occurs to DNA as a result of radiation becomes "fixed" by oxygen. This is borne out by clinical data which show good correlation between treatment outcome and pretreatment pO_2 measurements with less well oxygenated tumors showing the worst results. It has also been shown that a low pretreatment hemoglobin level is associated with poorer locoregional control rates after RT, although this observation may, at least in part, be related to the fact that patients with low hemoglobin levels may have biologically more aggressive disease (51–54). These observations have led to a number of different therapeutic interventions to optimize the oxygenation of tumors and, hence, increase radiosensitivity.

Modification of Hemoglobin Level

Hemoglobin concentration is an important prognostic factor for response to RT in head and neck cancer. Trials evaluating the effects of blood transfusion during treatment to maintain hemoglobin levels above a certain threshold have not shown a great benefit, although it is still considered standard practice in many centers to monitor levels weekly during RT and to transfuse to maintain a haemoglobin level above 12g/dl. The use of erythropoietin (EPO) is another method that has been used to maintain haemoglobin levels during treatment. In a large randomized trial, 351 patients with head and neck cancer were randomized to receive epoetin-β or placebo during a course of radical RT. There was a statistically significant difference in locoregional control and survival between the two groups; but, surprisingly,

this was in favor of the placebo group (55). One possible explanation of this finding is that head and neck cancer cells may express EPO receptors that may stimulate anti-apoptotic intracellular signalling pathways and, hence, increase cell survival during a course of RT. Another large randomized trial of EPO-α has been completed; however, as yet, the results are not available. At present, the use of EPO during radical RT or radical chemoradiotherapy for head and neck cancer cannot be recommended.

Hypoxic Cell Radiosensitizers

Chemical radiosensitization of hypoxic cells is possible using compounds that mimic the biological effects of oxygen. These agents act by diffusing within the tumor from blood vessels to areas that contain hypoxic cells. Unlike oxygen, these agents are not metabolized before reaching the hypoxic cells. Their radiosensitization effect has been shown to be directly related to the electron affinity of the compounds. The first compounds selected that had good efficacy in vitro and in animal models were the nitroimidazoles. Results in clinical trials were disappointing due to the occurrence of dose-limiting neurotoxicity, such that doses shown to be effective in laboratory studies could not be used in humans. A less toxic drug nimorazole was developed in Denmark and was shown that this could be given at a clinically relevant dose alongside conventional fractionated RT. In the DAHANCA-5 trial, 422 patients with pharyngeal or supraglottic laryngeal cancers were randomized to receive nimorazole or placebo 90 minutes prior to RT. The results showed a highly significant benefit in terms of improved locoregional tumor control (49% vs. 33% at 5 years) and disease-specific survival (52% vs. 41% at 5 years) in favor of those treated with nimorazole (56). Despite these impressive benefits nimorazole is currently not used as a standard treatment outside Denmark due to logistical constraints.

Alteration of Inspired Oxygen Content

Other strategies to modify tumor hypoxia and, hence, improve radiosensitivity have included raising the oxygen content of the inspired gas during RT—either through breathing oxygen in hyperbaric conditions or through high-oxygen-gas breathing. A recent Cochrane database review of the effect of hyperbaric oxygen (HBO) therapy on tumor sensitization to RT has shown a reduced mortality for head and neck cancers (relative risk 0.82, $p = 0.03$) and an improvement in local tumor control. However, the trials concerned used unusual hypofractionated regimens (a small number of relatively large fractions) due to the practical constraints of delivering HBO during RT. The benefit of HBO therapy was at the cost of significant adverse effects including oxygen-toxic seizures and severe radiation tissue injury that, in conjunction with the impracticalities, has severely limited its use (57).

Accelerated radiotherapy with carbogen and nicotinamide (ARCON) is a treatment strategy that aims to combat accelerated repopulation and hypoxia. Accelerated RT is combined with inhalation of hyperoxic gas (carbogen, 95% oxygen + 5% carbon dioxide) and the vaso-active drug nicotinamide that decreases perfusion-limited hypoxia. Phase II trials have shown good locoregional control rates in all head and neck sites (except the oral cavity) (58). Phase III trials of ARCON are now under way.

Bioreductive Drugs

An alternative approach to tumor hypoxia aims to exploit, rather than overcome, tumor hypoxia using drugs that are preferentially cytotoxic to hypoxic cells (so-called bioreductive agents). Tirapazamine is a prodrug (i.e., an inactive agent that is metabolized to an active form) that is reduced in conditions of hypoxia to its active free radical moiety that produces DNA strand breaks. In normoxic conditions, such as those found in normal tissues, it remains in its inactive form. The greatest clinical efficacy for tirapazamine has been seen in lung cancer patients. A randomized phase II trial in patients with advanced HNSCC has shown a trend for better locoregional control and failure-free survival in patients who received tirapazamine (59). Based on the promising results of this trial, a large international phase III trial [Head and Neck Cancer Study of Tirapazamine, Cisplatin and Radiation Therapy (HEADSTART)] is in progress. This study is comparing the tirapazamine regimen (70 Gy conventionally fractionated radiation, tirapazamine and cisplatin) to a control arm of radiation (70 Gy conventionally fractionated) and cisplatin.

Meta-Analysis of Hypoxia Modification Trials

A meta-analysis of hypoxia modification in head and neck cancers has been reported. Data in this report were compiled by combining 27 trials in 4250 patients. This meta-analysis demonstrated a 7% benefit in terms of locoregional control for patients who were treated with a regimen that involved hypoxia modification plus radiation compared with RT alone (46% vs. 39%). This finding translates to an odds ratio of 1.35 (95% confidence intervals 1.20–1.53) in favor of hypoxia modification (60).

ANTIEPIDERMAL GROWTH FACTOR RECEPTOR TARGETED THERAPY

Epidermal growth factor receptor (EGFR) is overexpressed in 90% of HNSCC and is known to promote tumor cell growth, invasion, evasion of apoptosis (programmed cell death) in response to RT and/or chemotherapy, and the development of new blood vessels (angiogenesis). EGFR signalling also plays a role in repair of DNA damage. Anti-EGFR therapy has been shown to be a rational strategy for combination therapy with radiation in preclinical and early stage clinical trials. More recently a large randomized phase III trial in patients with stage III/IV HNSCC confirmed the potential of this approach. Patients received primary radical RT with or without concomitant cetuximab (an inhibitory monoclonal antibody against EGFR). Patients in the cetuximab treatment arm had a statistically significant increase in median overall survival (49 vs. 29.3 months, $p = 0.03$). In addition, the median duration of locoregional control was significantly improved in the cetuximab arm (24.4 vs. 14.9 months, $p = 0.005$) (61). These data are extremely encouraging; however, unfortunately, at the time that the trial was set up concomitant chemoradiotherapy was not the standard of care. A further follow-on phase III study is examining the role of cetuximab in combination with concomitant chemoradiotherapy and these results are awaited with interest. Other EGFR-targeted agents are also being evaluated. These include the small-molecule tyrosine kinase inhibitors gefitinib (Iressa) and lapatinib (Tykerb).

As yet, these drugs can not be considered to be part of the standard of care, and their use should be restricted to clinical trials or to patients in whom concomitant chemoradiotherapy is contra-indicated (elderly patients, poor renal function, poor performance status).

RADIOPROTECTORS IN HEAD AND NECK CANCER

An alternative approach to enhancing the therapeutic index of RT is to protect normal tissues form the deleterious effects of radiation. The concern about the use of such agents is the danger that they may also protect tumor cells from radiation-induced damage.

Sulphydryl-Containing Agents

This group of drugs act as free-radical scavengers and tend to make cells more resistant to the effects of radiation. The clinical development of these agents can be traced back to the 1950s, and attempts by the military to design agents that would allow soldiers to withstand the effects of radiation doses received during a nuclear conflict. Amifostine (WR-2721) is the best studied drug of this group. In randomized controlled clinical trials it has been shown to reduce treatment-related xerostomia and cisplatin-induced nephrotoxicity (62,63). However, this agent is also associated with significant toxicity (largely in the form of nausea and hypotension) and is expensive—both considerations that have limited its use in U.K. (64). Concern has also been expressed about the fact that the randomized trials lacked the necessary statistical power to detect a protective effect on the tumor (65). Until such concerns have been addressed it is unlikely that this drug will find a place in routine practice in the U.K.

Human Keratinocyte Growth Factor (huKGF)

Human keratinocyte growth factor (huKGF) is a specific growth factor that has the potential to accelerate cell division in keratinocytes and squamous cell precursors. A large randomized trial of huKGF in 212 patients receiving intensive therapy for hematological malignancies has confirmed the ability of this agent to reduce the maximum grade and overall duration of oral mucositis (66). This agent is currently undergoing evaluation in a randomized trial in patients receiving concomitant chemoradiotherapy for HNSCC. The obvious concern in this approach is the possibility that huKGF will also act as a growth factor for the malignant squamous cell population. The results of the trial will be awaited with interest.

CONCLUSION

In this chapter we discussed the avenues of research into optimization of RT delivery as a means of improving the outcome of patients treated for head and neck cancer. In particular, we have focused on the specific issues of the technique of radiation delivery, the role of advanced imaging modalities in treatment planning, and the selection of the optimal fractionation schedule. In addition, we discussed ways in which agents other than cytotoxic chemotherapy drugs may interact with radiation and enhance (oxygen, hypoxic cell sensitizers, bioreductive drugs, growth factor inhibitors) its effect in tumor tissues or reduce (amifostine, huKGF) its effect in normal tissues.

REFERENCES

1. Mendenhall WM, Amdur RJ, Morris CG et al. T1-T2N0 squamous cell carcinoma of the glottic larynx treated with radiation therapy. J Clin Oncol 2001; 19: 4029–36.
2. Bourhis J AC, Pignon JP. Update of MACH-NC (Meta-analysis of chemotherapy in head and neck cancer) database focussed on concomitant chemotherapy. J Clin Oncol 2004; 22(14S): 5505.
3. Pignon JP, Bourhis J, Domenge C et al. Chemotherapy added to locoregional treatment for head and neck squamous-cell carcinoma: three meta-analyses of updated individual data. MACH-NC Collaborative Group. Meta-Analysis of Chemotherapy on Head and Neck Cancer. Lancet 2000; 355: 949–55.
4. Bernier J, Cooper JS, Pajak TF et al. Defining risk levels in locally advanced head and neck cancers: a comparative analysis of concurrent postoperative radiation plus chemotherapy trials of the EORTC (#22931) and RTOG (#9501). Head Neck 2005; 27: 843–50.
5. Bentzen SM. Dose-response relationships in radiotherapy. In: Gordon Steel, ed. Basic Clinical Radiobiology, 3rd ed. London: Arnold, 2002: 94–104.
6. Steel GG, McMillan TJ, Peacock JH. The 5Rs of radiobiology. Int J Radiat Biol 1989; 56: 1045–8.
7. Salama JK, Seiwert TY, Vokes EE. Chemoradiotherapy for locally advanced head and neck cancer. J Clin Oncol 2007; 25: 4118–26.
8. Seiwert TY, Salama JK, Vokes EE. The chemoradiation paradigm in head and neck cancer. Nat Clin Pract Oncol 2007; 4: 156–71.
9. Ang KK, Trotti A, Brown BW et al. Randomized trial addressing risk features and time factors of surgery plus radiotherapy in advanced head-and-neck cancer. Int J Radiat Oncol Biol Phys 2001; 51: 571–8.
10. Yamazaki H, Inoue T, Teshima T et al. Tongue cancer treated with brachytherapy: is thickness of tongue cancer a prognostic factor for regional control? Anticancer Res 1998; 18: 1261–5.
11. Yamazaki H, Inoue T, Koizumi M et al. Comparison of the long-term results of brachytherapy for T1-2N0 oral tongue cancer treated with Ir-192 and Ra-226. Anticancer Res 1997; 17: 2819–22.
12. Lapeyre M, Hoffstetter S, Peiffert D et al. Postoperative brachytherapy alone for T1-2 N0 squamous cell carcinomas of the oral tongue and floor of mouth with close or positive margins. Int J Radiat Oncol Biol Phys 2000; 48: 37–42.
13. Hall CE, Harris R, A'Hern R et al. Le Fort I osteotomy and low-dose rate Ir192 brachytherapy for treatment of recurrent nasopharyngeal tumours. Radiother Oncol 2003; 66: 41–8.
14. Gregoire V, Eisbruch A, Hamoir M et al. Proposal for the delineation of the nodal CTV in the node-positive and the post-operative neck, Radiother Oncol 2006; 79: 15–20.
15. Gregoire V, Levendag P, Ang KK et al. CT-based delineation of lymph node levels and related CTVs in the node-negative neck: DAHANCA, EORTC, GORTEC, NCIC, RTOG consensus guidelines. Radiother Oncol 2003; 69: 227–36.
16. Chao KS, Deasy JO, Markman J et al. A prospective study of salivary function sparing in patients with head-and-neck cancers receiving intensity-modulated or three-dimensional radiation therapy: initial results. Int J Radiat Oncol Biol Phys 2001; 49: 907–16.
17. Eisbruch A, Marsh LH, Martel MK et al. Comprehensive irradiation of head and neck cancer using conformal multisegmental fields: assessment of target coverage and noninvolved tissue sparing. Int J Radiat Oncol Biol Phys 1998; 41: 559–68.
18. Butler EB, Teh BS, Grant WH 3rd et al. Smart (simultaneous modulated accelerated radiation therapy) boost: a new accelerated fractionation schedule for the treatment of head and neck cancer with intensity modulated radiotherapy. Int J Radiat Oncol Biol Phys 1999; 45: 21–32.
19. Creak AL, Harrington K, Nutting C. Treatment of recurrent head and neck cancer: re-irradiation or chemotherapy? Clin Oncol (R Coll Radiol) 2005; 17: 138–47.
20. Costleigh BJ, Miyamoto CT, Micaily B et al. Heightened sensitivity of the esophagus to radiation in a patient with AIDS. Am J Gastroenterol 1995; 90: 812–14.
21. Formenti SC, Chak L, Gill P et al. Increased radiosensitivity of normal tissue fibroblasts in patients with acquired immunodeficiency syndrome (AIDS) and with Kaposi's sarcoma. Int J Radiat Biol 1995; 68: 411–12.
22. Symonds RP. Treatment-induced mucositis: an old problem with new remedies. Br J Cancer 1998; 77: 1689–95.
23. Bensinger W, Schubert M, Ang KK et al. NCCN Task Force Report. prevention and management of mucositis in cancer care. J Natl Compr Canc Netw 2008; 6(Suppl 1): S1–21; quiz S22–4.
24. Feber T. Management of mucositis in oral irradiation. Clin Oncol (R Coll Radiol) 1996; 8: 106–11.
25. Ferraro JM, Mattern JQ 2nd. Sucralfate suspension for stomatitis. Drug Intell Clin Pharm 1984; 18: 153.
26. Epstein JB, Stevenson-Moore P. Benzydamine hydrochloride in prevention and management of pain in oral mucositis associated with radiation therapy. Oral Surg Oral Med Oral Pathol 1986; 62: 145–8.
27. Pillsbury HC 3rd, Webster WP, Rosenman J. Prostaglandin inhibitor and radiotherapy in advanced head and neck cancers. Arch Otolaryngol Head Neck Surg 1986; 112: 552–3.
28. Abdelaal AS, Barker DS, Fergusson MM. Treatment for irradiation-induced mucositis. Lancet 1989; 1: 97.
29. Rothwell BR, Spektor WS. Palliation of radiation-related mucositis. Spec Care Dentist 1990; 10: 21–5.
30. Spijkervet FK, van Saene HK, van Saene JJ et al. Mucositis prevention by selective elimination of oral flora in irradiated head and neck cancer patients. J Oral Pathol Med 1990; 19: 486–9.
31. Dorr W, Jacubek A, Kummermehr J et al. Effects of stimulated repopulation on oral mucositis during conventional radiotherapy. Radiother Oncol 1995; 37: 100–7.

32. Maciejewski B, Zajusz A, Pilecki B et al. Acute mucositis in the stimulated oral mucosa of patients during radiotherapy for head and neck cancer. Radiother Oncol 1991; 22: 7–11.

33. LeVeque FG, Montgomery M, Potter D et al. A multicenter, randomized, double-blind, placebo-controlled, dose-titration study of oral pilocarpine for treatment of radiation-induced xerostomia in head and neck cancer patients. J Clin Oncol 1993; 11: 1124–31.

34. Fernando IN, Patel T, Billingham L et al. The effect of head and neck irradiation on taste dysfunction: a prospective study. Clin Oncol (R Coll Radiol) 1995; 7: 173–8.

35. Chung NN, Ting LL, Hsu WC et al. Impact of magnetic resonance imaging versus CT on nasopharyngeal carcinoma: primary tumor target delineation for radiotherapy. Head Neck 2004; 26: 241–6.

36. Emami B, Sethi A, Petruzzelli GJ. Influence of MRI on target volume delineation and IMRT planning in nasopharyngeal carcinoma. Int J Radiat Oncol Biol Phys 2003; 57: 481–8.

37. Ling CC, Humm J, Larson S et al. Towards multidimensional radiotherapy (MD-CRT): biological imaging and biological conformality. Int J Radiat Oncol Biol Phys 2000; 47: 551–60.

38. Schoder H, Yeung HW, Gonen M et al. Head and neck cancer: clinical usefulness and accuracy of PET/CT image fusion. Radiology 2004; 231: 65–72.

39. Chao KS, Bosch WR, Mutic S et al. A novel approach to overcome hypoxic tumor resistance: Cu-ATSM-guided intensity-modulated radiation therapy. Int J Radiat Oncol Biol Phys 2001; 49: 1171–82.

40. Nishioka T, Shiga T, Shirato H et al. Image fusion between ^{18}FDG-PET and MRI/CT for radiotherapy planning of oropharyngeal and nasopharyngeal carcinomas. Int J Radiat Oncol Biol Phys 2002; 53: 1051–7.

41. Scarfone C, Lavely WC, Cmelak AJ et al. Prospective feasibility trial of radiotherapy target definition for head and neck cancer using 3-dimensional PET and CT imaging. J Nucl Med 2004; 45: 543–52.

42. Hoskin PJ, Saunders MI, Goodchild K et al. Dynamic contrast enhanced magnetic resonance scanning as a predictor of response to accelerated radiotherapy for advanced head and neck cancer. Br J Radiol 1999; 72: 1093–8.

43. Hermans R, Meijerink M, Van den Bogaert W et al. Tumor perfusion rate determined noninvasively by dynamic computed tomography predicts outcome in head-and-neck cancer after radiotherapy. Int J Radiat Oncol Biol Phys 2003; 57: 1351–6.

44. Bentzen SM, Thames HD. Clinical evidence for tumor clonogen regeneration: interpretations of the data. Radiother Oncol 1991; 22: 161–6.

45. Withers HR, Taylor JM, Maciejewski B. The hazard of accelerated tumor clonogen repopulation during radiotherapy. Acta Oncol 1988; 27: 131–46.

46. Fowler JF. Is there an optimum overall time for head and neck radiotherapy? A review, with new modelling. Clin Oncol (R Coll Radiol) 2007; 19: 8–22.

47. Horiot JC, Le Fur R, N'Guyen T et al. Hyperfractionation versus conventional fractionation in oropharyngeal carcinoma: final analysis of a randomized trial of the EORTC cooperative group of radiotherapy. Radiother Oncol 1992; 25: 231–41.

48. Horiot JC, Bontemps P, van den Bogaert W et al. Accelerated fractionation (AF) compared to conventional fractionation (CF) improves loco-regional control in the radiotherapy of advanced head and neck cancers: results of the EORTC 22851 randomized trial. Radiother Oncol 1997; 44: 111–21.

49. Dische S, Saunders M, Barrett A et al. A randomised multi-centre trial of CHART versus conventional radiotherapy in head and neck cancer. Radiother Oncol 1997; 44: 123–36.

50. Bourhis J, Overgaard J, Audry H et al. Hyperfractionated or accelerated radiotherapy in head and neck cancer: a meta-analysis. Lancet 2006; 368: 843–54.

51. Brizel DM, Dodge RK, Clough RW et al. Oxygenation of head and neck cancer: changes during radiotherapy and impact on treatment outcome. Radiother Oncol 1999; 53: 113–17.

52. Gatenby RA, Kessler HB, Rosenblum JS et al. Oxygen distribution in squamous cell carcinoma metastases and its relationship to outcome of radiation therapy. Int J Radiat Oncol Biol Phys 1988; 14: 831–8.

53. Nordsmark M, Bentzen SM, Rudat V et al. Prognostic value of tumor oxygenation in 397 head and neck tumors after primary radiation therapy. An international multi-center study. Radiother Oncol 2005; 77: 18–24.

54. Nordsmark M, Overgaard M, Overgaard J. Pretreatment oxygenation predicts radiation response in advanced squamous cell carcinoma of the head and neck. Radiother Oncol 1996; 41: 31–9.

55. Henke M, Laszig R, Rube C et al. Erythropoietin to treat head and neck cancer patients with anaemia undergoing radiotherapy: randomised, double-blind, placebo-controlled trial. Lancet 2003; 362: 1255–60.

56. Overgaard J, Hansen HS, Overgaard M et al. A randomized double-blind phase III study of nimorazole as a hypoxic radiosensitizer of primary radiotherapy in supraglottic larynx and pharynx carcinoma. Results of the Danish Head and Neck Cancer Study (DAHANCA) Protocol 5–85. Radiother Oncol 1998; 46: 135–46.

57. Bennett M, Feldmeier J, Smee R et al. Hyperbaric oxygenation for tumour sensitisation to radiotherapy. Cochrane Database Syst Rev 2005:CD005007.

58. Kaanders JH, Pop LA, Marres HA et al. ARCON: experience in 215 patients with advanced head-and-neck cancer. Int J Radiat Oncol Biol Phys 2002; 52: 769–78.

59. Rischin D, Peters L, Fisher R et al. Tirapazamine, cisplatin, and radiation versus fluorouracil, cisplatin, and radiation in patients with locally advanced head and neck cancer: a randomized phase II trial of the Trans-Tasman Radiation Oncology Group (TROG 98.02). J Clin Oncol 2005; 23: 79–87.

60. Overgaard J, Horsman MR. Modification of hypoxia-induced radioresistance in tumors by the use of oxygen and sensitizers. Semin Radiat Oncol 1996; 6: 10–21.

61. Bonner JA, Harari PM, Giralt J et al. Radiotherapy plus cetuximab for squamous-cell carcinoma of the head and neck. N Engl J Med 2006; 354: 567–78.

62. Brizel DM, Wasserman TH, Henke M et al. Phase III randomized trial of amifostine as a radioprotector in head and neck cancer. J Clin Oncol 2000; 18: 3339–45.

63. Buentzel J, Micke O, Adamietz IA et al. Intravenous amifostine during chemoradiotherapy for head-and-neck cancer: a randomized placebo-controlled phase III study. Int J Radiat Oncol Biol Phys 2006; 64: 684–91.

64. Rades D, Fehlauer F, Bajrovic A et al. Serious adverse effects of amifostine during radiotherapy in head and neck cancer patients. Radiother Oncol 2004; 70: 261–4.

65. Brizel DM, Overgaard J. Does amifostine have a role in chemoradiation treatment? Lancet Oncol 2003; 4: 378–81.

66. Spielberger R, Stiff P, Bensinger W et al. Palifermin for oral mucositis after intensive therapy for hematologic cancers. N Engl J Med 2004; 351: 2590–8.

5

Chemotherapy for Squamous Cell Carcinoma of the Head and Neck

Jill Gilbert and Arlene A Forastiere

INTRODUCTION

The role of chemotherapy in head and neck squamous cell cancer (HNSCC) continues to evolve. This chapter focuses on chemotherapy for SCCs of the head and neck region, including tumors of the oral cavity, oropharynx, larynx, and hypopharynx. SCCs account for more than 90% of tumors arising in this region. Other epithelial malignancies including adenocarcinomas and neuroendocrine cancers as well as nonepithelial lesions such as sarcomas have distinct biological features and are beyond the scope of this discussion.

Over the last two decades, the role of chemotherapy has broadened. The Meta-Analysis of Chemotherapy in Head and Neck Cancer (MACH-NC) by Pignon et al. further emphasized the significance of chemotherapy in HNSCC (1). A total of 87 trials were evaluated (50 concurrent, 32 neoadjuvant, 9 adjuvant trials) and demonstrated an absolute survival benefit of 4.4% at 5 years, hazard ratio 0.88, with the use of chemotherapy. When the trials of concurrent chemoradiotherapy (CCR) were evaluated separately, the hazard ratio was 0.81 with an absolute benefit of 8% at 5 years ($p < 0.0001$). In fact, the use of CCR has gained widespread acceptance in a variety of HNC settings including: function preservation, unresectable disease, nasopharyngeal primaries, and in the high-risk postoperative patient (1).

Insights into the molecular basis of HNSCC have led to the investigation of novel targeted agents for early- and advanced-stage disease. Promising results have been demonstrated in combination with radiation therapy (RT) in initial curative therapy and in the setting of metastatic or recurrent disease. With the use of targeted agents, clinical investigators are finding new challenges in the design of meaningful clinical trials, including definition of response, evaluation of quality of life, and improvement in symptom burden. This chapter discusses the traditional cytotoxic chemotherapy agents, common chemotherapy-based strategies in HNSCC, and the use of targeted agents for this disease.

CYTOTOXIC CHEMOTHERAPY AGENTS

Multiple cytotoxic agents have demonstrated efficacy as single agents in HNSCC. The response rate for these agents often stems from clinical trials in patients with incurable recurrent or metastatic disease. Many different cytotoxic drugs have been identified as having activity in recurrent or metastatic HNSCC, giving single agent response rates of up to 30%. Responses achieved in recurrent or metastatic disease are generally short lived, and the median survival of treated patients remains unaltered at 6–9 months (2). Because many of these patients have been previously treated with chemotherapy or RT, the single-agent response rates may underestimate the true effect of the chemotherapy in a previously untreated or newly diagnosed population. While multiple cytotoxic agents have demonstrated the ability to produce a tumor response, the most commonly used agents are discussed below (Table 5.1).

Cisplatin

Cisplatin inhibits DNA synthesis by forming intrastrand and interstrand crosslinks between guanine–guanine pairs of DNA. It is currently regarded as the most active agent in HNSCC giving response rates of approximately 20–50% in phase II trials (3). The dose range most often used is 80–120 mg/m² every 3–4 weeks. Comparison of standard and higher doses has not demonstrated any advantage to use of higher doses in terms of response or survival. This finding was confirmed in a randomized study comparing 60 mg/m² and 120 mg/m² (15). Although pilot studies evaluating the use of very high doses (200 mg/m²) as a single agent demonstrated higher response rates for the higher dose, use of this dose level carried a considerable risk of irreversible toxicity (4).

Toxicities associated with use of conventional-dose cisplatin are considerable and include effects on the kidney, bone marrow, gut, and peripheral nervous system. This makes the drug difficult to use in patients with poor performance status or with comorbid disease. Cisplatin analogues have been widely tested in HNSCC with the aim of maintaining efficacy with less toxicity. The most successful is carboplatin, which has less renal, neurologic, otologic, and gastrointestinal (GI) toxicity but is dose limited by myelosuppression. The response rate in HNSCC is slightly lower than cisplatin at 14–30% with a pooled average from single agent studies of 22% (16). The lower efficacy of carboplatin compared to cisplatin has been suggested in a randomized trial evaluating its use in combination with 5-fluorouracil (17). However, though not directly compared to cisplatin in clinical study, recent published trials demonstrate encouraging efficacy of carboplatin-based CCR as therapy for locally advanced disease (18,19). However, cisplatin therefore remains one of the reference agents in the treatment of HNSCC. Oxaliplatin is the newest of the platinum compounds to come into clinical use and has an established role in GI cancers. Although no head to head comparison with cisplatin has been reported,

Table 5.1 Activity of Single Agent Cytotoxic Chemotherapy in HNSCC

Drug	Mechanism	Response rate
Cisplatin	Inhibits DNA synthesis by forming intra- and interstrand crosslinks	20–50% Common dosing regimen 75–100 mg/m^2 IV every 21 days
Methotrexate	Inhibits DNA synthesis and repair; interferes with use of folate for DNA synthesis and repair; inhibits dihydrofolate reductase	10–30% 40–60 mg/m^2 IV weekly Does not usually require leucovorin rescue; usually well tolerated
5-Fluorouracil	Antimetabolite that inhibits thymidine synthase	15% Commonly given as 1000 mg/m^2 day by continuous infusion over 96–120 hrs
Paclitaxel	Promotes formation of tublin dimers, stabilizes microtubules, and leads to cell cycle arrest in G2/M	37% Requires premedication with steroids, diphenhydramine and H2-blocker to prevent allergic reaction
Docetaxel	Promotes formation of tublin dimers, stabilizes microtubules, and leads to cell cycle arrest in G2/M	22–45% May require dexamethasone to prevent associated fluid retention
Gemcitabine	Structurally similar to deoxycytidine and inhibits DNA synthesis by competing with deoxycytidine during DNA synthesis	13%
Capecitabine	Oral fluoropyrimidine prodrug; Ultimately transformed by a series of enzymatic steps to 5-fluorouracil; simulates continuous infusion 5-fluorouracil	24% response rate in nasopharyngeal population

Source: From Refs. 3–14.
Abbreviation: HNSCC, head and neck squamous cell carcinoma.

oxaliplatin remains of interest for further investigation in HNSCC, due to its favorable toxicity profile (20).

Methotrexate

Methotrexate is the 4-amino 10-methyl analogue of folic acid. It binds and inhibits dihydrofolate reductase (DHFR) that is a critical enzyme in the maintenance of intracellular folates in their reduced form as tetrahydrofolates. These reduced folates are vital for the synthesis of nucleic acids and their depletion interferes with cellular capacity to repair DNA, resulting in DNA strand breaks. The mode of action of methotrexate is extremely complex, and drug-mediated inhibition of DHFR is only one of several mechanisms of its action. It also acts by direct inhibition of folate-dependent enzymes and by incorporating aberrant nucleotides into DNA, resulting in inhibition of DNA synthesis. In palliative therapy for recurrent or metastatic HNSCC, single-agent methotrexate has been regarded as a minimally toxic drug and has been widely used for many years. Different doses and schedules have been tested, but the most commonly used schedule is weekly intravenous bolus treatment, using a dose of 40–60 mg/m^2. The objective response rate to methotrexate given in this dose range is 10–30%. A degree of dose dependence is apparent from several nonrandomized studies in the literature in which doses up to 500 mg/m^2 have been used (5,6). However, the toxicity of higher doses is considerable, negating any benefit in the palliative setting.

Moreover, higher doses require specific hydration and urine alkalinization regimes, making administration more cumbersome.

Use of folinic acid (leucovorin) can reverse many of the cytotoxic effects of methotrexate on normal and malignant cells. Leucovorin can enhance the therapeutic index of methotrexate by limiting the toxicity of higher doses of methotrexate. Doses greater than 70 mg/m^2 require folinic acid rescue. Randomized trials comparing high-dose methotrexate with folinic acid rescue with standard-dose methotrexate have failed to show any survival advantage to the higher doses (21,22). Over the last decade, a number of methotrexate analogues have been evaluated including trimetrexate, edatrexate, and piritrexin (23–25). To date, these have not been shown to have any advantage over methotrexate, and edatrexate in particular has a worse toxicity profile. Within this class of drug, the multitargeted antifolate pemetrexed is the most recent to undergo study in cancers of the upper aerodigestive tract. Activity has been demonstrated in head and neck cancer. Whether this compound has advantages over methotrexate remains to be demonstrated (26–28).

5-Fluorouracil

5-Fluorouracil is an antimetabolite that exerts its cytotoxic effects in several different ways. The predominant effect is through the inhibition of thymidine synthase, leading to depletion of nucleotides required for DNA synthesis and repair. Early studies with 5-fluorouracil in patients with advanced, multiply relapsed HNSCC indicated a single-agent response rate of 15%. Randomized trials have demonstrated that higher response rates are obtained when 5-fluorouracil is given by continuous infusion over 96 or 120 hours. Delivery of 5-fluorouracil by continuous infusion may be associated with a different spectrum of toxicity with mucositis and diarrhea gaining predominance over myelosuppression (8). 5-Fluorouracil assumed increasing importance in the management of HNSCC following the discovery of synergy with cisplatin, which was shown to result in an increase in objective response rates up to 70% including a reported complete remission rate of up to 27% in recurrent HNSCC in the original study (7).

Taxanes

Paclitaxel and its semisynthetic derivative, docetaxel, are drugs with broad anticancer activity that have a novel mechanism of action. They act by promoting the formation of tubulin dimers, stabilizing microtubules during cell division and thereby leading to arrest of cells in the G2/M phase of the cell cycle. Docetaxel is twice as active as paclitaxel in promoting tubular polymerization. This greater cytotoxicity may be related to its higher affinity for microtubules or to greater intracellular accumulation (9,11,29).

Multiple-dose and schedule regimens of pachtaxel have been studied. The original phase I and II studies used a 24-hour infusion, and there is evidence that paclitaxel is schedule dependent, with greater activity seen with use of prolonged treatments. Delivery by 24-hour infusion may be more effective than the currently used 3-hour or 1-hour infusion schedules, but any incremental benefit of higher doses or longer infusion times comes at the cost of increased toxicity, particularly severe and life-threatening myelosuppression. The results of a phase II trial of 24-hour infusion paclitaxel carried out by the Eastern Cooperative Oncology Group (ECOG) to evaluate the single-agent activity reported a 40% overall response rate and median survival of 9.2 months in 34 patients with relapsed HNSCC making it one of the most effective single agents in this disease (10). A subsequent trial (E1393) compared high- (200 mg/m^2) and low-dose (135 mg/m^2) paclitaxel administered by 24-hour infusion combined with cisplatin. No advantage was found for the high-dose regimen, and the toxicity associated with both regimens was severe (30). Trials conducted within the ECOG after this latter study utilized the 3-hour infusion of paclitaxel that is associated with less myelotoxicity but more neuropathy. In contrast to paclitaxel, the activity of docetaxel remains schedule dependent and is given as a single dose (standard 75 mg/m^2) over 1-hour every 3 weeks (31). Clinically, use of docetaxel in recurrent/metastatic HNSCC results in objective responses in 22–45% of patients, with a median duration of response of 5 months, which compares favorably with currently used combination treatments. The major toxicities of docetaxel are neutropenia, mucositis, and fluid retention, which can be prevented by premedicating patients with corticosteroids and diphenhydramine (11).

Taxanes are also potent radiosensitizers because G2/M is the cellular phase at which cells exhibit greatest radiosensitivity. Data derived from Tishler and colleagues showed that paclitaxel potentiated the effect of radiation in vitro in many cell lines at clinically achievable paclitaxel concentrations (<10 nmol/L), indicating potential for developing a chemoradiation regimen simultaneously utilizing paclitaxel or docetaxel (18,32–35).

USES OF CYTOTOXIC CHEMOTHERAPY FOR HNSCC
Palliative Chemotherapy for Recurrent or Metastatic Disease

The rationale for using multiple drugs in combination is to develop regimens that produce higher response rates and increase overall survival because of differing mechanisms of the component drugs. However, results of the combination of agents have been largely disappointing. Additionally, trials comparing combination to single-agent chemotherapy did not demonstrate improvements in survival or time to progression for the combination over the single agent. Moreover, although toxicity was increased with combination therapy. In general, combination cytotoxic therapy can lead to improved overall response rates but without an improvement in survival. This is largely due to the limited proportion of patients showing response (30–40%) and the paucity of complete responses. In a study by Jacobs and colleagues, 40 response rates were higher for cisplatin in combination with 5-fluorouracil compared with either single-agent (32% vs. 17% and 13% for cisplatin and 5-fluorouracil, respectively) (36,37). In a study comparing single-agent methotrexate with cisplatin/5-fluorouracil and carboplatin/5-fluorouracil, the superior response rate of the combination treatments was clear, but increased toxicity was observed for the combinations (38,42). However, overall survival was not different between the three treatment arms. Many other randomized studies of single agents versus combination chemotherapy in recurrent or metastatic HNSCC confirm the findings of higher response rate without impact on survival (Table 5.2). Thus, the utility of these combinations in the palliative setting must be examined carefully in population with a very limited life expectancy. Based on numerous trials, the regimen of cisplatin and 5-fluorouracil has remained the reference regimen for testing new combinations.

Concurrent Chemoradiotherapy (CCR)
Primary Treatment Modality

The rationale for the concurrent administration of chemotherapy and RT stems from the ability of certain chemotherapeutic agents to enhance the radiation sensitivity of tumors and ultimately improve efficacy. Several reasons for this observation are likely play a role including

1. inhibition of the repair of sublethally damaged cells after radiation
2. improved blood supply to tumor with cytoreduction, leading to improved tumor tissue oxygenation and radiosensitivity (42).

As chemotherapy in general does not have overlapping toxicities with RT, delivery of this combined modality is usually feasible. However, it should be remembered that

Table 5.2   Randomized Trials Comparing Combination Cytotoxic Regimens in Recurrent HNC

Authors	Schema	Results
Gibson et al. ECOG 1395	CDDP 100 mg/m² d 1 and 5FU 1000 mg/m²/24 hr by continuous IV infusion Versus CDDP 75 mg/m² d 1 and P 175 mg/m² IV over 3 hrs d 1 Cycles of both arms repeated every 21 days	RR 27% CDDP/5FU RR 26% CDDP/P Median survival 8.7 mos CDDP/5FU and 8.1 mos CDDP/P group No significant difference in overall survival or response rate
Forastiere et al. ECOG 1393	P 200 mg/m²/24-hr continuous infusion d 1 plus CDDP 75 mg/m² d 1 plus G-CSF versus P 135 mg/m²/24-hr continuous infusion d 1 plus CDDP 75 mg/m² d 1 Cycles of both arms repeated every 21 days	RR 35% for high-dose arm and 36% for low-dose arm In both arms, estimated median survival 7.3 mos, and 1-year survival 29% Overall, no advantage for high-dose P Significant hematological toxicity noted in both arms
Fountzilas et al.	P 175 mg/m² day 1 (3-hr) and Gemcitabine 1000 mg/m² d 1 and 8, every 21 days versus P 175 mg/m² day 1 (3-hr) and Do 40 mg/m² on d 1 every 28 days	RR 20% P/G RR 29% P/Do (NS) TTP 4.4 mos P/G TTP 6.0 mos P/Do (NS) Median overall survival: 8.6 mos P/G 11 mos P/Do (NS)
Clavel et al. (41)	Methotrexate 40 mg/m² d 1 and 15 plus bleomycin 10 mg d 1, 8, 15, vincristine 2 mg d 1, 8, 15, plus CDDP 50 mg/m² d 4 (repeated every 21 days) = CABO versus CDDP 100 mg/m² d 1 and 5 FU 1000 mg/m²/day × 4 per continuous infusion, every 21 days: CF versus CDDP 50 mg/m² d 1 and 8, every 28 days	Overall RR to CABO and CF superior to C (34% and 31% vs. 15%, respectively, *p* = 0.003) No significant difference in progression-free survival or overall survival between the three arms

Source: From Refs. 30, 39–41.
Abbreviations: ECOG, eastern cooperative oncology group; RR, response rate; 5FU, 5-Fluorouracil; TTP, time to progression; Do, pegylated liposomal doxorubicin; P, paclitaxel; CDDP, cisplatin; G-CSF; CABO, cisplatin, methotrexate, bleomycin and vincristine; CF, cisplatin and 5FU; C, cisplatin.

just as sensitivity of tumor tissue to RT is enhanced, sensitivity of normal tissue to RT is also enhanced by the addition of chemotherapy. Thus, acute and chronic, late toxicity may be increased with CCR. Multiple randomized trials of CCR versus RT alone have been reported in the literature (Table 5.3).

CCR has demonstrated improvements in clinical outcomes in the resectable and unresectable locally advanced patient population. In general, the addition of chemotherapy results in improved locoregional control, disease-free survival, and overall survival. The Intergroup Trial (RTOG 91-11) serves as a landmark trial, supporting the use of CCR for organ preservation in larynx cancer; moreover, results from this trial have been extrapolated to other sites in the head and neck. A total of 547 patients with locally advanced, resectable laryngeal cancer were randomized to one of three treatment groups. Arm 1 consisted of induction chemotherapy that was identical to the VA laryngeal trial regimen of three cycles of cisplatin and 5-fluorouracil, followed by definitive standard fractionation radiotherapy (RT) in responding patients. Arm 2 consisted of CCR using cisplatin 100 mg/m² IV on days 1, 22, and 43 during definitive standard fractionation RT (2 Gy per day to total of 70 Gy). Arm 3 consisted of single-modality standard fractionation radiation therapy alone to 70 Gy. The neck was managed uniformly with a planned neck dissection at the completion of the assigned treatment for patients with N2 or N3 disease at study entry. After a median follow-up of 6.9 years, the 5-year rates of laryngectomy free survival (44.6%, 46.6%, and 33.9%, respectively) and disease-free survival (38.6% and 39% vs. 27.3%) were significantly better with either induction chemotherapy or CCR compared to RT alone. The rates of laryngeal preservation and locoregional control, however, were significantly better in the CCR arm compared to the induction chemotherapy and RT-alone arms, and there was no significant difference for these end points when induction was compared to RT alone. There was no significant difference

Table 5.3 Selected Trials of Concurrent Chemoradiotherapy versus Radiotherapy Alone in Locally Advanced HNSCC

Author	Disease site	Resectability	Schema	Results
Merlano et al.	OC, OP, H, L, NP	Unresectable	Group 1: 70 Gy/2 Gy per d/35 Fx Group 2: Three courses of 20 Gy each, 2 Gy/d given daily for 5 consecutive days, wks 2–3, 5–6, 8–9 plus CDDP 20 mg/m^2 and 5 FU 200 mg/m^2 for 5 consecutive days, wks 1, 4, 7, and 10	5-year follow-up: CRT 43% vs. 22% RT ($p = 0.037$) CRT OS 24% vs. 10% RT ($p = 0.01$) CRT PFS 21% vs. 9% RT ($p = 0.008$) CRT LRC 64% vs. 32%RT ($p = 0.038$)
Denis et al.	OP	Unresectable	Group 1: 70 Gy/2 Gy per day/35 Fx Group 2: 70 Gy/2 Gy per day/35 Fx plus CBA 70 mg/m^2/d and 5 FU 96 hr CIV 600 mg/m^2/d on days 1–4, 22–25, 43–46	5-year follow-up: CRT OS 22% vs. 16% RT ($p = 0.05$) CRT Specific DFS 27% RT vs. 15% ($p = 0.01$) CRT LRC 48% vs. 25% RT ($p = 0.002$)
Forastiere et al.	L	Resectable	Group 1: Induction: CDDP 100 mg/m^2 d 1, 22 and 5 FU 1000 mg/m^2/d CIV for 120 hrs, day 1, 22 After induction completion: RT 70 Gy/2 Gy/d for 35 Fx Group 2: RT 70 Gy/2 Gy/d for 35 Fx plus CDDP 100 mg/m^2 on d 1, 22, 43 Group 3: RT 70 Gy/2 Gy/d for 35 Fx	5-year follow-up: LFS Group 1: 45% Group 2: 47% Group 3: 34% ($p = 0.011$ for 1 or 2 compared to 3) LP Group 1: 71% Group 2: 84% Group 3: 66% ($p = 0.0029$ 2 vs. 1 and 0.00017 for 2 vs. 3C) LRC Group 1: 55% Group 2: 69% Group 3: 51% ($p = 0.0018$ 2 vs. 1 and $p = 0.0005$ for 2 vs. 3) DFS Group 1: 39% Group 2: 39% Group 3: 27% ($p = 0.016$ and 0.0058 for 1 or 2 vs. 3) OS Group 1: 59% Group 2: 55% Group 3: 54% NS trend toward improved survival in Arm 1
Brizel et al.	OC, OP, H, L, NP, S	Resectable and unresectable	Group 1: 1.25 Gy BID to total 75 Gy/6 wks Group 2: 1.25 Gy BID to total 70 Gy/7 wks plus CDDP 12 mg/m^2/d for 5 d and 5 120-hr CIV 5 FU 600 mg/m^2/on wk 1 and 6 of RT 2 adjuvant cycles of CDDP and 5 FU given	3-year follow-up: CRT OS 55% vs. 34% RT($p = 0.07$) CRT RFS 61% vs. 41% RT($p = 0.08$) CRT LRC 70% vs. 44% RT($p = 0.01$)
Adelstein et al.	OC, OP, H, L	Unresectable	Group 1: 70 Gy/2 Gy per day/35 Fx Group 2: 70 Gy/2 Gy per day/35 Fx plus CDDP 100 mg/m^2 d 1, 22, 43 Group 3: 2 Gy/d split course for a total dose of 60–70 Gy plus CDDP 75 mg/m^2 d 1 and 5 FU 1000 mg/m^2 96 hr CIV d 1 every 4 wks for 3 cycles	3-year follow-up: OS 23% vs. 37% ($p = 0.014$) vs. 27% (NS) CRT CCR 27.4% vs. 40.2% vs. 49.4% ($p = 0.02$ for 1 vs. 3, NS 1 vs. 2) CRT specific DFS 33% vs. 51% vs. 41% ($p = 0.01$ for 1 vs. 2)

Source: From Refs. 43–47.
Abbreviations: OC, oral cavity; H, hypopharynx; L, larynx; NP, nasopharynx; CCR, concurrent chemoradiotherapy; RT, radiotherapy; CDDP, cisplatin; PFS, progression free survival; FU, fluorouracil; LRC, locoregional control; OS, overall survival; CBA, carboplatin; CIV, contmuous intravenous infusion; LP, laryngeal preservation; DFS, disease free survival; LFS, laryngectomy free survival; BID, twice per day; CCR, concurrent chemoradiotheraphy.

among the three treatments in overall survival (55% at 5 years) (45). Based on these results, concurrent cisplatin and RT is the standard of care to achieve larynx preservation.

Postoperative Concurrent Chemoradiotherapy in High-risk Patients

Given the excellent rates of locoregional control using CCR, the question arises whether the use of CCR in the adjuvant, postoperative setting can improve clinical outcomes in patients at high risk of relapse after complete resection. Two well designed randomized trials that used the same treatment, but with some variation in definition of high risk, demonstrated that the addition of cisplatin, given concurrently, does enhance the efficacy of RT after curative resection (Table 5.4).

Bernier et al. reported for the EORTC a randomized trial of 334 patients enrolled following curative resection of SCC of the oropharynx, oral cavity, larynx, or hypopharynx. The treatments were Arm 1—adjuvant standard fractionation RT to a total of 66 Gy; Arm 2—the same RT with the addition of cisplatin 100 mg/m² on days 1, 22, and 43, currently with RT. This trial defined high-risk features as pT3 or pT4 disease, extranodal spread, positive resection margins, perineural or vascular involvement, or oral cavity or oropharyngeal tumors with involvement of level IV or V lymph nodes. Overall survival and progression-free survival significantly favored the CCR arm with hazard ratios of 0.75 and 0.70, respectively. The 5-year cumulative incidence of local or regional relapse showed a significant benefit for the CCR arm as well (18% vs. 31%, $p = 0.007$) (48). A second randomized trial, reported by Cooper et al. for the Radiation Therapy Oncology Group (RTOG) and U.S. Intergroup, compared the same two treatments in patients with primaries of the oral cavity, oropharynx, larynx, or hypopharynx who had gross total resection of disease (49). In this trial, *high risk* was defined as the presence of two or more positive lymph nodes, extracapsular extension of disease, or microscopically involved mucosal margins.

Other important differences, in addition to the definition of high risk, should be noted about the two trials. The end points of the two trials differed; although the Bernier trial was designed to detect a 15% improvement in progression-free survival, the U.S. Intergroup trial was designed to detect an improvement in local and regional control. Although Bernier noted a significant improvement in progression-free survival and overall survival, the U.S. Intergroup trial did not detect a difference in overall survival. Mature results at 5 years were reported by the EORTC while the Radiation Therapy Oncology Group (RTOG)/Intergroup trial reported 2-year results. CCR did result in a significant improvement in disease-free survival and locoregional control in both trials. The discrepant survival results may be due to differences in study design, definition of *high risk* and more advanced nodal disease in the RTOG/Intergroup trial. In an attempt to reconcile the differing results, a pooled data analysis of the two trials was performed that showed a reduction in death of 28% in favor of CCR over adjuvant RT alone. The impact of CCR for both trials was greatest in the group of patients with extracapsular extension and/or positive surgical margins (50).

The 5-year results of the U.S. Intergroup/ECOG trial were recently reported in abstract form by Cooper et al (51). Surprisingly, with longer follow-up none of the previously reported end points (overall survival, disease-free survival, low control) are significantly different in the overall comparison of the two treatment groups. The authors hypothesize that this may reflect statistical "noise" induced by the inclusion in the trial of 4% of entries whose disease was not high enough risk. Given the results of the pooled analysis discussed above, unplanned subset analyses of these long-term results were performed and showed a significant benefit for disease-free survival and locoregional control but not overall survival, for patients with either extracapsular extension of disease or a microscopic margin treated with postoperative RT and cisplatin. There was no benefit for patients with neither of these two high-risk features (e.g., multiple positive nodes only). Although the results of

Table 5.4 Phase III Trials or Adjuvant Therapy in High Risk Disease

Author	High Risk Features	Therapy	Outcomes
Bernier et al.	pT3 or pT4 or extranodal spread, positive resection margins, perineural involvement or vascular tumor embolism	Group 1: Total resection →RT 66 Gy over 6.5 wks Group 2: Total resection →RT 66 Gy over 6.5 wks plus CDDP 100 mg/m² d 1, 22, 43	PFS: hazard ratio 0.75, favoring combined therapy ($p = 0.04$) OS: hazard ratio 0.70, favoring combined therapy ($p = 0.02$) 5-year cumulative incidence of local or regional relapses: Group 1: 31% Group 2: 18%, $p = 0.007$
Cooper et al.	Histologic evidence of invasion of two or more regional lymph nodes, extracapsular extension of nodal disease, microscopically involved mucosal margins of resection	Group 1: Total resection →RT 60–66 Gy over 6–6.6 wks Group 2: Total resection →RT60–66 Gy over 6–6.6 weeks Plus CDDP 100 mg/m² d 1, 22, 43	Local regional recurrence: Hazard ratio 0.61, favoring combined therapy group, $p = 0.01$ DFS: Hazard ratio for disease or death 0.78, favoring combined therapy group, $p = 0.04$ OS: No significant difference

Source: From Refs. 48, 49.
Abbreviations: PFS, progression free survival; RT, radiation therapy; OS, overall survival; CDDP, cisplatin; DFS, disease free survival.

the subset analyses are considered hypothesis generating, they are consistent and supportive of the findings of the pooled EORTC and RTOG/Intergroup data. Thus, postoperative concurrent cisplatin and RT is recommended for patients whose pathology shows either a positive margin or involved nodes with extracapsular extension of disease.

Induction Chemotherapy

Induction chemotherapy for locally advanced HNSCC was a common area of investigation in the 1970s and 1980s. The hypothesis behind induction chemotherapy stems from the potential (1) to improve local control and survival by reducing the tumor burden prior to local therapy, (2) to eradicate micrometastatic disease, (3) improve chemotherapy delivery to viable remaining tumor, and (4) early palliation of symptoms. In 1985, the Department of Veterans Affairs (VA) Laryngeal Cancer Study Group initiated a landmark multicenter randomized trial of induction chemotherapy followed by definitive RT versus total laryngectomy followed by RT (52). The study enrolled 332 patients with locally advanced (stage III and IV, nonmetastatic) laryngeal cancer. The induction chemotherapy consisted of cisplatin and 5-fluorouracil followed by definitive RT to a total dose of 66–76 Gy. Patients in the chemotherapy arm were assessed for response after two cycles and those who demonstrated a partial response (PR) (>50% response) received a third course of chemotherapy followed by RT. Those patients who demonstrated less than a partial response received a total laryngectomy followed by adjuvant RT. Several important findings have resulted from this trial:

1. The 3-year laryngeal preservation rate was 62%.
2. There was no difference in overall survival between the two arms. Thus, laryngeal preservation does not compromise this end point.
3. Patients who received induction chemotherapy had a decreased rate of distant failure as compared to the surgery arm.
4. Patients in the surgery arm demonstrated improved locoregional control over the chemotherapy arm.
5. Long-term quality of life study showed that patients in the organ preservation arm had significantly better scores on mental health domain survey, better pain scores, and better scores in the domains related to patient impression of treatment success (52,53).

The EORTC also conducted a clinical trial using an identical approach. In this clinical trial, 202 patients with locally advanced, resectable cancer of the hypopharynx were randomized to induction chemotherapy with cisplatin and 5-flourouracil followed by definitive RT versus immediate surgery followed by RT. This trial differed from the VA trial in that patients were required to demonstrate a complete response to receive all three cycles of induction chemotherapy. At 5 years follow-up, there was no significant difference in survival between the two arms. However, chemotherapy was associated with decreased distant failure. The 3- and 5-year estimates of retaining a functional larynx in patients on the induction arm were 42% and 35%, respectively (54). Many other randomized controlled trials were performed, principally in the 1980s, of induction chemotherapy followed by surgery and/or RT compared

to locoregional therapy alone. With the exception of two trials, no differences in survival were observed, and this was consistent with the results of meta-analyses (55–57).

With the improved locoregional control realized with CCR, induction chemotherapy has garnered a renewed interest. As local failure rates have improved with CCR, distant failure rates appear to have increased. The questions that have arisen from these observations are whether local failure and distant failure can be controlled with either more effective induction chemotherapy or the addition of induction chemotherapy to CCR (termed sequential therapy). Multiple clinical trials have evaluated intensification of induction chemotherapy (Table 5.5). One of the most promising regimens is the combination of docetaxel, cisplatin, and 5-flurorouricil (TPF). In the TAX 324 trial, Posner et al. compared cisplatin, docetaxel, 5-fluorucil with the standard regimen of cisplatin and 5FU as induction chemotherapy in patients with stage III or IVA, IVB HNSCC (nonmetastatic). Five hundred one patients were randomized to the two arms. After induction chemotherapy, patients in both treatment groups received RT and concurrent weekly carboplatin. The primary end point of the trial was overall survival. At a minimum follow-up of 2 years, the TPF arm demonstrated a significantly better median overall survival of 71 months versus 30 months, respectively ($p = 0.006$). Although significantly improved locoregional control was noted in the TPF arm (62% vs. 60%, $p = 0.04$), there was no difference in distant metastatic disease rates. It should be noted that the rates of distant failure for both arms were low at 5% and 9%, perhaps reflecting an effect of induction chemotherapy, not the intensity of this therapy (58). Trials evaluating the use of TPF followed by CCR versus chemoradiotherapy alone are ongoing.

Cytotoxic Chemotherapy for Nasopharyngeal Carcinoma

Although nasopharyngeal carcinoma (NPC) is a rare malignancy worldwide, this disease is endemic in Southern China, South-East Asia, and the Mediterranean basin with approximately 10–50 cases per 100,000 population. In endemic areas, undifferentiated NPC (World Health Organization types II and III) predominates, whereas type I (SCC) is more commonly noted in Western countries. Although two randomized trials of adjuvant chemotherapy did not demonstrate a survival advantage over radiotherapy alone, multiple randomized trials have demonstrated the superiority of CCR over RT alone in this disease. In the Intergroup trial by Al-Sarraf et al., 147 patients with stage III or IV NPC were randomized to standard fractionation RT alone versus RT with cisplatin 100 mg/m^2 on day 1, 22, 43 followed by three cycles of adjuvant cisplatin and continuous infusion 5-fluorouracil (5 FU). The results demonstrated significantly improved progression-free survival, median survival, and 3-year survival in the chemotherapy arm over RT alone. Yet the contribution of adjuvant therapy to these outcomes is debated (61). An identical trial, performed by the Hong Kong Nasopharyngeal Cancer Study Group, confirmed the locoregional control benefit of CCR in an Asian population with predominantly type II and III disease. However, no survival benefit was noted at a median follow-up of 2.3 years. This discrepancy may be due to the favorable results in the RT arm, the more advanced stages

Table 5.5   Selected Randomized Trials of Induction Chemotherapy in Locally Advanced HNSCC

Author	Resectable	Site	Schema	Outcomes
Zorat et al.	Resectable and Unresectable	OC, OP, H, paranasal sinus	**Group 1:** Resectable: CDDP 100 mg/m² d 1, 5 FU 1000 mg/m² d1-5 every 3 wks for 4 cycles → surgery → adjuvant RT (40–50 Gy) Unresectable: CDDP 100 mg/m² d 1, 5 FU 1000 mg/m² d1-5 every 3 wks for 4 cycles → radical RT (65–70 Gy) **Group 2:** Resectable: Surgery → adjuvant RT (40–50 Gy) Unresectable: Radical RT (65–70 Gy)	10-year follow-up: All patients 10 year OS: 19% vs. 9% Group 1 vs. Group 2 ($p = 0.13$) Operable patients 10-year OS: 23% vs. 14% Group 1 vs. Group 2 ($p = 0.73$) Inoperable patients 10-year OS: 16% vs. 6% Group 1 vs. Group 2 ($p = 0.04$)
Hitt et al.	Resectable and Unresectable	OC, OP, H, L	**Group 1:** CDDP 100 mg/m² d 1, 5 FU 1000 mg/m² d 1–5 CIV for 3 cycles every 3 wks → CDDP 100 mg/m² d 1, 22, 43 and RT (70 Gy) **Group 2:** Paclitaxel 175 mg/m² d 1, CDDP 100 mg/m² d2, 5 FU 500 mg/m² CIV d 1–5, every 3 wks for 3 cycles → CDDP 100 mg/m² d 1, 22, 43 and RT (70 Gy)	RR: 14% vs. 33% ($p < 0.001$) MTTF: 12 mo vs. 20 mo Group 1 vs. 2 ($p = 0.006$) OS: 37 mo vs. 43 mo Group 1 vs. 2 ($p = 0.06$) OS significantly favored Group 2 over Group 1 if consider only unresectable patients ($p = 0.04$)
Remenar and Vermorken et al.	Unresectable	OC, OP, H, L	**Group 1:** CDDP 100 mg/m² d 1 and 5 FU 1000 mg/m² d 1–5 CIV q 3 wks for 4 cycles → RT 66–74 Gy +/− surgery **Group 2:** Docetaxel 75 mg/m² d 1, CDDP 75 mg/m² d 1, 5 FU 750 mg/m²/d d1–5 CIV every 3 wks for 4 cycles → RT 66–74 Gy +/− surgery	32-mo follow-up PFS: 8.2 mo vs. 11.0 mo Group 1 vs. 2 ($p = 0.071$) OS (at 51 mo): 14.2 mo vs. 18.6 mo Group 1 vs. 2 ($p = 0.0052$) RR: Group 1: 54% Group 2: 68% ($p = 0.006$)
Posner et al.	Unresectable and Resectable	OC, L, OP, H	**Group 1:** Docetaxel 75 mg/m² on d 1, CDDP 100 mg/m² IV d 1, 5 FU 1000 mg/m²/d CIV days 1–5 q 3 wks for 3 cycles → RT 70–74 Gy with concurrent CBA AUC 1.5 weekly × 7 **Group 2:** CDDP 100 mg/m² IV d 1, 5 FU 1000 mg/m²/d CIV days 1–5 q 3 wks for 3 cycles → RT 70–74 Gy with concurrent CBA AUC 1.5 weekly × 7	Hazard ratio for death 0.70, $p = 0.006$ favoring TPF (Group 1) Overall 3-year survival 62% vs. 48% ($p = 0.006$) Locoregional control favored TPF (Group 1), $p = 0.04$

Source: From Refs. 56, 58–60.
Abbreviations: OC, oral cavity; OP, oropharynx; H, hypopharynx; L, larynx; NP, nasopharynx; NS, not specified; CDDP, cisplatin; CIV, continuous IV infusion; CR, complete response; OS, overall survival; RT, radiation therapy; MTTF, median time to treatment failure; PFS, progression-free survival; RR, response rate; FU, fluorouracil; CBA, carboplatin; AUC, Area Under the Curve; TPF, docetaxel, cisplatin, 5-fluorouracil.

at presentation, or the relatively short follow-up (62). The MACH-NC further demonstrated the benefit of chemotherapy in this disease with an absolute survival benefit of 6% at 5 years from the addition of chemotherapy. Moreover, a significant interaction was noted between the timing of chemotherapy and overall survival ($p = 0.005$) with the largest benefit resulting from CCR (1) (Table 5.6).

TARGETED DRUG THERAPY FOR HNSCC

Elucidation of the mechanistic basis of tumor proliferation, growth and survival in HNSCC has allowed the rational development of molecularly targeted agents for this disease. Although multiple facets of the complex biology of HNSCC are currently under investigation, several areas of research have led to the translation of the science into drug development as pertains to HNSCC. As drug discovery progresses, the arsenal of therapeutic agents for HNSCC now includes a number of novel therapies. It remains prudent to understand the basic mechanistic underpinnings of these drugs.

Molecular targets in HNSCC
Epidermal Growth Factor Receptor
Although multiple signaling pathways and molecular targets are under investigation, the largest body of clinical data resides in the use of agents that target the epidermal growth factor receptor (EGFR) in HNSCC. One of the most important recent discoveries in HNSCC is the elucidation of the role of the EGFR in HNSCC. The EGFR (*erb*B-1) is a member of the *erb*B subfamily of receptors and is overexpressed in the majority of HNSCC. The EGFR resides in

Table 5.6 Phase III Randomized Trials in Locally Advanced Nasopharyngeal Carcinoma

Author	World Health Organization classification	Stage	N	Therapy	Outcomes
Chan et al.	I,II, III (predominant III)	Stage II–IV T1–4, N2, N3, or N1 of at least 4 cm	Group 1: 176 Group 2: 174	Group 1: RT 66 Gy/33 Fx per 6.5 wks Group 2: RT 66 Gy/33 Fx per 6.5 wks plus CDDP 40 mg/m^2 weekly during RT	5-year follow-up: PFS: Group 1: 52% Group 2: 60% Not significant (except significant for T3/T4 only 0.012) OS: Group 1: 59% Group 2:70% (p = 0.065 but significant for T3/T4 p = 0.013) LRC: Trend favoring Group 2 in T3/T4 (p = 0.051) Distant metastases: NS
Ma et al.	I, II, III (predominant II, III)	Stage III–IV T1–T4, N0–N3	Group 1: 228 Group 2: 228	Group 1: RT 68–72 Gy, 2 Gy/d Group 2: RT 68–72 Gy, 2 Gy/d plus CDDP 100 mg/m^2 IV on d 1, bleomycin 10 mg/m^2 d 1–5, 5 FU CIV 800 mg/m^2 d 1–5, repeated q 21 days	6-year follow-up: 5 year OS: 56% vs. 63% favoring group 2 (p = 0.11) 5-yr RFS: 50 mo vs. not reached favoring Group 2 (p = 0.05) FLR: 74% vs. 82% (p = 0.04)
Al-Sarraf et al.	I, II, III	Stage III, IV T1–4, N0–3	Group 1: 69 Group 2: 78	Group 1: RT 1.8–2.0 Gy/d Fx total dose Gy Group 2: RT 1.8–2.0 Gy/d Fx total dose Gy plus CDDP 100 mg/m^2 d 1, 22, 43; Upon completion of RT, CDDP 80 mg/m^2 IV d 71, 99, 127 and 5 FU 1000 mg/m^2 96 hr CIV d 71–74, 99–102, 127–130	5-year follow-up: 3-yr PFS: Group 1: 24% Group 2: 69% (p < 0.001) 3-year survival; Group 1: 47% Group 2: 78% (p = 0.005)

Source: From Refs. 61, 63, 64.
Abbreviations: CDDP, cisplatin; CIV, continuous IV infusion; OS, overall survival; RT, radiation therapy; PFS, progression-free survival; LRC, locoregional control; FU, fluorouracil; RFS, relapse free survival; FLR, freedom from local recurrence.

the plasma membrane and is composed of three domains: an extracellular ligand binding domain, the transmembrane segment, and the intracellular tyrosine kinase domain. Binding of the receptor's ligands [EGF, amphiregulin, and Tumor Growth Factor (TGF)-alpha] lead to homo- and heterodimerization with other members of the *erb*B family. This results in activation of the EGFR tyrosine kinase and phosphorylation of multiple downstream targets. Activation of the receptor promotes cellular processes including cell proliferation, motility, adhesion, invasion, and angiogenesis. In HNSCC, increased EGFR gene copy number is associated with a worse progression-free survival and overall survival (65). Given this, the EGFR provides an attractive therapeutic target for HNSCC.

Angiogenesis

Vascular endothelial growth factor (VEGF) and its receptors play key roles in cancer angiogenesis. The VEGF family of molecules includes six growth factors (VEGF-A, VEGF-B, VEGF-C, VEGF-D, VEGF-E, VEGF-F) and three receptors (VEGFR-1, VEGFR-2, VEGFR-3, also known as Flt-1, KDR/Flk-1, and Flt-4, respectively. VEGF is overexpressed in head and neck cancer, and high circulating VEGF levels have been associated with a decreased progression-free survival, overall survival, and response to chemotherapy (66). The VEGF receptors (VEGFR) are tyrosine kinases, and binding of ligand to the receptors result in a complex signaling cascade, ultimately leading to angiogenesis, endothelial cell survival, and vascular permeability. VEGFR-2 is predominantly expressed in endothelial cells and has been a key VEGFR associated with tumor vascularization, proliferation, and metastasis. In vitro, VEGF production by tumor cells can be induced by radiation and can protect tumor cells from RT. Additive or synergistic effects are also noted with chemotherapy (67–70). As tumor formation and survival is dependent on angiogenesis, the VEGF pathway provides a novel target for therapeutic gain.

Tumor Hypoxia

In HNSCC, the tumor microenvironment has proven to be particularly important in terms of response to therapies, including surgery, chemotherapy, and radiation-based therapies. Although the reason for this observation is not entirely clear, several factors likely play a role. First, tumor hypoxia contributes to genomic instability and may promote survival of cells that lack the ability to undergo apoptosis. Although hypoxia can delay progression through the cell cycle, cells that are "hypoxia resistant" may be selected out for a growth advantage, providing a clone that is able to repopulate under hypoxic conditions. Hypoxia inducible factor (HIF)-alpha, a transcription factor, is upregulated under hypoxic conditions and stimulates neovascularization (71). In fact, HIF-1-alpha expression activates VEGF transcription (72). HNSCCs demonstrate increased expression of HIF-1-alpha protein (73–75). Overexpression has been associated with locoregional failure and shortened disease-free and overall survival in HNSCC treated with CCR. Other potential markers of a hypoxic tumor environment in HNSCC include carbonic anhydrase IX, glucose transporters 1 and 3 (GLUT-1 and GLUT-3), and the erythropoietin receptor (76).

Clinical Experience Using Molecularly Targeted Agents
EGFR-inhibitor Therapy

Although the available anti-EGFR therapies include monoclonal antibodies that target the EGFR and small molecule tyrosine kinase inhibitors, only cetuximab is U.S. Food and Drug Administration (FDA) approved for the treatment of HNSCC (77,78) (Table 5.7).

Cetuximab, a recombinant human/mouse chimeric monoclonal antibody, is one of the first EGFR inhibitors to be studied in HNSCC. Cetuximab binds specifically to the extracellular domain of the EGFR and competitively inhibits the binding of ligands to the receptor. Human oral SCC cell lines treated with cetuximab demonstrate cell accumulation in the radiosensitive G1 phase, which is associated with increased expression of the cell cycle inhibitors p27 (KIP1) and p15 (INK4B) (82). Furthermore, cetuximab treatment results in a decrease of cells in the S phase of the cell cycle, the phase during which sublethal damage repair in response to RT occurs. In vitro, treatment with cetuximab inhibits ERK1/2 activation, a downstream effector of the MAP kinase pathway. Preclinically, cetuximab is synergistic with RT and with chemotherapy, especially platinum-based cytotoxic chemotherapy (83,84). These findings have served as the basis for the clinical investigation of cetuximab in HNSCC, in a monotherapy and combined modality setting.

Monotherapy. As a single agent, activity has been demonstrated in platinum-refractory patients with recurrent or metastatic disease. Vermorken et al. reported the results of a single-arm, multicenter clinical trial of 103 patients with recurrent or metastatic HNSCC with documented progression within 30 days after two to six cycles of a platinum-based chemotherapy. Cetuximab was administered intravenously at a loading dose of $400 \, mg/m^2$ followed by weekly doses of $250 \, mg/m^2$. The objective response rate of single agent cetuximab was 13%, with a disease control rate (complete response/partial response/stable disease) rate of 46%. Median time to progression was 70 days (79).

Table 5.7 Trials of Single-Agent Epidermal Growth Factor Receptor Inhibitor Therapy in Advanced HNSCC

Authors	Drug	Mechanism	Population	Design	Results
Vermorken et al.	Cetuximab	Monoclonal antibody	Recurrrent or metastatic HNSCC who failed to respond to platinum-based therapy N = total of 103 patients enrolled and treated with cetuximab	Cetuximab $400 \, mg/m^2$ on wk 1 followed by $250 \, mg/m^2$ weekly for at least 6 wks At time of progression, patients could receive same dose of cetuximab plus platinum (N = 53 patients who received combination therapy)	Single-agent response rate 13% Disease control rate 46% TTP 70 days 0% response rate for combination therapy Disease control rate 26% TTP 50 days Median survival for both arms 178 days
Cohen et al.	Gefitinib	Oral small molecule EGFR tyrosine kinase inhibitor	Recurrent or Metastatic HNSCC considered ineligible for curative surgery or radiation therapy N = 52 patients enrolled	Gefitinib administered at a fixed dose of $500 \, mg/day$	Overall response rate 10.6% Disease control rate 53% TTP 3.4 mo Median survival 11.4 mo
Soulieres et al.	Erlotinib		Recurrent or metastatic HNSCC considered ineligible for curative surgery or radiation therapy N = 115 patients	Erlotinib administered at a dose of $150 \, mg/day$	Overall response rate 4.3% Median duration of response 9.7 wks Median PFS 9.6 wks Median overall survival 6.0 mo

Source: From Refs. 79–81.
Abbreviations: HNSCC, head and neck squamous cell carcinoma; TTP, time to progression; PFS, progression-free survival; EGFR, epidermal growth factor receptor; TIP, Time to Progression.

Other trials evaluated cisplatin plus cetuximab in patients who did not achieve complete or partial response to a platinum-based doublet testing the hypothesis that cetuximab may overcome platinum resistance. Trials in this patient population consistently showed a response rate of 10% (85,86). Thus, one can conclude that cetuximab does not overcome platinum resistance but used as monotherapy, second-line, has a response rate of 10–13%.

In combination with cytotoxic chemotherapy. The results of two trials show improved outcomes when cetuximab is added to platinum-based chemotherapy as first-line treatment of patients with recurrent or metastatic disease (87). A randomized, placebo-controlled trial reported by Burtness et al. compared cetuximab and cisplatin with placebo and cisplatin. The addition of cetuximab to cisplatin improved the response rate from 10% (placebo and cisplatin) to 26% (cetuximab and cisplatin), $p = 0.03$. Interestingly, EGFR expression was not predictive of response. In fact, patients with the highest density and intensity of staining of the EGFR (by immunohistochemistry) demonstrated a relative resistance to the addition of cetuximab, perhaps related to undersaturation of the EGFR by the monoclonal antibody, or to the activation of alternate signaling pathways that allow biological "escape" from receptor blockade. The second trial, by Vermorken et al., randomized patients to the combination of carboplatin/cisplatin plus 5-fluorouracil with or without the addition of cetuximab. Until recently, no single agents or combination of agents have demonstrated a survival advantage in the metastatic or recurrent disease setting. The results of this trial show a statistically significant improvement in response rate, progression-free survival and overall survival with cetuximab added to the standard platinum plus 5-fluorouracil combination regimen (88). These studies leave the following questions to be addressed in future trials:

1. Is a survival advantage dependent on a particular cytotoxic chemotherapy regimen in combination with cetuximab?
2. Will the survival advantage observed in the trial reported by Vermorken persist once follow-up matures?
3. What is the cost-effectiveness of an expensive intervention in patients with a limited life expectancy?

In combination with radiation therapy. The safety and efficacy of cetuximab plus radiation compared to radiation therapy alone for curative treatment of locally advanced HNSCC has been reported. In a multicenter, controlled clinical trial, 424 patients with stage III/IV HNC (multiple primary sites) were randomized (1:1) to receive cetuximab plus RT versus RT alone. Stratification factors were Karnofsky score (60–80 vs. 90–100), nodal stage (N0 vs. N+), tumor stage [T1–3 vs. T4 using American Joint Committee on Cancer (AJCC) criteria] and RT fractionation (concomitant boost vs. once daily vs. twice-daily). RT was administered for 6–7 weeks. Starting one week before RT, cetuximab was administered as a 400 mg/m² loading dose, followed by 250 mg/m² weekly for the duration of RT. Of the 424 randomized patients, the majority were male, White, and had Karnofsky performance status >80. The majority of patients had oropharyngeal primary tumors. Patient characteristics were similar across study arms. Fifty-six percent of patients received RT therapy with concomitant boost, 26% once

daily RT and 18% twice-daily RT. The primary endpoint of the trial was locoregional control. The results were a statistically significant improvement in locoregional control for the cetuximab plus RT group vs. RT alone (24.4 months vs. 14.9 months, hazard ratio 0.68, $p = 0.005$). The median duration of overall survival also favored the combination arm (49.0 months vs. 29.3 months, hazard ratio 0.74, $p = 0.03$) (89). There was no significant difference in the distant metastatic rate, and it should be noted that local-regional control using the standard definition of event was not reported. These results represent a proof of principle. Interpretation of the results is confounded by the multiple primary sites, inclusion of resectable and unresectable patients, and multiple radiation regimens. It should be emphasized that this novel combination has not been directly and prospectively compared to what is considered the "gold standard" for chemoradiotherapy in locally advanced HNSCC, cisplatin in combination with radiation therapy. Presently, the only indication for using this combination is in patients who are not suitable for treatment with platinum-based chemoradiotherapy due to poor performance status or comorbidities. Otherwise, cetuximab should not be substituted for platinum-based chemoradiotherapy.

Toxicities. Although the toxicity of cetuximab is generally less severe than toxicity associated with cytotoxic chemotherapy, the adverse effects can still be significant. Dermatologic toxicities remain the most common side effect of cetuximab. These include acneform rash, skin drying, and fissuring and inflammatory and infectious sequalae (blepharitis, cellulitis). The rate of acneform rash is approximately 87% with severe rash in 10–17%. Severe hypersensitivity reaction occurs in 3–4% of patients nationally. However, the incidence is substantially higher in certain geographic areas of the country. In some cases, these reactions may be life threatening, (including anaphylaxis, bronchospasm, urticaria, or hypotension). Less severe, Grade 1 or 2 infusion reactions occur in approximately 19% of patients. Other toxicities of single agent cetuximab include hypomagnesemia in 10–15%, pulmonary toxicity (interstitial lung disease) in <0.5% (90).

Angiogenesis Inhibitors

Although experience using anti-VEGF strategies in HNSCC is limited, multiple clinical trials investigating this approach are ongoing. Bevacizumab, a recombinant humanized monoclonal antibody to VEGF, is the most common agent studied as an anti-angiogenic agent for HNSCC. Bevacizumab is FDA approved for the treatment of metastatic colorectal carcinoma and for advanced, incurable non-small-cell lung cancer (91). Because EGFR activation also upregulates VEGF, investigators have completed a phase I/II study of the combination of a small-molecule EGFR tyrosine kinase inhibitor (erlotinib) in combination with bevacizumab (92). Compared to erlotonib alone, the combination reduced expression of endothelial Kinase Domain Region (KDR), EGFR, and VEGF levels. The reported median overall survival of 7.3 months and progression-free survival of 3.9 months compare favorably to historical controls (93). Bevacizumab in combination with RT, 5-flurorouracil, and hydroxyurea was shown to be tolerable and had evidence of potential efficacy in a high-risk HNSCC population. However, these results need to be confirmed in a larger investigation. Clinical investigations that examine the role for bevacizumab in locally advanced curable and metastatic HNSCC are ongoing.

Hypoxia Cell Sensitizers

Tirapazamine, a hypoxic cytotoxin, forms cytotoxic-free radicals which lead to DNA breaks, chromosome aberrations, and cell death in the setting of hypoxia. This agent has garnered significant attention in HNSCC as a concurrent therapy with radiation or chemoradiotherapy. In a multi-institutional phase II trial of concurrent tirapazamine and RT for locally advanced HNSCC, the 1- and 2-year local control rates were 64% and 59%, respectively. These results proved encouraging given that 72% of patients had T3–4 and N2–3 disease (94). In a study from the Trans-Tasman Radiation Oncology Group, 122 previously untreated patients with locally advanced HNSCC were enrolled in a randomized phase II evaluation of tirapazamine, cisplatin, and radiation or 5-fluorouracil, cisplatin, and radiation. Although no difference was noted in 3-year overall failure-free survival rates, the tirapazamine arm noted a trend toward significance for the outcome of 3-year locoregional failure-free rates. In a substudy, pretreatment and midtreatment [^{18}F]-Misonidazole positron emission tomography (PET) scans, a method of imaging hypoxic areas of tumor, were performed. Patients who demonstrated hypoxia on PET scan had significantly reduced risk of locoregional failure with the addition of tirapazamine (95,96). The efficacy of tirapazamine is presently being investigated in a randomized phase III study.

Integration of Targeted Agents into Induction or Concurrent Chemoradiotherapy Regimens

One of the most important questions currently is how to integrate targeted therapy into the standard backbone of established treatments for HNSCC: chemotherapy for metastatic disease, CCR with curative intent for locally advanced disease, and induction chemotherapy. Although many trials are ongoing, few studies to date have been published in the literature. The goal remains to improve treatment efficacy without increasing toxicity. Moreover, as trials are designed, it will be important to understand which subsets of patients ultimately benefit from the integration of these agents.

CLINICAL CHALLENGES WITH CHEMOTHERAPY OR TARGETED AGENTS FOR HNSCC
Measurement of Objective Response

Measurement of objective response, an important means of evaluating the success of treatment, remains difficult in HNSCC. Moreover, the use of targeted agents may not result in traditional tumor response rates. In fact, many of these agents demonstrate cytostatic properties, making the determination of treatment success challenging.

Historically, assessment by conventional radiological methods [such as computed tomography (CT) scan] or direct visualization can be hampered by the anatomic complexity of the region, the presence of ulceration, treatment-related edema, and the frequent occurrence of bacterial superinfection (Table 5.3). Thus, in the head and neck,

accurate tumor measurements using conventional imaging methods can be difficult. Another challenge is the definition of objective response: The Response Evaluation Criteria in Solid Tumors (RECIST) is widely accepted as a method of measuring tumor response. However, several limitations to RECIST should be noted. RECIST relies on a single-diameter measurement that works best for spherical masses. In the head and neck, a lesion may clinically shrink or flatten, but using RECIST criteria, the longest diameter remains the same. Moreover, traditional response rates determined by measurement of size do not apply to targeted agents, which may cause central tumor necrosis or reduction in metabolic activity without change in size. Thus, time to progression or progression-free survival may be more valid "measurements" of efficacy than traditional criteria of size reduction. Traditional trial designs, which rely on response rate, can underestimate or miss the efficacy and utility of a targeted agent.

The use of F2-18 fluorodeoxyglucose positron emission tomography (FDG-PET) has gained considerable interest in the evaluation of response in HNSCC. This technique provides tumor imaging by measuring metabolic activity of tissues and, by identifying changes in their metabolism after a course of therapy, possibly predicting for response. Importantly, the ability of PET to detect residual disease in HNSCC patients treated with definitive RT (with or without chemotherapy) is under study and appears promising. Posttreatment PET imaging with fused CT scan was performed on 28 patients approximately 8 weeks after completing definitive RT for locally advanced HNSCC. In comparison to CT alone, the overall sensitivity and specificity of FDG-PET/CT was 76.9% and 93.3%, compared to 92.3% and 46.7% for CT alone. The accuracy of FDG-PET/CT was 85.5% versus 67.9% for CT alone (97). However, several points should be made concerning this imaging modality:

1. The specificity of PET increases as time from completion of RT-based therapy increases (97,98).
2. All HNSCC are not FDG avid. The sensitivity of FDG-PET is 85% for the baseline diagnosis and staging of HNSCC (99).
3. The role of FDG-PET in evaluation of response by targeted agents is presently under investigation.

Toxicity

Toxicity of chemotherapy is another important consideration in the treatment of HNSCC. Acute and chronic toxicities of therapy can have a significant impact on quality of life. Failure to provide adequate supportive measures may

1. compromise the delivery of curative therapy
2. diminish quality of life
3. lead to excessive morbidity of treatment
4. in some cases may also negatively impact survival.

The late effects of therapy are often poorly captured in contrast to acute effects but may be just as important. If unattended to, these toxicities can significantly diminish the quality of survivorship. One potential benefit to the use of targeted agents is the relatively favorable toxicity profile of these drugs. However even as single agents, dose-limiting toxicity may occur. A common misconception is that targeted agents are better tolerated than a traditional cytotoxic chemotherapy. Although this may be the case with some agents, targeted agents can have significant associated morbidity, especially when combined with other therapies. The potential for negative impact on quality of life must not be underestimated and should be a focus of research in conjunction with standard measurements of efficacy such as response rates and survival. This ability to maximize the risk–benefit ratio of a regimen becomes especially important when treating the patient with incurable recurrent or metastatic disease. Given that the benefit of targeted agents may not be demonstrable with traditional response criteria, it is critical to evaluate the contribution of these agents to symptom control and the quality of survivorship as their "efficacy" may ultimately be demonstrated in these areas. Although few quality-of-life (QOL) studies of targeted agents have been reported in the literature, encouraging results were noted by Curran et al (100). In this QOL analysis of a randomized trial of RT versus RT plus cetuximab in a locally advanced HNSCC population, the addition of cetuximab did not affect negatively the QOL. Investigations of QOL for patients receiving targeted agents alone and in combination with cytotoxics are ongoing.

The Role of Human Papillomavirus (HPV) and Chemotherapy for Oropharyngeal Primaries

The role of human papillomavirus (HPV) in the epidemiology and prognosis of orpharyngeal primary tumors has recently been elucidated. Although HPV demonstrates multiple serotypes, the high-risk serotypes for the development of malignancy include types 16, 18, 31, and 33. These high-risk serotypes produce two viral oncoproteins, E6 and E7, which inactivate TP53 and the retinoblastoma gene product, respectively. Oncogenic HPV causes virtually all cervical SCC. HPV is associated with approximately 60% of oropharyngeal HNSCC (101,102). D'Souza et al. performed a case-control study of HPV in 100 newly diagnosed patients with oropharyngeal SCC and 200 control patients without cancer. Oropharyngeal cancer was significantly associated with HPV type 16, seropositivity for the HPV-16 L1 capsid protein, number of vaginal sex partners, and a high lifetime number of oral sex partners. Importantly, HPV-positive patients with oropharyngeal cancer were more likely to have significantly less tobacco and alcohol use as compared to HPV-negative patients (103).

While an epidemiological association has been noted, the question remains whether HPV positivity affects clinical outcomes in patients with oropharyngeal carcinoma. ECOG 2399, a phase II trial of chemoradiation for organ preservation in respectable stage III or IV SCC of the larynx or oropharynx stratified patients into HPV-positive (determined by in situ hybridization of formalin fixed paraffin embedded tumors) and HPV-negative patients. Response rates after induction chemotherapy and CCR were significantly higher in HPV-positive patients (81.6% vs. 55.2% and 84.2% vs. 56.9%, respectively). HPV-positive patients demonstrated a 72% lower risk of progression and a 79% lower risk of death than the HPV-negative subset (34,104). However, these findings were only demonstrated for the oropharyngeal primaries. Interestingly, in the Bonner trial of cetuximab plus RT versus RT alone for

locally advanced HNSCC, the subset that demonstrated a significant survival advantage was the oropharyngeal primary site (89). Although HPV status was not evaluated in this trial, the question arises whether targeted therapy may be used with equivalent efficacy to cytotoxic chemotherapy in the oropharyngeal primaries that are HPV positive.

CONCLUSIONS

The successful treatment of HNSCC remains a challenging goal. Importantly, survivals and outcomes have improved with recent treatment modalities, including CCR. The elucidation of molecular pathways in HNSCC is expected to further improve on these outcomes. Despite recent advances in therapy, a significant portion of patients still die of this disease each year. Thus, further investigation is warranted to effectively combat this disease and its morbidities.

REFERENCES

1. Pignon JP, le Maitre A, Bourhis J. Meta-analyses of chemotherapy in head and neck cancer (MACH-NC): an update. Int J Radiat Oncol Biol Phys 2007; 69(2 Suppl): S112–4.
2. Vokes EE, Weichselbautn RR, Lippman SM, Hong WK. Head and neck cancer. N Engl J Med 1993; 328: 184–94.
3. Al-Sarraf M. Chemotherapeutic management of head and neck cancer. Cancer Metastasis Rev 1987; 6: 181–98.
4. Forastiere AA, Takasugi BJ, Baker SR et al. High-dose cisplatin in advanced head and neck cancer. Cancer Chemother Pharmacol 1987; 19: 155–8.
5. Mitchell MS, Wawro NW, DeConti RC et al. Effectiveness of high-dose infusions of methotrexate followed by leucovorin in carcinoma of the head and neck. Cancer Res 1968; 28: 1088–94.
6. Kirkwood JM, CanelJos GP, Ervin TJ et al. Increased therapeutic index using moderate dose methotrexate and leucovorin twice weekly vs. weekly high dose methotrexate-leucovorin in patients with advanced squamous carcinoma of the head and neck: a safe new effective regimen. Cancer 1981; 47: 2414–21.
7. Kish JA, Weaver A, Jacobs J et al. Cisplatin and 5-fluorouracil infusion in patients with recurrent and disseminated epidermoid cancer of the head and neck. Cancer 1984; 53: 1819–24.
8. Tapazoglou E, Kish J, Ensley J et al. The activity of a single-agent 5-fluorouracil infusion in advanced and recurrent head and neck cancer. Cancer 1986; 57: 1105–9.
9. Forastiere AA. Use of paclitaxel (Taxol) in squamous cell carcinoma of the head and neck. Semin Oncol 1993; 20(4 Suppl 3): 56–60.
10. Forastiere AA, Shank D, Neuberg D et al. Final report of a phase II evaluation of paclitaxel in patients with advanced squamous cell carcinoma of the head and neck: an Eastern Cooperative Oncology Group trial (PA390). Cancer 1998; 82: 2270–4.
11. Dreyfuss AI, Clark JR, Norris CM et al. Docetaxel: an active drug for squamous cell carcinoma of the head and neck. J Clin Oncol 1996; 14: 1672–8.
12. Samlowski WE, Gundacker H, Kuebler JP et al. Evaluation of gemcitabine in patients with recurrent or metastatic squamous cell carcinoma of the head and neck: a Southwest Oncology Group phase II study. Invest New Drugs 2001; 19: 311–15.
13. Catimel G, Vermorken JB, Clavel M et al. A phase II study of gemcitabine (LY 188011) in patients with advanced squamous cell carcinoma of the head and neck. EORTC Early Clinical Trials Group. Ann Oncol 1994; 5: 543–7.

14. Chua DT, Sham JS, Au GK. A phase II study of capecitabine in patients with recurrent and metastatic nasopharyngeal carcinoma pretreated with platinum-based chemotherapy. Oral Oncol 2003; 39: 361–6.

15. Veronesi A, Zagonel V, Tirelli U et al. High-dose versus low-dose cisplatin in advanced head and neck squamous carcinoma: a randomized study. J Clin Oncol 1985; 3: 1105–8.

16. Al-Sarraf M. New approaches to the management of head and neck cancer. The role of chemotherapy. Adv Oncol 1990: 11–14.

17. Forastiere AA, Metch B, Keppen M et al. Randomised comparison of cisplatin +5-FU vs carboplatin +5 FU vs methotrexate in advanced squamous cell carcinoma of the head and neck. J Clin Oncol 1992; 10: 1245–51.

18. Cmelak AJ, Murphy BA, Burkey B et al. Taxane-based chemoirradiation for organ preservation with locally advanced head and neck cancer: results of a phase II multi-institutional trial. Head Neck 2007; 29: 315–24.

19. Chougule PB, Akhtar MS, Rathore R et al. Concurrent chemoradiotherapy with weekly paclitaxel and carboplatin for locally advanced head and neck cancer: long-term follow-up of a Brown University Oncology Group Phase II Study (HN-53). Head Neck 2008; 30: 289–96.

20. Zhang L, Zhao C, Peng PJ et al. Phase III study comparing standard radiotherapy with or without weekly oxaliplatin in treatment of locoregionally advanced nasopharyngeal carcinoma: preliminary results. J Clin Oncol 2005; 23: 8461–8.

21. Taylor SG 4th, McGuire WP, Hauck WW et al. A randomized comparison of high-dose infusion methotrexate versus standard-dose weekly therapy in head and neck squamous cancer. J Clin Oncol 1984; 2: 1006–11.

22. Woods RL, Fox RM, Tattersall MH. Methotrexate treatment of squamous-cell head and neck cancers: dose-response evaluation. Br Med J (Clin Res, ed) 1981; 282: 600–2.

23. Robert F. Trimetrexate as a single agent in patients with advanced head and neck cancer. Semin Oncol 1988; 15(2 Suppl 2): 22–6.

24. Schornagel JH, Verweij J, de Mulder PH et al. Randomized phase III trial of edatrexate versus methotrexate in patients with metastatic and/or recurrent squamous cell carcinoma of the head and neck: a European Organization for Research and Treatment of Cancer Head and Neck Cancer Cooperative Group study. J Clin Oncol 1995; 13: 1649–55.

25. Degardin M, Domenge C, Cappelaere P et al. A phase II study of piritrexim in patients with advanced squamous cell carcinoma of the head and neck. Eur J Cancer 1994; 30A: 1044–5.

26. Paz-Ares L, Ciruelos E, Garcia-Carbonero R et al. Pemetrexed in bladder, head and neck, and cervical cancers. Semin Oncol 2002; 29(6 Suppl 18): 69–75.

27. Pivot X, Raymond E, Laguerre B et al. Pemetrexed disodium in recurrent locally advanced or metastatic squamous cell carcinoma of the head and neck. Br J Cancer 2001; 85: 649–55.

28. Adjei AA. Preclinical and clinical studies with combinations of pemetrexed and gemcitabine. Semin Oncol 2002; 29(6 Suppl 18): 30–4.

29. Ringel I, Horwitz SB. Studies with RP 56976 (taxotere): a semisynthetic analogue of taxol. J Natl Cancer Inst 1991; 83: 288–91.

30. Forastiere AA, Leong T, Rowinsky E et al. Phase III comparison of high-dose paclitaxel + cisplatin + granulocyte colony-stimulating factor versus low-dose paclitaxel + cisplatin in advanced head and neck cancer: Eastern Cooperative Oncology Group Study E1393. J Clin Oncol 2001; 19: 1088–95.

31. Bissery MC, Guenard D, Guéritte-Voegelein F et al. Experimental antitumor activity of taxotere (RP 56976, NSC 628503), a taxol analogue. Cancer Res 1991; 51: 4845–52.

32. Tishler RB, Geard CR, Hall EJ et al. Taxol sensitizes human astrocytoma cells to radiation. Cancer Res 1992; 52: 3495–7.

33. Tishler RB, Schiff PB, Geard CR et al. Taxol: a novel radiation sensitizer. Int J Radiat Oncol Biol Phys 1992; 22: 613–17.

34. Cmelak AJ, Li S, Goldwasser MA et al. Phase II trial of chemoradiation for organ preservation in resectable stage III or IV squamous cell carcinomas of the larynx or oropharynx: results of Eastern Cooperative Oncology Group Study E2399. J Clin Oncol 2007; 25: 3971–7.

35. Willey CD, Murphy BA, Netterville JL et al. A Phase II multi-institutional trial of chemoradiation using weekly docetaxel and erythropoietin for high-risk postoperative head and neck cancer patients. Int J Radiat Oncol Biol Phys 2007; 67: 1323–31.

36. Jacobs C, Meyers F, Hendrickson C et al. A randomized phase III study of cisplatin with or without methotrexate for recurrent squamous cell carcinoma of the head and neck. A Northern California Oncology Group study. Cancer 1983; 52: 1563–9.

37. Chauvergne J, Cappelaere P, Fargeot P et al. [A randomized study comparing cisplatin alone or combined in the palliative treatment of carcinoma of the head and neck. Analysis of a series of 209 patients]. Bull Cancer 1988; 75: 9–22.

38. Forastiere AA, Metch B, Schuller DE et al. Randomized comparison of cisplatin plus fluorouracil and carboplatin plus fluorouracil versus methotrexate in advanced squamous-cell carcinoma of the head and neck: a Southwest Oncology Group study. J Clin Oncol 1992; 10: 1245–51.

39. Gibson MK, Li Y, Murphy B et al. Randomized phase III evaluation of cisplatin plus fluorouracil versus cisplatin plus paclitaxel in advanced head and neck cancer (E1395): an intergroup trial of the Eastern Cooperative Oncology Group. J Clin Oncol 2005; 23: 3562–7.

40. Fountzilas G, Papakostas P, Dafhi U et al. Paclitaxel and gemcitabine vs. paclitaxel and pegylated liposomal doxorubicin in advanced non-nasopharyngeal head and neck cancer. An efficacy and cost analysis randomized study conducted by the Hellenic Cooperative Oncology Group. Ann Oncol 2006; 17: 1560–7.

41. Clavel M, Vermorken JB, Cognetti F et al. Randomized comparison of cisplatin, methotrexate, bleomycin and vincristine (CABO) versus cisplatin and 5-fluorouracil (CF) versus cisplatin (C) in recurrent or metastatic squamous cell carcinoma of the head and neck. A phase III study of the EORTC Head and Neck Cancer Cooperative Group. Ann Oncol 1994; 5: 521–6.

42. Gilbert J, Forastiere AA. Organ preservation trials for laryngeal cancer. Otolaryngol Clin North Am 2002; 35: 1035–54, vi.

43. Merlano M, Benasso M, Corvó R et al. Five-year update of a randomized trial of alternating radiotherapy and chemotherapy compared with radiotherapy alone in treatment of unresectable squamous cell carcinoma of the head and neck. J Natl Cancer Inst 1996; 88: 583–9.

44. Denis F, Garaud P, Bardet E et al. Final results of the 94–01 French Head and Neck Oncology and Radiotherapy Group randomized trial comparing radiotherapy alone with concomitant radiochemotherapy in advanced-stage oropharynx carcinoma. J Clin Oncol 2004; 22: 69–76.

45. Forastiere AA, Goepfert H, Maor M et al. Concurrent chemotherapy and radiotherapy for organ preservation in advanced laryngeal cancer. N Engl J Med 2003; 349: 2091–8.

46. Brizel DM, Leopold KA, Fisher SR et al. A phase I/II trial of twice daily irradiation and concurrent chemotherapy for locally advanced squamous cell carcinoma of the head and neck. Int J Radiat Oncol Biol Phys 1994; 28: 213–20.

47. Adelstein DJ, Li Y, Adams GL et al. An intergroup phase III comparison of standard radiation therapy and two schedules of concurrent chemoradiotherapy in patients with

unresectable squamous cell head and neck cancer. J Clin Oncol 2003; 21: 92–8.

48. Bernier J, Domenge C, Ozsahin M et al. Postoperative irradiation with or without concomitant chemotherapy for locally advanced head and neck cancer. N Engl J Med 2004; 350: 1945–52.

49. Cooper JS, Pajak TF, Forastiere AA et al. Postoperative concurrent radiotherapy and chemotherapy for high-risk squamous-cell carcinoma of the head and neck. N Engl J Med 2004; 350: 1937–44.

50. Bernier J, Cooper JS, Pajak TF et al. Defining risk levels in locally advanced head and neck cancers: a comparative analysis of concurrent postoperative radiation plus chemotherapy trials of the EORTC (#22931) and RTOG (#9501). Head Neck 2005; 27: 843–50.

51. Cooper JS, Pajak TF, Forastiere A et al. Long term survival results of a phase III integroup trial (RTOG 95–01) of surgery followed by radiotherapy vs. radiochemotherapy for resectable high risk squamous cell carcinoma of the head and neck. N Engl J Med 2004; 350: 1937–44.

52. Induction chemotherapy plus radiation compared with surgery plus radiation in patients with advanced laryngeal cancer. The Department of Veterans Affairs Laryngeal Cancer Study Group. N Engl J Med 1991; 324: 1685–90.

53. Terrell JE, Fisher SG, Wolf GT. Long-term quality of life after treatment of laryngeal cancer. The Veterans Affairs Laryngeal Cancer Study Group. Arch Otolaryngol Head Neck Surg 1998; 124: 964–71.

54. Lefebvre JL, Chevalier D, Luboinski B et al. Larynx preservation in pyriform sinus cancer: preliminary results of a European Organization for Research and Treatment of Cancer phase III trial. EORTC Head and Neck Cancer Cooperative Group. J Natl Cancer Inst 1996; 88: 890–9.

55. Domenge C, Hill C, Lefebvre JL et al. Randomized trial of neoadjuvant chemotherapy in oropharyngeal carcinoma. French Groupe d'Etude des Tumeurs de la Tete et du Cou (GETTEC). Br J Cancer 2000; 83: 1594–8.

56. Zorat PL, Paccagnella A, Cavaniglia G et al. Randomized phase III trial of neoadjuvant chemotherapy in head and neck cancer: 10-year follow-up. J Natl Cancer Inst 2004; 96: 1714–17.

57. Paccagnella A, Orlando A, Marchiori C et al. Phase III trial of initial chemotherapy in stage III or IV head and neck cancers: a study by the Gruppo di Studio sui Tumori della Testa e del Collo. J Natl Cancer Inst 1994; 86: 265–72.

58. Posner MR, Hershock DM, Blajman CR et al. Cisplatin and fluorouracil alone or with docetaxel in head and neck cancer. N Engl J Med 2007; 357: 1705–15.

59. Hitt R, Lopez-Pousa A, Martinez-Trufero J et al. Phase III study comparing cisplatin plus fluorouracil to paclitaxel, cisplatin, and fluorouracil induction chemotherapy followed by chemoradiotherapy in locally advanced head and neck cancer. J Clin Oncol 2005; 23: 8636–45.

60. Vermorken JB, Remenar E, van Herpen C, et al. Cisplatin, fluorouracil and docetaxel in unresectable head and neck cancer. N Engl J Med 2007; 357: 1695–704.

61. Al-Sarraf M, LeBlanc M, Giri PG et al. Chemoradiotherapy versus radiotherapy in patients with advanced nasopharyngeal cancer: phase III randomized Intergroup study 0099. J Clin Oncol 1998; 16: 1310–17.

62. Lee AW, Lau WH, Tung SY et al. Preliminary results of a randomized study on therapeutic gain by concurrent chemotherapy for regionally-advanced nasopharyngeal carcinoma: NPC-9901 Trial by the Hong Kong Nasopharyngeal Cancer Study Group. J Clin Oncol 2005; 23: 6966–75.

63. Chan AT, Teo PM, Ngan RK et al. Concurrent chemotherapy-radiotherapy compared with radiotherapy alone in locoregionally advanced nasopharyngeal carcinoma: progression-free

survival analysis of a phase III randomized trial. J Clin Oncol 2002; 20: 2038–44.

64. Ma J, Mai HQ, Hong MH et al. Results of a prospective randomized trial comparing neoadjuvant chemotherapy plus radiotherapy with radiotherapy alone in patients with locoregionally advanced nasopharyngeal carcinoma. J Clin Oncol 2001; 19: 1350–7.

65. Baselga J, Arteaga CL. Critical update and emerging trends in epidermal growth factor receptor targeting in cancer. J Clin Oncol 2005; 23: 2445–59.

66. Kyzas PA, Stefanou D, Batistatou A et al. Prognostic significance of VEGF immunohistochemical expression and tumor angiogenesis in head and neck squamous cell carcinoma. J Cancer Res Clin Oncol 2005; 131: 624–30.

67. Rosen LS. VEGF-targeted therapy: therapeutic potential and recent advances. Oncologist 2005; 10: 382–91.

68. Caballero M, Grau JJ, Blanch JL et al. Serum vascular endothelial growth factor as a predictive factor in metronomic (weekly) paclitaxel treatment for advanced head and neck cancer. Arch Otolaryngol Head Neck Surg 2007; 133: 1143–8.

69. Tae K, El-Naggar AK, Yoo E et al. Expression of vascular endothelial growth factor and microvessel density in head and neck tumorigenesis. Clin Cancer Res 2000; 6: 2821–8.

70. McMahon G. VEGF receptor signaling in tumor angiogenesis. Oncologist 2000; 5(Suppl 1): 3–10.

71. Forsythe JA, Jiang BH, Jyer NV et al. Activation of vascular endothelial growth factor gene transcription by hypoxia-inducible factor 1. Mol Cell Biol 1996; 16: 4604–13.

72. Wouters A, Pauwels B, Lardon F et al. Review: implications of in vitro research on the effect of radiotherapy and chemotherapy under hypoxic conditions. Oncologist 2007; 12: 690–712.

73. Mohamed KM, Le A, Duong H et al. Correlation between VEGF and HIF-1alpha expression in human oral squamous cell carcinoma. Exp Mol Pathol 2004; 76: 143–52.

74. Gross J, Fuchs J, Machulik A et al. Apoptosis, necrosis and hypoxia inducible factor-1 in human head and neck squamous cell carcinoma cultures. Int J Oncol 2005; 27: 807–14.

75. Kyzas PA, Stefanou D, Batistatou A et al. Hypoxia-induced tumor angiogenic pathway in head and neck cancer: an in vivo study. Cancer Lett 2005; 225: 297–304.

76. De Schutter H, Landuyt W, Verbeken E et al. The prognostic value of the hypoxia markers CA IX and GLUT 1 and the cytokines VEGF and IL 6 in head and neck squamous cell carcinoma treated by radiotherapy +/- chemotherapy. BMC Cancer 2005; 5: 42.

77. Pomerantz RG, Grandis JR. The role of epidermal growth factor receptor in head and neck squamous cell carcinoma. Curr Oncol Rep 2003; 5: 140–6.

78. Ciardiello F, Tortora G. Anti-epidermal growth factor receptor drugs in cancer therapy. Expert Opin Investig Drugs 2002; 11: 755–68.

79. Vermorken JB, Trigo J, Hitt R et al. Open-label, uncontrolled, multicenter phase II study to evaluate the efficacy and toxicity of cetuximab as a single agent in patients with recurrent and/or metastatic squamous cell carcinoma of the head and neck who failed to respond to platinum-based therapy. J Clin Oncol 2007; 25: 2171–7.

80. Cohen EE, Rosen F, Stadler WM et al. Phase II trial of ZD1839 in recurrent or metastatic squamous cell carcinoma of the head and neck. J Clin Oncol 2003; 21: 1980–7.

81. Soulieres D, SenzerNN, Vokes EE et al. Multicenter phase II study of erlotinib, an oral epidermal growth factor receptor tyrosine kinase inhibitor, in patients with recurrent or metastatic squamous cell cancer of the head and neck. J Clin Oncol 2004; 22: 77–85.

82. Kiyota A, Shintani S, Mihara M et al. Anti-epidermal growth factor receptor monoclonal antibody 225 upregulates

p27(KIP1) and p15(INK4B) and induces G1 arrest in oral squamous carcinoma cell lines. Oncology 2002; 63: 92–8.

83. Huang SM, Li J, Harari PM. Monoclonal antibody blockade of the epidermal growth factor receptor in cancer therapy. Cancer Chemother Biol Response Modif 2001; 19: 339–52.

84. Bonner JA, Raisch KP, Trummell HQ et al. Enhanced apoptosis with combination C225/radiation treatment serves as the impetus for clinical investigation in head and neck cancers. J Clin Oncol 2000; 18(21 Suppl): 47S–53S.

85. Baselga J, Trigo JM, Bourhis J et al. Phase II multicenter study of the antiepidermal growth factor receptor monoclonal antibody cetuximab in combination with platinum-based chemotherapy in patients with platinum-refractory metastatic and/or recurrent squamous cell carcinoma of the head and neck. J Clin Oncol 2005; 23: 5568–77.

86. Herbst RS, Arquette M, Shin DM et al. Phase II multicenter study of the epidermal growth factor receptor antibody cetuximab and cisplatin for recurrent and refractory squamous cell carcinoma of the head and neck. J Clin Oncol 2005; 23: 5578–87.

87. Burtness B, Goldwasser MA, Flood W et al. Phase III randomized trial of cisplatin plus placebo compared with cisplatin plus cetuximab in metastatic/recurrent head and neck cancer: an Eastern Cooperative Oncology Group study. J Clin Oncol 2005; 23: 8646–54.

88. Vermorken J, Mesia R, Rivera F et al. Platinum-based chemotherapy plus cetuximab in head and neck cancer. N Engl J Med 2008; 359: 1116–27.

89. Bonner JA, Harari PM, Giralt J et al. Radiotherapy plus cetuximab for squamous-cell carcinoma of the head and neck. N Engl J Med 2006; 354: 567–78.

90. ERBITUX (cetuximab) [package insert]. New York, NY: Imclone Systems Inc. and Princeton, NJ Bristol-myers squibb co.; November 2008.

91. Chen HX. Expanding the clinical development of bevacizumab. Oncologist 2004; 9 Suppl 1: 27–35.

92. Seiwert TY, Davis DW, Yan AM, et al. pKDR/KDR ratio predicts response in a phase I/II pharmacodynamic study of erlotinib and bevacizumab for recurrent or metastatic head and neck cancer (HNC). Journal of Clinical Oncology 2007; 25, 18S(June 20 Suppl): 6021.

93. Seiwert TY, Haraf DJ, Cohen EE et al. A phase I study of bevacizumab (B) with fluorouracil (F) and hydroxyurea (H) with concomitant radiotherapy (X) (B-FHX) for poor prognosis head and neck cancer (HNC). J Clin Oncol 2008; 26: 1732–41.

94. Le QT, Taira A, Budenz S et al. Mature results from a randomized Phase II trial of cisplatin plus 5-fluorouracil and radiotherapy with or without tirapazamine in patients with resectable Stage IV head and neck squamous cell carcinomas. Cancer 2006; 106: 1940–9.

95. Rischin D, Peters L, Fisher R et al. Tirapazamine, cisplatin, and radiation versus fluorouracil, cisplatin, and radiation in patients with locally advanced head and neck cancer: a randomized phase II trial of the Trans-Tasman Radiation Oncology Group (TROG 98.02). J Clin Oncol 2005; 23: 79-87.

96. Rischin D, Hicks RJ, Fisher R et al. Prognostic significance of [18F]-misonidazole positron emission tomography-detected tumor hypoxia in patients with advanced head and neck cancer randomly assigned to chemoradiation with or without tirapazamine: a substudy of Trans-Tasman Radiation Oncology Group Study 98.02. J Clin Oncol 2006; 24: 2098–104.

97. Andrade RS, Heron DE, Degirmenci B et al. Posttreatment assessment of response using FDG-PET/CT for patients treated with definitive radiation therapy for head and neck cancers. Int J Radiat Oncol Biol Phys 2006; 65: 1315–22.

98. Kim SY, Lee SW, Nam SY et al. The feasibility of 18F-FDG PET scans 1 month after completing radiotherapy of squamous cell carcinoma of the head and neck. J Nucl Med 2007; 48: 373–8.

99. Dammann F, Horger M, Mueller-Berg M et al. Rational diagnosis of squamous cell carcinoma of the head and neck region: comparative evaluation of CT, MRI, and 18FDG PET. AJR Am J Roentgenol 2005; 184: 1326–31.

100. Curran D, Giralt J, Harari PM et al. Quality of life in head and neck cancer patients after treatment with high-dose radiotherapy alone or in combination with cetuximab. J Clin Oncol 2007; 25: 2191–7.

101. Ringstrom E, Peters E, Hasegawa M et al. Human papillomavirus type 16 and squamous cell carcinoma of the head and neck. Clin Cancer Res 2002; 8: 3187–92.

102. Gillison ML, Koch WM, Capone RB et al. Evidence for a causal association between human papillomavirus and a subset of head and neck cancers. J Natl Cancer Inst 2000; 92: 709–20.

103. D'Souza G, Kreimer AR, Viscidi R et al. Case-control study of human papillomavirus and oropharyngeal cancer. N Engl J Med 2007; 356: 1944–56.

104. Fakhry C, Westra WH, Li S et al. Improved survival of patients with human papillomavirus-positive head and neck squamous cell carcinoma in a prospective clinical trial. J Natl Cancer Inst 2008; 100: 261–9.

6

Anesthesia for Head and Neck Cancer

Colm Irving

INTRODUCTION

The peri-operative anesthetic management of patients undergoing resection of tumors of the head and neck presents the anesthetist with a unique set of challenges (1,2), which can be grouped into seven main categories:

1. Preoperative assessment
2. The difficult airway
3. The shared airway
4. Pharyngolaryngo-oesophagectomy
5. Anesthetic complications and techniques in head and neck surgery
6. Management of the free flap
7. Postoperative care

The goal of this chapter is to give the surgeon a basic knowledge of those aspects of anesthetic management that have either a direct bearing on surgical access and technique or contribute overall to a good outcome.

PREOPERATIVE ASSESSMENT
Concurrent Disease

The vast majority of patients will be in their sixth or seventh decade, many with a history of smoking and heavy alcohol intake and are therefore likely to have significant concurrent disease that will require evaluation and possible remedial treatment. It is beyond the scope of this chapter to discuss individual conditions in detail, but certain key factors should be taken into account when considering the extent of preoperative investigation and preparation (Tables 6.1 and 6.2).

Airway Assessment

A detailed assessment of the airway is mandatory in this population of patients to predict difficult intubations. The essence of the dilemma that faces the anesthetist is that some patients who are difficult to intubate may become totally obstructed and therefore impossible to ventilate by facemask following the induction of general anesthesia due to the attendant loss of supportive muscle tone in an already partially obstructed airway. This is the classic "can't intubate can't ventilate" scenario with rapid onset of hypoxia and ultimately cardiac arrest if the airway is not secured. The induction of general anesthesia in this subgroup of patients is therefore potentially life threatening, and the anesthetist should attempt to identify these patients beforehand and have a clear plan for securing the airway.

History

The anesthetic record of any preliminary direct or indirect endoscopy will give valuable information about the ease or difficulty of airway management. Previous resection may distort and scar normal anatomy, and previous irradiation of the head and neck can cause fibrosis. All of these factors will render tissues inflexible and difficult to displace during direct laryngoscopy. The presence of a tracheostomy will naturally simplify airway management but it is advisable to ascertain whether the tracheostomy tube may be attached directly to the anesthetic circuit, if not it will require replacement.

Examination and Predictive Tests

Conventional methods of tracheal intubation depend on the ability of the anesthetist to view the glottis directly under general anesthesia with a rigid laryngoscope. The glottis can only be visualized directly if the patient can open his or her mouth sufficiently wide, there is enough mandibular space into which the soft tissues may be displaced anteriorly by the instrument, and the patient can extend the head on the neck to line up the mouth with the glottis. Several simple bedside tests for these factors have been devised that may be used to predict the likelihood of a difficult intubation (Table 6.3).

More elaborate tests involving either a combination of risk factors such as the Wilson test (12) or radiological assessment of the mandible or the cervical spine exist but are not practical enough to perform routinely.

A problem common to all of these predictive tests used either alone or in combination (13) is that although sensitivity can be up to 90% (i.e., 90% of difficult intubations are correctly predicted) positive predictive value is poor. Because difficult intubation is rare compared to the very large number of "easy" intubations any predictive test with a specificity less than 100% will yield a large number of false positives compared to the number of true positives. This means that many patients predicted to be difficult will in fact be easy (14). Another fundamental problem with these tests in this group of patients is that they cannot give any indication of potential obstruction from tongue base or supraglottic tumors that can block the airway when pharyngeal tone is lost on induction of anesthesia (15).

Investigations

These tests are therefore at best useful indicators, and a true picture of the airway can only be built up by combining

Table 6.1   Key Factors in Preoperative Assessment

Tumor progression with or without encroachment into the airway may limit the time available for medical improvement.

It is essential to optimize any unstable cardiac condition such as ischemia or dysrhythmia

Surgery confined to the head and neck, even that involving major reconstruction, is generally speaking less likely to interfere with postoperative respiratory function than surgery to the chest and abdomen and therefore the potential for postoperative cardiorespiratory complications is less. Intracavity surgery involving the chest or abdomen carries a higher risk. Cardiopulmonary exercising (CPX) testing is proving to be a useful method of risk stratification for this higher risk group with significant morbidity and mortality in those with an anaerobic threshold below 11 mls/kg/mn.

Patients with a history of alcohol abuse may have alcoholic liver disease or alcoholic cardiomyopathy that will require further investigation prior to surgery.

Preoperative serum albumin is a good predictor of surgical outcome. A level below 21 g/dl is associated with an increase in morbidity and mortality rates to 65% and 29%, respectively, in surgery of all types. Nutritional must be optimized in the time available preferably using the enteral route.

Source: From Refs. 3–5.

Table 6.2   Preoperative Investigations

FBC	All patients for general anesthesia
Sickle screen	All patients of African descent (A positive sickle test must be followed up with hemoglobin electrophoresis)
U&E	All patients for intermediate/major surgery
	All patients on diuretics
	All patients with a history of renal impairment
Calcium	Any patient with a history of thyroid or parathyroid surgery or undergoing laryngectomy
ECG	All patients with a history of cardiovascular disease
	As a baseline investigation in all patients older than age 40 years for general anesthesia
LFTs	Patients with a history of heavy alcohol consumption
Clotting screen	All patients on anticoagulants
	All patients with abnormal LFTs.
	All patients undergoing major/complex surgery.
Chest X-ray	All patients with acute respiratory symptoms or suspected tuberculosis
	All patients with chronic cardiorespiratory disorders who have not been x-rayed in the last 6 months
PFTs	All patients undergoing thoracotomy
	All patients with chronic airways disease

Source: From Refs. 6 and 7.
Abbreviations: U&E, urea and electrolytes; ECG, electrocardiogram; LFTs, liver function tests; PFTs, pulmonary function tests.

their results with the results of previous laryngoscopic examination and computed tomography (CT) or magnetic resonance imaging (MRI) imaging (Table 6.4). Cervical spine flexion and extension views are indicated in rheumatoid arthritis to assess the stability of the atlanto-axial joint.

Table 6.3   Tests to Predict Difficult Intubation

Mallampati described a test, subsequently modified, which grades the visibility of pharyngeal structures (Fig. 6.1); a high grade suggests a lack of mandibular space and a potential difficult intubation.

Patients with trismus will be unable to open their mouths wide enough to view any pharyngeal structures and mouth opening should then be recorded in centimeters.

The Patil test measures the mandibular space and the ability to extend the head (Fig. 6.2). The thyromental distance is the distance from the inside of the mentum to the thyroid cartilage with the head fully extended on the neck. A distance of less than 6.5 cm is predictive of a difficult intubation.

Mandibular protrusion is a useful indicator of mandibular mobility. Class C protrusion, the inability to protrude the lower incisors beyond the upper, being associated with a high incidence of difficult laryngoscopy

Source: From Refs. 8–11.

THE DIFFICULT AIRWAY

Management of the difficult airway is a complex area, which many authors have attempted to rationalize in the form of management algorithms (16). These algorithms are rather unwieldy for everyday use particularly in the emergency situation but are useful in that they outline the general principles around which the anesthetist must formulate a plan for each particular patient in cooperation with the surgical team. A simplified airway management algorithm is shown (Fig. 6.3). The first step in this algorithm is to predict the difficulty of intubation, notwithstanding the shortcomings of our present methods it is possible to construct a list of fairly reliable predictors of difficult intubation (Table 6.5). In practice the purpose of these predictors is to identify those patients who require an awake intubation. *Awake intubation* refers to any method of intubating the trachea before the induction of general anesthesia thus ensuring the maintenance of airway tone, self-ventilation of the lungs, and therefore oxygenation in the event that orotracheal or nasotracheal intubation cannot be achieved. In the opinion of the author trismus, mandibular immobility and tongue base or supraglottic masses are absolute indications for awake intubation.

High Degree of Predicted Difficulty: Awake Intubation

The most commonly employed method is awake intubation using a flexible fiber optic bronchoscope after preparing the patient with a combination of conscious sedation and local anesthesia of the airway, in skilled hands it is well tolerated and is associated with cardiovascular stability and good oxygen saturation (17,18). A variety of agents have been used alone or in combination to provide conscious sedation including benzodiazepines, propofol, and opiates. Remifentanil is a potent, short-acting opiate that provides excellent conscious sedation while possessing the advantage of rapid offset in the event of airway obstruction (18). Local anesthesia of the nasopharynx, oropharynx, and larynx will provide analgesia and depress airway reflexes such as gagging, laryngospasm, and coughing that will hinder the passage of the scope and obscure the view. Lignocaine can be administered directly to mucosal surfaces as 2% gel, 4% solution, or a 10% aerosol spray or can be inhaled via a nebulizer taking care not to exceed the maximum dose of 3 mg/kg.

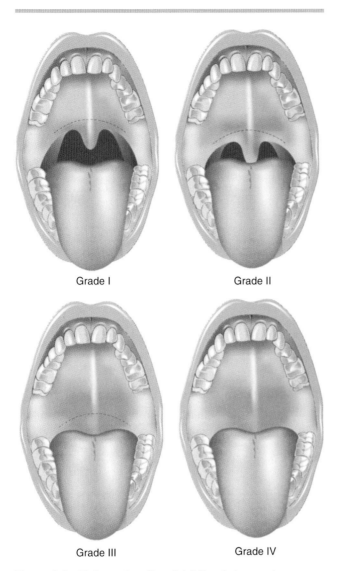

Grade I — Grade II

Grade III — Grade IV

Figure 6.1 Mallampati grading of visibility of pharyngeal structures. The posterior pharyngeal wall is visible below the soft palate in grades I and II, posterior pharyngeal wall not visible in grades III and IV. *Source*: Adapted from Ref. 9.

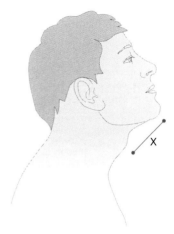

Figure 6.2 The Patil test of thyromental distance. A distance of less than 6.5 cm is predictive of a difficult intubation. *Source*: Adapted from Ref. 10.

attempt to preserve airway tone and spontaneous breathing until adequate mask ventilation can be established at which point the patient can be paralyzed or anesthesia deepened to facilitate intubation. If intubation proves difficult but the lungs can still be ventilated (can ventilate cannot intubate) endotracheal intubation will be achieved in the majority of cases using one of the following techniques for difficult asleep intubation (Table 6.7).

If one finds that the lungs cannot be ventilated nor the trachea intubated (can't ventilate can't intubate) there are several techniques (Table 6.8) that may help to achieve adequate ventilation of the lungs. However these are temporizing measures only, and the safest option is to wake the patient up and then attempt an awake fiber optic intubation or tracheostomy under local anesthetic. If it is thought that the patient will not wake before hypoxia or hypercarbia cause a cardiac arrest one must proceed immediately to an emergency tracheostomy or cricothyroidotomy.

The Management of Stridor

The presence of stridor is indicative of a 50% reduction in airway diameter and can result from tumor progression or postoperative/postextubation airway swelling. Stridor is a medical emergency, and the anesthetic team should always be notified and intensive care warned of a potential admission. If the cause is tumor progression, management involves securing the airway with an endotracheal tube or tracheostomy (vide infra) before the tumor causes complete obstruction. Medical management can buy valuable time by reducing the degree of stridor or temporarily eliminating it allowing definitive intervention in less pressured circumstances. Postoperative stridor management depends on the underlying cause and may occasionally require an anesthetic or surgical airway.

Heliox

Helium is markedly less dense than oxygen and nitrogen. The density of a gas determines its ability to maintain

The vocal cords and trachea can be anesthetized by spraying lignocaine 4% solution through the suction channel of the bronchoscope ("spray as you go") or injecting through the cricothyroid membrane. Table 6.6 outlines a simple technique for awake fiber optic intubation under remifentanil sedation. Tracheostomy or cricothyroidotomy under local anesthetic is the recommended technique for securing the airway in cases of severe acute airway obstruction. Indeed it is one situation where awake fiber optic intubation is absolutely contraindicated (19) because of the risk of precipitating complete obstruction as a result of irritation of the airway, bleeding, or dislodging friable tumor.

Lesser Degrees of Predicted Difficulty

For these patients conventional asleep intubation is indicated. Anesthesia should be induced either with a slow intravenous injection or with an inhalational agent in an

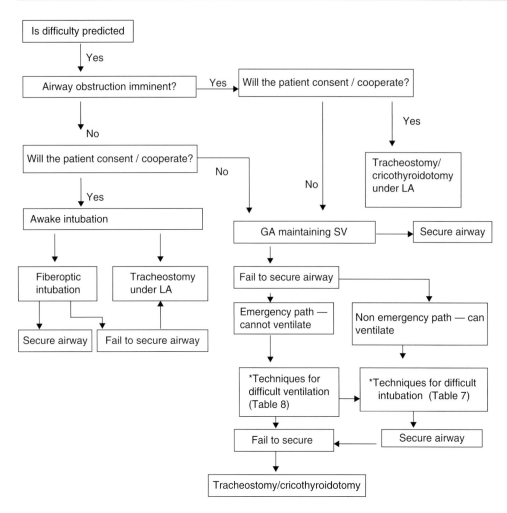

Figure 6.3 Algorithm for management of the difficult airway. *Abbreviations*: LA, local anesthesia; GA, general anesthesia; SV, spontaneous ventilation. *If the airway cannot be secured rapidly at this point with an anesthetic technique proceed immediately to a surgical airway, repeated instrumentation will precipitate complete obstruction.

Table 6.4   Summary of Preoperative Airway Assessment

History	Recent anesthetic record
	Previous surgery/tracheostomy
	Previous irradiation
Examination	Mallampati test
	Patil test
	Mouth opening
	Mandibular protrusion
	Neck extension
Investigation	Direct/fiber optic laryngoscopy
	CT/MRI
	Cervical spine X-ray in rheumatoid arthritis

Abbreviations: CT, computed tomography; MRL, magnetic resonance imaging.

Table 6.5   Findings Suggestive of Difficult Intubation. Those Marked[a] are Absolute Indications for Awake Intubation

Class C mandibular protrusion
Trismus (interincisor distance of less than 3 cm)[a]
Mallampati grade greater than II
Thyromental distance less than 6.5 cm (or less than three finger breadths)
Immobile mandibular space due to tumor, previous surgery, or irradiation[a]
Inability to extend neck or touch chin on chest
Tongue base or supraglottic masses on imaging[a]

laminar flow, the lower the density the greater the likelihood that flow will be laminar. Laminar flow allows a greater flow rate for a given pressure difference. Low density also improves flow rates when flow is turbulent.

Heliox (20) is a mixture of helium and oxygen in the ratio of 79%:21%, it is 3 times less dense than air. This means that in the turbulent flow conditions likely to be encountered in upper airway obstruction. Heliox will facilitate the transfer of oxygen and reduce the work of breathing. One limiting factor in the use of helium/oxygen mixtures is the necessity to keep the concentration of oxygen less than 40% to maintain the advantages of low density, for some patients an oxygen concentration of 21% may be too low despite the improved flow characteristics.

Table 6.6 Technique for Awake Intubation Using the Intubating Bronchoscope

1	Give a glycopyrronium premedication to reduce secretions
2	Secure intravenous access
3	Otrivine (xylometazoline 0.1%) drops and lignocaine 2% gel to nares for nasal intubation
4	Administer oxygen via a nasal cannula in opposite nostril
5	Sedation with a continuous infusion of remifentanil starting at 0.3 mcg/kg/min. Adjust the rate according to respiratory rate and level of sedation. Conditions are optimal in 4 to 5 minutes (Another advantage of remifentanil is its LA sparing due to marked antitussive effect.)
6	Mount a size 6.0 cuffed reinforced endotracheal tube onto the bronchoscope
7	Advance the scope until the epiglottis and vocal cords are visualized. The nasal route provides a better angle of attack and produces less gagging.
8	Spray the vocal cords with 2–3 mls 4% lignocaine via the suction channel of the scope
9	Pass the scope through the cords
10	Pass the tube with a continuously rotating motion to avoid catching the bevel on vocal cords or tumor.
11	After confirming correct positioning of the tube in the trachea and above the carina with the bronchoscope induce general anesthesia

Source: From Ref. 18.

Table 6.7 Techniques for Difficult Asleep Intubation. Where the Lungs can be Ventilated but Intubation is Difficult

Bougie: Passing a gum elastic bougie through the vocal cords and railroading the endotracheal tube over the bougie
Alternative laryngoscope blades: Using a straight blade, anterior commisure or McCoy laryngoscope to elevate the epiglottis
Fiber optic intubating bronchoscope
Retrograde intubation: Passing a guide wire or catheter retrograde through the cricothyroid membrane and through the vocal cords and then railroading the endotracheal tube over the guide

Table 6.8 Techniques for Difficult Lung Ventilation. When the Lungs cannot be Ventilated Using a Facemask and the Trachea cannot be Intubated

Oro/nasopharyngeal airways
Laryngeal mask airway
Two-person mask ventilation
Rigid bronchoscopy and jet ventilation

Nebulized Adrenaline

Adrenaline is believed to reduce edema by alpha–adrenergic–mediated vasoconstriction of inflamed mucosa. 1–2 ml of 1/1000 adrenaline (1 ml of 1/1000 contains 1 mg of adrenaline) can be administered every 30 minutes as required.

Electrocardiogram (ECG) monitoring is advisable in the elderly or those with a history of cardiovascular disease.

Corticosteroids

Steroids are known to reduce stridor in a number of situations ranging from croup to postextubation stridor and including airway obstruction secondary to tumor (21). The latter is presumably a result of a reduction in peri-tumor edema secondary to their anti-inflammatory action. Dosing regimes vary, and the route of administration will be dictated by the severity of the stridor; but dexamathasone 0.1 mg/kg four times a day would be a sensible and reliable starting point. It will take 15 to 30 minutes for an effect to be seen after parenteral administration so it would be advisable to administer either Heliox or adrenaline concurrently. Treatment is usually required for a relatively short period of time so the risk of serious side effects is reduced.

Emergency Intubation

In an emergency where complete airway obstruction is imminent awake fiber optic intubation is not a recommended option for the reasons discussed above.

In this situation the safest options are

1. Tracheostomy under local anesthetic.
2. Cricothyroidotomy under local anesthetic using a large-gauge cannula and jet ventilation. A 13- or 14-gauge cannula will allow sufficient flow rates to adequately oxygenate the lungs and there are several custom-made cannulae (e.g., Ravussin needle). This method of ventilating the lungs is essentially a short-term measure that buys time to establish a more secure airway, either by endotracheal intubation or tracheostomy. Although good oxygenation is usually achieved, adequate carbon dioxide (CO_2) elimination cannot be guaranteed. To avoid barotrauma always ensure that there is egress for the expired gas either through the glottis or through another cannula inserted through the cricothyroid membrane.
3. If it is felt that the patient would not tolerate either of the above the anesthetist should attempt inhalational or intravenous induction of anesthesia in the operating theatre with the surgeon scrubbed ready to perform an emergency tracheostomy.

THE SHARED AIRWAY
Elective Tracheostomy

Where surgery involves the fashioning of a permanent or temporary tracheostomy before the end of the operation the endotracheal tube is replaced with a laryngectomy tube (Fig. 6.4) to maintain the airway and facilitate ventilation while ensuring as little encroachment as possible into the surgical field. At the end of the operation this is in turn replaced with a dual cannula tracheostomy tube intended for postoperative ward use such as the Shiley tube; the inner tube can be removed for cleaning.

Tracheostomy is a procedure that requires close cooperation between surgeon and anesthetist and should be carried out in controlled stages. Once the surgeon exposes the anterior tracheal wall, preferably after division of the thyroid isthmus, a stay silk safety suture is placed through the tracheal ring below the intended tracheostomy site, and the long suture ends are brought out onto the chest skin where they are taped. The purpose of the stay suture is to help find the tracheal opening again if the tube becomes

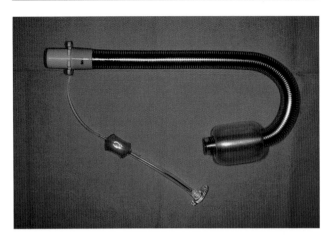

Figure 6.4 The Rusch laryngoflex tracheostomy tube. The curvature and length of the tube allow the breathing circuit and attachments to be kept away from of the surgical field. This tube is reinforced.

dislodged, by gently pulling on the long stay suture the tracheal opening above it will be more easily identified. The tracheal opening is then made, and the tracheostomy tube is carefully inserted taking care not to rupture the endotracheal tube cuff. To allow insertion of the tracheostomy tube the endotracheal tube should be withdrawn so that its tip lies just proximal to the tracheostome and only when correct positioning of the tracheostomy tube is confirmed should it be withdrawn completely. Airway fire is a complication that is that is commonly associated with laser airway surgery (vide infra); however, it is also a risk when using diathermy to open the trachea or for hemostasis once the trachea is opened. The combination of the high temperature achieved by the diathermy tip, and the often obligatory high-inspired concentrations of oxygen is a potent trigger for ignition. If diathermy is necessary the anesthetist can lessen the risk by advancing the cuff of the endotracheal tube distal to the tracheal opening thus separating the two components and by using as low a concentration of oxygen as possible.

Incorrect placement of the tracheostomy tube will be detected first by the anesthetist and potential hazards include extratracheal placement, endobronchial intubation, and herniation of the cuff. Failure to inflate the lungs, the absence of an end-tidal CO_2 trace and a gross elevation of airway pressure all indicate that the tube is extratracheal. A fall in oxygen saturation is a relatively late sign. If positioning outside the airway is suspected, stop ventilation, remove the tracheostomy tube, and regain control of the airway by advancing the endotracheal tube so that its cuff lies distal to the tracheostome. Because of the shorter tracheal length compared to the nontracheostomized patient it is easy for tracheostomy tube that is advanced too far to enter a main bronchus. Endobronchial intubation is detected by observing unequal ventilation of the lungs; a fall in end-tidal CO_2, a moderate rise in airway pressure and a late fall in oxygen saturation. This situation is easily rectified by withdrawing the tube slightly until equal ventilation of the lungs is observed and suturing the tube securely in place. Herniation of the tube cuff over the end of the tube or abutment of the tip of the tube against the tracheal mucosa

can partially or completely occlude the lumen. The picture produced is one of inadequate or absent lung inflation, failure to detect end-tidal CO_2; elevation of airway pressure and again a late fall in oxygen saturation. This can be remedied by deflating and then gently reinflating the cuff with only as much air as is needed to achieve an airtight seal. Overinflation of the cuff not only predisposes to cuff herniation but also will damage tracheal mucosa leading to either perforation of the back wall or necrosis and later stenosis.

Indications for Elective Tracheostomy

There are certain absolute indications for the provision of a temporary tracheostomy following head and neck surgery (Table 6.9), these are operations following which postoperative swelling, hemorrhage or secretions in the upper airway will almost certainly lead to either respiratory obstruction or soiling of the lower airway (1,2).

There are other situations (Table 6.10) where the indication is not clear-cut but where a tracheostomy would have certain advantages such as the facilitation of postoperative ventilation and airway toilet or the optimization of oxygen delivery to free flaps. There is a strong case for performing a tracheostomy at the end of surgery in patients who were found to be difficult intubations in the anesthetic room; if these patients obstruct in the postoperative period, airway swelling or soiling and the difficult working conditions of a ward environment will turn a difficult intubation into an impossible one. The decision to perform a tracheostomy in these cases is a balance between the potential for present or future airway obstruction or soiling and the potential morbidity of the tracheostomy and will depend largely on the postoperative care facilities available. A possible alternative in some cases is to leave the endotracheal tube in place for 24 to 48 hours and extubate when the swelling has subsided but only where intensive care facilities are available staffed by a resident anesthetist of sufficient experience who can resecure the airway in the event of an accidental extubation.

Endoscopy and Microsurgery

Endoscopy of the aero-digestive tract and microsurgery of the larynx require an unimpeded surgical view. This can be achieved in one of two ways.

Table 6.9   Absolute Indications for Elective Tracheostomy

Partial laryngectomy
Total pharyngectomy
Total glossectomy
Disrupted mandible
Bilateral radical neck dissection

Table 6.10   Relative Indications for Elective Tracheostomy

Partial pharyngectomy
Partial glossectomy.
Free flap reconstruction
Patient likely to need postoperative respiratory support.
Difficult intubation

First, by using small-bore microlaryngoscopy endotracheal tubes with an internal diameter of 4 to 5 mm. These can be passed orally or nasally depending on the site of the lesion and anesthetic preference. Their diameter is large enough to permit adequate minute ventilation but small enough to allow the surgeon good access. These tubes are suitable only for short-term anesthesia (up to 1 hour) as their narrow bore predisposes them to blocking and kinking during more prolonged procedures.

Second, where a completely unimpeded view is required as for laser microsurgery, and in particular for posterior commissure lesions, the endotracheal tube can be dispensed with by using high-frequency jet ventilation (HFJV) (22). Ventilation of the lungs is achieved using high frequency (60–300 cycles per minute) small volume bursts of gas delivered at a pressure of 0.4 to 2 bar via a small-bore catheter or needle. The jet of gas can be delivered from above or below the vocal cords. A jet from above the cords (supraglottic) is delivered via a Venturi needle attached to a suspension laryngoscope or a built in ventilation channel (Fig. 6.5). A jet from below the cords is delivered from a catheter passed through the cords (transglottic) or percutaneously through the cricothyroid membrane (transtracheal).

This is an elegant technique in that it provides optimal access for the surgeon but requires greater vigilance from the anesthetist than standard techniques with an endotracheal tube (Table 6.11). If the jet is supraglottic the scope and needle must be in line with the airway or ventilation will be inadequate, and there is a risk of barotrauma to paralaryngeal tissues. Obese patients are not suitable for this technique as ventilation is invariably inadequate due to the excessive weight of the chest wall and pressure from abdominal contents. Barotrauma, that is pneumothorax and pneumomediastinum, are constant risks, modern jet ventilators have pressure sensing that will deactivate the ventilator if end-expiratory pressure does not fall below a preset level. Conventional anesthetic circuits cannot be employed, and anesthesia must be maintained via the intravenous route. Although ventilation and CO_2 elimination are usually adequate tidal volume is impossible to measure because of the open nature of the system and during prolonged procedures arterial blood gas sampling, or gas sampling through a separate sampling tube, is required to determine CO_2 levels.

Laser Surgery

The CO_2 laser offers several advantages over conventional surgical methods in the treatment of certain lesions of the oral cavity, pharynx, and larynx (23,24). Laser surgery poses problems for the anesthetist (25), which can be grouped into two main categories.

Competition for the Airway: Endotracheal Tubes and Jet Ventilation

Lesions of the oral cavity and pharynx can be managed with a laser-resistant endotracheal tube in situ. The advantages of a tube are that it ensures adequate ventilation at all times and protects the lower airway from blood, smoke, and debris. The disadvantages being the possibility of tube ignition and partially impeded surgical access. If a completely unimpeded view of the vocal cords is required as for posterior laryngeal lesions the ideal method is HFJV. In addition to the usual precautions that must be taken with this technique it is necessary to remove smoke with an adequate suction system (Fig. 6.6) to avoid contamination of the lower airways and the theatre atmosphere.

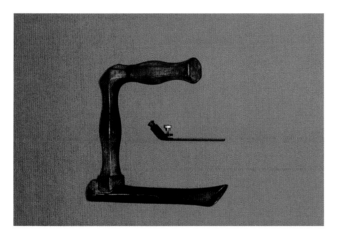

Figure 6.5   Venturi needle for jet ventilation and a Downs (Rhys Evans) microlaryngoscope.

Table 6.11   The Advantages and Disadvantages of Jet Ventilation

Advantages
  Best surgical access especially posterior commisure lesions
  Ideal for laser microsurgery

Disadvantages
  Not suitable for obese patients
  CO_2 elimination and tidal volume difficult to monitor
  Increased risk of barotrauma
  Suitable only for short-term procedures
  Airway not protected from soiling

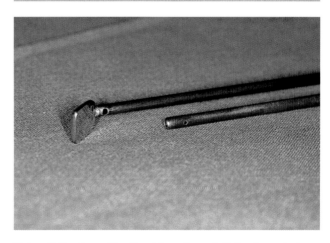

Figure 6.6   Downs (Rhys Evans) laser gas-aspirating sucker and mirrors.

Fire Hazards: Anesthetic Agents and Tracheal Tube Ignition

Three components are necessary for an airway fire to occur (1) a combustible material, usually the endotracheal tube; (2) an oxidizing agent, oxygen, or nitrous oxide; and (3) a source of ignition, usually laser light or diathermy. Nitrous oxide supports combustion and should be avoided in laser surgery and replaced with air. Oxygen, naturally, cannot be avoided, but the inspired concentration should be kept as low as possible while maintaining adequate oxygen saturation. Modern volatile anesthetic agents are not flammable at the concentrations likely to be found in clinical practice.

Laser radiation will ignite most nonglass and nonmetal material and standard endotracheal tubes made of polyvinyl chloride (PVC) or rubber will readily ignite when exposed to a laser beam and should never be used for laser surgery. Several methods of providing a laser-resistant tube have been devised. These range from the protection of standard red rubber and PVC tubes with aluminium tape (23) to the use of all metal flexible tubes, for example. Mallinckrodt laserflex (Fig. 6.7). An intermediate solution is the use of a cuffed tracheal tube made of silicone that is less flammable than rubber or PVC that possesses an outer metallic coating, for example the Xomed lasershield (Fig. 6.8). The thin walled cuffs of these tubes are unprotected and the subglottis must be packed off with saline-soaked gauze to protect them from the laser beam. The cuff should be inflated with saline so that if it is penetrated the saline will act as a heat sink and lessen the likelihood of ignition. Some tubes have a double cuff so that if the upper cuff is penetrated an airtight seal is still provided by the lower cuff. A further refinement is to add methylene blue to the saline so that a cuff penetration is more readily detected.

Operations on the Trachea

Greatest competition for the airway undoubtedly occurs during operations for resection and reconstruction of the trachea and for surgery on an end tracheostome. The anesthetist has the following options.

Endotracheal Intubation/Tracheostomy

It is possible for the surgeon to operate around a tube placed in the trachea with its cuff distal to the site of surgery provided it is of a small diameter. It is even feasible for the tube to be removed from the airway for short periods provided the patient remains well oxygenated, there is no soiling of the airway with blood or debris, and the tube is reinserted before arterial desaturation begins. The disadvantage to this technique is that ventilation is necessarily interrupted and the lower airway is not protected.

Jet Ventilation

Perhaps the most satisfactory method of providing adequate ventilation while allowing optimal surgical access is to ventilate the patient using HFJV through a small-diameter catheter placed with its tip distal to the site of surgery.

Intra-operative Tracheal Injury

The management of intra-operative tracheal injury depends on the level of the tear. A tear proximal to the cuff of the endotracheal tube can be repaired with the tube in situ. However if the surgeon requires more complete access or if the tear extends distal to the endotracheal tube the situation is best managed with HFJV down a suitable catheter such or a Cook airway exchange catheter, which may be passed down an existing endotracheal tube (26). In very low tracheal tears individual intubation of the bronchi may be necessary.

PHARYNGOLARYNGO-OESOPHAGECTOMY

Continuity of the gastrointestinal tract following circumferential excision of the pharynx or upper esophagus can be restored using a pedicled flap, jejunal free flap, or gastric transposition. The latter two procedures, because of the encroachment into the abdomen and thorax, represent a greater physiological insult than other head and neck procedures with greater potential for postoperative

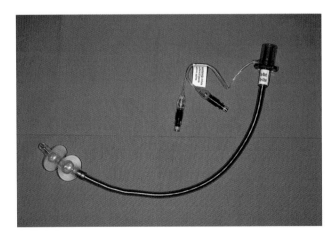

Figure 6.7 The Malinckrodt laserflex tube. A metal tube with a nonreflective matte surface. Note the double cuff inflated with saline.

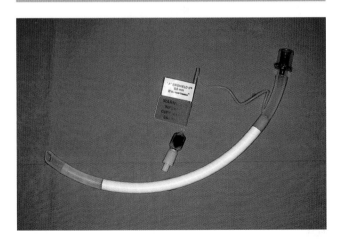

Figure 6.8 The Xomed Lasershield. A silicone tube with an outer metallic coating. Note the methylene blue in the pilot balloon.

cardorespiratory complications and death. Most studies report morbidity and in hospital mortality figures in the region of 35% and 5%, respectively, for both procedures (27–29). In terms of age, coexisting illness and potential for postoperative complications these patients closely resemble those with esophageal cancer undergoing esophagectomy. It would seem sensible therefore to follow the same guidelines for preoperative assessment and peri-operative management (30).

Preoperative Assessment

Preexisting pulmonary disease predisposes to the development of postoperative pulmonary complications. Those with a preoperative forced vital capacity (FVC) less than 90% of predicted, an forced expiratory volume in one second (FEV1) less than 70% of predicted or with a low preoperative Pa02 are more likely to develop pulmonary complications (31). Preoperative cardiac and hepatic dysfunction are also significant risk factors. Bartels and coworkers (32) devised a scoring system that grouped patients into low, moderate, and high-risk groups depending on preoperative findings in four systems (Table 6.12).

The minimum set of investigations should include baseline hematological and biochemical profiles, arterial blood gases on air, pulmonary function tests, electrocardiogram, and chest X-ray (30) (Table 6.13).

Table 6.12   Risk Factors in Esophagectomy

System (risk factor)	Health status of a system (risk factor)		
	Normal (x1)	Compromised (x2)	Severely impaired (x3)
System (risk factor)			
General status (x4)	4	8	12
Cardiovascular (x3)	3	6	9
Pulmonary (x2)	2	4	6
Hepatic (x2)	2	4	6
Total Risk Score	Risk		30-day mortality
11–15	Low		2%
15–21	Moderate		5%
22–33	High		25%

Each system is scored as normal, compromised, or severely impaired and multiplied by a risk factor (30) thus: The risk score for each system is obtained by multiplying the particular system risk factor by the health status risk factor, that is, 1, 2, or 3. The total risk score is derived by adding up the individual risk scores.

Table 6.13   Minimum Preoperative Investigations for Gastric Transposition or Jejunal Free-Flap Reconstruction

FBC
Clotting screen
Urea and electrolytes
Liver function tests
Artcrial blood gases on air
Pulmonary function tests
ECG
Chest X-ray

Source: Ref. 18.
Abbreviations: FBC, full blood count; ECG, electrocardiogram.

Patients deemed high risk on the basis of these preliminary investigations can be further risk stratified with cardiopulmonary exercise testing (4). Patients with ischemic heart disease will need a cardiology assessment that may include an exercise stress test, echocardiography, or thallium perfusion (30).

Intraoperative Management

The complex nature of the surgery and the high rate of comorbidity dictate that invasive monitoring, that is, direct arterial blood pressure and central venous pressure is essential. Cardiac output monitoring gives useful information in patients with cardiovascular risk factors, but most current methods of measurement are difficult to use in the theater setting, and it should be reserved for the very high-risk patient. Thoracic epidural analgesia, used in conjunction with general anesthesia as part of the anesthetic technique and continued into the postoperative period, has been shown to decrease the incidence of respiratory complications and provide superior pain relief after major surgery (33).

It has been known for some time that limiting intraoperative fluids during esophagectomy is associated with a decrease in the incidence of respiratory complications (31). The anesthetist should aim to use crystalloid to replace the preoperative deficit and for maintenance requirements and replace any blood loss with colloid or blood in an effort to keep fluid in the intravascular space. However there is a unique feature of gastric transposition that may limit the degree to which fluids may be restricted (34,35), Digital dissection of the esophagus and transfer of the stomach to the neck interferes with venous return, which may lead to gross hypotension and initiates ventricular dysrhythmias as a result of direct mechanical stimulation of the myocardium. Ensuring adequate hydration prior to this phase of the operation can attenuate the fall in blood pressure.

Postoperative Management

These patients must be managed postoperatively in a high-dependency area with the ability for escalation or transfer to intensive care if a higher level of organ support (e.g., mechanical ventilation) is required. Major postoperative complications such as chest infection, myocardial ischemia, or anastomotic breakdown do not declare themselves for 2 to 3 days and therefore the patient should stay for at least 78 hours.

The continuance of epidural analgesia into the postoperative period is associated with a reduction in postoperative pulmonary complications (33,36). Crystalloids should be administered at a rate of 1.5 to 2 mls/kg/hr (29) to cover maintenance requirements, and colloid given to correct hypovolemia or to replace drain losses of pleural fluid or blood.

An early return of spontaneous breathing will cut down on the rate of ventilation-associated pneumonias and aid early mobilization. Intensive prophylactic chest physiotherapy is mandatory; the presence of a tracheostomy greatly facilitates early weaning and physiotherapy.

When total thyroidectomy is performed serum calcium should be checked postoperatively, and any deficiency corrected (see below). Nutrition can be provided either enterally via a jejunostomy tube placed at surgery or intravenously as total parenteral nutrition.

ANESTHETIC COMPLICATIONS AND TECHNIQUES IN HEAD AND NECK SURGERY

Air Embolism

The head-up position is employed in head and neck surgery to reduce bleeding in the surgical field. In this position the veins of the head and neck are above the level of the right atrium; and if the difference in height is greater than the central venous pressure air will enter the venous circulation if a vein is breached. The danger from venous air embolism lies not just in its obstructive effects on the right side of the circulation with a reduction in cardiac output and resulting hypotension but also in the possibility of air entering the arterial side of the circulation via a patent foramen ovale or right to left shunt and embolizing a coronary or cerebral artery (so-called paradoxical embolism). Up to 30% of the population have a probe patent foramen ovale at postmortem (37).

The precordial Doppler is a highly sensitive ultrasonic probe, which is used in neurosurgery to detect air emboli as small as 0.12 ml; however, it is prone to interference from surgical diathermy and is highly dependent on operator experience. The most sensitive clinical sign is a fall in end-tidal CO_2 as detected by the capnograph (Table 6.14), the other signs depend on the presence of large volumes of air or occur relatively late.

Management (Table 6.14) is directed at preventing the ingress of further air and aspirating or minimizing the effects of air already embolized. Nitrous oxide replaces nitrogen in air containing spaces and diffuses in 35 times more rapidly than nitrogen diffuses out causing the embolus to expand. The administration of 100% oxygen not only improves oxygen saturation but also has the effect of decreasing the embolus size.

Carotid Sinus Reflex

Surgical manipulation of the carotid sinus can lead to profound bradycardia and hypotension. This is most likely to occur in hypertensive men older than age 50, and though the above response is the most common hypotension alone, bradycardia alone or even hypotension and tachycardia can occur (2). The anesthetist should immediately inform the surgeon who can then stop temporarily while either an anticholinergic such as atropine or glycopryrrlate is administered to restore the heart rate or local anesthetic is applied directly onto the sinus thus blocking the afferent limb of the reflex.

Cerebral Edema

The internal jugular veins constitute the major venous drainage from the head, and these vessels are commonly subjected to manipulation and temporary occlusion if not sacrifice, as in radical neck dissection. The resultant interference with venous drainage in addition to the hypotension and reduction in cerebral perfusion pressure caused by anesthesia and the head-up position can lead to cerebral edema (38).

Cerebral edema can be difficult to detect under the masking effect of general anesthesia but unexplained changes in pulmonary and cardiac function should alert one to the possibility of raised intracranial pressure. Neurogenic pulmonary edema and the neurogenic myocardial damage syndrome may account for these changes. The latter is thought to be due to hypothalamic sympathetic discharge causing focal coronary artery spasms leading in turn to areas of myocardial ischemia.

For these reasons it is recommended that a bilateral radical neck dissection be undertaken as a staged procedure with an interval of at least 3 weeks between each operation. If a staged procedure is not possible or if a radical neck dissection is carried out in a patient known to have an absent or thrombosed internal jugular vein on the opposite side, a tracheostomy should be performed or overnight intubation and ventilation be considered to prevent airway obstruction until the vertebral veins accommodate.

Postoperative facial edema and petechiae, cyanosis and airway obstruction are all signs of raised intracranial pressure. The management of cerebral edema is outlined in Table 6.15.

Positioning

Head and neck surgery can be prolonged and care should be taken when positioning the patient to avoid causing injury (39). The ulnar and common peroneal nerves are particularly susceptible to damage because they lie in a superficial position close to bony prominences, all bony pressure points should be protected with gauze or gel padding. Head rings should be firm enough to prevent the head from moving but soft enough to avoid excessive pressure on the scalp. Eyes should be taped shut and covered with gauze pads or a hard plastic shield. The reverse Trendelenburg (head-up) position not only increases the risk of

---

Table 6.14 The Detection and Management of Air Embolism

Detection
  Fall in end tidal CO_2
  Hypotension
  Fall in oxygen saturation
  Elevation of central venous pressure
  Millwheel murmur
  ECG evidence of right heart strain

Management
  Flood the area with saline
  Head down position
  Discontinue nitrous oxide
  100% O_2
  Aspirate air from right heart via central line with patient in left lateral position

Abbreviation: ECG, electrocardiogram.

Table 6.15 The Management of Cerebral Edema

Head up position 20–30 degrees
Increase blood pressure to elevate cerebral perfusion pressure
Mannitol or frusemide to reduce edema
Tracheal intubation to protect the airway
Hyperventilate to a PaCO2 of 3.5–4.5 kPA

Abbreviation: kPA, kilopascales.

air embolism but also potentiates the hypotensive action of general anesthesia by allowing blood to pool in the lower half of the body, the latter can be attenuated by placing the patient in a head-up legs-up (deckchair) position.

Hypotensive Anesthesia

This refers to the technique of deliberately lowering the blood pressure during general anesthesia to reduce blood loss to improve visibility in the surgical field and reduce the likelihood of blood transfusion with its attendant risks. This is advantageous in head and neck tumor surgery, in particular maxillofacial surgery, where the surgical field is restricted and blood loss can be great. A recent systematic review (40) concluded that hypotensive anesthesia was effective in reducing blood loss, transfusion rate, and operating time. No significant changes in cerebral, cardiovascular, renal, or hepatic function were seen in patients receiving hypotensive anesthesia compared to controls, but it also stated that careful patient selection was mandatory. The key to safe hypotensive anesthesia lies in careful patient selection; contraindications to hypotensive anesthesia are listed in Table 6.16. Adequate monitoring should be employed for longer cases or the higher risk patient, this mean direct blood pressure monitoring with an arterial line and central venous pressure monitoring to gauge the state of filling. It is best to aim for a reduction in mean arterial pressure (MAP) of 30% compared to normal preoperative blood pressure rather than trying to achieve a specific target pressure with a lower MAP limit of 50 mm Hg for American Society of Anesthesiologists (ASA) class 1 patients and 80 mm HG in the elderly.

A variety of pharmacological agents have been used to induce hypotension ranging from vasodilators such as nitoglycerine and sodium nitroprusside to inhibitors of the sympathetic nervous system such as clonidine and beta blockers, but few if any of these drugs satisfy the ideal criteria of rapid onset and offset, lack of toxicity, and predictable dose-dependent effect. Modern techniques rely on the natural hypotensive effect of most anesthetic agents, many of which do satisfy these criteria, to achieve adequate hypotension at normal anesthetic concentrations (41). A combination of remifentanil (a potent short-acting opiate)

with an intravenous (e.g., propofol), or inhalational anesthetic agent (sevoflurane, desflurane, or isoflurane) will produce acceptable results in the vast majority of cases.

Tilting the head up by 20 to 25 degrees will help to lower blood pressure by a reduction in venous return to the heart.

MANAGEMENT OF THE FREE FLAP

Free tissue transfer is often required in head and neck cancer surgery to repair the defects left following tumor excision. The general principles that govern the anesthetic management of free-flap surgery are neatly encapsulated in the Poiseuille-Hagen equation.

$$Flow = \frac{Pressure \times Radius^4 \times \pi}{Length \times viscosity \times 8}$$

This formula describes laminar flow through a tube for a Newtonian fluid, and although blood is not a Newtonian Fluid (its viscosity changes with flow) it usefully relates the factors that will determine flow to a transplanted flap, that is, maximum flow, and therefore maximum oxygen transport, is achieved with blood of low viscosity under a high-perfusing pressure through nonconstricted vessels.

The goals of the anesthetic technique are to maintain a state of vasodilatation, achieve an adequate perfusion pressure, and lower the viscosity of the blood (Table 6.17) (42,43).

Vasodilatation

The relationship between flow and the fourth power of the radius means that vessel diameter is the major determinant of flow. The patient must be kept warm at all costs to avoid vasoconstriction. If possible start actively warming before theater using a warm air blanket, raise the ambient temperature of the theatre to 22 to 24°C, place the patient on a warming mattress, or cover him or her with a warm air blanket and warm all intravenous fluids. Monitor core and peripheral temperature throughout the procedure.

Hypovolemia is a potent cause of vasoconstriction. Crystalloids should be used to replace the preoperative deficit (10–20 ml/kg) and ongoing insensible losses (4–8 ml/kg) and colloid should be used to replace blood loss (42).

Table 6.16 Contraindications to Hypotensive Anesthesia

Cardiac disease
  Ischemic heart disease
  Untreated hypertension
  Symptomatic aortic or mitral stenosis
  Congestive cardiac failure
  Peripheral vascular disease
  Anemia and hemoglobinopathies

Cerebrovascular disease
  History of TIA/CVA
  Greater than 70% carotid artery stenosis
  Raised intracranial pressure
  Spinal cord compression

Hepatic disease

Renal disease

Abbreviations: TIA, transient ischaemic attack; CVA, cerebrovascular accident.

Table 6.17 Principles of Anesthesia for Free-Flap Surgery

Maintain perfusion pressure
  Adequate hydration
  Adequate urine output (1–2 ml/kg/hr)
  Direct blood pressure monitoring

Vasodilate
  Normothermia
  Adequate hydration
  Avoid acidosis
  Effective analgesia
  Avoid vasoconstrictors

Maximize oxygen delivery
  Hematocrit 30–35%
  Maintain good oxygen saturation

Central venous pressure monitoring will help guide fluid management to achieve a state of adequate hydration and normovolemic hemodilution (see below) without fluid overload. Postoperative edema will compromise flap perfusion not only by restricting flow but also by predisposing to pulmonary edema and consequent hypoxemia. Metabolic acidosis may occur as a result of hypovolemia and hypoperfusion, therefore regular arterial blood gas analysis may help to guide fluid management.

Perfusion Pressure

Perfusion pressure should be maintained with appropriate fluid management as above. Inotropes and vasopressors are a last resort, as the majority will cause vasoconstriction at therapeutic doses. If an inotrope is required those that improve cardiac output by inodilation, for example, dobutamine or dopexamine, have theoretical advantages. Direct blood pressure measurement using an arterial line not only allows for continuous monitoring but also enables the anesthetist to monitor blood gases and hematocrit. The maintenance of an adequate urine output (1–2 ml/kg/hr) is a reassuring indicator of adequate volume status.

Viscosity

An hematocrit in the range 30 to 35% will lower the viscosity of blood and improve flow (Fig. 6.9). A level lower than this produces very little reduction in viscosity, and any advantage gained will be offset by the lower oxygen carrying capacity. This is achieved by replacing initial blood loss with colloid until the hematocrit is in the desired range (normovolemic hemodilution) the aim being to reduce viscosity and hence improve blood flow in small vessels. Some workers have recommended hypervolemic hemodilution, that is, the administration of fluids at a rate greater than

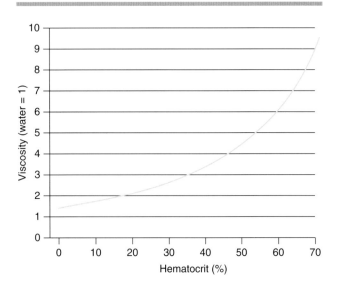

Figure 6.9 The relationship between hematocrit and blood viscosity. A hematocrit of 30–35% will lower viscosity and improve blood flow. *Source:* From Ref. 43.

blood loss to elevate the central venous pressure (CVP) to >10 cm H_2O (43). There is no evidence to suggest that either approach is more beneficial than the other, and it would seem prudent, in a population of patients likely to have concurrent cardiac or pulmonary disease, to adopt the normovolemic approach.

Postoperative Management

Postoperative care is an extension of intra-operative management. Keep the patient warm, well hydrated, and with an adequate urine output. Pain causes vasoconstriction, and morphine by continuous infusion or a patient-controlled system will control pain from the donor and recipient sites. Regular observations of flap color, temperature, and blood flow using a Doppler ultrasound probe should be carried out. The close observation required in the postoperative period is best carried out in a high dependency area.

Postoperative mechanical ventilation is rarely necessary unless there has been a laparotomy (e.g., jejunal free flap) or the patient has cardiorespiratory comorbidity. Mechanical ventilation drops the blood pressure and therefore interferes with flap perfusion, as a result of raised intrathoracic pressure and obligatory sedation.

POSTOPERATIVE CARE
Level of Care

Following surgery confined to the head and neck with or without a tracheostomy the vast majority of patients may be cared for in the general ward setting by nurses with specialist head and neck training. As discussed above patients undergoing pharyngolaryngo-esophagectomy must be cared for in high-dependency or intensive care.

Fluid and Electrolyte Management

The fluid management of patients undergoing pharyngo-laryngo-esophagectomy or free-flap reconstruction has already been discussed. Fluid management in surgery confined to the head and neck is much simpler as there will be no occult or third-space losses, the site is relatively superficial, hemostasis and drainage are given a high priority, and any losses of blood or fluid will be readily apparent. Hence in this group it is acceptable to prescribe maintenance fluids only for the first 24 hours and replace any drain losses as they occur with colloid. A range of 1–1.5 ml/kg/hr of a balanced salt solution such as Hartmanns should ensure adequate hydration without the risk of fluid overload.

Feeding

In patients with anastomoses in the upper aerodigestive tract enteral feeding via nasogastric or jejunostomy tube should commence on the first postoperative day unless there is an ileus or lower gastrointestinal anastomosis in which case parenteral nutrition should be commenced.

Calcium

Follow total thyroidectomy it is essential to monitor calcium commencing on the first postoperative night. An adjusted level must be obtained as serum albumin is often low as a result of hemodilution or poor preoperative nutritional status (for every 1g/l difference between the patient's serum albumin and a figure of 40g/l add 0.02mmol/l to the patient's serum calcium to arrive at the corrected value). To correct a low calcium give a bolus of 10ml of 10% calcium gluconate or an infusion of 40mls in 500mls saline over 2 to 8 hours and repeat the level.

Pain Relief

Minor to intermediate surgery confined to the head and neck will generally be controlled with enteral or intravenous paracetamol or opiates (codeine, tramadol, morphine) administered via the enteral or intramuscular routes. Major to complex surgery will generally require a strong intravenous opiate such as morphine; this can be given as a continuous infusion or via a patient controlled analgesia (PCA) system. The great risk with intravenous opiate is the potential for respiratory depression in a population of patients with already at-risk airways. A continuous infusion should only be considered in the high-dependency or intensive care setting. PCA has a better safety profile and can be given in the general ward but only where the nursing staff have received appropriate education and with the support of an acute pain team. Vomiting and retching are undesirable in patients with anastomoses in the upper aerodigestive tract and adequate anti-emesis should be prescribed when opiates are used.

The advantages of thoracic epidural analgesia for chest wall and abdominal surgery have already been discussed, but local anesthetic epidurals will cause hypotension that may impair blood flow to tissues, particularly those above the level of the block where any free-flap reconstruction is likely to be sited. The epidural administration of opiates such as fentanyl or diamorphine may help attenuate the fall in blood pressure without compromising the quality of analgesia. Nonsteroidal analgesics are best avoided in head and neck surgery because of their deleterious effects on platelet function, but they can be a useful adjunct to other analgesics where pain control is inadequate.

CONCLUSION

Head and neck surgery is unique in that the surgeon and anesthetist share a common pathway, it is not so much that they compete for the airway but that they cooperate closely to maintain it, and both should respect the others role in airway management. The flexible fiber optic intubating bronchoscope has revolutionized the management of the difficult intubation in anesthesia for head and neck surgery, and many patients are now intubated using this technique who formerly would have required a tracheostomy either awake or asleep after failed attempts at intubation. It is not, however, the answer in all situations, and the anesthetist must know when to request a surgical airway. The role of the anesthetist is not confined to the airway; involving them early in the assessment and preparation of patients for major head and neck surgery as part of the multidisciplinary team will help to minimize peri-operative morbidity and mortality.

REFERENCES

1. Robbie DS. Anaesthesia for surgeryin malignant disease of the head and neck. In: Filshie J, Robbie DS, eds. Anaesthesia and malignant disease. London: Edward Arnold, 1989; 135–49.
2. Howland WS, Rooney SM, Goldiner PL. Manual of Anaesthesia in Cancer Care. New York: Churchill Livingstone, 1986.
3. ACC/AHA 2007 Guidelines on Perioperative Cardiovascular Evaluation and Care for Noncardiac Surgery. A Report of the American College of Cardiology/American Heart Association Task Force on Practice Guidelines (Writing Committee to Revise the 2002 Guidelines on Perioperative Cardiovascular Evaluation for Noncardiac Surgery) Circulation 2007; 116: 1971–96.
4. Older P, Hall A. Clinical review: how to identify high-risk surgical patients. Critical Care 2004; 8: 369–72.
5. Gibbs J, Cull W, Henderson W et al. Preoperative serum albumin level as a predictor of operative mortality and morbidity: results from the National VA Surgical Risk Study. Arch Surg. 1999; 134: 36–42.
6. The British Association of Otorhinolaryngologists – Head and Neck Surgeons. Pre-op tests – Guidelines for ENT. 2006; www.entuk.org.
7. Royal College of Radiologists. Making the best use of a department of Clinical Radiology: guidelines for doctors (5th edition). London: RCR, 2004.
8. Mallampati SR, Gatt SP, Gugino LD et al. A new sign for predicting difficult intubation. Can Anaes Soc J 1985; 32: 429–34.
9. Samsoon JLT, Young JRB. Difficult tracheal intubation: a retrospective study. Anaesthesia 1987; 42: 487–90.
10. Patil V, Stehling LC, Zaunder HL. Fibreoptic endoscopy in anaesthesia: Chicago: Year Book Medical Publishers, 1983.
11. Calder I. Predicting difficult intubation. Anaesthesia 1992; 47: 528–9.
12. Wilson ME, Speighalter D, Robertson JA et al. Predicting difficult intubation. Brit J Anaes 1988; 61: 211–16.
13. Lewis M, Keramati S, Benumof JL, Berry CC. What is the best way to predict oropharyngeal classification and mandibular space length to predict difficult laryngoscopy. Anesthesiology 1994; 81: 69–75.
14. Yentis SM. Predicting difficult intubation – worthwhile exercise or pointless ritual? Anaesthesia 2002; 57: 105–9.
15. Editorial. Br J Anaesth 1996; 77: 309–11.
16. Practice guidelines for management of the difficult airway. An updated report by the American Society of Anesthesiologists Task Force on Management of the Difficult Airway. Anesthesiology 2003; 98: 1269–77.
17. Sidhu VS, Whitehead EM, Ainsworth QP et al. A technique of awake fibreoptic intubation. Experience in patients with cervical spine disease. Anaesthesia 1993; 48: 910–14.
18. Mingo OH, Ashpole KJ, Irving CJ et al. Remifentanil sedation for awake fibreoptic intubation with limited application of local anaesthetic in patients for elective head and neck surgery. Anaesthesia 2008; 63: 1065–9.
19. Mason RA. Learning fibreoptic intubation: fundamental problems. Anaesthesia 1992; 47: 729–31.
20. Wigmore T, Stachowski E. A review of the use of Heliox in the critically Ill. Critical Care and Resuscitation 2006; 8: 64–72.
21. Elsayem A, Bruera E. High-dose corticosteroids for the management of dyspnea in patients with tumor obstruction of the upper airway. Support Care Cancer 2007; 15: 1437–9.
22. Evans KL, Keene MH, Bristow AS. High-frequency jet ventilation—a review of its role in laryngology. J Laryngol Otol 1994; 108: 23–5.
23. Rhys Evans PH, Frame JW, Brandrick J. A review of carbon dioxide laser surgery in the oral cavity and pharynx. J Laryngol Otol 1986; 100: 69–77.

24. Frame JW, Das Gupta AR, Dalton GA et al. Use of the carbon dioxide laser in the management of premalignant lesions of the oral mucosa. J Laryngol Otol 1984; 98: 1251–60.

25. Paes ML. General anaesthesia for carbon dioxide laser surgery within the airway: a review. Br J Anaesth 1987; 59: 1610–20.

26. Montgomery PQ, Mochloulis G, Sidhu VS. A Cook airway exchange catheter in the management of intraoperative tracheal injury. Anaesth Intensive Care 1996; 24: 617.

27. Spiro RH, Bains MS, Shah JP et al. Gastric transposition for head and neck cancer: A critical update. Am J Surg 1991; 162: 348–52.

28. Triboulet JP, Mariette C, Chevalier D et al. Surgical management of carcinoma of the hypopharynx and cervical esophagus: analysis of 209 cases. Arch Surg 2001; 136: 1164–70.

29. Daiko H, Hayashi R, Saikawa M et al. Surgical management of carcinoma of the cervical esophagus. J Surg Oncol 2007; 96: 166–72.

30. Allum WH, Griffin SM, Watson A et al. Association of Upper Gastrointestinal Surgeons of Great Britain and Ireland; British Society of Gastroenterology; British Association of Surgical Oncology. Guidelines for the management of oesophageal and gastric cancer. Gut 2002; 50(Suppl 5): v1–23.

31. Nishi M, Hiramatsu Y, Hioki K, et al. Pulmonary complications after subtotal oesophagectomy. Br J Surgery 1998; 75: 527–30.

32. Bartels H, Stein HJ, Siewert JR. Preoperative risk analysis and postoperative mortality of oesophagectomy for resectable oesophageal cancer. Br J Surg 1998; 85: 840–4.

33. Rigg JRA, Jamrozik K, Myles PS et al. Epidural anaesthesia and analgesia and outcome of major surgery: a randomised trial. Lancet 2002; 359: 1276–82.

34. Plant M. Anaesthesia for pharyngolaryngectomy with extrathoracic oesophagectomy and gastric transposition. Anaesthesia 1982; 37: 1211–13.

35. Condon HA. Anaesthesia for pharyngo-laryngo-oesophagectomy with pharyngo-gastrostomy. Brit J Anaesth 1971; 43: 1061–5.

36. Watson A. Influence of thoracic epidural analgesia on outcome after resection for oesophageal cancer. Surgery 1994; 115/4: 429–32.

37. Hagen PT, Scholtz DG, Edwards WD. Incidence and size of patent foramen ovale during the first 10 decades of life: an autopsy study of 965 normal hearts. Mayo Clin Proc 1984; 59: 17–20.

38. Donham RT. Complications of anaesthesia. In: Johns ME, ed. Complications in otolaryngology. Vol 2. Head and neck. Philadelphia: BC Decker; 1986; 29–52.

39. Aitkenhead AR. Injuries associated with anaesthesia. A global perspective. Br J Anaesth 2005; 95: 95–109.

40. Choi WS, Samman N. Risks and benefits of deliberate hypotension in anaesthesia: a systematic review. Int J Oral Maxillofac Surg 2008; May 27. [Epub ahead of print]

41. Degoute CS. Controlled hypotension: a guide to drug of choice. Drugs 2007; 67: 1053–76.

42. Quinlan J. Anaesthesia for reconstructive surgery. Anaesthesia and Intensive Care Medicine 2006; 7: 31–5.

43. McDonald DJF. Anaesthesia for microvascular surgery: a physiological approach. Brit J Anaes 1985; 57: 904–12.

7

Nursing Care of Head and Neck Cancer Patients

Nicola Tinne, Catherine South, Kevin Russell, Pauline Doran-Williams,
Annabel Hooper and Frances Rhys Evans

INTRODUCTION

The head and neck is perhaps one of the most complex sites for cancer treatment, not only because of the difficult management problems, but also because of the many physical and psychological traumas potentially affecting the patient. Nowhere else in the body does an area have tissue with such diversity. Disease and its progression can dramatically alter the patient's appearance, as well as his or her basic functions, such as breathing, eating, speech, hearing, and sight. With such physical and functional changes comes the emotional trauma of reintegrating back into everyday life following treatment.

It is vital that head and neck nurses have sound theoretical knowledge of the anatomy and physiology of the area, the disease process, and treatment options. When complex surgical reconstruction procedures are necessary to restore appearance and function a comprehensive rehabilitation service to support this work is essential.

Radiotherapy, with or without chemotherapy, has reduced the need for functionally damaging surgery (1,2). Combining chemotherapy and radiotherapy has improved disease-free survival but has associated treatment toxicities that can lead to hospital admissions (3,4). Although chemotherapy is still used in the palliative setting it can enhance curative treatments, and most patients receive combined modality regimens depending upon their presenting health and fitness. Induction or neoadjuvant chemotherapy is often used initially to shrink disease and improve symptoms (4,5). Chemotherapy can be started within a week of patients being told their diagnosis and has immediate benefit in some cases that gives their morale a boost. Although this chapter is written from the perspective of the United Kingdom it is hoped it demonstrates the underlying principles of the nursing care of head and neck cancer patients.

NURSING CARE AND THE MULTIDISCIPLINARY TEAM

Caring for the head and neck cancer patient is one of the most challenging and exciting areas for nurses. Owing to the multifaceted nature of the work, one is constantly reviewing and learning to try to improve the delivery of care. A multidisciplinary team (MDT) approach is necessary to provide quality care throughout the course of treatment, as well as during the rehabilitation period. Better survival outcomes and more robust treatment decisions are made in the MDT meeting (6) thus improving survival rates for head and neck patients (7). MDT meetings are made up of healthcare professionals with all the relevant skills, knowledge, and expertise to care for the complex needs of head and neck cancer patients (8).

The MDT is responsible for making decisions about treatment (8); however, the decisions made only stand in that present moment and under the particular circumstances presented (9). Multidisciplinary working and shared decision making benefits the patients by increasing the probability that the most appropriate interventions will be offered to the patients (9,10). Even if those present do not meet the patient they still have a duty to exercise their judgment with reasonable care (6). Members of the supporting multidisciplinary care team should include those listed in Box 7.1.

The relevant core members of the team should meet the patient and family prior to treatment so that introductions can be made and needs assessed for the course of care, thus facilitating a cohesive approach. The United Kingdom National Institute for Clinical Excellence (NICE) recommends that each patient has a 'key worker' which is usually a Clinical Nurse Specialist (CNS). The CNS aims to meet the patient and family at the point of diagnosis, be involved in treatment decisions, provide an individualized approach to psychological and social support (8), and have a central role in the MDT.

The patient's general condition and any comorbidities must be taken into account when deciding the treatment plan (1). Patients living on their own with few social contacts and communication difficulties are vulnerable (11,12). Additionally, helping patients with alcohol and tobacco problems are priorities for the CNS prior to commencing treatment (13). The CNS can also be the link person to further decisions made in the MDT to the patient and members of the family.

Box 7.1 The Supporting Multidisciplinary Care Team

Clinical nurse specialist	Nursing staff
Dietitian	Speech and language therapist
Physiotherapist	Pain management specialist
Pharmacist	Dentist
Dental hygienist	Maxillofacial prosthedontist
Occupational therapist	Community liaison nurse
Social worker	Psychotherapist
Palliative care team	Chaplain

PSYCHOLOGICAL SUPPORT AND COMMUNICATION

When a patient is first diagnosed as having cancer, a potentially life-threatening disease, the initial shock, anger, sense of loss, lack of control, and grief are virtually the same feelings one experiences after bereavement (14,15). It is therefore important to recognize that the patients will be in need of the appropriate support. They are grieving the loss of part of themselves and the life they once had, which will never be quite the same again.

Feelings of anger and spiritual questioning "why did God allow this to happen to me?," "why me, what have I done to deserve this?" are common and entirely normal. It is a rare person who can live contentedly with an uncertain and unpredictable life. The patient and family will be desperate to alleviate that uncertainty and in doing so will cling to the medical staff's every verbal and nonverbal response to elicit a hint or shred of reassurance for the future.

It is best to give clear and honest answers to questions asked by the patients concerning their future survival and quality of life. However, it should be sensitively done as maintaining hope can give the patient a sense of strength and security. Often the patients will give a direct or indirect indication of how much information they want to be told. For some, the prospect that they will still be able to enjoy some quality of life, pursue a hobby, travel, be free from pain, and so forth is tremendously reassuring. Care must be individualized and take into account patients' personality, age, gender, social support, previous experience of illness, health information processing style, physical condition, mood, and emotional stability (16).

If the patient's symptoms are controlled and are minimal then hopefully a relatively normal lifestyle can be resumed. Various studies have found that patients who maintain close relationships with their family and friends are more likely to cope with the course of their treatment and rehabilitation (17,20).

Patients will experience a degree of depression at some stage in their illness, and this too must be recognized as a normal response to the threat of disfigurement, dysfunction, and possibly death. Massie described a higher incidence of depression in oropharyngeal cancers: The patient and family must be given the opportunity, time, and privacy to express their anxiety and fears (21,84). Initially managing depression involves maintaining a good relationship, listening attentively, and helping them adjust their emotions with the help of available support (16).

Once the period of grieving has begun, the diagnosis of cancer can also precipitate the onset of the patient's coping mechanisms as recognized by Caplan (22). Often these are strategies patients have used previously to deal with difficult circumstances (23), and it can be helpful to ask about these (16). Most patients demonstrate an extraordinarily brave determination to get on with their life, whatever their dysfunction and/or disfigurement, especially if the alternative is death (24). Most patients employ a coping mechanism, which we all practice to some extent in our lives, that of social comparison. They frequently compare themselves to others, with the subconscious intent to be in a stronger, more positive position. By comparing their handicaps with others, they will reason that to lose their ear or voice or part of their tongue, for example, is better

than to lose an eye or to be confined to a wheelchair for life (25). By making these comparisons, the patients try to relieve some of their feelings about their fate and enhance the value and quality of their life.

Helping patients and their families to express themselves and feel comfortable to interact with the staff involved with their care will foster trust and reassurance with the knowledge that everyone is seen to be working together to achieve an acceptable quality of life. Some patients and families may want to talk to someone who is not involved in their immediate care. Often referral to a mental health professional or support group can be helpful (16).

Specifically an important area of concern are the psychological effect of head and neck cancer and its treatment, on aspects of sexuality. Sexuality is a concept that embraces many aspects of an individuals' sexual personality. It includes gender identity, sexual expression and orientation, intimacy and reproduction, and how we perceive our physical self. Although it is a constant part of our being it changes throughout life and can be altered by such events as cancer diagnosis and surgery and altered body image. Clearly this is very relevant to people with head and neck cancer.

There is limited direct research into the extent to which people with head and neck cancer have problems with sexuality, but some evidence can be gleaned from quality of life studies using tools such as the European Organization for Research and Treatment of Cancer head and neck cancer-specific questionnaire and Functional Assessment of Cancer Therapy for Head and Neck Cancer. Bjordal et al. found that problems with sexuality were the second worse symptom after dry mouth after a year in a cohort of head and neck patients receiving concomitant chemoradiation therapy (26). All other symptoms, for example, pain improved over the year, but problems with sexuality and dry mouth did not.

When addressing sexuality issues with patients healthcare professionals need to know their own limitations when discussing the subject and refer to specialist practitioners where appropriate. It is helpful if they are aware of some of the barriers which might prevent a successful outcome such as ageism, that is, an older woman will not have sexuality problems because she is postmenopausal (27). Specific examples of problems may relate to surgical interventions such as exploring how a person postlaryngectomy kisses, or how to wear jewelery if the patient has skin reactions to radiotherapy treatment. Consider also the how an individual post-partial glossectomy communicates with a partner or potential partner. A cosmetic camouflage service and good prosthetics departments are also vital for some patients in helping them to regain their identity and confidence in facing their partner, family, and the public.

With respect to communication most patients at some stage in their course of treatment have their ability to communicate interrupted. This can be temporary due to a tracheostomy, laryngeal edema from tumor, or surgical inflammation postoperatively. Speech will also be affected following laryngectomy, glossectomy, and other oral and pharyngeal reconstructions for varying periods of time.

To help the patient, the nurse may ask questions in such a way that a "yes" or "no" or "nod" of the head would suffice in the initial postoperative period. Written communication is always made available such as pen and paper or a magic slate. Flash cards depicting areas of care are also useful as a temporary measure or for the illiterate patient. Attempting to communicate will be extremely frustrating at times for the patients especially if they are feeling depressed or unwell and it is vital that the nurse is gentle, encouraging, and patient in helping the persons to communicate so that they do not regress or become mute.

Often conversation has to be repeated several times before it is understood, but practice at communication must be encouraged in a safe and private environment, especially in the early postoperative period where the patients may be upset at the sound of their initial voice. Nothing irritates a patient more than if the rushed nurse, doctor, or frustrated family member finishes the patient's sentence for him or her in their desire to be helpful, particularly if it has been interpreted incorrectly. Family and friends should be reassured and educated on these points.

SPECIFIC ISSUES OF CARE PRIOR TO TREATMENT
Information
Patients with head and neck cancer should have their information needs individually assessed but most need and want written information (28). Patients can also access information via the internet about investigations and treatment [National Health Service (NHS) Direct Online, www.nhsdirect.nhs.uk] and NICE also has online guidance (www.nice.org.uk) for head and neck cancer (8). The CNS will offer support and guidance, while acting as a key worker for patients at diagnosis, throughout and after their treatment (8,13). The use of Cancer Backup (www.cancer-backup.org.uk/Home) that has site-specific printable information on side effects can be a very useful supplementation along with local hospital resources. The British Thyroid Association (http://www.btf-thyroid.org/) and Ear, Nose and Throat (ENT) UK (www.entuk.org/) and the National Association Laryngectomy Club (NALC; www.laryngectomy.org.uk/) also offer comprehensive patient information booklets. It is also important to guide patients who find, or are given, information of unknown quality.

Nutrition
The dietitian will assess the patient's nutritional status and may prescribe a tailored regime straight away, especially if the patient has been experiencing dysphagia or is otherwise nutritionally debilitated. A nasogastric tube or parenteral nutrition via a radiologically guided (RIG) or endoscopically placed PEG may be required prior to commencement of definitive treatment (29). Around 40% of head and neck patients at diagnosis are malnourished (30), and the treatment process must be monitored to ensure that dietetic intervention is optimized (31). This is especially true of radiotherapy patients as their custom-made mask must fit well throughout the treatment, and weight loss affects the contours of the face.

Oral Care
Good oral hygiene is essential for any head and neck cancer treatment regimen. The maxillofacial team and dental hygienist will assess the patient and advise routine dentistry or extractions. Good oral hygiene, supportive care, and

improvements in radiotherapy techniques have reduced the incidence of osteoradionecrosis (32). The dental hygienist will ensure that dentition is in the best possible order prior to starting radiotherapy, and instructions for using fluoride gel with rationale will also be provided. A maxillofacial prosthodontist should also be available to take any intraoral and facial impressions prior to surgery.

Speech Therapy
The speech therapist will meet any patient who has or may have any speech, swallowing, or hearing impairment. It is vital that the patients see the speech therapist while they are still able to communicate freely to get to know each other, make assessments, and discuss the rehabilitation program. The Speech and Language Therapist (SLT) is a key worker for patients undergoing laryngectomy and will discuss surgical voice restoration (or alternative methods of communication such as an electro larynx or esophageal speech) if it seems that the patient will not be a suitable candidate for tracheo-esophageal puncture) prior to surgery. Ideally the patient will meet a current laryngectomee patient and hear him or her using tracheo-esophageal speech or alternative, along with his or her story of recovery (33).

Any patient who is experiencing swallowing difficulties prior to treatment should be evaluated by a SLT to identify any sign of aspiration, ascertain whether he or she can maintain a good standard of nutrition orally, and to plan care during treatment as well as posttreatment rehabilitation (8,34).

Audiological evaluation is a valuable base line and assists in comparing changes that may occur following surgery, radiotherapy, or chemotherapy.

Social Worker
The social worker can meet the patient and make an assessment and advise and help with any necessary documentation and employment benefits. The CNS also participates with benefits liaison and completes charitable grant applications for patients with specific needs.

Physiotherapy
Physiotherapists assess preoperatively and teach patients to clear secretions and cough effectively postoperatively to maintain a clear airway (35). Those patients with pulmonary problems or due to undergo a radical neck dissection can be seen by the physiotherapist for preoperative assessment of muscle strength and range of movement. Exercises can be given, and an explanation of a postoperative exercise program to decrease the degree of shoulder drop and limitation of movement following a radical neck dissection.

Research Nurse
Clinical trials often run concurrently with standard treatment, and patients recruited need support from the research nurse and often the CNS as they are closely linked. The research nurse helps the patient interpret the information and monitors patients throughout the screening phase, treatment, and follow-up. They are also a resource for the head and neck ward providing teaching advice and

explanations as needed. Referral for additional help from other members of the team will also follow as appropriate.

NURSING INTERVENTIONS PRIMARILY RELATING TO SURGERY

In view of the multiple aspects of care that may be required for each individual patient, the main nursing interventions have been subdivided for clarity.

Airway Management

Airway management and tracheostomy maintenance are some of the most demanding and anxious aspects of any nursing care. This mostly stems from fear of potentially acute and life-threatening situations, particularly in head and neck oncology because of the complex surgery involved and the unpredictable nature of any possible emergency.

For this reason it is imperative that nurses caring for this group of patients have a thorough clinical and theoretical knowledge of airway management. The patient and family will experience feelings of apprehension and uncertainty over an altered airway. Therefore it is vital that the nursing staff manage and teach the patient and family how to care for the airway in a calm, sensible and logical way. By sharing one's knowledge and adopting this manner, it will reduce anxiety and build confidence and trust for the patient and family. There should be a comprehensive and illustrated care plan for staff and relatives to follow while the patient is in hospital and written instructions for home to assist the community support team.

Those patients who are temporarily stridulous or who have a compromised airway, not necessitating a tracheostomy, can gain respiratory relief from humidified oxygen or from heliox (helium and oxygen). The helium gas in heliox has a lower viscosity than nitrogen and therefore produces less airway resistance so that the patient can ventilate more easily. Adrenaline nebulizers can also provide relief.

A tracheostomy may be a permanent or, more likely, temporary procedure to provide and maintain a patient's airway. In the latter situation obstruction such as tumor or edema caused by surgery or radiotherapy are bypassed. A tracheostomy can also be performed to enable the removal of tracheobronchial secretions when the patient is too weak to expectorate independently. Many patients with head and neck cancer do also have chronic obstructive airway disease or chronic bronchitis and may benefit from a tracheostomy to assist in reducing dead space and removal of secretions.

Tracheostomy Care

Equipment. It is essential that a patient who has a tracheostomy should always have at his or her bedside (or easily accessible if the patient is self-caring or ambulant) the items mentioned in Table 7.1 and Figure 7.1.

Assessment. The airway should be kept free of secretions at all times, and this is most effectively accomplished by encouraging the patient to cough. Not only is the airway cleared but the lungs expand to prevent atelectasis and pneumonia. Any nurse who is starting a span of duty should always do a baseline assessment of the airway and

Table 7.1 Equipment for Tracheostomy Care at the Bedside

Check emergency equipment is by bedside every shift

Emergency Tracheostomy Box	Bedside
• 2 x spare cuffed tracheostomy tubes, one same size and one a size smaller	• Scissors, gloves, aprons, goggles, and mask
• Tracheal dilators	• Sterile water labeled to flush suction tubing
• 10 ml syringe and lubrication jelly (KY jelly/Aquagel)	• Sodium bicarbonate
• Stitch cutter	• Oxygen outlet functioning
• Catheter mount and disconnection wedge	• Suction unit functioning and suction catheters of appropriate size available
• Percutaneous tracheostomy guidewire	• Oxygen saturation monitor

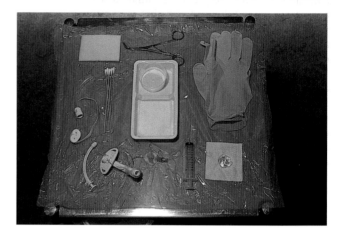

Figure 7.1 Equipment for changing a tracheostomy tube and cleaning of the stoma.

tube to check on the type and amount of secretions and the need for humidification or nebulizing spray. Listening to the breathing is vital for early signs of obstruction. This should be documented in the care plan that should detail the size and type of tube, cleaning the inner tube instructions (if not using a disposable inner tube), and frequency of suctioning required. The patient should have humidification, nebulizers guidelines recorded, and oxygen saturation monitoring available.

Suctioning. With a newly formed tracheostomy or if the patient is too weak to cough, the secretions must be suctioned from the trachea. This is a clean procedure, and sterilized equipment must be used. Choosing the right-sized catheter is essential for safe and effective suctioning (see below for a formula). The catheter should be inserted to the depth of the carina or until resistance is felt, or a cough is produced (36) withdraw the catheter 1 cm and then apply suction on withdrawal of catheter (37). Rapid release of folded tubing is traumatic, and suction catheters with a port to occlude digitally are best practice. (Feber 2000). The suction pressure should be between 13.5 and 20 kPa with the port uncovered (38). The whole procedure should not take longer than 10 seconds to reduce the risk of mucosal damage and hypoxaemia. However, as soon as patients are able to cough effectively, suctioning should be limited to the length of the tracheostomy tube plus 1 cm unless contraindicated by other factors (39). Ensure that oxygen saturation is monitored and if required reattach oxygen to limit hypoxia (40). Suctioning should be performed only when needed and not as part of routine, so that damage to the trachea is avoided.

Formula for deciding appropriate tracheostomy suction catheter:

External diameter of tracheostomy tube	Multiplied by 3	Divided by two = suction catheter size
Example: 8 mm	24	12
6 mm	18	10 (as per available number sequence)

Type of tube. Various types of tracheostomy tube are available, but for safety it is essential to use one that has a separate inner tube and one that is comfortable for the patient. These are available in cuffed, noncuffed, fenestrated, and nonfenestrated forms in different sizes, the use of each of them being indicated in different clinical situations. Disposable inner tubes are useful for reducing infection and saving time on cleaning especially in the ward setting. Nondisposable inner tubes may initially have to be cleaned every half an hour, but every patient should be carefully assessed on a continual basis. The outer tube needs changing less frequently according to the amount of secretions and manufacturers' guidelines. It is common for acute airway obstruction to occur because of a build-up of crusts at the bottom end of a tracheostomy tube, which is not recognized unless the whole tube is changed. The tube manufacturer should state when the tube should be changed (usually 28 days); however, this is open to individual preference and requirement along with safety issues (for instance if the patient is having bleeding or tumor invading the stoma). A cuffed tube should be inserted for bleeding stomas as tolerated or the situation allows. A tracheostomy bypasses the body's natural ability to warm, humidify, and filter the air we breathe (41) that if not corrected causes drying of the tracheal mucosa and thickening of secretions. This will increase the risk of tracheitis, atelectasis, infection, and airway obstruction. The tracheostomy also prevents them from increasing their intrathoracic pressure that enables the normal physical capacity to cough and clear secretions (42). In the immediate postoperative period mechanical humidifiers allow delivery of warm, moist oxygen through the tracheostomy tube. They can reduce the requirement for suctioning and are recommended as treatment of choice. Heat Moisture Exchangers are a range of products designed to conserve heat and moisture during expiration with a small amount of resistance once placed on the end of the tracheostomy tube. Other groups of humidification include stoma filters, bibs, and nebulizers.

Communication. Tracheostomy tubes should be fitted with speaking valves as soon as possible to help ease feelings of isolation for the patient and facilitate practice of speech.

Laryngectomy patients may have had a tracheoesophageal puncture performed either as a primary or

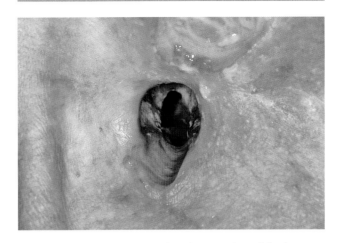

Figure 7.2 Large stomal tracheo-oesophageal fistula.

secondary procedure. They will wear a Foley catheter in the puncture site until they are ready to be fitted with the surgical voice prosthesis. If this is done primarily at the time of laryngectomy, the valve is usually fitted after normal swallowing has been started after 7 to 10 days. As a secondary procedure the valve can usually be fitted within 2 to 3 days (38). If this procedure is not possible patients should be introduced to an artificial device for communication, such as the use of electronic Speech-Generated Devices although some prefer to use pen and paper and write in advance or use gestures initially (43). Patients who are unable to produce a voice are vulnerable to depression and need continued psychological support especially if they live alone or are elderly. The electronic larynx that is battery powered and produces sound through vibration can be loud and embarrassing and takes practice with support from the SLT (44).

Laryngectomy tubes or stoma buttons. Some of these do not have an inner tube and therefore will need to be changed frequently especially when they are first used. Whenever the tube is removed it is essential that the airway is checked with a torch to make sure that there are no crusts building up below the tube. These can be removed carefully with angled forceps.

Peristomal wounds. Those patients with wounds in or around the stoma (Fig. 7.2) will need to have their tube removed to get good visualization of the wound and access for toileting.

Tracheostomy dressing. The tracheostomy dressing should be renewed, and the circumference of the stoma cleaned and dried at least once, if not twice, a day or more frequently depending on mucus production, to ensure secretions are cleared and do not lie wet against the skin causing excoriation. Using an appropriate barrier cream (i.e., Cavilon) can aid in preventing excoriation of the surrounding skin and any signs on infection should be documented and a swab taken if appropriate.

Self-care. Gradually as the patient and family members feel ready, tracheostomy care can be taught to them.

The main focus is to help the patients feel confident in keeping their tracheostomy tube patent by themselves by teaching the three basic aspects of tracheostomy care: changing the inner tubes of their tracheostomy tube, humidifying with a nebulizing spray, and expectorating secretions. This is obviously the patients' main priority, and they must be supported and encouraged. It must be recognized that each patient and his or her circumstances are different: some patients feel ready to learn all aspects of care from changing the tracheostomy dressing to doing a complete tube change, whereas others need considerable support.

Laryngectomy. The laryngectomy patient will need to learn all aspects of stomal toilet care and what to do in the event of an emergency. The permanency of their condition makes a laryngectomy patient realize that their freedom, independence, and survival depend on their knowledge and practical care. However, this type of permanent stoma is easier to manage, and laryngectomy tubes are very rarely needed in the long term. Stoma buttons or stoma vents (2) are much easier to use but may not be necessary for permanent use. The local ambulance service within their primary care trust should be notified that the patient has an altered airway in case of emergency, and lifelong links should be formed with their local NALC group through the CNS or SLT.

Postoperative Wound Care
Flap Care

General comments. Astute and skilled specialist head and neck nursing is necessary for the care of head and neck patients who have often had intricate reconstructions often involving free and pedicled flaps.

In the first 24 to 48 hours the patient will be nursed on a one-to-one basis for close observation and monitoring, sometimes in a high-dependency unit, particularly if he or she has a flap repair. The patient needs to be nursed in a semisitting position because gravity will help to reduce edema. Basic wound observation remains the same, but specific observations are necessary for flaps. The aim of the role of the high-dependency nurse is to monitor the flap frequently during the first 48 hours after the operation. An in-depth patient handover, with the surgeon, anesthetist, and the patients' named nurse is indispensable (45). This handover information should include the type of flap, area of origin, blood supply used, and areas to listen for the anastamosis with a doppler, if required. It is important that all involved in the patient's care are aware of what to look for and what potentially could go wrong. Blood flow into the flap must be adequate, and blood draining from the flap must also be unobstructed. The skin flap should be pink, warm, and blanch, showing a normal capillary return of 2 to 3 seconds when touched. A skilled practitioner with a high level of observational skills is therefore required.

The physiological reasons why flaps are at a high risk of failure in the immediate postoperative period, while the patient is in the high-dependency environment are

1. Hypothermia, in which a lower-than-normal core temperature encourages vasoconstriction and reduced blood flow in the flap.

2. Mechanical obstruction, such as kinking of the vessels through poor patient positioning, edema, or hematoma all of which impose pressure on the vessels resulting in arterial or venous occlusions.

3. A failure to provide adequate pain relief may also add to vasoconstriction and a threat to the circulating volume in the flap.

Flap monitoring. A white skin paddle color indicates a dearterialized flap where the blood supply is inadequate. When pricked by a member of the surgical team the flap should bleed if the circulation is adequate but not if the arterial supply is compromised. It must be remembered however that the normal color for the flap is the same as its original donor site, which is often paler than mucosal areas within the mouth (Fig. 7.3). Arterial devascularization is more commonly seen in the first 24 hours after operation. A blue or dusky discoloration indicates venous congestion, and this may occur later, after several days.

As previously described a skilled practitioner in a high-dependency unit should look after the patient postoperatively in which regular and objective observation must be performed for the first 0 to 72 hours. Studies (46) have shown that the following frequency for flap observations is acceptable:

- Quarter hourly for the first 4 hours postoperatively
- Half hourly for the subsequent 20 hours
- Hourly for the next 48 hours
- For the remaining hours this can be assessed according to clinical need

The practitioner will be assessing the color, turgidity, temperature, and capillary refill of the flap (Table 7.2).

The critical care nurse must monitor the patient's temperature, fluid balance, pain relief requirements, position, nutrition, and comfort, but overall a confident skilled practitioner is required.

Tapes and dressings. There must be no kinking, tension, or pressure on the flap. Vigilant attention must be given to ensure that tracheostomy tapes, dressing tapes, and

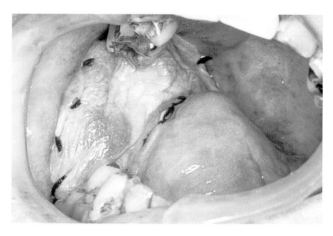

Figure 7.3 Free radial forearm flap in the oral cavity.

Table 7.2 Flap Monitoring Observations

Observations	Venous congestion	Normal	Arterial occlusion
Capillary refill	Brisk: under 2 seconds	2–3 seconds	Absent or longer than 6 seconds
Temperature	Colder than surrounding	Warm	Cold
Colour	Mottled or purple tissue	Pink usual skin tone	Paler than the patients skin tone
Turgidity	Turgid	Soft	Flaccid

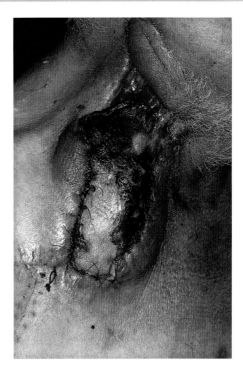

Figure 7.4 Partial loss of a latissimus dorsi flap.

bandages are not tied too tightly around the flap or wound. Some cosmetic surgeons prefer to stitch the tracheostomy tube in situ so that neck tapes are not required. Care should also be taken with Hudson or tracheostomy mask tapes that they are not too tight around the neck thus impeding blood flow. Oxygen tubing and other lines should not lie over the wound or flap site causing pressure.

Observation of mottling, duskiness, or sudden tightness of the neck dressing can be indicative of hematoma formation and possibly impending flap failure. Bandages used around the neck can also have the disadvantage of preventing visualization of important signs of skin changes and are generally not needed when suction drainage is used. The patient should be kept warm to avoid vasoconstriction.

Drainage bottles. All drainage bottles must be patent and checked regularly because a devacuumed or clamped bottle can cause flap failure, through the build-up of excess fluid that creates pressure on the capillaries. If the Redivac tubing is temporarily clamped for movement of the patient, it is essential that it is reopened.

Patency of the drainage bottle means that the connections are secure and the suction element (e.g. *Redivac drains* are inserted routinely and kept until their drainage decreased to less than 50 mL per 24 hours) is intact. The drain should be primed so that the suction pump is continuous, as ineffective drainage can result in haematoma or oedema.

Fluid balance. The patient must have an adequate fluid balance with the aim of being neither overloaded, nor dehydrated. The hemoglobin should be ideally over 10 g/dL, and if below this, the patient should be transfused to ensure that sufficient oxygen is perfusing all wound areas. When a flap is being used, the hemoglobin should not be too high as the blood circulation may become more sluggish, and this may jeopardize the circulation particularly in the first few days after operation.

Flap failure. The medical team must be notified immediately if the flap is showing any signs of failure. Flaps can tolerate approximately 4 hours of ischemia before irreversible tissue necrosis occurs. The team will assess the situation and start medical intervention to save the flap if necessary. Such measures may include releasing one or two vital sutures to ease pressure or tension or evacuating a hematoma, which can be done either on the ward or may necessitate the patient going back to theater. Pedicled

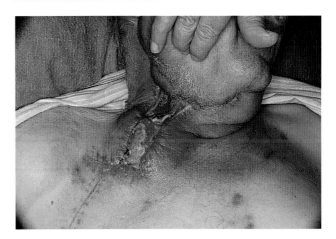

Figure 7.5 Satisfactory healing after 2 weeks.

latissimus dorsi flaps sometimes can suffer circulation problems if the axilla is compressed, but this can be relieved if the arm is abducted and supported.

In general the survival of free flaps is an "all-or-nothing" phenomenon because the circulation failure is usually in the main artery or vein. Salvage of a compromised flap is an emergency procedure to evacuate the clot and/or redo the anastomosis. For pedicled cutaneous or myocutaneous flaps, tissue loss is usually partial and a "wait-and-see" policy is adopted to allow demarcation. The underlying muscle is normally viable and will eventually granulate well (Figs. 7.4 and 7.5).

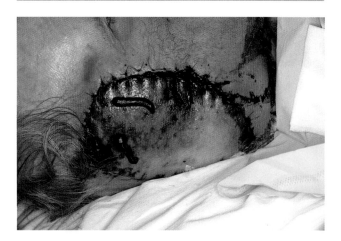

Figure 7.6   Leeches on a congested flap.

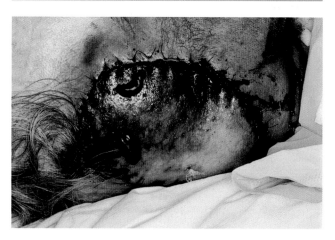

Figure 7.7   After 30 minutes.

Necrosis can take several days to develop, and during this immediate period it can be difficult to determine whether the flap is going to recover (47). A time of high psychological anxiety for the patient ensues, and the therapeutic relationship between members of the multidisciplinary team is key to their well-being and ongoing development.

Leeches. Another simple, noninvasive, and painless measure to reduce congestion in a flap is by the application of leeches. Each leech can remove approximately 10 ml of blood. Three or four leeches can be applied as necessary in the acute situation to the congested area and may be all that is necessary to ease the tension and improve blood flow (Figs. 7.6 and 7.7). Improvements in the skin color are noticed almost immediately. With a skilled, professional, and empathetic approach, patients will understand and comply especially as the alternative could be a lengthy surgical procedure. Frodel et al. have suggested utilizing leeches in the salvage of compromised facial soft tissue avulsions (48). In summary, leeches provide another mechanism to reduce venous congestion by bleeding out from the flap, utilizing their own intrinsic anticoagulant.

Skin Grafts Care

Skin grafts are composed of epidermal tissue and a thin layer of dermis. Skin grafts vary in thickness dependent on the recipient area to be covered. It may be a full thickness (Wolfe) graft, which is often taken from the postauricular sulcus or the inguinal region. The most commonly used type of skin graft is a split thickness (Thiersch) graft, which may be taken from the upper arm or from the thigh. The skin graft is removed from the donor site and sutured or laid on the recipient area. It acts as a dressing to cover the wound site and eventually becomes incorporated as skin epidermis. A Thiersch graft may also be taken from the buttocks as this is a useful area especially if the patient is worried about the potential scarring and disfigurements at the donor site.

Nursing observation and care will include the donor site and the recipient site. The protective covering of the donor site will depend on the surgeon's preference.

The pain often experienced by the patient is due to exposure of nerve endings that necessitates an occlusive dressing (49). If the wound leaks excessive exudate the top dressing can be taken down and rebandaged. However if the exudate looks or smells infected the dressing should be irrigated thoroughly to ease removal and assess the wound bed.

The most common complications of donor sites are infection and slippage of dressings. Beldon researched appropriate dressings and found that an alginate with film dressing promoted comfort and healing (50). Mepitel silicone primary dressing is also recommended as it can be left intact over the wound bed while saturated secondary dressings are replaced. The inflammatory and highly exuding phase occurs during the first 48 to 72 hours. Typically healing occurs within 10 to 14 days (49). When it is time for the dressing to be removed it should be gently soaked off in the bath or shower. Re-epithelialization occurs in the donor site area as the healing process takes place. For this reason the dressing must never be forced off as the neo-epithelium tissue will be damaged.

Patients often complain of most of their pain being in the donor site area postoperatively. Some anesthetists give a regional nerve block to ease the pain on the donor limb particularly if it has been bilateral. A local injection of Marcain can also dull the pain in the early postoperative period. The pain is due to exposure of nerve endings. Regular analgesia and avoidance of friction from night clothes and bedding is essential.

The recipient site is often exposed to air while healing occurs. If this is too painful in the early days, a nonadherent dressing such as mepitel or geliperm can be used. It is essential that the area is reassessed every day with a view to exposing it to the air to dry as soon as the patient can tolerate this. If it is covered for too long, the area becomes wet and infected. Once the area has begun to dry, moisturizing cream can be applied to prevent crust formation and to ease any discomfort. The massaging effects of the moisturizing are very beneficial in preventing taught scar tissue and facilitating a smooth supple skin.

If a radial forearm flap has been used the donor arm is usually immobilized in a sling and plaster until the graft "takes" at around 5 days.

Wound Care

Wound complications. A wound complication is not only distressing and discouraging for the patient and medical staff but also invariably means a prolonged stay in hospital.

Fistulae. These require patience and perseverance and will often gradually close spontaneously but if larger may need surgical intervention. Keeping the fistula clean, free from infection. and as dry as possible may at times be very demanding but will encourage healing (Figs. 7.8 and 7.9).

Sloughing wounds. These may require surgical debridement although hydrogels (with an absorbent secondary dressing) are a less invasive technique that utilize the body's natural mechanisms for debriding devitalized tissue and a holistic wound assessment should be made (51).

Fungating wounds. These are cancerous wounds that break through the skin surface and can be ulcerative and crater-like or nodular. The main aim in caring for these is to improve the patient's quality of life (52): managing any pain systemically, containing exudates, and preventing malodor. Minimizing the time it takes to dress the wound and keeping the dressings simple is important, particularly if the patient wants to manage his or her own care. Malodorous wounds can be covered with carbon-impregnated dressings, and topical antibiotics can be applied such as metronidazole that is an excellent deodorizer. Metronidazole taken systemically is also effective or the use of aromatherapy diffusers (Figs. 7.10 and 7.11). The use of silver-impregnated dressings has also been beneficial in controlling odor and multiresistant infections. There is a wide variety of combined dressings available that tackle malodor, bleeding, and exudates (53,54).

Vascular wounds. These can be dressed with alginate products such as Kaltostat.

Hemorrhage

Intraoral bleeding. Minor bleeding can be controlled by rinsing with tranexamic acid. Patients should also be shown how to roll up gauze and apply pressure to the site

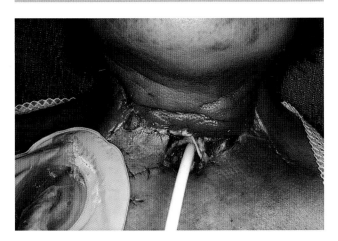

Figure 7.8 Pharyngocutaneous fistula postjejunum anastomosis requiring stoma bag for secretions.

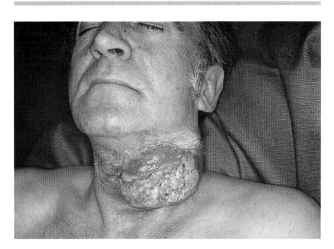

Figure 7.10 Fungating neck wound.

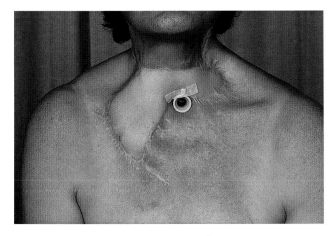

Figure 7.9 Six months later after complete healing using a latissimus dorsi flap.

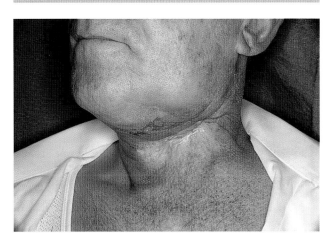

Figure 7.11 Eight months later after chemoradiation.

for around 20 minutes, during which time they should sit still and minimize activity.

Major arterial bleeds. These are potentially fatal for some patients, but even minor bleeds can be very distressing. A massive hemorrhage is usually heralded over preceding hours by more minor episodes of bleeding, and the source of any minor bleeding must be very carefully investigated. Patients with a previous history of radiation therapy and who have had a fistula or infection are most at risk if the wound has broken down or those with a tumor fungating within the neck. If active resuscitation is considered appropriate, the patient should be cannulated for administering volume expanders and blood .When bleeding occurs, the nurse must apply firm pressure with large pads and call for emergency assistance. The rest of the team can administer resuscitation and coordinate theatre staff if appropriate (55,56).

When the patient has advanced untreatable head and neck disease and is thought to be at risk of carotid artery rupture, a multiprofessional approach must be taken to the consideration of how best to manage a catastrophic bleed and when and how to inform patient and relatives (56). In general, authors agree that an open and honest approach is most helpful to patient and family (36,57), in which each case should be decided on an individual basis. A plan of action should be agreed as per the British Association of Head and Neck Oncology Nurses (BAHNON, 1995) and hospital guidelines (36); a "Do Not Attempt Resuscitation" Order should be signed and held in the patient's notes. A similar approach should be taken with close cooperation between hospital and community teams if the patient is to be in his own home (58). The intravenous, or if unavailable, the subcutaneous or intramuscular, route can be used to deliver a sedative such as midazolam to relieve the anxiety associated with a carotid blowout. Opioids may be indicated only if there is concurrent pain (59). A supply of gloves and dark towels should be available, and the patient nursed in a side room if in hospital. Gentle suctioning, insertion of a cuffed tube if the patient has a tracheostomy, and appropriate positioning of the patient can help to maintain a clear airway and minimize the discomfort and fear associated with sensations of choking (56,58). Support is essential for all those present at this distressing event (56).

PAIN MANAGEMENT

Pain is experienced by 40 to 80% of patients suffering from head and neck cancer (60,61) in various phases of the disease and its treatment. It is often difficult to assess and not always easy to elicit the exact cause due to the complex structure of the head and neck and diverse sensory innervations. Ruzicka et al. subdivide pain sources as 65 to 80% related to disease and tumor, 25% cancer therapies and investigations, and 3 to 10% have concurrent conditions unrelated to their cancer (62). Medical expertise from a specialist in pain management, who has a good understanding of head and neck disease and treatment, is imperative in helping to control this symptom. Access for administration of analgesia is an important issue for the head and neck patient because swallowing is often difficult or inadvisable during the early postoperative phase. Once the patient's controlled intravenous analgesia has been

discontinued, a nasogastric or gastrostomy tube is the preferred option. Aspirin-based products should not be used preoperatively, and if used postoperatively with great caution as they interfere with hemostasis in surgery and may predispose to postoperative hematoma formation (55). Complementary methods are also of value in pain management such as acupuncture, diversional therapy, massage, and aromatherapy as well as the prescribed regular analgesic medication. Monitoring the effectiveness and evaluating the pain management regimen should be continued throughout the patient's course of treatment and at follow-up appointments. Please refer to the chapter in this book on palliation of advanced head and neck cancer for further information.

MOUTH CARE

The aim of comprehensive mouth care is to maintain good oral hygiene, to prevent plaque build-up, dental decay, and infection. It also is essential to keep the oral mucosa moist and intact and to promote patient comfort and well-being. To help achieve good oral status, the patient must be adequately hydrated and the appropriate instruments, solutions, and methods used.

Incapacitated patients and those unable to perform their own oral toilet are most at risk of developing mouth-care problems. It is essential that the nurse makes a thorough assessment of the patient's oral status and assists them in the most appropriate regimen. Irrigation of the oral cavity is very beneficial when the patient has an intraoral lesion or surgical site. Irrigation helps to keep the mouth or any cavities fresh and clean. It stimulates blood supply, reduces edema, helps to alleviate pain and discomfort, controls odor, and helps to prevent and clear debris and infection. When the patient is learning to irrigate, the nurse assists by offering support and advice. The patient is guided and helped to avoid trauma to exposed tissues, flaps, or grafts.

If the oral cleaning is painful or uncomfortable, the patient must be offered analgesia half an hour prior to his or her oral hygiene regimen. Rinsing with warm saline every 3 to 4 hours and using a soft-bristle or baby toothbrush can facilitate mouth care (63).

There will be periods when the patients feel inundated and overwhelmed at the many aspects of their care rehabilitation that they are trying to manage, such as tracheostomy care and enteral feeding. It is therefore practical and sensible to keep all of these regimens as simple and as logical as possible for optimum patient compliance, especially if they are going to be long term.

NURSING CONSIDERATIONS FOR RADIOTHERAPY AND CHEMOTHERAPY TREATMENTS IN HEAD AND NECK CANCER PATIENTS

The use of radiotherapy to treat head and neck cancer patients, postoperatively and as first-line treatment is common and necessitates nurses understanding of it (64,65). Quality of life studies clearly demonstrate that the lowest point in the patient's treatment experience is radiotherapy (66).

There is a more common trend toward treating advanced head and neck cancer patients with radiotherapy and chemotherapy in the curative setting to preserve organ function and reserve surgery for the relapsed or recurrent disease setting (2). Randomized controlled trials have found that concurrent chemotherapy with radiotherapy was better than radiotherapy alone or induction chemotherapy followed by radiotherapy (5) and similarly post-operative chemo-radiation has also improved disease-free survival (67–69).

The chemotherapy agents enhance cell kill during radiotherapy and cisplatin and fluorouracil, commonly used in head and neck cancer, are from this radiosensitizer group (4). Although improving survival, however, concomitant treatment increases toxicities that can lead to patients needing longer hospital stays for nutritional support and hydration (70).

The severity of mucosal and skin reactions is influenced by the radiation or combined chemotherapy and radiation therapy, genetic and personal factors (71). The total dose per fraction of radiotherapy and the volume of normal tissue included in the treatment field is also a factor (1). The side effects of radiotherapy are enhanced by the addition of chemotherapy, and smoking further enhances these (72). Side effects include dry mouth, difficulty with speech and swallowing, and increased pain (12,36,72,73). Brief interventions delivered at a "teachable moment" postdiagnosis/pretreatment are recommended to strongly advise that patients stop smoking as patients will be motivated to adhere to advice at this time.

An understanding of the impact of having a cancer diagnosis and therapies is vital to guide practice. Providing consistently accurate information about the likely consequences of treatment is essential for effective management of their side effects (64). The ability to accurately determine the severity of symptoms can enhance trust, reduce anxiety, and improve patient satisfaction with care (71). All nurses in outpatient and inpatient ward nurses have a responsibility to understand and manage the side effects of treatment.

Nutritional Support

The head and neck team need to incorporate nutritional assessment and monitoring into each stage of the cancer treatment process to ensure that dietetic intervention is optimized (31). Pain on eating, ulcerated mouth, presence of dysphagia, and poor fitting dentures are all additional factors that may interfere with an individual's ability to chew and swallow a nutritionally balanced diet. As around 40% of patients at diagnosis are malnourished (30) and likely, while undergoing radical radiotherapy, to develop nutritional complications due to mucositis, taste, and appetite changes, dysphasia, and a build-up of difficult-to-clear secretions near the end of treatment all lead to weight loss. This particularly affects those having treatment to the oral cavity and pharynx with premorbid conditions. These patients could also benefit from prophylactic PEG placement prior to commencing therapy (29). Tube placement minimizes the active weight loss during treatment and helps maintain weight (30). RIG/PEG tubes are more aesthetically pleasing for patients than the alternative nasogastric tube that is taped to the nose and is at risk of accidental displacement and potentially aspiration (74). There can, however, be complications associated with their placement that could delay treatment if placed prophylactically, and these include tube migration, gastrointestinal bleeding, pain, infection, and leakage (75). There can be difficulty weaning patients off their enteral feeding tube and returning to normal swallow following treatment, and SLT assessment and input is vital to recovery and rehabilitation.

Mucositis and Oral Care

Patients who smoke during induction chemotherapy and those with a poor diet are more likely to suffer mucositis during radiotherapy or chemo-radiation (76). Stopping smoking and working out a regimen during radiotherapy treatment with the specialist oral surgeon and dental hygienist is an important preparatory step. Radiation affects the bones ability to repair itself following a dental extraction and can lead to osteoradionecrosis. The salivary glands are often included within the treatment field and do not function as well following radiotherapy. If only one side of the face is treated the other often compensates, but it is the saliva that naturally cleans the teeth and helps remove debris to prevent caries. Following radiotherapy the saliva is thicker and less effective and dental decay is secondary to xerostomia [p.464 (64)]. Prescription fluoride gels and regular mouthwashes along with adequate hydration will promote comfort and help maintain the mucosa, although radiotherapy will lead to mucositis as the treatment continues in around the 3rd week (63,76).

Best management of mucositis also involves adequate pain relief, and though some patients manage on soluble aspirin gargles and paracetamol with a mixed local anaesthetic solution (63). Often referral to the specialist pain team is necessary and opiates are required. Close monitoring of nutritional intake and appropriate interventions to rehydrate or refer to the SLT for swallow assessment will prevent the risk of aspiration due to edema and subsequent loss of function. If patients are using a feeding tube nurses must reinforce the teaching of oral hygiene, especially monitoring their temporomandibular joint function that may be impaired and that may in turn limit oral hygiene (36).

Skin Care

Irradiation inhibits the production of keratinized epithelium by damaging the dividing cells in the basal layer of the skin, causing initially a sunburn-like effect (77). The severity of symptoms depends on the relationship between: time, dose, and volume of tissue treated (78). Radiation-induced skin reactions are influenced additionally by general health, adequate nutrition, chronic illness, and combined treatment modalities (71,79).

Head and neck cancer patients are treated in an individually cast shell, which is fixed to the radiation treatment couch to ensure that daily setup is accurate (64,80). Skin reactions also increase, the closer the tumor is to the skin surface (79,80).

Surveys of skin care practice for radiotherapy reactions in the U.K. and abroad have concluded that there are a variety of approaches and products in use based largely on historical precedent and personal preference rather than clinical evidence (81,82).

Table 7.3 Management of Radiation Induced Skin Reactions

Causes of skin reactions to radiotherapy
* The skin is radiosensitive and undergoes rapid mitosis
* Radiation causes biochemical changes within the DNA molecules and damages the basal layer (cell-renewal takes 2–3 weeks)
* 5-fluorouracil is a radio-sensitizing drug and increases reactions in many head and neck treatment regimens

Minimizing the damage of radiation induced skin reactions
* Skin care guidelines and patient teaching (premoisturizing, shaving, loose collars and cotton clothing, etc.)
* On-treatment clinics and weekly audit
* Linear Accelerators have reduced skin reaction incidence and severity as they deliver maximum dosage below the skin.
* Treatment shell "cut-outs" during radiotherapy

Levels of skin reaction
* Erythema: loss of moisture leads to a "sunburn," which occurs gradually and becomes noticeable at around 2–3 weeks, dependingon dosage and fractionation
* Dry desquamation: dryness, cracking, and scaling starts to appear in patches, with the erythema, often accompanied by a build-up of emollient cream
* Moist desquamation: blistering, broken, and weeping skin with a light to moderate exudate (could occur at the very end of or following radiotherapy)

Management of skin reaction
* Erythema and dry desquamation:
    Regular application of aqueous cream being careful to avoid build-up in skin creases
* Moist desquamation during treatment:
    Low exudate: use hydrogel sheets or gel with pad/foam and light bandage
    Moderate exudate: as above, or more absorbent alginate/hydrocolloid/foam

NB as healing progresses and exudates decrease dressings can be reduced for comfort (i.e., mepitel with light secondary dressing, secured with a bandage or tape to healthy skin outside the treatment area)

Recommended nursing care of skin reactions is careful monitoring and use of emollients during treatment while the skin is intact (Table 7.3).

CONTINUING SUPPORT

Information on support services and groups must also be made available for those patients in the follow-up phase of treatment (19). It is important to continue to inquire in the follow-up clinics how the patients are coping at home and if they have any relationship or personal worries as many problems sometimes manifest only when the patients are back at home. It may be appropriate for the patient to be followed up in the clinical nurse specialist (or equivalent) led clinic for ongoing psychological, social, or sexual health support, which also ensures continuity for the patient. In the general follow-up clinic where the patient may meet a new or different member of the medical team it is often difficult or inappropriate to discuss personal matters. The patient is usually only concerned with one vital medical issue: that he or she is still free of cancer.

CONCLUSION

Intensive and comprehensive nursing and a unified approach to care with the medical staff and multidisciplinary team offers the patient an optimum opportunity to regain, in his or her perception, a quality of life that is acceptable after the impact of head and neck cancer and its treatment. The delivery of this care should be with total empathy and consideration at all times.

REFERENCES

1. Kelly LE, Ward EC, Van As Brooks eds. Radiation and chemotherapy. In: Head and neck cancer: treatment, rehabilitation and outcomes. San Diego, CA: Plural Publishing, 2007: 57–86.
2. Scarpa R. Advanced practice nursing in head and neck cancer: implementation of five roles. Oncology Nursing Forum 2004; 31: 579–83.
3. Posner MR. Adjuvant post-operative chemoradiotherapy in head and neck cancer patients: A standard of care? Editorial. The Oncologist 2005; 10: 174–5. Retrieved March 28, 2008, from www.theoncologist.com
4. Hilderley LJ. Radiation therapy. In: Gates RA, Fink RM, ed. Oncology nursing secrets, 2nd ed. Philadelphia: Hanley and Belfus, 2001; 35–43.
5. Forastiere AA, Goepfert H, Maor M et al. Concurrent chemotherapy and radiotherapy for organ preservation in advanced laryngeal cancer. The New England Journal of Medicine 2003; 349: 2091–8.
6. Sidholm MA, Poulsen MG. Multidisciplinary care in oncology: medicolegal implications of group decisions. Lancet Oncology 2006; 7: 951–4.
7. Birchall M, Bailey D, King P. Effect of process standards on survival of patients with head and neck cancer in the south and west of England. The British Journal of Cancer 2004; 91: 1477–81.
8. National Institute for Clinical Excellence. Health care services for head and neck cancers, understanding NICE guidance-information for the public. November 2004. Retrieved 12/24/2007, from www.nice.org.uk/nicemedia/pdf/csghn_publicinfoenglish.pdf
9. Randall F, Downie RS. Teamwork. In: Palliative care ethics, a good companion. Oxford, UK: Oxford Medical Publications, 1996: 40–59.
10. National Institute for Clinical Excellence. Improving outcomes in head and neck cancers. London: National Institute for Clinical Excellence, 2004; 43–7.

11. Feber T. Mouthcare. In: Head and neck oncology nursing. Oxford, UK: Whurr Publishing, 2000: 2.2, 121–46.

12. Sharp L, Tishelman C. Smoking cessation for patients with head and neck cancer: a qualitative study of patients' and nurses' experiences in a nurse-led intervention. Cancer Nursing 2005; 28: 226–35.

13. Semple Jane CJ. The role of the CNS in head and neck oncology. Nursing Standard 2001; 15: 39–42.

14. Kubler-Ross E. On death and dying. New York: Scribner Classics, 1969.

15. Massie MJ, Holland J. Overview of normal reactions and prevalence of psychiatric disorders. In: Holland JC, Rowland JH, ed. Handbook of psychooncology: psychological care of the patient with cancer. New York: Oxford University Press, 1989: 273–82.

16. Furlong E, O'Toole S. Psychological care for patients with cancer. In: Kearney N, Richardson A, eds. Nursing patients with cancer. Oxford, UK: Churchill Livingstone, 2005; 1717–35.

17. Wortman CB, Dunkel-Schetter C. Interpersonal relationships and cancer: a theoretical analysis. J Clin Issues 1979; 39: 120–55.

18. Mesters I, Van den Borne H, McCormick L et al. Openness to discuss cancer in the nuclear family: scale, development and validation. Psychosomatic Medicine 1997; 59: 269–79.

19. Edwards D. Face to face. Patient, family and professional perspectives of head and neck cancer care. London: King's Fund Publishing, 1997.

20. Kugaya A, Akechi T, Okamura H et al. Correlates of depressed mood in ambulatory head and neck cancer patients, Psycho oncology 1999; 8: 494–9.

21. Houldin A. Patients with cancer: understanding the psychological pain. Philadelphia: Lippincott, 2000.

22. Caplan G. Principles of preventative psychiatry. London: Basic Books, 1966.

23. Holland J, Lewis S. The human side of cancer: living with hope, coping with uncertainty. New York: Harper Collins, 2000.

24. Rhys Evans F. An investigation into functional problems following major oral surgery in head and neck cancer patients, and coping mechanisms employed by the patient. MSc Thesis, University of Surrey, 1993.

25. Harcourt D, Rumsey N. Altered body image. In: Kearney N, Richardson A, eds. Nursing patients with cancer. Oxford, UK: Churchill Livingstone, 2005; 701–16.

26. Bjordal K, de Graeff A, Fayers PM, et al. A prospective study of quality of life in head and neck cancer patients. Part II: longitudinal data. Laryngoscope 2001; 111: 1440–52.

27. Quinn B. Sexual health in cancer care. Nursing Times 2003; 99: 32–4.

28. Semple CJ, McGowan B. Need for appropriate written information for patients, with particular reference to head and neck cancer. J Clin Nurs 2002; 11: 585–93.

29. Cady J. Nutritional support during radiotherapy for head and neck cancer: the role of prophylactic feeding tube placement. J Clin Oncol Nurs 2006; 11: 875–80.

30. Manger S, Slevin N, Mais K et al. Evaluating predictive factors for determining enteral nutrition in patients receiving radical radiotherapy for head and neck cancer: a retrospective review. Radiother Oncol 2006; 78: 152–78.

31. Batty J. Nutrition. In: Feber T, ed. Head and neck oncology nursing. London: Whurr Publishing, 2000: 171–88.

32. Chambers M, Garden A, Lemon J et al. Oral complications of cancer treatment. In: Davies A, Finlay I, eds. Oral care in advanced disease. Oxford, Oxford University Press 2005: 171–83S.

33. Harvey M. Altered communication. In: Feber T, ed. Head and neck oncology nursing. Oxford, UK: Whurr Publishing, 2000: 189–218.

34. Sievers AEF. Postoperative management of the head and neck surgical patient. In: Clarke LK, Dropkin MJ, eds. Head and neck cancer. Pittsburgh, PA: Oncology Nursing Society, 2006: 85–102.

35. Saunders NA, Coman WB, Guminski AD. Cancer of the head and neck. In: Ward EC, Van As Brooks eds. Head and neck cancer: treatment, rehabilitation and outcomes. San Diego, CA: Plural Publishing, 2007: 2–26.

36. Feber T. Carotid Haemorrhage. In: Head and neck oncology nursing. Oxford, UK: Whurr Publishing, 2000: 245–52.

37. Wood CJ. Endotracheal suctioning: a literature review. Intensive and Critical Care Nursing 1998; 14: 124–36

38. Russell C, Matta B, eds. Tracheostomy: a multiprofessional handbook. Cambridge, UK: Cambridge University Press, 2004.

39. Griggs A. Tracheostomy: suctioning and humidification. Nursing Standard 1998; 13: 49–53.

40. Day T. Tracheal suctioning: when, why and how. Nursing Times 2000; 96: 13–15.

41. Harkin H, Russell C. Tracheostomy patient care. Nursing Times 2001; 97: 34–6.

42. Docherty B. Respiratory Care. Professional Nurse 2001; 16: 1020.

43. Happ MB, Roesch TK, Kagan SH. Patient communication following head and neck cancer surgery: a pilot study using electronic speech-generating devices. Oncology Nursing 2005; 32: 1179–87.

44. Coltart L. Voice restoration after laryngectomy. Nursing Standard 1998; 13: 36–40.

45. Storch J, Rice J. Reconstructive plastic surgical nursing clinical management and wound care. Oxford, Blackwell Publishing 2005: 300–5.

46. Hitchinson CR, Williams KD. Post operative free flap monitoring: clinical guidelines. 2000. Available at http://www.bahnon.org.uk/professional%20guidelines/flpa%20guidelines.doc

47. Mc Gregor A, Mc Gregor I. Fundamental techniques of plastic surgery. Churchill, UK: Livingstone, 2000.

48. Frodel JL Barth P, Wagner J. Salvage of partial facial soft tissue avulsions with medicinal leeches. Otolaryngal Head and Neck Surgery 2004; 131: 934–6.

49. Jones C, Robinson D. Wound care after head and neck surgery. In: Feber T, ed. Head and neck oncology nursing. Oxford, UK: Whurr Publishing, 2000: 239.

50. Beldon P. Comparison of four different dressings on donor site wounds. Br J Nurs 2003; 13(Tissue Viability Suppl): S38–45.

51. Davies P. Current thinking on the management of necrotic and sloughy wounds. Professional Nurse 2004; 19: 34–6.

52. Laverty D. Complex wounds in head and neck cancer. In: Booth S, Davies A, eds. Palliative care consultations in head and neck cancer. Oxford, UK: Oxford University Press, 2006: 121–37.

53. Kelly N. Malodorous fungating wounds: a review of current literature. Professional Nurse 2002; 17: 323–6.

54. Naylor W. Malignant wounds: aetiology and principles of management. Nursing Standard 2002; 16: 45–53.

55. Rhys Evans F. Tumours of the head and neck. In: Tshudin V, ed. Nursing the patient with cancer. London: Prentice Hall, 1996: 178–201.

56. Frawley T, Begley CM. Caring for people with carotid artery rupture. Brit J Nurs 2006; 13: 24–28.

57. Forbes K. Palliative care in head and neck cancer. Clinical Otolaryngology 1997; 22: 117–22.

58. Potter E. The management of carotid artery rupture. British Association of Head and Neck Oncology Nurses. Retrieved September 7, 2008, from http://www.bahnon.org.uk/professional guidelines/carotid haemorrhage guidelines

59. Twycross R, Wilcock A, Charlesworth S et al. Palliative care formulary, 2nd ed. Abingdon: Radcliffe Medical Press Oxford, England, 2002.

60. Bonica JJ. Treatment of cancer pain: current status and future needs. In: Fields HL, ed. Advances in pain and therapy. Vol. 9. New York: Raven Press, 1985: 589–617.

61. Webster M, Hagen NA. Pain management in advanced and recurrent disease. In: Booth S, Davies A, eds. Palliative care consultations in head and neck cancer. Oxford, UK: Oxford University Press, 2006: 139–60.

62. Ruzicka D, Gates RA, Fink RM. Pain management. In: Gates RA, Fink RM, eds. Oncology nursing secrets, 2nd ed. Philadelphia: Hanley and Belfus, 2001: 391–415.

63. Jennings RL, Harris LL. Cancers of the head and neck. In: Gates RA, Fink RM, eds. Oncology nursing secrets, 2nd ed. Philadelphia: Hanley and Belfus, 2001: 251–62.

64. Edwards S. Radiotherapy for head and neck cancer. In: Feber T, ed. Head and neck oncology nursing. Oxford, UK: Whurr Publishing, 2000: 453–77.

65. Wells M. What's so special about radiotherapy nursing? European Journal of Oncology Nursing 1998; 2: 162–8.

66. Campbell BC, Marbella A, Layde PM. Quality of life and recurrence concern in survivors of head and neck cancer. The Laryngoscope 2000; 110: 895–906.

67. Cooper J, Pajak TF, Forastiere A et al. Postoperative concurrent radiotherapy and chemotherapy for high risk squamous cell carcinoma of the head and neck. The New Engl J Med 2004; 350: 1937–44.

68. Bernier J, Domenge C, Ozsahin M et al. Postoperative irradiation with or without concomitant chemotherapy for locally advanced head and neck cancer. New Engl J Med 2004; 350: 1945-1952.

69. Bernier J, Cooper JS. Chemoradiation after surgery for high risk head and neck cancer patients: How strong is the evidence? The Oncologist 2005; 10: 215–24.

70. Adelstein DJ, Li Y, Adams GL et al. An intergroup phase iii comparison of standard radiation therapy in patients with unresectable squamous cell head and neck cancer. J Clin Oncol 2003; 21: 92–8.

71. Porock D. Factors influencing the severity of radiation skin and oral mucosal reactions, Eur J Cancer Care 2002; 11: 33–43.

72. Browman GP, Wong G, Hodson I et al. Influence of cigarette smoking on the efficacy of radiation therapy in head and neck cancer. The New Engl J Med 1993; 328: 59–63.

73. Gritz ER, Schacherer C, Koehly L et al. Smoking withdrawal and relapse in head and neck cancer patients. Head & Neck 1999; 21: 420–7.

74. Ziegler L, Newell R, Stafford N et al. A literature review of head and neck cancer patients information needs, experiences and views regarding decision-making. Eur J Cancer Care 2004; 13: 119–26.

75. Williams E, Sabol DA, DeLegge M. Small bowel obstruction caused by bowel wall haematoma following PEG. Gastrointest Endosc 2003; 57: 273–4.

76. Porock D, Nikoletti S, Cameron F. The relationship between factors that impair wound healing and the severity of acute radiation skin and mucosal toxicities in head and neck cancer, Cancer Nurs 2004; 27: 71–8.

77. Campbell J, Lane C. Developing a skin care protocol in radiotherapy. Professional Nurse 1996; 12: 105–8.

78. Noble-Adams R. Radiation-induced skin reactions 2: development of a measurement tool. Br J Nurs 1999; 8: 1208–11.

79. Sitton E. Managing side effects of skin changes and fatigue. In: Nursing care in radiation oncology, 2nd ed. Philadelphia: WB Saunders Company, 1997: 79–88.

80. Dobbs J, Barrett A, Ash D. Practical radiotherapy planning, 3rd ed. Bristol, UK: Arnold, 1999.

81. D'Haese S, Bate T, Claes S et al. Management of skin reactions during radiotherapy: a study of nursing practice. Eur J Cancer Care 2005; 14: 28–42.

82. Nystedt KE, Hill JE, Mitchell AM et al. The standardization of radiation skin care in British Columbia: a collaborative approach. Oncology Nurs Forum 2005; 32: 1199–206.

83. Randall F, Downie RS. Clinical treatment decisions. In: Palliative care ethics, a good companion. Oxford, UK: Oxford Medical Publications, 1996: 110–38.

84. Massie MJ. Prevalence of depression in patients with cancer. J Natl Cancer Inst Monogr 2004; 32: 51–7.

8

Nutritional Support of Head and Neck Cancer Patients

Clare Shaw

INTRODUCTION

Up to 60% of head and neck cancer patients may be malnourished at diagnosis (1). Weight loss and malnutrition in head and neck cancer patients are primarily caused by a reduced food intake that may be due to physical or psychological factors. Metabolic changes due to malignant disease may also contribute to the development of malnutrition. Treatment of head and neck cancer may further exacerbate a poor dietary intake thereby increasing the risk of complications during treatment (2,3).

CAUSES OF POOR DIETARY INTAKE AND WEIGHT LOSS

The causes of a poor diet and weight loss are complex (Table 8.1) and are exacerbated by the metabolic effects of the tumor. These include increased glucose–carbon cycling, elevated protein turnover, and possibly increased fat oxidation (4,5). These metabolic changes may be mediated by cytokines including Interleukin-1, Interleukin-6, and tumor necrosis factor (6). Surgery, trauma, and sepsis cause an elevation in metabolic rate, increased protein breakdown, and nitrogen excretion resulting in a loss of lean body mass. Increasing use of chemo-radiation treatment plans or hyperfractionated radiotherapy treatment regimens may enhance weight loss during treatment (7,8).

BENEFITS OF NUTRITIONAL SUPPORT

Although nutritional support may be able to maintain or improve body weight, body fat, and lean body mass, the effect may not be as great as in those who do not have underlying malignant disease (9). Studies have shown that long-term enteral nutrition have can maintain or improve nutritional status among head and neck cancer survivors (10). Nutritional support has been shown to be of benefit in several ways.

Perioperative Nutritional Support

Perioperative nutritional support may reduce morbidity and mortality (11). Studies that have failed to show the benefit of perioperative nutritional support have often not distinguished between patients with a good nutritional status and those who are malnourished. It is likely that severely malnourished patients benefit more from nutritional support than those patients who are already well nourished. For preoperative nutritional support to be effective in influencing clinical outcome malnourished patients should receive perioperative nutrition for 7 to 15 days before surgery (12). Preoperative enteral nutrition is as effective as parenteral nutrition and should always be the method of choice when there is a functioning gastrointestinal tract and this can be accessed safely. Postoperative parenteral nutrition, enteral nutrition, or adequate oral nutrition are equally effective in reducing nutrition-related postoperative complications.

Tolerance to Treatment

Studies of the nutritional support of patients undergoing treatment have provided varying results. Some studies, but not all, have shown the benefits of nutritional support with respect to chemotherapy or radiotherapy toxicity in patients (9). The benefits included a decrease in medications given for symptom control, a reduction in the duration of chemotherapy-induced nausea and vomiting, better tolerance of chemotherapy, and fewer treatment delays. This may have an impact in terms of control of disease as it is recognized that delays in treatment may contribute to a poorer outcome for the patient.

Malnutrition in head and neck cancer patients has been shown to be associated with immunoincompetence although studies have failed to show a significant improvement in immune function on feeding such patients (13).

Intensive nutritional support of head and neck patients undergoing radiotherapy treatment, in the form of gastrostomy feeding, helps patients maintain their nutritional status and quality of life during and after treatment (10,14).

NUTRITIONAL SCREENING AND ASSESSMENT

All patients with head and neck cancer must undergo a nutritional assessment at first contact with the hospital. All patients who are assessed as being malnourished or at risk of developing malnutrition must be referred to a dietitian. It is likely that nearly all head and neck cancer patients will require dietary advice during the course of their disease and treatment. The use of locally developed guidelines may lead to an improvement in the nutritional management of patients, particularly where a dietitian is present at the multidisciplinary clinic (15). Some disease and treatment factors are associated with the increased use of enteral nutrition and these include increasing age, poor World Health Organization performance status, and advanced stage (16).

Nutritional screening and early identification of problems can be quick and easy to perform. The dietitian will then undertake a more detailed assessment. The following criteria may be used for a rapid screening of whether a dietetic referral is required.

Table 8.1   Causes of Poor Dietary Intake and Weight Loss

Anorexia	Cytokines produced by the body in response to the presence of a tumor, such as interleukin and tumor necrosis factor, may depress appetite (3)
Psychological factors	Depression and anxiety
Excessive alcohol intake	Depression of appetite Displacement of foods from the diet Thiamin deficiency and Wernicke–Korsakoff syndrome may occur in chronic alcoholics
Dysphagia and/or trismus	Dietary deficiency of all nutrients particularly energy
Poor oral hygiene and oral infection	Tumor burden and opportunistic infection
Taste changes	May occur in up to 70% of patients and can be due to tumor, radiotherapy, or chemotherapy (4)
Stomatitis or mucositis	Caused by radiotherapy or chemotherapy (4)
Pain on chewing or swallowing	Caused by presence of tumor, treatment or infection
Xerostomia	Often occurs after radiotherapy to salivary gland (4)

Have You Lost Weight?

An unintentional weight loss of 10% of normal body weight should be regarded as being clinically significant and requires nutritional input. It may be obvious on examination that the patient exhibits muscle wasting and depletion of fat stores, but it should also be remembered that patients who are overweight but who are losing weight may still becoming malnourished if they are not given sufficient support.

Do You Have Any Eating Difficulties?

Difficulties with eating may include loss of appetite or difficulty with chewing or swallowing. A good guide is to ask patients whether they can eat food of a normal consistency and how much of their usual portions they can manage. Patients who have not eaten for more than 24 hours require an urgent referral to a dietitian.

Patients should be reassessed on a weekly basis as nutritional status and ability to eat can change rapidly. Additional methods of assessing nutritional status are available such as calculation of body mass index, triceps skinfold thickness, midarm muscle circumference, and measurements of muscle function; however, these are often time-consuming and not necessary to identify patients who need a referral to a dietitian. Patients must have their nutritional status monitored, preferably by a dietitian, throughout the course of their disease and treatment. Nutritional intake and changes in nutritional status can occur rapidly in this group of patients, and appropriate intervention must be implemented quickly to avoid weight loss. Frequency of monitoring will depend on the patient's clinical condition, treatment, and frequency of hospital visits. The parameters that should be monitored are shown in Table 8.2.

NUTRITIONAL REQUIREMENTS

Cancer patients may have elevated energy requirements due to the metabolic changes that occur in cancer cachexia, surgery, trauma, and sepsis (5,6).

Energy requirements. Energy requirements may range from 30 kcal/kg to 40 kcal/kg although requirements may exceed this range for patients who are particularly cachectic (9). To determine initial energy requirements a figure of

Table 8.2   Nutritional Parameters

Appearance
Weight and height
Difficulties with eating and drinking
Nutritional intake
Fluid intake
Biochemistry: urea and electrolytes, liver function tests, blood glucose, urinalysis, vitamin and mineral status

30 to 35 kcal/kg may be used or basal requirements may be calculated using the Schofield equation (17). The dietitian may carry out a detailed assessment of requirements.

Nitrogen requirements. Adequate dietary nitrogen and energy are required for patients to maintain nitrogen balance. Immediately postoperative patients may be unable to maintain nitrogen balance due to the metabolic effects of trauma. Nitrogen requirements range from 0.17 g/kg to 0.30 g/kg/day (1 g protein per kg body weight to 1.9 g protein per kg body weight). Hypoalbuminemia may arise as a result of the metabolic response to injury and infection and therefore may not respond to an increase in dietary protein (18). A decrease in plasma albumin due to trauma is associated with a rise in acute phase proteins such as C-reactive protein. Measurement of acute phase proteins may give an indication of the distinction between hypoalbuminemia due to trauma and that due to malnutrition.

Fluid requirements. Normal fluid requirements may range from 30 to 35 ml/kg per day. Requirements may be increased in patients requiring ventilation, during sepsis, or where output is high, for example, in diarrhea.

Vitamins and minerals. Dietary intake should aim to meet the daily requirements for all vitamins and minerals (19). Vitamin and mineral supplementation may be indicated in a number of patients where dietary intake is poor or requirements for particular nutrients may be increased. Head and neck cancer patients may require a liquid preparation. Some studies have shown the benefit of additional vitamin C and zinc in the healing of pressure sores and leg ulcers in nutritionally depleted noncancer patients (20,21).

The potential benefit in cancer patients has been more difficult to demonstrate due to the lack of studies and evidence that cancer patients may have abnormally low plasma levels of some vitamins and minerals (22). Supplementation with individual vitamins or minerals at high doses may affect the metabolism of other nutrients, for example, supplementation with high doses of zinc may cause alterations in copper metabolism; and it is therefore important not to exceed safe upper limits for vitamin and mineral intake (23,24). It has also been suggested that supplementation with some vitamins, for example, alpha-tocopherol and beta carotene may increase the rate of second primary cancers in head and neck cancer patients (25). It is often more appropriate to ensure an adequate supply of vitamins and minerals with diet and enteral feeds and use a multivitamin and mineral preparation when intake continues to be inadequate. Parenteral thiamin (vitamin B1) may be required for patients with thiamin deficiency due to a high alcohol intake.

METHODS OF NUTRITIONAL SUPPORT
Oral Nutrition
Patients who can swallow sufficient food and fluids safely may be able to meet their requirements orally. Patients who are at risk of aspiration should be referred to a Speech and Language Therapist to assess swallowing and whether it is safe to proceed with oral intake. The dietitian may advise the patient on the following:

1. Suitability and consistency of food
2. Fortification of food to increase energy and/or protein
3. Adequacy of energy intake
4. Adequacy of fluid intake
5. Vitamin and mineral supplementation where appropriate
6. Use of nutritional supplements where appropriate.

Dietary management of eating difficulties and nutritional supplement strategies are listed in Tables 8.3 and 8.4. Patients who are particularly anorexic may benefit from an appetite stimulant such as progestational agents and corticosteriods (26).

Enteral Tube Feeding
Enteral tube feeding may need to be considered for the following situations:

1. Patients with dysphagia
2. Patients with severe mucositis
3. Patients who are at risk of aspiration

Table 8.3   Dietary Management of Eating Difficulties

Symptom	Dietary management
Anorexia	Small portions Increase frequency of eating Encourage foods that are enjoyed Make use of best meal of the day (e.g., this may be breakfast) Encourage high-energy foods Fortify food to increase energy intake (e.g., use full cream milk, use extra butter, cheese, cream) Use alcohol as an appetite stimulant (in moderation) Medroxyprogesterone acetate or megestrol acetate as appetite stimulant
Dysphagia	Small frequent meals Modify consistency of food so all food is soft. Food may need to be pureed or liquidized Fortify food to increase energy intake May require additional nutritional supplements May need to use commercial thickening agent for thin liquids if risk of aspiration (needs assessment from speech and language therapist)
Mucositis	Modify consistency of food so all food is soft Avoid rough, coarse, or dry food Avoid acidic, salty, or highly spiced food Avoid alcohol Avoid hot food, foods that are cold or at room temperature may be better tolerated May require additional nutritional supplements Take food after taking analgesia
Xerostomia	Moist foods, use sauces, gravies, butter, custard, cream and milk to make food moist Food may need to be soft or pureed May require additional nutritional supplements Take frequent small sips of water Try sour or tart foods (e.g., lemon, acid drops, pineapple [only if no stomatitis]) Try sugar free chewing gum to stimulate saliva Avoid dry or crisp foods (e.g., bread, nuts, crackers) Try artificial saliva Refer to a dental hygienist

Table 8.4 Nutritional Supplements Suitable for Head and Neck Patients

Type of supplement	Nutritional value and use of supplement
Nutritionally complete	Designed to replace all food if sufficient volume is consumed, usually 1.5–2 liters depending on energy density Contains protein, fat, carbohydrate, vitamins and minerals in a liquid form May be used as a supplement to food when total food intake is poor. Available in a variety of flavors both sweet and savory Often based on milk protein Usually provide 1–1.5 kcal/ml Some may contain dietary fiber
Energy and protein supplements	Often available as milk protein-based drinks or fruit juice-flavored drinks Provide protein and energy but may not meet vitamin and mineral requirements Used as a supplement to a poor food intake Usually provide 1–2 kcal/ml
Carbohydrate supplement	Available as a powder or liquid Provides 3.75 kcal/g for powder and up to 2.25 kcal/ml for liquid Can be added to ordinary food and drinks Provides energy but no vitamins and minerals
Protein supplement	Available as a powder Can be added to ordinary food to increase protein content Rarely used in isolation in cancer patients who often require energy, vitamins and minerals in addition to protein
Fat supplement	Available as a long chain triglyceride fat emulsion as a liquid Can be added to food or liquids to increase energy content Provides energy but no vitamins or minerals

4. Patients who are required to be nil by mouth, for example, postoperatively
5. Patients who can swallow but are unable to take sufficient to meet their nutritional requirements.

Methods of Tube Feeding

Nasogastric feeding. Nasogastric feeding may be the route of choice for patients requiring relatively short-term feeding such as for periods of fewer than 4 weeks. Fine-bore tubes made from soft polyurethane or silicone are less likely to cause complications such as rhinitis, esophageal irritation, and gastritis (27). The position of the nasogastric tube must be checked before feeding is started to avoid accidental intrapulmonary aspiration in accordance with local guidelines. It may be advisable to radiograph all nasogastric tubes in patients who have altered anatomy of the head and neck or have altered swallowing or gag reflex. Radiographs may also be used to assist with the difficult insertion of nasogastric tubes. All tubes should be secured to the nose and face with adhesive tape to help prevent accidental removal.

Patients who may require periods of nasogastric feeding include those having undergone surgery such as a partial glossectomy, mandibulectomy, or maxillectomy. Patients receiving brachytherapy or conventional radiotherapy where there have not been swallowing problems prior to treatment may also require periods of nasogastric feeding. Patients who undergo surgery followed by a course of radiotherapy may require a gastrostomy inserted at the time of their initial surgery. This would be appropriate for patients who may have a number of short periods of time when they require enteral tube feeding. This avoids the patient undergoing multiple insertions of a nasogastric tube and avoids delay in being able to feed the patient when side effects develop.

Tracheo-esophageal catheter feeding. Patients who have a tracheo-esophageal puncture as a primary procedure for the fitting of a voice valve may be fed immediately postoperatively via a catheter inserted through the puncture site. This route for feeding would include patients who had undergone a laryngectomy or pharyngolaryngectomy. The catheter would be expected to be used for feeding for approximately 7 days in patients who had not undergone previous radiotherapy and approximately 10 days in patient who had undergone previous radiotherapy treatment. Once swallowing and oral intake has been established postoperatively the catheter is removed and replaced with a voice prosthesis, for example, a Blom–Singer valve.

Gastrostomy feeding. Gastrostomy feeding may be appropriate for patients requiring enteral feeding for periods of longer than 3 to 4 weeks (Table 8.5). Patients who are at high risk of having a prolonged period of establishing oral intake should be considered for insertion of a gastrostomy

Table 8.5 Indications for Insertion of PEG

Poor nutritional intake and deteriorating nutritional status despite dietary advice on fortifying foods and dietary supplements
Dysphagia – unable to take adequate oral nutrition
Aspiration of food or fluids
Fistulae where patient is required to be nil by mouth for a period of greater than 3–4 weeks
Enteral tube feeding required for period of longer than 3–4 weeks
At the time of surgery where resumption of oral intake is anticipated to be slow, e.g., total glossectomy
At the time of oropharyngeal resection to avoid irritation by nasogastric tube
Prior to hyperfractionated radiotherapy

tube at the time of their initial surgery (14). Examples include total glossectomy, hemilaryngectomy, or extensive or hyperfractionated radiotherapy or chemo-radiation. It may also be preferable for patients who have undergone oropharyngeal resection and repair as this avoids a nasogastric tube causing irritation to the site of repair. Gastrostomy tubes are cosmetically more acceptable to patients and avoid some of the complications that may arise with the long-term use of nasogastric tubes.

Gastrostomy tubes may be inserted surgically, radiologically, or more commonly via endoscopy. Tubes inserted via endoscopy are percutaneous endoscopic gastrostomy tubes and are commonly known as a PEG. Tubes may vary in size from 9 French to 22 French and are retained within the stomach with a flange or balloon. This procedure may be difficult in patients with extensive disease or a stricture that prevents the passage of an endoscope. In such patients a tube may be placed radiologically or as an open gastrostomy. Radiologically placed tubes require the insertion of a nasogastric tube to inflate the stomach with air prior to the tube placement. This may be difficult in some patients due to the presence of tumor or fibrotic tissue.

Morbidity associated with PEG insertion is usually less than 10% with the most common complications including local site infection, leakage, or bleeding although some centers have identified that complication rates may be higher in head and neck cancer patients (28, 29). Major complications that can occur include necrotizing fasciitis and intra-abdominal wall abscesses. A potential complication is the metastatic spread from the original head and neck tumor to the gastrostomy site associated with the pull-through method of gastrostomy tube insertion, although this does appear to be rare (30). Once the gastrostomy tract has become established it may be replaced with a "button." This serves the same purpose as a gastrostomy but lies flush with the patient's abdomen. Care of the gastrostomy site is important in maintaining the tract and reducing the risk of infection (31) (Table 8.6).

Jejunostomy feeding. Fine-bore feeding jejunostomy tubes may be inserted with a fine catheter to access the jejunum through the anterior abdominal wall. Jejunostomy tubes may be used in patients who have had upper gastrointestinal surgery making the use of a gastrostomy tube inappropriate or where gastric emptying is severely compromised. Such patients would include those who have undergone a stomach pull up. Jejunostomy feeding often requires the use of a feeding pump for continuous feeding.

Table 8.6 Care of the PEG Site

PEG tube and retention device should be left in position for 24 hours postinsertion
Commence care of PEG site 24–48 hours postinsertion
Note the position of external fixation device on PEG tube
Release exterior retention device and clean skin with sterile saline
Rotate PEG tube through 360° to maintain stoma tract
Dry skin surrounding PEG tube
Replace external fixation device to usual position; the position of the external fixation device may change if the patient gains weight
Seven days postinsertion it is no longer necessary to use sterile saline and a clean technique may be used to care for the skin

Enteral Feeds

Commercially prepared enteral feeds should be used for nasogastric, gastrostomy, or jejunostomy feeding as they are sterile when packaged and are of known nutritional composition (Table 8.7).

Details of the exact composition of commercially produced enteral feeds can be obtained from the manufacturers. For the vast majority of head and neck cancer patients a whole-protein polymeric feed can be used. Energy-dense feeds may be required for patients with increased energy requirements.

Some enteral preparations include ingredients such as arginine or omega-3 fatty acids that are designed to improve nutritional variables as well as clinical outcome, postoperative infections, and wound complications. Studies have, as yet, failed to show the benefit of these specialized feeds in head and neck cancer patients (32,33).

Feeding regimens. Enteral feeding regimens must be devised to fit in with the patient's lifestyle and tolerance to feed. Various regimens may be used (Table 8.8).

During the postoperative period feed may be started at full strength and in a small volume such as 50 ml/hour. The rate of feed can gradually be increased according to tolerance with the aim of meeting nutritional requirements within 24 to 48 hours. During this period additional intravenous fluid may be required to meet the patient's fluid requirements. As enteral feeding is established the intravenous fluids must be decreased, but fluid requirements should be met at all times, taking into account any additional fluid losses. Where feed tolerance appears to be poor, gastric emptying may be assessed by gastric aspiration. Gastric stasis may require the use of prokinetics. The incidence of pharyngocutaneous fistula after laryngectomy may be reduced with the use of a gastro-esophageal reflux prophylaxis regimen based on metoclopramide and ranitidine (34).

Patients with dysphagia, aspiration, or mucositis who require enteral tube feeding may be able to tolerate their full nutritional and fluid requirements within the first 24 hours.

Complications of enteral tube feeding may occur. These should be managed with dietetic and medical management (Table 8.9).

Monitoring of enteral tube feeding. Patients on enteral tube feeds should be monitored regularly (Table 8.10). The frequency of monitoring such parameters will vary on the clinical condition of the patient and if the enteral feed is being established or being monitored while the patient is at home. The frequency of monitoring will decrease with time but should continue with patients after discharge from hospital.

Changes in nutritional status may require nutritional requirements to be recalculated and the feeding regimen changed.

Withdrawal of enteral tube feeding. Enteral tube feeding should only be stopped when sufficient oral diet and fluids are being taken. There may need to be a weaning period during which enteral feeding is reduced and oral intake is increased. The dietitian should assess oral intake during this period, and the enteral tube feed stopped only when oral intake is considered to be adequate. Method of removal of PEG tubes depends on the type of tube used and may require a repeat endoscopy. It is necessary to refer to the manufacturer's guidelines.

Table 8.7 Enteral Feeds

Type of feed	Features of feed
Whole protein/polymeric containing protein, hydrolysed fat and carbohydrate	Requires digestion Generally provides 1–1.5 kcal/ml feed Usually adequate intake of vitamins and minerals when 1000–1500 ml taken May contain dietary fiber
Isotonic whole protein but containing protein, hydrolysed fat, medium chain triglycerides and maltodextrins	Requires digestion Suitable for patients with suspected gastrointestinal intolerance May contain dietary fibre
Chemically defined peptide or elemental	Does not require digestion, may be absorbed directly into bloodstream May be low in fat or contain medium chain triglycerides Suitable for patients with impaired gastrointestinal function Hyperosmolar and low in residue
Special application feeds May have altered levels of energy, protein, electrolytes, vitamins and minerals to suit particular conditions such as renal failure	Require digestion as for whole protein/polymeric feeds Rarely required in head and neck cancer patients The value of glutamine, arginine, omega-3 fatty acid enriched feeds to promote immune function has yet to be demonstrated

Table 8.8 Feeding Regimens

Feeding regimen	Advantages	Disadvantages
Continuous feeding via a pump	Easily controlled rate Reduction of gastrointestinal complications Minimizes stress on cardiac, respiratory, and renal function	Patient connected to feeding pump for majority of day
Intermittent feeding via a pump or gravity drip	Patient has periods of time free of feeding Some patients may find gravity feeding easier than managing a pump Some feed may be given overnight	May have an increased risk of gastrointestinal symptoms (e.g., early satiety) Overnight feeding may not be suitable for those at high-risk of aspiration
Bolus feeding	May reduce time connected to feed	Increased risk of gastrointestinal side effects Administration of feeds time consuming

Table 8.9 Complications of Enteral Tube Feeding

Complication	Possible cause	Suggested management
Diarrhea	Antibiotics Bacterial infection Hypoalbuminemia Hyperosmolar feed Impaired intestinal function Drugs (e.g., magnesium salts, chemotherapy) Overuse of laxatives Use of sorbitol-based drugs	Review antibiotic administration Stool culture if persistent Reduce rate of feed Reduce osmolarity of feed Use fiber containing feed Anti-diarrhea medication
Constipation	Opioid drugs Lack of dietary fibre Lack of fluid	Laxatives or enema Use fiber-containing feed Increase fluid intake
Nausea	Drugs Rapid administration of feed Hyperosmolar feed	Anti-emetics Reduce rate of feed Use isotonic feed
Aspiration	Patient unconscious Displacement of nasogastric tube	4-hourly aspiration Postpyloric feeding (e.g., nasoduodenal or jejunal feeding) Drugs to encourage gastric emptying, (e.g., metoclopramide) Prop patient's head so there is a minimum 45° elevation between head and neck and thorax

Table 8.10 Monitoring of Enteral Tube Feeding

Body weight
Urea and electrolytes
Full blood count
Tolerance to feed (e.g., nausea, fullness, bowels)
Quantity of feed taken
Care of tube
Stoma site (in case of PEG and jejunostomy)

Home enteral feeding. Patients who are unable to resume an adequate oral intake can be taught to manage enteral tube feeding at home. Ten percent of long-term head and neck cancer survivors require permanent enteral nutrition (10). Adequate time should be allowed in the hospital setting for patients to become fully accustomed to the techniques of administration of feed and care of the gastrostomy tube prior to discharge home. The feeding regimen should be planned to fit into the home circumstances, feed tolerance, and patient choice (Table 8.8).

Home support in the form of the general practitioner, community nursing, and community dietetic services should be established although the amount of support may vary depending on local resources. Patients at home should be monitored from a nutritional perspective. Patients with a PEG should have the site monitored regularly by the community nurse and by the doctor at outpatient appointments.

Many of the enteral feed manufacture companies have a home delivery service that may be of help to patients as this avoids having to carry heavy feed and bulky equipment. The hospital or community dietitian can arrange this.

Management of a Chylous Fistula

A chylous fistula as a complication of a neck dissection may be treated conservatively if the output remains below 600 ml (35). Some clinicians have advocated the use of a low-fat diet, use of medium-chain triglycerides, or the use of parenteral nutrition in supporting patients with this complication (36–38). Nutritional and electrolyte support is essential in the conservative management of low-volume chylous fistulae, and this may be achieved with the administration of a low long chain triglyceride enteral feed (39).

Parenteral Nutrition

Parenteral nutrition should only be used when it is not possible to feed patients via the enteral route. Its use carries the risk of life-threatening complications, such as sepsis and metabolic disorders, and therefore it must be administered and monitored correctly. It is rarely used in head and neck cancer patients as the gastrointestinal tract is usually accessible.

It may be considered for the following patients (40):

1. When all methods and routes of enteral nutrition have been considered but are not deemed appropriate
2. When the gastrointestinal tract is inaccessible and it is not possible to insert an enteral feeding tube
3. When complete rest of the gastrointestinal tract is required.

REFERENCES

1. Guo C-B, Ma D-Q, Zhang K-H. Nutritional status of patients with oral and maxillofacial malignancies. J Oral Maxillofac Surg 1994; 52: 559–62.
2. Lopez MJ, Robinson P, Madden T et al. Nutritional support and prognosis in patients with head and neck cancer. J Surg Oncol 1994; 55: 33–6.
3. von Meyenfeldt MF, Fredrix EWHM, Haagh WAJJM et al. The aetiology and management of weight loss and malnutrition in cancer patients. Bailliere's Clin Gastroenterol 1988; 2: 869–85.
4. Thiel H-J, Fietkau R, Sauer R. Malnutrition and the role of nutritional support for radiation therapy patients. Recent Results Cancer Res 1988; 108: 203–26.
5. Hyltander A, Drott C, Korner U et al. Elevated energy expenditure in cancer patients with solid tumours. Eur J Cancer 1991; 27: 9–15.
6. Espat NJ, Moldawaer LL, Copeland EM. Cytokine-mediated alterations in host metabolism prevent nutritional repletion in cachetic cancer patients. J Surg Oncol 1995; 58: 77–82.
7. Allen AM, Elshaikh M, Worden FP et al. Acceleration of hyperfractionaed chemoradiation regimen for advanced head and neck cancer. Head and Neck 2007: 29: 137-42.
8. Lin A, Jabbari S, Worden FP et al. Metabolic abnormalities associated with weight loss during chemoirrdiation of head and neck cancer. Int J Radiat Oncol Biol Phys 2005; 63: 1413–18.
9. Bozzetti F. Nutrition support in patients with cancer. In: Payne-James J, Grimble G, Silk D, eds. Artificial nutrition support in clinical practice. London: Edward Arnold, 1995; 511–33.
10. Schattner MA, Willis HJ, Raykher A et al. Long-term enteral nutrition facilitates optimization of body weight. JEPN 2005; 29: 198–203.
11. Heys SD, Park KGM, Garlick PJ et al. Nutrition and malignant disease: implications for surgical practice. Br J Surg 1992; 79: 614–23.
12. Campos ACL, Meguid MM. A critical appraisal of the usefulness of perioperative nutritional support. Am J Clin Nutr 1992; 55: 117–30.
13. Brookes GB, Clifford P. Nutritional status and general immune competence in patients with head and neck cancer. J R Soc Med 1981; 74: 132–9.
14. Fietkau R, Iro H, Sailer D et al. Percutaneous endoscopically guided gastrostomy in patients with head and neck cancer. Recent Results Cancer Res 1991; 121: 269–82.
15. Wood K. Audit of nutritional guidelines for head and neck cancer patients undergoing radiotherapy. J Hum Nutr Dietet 2005; 18: 343–51.
16. Mangar S, Slevin N, Mais K et al. Evaluating predictive factors for determining enteral nutrition in patients receiving radical radiotherapy for head and neck cancer: a retrospective review. Radiotherapy and Oncology 2006; 78: 152–8.
17. Schofield WN, Schofield C, James WPT. Basal metabolic rate: review and prediction. Hum Nutr Clin Nutr 1985; 39c(Suppl 1): 5–96.
18. Rothschild MA, Oratz M, Schreiber SS. Serum albumin. Hepatology 1988; 8: 385–401.
19. Department of Health. Dietary reference values for food energy and nutrients in the United Kingdom. Department of Health report on health and social subjects. Report No. 41. London: HMSO, 1991.
20. Taylor TV, Rimmer S, Day B et al. Ascorbic acid supplementation in the treatment of pressure sores. Lancet 1974; ii: 544–6.
21. Hallbook T, Lanner E. Serum zinc and healing of venous leg ulcers. Lancet 1972; ii: 780–2.
22. Doerr TD, Prasad AS, Marks SC et al. Zinc deficiency in head and neck cancer patients. J Am Coll Nutr 1997; 16: 418–22.
23. Food Standards Agency. Food standards agency expert group on vitamins and minerals. Safe upper levels for vitamins and minerals. London: Food Standards Agency, 2003.

24. Walsh CT, Sandstead HH, Prasad AS et al. Zinc: health effects and research priorities for the 1990s. Environ Health Perspect 1994; 102(Suppl 2): 4–46.

25. Bairati I, Meyer F, Gelinas M et al. A randomised trial of antioxidant vitamins to prevent second primary cancers in head and neck cancer. JNCI 2005; 97: 481–8.

26. Behl D, Jatoi A. Pharmacological options for advanced cancer patients with loss of appetite and weight. Expert Opin Pharmacother 2007; 8: 1085–90.

27. Payne-James J. Enteral nutrition: tubes and techniques of delivery. In: Payne-James J, Grimble G, Silk D, eds. Artificial nutrition support in clinical practice. London: Greenwich Medical Media Ltd., 2001: 281–302.

28. Bailey CE, Lucas CE, Ledgerwood AM et al. A comparison of gastrostomy techniques in patients with advanced head and neck cancer. Arch Otolaryngol Head Neck Surg 1992; 118: 124–6.

29. Walton GM. Complications of percutaneous gastrostomy in patients with head and neck cancer: an analysis of 42 consecutive patients. Ann R Coll Surg Engl 1999; 81: 272–6.

30. Mincheff TV. Metastatic spread to a percutaneous gastrostomy site from head and neck cancer: case report and literature review. J Soc Laparoendosc Surgeons 2005; 9: 466–71.

31. Löser C, Aschl G, Hēbuterne X et al. ESPEN guidelines on artificial enteral nutrition – Percutaneous endoscopic gastrostomy (PEG). Clin Nutr 2005; 24: 848–61.

32. de Luis DA, Izaola O, Aller R et al. A randomized clinical trial with oral Immunonutrition (omega 3-enhanced vs. arginine enhanced formulae) in ambulatory head and neck cancer patients. Ann Nutr Metab 2005; 49: 95–9.

33. Van Bokhorst-De Van Der Schuer MAE, Langendoen SI et al. Perioperative enteral nutrition and quality of life of severely malnourished head and neck cancer patients: a randomised clinical trial. Clin Nutr 2000; 19: 437–44.

34. Seikaly H, Park P. Gastroesophageal reflux prophylaxis decreases the incidence of pharyngocutaneous fistula after total laryngectomy. Laryngoscope 1995; 105: 1220–2.

35. Spiro JD, Spiro RH, Strong EW. The management of chyle fistula. Laryngoscope 1990; 100: 771–4.

36. Izzard ME, Crowder VL, Southwell KE. The use of monogen in the conservative management of chylous fistula. Otolaryngol Head Neck Surg 2007; 136: S 50–53.

37. Martin IC, Marinho LH, Brown AE et al. Medium chain triglycerides in the management of chylous fistulae following neck dissection. Br J Oral Maxillofac Surg 1993; 31: 236–8.

38. Younus M, Chang RWS. Chyle fistulae. Treatment with total parenteral nutrition. J Laryngol Otol 1988; 102: 384.

39. Al-Khayat M, Kenyon GS, Fawcett HV et al. Nutritional support in patients with low volume chylous fistula following radical neck dissection. J Laryngol Otol 1991; 105: 1052–6.

40. Thomas B, Bishop J, eds. Parenteral nutrition. In: Manual of dietetic practice. Oxford, UK: Blackwell Scientific, 2007: 113–19.

9

Dental Management of the Head and Neck Patient

Robert E Wood

INTEGRATION OF DENTAL TREATMENT WITH MEDICAL AND SURGICAL TREATMENT

The goal of dental management of the head and neck oncology patient is to ensure the patient enters his or her active treatment phase without delay and in possession of a healthy, functional, and well-maintained dentition. If possible, all potential sources of infection should be removed prior to cancer treatment. The dental treatment plan will be decided with consideration given to the types of anticancer treatment, the patient's wishes, and the dentist's experience and knowledge in the management of other similar patients. Close cooperation between the dental team and the responsible physician is imperative.

PRE-TREATMENT ASSESSMENT

The dental assessment of the head and neck cancer patient commences in the same manner as the conventional dental patient. A myriad of intercurrent disorders may affect the type and method of dental service delivery. Concomitant serious systemic disease may ultimately alter the oncologic treatment plan. Part of the medical history should include inquiries as to the value the patients place on their teeth, how well they care for their teeth, whether they have and wear dental prostheses, and whether they are under the regular care of a dentist. If patients are under the care of a family dentist it is likely that they will overestimate the frequency and quality of care received at their routine visits. Further, many conditions that may be safely monitored in a general dental practice, without intervention, must be dealt with in the oncology patient.

Following review of the medical history it is imperative that a thorough clinical examination of the teeth, their supporting structures, and the remainder of the oral cavity be completed. This assessment includes charting of the patient's teeth, measurement of the quantity of saliva, evaluation of temporomandibular joint function, and description of the periodontal status. Biopsy of oral sites suspicious of malignancy is necessary as upper aerodigestive tract malignancies may be multiple in nature, that is, field cancerization (1). The use of direct fluorescence visualization technology has become popular; however, it is unproven technology for routine use in the general population as a means of detecting occult cancers. Finally an objective assessment of oral hygiene level and the presence of plaque and calculus deposits should also be done.

As part of the overall assessment a dental radiographic examination must be completed (2). At the author's institution this is composed minimally of a pantomographic examination supplemented with intraoral bite-wing and periapical radiographs as clinically indicated. Frequently, a full mouth series of 16 or more intraoral radiographs is exposed. This is done to afford the dental surgeon and the oncologist as much information as possible on the health of the dentition (Fig. 9.1). The amount of radiation received in this procedure is trivial when compared to the prescribed dose and use of direct digital radiography for panoramic and intraoral images reduces this burden further and moreover provides images that are readily shared with the care team.

PRE-RADIATION TREATMENT

The twin primary goals of dental care for radiation patients are the prevention of postradiation caries and osteoradionecrosis. A secondary goal is communicating to the patient the complications of radiation therapy treatment of the head and neck, which may include mucositis, xerostomia, trismus, dysgeusia, dysphagia, pain, and susceptibility to fungal infection and postradiation caries. After consultation with the radiation oncologist concerning field sizes and prescribed doses of radiation, an adequate amount of time should be spent with each patient discussing how his or her individualized radiation treatment will affect the mouth. Presently the management of head and neck cancers is trending towards routine use of intensity modulated radiation treatment (IMRT) designed to reduce adjacent tissue toxicity. This however has not eliminated many of the short-, medium-, and long-term side effects in this patient group.

Dental extractions should be done as soon as possible in those patients that require them. Teeth may be extracted because they are decayed and unrestorable, lack opposing teeth, are prosthetically useless, are likely to be lost during the course of treatment, or in patients who are unwilling to carry out the rigorous oral hygiene regimen required. In addition, partly erupted third molar teeth and teeth with severe periodontal disease should be removed to prevent pericorinitis or other infections. Teeth with periapical inflammatory disease or nonvital teeth may be kept if the patient is willing to undergo root canal treatment. The author is generally more aggressive with respect to extractions "in the field: and in the posterior mandible. If a large number of teeth are to be removed it is important for the dentist to liaise with the radiation oncologist to ensure that any

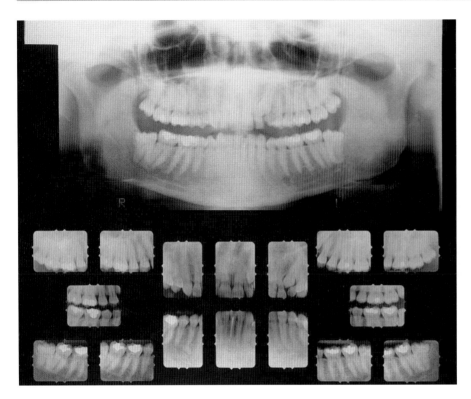

Figure 9.1 Panoramic radiograph of jaws with 4 bitewings supplies the dentist and the surgeon with more information on which to base a treatment decision.

such extractions do not interfere with radiation positioning device fabrication or treatment planning.

Restorative dentistry should, if possible, be completed prior to radiation treatment; however, it may be delayed until after cancer treatment because it is imperative that the dental treatment be completed in as short a time as possible. Dentistry should not delay radiation treatment. To permit this, patients should be referred immediately after their first hospital consultation so that their dental work may be done while the radiation planning, mask, and simulator appointments are being done. Ill-fitting dentures may be adjusted or adapted, but new prostheses are generally not fitted until well after completion of radiation.

Sanative periodontal treatment and institution of appropriate oral hygiene care are pivotal and may involve the services of the dentist, preventive dental assistant, or dental hygienist. The patient's teeth are cleaned thoroughly, and oral hygiene instruction is given. Fluoride trays are made for most patients, and the need for daily topical fluoride use has not been eliminated by IMRT. This is done by fabricating dental stone models and making vinyl athletic mouth guards. When the mouth guards are finished, they are delivered to the patient along with a prescription for neutral sodium fluoride gel, written instructions for their correct use, and a clear warning that they must be used as directed for life. An example of fluoride instructions is provided in Table 9.1. The use of topical fluoride has been proven to markedly reduce the incidence of postradiation caries (3). The fluoride tray has an additional use in the patient with fixed cast-metal bridgework in that it may be placed in the mouth during the radiation treatment. When this is done it displaces the adjacent soft tissue off

Table 9.1 Oral Hygiene Recommendations

The life-long daily application of the topical neutral sodium fluoride gel is mandatory if you wish to keep your teeth and prevent serious health consequences. Use only the fluoride gel prescribed by your dentist or physician. Make sure that before you leave the cancer center that you are shown how to use the trays and you understand that this is a lifelong commitment. Never discontinue its use unless advised by your doctor or physician at the cancer center.

Daily procedure

Select a time of day when you will not need to rinse, eat, or drink for a minimum of 1 hour. Many people apply the fluoride before retiring to bed.

Brush and floss your teeth thoroughly. If you are having problems mechanically removing the plaque from your teeth ask the advice of your dental hygienist.

Using the custom trays provided to you by your dentist, place a small quantity of fluoride gel in each of the upper and lower trays. The trays are custom made for you so there is no need to "fill them up."

Using a cotton swab distribute the gel throughout the tray so all teeth will be covered with a thin film of fluoride when the tray is placed on the teeth.

Place one, if possible both trays on the upper and lower arches and leave in place for 5 minutes. The 5 minutes must be rigidly adhered to.

After 5 minutes has elapsed remove the trays and spit out the excess. Do not rinse, eat, or drink for 1 hour.

Rinse the trays out with cool water and let them dry. Do not store them on the stone models and do not clean them with denture cleaners or subject them to heat.

If you have any questions about their correct use contact your dentist or physician at the cancer center.

the bridgework and avoids radiation "hotspots" thereby preventing undue radiation mucositis.

PERI-RADIATION TREATMENT

Patients should be seen as required, but minimally at least once by the dental team during the course of their radiation treatment. This visit serves to assess the presence of radiation-related side effects and provides an opportunity to ameliorate or remove them.

The patient will undoubtedly experience some degree of radiation mucositis (Fig. 9.2). This is part of the treatment and is troublesome because it is painful and prevents patients from maintaining adequate nutrition (4). It may be managed through use of topical anesthetic agents; ice chips; rinsing with cool, weak, sodium bicarbonate; and water rinses and by using systemic analgesics. The type of antimucositis therapy may range from simple bicarbonate of soda and water rinses, to topical anesthetics and systemic

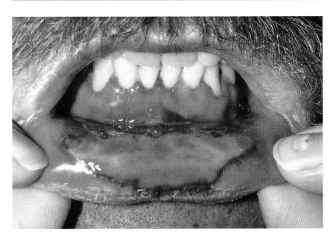

Figure 9.2   Typical appearance of intraoral radiation mucositis.

analgesics. The occasional patient will complain that the vestibular and lingual soft tissues are sore as a result of roughened or sharp tooth edges. These teeth may be smoothed using a dental hand piece or they can be covered with a thin form-fitting acetate layer (Fig. 9.3), which provides a smooth contacting surface and allows the soft tissues to glide across the teeth. Presently there is no completely effective means of treating mucositis.

Candidiasis occurs in most radiation patients some time during the course of their treatment (Fig. 9.4). It presents clinically as a whitish plaque present on the oral mucosa that may be removed with gentle pressure on a wet gauze. In some cases the oral mucosa may appear red and atrophic. Most cases of candidiasis can be managed by the judicious use of topical, or more rarely systemic antifungal agents. Topically applied mycostatin ointment, rinses, or medicated antifungal lozenges can be used directly or on the tissue surface of dentures according to manufacturers (1) instructions for the particular agent chosen. Alternately systemic fluconazole can be administered if there is no response to topical agents.

Mastication and swallowing may be altered or hindered during radiation treatment. Patients should be encouraged to follow a soft diet, and the services of a clinical dietician should be employed to ensure that the patient is receiving an adequate caloric and nutrient intake. For patients in whom the tongue is involved, dysgeusia may occur making the motivation to eat less. This lack of taste will resolve itself over time but is troubling to the patient. The patient should be reassured that he or she will regain his or her sense of taste; however, it may be a period of months before foods taste as they should. Many oncology patients alter their diet to a cariogenic one. Early nutritional counseling by a qualified dietitian occurs at the author's institution to ameliorate this. If there is a shift in a patient toward a cariogenic diet this needs to be offset by scrupulous oral hygiene measures, daily topical fluoride gel use, and more frequent dental examinations and intra-oral dental radiographs.

Xerostomia is the side effect of radiation treatment that patients find most troubling. The use of parotid-sparing

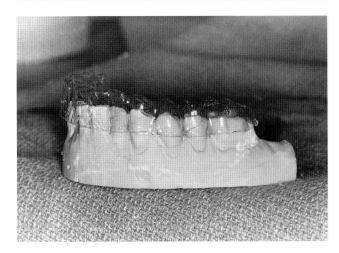

Figure 9.3   Acetate dental splint allows smooth movement of buccal mucosa and tongue across dental surfaces. It may be fabricated from study models or fluoride tray models.

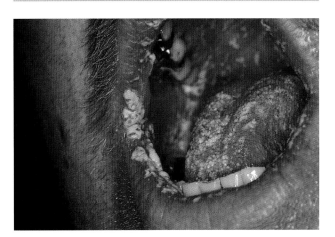

Figure 9.4   Intraoral candidiasis as seen here is a common occurrence in the mouths of head and neck cancer patients.

radiation may in the future prove to be one means of improving salivary outcomes; however, even if patient's comfort improves most are still at risk of developing postradiation caries. Although saliva substitutes are helpful most patients tend to carry a small supply of water with them. In some jurisdictions salivary substitutes are supplied at no cost to the patient on prescription whereas in other locales patients must pay for them out of pocket. Many of these salivary substitutes contain fluoride, but it has been the experience of the author that none is as effective at caries reduction as daily topical fluoride gel applications in a custom carrier. Custom-carrier fluoride gel application is also superior to brushing the fluoride gel on the teeth. Patients should be firmly discouraged from relying on sugar-containing sweets/candies or chewing gum to stimulate salivary flow because these substances will markedly hasten the caries process (5). Salivary stimulants such as pilocarpine may stimulate salivary flow and are suitable in a few selected patients (6).

In a few patients, dental sensitivity occurs. This manifests as marked tooth sensitivity to cold, and occasionally hot. The daily topical fluoride applications help to lessen this, but some patients may benefit from desensitizing dentifrices, alteration in the temperature of their fluids, and, in many cases, professional application of desensitizing agents.

Finally denture prostheses may become loose when body mass is lost during treatment. Dentures may also become irritating. If this occurs, temporary soft-tissue conditioning relines may be used to reversibly alter the fit of the denture. Permanent changes to the dentures should be avoided until well after the radiation treatment. Inevitably patients will regain their body weight, and prematurely refitted dentures will no longer fit.

POST-RADIATION TREATMENT

It is anticipated in most cases that the head and neck cancer patient will have a long life following completion of the radiation treatment. For this reason it is important to liaise with the family dentist and provide either an information package or a list of references, which he or she may consult. The cancer center dental unit should see the patients annually to see that they are compliant with respect to their oral hygiene measures and to see that they are free of postradiation caries and are receiving the appropriate level of care in the community setting. Teeth affected by postradiation caries (Fig. 9.5) are difficult to restore. In the author's institution direct restorative materials such as amalgam and resin-modified glass ionomer are used to treat postradiation caries (7,8).

Teeth, which are unrestorable due to postradiation caries, may require extraction. Alternatively they may be treated with root canal therapy and then allowed to exfoliate on their own. If extractions are required, it is important to discuss the location of the teeth with respect to the radiation fields with the radiation oncologist. Teeth that are well outside the field do not require any special management. Teeth within the field should be extracted without raising a surgical flap when possible. In addition the use of a low epinephrine-containing local anesthetic and systemic antibiotics are recommended (9). Very few patients, in the author's experience, require prophylactic hyperbaric oxygen (HBO) unless there is preexisting osteoradionecrosis or the radiation

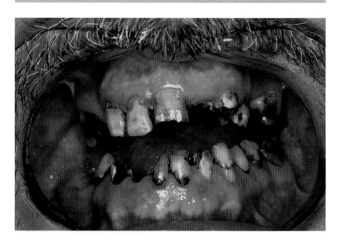

Figure 9.5 Rampant post-radiation caries as pictured here almost always occurs in those patients who are xerostomic, have poor oral hygiene and neglect to use daily sodium fluoride gel as directed.

dose at the site of the extractions was high. Generally the mandible is more susceptible to osteoradionecrosis than the maxilla. Minor cases of osteoradionecrosis can be handled by the dental team (10). The determination of what constitutes a minor case of osteoradionecrosis rests in the hands of the surgeon. With the advent of IMRT there is a move to spare bone, and cortical bone particularly. The use of HBO prophylactically prior to all dental extractions is not warranted without knowing whether the tooth was in the field irradiated. Additionally in this author's experience it is better to not extract all the teeth at one appointment. Serial extraction of teeth a few at a time allows the practitioner to observe the progression of wound healing. Generally in postirradiated patients it is better to manage a small wound rather than many small wounds or several large ones. This is inconvenient to the patient; however, it is also safer.

Postradiation trismus and lack of biting power has been seen in many patients and is likely to be a problem in the future as radiation doses escalate. This may be offset in part by IMRT radiation techniques that spare the temporomandibular apparatus. Current dental therapy is not satisfactory in preventing or altering these sequelae although physiotherapy or massage therapy may assist in diminishing the symptoms. There are numerous products available that use active mobilization techniques and dynamic splinting (24). If a patient has planned combined mandibular surgery followed by radiation treatment or radiation/chemotherapy treatment any forceful opening of the mouth must be done with caution lest the jaw be fractured or retention bars be loosened.

IMPLICATIONS OF CHEMOTHERAPY

Concommitant use of chemotherapy with radiation treatment presently plays a large role in the management of head and neck malignancy (11). The same general rules of management as seen in the head and neck radiation patients apply to the patient receiving chemotherapy. It is known that dental sepsis is responsible for many febrile episodes (12) and may be entirely avoided by implementing the same general treatment planning principles described above. An additional consideration with the chemotherapy candidate is the concept of zero tolerance for sources of infection, the requisite need to know current blood count values, and the use of prophylactic antibiotic coverage when appropriate.

PROSTHETIC REHABILITATION FOR SURGICAL ONCOLOGY PATIENTS

The dental management of the prosthetic patient includes the general principles of diagnosis and treatment detailed above. The dentition should be in a good state of repair, and the patient must be motivated to care for it.

Prosthetic rehabilitation should begin prior to the cancer surgery. It is pivotal that the treating dentist or prosthodontist assess the patient prior to surgery and devise the appropriate prostheses to suit the individual patient and the surgeon. In addition a thorough physical record of what was present prior to the surgery will allow a better postsurgical prosthetic result. The initial appointment also serves as an opportunity to develop a working rapport with the patient and allows the patient to express his or her expectations and for the practitioner to communicate what can and cannot be accomplished as an end result. The dentist and patient must know what can realistically be expected from an appliance. Surgeons should be cautioned against promising the patient that the dentist will replace and relieve all his or her problems with a prosthetic device. This sets the patient, the dentist, and the surgeon up for certain failure. No dental prosthesis is as good as one's own dentition. If patients' expectations are at the same level as what can be delivered postoperatively and if they understand when each event is likely to occur there is a greater likelihood of clinical success.

Maxillectomy Candidate

The candidate for maxillectomy should be assessed with the surgeon. The surgeon should indicate the proposed limits of the surgery and structures to be removed and those that will remain. If possible the surgery should take into account three important principles, which ultimately govern the success or failure of prosthetic rehabilitation: support, stability, and retention. Support is the feature of the residual anatomy that will contribute the resistance to intrusion of the denture. Leaving horizontal bony areas on which the denture sits, if this does not compromise the surgical/oncological result, maximizes support. Stability is that feature of the denture base that makes the denture resistant to side-to-side and front-to-back movement. Teeth and vertical bony elements, such as alveolar processes of the maxilla that possess suitable mucosal coverage, contribute to the stability of the denture. Retention of a denture is that property of the denture that keeps the denture affixed to the supporting structures. It is derived in the partially edentulous patient by placing clasp elements about residual teeth. In partially and completely edentulous patients the patients' ability to mechanically adapt and learn to wear their prostheses may be the biggest contributing factor to the denture's overall stability

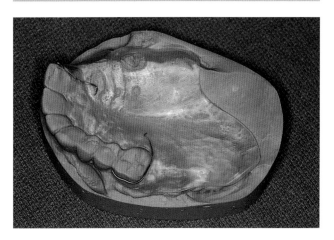

Figure 9.6 Irreversible hydrocolloid impression made prior to excision of a palatal tumour. Note the posterior extent of the impression onto the soft palate. In addition to these impressions a vinyl polysiloxane bite registration is often taken to orient the upper and lower jaws.

At the time of the presurgical planning session it is impossible to give the exact location of the surgical margins to the dentist; however, a best estimate should be provided after physical examination and assessment of diagnostic images. Immediately subsequent to this, the patient should be brought to the dental suite and be assessed. The usual history and conservative dental treatment should be done as outlined above, and the patient should know in as much detail as possible what the dentist is going to do and when it is going to be done. The dentist should deduce how much the patient expects from the prostheses with respect to speech, mastication, and cosmetics.

In most instances irreversible hydrocolloid impressions and stone models should be made of the upper and lower jaws. In the maxillectomy patient the standard impression material may need to be extended posteriorly to allow a wide impression of the posterior hard and soft palate (Fig. 9.6). This is uncomfortable for most patients, and the purpose of the procedure, if properly explained, will be accepted. If teeth are to form part of the appliance a tooth shade and mold should be selected and recorded, and a bite registration should be obtained in a permanent material such as polyvinyl siloxane. If soft palate is to be resected, allowances may be made in the appliance to prevent velopharyngeal insufficiency.

In some instances it is wise to pour the impressions twice in crown and bridge stone reserving a duplicate set of models for use or study at a later date. The patient's models are then brought back to the surgeon, and the margins of the excision are scribed on the cast. The surgical splint obturator is then fabricated out of clear acrylic with the bulb portion slightly shy of the surgeon's margins. After a surgeon and a dentist have worked together for some time the latter will have a greater appreciation of the slight variations in surgical techniques of the former. The appliance must be ready for the date of surgery, which should be noted in the chart. In the author's institution the prosthodontist or dentist attends the latter portion of the operation and adapts the borders of the surgical splint with one of the cold-cure soft-tissue conditioning materials or a thermoplastic adaptable material, after the surgeon has completed his or her resection. When the dentist has positioned the device in its appropriate final position the surgeon fixes the appliance in place over the packing (13). The prosthesis may be self-retentive in patients with a large number of teeth but more likely needs to be fixed with circumzygomatic wiring, wiring into preprepared holes, or held in place with a lag screw directly into the hard palate. If a lag screw is used it is important to ensure that the screw is readily removable via the oral aperture postoperatively. It must be positioned and angled in a manner that allows placement of the screwdriver head for removal. The patient is then taken to the recovery room and is seen by the dentist and surgeon about 1 to 2 weeks postoperatively. The purpose of the surgical splint is to allow the patient to take oral sustenance quickly, facilitate speech, and provide a matrix for healing. The splint minimizes the length of the hospital stay and allows the patient to function well during the immediate postoperative period.

At the first postoperative appointment it is prudent to provide an appropriate level of systemic analgesia for the patient. This should be given about 1 hour prior to the contemplated removal of the appliance. It is preferable to have the surgeon who placed the fixation devices remove them as well as the packing. The appliance and the patient are then brought to the dental suite where the defect is debrided gently with moistened gauze. At this time the dentist explains to the patient and the caregiver the method of cleaning the defect and the importance of keeping the surgical site clean. At the author's institution this is done with hemostats and 2 x 2 moist gauze. The gauze is folded in half and fixed in the end of the hemostat. It is then rolled against the outer border of the defect to remove the hardened nasal secretions and clotted blood (Fig. 9.7). This procedure may be facilitated by using a 3% hydrogen peroxide solution. The appliance and the cavity are cleaned thoroughly and then the appliance is adapted to

the developing scar band using cold-cure soft-tissue conditioning material. Many choices of material are available depending on the geographic location of the dentist as well as the dentist's personal preference. Patients may be seen on a weekly or bi-weekly basis for 8 to 10 weeks. At each appointment the bulb of the appliance may be cleaned and readapted to the changing defect. Patients are then seen monthly for another 2 to 3 months at which time an interim or in some cases final appliance is fabricated. The timeline for implementation of each stage of treatment varies from patient to patient and is highly dependent on the surgical procedure.

After 4 months and in some cases before, the surgical splint outlives its usefulness. The soft-tissue conditioning material has deteriorated, and the porous nature of the adapted appliance becomes inadequate from a fit and an olfactory standpoint. At this time an interim appliance can be fabricated. The interim appliance is designed to improve cosmetics and address the masticatory as well as the speech concerns of the patient. It is generally made of tissue-colored acrylic with wrought wire clasps and appropriately colored and shaped denture teeth. It may be made from irreversible hydrocolloid impressions or with polyvinyl siloxane impressions made using custom impression trays from the reserved presurgical casts. A number of things need to be assessed at this point including the lip position and height, phonetics, the location of the denture neutral zone, and the degree of healing. The neutral zone is the three-dimensional space in between the tongue and the cheeks and lips where one can place the teeth without fear that the patient will bite his or her cheek or lips. On occasion the interim appliance will serve as a final prosthesis whereas in other cases it allows completion of healing for another 6 to 8 months until the denture base is ready to accept a final prosthesis. The hard, nonporous surface of the interim appliance and its bulb allows for a cleaner oral environment. In addition the revised appliance is made to more closely approximate the defect as well as the surrounding structures. It may, for this reason, be made thinner, smaller, and lighter than the surgical splint. The general principles of denture construction for the normal patient can be adapted to prosthesis fabrication for this group of patients.

If the interim appliance is satisfactory for the long-term (greater than 1 year) cancer survivor there is no need to fabricate a "final" prosthesis. If a patient has adapted well to the interim appliance and is pleased with chewing ability, cosmetics, and speech it may not be advisable to place a new, now-foreign appliance and require another period of adaptation. After a prolonged period of healing and assurances that no further surgery is planned a final prosthesis can be fabricated. An assessment of the patient's desires with respect to cosmetics, chewing, and speech is then undertaken with recommendations by the patient with respect to which is most important to him or her. The dentist, while doing the physical intra-oral examination again evaluates the areas of the denture base that will afford stability, support, and retention.

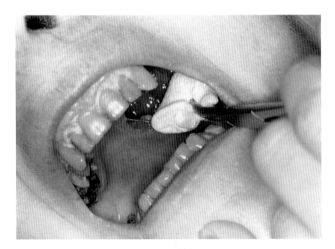

Figure 9.7 Figure depicting a gauze positioned in a hemostat or snap for use in cleaning the intra-oral defect of a maxllectomy patient. Patients must be encouraged to commence cleaning and looking after their defect to allow proper healing and general wound cleanliness.

The Final Appliance: Timing and Function

When the final appliance is being planned the patient must be capable of cleaning and caring for his or her oral defect (Fig. 9.8). In addition, patients will be used to having an

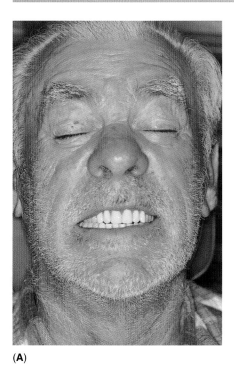

(A)

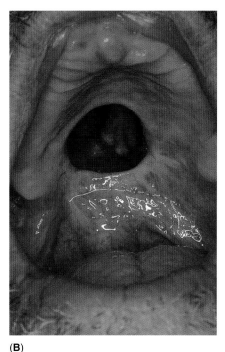

(B)

Figure 9.8 Example of a final obturator appliance in situ (**A**) and removed to show the defect (**B**).

appliance present in their mouth and be ready for fabrication of a final appliance. If the patient is dentate it is very important to ensure that the abutment teeth are healthy, vital, and have good periodontal support. Teeth requiring root canal treatment and restorations should be managed during the phase the patient is wearing his or her interim appliance. Often teeth that would normally be extracted in a conventional patient will be retained in the oncology patient if they are, at all, prosthetically useful from the standpoint of offering stability, support, or retention. Once the patient's dentition is appropriately restored and the patient is demonstrating good oral hygiene practice, the patient is ready for a final appliance. All soft tissues visible to the dentist should be examined for any sign of mucosal abnormality, which, if present should be brought to the surgeon's attention.

At this time patients should be questioned with respect to what they expect and want from their new appliance. There should be a firm and frank discussion with patients to explain, once again what may be accomplished and what may not be feasible. This discussion should be done with the dentist sitting in front of the patient and taking an adequate amount of time to listen to the patient's concerns and be assured that the patient fully comprehends what the dentist can do. The results of this conversation should be recorded in the chart, and the dentist may elect to read them back to the patient. Taking an adequate amount of time at this appointment avoids the possibility of failure later, assures the patient that the dentist is genuinely interested in the outcome, and, in some instances, lowers the patient's expectations to an achievable level.

In the partly dentate patient the final appliance is frequently made of a combination of cast chrome-cobalt with cast or wrought wire clasps, rests, and an acrylic bulb with teeth of appropriate shade and a soft tissue-colored denture acrylic base. The bulb and the periphery of the denture must extend to the margin of the scar band and put slight pressure on this band. This gentle pressure will form a seal when the patient swallows and will prevent nasal regurgitation. The amount of pressure varies, but an obturator bulb that is too large will cause ulceration and pain. An obturator bulb that is inadequate in size will not prevent nasal escape of fluids. The nasal aspect of the obturator bulb may be made hollow from above or be entirely hollow to lighten the weight of the appliance. Alternatively it may be made entirely of acrylic. The nasal portion should avoid contact with any nasal bones left by the surgeon because they will invariably be irritated and hemorrhage. If the entire nasal and sinus contents are removed at surgery the bulb may be extended upwards to allow more normal sounding speech, obtain bony support from horizontal bony surfaces and stability from vertical surfaces with the caveat that the bulb can only be extended as far as the oral aperture will accommodate the appliance. Occasionally a two-part appliance may be used with an upper portion fitted to the nasal/sinus cavity and extending up to the orbital floor and a lower denture portion that keys into this. The oral portion of the obturator should allow placement of the teeth in the prosthetic neutral zone, that is, altered by surgery. Additionally it should extend as far as possible for support but should not cause ulceration nor interfere with normal occlusion or mastication. The vestibular surface and palatal surfaces should be shaped in a manner that allows the oral musculature to assist in holding the appliance in place. In a posterior appliance this may mean having a

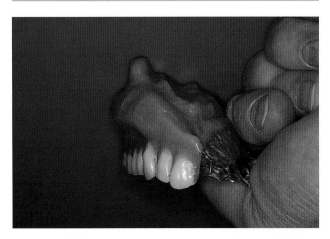

Figure 9.9 Vestibular concavity of the obturator allows, in some patients, the buccinator muscle to assist in keeping the denture in place.

concave vestibular surface (Fig. 9.9). The oral surfaces should also be highly polished to allow the soft tissues to glide across them.

The spectrum of appliances for rehabilitation of maxillary defects is huge, and for more comprehensive information in treating this group of patients the reader is referred to the following reference articles (14,15).

Mandibulotomy Candidate

The mandibulotomy splint is used in instances where a mandibular "swing" approach is used to gain access to upper aerodigestive tract malignancies. It is an alternative to a mandibular resection and is usually used in cases where there is no underlying bony involvement of the mandible (16). During the course of the procedure an osseous cut is made, usually in the anterior, and preferably through either an edentulous area or an extraction socket. The distal ends of the right and left sides of the mandible are then rotated outwards allowing direct view of the tongue and adjacent structures.

Following removal of the tumor the mandibular segments are reapproximated and plated with rigid fixation devices. The mandibulotomy splint is used to orient the teeth in three planes (coronal, axial, and medial-lateral) so that when the segments are realigned the teeth and the temporomandibular joints are in virtually the same position they were in prior to the splitting of the mandible. If the mandible is reapproximated in the absence of an appropriate splint or rigorous attention to maintenance of the three-dimensional spatial relationships of the jaws, joint pain and malocclusion will result; and expensive fixed prosthetic or removable appliances may be required to alleviate what is an essentially iatrogenic condition. The competent surgeon should not underestimate the degree of discomfort associated with what are seemingly trivial changes in the three-dimensional position of teeth. In addition to occlusal disharmony, teeth may become nonvital if excessively stressed; and some patients will suffer severe clinically significant impairment to their ability to masticate food and the function of their temporomandibular apparatus. Although it is best if dentate and edentulous patients are managed with the use of a splint it is particularly important in the former.

Mandibulotomy splints require about 5 working days to complete. At the first appointment the status of the dentition is assessed and irreversible hydrocolloid impressions are made from which dental stone models are poured. Impressions of the upper and lower arches are done and kept for occlusal analysis postoperatively. The lower model is used to fabricate the mandibulotomy splint. The splint may be made of either orthodontic wire embedded in acrylic resin or alternatively it may be cast from chrome-cobalt alloy. In the author's experience the latter are difficult to adjust and less forgiving than the acrylic ones. Prior to the mandibulotomy operation the splint is tried-in clinically (Fig. 9.10) to make sure it fits the lower teeth and is not causing occlusal disharmony with the upper teeth. At the time of operation the surgeon makes the osseous cut and removes the tumor. It is extremely important that any surgical cut through tooth-bearing portions of the jaw completely avoids the remaining teeth and their periodontal support apparatus. In the lower anterior mandible it is technically very difficult to section the right and left mandible without devitalizing an incisor tooth. When any tooth becomes nonvital or any periodontal support is compromised in the line of section, wound infection will almost always follow. After the operation the right and left mandibular segments are swung back into position and the splint is applied. If necessary it may be cemented or bonded to the teeth temporarily using zinc phosphate cement or light-cured acrylic

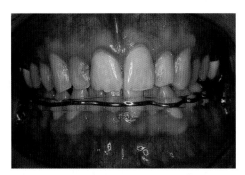

(A)

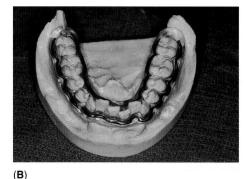

(B)

Figure 9.10 Mandibulotomy splint at the try-in appointment on the patient's teeth (A) and on a model (B).

resin. When it is firmly in place, the right and left mandibular segments are plated with the surgeon's preferred plating system. Compression plating will tend to move the segments closer together disrupting occlusion whereas passive plating may leave a saw-cut width gap of bone between the segments. The splint may then be removed or left for removal at a later date. The attending dentist may do this postoperatively.

Mandibulectomy/Glossectomy Patient

In general mandibular appliances are less well tolerated than upper ones. This is most likely due to the presence of the tongue and paramandibular musculature, which makes prosthetic restoration of the lower jaw a functional challenge. Following tongue or mandibulectomy surgery this challenge is heightened.

Patients with uncomplicated marginal mandibulectomy may be treated using variations of partial or complete lower dentures. Remembering the triad of support, stability, and retention the surgeon should plan ahead to leave as much horizontal bony surface as possible for denture support. Stability can be improved by ensuring that the buccal and lingual vestibules are not obliterated but are deep. Ablation of the buccal or lingual vestibules is a prime cause for denying patients prosthetic rehabilitation. Stability and support are highly dependent on the surgeon's ability to provide the dentist with tissue that is firmly bound down to bone. Large bulky grafts are not amenable to prosthetic rehabilitation. In this era of increased primary closure of mandibular and maxillary defects too many patients achieve primary closure but in doing so are turned into oral cripples because vestibules are ablated, and support, stability, and retention have been forever lost. Retention is improved by ensuring that as many dental units are kept as possible and that they are well cared for. Seemingly hopeless teeth can be used in some cases for improving stability and retention. A large bulky graft also reduces the retention of the denture by obliterating the neutral zone in which teeth may be placed.

Patients with partial mandibulectomy and osseous/rigid fixation plate reconstruction may also be rehabilitated using variations of removable partial and full dentures if adequate support, stability, and retention are present postoperatively. It is generally not acceptable to rest a denture on a fixation plate so some osseous support should be made available. In some instances a three-quarters or unilateral partial denture may be used if particular patient anatomy is conducive to it. Often, providing a patient with a single side of contacting functional teeth is adequate to meet his or her needs. In many patients with well-performed, unilateral mandibular surgery and one side of occluding teeth, they are often better left without a prostheses. Once again communication between the practitioner and the patient is pivotal in reaching a satisfactory result.

The glossectomy patient presents different problems for the dentist in that, depending on the amount of tongue removed and the results of reconstruction, there may be serious speech impairment. Following glossectomy the tongue may be physically smaller and deviated to one side. There are also usually clinically significant sensory and motor neural deficits that make speech more difficult. Patients may be unable to make certain sounds such as *t*,

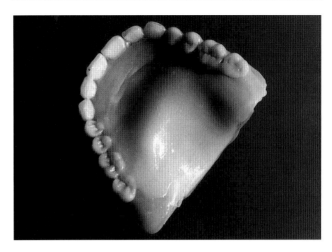

Figure 9.11 Addition of material to a maxillary appliance allows a deficient tongue to achieve contact with the palate so that a partial glossectomy patient can make speech sounds they normally would not be able to do.

k, hard g or **s**. In these patients alterations to upper and lower dentures or purposeful fabrication of a maxillary appliance with a lowered palate may allow many of these sounds to be made (Fig. 9.11). In these cases it is imperative that the dentist work closely with surgeon and the speech/language pathologist.

IMPLANTS

Osseointegrated implants are playing a greater role in the rehabilitation of surgical oncology patients [20]. Previous radiation therapy techniques precluded their use, but with the advent of IMRT, precise mapping of bone dose can be done and implants can and have been placed. No implant should be placed without consulting the radiation oncologist and determining the radiation dose at the proposed implant site. The lower the dose the safer it is to place implants. The success rate of implants appears to be improved by using HBO. In addition implants should be placed only if they are prosthetically useful. For this reason it is wise for the surgeon to contact the prosthodontist prior to placing the implant to ensure that it can form an integral part of the final prosthesis.

Unfortunately implants are expensive, and this may make them unfeasible for many patients. Implants are placed following a thorough radiological examination and treatment planning session to ensure that there is adequate bone to allow their placement. Cone-beam computed tomography is adequate to ascertain bone volume in three dimensions and guide implant placement [21]. If implants are to be placed in a site previously covered with grafted skin it is imperative that the implant fixture is covered by a reasonably thin skin or mucosal covering. Implants can be placed in free vascularized grafts or residual bone; however, these areas must not be covered with large bulky skin grafts because this causes unfavorable loading of the implant (Fig. 9.12).

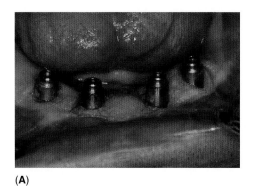

(A)

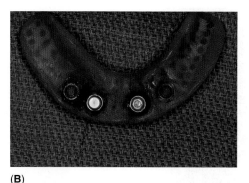

(B)

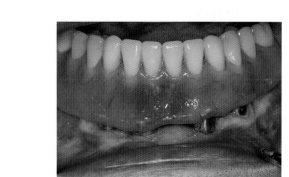

(C)

Figure 9.12 Photograph of a floor-of-mouth cancer patient that had a resection and rehabilitation consisting of a radial fore-arm free vascularized graft. Osseo-integrated implant prosthetic rehabilitation was then undertaken with **(A)** four Straumann tissue-level implant RN (4.1 mm implant diameter) and 4.8 mm diameter restorative platform **(B)** female receptacles for implant platform on the tissue-surface of the lower prostheses and **(C)** shows the final prostheses in place. [Case courtesy of Dr. D. Somerville, Princess Margaret Hospital and Straumann Canada].

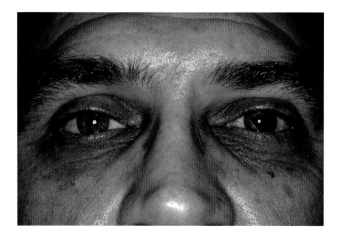

Figure 9.13 This patient has a well-fitting custom-made ocular prosthesis designed and made by a certified ocularist. It is difficult to tell which eye is the real one and which is the prosthetic one.

ANAPLASTOLOGY/OCULAR PROSTHETICS

A complete maxillofacial oncology service should ideally include as part of the restorative team an anaplastologist and an ocularist. The ocularist, among other services, fits ocular prostheses in patients who have had surgical enucleation of the globe or surgical removal of the eye and surrounding structures. This is done using modified impressions of the residual eye contents. The ocularist may modify the socket or globe by adding and removing prosthetic material. Judicious use of progressively larger implants can shape the size of the orbital bony architecture in young patients. Ocularists must select the correct pupil size, custom paint the iris to ensure that the eye is compatible with the remaining anatomy, is comfortable, is attractive, and allows the patient to maintain hygiene of the eye region (Fig. 9.13). This is a gross oversimplification of the talents of the ocularist. A more detailed description of the many functions of the ocularist may be found elsewhere (17). In maxillofacial prosthetics the ocularist works with the surgeon, prosthodontist, and anaplastologist to ensure that any patients requiring prosthetic eyes receive a high-quality ocular prosthesis, which can function as an integral part of the prosthetic rehabilitation. The role of the surgeon in these cases is to place craniofacial osseo-integrated implants that are smaller and shorter than conventional dental implants into the bed. They are well tolerated by skin, and HBO use appears to increase their success rate.

The anaplastologist performs a similar function as the ocularist and prosthodontist. He or she fabricates facial prostheses including nasal, periorbital, auricular, and facial prostheses to replace facial components that are lost as a consequence of cancer surgery or radiation treatment. The anaplastologist like the ocularist must be part anatomist, part artist, and part materials expert (Fig, 9.14). The anaplastologist, prosthodontist, dentist, and ocularist work together with the surgeon to reconstitute the patient back to a level that allows him or her to function normally.

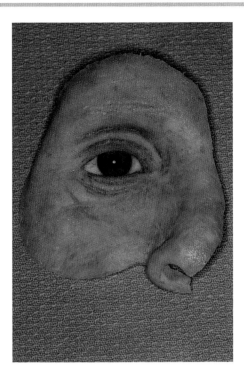

Figure 9.14 Integrated effort of anaplastologist, prosthodontist and ocularist results in an appliance which will reconstitute the missing portions of a patient's anatomy.

THE LONG-TERM CANCER SURVIVOR

The long-term head and neck cancer survivor can be integrated back into a general dental practice if the general practitioner is provided with either a resource person or obtains appropriate information for his or her care. Postradiation patients should be kept under close observation with a 3- to 6-month recall schedule and prompt management of any problem that may arise. These patients should be on life-long topical neutral sodium fluoride gel application in custom fluoride trays as well as strict self-directed oral hygiene measures. Failure to do so will result in the development of postradiation caries. If any invasive or extensive dental work is contemplated it is wise for the general practitioner to discuss the patient with the radiation oncologist or the dentist at the oncology center. At the author's institution, the patients are seen yearly to assess the general condition of the mouth. The patient must be cautioned to maintain his or her tobacco abstinence or if he or she still smokes be directed to their family physician or community resource person in an effort to get them to stop.

Because oral cancer can recur, each follow-up examination should include an evaluation of the neck nodes and the oral and paraoral soft tissues. Visual examination by an experienced practitioner is the best method for spotting early cancers although toluidine-blue rinses, and fluorescence visualization have been postulated as methods for diagnosing early cancers (18). This author does not favor the use of these agents or devices in the general dental practice. Although they may be of use in patients susceptible to oral cancers due to the high incidence of false positives,

the likelihood that numerous unnecessary biopsies may be undertaken, and the generation of unnecessary fear in the public (19,22).

There is a temptation to avoid exposing radiographs on postradiation patients because of the misperception that these patients have had "too much radiation already" or that the diagnostic radiation will "cause: another cancer. Radiographs should be used when there is a probability that they will add to the diagnostic capability. The cancer patient, who is xerostomic, eating more highly refined carbohydrates, and may not be exercising optimal oral hygiene is at greater risk of developing dental disease. For this reason, more, rather than fewer radiographs may need to be exposed.

Many patients with osteoporosis or with cancers other than head and neck cancers may be on parenteral or oral bisphosphonate treatment. In a small number of these patients oral surgical procedures may lead to osteonecrosis of the jaws. Osteonecrosis of the jaws, unlike osteoradionecrosis, which it superficially resembles, is not currently amenable to treatment. Any head and neck cancer patient taking bisphosphonates of any kind should be approached with caution when oral surgical procedures are contemplated. The initial case reports of bisphosphonate-imbibing head and neck cancer patients, and the complications that are occurring are beginning to appear in the literature (23). It is tempting to think that bisphosphonate-induced osteonecrosis of the jaws is only associated with intravenous (nitrogen-containing bisphosphonates) used in the management of cancers such as multiple myeloma, metastatic breast cancer, and metastatic prostate cancer. This may in the future prove to be untrue.

In evaluating the postsurgical patient the prosthetic appliance should be examined for signs of deterioration, wear, and discoloration. The defect should be evaluated for cleanliness, and recurrence and an assessment of fit and occlusion should be made. Appliances may wear out or require relining. If a patient is content with his or her appliance it may be best to leave well enough alone. It is the patient who is the final arbiter of satisfaction with respect to fit and function—not the dentist. Although an appliance may not be "prosthetically ideal," if a patient is content, and the appliance is not damaging adjacent hard or soft oral structures, there is no need to fabricate a new one.

REFERENCES

1. Hughes CJ, Spiro RH. Carcinoma of the oropharynx. A NZ J Surg 1994; 64: 302–6.
2. Bishay N, Petrikowski CG, Maxymiw WG et al. Optimum dental radiography in bone marrow transplant patients. Oral Surg Oral Med Oral Pathol Oral Radiol Endod 1999; 87: 375–9.
3. Myers RE, Mitchell DL. Fluoride for the head and neck radiation patient. Mil Med 1988; 153: 411–13.
4. Backstrom I, Funegard U, Andersson I et al. Dietary intake in head and neck irradiated patients with permanent dry mouths. Eur J Cancer 1995; 31B: 253–7.
5. Tatum RC, Daniels R. The correlation of radiotherapy to salivary gland production and increased caries incidence: a caries control method. Oral Med Oral Pathol Oral Radiol Endod 1982; 52: 9–11.
6. Niedermeier W, Matthaues C, Meyer C et al. Radiation-induced hyposalivation and its treatment with oral pilocarpine. Oral Med Oral Pathol Oral Radiol Endod 1998; 86: 541–9.

7. Wood RE, Maxymiw WG, McComb D. A clinical comparison of glass ionomer (polyalkenoate) and silver amalgam restorations in the treatment of class V caries in xerostomic head and neck cancer patients. Oper Dent 1993; 18: 94–102.

8. McComb D, Erickson RL, Maxymiw WG et al. A clinical comparison of glass ionomer, resin-modified glass ionomer and resin composite restorations in the treatment of cervical caries in xerostomic head and neck radiation patients. Oper Dent 2002; 27: 430–7.

9. Maxymiw WG, Liu F-F, Wood RE. Post-radiation dental extractions without hyperbaric oxygen. Oral Med Oral Pathol Oral Radiol Endod 1991; 72: 270–4.

10. Wong JK, Wood RE, McLean M. Conservative management of osteoradionecrosis. Oral Med Oral Pathol Oral Radiol Endod 1997; 84: 16–21.

11. Merlano M, Benasso M, Cavallari M et al. Chemotherapy in head and neck cancer. Eur J Cancer 1994; 30B: 283–9.

12. Greenberg MS, Cohen SG, McKitrick JC et al. The oral flora as a source of septicemia in patients with acute leukemia. Oral Med Oral Pathol Oral Radiol Endod 1982; 52: 32–6.

13. Maxymiw WG, Wood RE, Anderson JD. The immediate role of the dentist in the maxillectomy patient. J Otolaryngol 1989; 18: 303–5.

14. Adisman IK, Minsley GE. Maxillofacial prosthetics. In: Owall B, Kayser AF, Carlsson GE, eds. Prosthodontics, principles and management strategies. London: Mosby-Wolfe, 1996: 201–21.

15. Laney WR. Restoration of acquired oral and perioral defects. In: Laney WR, Gibilisco JA, eds. Diagnosis and treatment in prosthodontics. Philadelphia: Lea and Febiger, 1983: 129–40.

16. Spiro RH, Gerold FP, Shah JP et al. Mandibulotomy approach to oropharyngeal tumors. Am J Surg 1985; 150: 466–9.

17. McFall JD. The role of the ocularist. Adv Opthalmic Plast Reconstr Surg 1990; 8: 53–4.

18. Epstein J, Oakley C, Millner A et al. The utility of toluidine blue application as a diagnostic aid in patients previously treated for upper oropharyngeal carcinoma. Oral Med Oral Pathol Oral Radiol Endod 1997; 83: 537–47.

19. Martin IC, Kerawal CJ, Reeds M. The application of toluidine blue as a diagnostic adjunct in the detection of epithelial dysplasia. Oral Med Oral Pathol Oral Radiol Endod 1998; 85: 444–6.

20. Nelson K, Heberer S, Glatzer C. Survival analysis and clinical evaluation of implant-retained prostheses in oral cancer resection patients over a mean follow-up period of 10 years. J Prosthet Dent 2007; 98: 405–10.

21. Nickenig HJ, Eitner S. Reliability of implant placement after virtual planning of implant positions using cone beam CT data and surgical (guide) templates. J Craniomaxillofac Surg 2007; 35: 207–11.

22. Poh CF, Ng SP, Williams PM et al. Direct fluorescence visualization of clinically occult high-risk oral pre-malignant disease using a simple hand-held device. Head Neck 2007; 29: 71–6.

23. Marunick M, Gordon S. Prosthodontic treatment during active osteonecrosis related to radiation and bisphosphonate therapy: a clinical report. J Prosthet Dent 2006; 96: 7–12.

24. Shulman DH, Shipman B, Willis FB. Treating trismus with dynamic splinting. Adv Ther 2008; 25: 9–16.

10

Palliation of Advanced Head and Neck Cancer

John E Williams and Karen E Broadley

INTRODUCTION

Head and neck malignancies are rare and constitute less than 5% of all cancers in the Western world with an average cure rate of about 50%. When the disease presents early, cure is possible in up to 90% of cases, but the patient may still be symptomatic as a result of treatment and may benefit from many of the management strategies discussed in this chapter.

If the cancer is more advanced, either when it presents or when disease recurs or progresses, then emphasis may be less on cure but more on good symptom control. The need to palliate the distressing symptoms associated with advanced malignancy is of utmost importance.

Palliative care is best described as

the active total care of a person whose disease is no longer responsive to curative treatment. Control of pain, of other symptoms and of psychological, social and spiritual problems is paramount. The goal of palliative care is achievement of the best quality of life for patients and their families. Many aspects of palliative care are also applicable earlier in the course of the illness in conjunction with anti-cancer treatment (1).

Although some of the common symptoms of head and neck malignancy may be due to treatment, they commonly occur as a result of disease progression. If further anticancer treatment is available this may be the most effective method of palliation. The potential benefits should be weighed up against the probable adverse effects, and this information should be shared with the patient and his or her family before embarking upon treatment.

This chapter is primarily concerned with the practical management of physical problems arising from the cancer and/or its treatment. However, it cannot be overstated how important it is to also manage the psychological problems from which these patients suffer. This is evident when reflecting how socially important the structures of the face and neck are from a functional (speech and swallow) and a psychosocial sense (aesthetic appearance). It is critical that the patient is treated holistically.

The main causes of symptoms in advanced head and neck cancer are

1. Local disease causing infiltration, pressure or ulceration
2. An incidental cause such as infection or coexisting illness
3. Side effects from treatment with chemotherapy, radiotherapy, surgery, or medication
4. Distant spread with metastases for example in the lungs and bone.

Symptom control may be synonymous with the treatment of the neoplastic process either with surgery, radiotherapy, or chemotherapy. Where these measures fail or are inappropriate, other symptom-specific measures need to be employed. This chapter addresses some of the more common symptoms and their management.

In all situations medication should be kept simple and easy to swallow. Patients generally prefer liquids as mouth opening may be difficult. In addition, tablets may get stuck because of mechanical problems or lack of saliva. Liquids are essential with tube feeding, and suppositories are useful where there is no upper gastrointestinal route of access. In other situations transdermal preparations or the subcutaneous route may be available and appropriate.

PAIN
General Considerations

Pain has been defined as "an unpleasant sensory and emotional experience associated with actual or potential tissue damage" (2). In patients with head and neck cancer, pain can occur following treatments such as surgery and radiotherapy (acute pain) or may be a longer term problem associated with the disease process itself (chronic pain). Chronic pain patients may be debilitated with advanced disease or may have a stable condition with long life expectancy.

Effective pain control is essential for all patients with head and neck cancer because pain diminishes activity, appetite, and sleep and may contribute to feelings of fear, anxiety, and depression (3). Head and neck cancer patients may also have the additional burden of difficulty in swallowing and talking and the presence of visible disease.

Recent developments in the understanding of pain physiology and pharmacology have indicated that pain transmission from the periphery to the brain is a complex process capable of modification and adaptation, known as "plasticity" (4). Prolonged nociceptive input into the dorsal horn of the spinal cord can result in sensitization of receptors, which then facilitates further pain transmission. This process is also known as "wind up." The N-methyl D-aspartate receptor is involved in this process and is a potential target for analgesics that can block this receptor such as methadone or ketamine. A summary of recently identified pain pathways and neurotransmitters is illustrated in Figure 10.1, and recent advances in pain pharmacology and physiology and their clinical relevance are given in Table 10.1.

Because of the many different processes involved in pain transmission effective analgesia is more likely if many different classes of analgesic drug are used to treat pain.

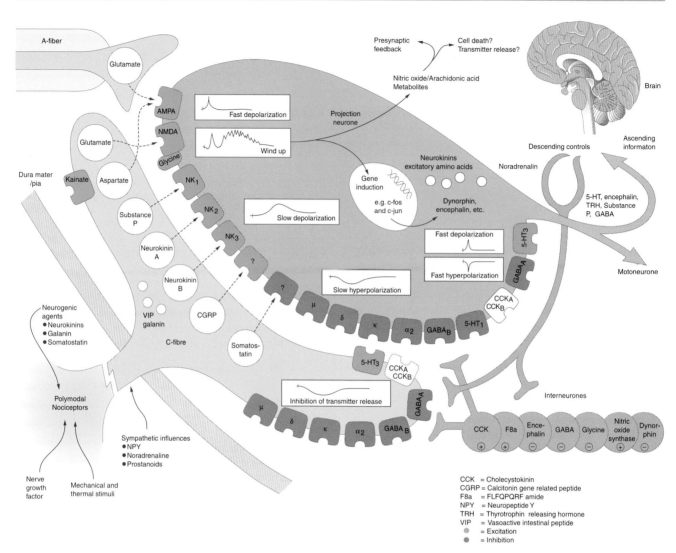

Figure 10.1   Cross-section through dorsal horn of spinal cord showing different stimulatory and inhibitory modulatory mechanisms.

Table 10.1   Recent Advances in Pain Pharmacology and Physiology and Clinical Relevance

Recent advance	Potential clinical relevance
Central nervous system plasticity and sensitization (wind up)	Treat pain early before long-term changes take place that may be difficult to reverse
NMDA receptor identified as being part of wind up process	NMDA-antagonist drugs such as methadone and ketamine may be effective
Evidence for the effectiveness of pre-emptive analgesia	Analgesic drugs given prior to a painful stimulus may be more effective
Evidence for the effectiveness of the multidisciplinary approach	Involve practitioners from other disciplines in treating chronic pain

Additionally it is likely that involvement of a multidisciplinary team approach including specialists from different disciplines such as psychology, physiotherapy, surgery, and palliative care would be beneficial (5).

Pain Assessment
Prior to commencement of analgesic therapy, patients with head and neck cancer pain should be investigated for the cause of the pain and the potential role of surgery,

radiotherapy, and chemotherapy in treating the cancer and relieving pain. This will involve a detailed history and examination and use of appropriate investigations such as magnetic resonance imaging scan.

Pain Syndromes in Head and Neck Cancer
Acute Pain
Acute pain can occur after surgery, radiotherapy, or chemotherapy. Postsurgical pain is usually treated in either the

postoperative recovery room or on the wards using opioids and other drugs such as nonsteroidal anti-inflammatory drugs (NSAIDs). Occasionally postsurgical pain may become a more persistent problem due to damage or bruising to nerves at the time of surgery or due to the formation of painful neuromata. In particular this may occur following radical neck dissection or following other major head and neck procedures.

It is essential to treat acute postoperative pain aggressively as it is usually responsive to analgesic medication, and there is some evidence that effective early treatment of acute pain may lead to a lower incidence of chronic pain problems (6).

Pain following radiation therapy or chemotherapy usually presents as oral mucositis that develops during the 2nd to 4th week after commencement of treatment. In patients who have difficulty in swallowing oral analgesics, this can be treated with either subcutaneous or intravenous opioids. Mucositis usually spontaneously resolves 3 to 4 weeks after cessation of therapy (7). Numerous different interventions have been evaluated for the prevention and treatment of oral mucositis including amifostine and ice chips (8,9).

Infection may play a role in exacerbating pain at any stage in the treatment of head and neck cancers. Infection may present as a worsening pain problem without any associated signs and symptoms such as fever, leukocytosis, or signs of local infection (10).

Chronic Pain

Chronic pain in head and neck cancer patients may be classified into nociceptive or neuropathic pain syndromes. Figure 10.2 shows three different pain transmission states: (1) physiological pain transmission, where the pain impulses travel from the stimulus to the brain with minimal dorsal horn wind up; (2) nociceptive pain where there is some peripheral and central sensitization; and (3) neuropathic pain where there is abnormal wind up resulting in altered pain transmission and supersensitivity.

Nociceptive pain may be due to tumor pressure or infiltration into the mucosa or submucosa, which may lead to ulceration and infection. This may be exacerbated by local irritation with alcohol or acid, edema, and movement especially in dynamic structures such as the tongue and soft palate.

Bony infiltration can result in localized pain or, if there is direct pressure on a sensory nerve, pain in the distribution of the nerve. Cervical spine lesions my be a cause of head and neck pain. Lesions may be as a result of cervical degeneration, metastases, or surgical trauma.

Neuropathic pain can result after tumor pressure on a nerve or infiltration of a nerve. Typically this type of pain is characterized by lancinating or shooting pains in the distribution of the nerve, pain in a numb area, burning pain, and dysaesthesiae such as "pins-and-needles." Neuropathic pain syndromes are listed in Table 10.2.

Drug Therapy

The majority of head and neck cancer pains can be managed using the World Health Organization (WHO) guidelines for the treatment of cancer pain (11). This involves

Table 10.2 Neuropathic Pain Syndromes in Head and Neck Cancer

Tumor	Neuropathic pain syndrome
Intraorbital	Sharp, lancinating pains in region of ophthalmic nerve
Maxillary antrum	Sharp, lancinating pains in distribution of maxillary nerve
Infratemporal fossa	Mandibular neuralgia, trismus, temporal pain
Nasopharynx, oropharynx, tonsillar region	Neuralgias in distribution of vagus and glossopharyngeal nerves
Postherpetic neuralgia	Commonly affects trigeminal nerve, stabbing pains, hyperaesthesia

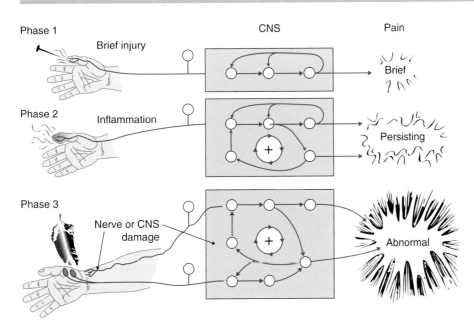

Figure 10.2 Three different pain transmiss machanisms; Phase 1, physiological pain; Phase 2, nociceptive pain; Phase 3, neuropathic pain (demonstrating "wind up" with nerve damage).

using noninvasive drug treatments according to a step-wise progression in drug dosages and by following the guidelines listed in Tables 10.3 and 10.4. Additional guidelines now exist for the treatment of neuropathic pain (12) that include the use of anticonvulsants, antidepressants, opioids, tramadol, and lidoderm patches.

Head and neck cancer patients who are unable to swallow tablets can take these drugs enterally via gastrostomy or nasogastric tubes or rectal route. Patients unable to use any enteral route may require these drugs to be given either subcutaneously or intravenously.

Step 1. Non-opioid Drugs

This group includes paracetamol, aspirin, and other NSAIDS such as ibuprofen, naproxen, and diclofenac.

NSAIDs work by inhibiting the cyclo-oxygenase enzyme responsible for producing prostaglandins, which contribute to the peripheral inflammatory response. NSAIDs are effective against nociceptive pain such as mucosal ulceration and bone pain. They are less effective for neuropathic pain.

All NSAIDs have the potential for adverse effects including hemorrhage, renal impairment, and gastric erosion. They should be used with caution in patients with renal dysfunction or with a history of peptic ulcer.

Recent developments have included the development of NSAIDs such as meloxicam. As specific cyclooxygenase (COX)-2 antagonists, they do not antagonize the production of prostaglandins responsible for normal physiological functioning, and thus have the potential for fewer adverse effects. However, recent studies have shown an increase in the incidence of cardiovascular adverse events associated with use of COX-2 antagonists, and the current recommendation is that a COX-2 nonspecific NSAID such as ibuprofen or diclofenac is used with a proton pump inhibitor such as lansoprazole to reduce gastrointesinal adverse effects (13).

Step 2. Opioids for Mild to Moderate Pain

Opioids for mild to moderate pain (formerly known as weak opioids) include codeine, dihydrocodeine and combinations of these drugs with paracetamol such as co-dydramol. Many of these combination preparations only have a small dose of weak opioid, and some practitioners pass directly from step 1 to step 3 in patients with pain resistant to nonopioids.

Tramadol is a relatively new step 2 drug. It works as an opioid agonist and as an activator of central nervous system descending inhibitory systems and is an alternative to codeine or dihydrocodeine (14).

Step 3. Opioids for Moderate to Severe Pain

Immediate release preparations include morphine tablets such as Sevredol or liquid morphine, Oramorph are opioids for moderate to severe pain (formerly known as strong opioids).

Sustained-release preparations such as the twice daily morphine sulphate tablets (MST) or the once daily MXL are used in stable long-term pain conditions. MST is available as a suspension that can pass down a feeding tube. In patients unable to take tablets, transdermal fentanyl may be an alternative. This preparation gives a sustained release of the strong opioid fentanyl and may be associated with fewer adverse effects compared to MST, specifically less constipation.

Alternative strong opioids in patients unable to take morphine, because of resistance or intolerance, include hydromorphone and oxycodone, which are available in immediate and sustained-release preparations, and oral methadone and parenteral alfentanil.

Opioid-induced Side Effects

The main side effects of opioid therapy include dry mouth, constipation, sedation, and nausea. Dry mouth is difficult to treat as it may in part have been caused by the underlying disease process. All patients should be prescribed a laxative on commencement of opioids. A combined bowel stimulant and stool softener may be appropriate. About one-third of patients will need an anti-emetic.

Adjuvant Drugs

This group of drugs can be used at all stages in the WHO ladder (15).They include drugs that have another primary indication, such as the treatment of depression or epilepsy, but which also have analgesic properties or may contribute to pain relief (Table 10.5).

Neuropathic pain syndromes are often treated with this group of drugs in the first instance (Table 10.6). Anticonvulsants such as gabapentin and pregabalin are now commonly used to treat neuropathic pain and are supported by a good evidence base (16). Additionally, the lidoderm patch has been shown to be effective in the treatment of neuropathic pain (17). This patch can be placed over a painful area and works by cooling, protecting a painful

Table 10.3 WHO Guidelines for Relief of Cancer Pain

"The right drug at the right dose at the right time intervals"
- By the mouth
- By the clock
- By the ladder
- For the individual
- Use of adjuvant medication
- Attention to detail

Table 10.4 WHO Analgesic Ladder

Step 1	Non-opioid +/- adjuvant
Step 2	Weak opioid for mild to moderate pain +/- non-opioid +/- adjuvant
Step 3	Strong opioid for moderate to severe pain +/- non-opioid +/- adjuvant

Table 10.5 Adjuvant Drugs Used for Neuropathic Pain

Drug class	Examples
Antidepressant	amitriptyline, nortriptyline
Anticonvulsant	gabapentin, pregabalin
Opioids	tramadol, oxycodone
Topical agents	lidoderm 5% patch

Table 10.6 Treatment of Neuropathic Pain

Nerve compression pain may respond to corticosteroids
Use adjuvant analgesics in first instance
Amitriptyline 10–25 mg at night, increase dose by 10–25 mg at
    weekly intervals according to response and side effects
Consider use of gabapentin or pregabalin in addition to amitriptyline
Consider use of opioids such as tramadol, oxycodone or fentanyl
    patch
Consider use of lidoderm patch applied topically to painful area

Table 10.7 Causes of Nausea and Vomiting

Metabolic
    Hypercalcemia
    Uremia
Raised intracranial pressure—cerebral metastases
Drug induced
Chemotherapy
Radiotherapy
Gastrointestinal cause
    Constipation
    Gastric distension and stasis
    Bowel obstruction
Pain
Anxiety

area of skin, and by releasing local anesthetic into the tissues beneath.

OTHER SYMPTOM PROBLEMS
Nausea and Vomiting
Nausea and vomiting occur in up to 50% of patients with advanced cancer, frequently together, although occasionally in isolation. Nausea and vomiting are generally multifactorial but there are commonly identifiable causes (Table 10.7). If a particular cause is thought to be reversible, it should be treated specifically. Frequently, however, this is not possible and anti-emetics are required.

There are many anti-emetics available, with different mechanisms of action and different uses (Table 10.8). Although in most cases the oral route is preferred, if intractable vomiting or mechanical problems prevent this, other routes must be considered. These include sublingual, rectal, subcutaneous, and intravenous administration. A subcutaneous infusion or regular subcutaneous injections can be useful when rapid control is needed. Most of the commonly used anti-emetics can be combined in a syringe driver with morphine or diamorphine. Once symptoms improve, the patient may be converted back onto oral preparations.

Nutritional Problems
Cachexia, a syndrome of anorexia and weight loss associated with cancer, is often multifactorial in nature. The syndrome is characterized by a chronic abnormal metabolic state with abnormalities in carbohydrate, fat, and protein metabolism. In patients with head and neck cancer there is often a relative decline in food intake, hypophagia. Decreased appetite is a frequent complaint and is often more of a concern to the family than for the patient.

Hypophagia may result from chronic nausea either due to chemotherapy or radiotherapy. The disease itself or previous anticancer treatment may have caused changes in taste and smell (Table 10.9). Diminished saliva production will be an aggravating factor, and there are often mechanical reasons due to tumor and treatment, which limit food intake (Table 10.10). The tumor may produce circulating products, which decrease the appetite. Cytokines, produced by the host in response to the tumor, probably have a large role to play.

Nausea should be treated and practical advice given such as avoidance of meal preparation where possible. Small frequent meals are often best, together with dietary supplements. Appetite stimulants can be used but should be avoided when hypophagia is due to a mechanical reason.

Studies in patients with non-endocrine-responsive cancer show that progestogens such as megestrol acetate improve appetite and food intake and have in some cases been shown to stimulate weight gain. Corticosteroids have a beneficial effect on appetite and well-being but rarely result in weight gain. Artificial cannabinoids also appear effective but their benefit has not been proven in clinical trials. All these drugs have side effects that may not be tolerable for the patient.

Tube feeding is common in head and neck cancer patients. Patients are frequently malnourished when they present due to a multitude of factors, and nasogastric feeding is used as a temporary measure while active treatment is being carried out. This allows for administration of medication in addition to nutritional intake. Generally nasogastric tubes are only used in the short term as the tube may cause chronic throat irritation, alar damage, and aggravate esophageal reflux. The appearance can be unacceptable to the patient, and in addition they can be easily dislodged. If a more long-term solution is required, then placement of a gastrostomy or jejunostomy tube can be performed using endoscopic- or radiological-guided placement (18). Where there is significant obstruction due to disease, then the latter method may be easier. If a fistula, previously used for speech, still exists between esophagus and trachea and is no longer being used, then a long tube can be placed this way. Enteral feeding can take place overnight to minimize disruption during the day.

In all cases there can be problems such as tube blockage, dislodgment, leakage, or skin infection. Patients may decide not to have a tube replaced if they have had many problems.

Mouth Care
Patients who have been treated for head and neck cancer often have a dry mouth (xerostomia) and are more susceptible to local infections such as *Candida*. Medication used for either analgesia or anti-emesis can also aggravate an already dry mouth.

As disease progresses, ulceration may occur, which can be painful. It may be difficult for patients to keep a dental plate in position due to pain, and cleansing may become impossible.

Many measures have been suggested to try and improve xerostomia. Water should be taken frequently, and ice chips can be soothing. Pilocarpine capsules have been used in xerostomia induced by radiation (19,20) and due

Table 10.8 Commonly Used Anti-Emetic Drugs, their Route of Administration and Uses

Drug	Usual dosages and route of administration	Typical dose in 24 hour subcutaneous infusion	Specific uses, apart from general anti-emetic
Cyclizine	50 mg PO/SC/IV tds	150 mg over 24 hours	Pharyngeal stimulation and vertigo
Haloperidol	1.5–3.0 mg PO/SC/IV od/bd	3–10 mg over 24 hours	Opioid-induced nausea and uremia
Domperidone	10–20 mg PO; 30–60 mg PR tds/qds	Not available	Gastric stasis
Metoclopramide	10 mg PO/SC/IV tds	30 mg over 24 hours	Gastric stasis
Prochlorperazine	5–10 mg PO tds 3–6 mg buccal – bd 5 mg tds, 25 mg bd –PR	Not suitable	Vertigo
Levomepromazine	6.25–12.5 mg PO/SC od/bd	12.5–25 mg over 24 hours	Where sedation is useful
Hyoscine	200–400 mg SC tds 1 mg transdermal, lasts 3 days	800–1200 µg over 24 hours	May improve sialorrhea
Granisetron	1 mg PO bd 3 mg IV	Not known	Chemotherapy-induced nausea
Dexamethasone	4–16 mg PO/IV/SC od	4–16 mg (tends to precipitate when mixed with other drugs at high doses)	Raised intracranial pressure, liver metastases

Abbreviations: od, once daily; bd, twice daily; tds, three times a day; qds, four times a day; stat, immediately; PO, by mouth; SC, subcutaneously; IV, intravenously; PR, per rectum.

Table 10.9 Causes of Taste Changes in Head and Neck Cancer

Surgical management of carcinoma of the oral cavity and tongue
Radiotherapy treatment for the same
Surgical or radiotherapeutic effect on the olfactory component of taste
Xerostomia
Stomatitis
Oral infections
Poor oral hygiene
Progressive local disease

Table 10.10 Causes of Hypophagia

Difficulty in mastication: edentulous, pain, dry mouth
Functional dysphagia: treatment related, progression of cancer
Chronic nausea
Changes in taste
Aspiration

to medication (21). Some of the lubricating sprays and gels such as Saliva Orthana or Oralbalance are also helpful but need to be used frequently. Recent studies suggest that chewing sugar-free gum can improve the symptoms.

Fungal infections should be treated either with topical therapy such as nystatin suspension or systemic treatment such as fluconazole. Dentures, if worn, should also be treated.

Patients should be encouraged to maintain as good mouth care as possible, to use a soft toothbrush and an antibacterial mouthwash. In some situations when ulceration is a problem, then mouthwashes, which often contain alcohol, may be extremely painful. In such situations, bicarbonate of soda solution can be helpful.

Infection

Infection is common in head and neck patients, with cellulitis, localized tumor infections, and orocutaneous fistulae contributing to more than 20% of febrile episodes in head and neck cancers (22).

In some situations, improving local mouth care by cleansing and reducing secondary bacterial infections may reduce the risk of developing overwhelming sepsis. In many situations, however, antibiotics are required because of clinical signs of infection or because of increasing pain and discharge. In this situation, broad-spectrum antibiotics such as metronidazole and a penicillin are commonly used.

Fungating Wounds

Fungating wounds occur as a result of local recurrence of disease, but may also be due to skin metastases or spread to the tracheostomy site or scar. A fungating tumor is distressing because of the appearance and the odor from necrotic tissue. Both of these can lead to social isolation and loss of intimacy between the patient and carers.

Pain can occur due to skin and muscle infiltration and may be aggravated as a result of inflammation due to treatment or supra-added infection. Pain can usually be managed effectively and treatment of infection may improve pain and also local swelling.

Where pain is a problem at the time of dressing changes, quick-acting opioid drugs given just prior to the procedure, for example, immediate-release morphine, may help. These need to be given about 20 to 30 minutes before. Where the skin is generally sore, then topical local anesthetic gels are useful as a short-term measure. These can be mixed with gel applied for wound debridement.

Odor

Necrotic tissue is susceptible to microbial colonization. Metronidazole gel has been shown to reduce odor and colonization but does not treat overwhelming infection (23). When odor is particularly offensive, then charcoal-containing dressings can be applied over the top of the wound dressing. Although it seems sensible to try and mask offensive smells with aromatherapy oils, this can make the unpleasant odor more noticeable, which may merely aggravate the problem.

Bleeding

Where there is capillary bleeding at the time of dressing changes, adrenaline soaks applied directly to the wound may reduce this. Many of the newer dressings such as the alginates are hemostatic. The dressings should be absorbent to prevent maceration of the surrounding skin, and fiber free to reduce infection and allow for ease of removal. Gentle pressure should be applied to the bleeding points. If bleeding becomes more of a problem, it is essential to check there are no aggravating factors (discontinue aspirin or anticoagulants, for example).

Tranexamic acid can be applied as a topical solution or given orally (0.5–1 g 4 times daily) to help with hemostasis. Where bleeding occurs from local lesions in the mouth, then tranexamic acid can be used as a mouth gargle. Where catastrophic bleeding is threatened and resuscitation is not appropriate, it may be appropriate to have medication to hand when the dressing is changed (crisis pack; Table 10.11).

Where there is continued severe bleeding and it is appropriate in the patient's condition, further management should be considered. Radiotherapy can be effective for superficial bleeding where there is still a possibility of its use. In some situations endovascular techniques and embolization have been used successfully (24,25). However, this is not without significant risks and should only be considered in patients who are relatively stable and are expected to have a fairly good quality of life for a while after the procedure.

Severe Hemorrhage

This complication is feared by all healthcare professionals and by those patients who are aware. A patient dying from exsanguination such as a "carotid blowout" is a traumatic event for everyone, and endovascular techniques should be considered if it is a likely occurrence (26). Severe bleeding though is not a common cause of death. In two series of head and neck patients referred for inpatient palliative care, two of 102 and one of 38 patients died in this manner (27,28). It is a more likely occurrence after surgery where radiotherapy has been used in the past. In the series of 38 patients, 11 patients had repeated episodes of bleeding, but these did not cause death. Most died as a result of pneumonia and general deterioration (27).

Blood loss can occur from either the tumor bed or from erosion of a large vessel. Where major bleeding is likely to be a problem, it is often heralded by several minor bleeds. These can be extremely worrying for the patient and carers, as the timing cannot be predicted. If small bleeds occur at dressing changes, at the time when healthcare practitioners are within the house, a crisis pack (Table 10.11) can be at the ready. It is always helpful for the patient to have a letter explaining his or her condition and how a bleed should be managed in accident and emergency department, as it is likely that they will be taken to their nearest hospital rather than to a specialist center. Should a bleed occur, then immediate pressure should be applied to the wound, and when the bleeding stops, a pressure dressing applied. When there

Table 10.11 Crisis Pack

In the event of distress caused by sudden acute bleed or by upper respiratory obstruction:
1. 10–20 mg IV/IM midazolam
2. Diamorphine IV/IM equivalent to 4-hourly dose (if not on opioids, give 10–20 mg)

If distress continues, commence a subcutaneous pump

is catastrophic bleeding such as a carotid blowout there is little time for medication to be drawn up and administered. In this situation it is important not to leave the patient alone but to remain at his or her side.

Fistulae and Secretions/Discharge

Where infection contributes to discharge, antibiotics may be appropriate. There may be excessive secretions, particularly where a fistula (or fistulae) has formed between the oral cavity and the skin. Liquid food and saliva can pour through, and the most absorptive dressings are needed to reduce contact with the skin to prevent irritation. Where there is excessive saliva production (particularly where it cannot be swallowed), the role of an anticholinergic such as hyoscine or glycopyrronium can be considered. Hyoscine is available as a transmucosal preparation (Kwells) or as a transdermal preparation that stays in place for 3 days (Scopaderm).

Lymphoedema

Lymphoedematous swelling of the face can occur in small areas or more generally. The lymphatics may be damaged as a result of cancer, radiotherapy, or surgery. In progressive disease there may be concomitant hypoalbuminaemia, and venous obstruction due to neck disease, which will exacerbate the condition. Infection can also be a causative factor as before. Lymphoedema is best managed when caught at an early stage. The skin should be protected by moisturizing it regularly, and care should be given to avoid skin damage. If infection occurs, this should be treated rapidly with antibiotics. If cellulitis causes the patient to be systemically unwell then prophylactic antibiotics should be considered after a second episode.

In moderate or severe lymphoedema, the face can be uncomfortable as well as unsightly due to pressure and skin tightness. It can be a particular problem after lying down at night. During the day the lymphoedema will slowly decrease through the effect of gravity. It can be minimized by raising the head at night.

Discomfort and pain should be treated with appropriate analgesia. Occasionally diuretics can reduce the tightness of the face though they rarely help with swelling. High-dose steroids may benefit, reducing tumor bulk and perivascular edema. If a trial of steroids fails to elicit any change, they should be stopped, as conversely they may also aggravate swelling and encourage candidal infection. Specialized massage of the face can improve lymphatic flow when there is no concomitant infection but should only be attempted by those experienced in its use. A compression dressing over absorbent dressings may be effective where skin is broken and weeping (lymphorrhoea), but comfort must not be compromised.

Dyspnoea

Dyspnoea may be due to concomitant disease such as bronchopneumonia or chronic obstructive airway disease, or may be due to cancer.

Many patients will have had a tracheostomy inserted during part of their cancer treatment. These can become blocked, with progression of local disease, secretions, or blood. It requires skilled nursing to care for a difficult and sometimes-distorted tracheostomy site. This is a common reason why such patients remain in hospital. When formation of a tracheostomy may give relief of symptoms in late-stage disease this should be considered. Whenever possible the patient and family should be involved in these discussions. It is always best to prevent a situation happening as an emergency but to plan it early as symptoms arise. Causes of dyspnoea and management are listed in Table 10.12.

Whatever the cause, breathlessness is a subjective symptom that is increasingly mentioned as a problem as a patient deteriorates. On occasions a specific cause cannot be found, and it may be attributed to generalized weakness and debility. Anxiety is frequently present, which can make the feeling worse. Fears of being suffocated and of breathing stopping during sleep are common and can make the night a worry. Reassurance is often needed, and simple things such as company, a night-light, and a fan can be helpful.

The general feeling of breathlessness can be improved by reducing anxiety and lowering the respiratory drive. Diazepam given in small doses (2–5 mg) morning and night together with regular oral morphine 2.5 to 5 mg may help to achieve this. Respiratory depression tends not to be a problem when the drugs are introduced in low doses and titrated up.

Sudden attacks of breathlessness or panic attacks can be eased by sublingual lorazepam (0.5–1 mg), which acts rapidly.

If acute airway obstruction occurs such as blockage of the tracheostomy tube or an acute bleed compromises the airway, then sedation should be administered (Table 10.12). Helium-oxygen mixture has been used with tracheal obstruction, the rationale being that it is less viscous than air and may require less respiratory effort.

Hypercalcaemia

This is common in patients with head and neck cancers. Occasionally, the hypercalcaemia may be picked up as an incidental finding, but the symptoms, such as thirst, constipation, and confusion, are likely indicators. Management of mild hypercalcaemia may involve encouragement of oral fluid intake. At a higher level particularly with dehydration, then intravenous fluids may be indicated, together with the use of bisphosphonates given intravenously. On some occasions resistant hypercalcaemia can be a terminal event.

Communication Problems

During early disease management, communication issues may have been a concern. In some situations, speech may just be understandable or the patient may use a mechanical device. As a patient becomes weaker or develops more extensive local disease, the patient may become harder to understand. In this situation, patients easily become frustrated, and there is a need to spend more time with them to try and develop some form of communication. Where writing has been relied on, it becomes more difficult as weakness progresses. The niceties of speech and conversation become lost. Liaison with a speech therapist is essential.

THE DYING PATIENT

When a patient is dying, all treatments, drugs, and investigations that are not necessary should be discontinued. Analgesia and anti-emetics should be continued. Analgesic requirements can increase at this time, and it is important that the patient is reviewed regularly. If terminal agitation or restlessness occurs it is important to exclude simple causes such as pain, urinary retention, or fecal impaction. If there is renal impairment, accumulation of drugs may be an aggravating factor. Agitation is, however, often due to the dying process. Medications such as midazolam (initially 20–30 mg in 24 hours) or levomepromazine (12.5–50 mg initially in 24 hours) given subcutaneously by continuous infusion have been used to good effect.

Respiratory distress can be reduced with opioids and benzodiazepines given subcutaneously. If excess secretions are a problem, parenteral fluids should be stopped and hyoscine or glycopyrronium be added to the syringe driver. In some circumstances patients may require suction.

Other terminal events should be anticipated. Even if an anti-emetic is not required regularly, one should be

Table 10.12 Common Causes of Dyspnea with Suggested Managements

Due to disease	Specific treatment
Upper airway obstruction	Humidified air to reduce sticky secretions
	Consider tracheostomy if due to disease progression
Nasal obstruction	Surgery, stenting, or laser treatment
SVCO	Radiotherapy or SVC stenting
Lung metastases	Symptomatic treatment
Lymphangitis carcinomatosis	Trial of high-dose steroids (12–16 mg dexamethasone a day)
Pleural effusion	Aspiration of effusion
Associated with the disease	
Pulmonary emboli	Anticoagulation as long as bleeding is not a problem
Bronchopneumonia	Antibiotics and bronchodilators
COAD	Bronchodilators

Abbreviations: SVCO, superior vena cava obstruction; SVC, superior vena cava; COAD, chronic obstructive airway disease.

prescribed in case it is needed. If hemorrhage is a possibility, then midazolam or another quick acting anxiolytic should be prescribed.

If the patient has expressed a wish about where he or she would like to die, efforts should be made to ensure the request is fulfilled. Most head and neck patients request to be on an inpatient unit where they are known. It may not be possible or appropriate, however, to move a sick person in his or her last days. In any event the patient has a right to peaceful and, if possible, private surroundings with his or her family near. They should be allowed to die with dignity, with respect given their religious beliefs and customs.

REFERENCES

1. World Health Organization. Cancer pain and palliative care Technical Report Series 804. Geneva, Switzerland: World Health Organization, 1990.
2. International Association for the Study of Pain, Subcommittee on Taxonomy. Part 2. Pain terms: a current list with definitions and notes on usage. Pain 1979; 6: 249–52 (updated 1982, 1986).
3. Moinpour CM, Chapman CR. Pain management and quality of life in cancer patients. In: Lehmann RKA, Zech D, eds. Transdermal fentanyl: A new approach to prolonged pain control. Berlin: Springer-Verlag, 1991: 42–63.
4. Dickenson AH. Recent advances in the physiology and pharmacology of pain: plasticity and its implications for clinical analgesia. J Psychopharmacol 1991; 5: 342–51.
5. Flor H, Fydrich T, Turk DC. Efficacy of multidisciplinary pain treatment centers: a meta-analytic review. Pain 1992; 49: 221–30.
6. McQuay HJ. Pre-emptive analgesia (Editorial). Br J Anaesth 1992; 69: 1–3.
7. Weisseman DE. Cancer-associated pain syndromes. Pain Digest 1991; 1: 92–9.
8. Worthington HV, Clarkson JE, Eden OB. Interventions for preventing oral mucositis for patients with cancer receiving treatment. Cochrane Database Syst Rev 2007 , Issue 4. Art. No.: CD000978. DOI: 10.1002/14651858. CD000978.pub3.
9. Rubenstein EB, Peterson DE, Schubert M et al. Mucositis Study Section of the Multinational Association for Supportive Care in Cancer. International Society for Oral Oncology. Clinical practice guidelines for the prevention and treatment of cancer therapy-induced oral and gastrointestinal mucositis. Cancer 2004; 100(9 Suppl): 2026–46.
10. Bruera E, MacDonald N. Intractable pain in patients with advanced head and neck tumours: a possible role of local infection. Cancer Treat Rep 1986; 70: 691–2.
11. World Health Organization. Cancer pain relief and palliative care. Geneva, Switzerland: World Health Organization, 1986.
12. Dworkin RH, O'Connor AB, Backonja M et al. Pharmacologic management of neuropathic pain: evidence-based recommendations. Pain 2007; 132: 237–51.
13. Jones R, Rubin G, Berenbaum F et al. Gastrointestinal and cardiovascular risks of nonsteroidal anti-inflammatory drugs. Am J Med 2008; 121: 464–74.
14. Desmeules JA. The tramadol option. Eur J Pain 2000; 4(Suppl A): 15–21.
15. World Health Organization. Cancer pain relief and palliative care. Report of a WHO expert committee. WHO Technical Report Series, 804. Geneva, Switzerland: World Health Organization, 1990.
16. Gilron I. Gabapentin and pregabalin for chronic neuropathic and early postsurgical pain: current evidence and future directions. Curr Opin Anaesthesiol 2007; 20: 456–72.
17. Gammaitoni AR, Alvarez NA, Galer BSJ. Safety and tolerability of the lidocaine patch 5%, a targeted peripheral analgesic: a review of the literature. Clin Pharmacol 2003; 43: 111–17.
18. Rustom IK, Jebreel A, Tayyab M et al. Percutaneous endoscopic, radiological and surgical gastrostomy tubes: a comparison study in head and neck cancer patients. J Laryngol Otol 2006; 120: 463–6.
19. LeVeque FG, Montgomery M, Potter D et al. A multicenter, randomized, double-blind, placebo-controlled, dose-titration study of oral pilocarpine for treatment of radiation-induced xerostomia in head and neck cancer patients. J Clin Oncol 1993; 11: 1124–31.
20. Davies AN, Shorthose K. Parasympathomimetic drugs for the treatment of salivary gland dysfunction due to radiotherapy. Cochrane Database Systematic Review 2007; CD003782.
21. Davies AN, Daniels C, Pugh R et al. A comparison of artificial saliva and pilocarpine in the management of xerostomia in patients with advanced cancer. Palliat Med 1998; 12: 105–11.
22. Hussain M, Kish JA, Crane L et al. The role of infection in the morbidity and mortality of patients with head and neck cancer undergoing multimodality therapy. Cancer 1991; 67: 716–21.
23. Finlay IG, Bowszc J, Ramlau C et al. The effect of topical 0.75% metronidazole gel on malodourous cutaneous ulcers. J Pain Symptom Manage 1996; 11: 158–62.
24. Bhansali S, Wilner H, Jacobs JR. Arterial embolization for control of bleeding in advanced head and neck carcinoma. J Laryngol Otol 1986; 100: 1289–93.
25. Chou WC, Lu CH, Lin G et al. Transcutaneous arterial embolization to control massive tumour bleeding in head and neck cancer: 63 patients' experience from a single medical centre. Support Care Cancer 2007; 15: 1185–90.
26. Chang FC, Lirng JF, Luo CB et al. Patients with head and neck cancers and associated postirradiated carotid blowout syndrome: endovascular therapeutic methods and outcomes. J Vasc Surg 2008; 47: 936–45.
27. Talmi YP, Bercovici M, Waller A et al. Home and inpatient hospice care of terminal head and neck cancer patients. J Palliat Care 1997; 13: 9–14.
28. Forbes K. Palliative care in patients with cancer of the head and neck. Clin Otolaryngol 1997; 22: 117–22.

11

Tumors of the Oral Cavity

Ian Ganly, Tihana Ibrahimpasic, Snehal G Patel and Jatin P Shah

INTRODUCTION

Tumors of the oral cavity are relatively less common compared to other head and neck sites such as the larynx, but the incidence and mortality rates for oral cancer, especially in younger men, have shown an increase in the U.K. and almost all the Eurpean community (EC) countries over the last few decades. The tumor and the consequences of its treatment can profoundly affect one or more of the several important functions that the oral cavity normally serves. Alteration of functions such as mastication, speech, taste, swallowing, oral sensation and continence, and of body image can have a devastating impact on quality of life. Apart from the obvious goal of disease-free survival, these factors must be considered in treatment planning.

SURGICAL ANATOMY

The oral cavity extends from the vermilion border of the lips to an arbitrary plane bound by the circumvallate papillae of the tongue inferiorly and the junction of the hard and soft palate superiorly. It can be divided into two functional units: that which is bathed constantly in saliva and is subject to salivary flow and that which is relatively dry. The significance of this division is of practical importance in that surgery on the inferior saliva-bathed structures runs the risk of developing the potential complication of postoperative salivary fistula formation and that to the superior relatively dry area may be complicated by postoperative wound contracture and residual deformity. There may also be some significance in the relative exposure of the mucosa to potential salivary carcinogens and the relative incidence of local recurrence of disease in these two areas (Fig. 11.1), an observation that is substantiated by an epidemiological study (1). The oral cavity is divided into several anatomical subsites (Fig. 11.2).

Lip

The lip includes only the vermilion surface or the portion that comes into contact with the opposing lip. This area is particularly vulnerable to cancer in the aged and those exposed to sun damage, the lower lip being more commonly affected. In European populations of spirit drinkers and cigarette smokers, squamous cancers at the commissures are more aggressive. At this site surgical excision involves difficult techniques for restoration of functional anatomy, and despite surgery and radiotherapy in combination, local recurrence is more common.

The lips are supplied by the superior and inferior labial branches of the facial artery. The upper lip is supplied by the infraorbital branch of the maxillary nerve (V^2) whereas the lower lip is supplied by the mental branch of the inferior dental nerve (V^3). The muscles of the lower lip are supplied by the cervical branch of the facial nerve and the marginal mandibular branch that leaves the lower border of the parotid gland and crosses the inferior border of the mandible superficial to the facial vessels to reach the face beyond the anterior border of the masseter muscle. The muscles of the upper lip and the orbicularis oris are supplied by the buccal branch of the facial nerve.

The upper lip drains lymph first into the buccal and parotid nodes, then into the prevascular facial node overlying the margin of the mandible and ultimately into the upper deep cervical nodes via the submandibular nodes. The lower lip drains into the submandibular nodes and then into the upper deep cervical nodes. The central portion of the lower lip drains first into the mental nodes and then to the submandibular and upper deep cervical nodes (level II) or directly to the omohyoid node (level III). Lesions of the central portions of the lips commonly metastasize to nodes at level I on both sides.

Buccal Mucosa

This site includes all the membrane lining of the inner surface of the cheeks and lips from the line of contact of opposing lips to the line of attachment of mucosa of the alveolar ridges and pterygomandibular raphe. The parotid (Stensen's) duct opens on a low papilla opposite the second upper molar tooth with the tiny openings of the ducts of the molar glands nearby.

The attached mucosa overlying the ascending ramus of the mandible from the level of the posterior surface of the last molar tooth to the apex superiorly, adjacent to the tuberosity of the maxilla constitutes the retromolar trigone. Tumors arising in this area are commonly not confined to it: indeed there is a quite common presentation of a tumor of the mandibular alveolus, often involving the posterior floor of mouth and passing superiorly to the maxillary tuberosity, thus in theory involving three primary sites. The buccal mucosa derives its blood supply from branches of the transverse facial artery that runs along the parotid duct from its origin from the superficial temporal branch of the external carotid artery. Much of the buccal mucosa is supplied by the buccal branch of the mandibular branch of the trigeminal nerve. Lymph drains into the parotid, submental, and submandibular lymph nodes, and ultimately into the upper deep cervical nodes or to the facial node on the

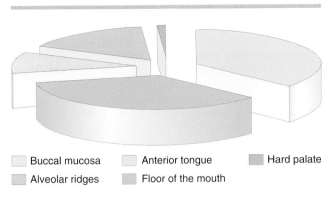

Buccal mucosa   Anterior tongue   Hard palate
Alveolar ridges   Floor of the mouth

Figure 11.1 Distribution of sites of squamous carcinoma of the oral cavity.

margin of the mandible and then to the submandibular lymph nodes.

Alveolar Ridges

The alveolar ridges include only the alveolar processes of the mandible and the maxilla, and their covering mucosa. As the mucosa is intimately fused to the underlying periosteum, tumors of both alveolar ridges may invade the alveolar bone of the jaws quite early in their natural history.

The lower alveolus receives its sensory innervation from the branches of the mandibular nerve (inferior alveolar, buccal, and lingual nerves) whereas the upper alveolus is innervated by branches of the maxillary nerve (superior alveolar, greater palatine, and nasopalatine nerves). The primary echelons of lymphatic drainage are the nodes in the submental and submandibular triangle. Tumors of the lower

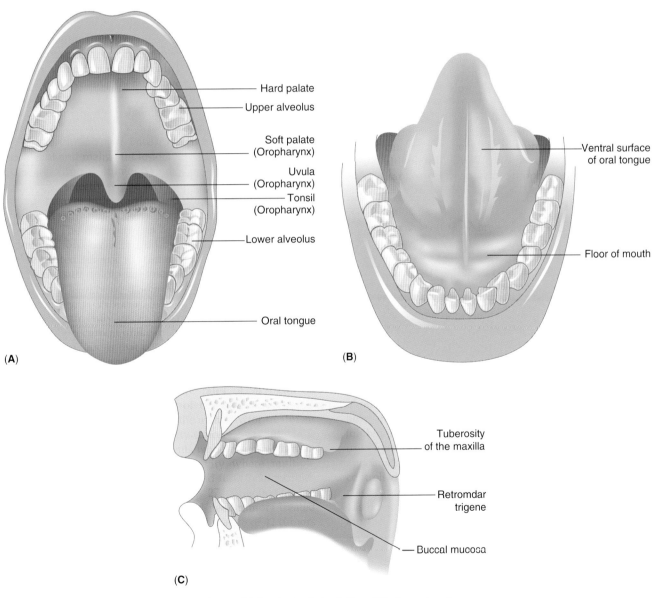

Figure 11.2 Anatomical subsites within the oral cavity.

jaw are much more likely to metastasize to the neck than those of the upper jaw.

Floor of the Mouth

The floor of the mouth is a horseshoe-shaped space overlying the mylohyoid and hyoglossus muscles, extending from the inner surface of the lower alveolar ridge to the undersurface of the tongue. Its posterior boundary is the base of the anterior pillar of the tonsil, and the space is divided into two sides by the frenulum of the tongue. The mylohyoid muscles form the partition between the mouth above and neck below. The floor of the mouth contains the openings of the submandibular and sublingual salivary gland ducts. Surgery or radiotherapy to the anterior floor of the mouth may interfere with free salivary flow and can result in salivary gland obstruction, which may mimic lymphadenopathy. Lymphatic channels from the floor of the mouth drain to the submental and submandibular lymph nodes.

Hard Palate

The hard palate is a semilunar area that extends from the inner surface of the superior alveolar ridge to the posterior edge of the palatine bone. Its mucosa is strongly united with the underlying periosteum, which in turn is secured to the bone by Sharpey's fibers. This mucoperiosteal fusion extends from the maxillary alveolus to the midline and ends posteriorly at the soft palate–hard palate junction. Over the horizontal plate of the palatine bone, however, the mucous membrane and periosteum are separated by a mass of mucous glands that may give rise to adenocarcinoma. The mucosa also contains numerous minor salivary glands from which minor salivary gland tumors may arise.

The hard palate is supplied by branches of the greater palatine artery, which emerges from the greater palatine foramen and passes laterally around the palate to enter the nose through the incisive foramen. The maxillary nerve supplies the greater part of the palate up to the incisive foramen by its greater palatine branch via the pterygopalatine ganglion whereas the premaxillary area between the incisors and incisive foramen is supplied by its nasopalatine branches. Lymphatic channels drain first to the retropharyngeal and then to the deep cervical nodes.

Anterior (Oral) Tongue

The freely mobile portion of the tongue extends anteriorly from the line of the circumvallate papillae to the undersurface of the tongue at the junction of the floor of mouth. It is composed of four areas: the tip, lateral borders, dorsum, and the nonvillous undersurface. The surface epithelium is keratinizing stratified squamous epithelium that is roughened by the presence of papillae. The dorsum of the anterior tongue bears no mucous or serous glands, these being concentrated mainly under the tip and the sides. Also under the tip, in a paramedian position on each side, open the tiny ducts of the anterior lingual glands.

The intrinsic muscles of the tongue (superior and inferior longitudinal, transverse, and vertical) are not attached to bone and serve to alter the shape of the tongue during chewing, swallowing, and articulation. The extrinsic muscles are attached to bone: genioglossus (mandible and hyoid), hyoglossus (hyoid), styloglossus (styloid process),

and palatoglossus (hard palate). The genioglossus is the largest and makes up the bulk of the tongue. The extrinsic muscles stabilize the tongue and by their contraction alter its position as well as its shape.

The major arterial supply is from branches of the lingual artery, which is the third branch of the external carotid artery. Minor contributions come from the tonsillar branch of the facial artery and the ascending pharyngeal artery. The midline of the tongue is an avascular plane due to the tough fibrous septum that prevents anastomosis of blood vessels of the two muscular halves.

The lingual vein accompanies the lingual artery and usually joins the internal jugular vein near the greater cornu of the hyoid. The tip of the tongue is drained by the deep lingual vein that is visible ventrally on each side of the midline. It runs backwards superficially on the hyoglossus and is joined at its anterior border by the vein from the sublingual gland to form the vena comitans of the hypoglossal nerve, draining into either the lingual, facial, or internal jugular veins. The hypoglossal nerve supplies all the muscles of the tongue except the palatoglossus, which is supplied by the pharyngeal plexus. The trigeminal component (cell bodies in the trigeminal ganglion) of the lingual nerve mediates common sensibility while the chorda tympani component (cell bodies in the geniculate ganglion of the facial nerve) mediates taste.

Although the lymphatic drainage of the tongue is extremely variable, as a general rule, the tip drains to the submental nodes whereas the rest of the anterior tongue drains to the submandibular nodes. A unique feature of these lymphatics is that lymph from one side may reach nodes of both sides of the neck, especially when ipsilateral channels are blocked. Patients may therefore require bilateral neck treatment to maximize locoregional control. Lymphatics from the tip of the tongue as from the anterior floor of the mouth may go directly from the submental nodes to the jugulo-omohyoid node at the junction of levels III and IV, thus missing out the submandibular and upper cervical nodes. This factor is extremely important in consideration of neck treatment for tumors at these sites.

PATHOLOGY

Squamous cell carcinomas (SCCs) account for more than 90% of malignant tumors of the oral cavity. However there is a variety of other types of pathology and these are classified by the World Health Organization (WHO) as shown in Table 11.1.

Epithelial Tumors

Malignant Epithelial Tumors

Squamous cell carcinoma. SCC typically presents as an obvious, exophytic, ulcerated lesion with a greyish necrotic base and an associated margin of induration (Fig. 11.3). Other morphological types include the flat, superficial type, the endophytic type that infiltrates deeply, and the verrucous type that is covered with filiform projections. Histologically, the tumor consists of irregular nests, columns, or strands of malignant epithelial cells infiltrating subepithelially. Verrucous carcinoma is an uncommon variant of SCC, and 75% of cases occur in the oral cavity. It is an exophytic warty

Table 11.1 Classification of Tumors of the Oral Cavity

A. Epithelial tumours
1. Malignant epithelial tumors
a. Squamous cell carcinoma
   Verrucous carcinoma
   Basaloid squamous cell carcinoma
   Papillary squamous cell carcinoma
   Spindle cell carcinoma
   Acantholytic squamous cell carcinoma
   Adenosquamous carcinoma
   Carcinoma cuniculatum
b. Lymphoepithelial carcinoma

2. Epithelial precursor lesions

3. Benign epithelial tumors
a. Papillomas
   Squamous cell papilloma
   Condyloma acuminatum
   Focal epithelial hyperplasia
b. Granular cell tumor
c. Keratoacanthoma

B. Salivary gland tumors
1. Malignant
   Acinic cell carcinoma
   Mucoepidemoid carcinoma
   Adenoid cystic carcinoma
   Polymorphous low grade adenocarcinoma
   Myoepithelial carcinoma
   Carcinoma ex pleomorphic adenoma
   Other carcinomas

2. Benign
   Pleomorphic adenoma
   Myoepithelioma
   Basal cell adenoma
   Canalicular adenomas
   Duct papilloma

C. Soft tissue tumors
   Kaposis sarcoma
   Lymphangioma
   Ectomesenchymal chondromyxoid tumor
   Focal oral mucinosis
   Congenital granular cell epulis

D. Haematolymphoid tumors
   Diffuse large B cell lymphoma (DLBCL)
   Mantle cell lymphoma
   Follicular lymphoma
   Extranodal marginal zone B cell lymphoma (MALT)
   Burkitt lymphoma
   T cell lymphoma
   Extramedullary plasmacytoma

E. Mucosal malignant melanoma

F. Tumors of bone
   Giant cell lesions
   Reparative granuloma
   Brown tumor of hyperparathyroidism
   Giant cell tumor of bone
   Fibro-osseous lesions
   Fibrous dysplasia
   Ossifying fibroma
   Periapical cemental dysplasia
   Chondrogenic neoplasms
   Chondroma
   Chondrosarcoma
   Osteogenic neoplasms
   Osteoid osteoma and osteoblastoma
   Ameloblastoma
   Osteogenic sarcoma
   Other tumours
   Histiocytosis X
   Multiple myeloma
   Ewing's sarcoma

G. Secondary tumors

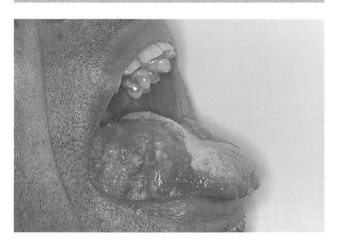

Figure 11.3 Squamous cell carcinoma of the tongue.

slow-growing variant. It usually affects older males, and human papillomavirus (HPV) has been found in 40% of cases. The tumor usually begins as a thin white keratotic plaque that then develops a papillary or verruciform appearance. It is broad based and spreads in a lateral fashion. It is usually asymptomatic. Histologically it consists of club-shaped papillae and blunt invaginations of well-differentiated epithelium with marked keratinization. The epithelium lacks the usual criteria for malignancy with few mitoses, and invasion of the stroma is with pushing margins rather than an infiltrating border. This can create diagnostic difficulties especially in superficial biopsy specimens.

Lymphoepithelial carcinoma. Lymphoepithelial carcinoma is a poorly differentiated SCC or undifferentiated carcinoma accompanied by a reactive lymphocytic infiltrate. It resembles nasopharyngeal nonkeratinizing carcinoma in its morphology. It is rare, accounting for 1 to 2% of all oral cavity and oropharynx cancers. More than 90% of these cancers occur in the tonsil and base of tongue with the remaining being found in the palate and buccal mucosa. Patients may present with an ulcerated mass, but often the mass may be submucosal. The tumor has a high propensity for regional cervical lymph nodes, and therefore many patients may present with a cervical lymph node mass. Histologically the tumor is invasive with clusters of cells surrounded by a rich lymphocytic infiltrate. The tumor cells are positive for pan-cytokeratin and epithelial membrane antigen. In Chinese patients Epstein-Barr virus encoded RNA is usually present on in situ hybridization.

EPITHELIAL PRECURSOR LESIONS (A DETAILED DISCUSSION FOLLOWS IN THE NEXT SECTION)
Benign Epithelial Tumors
Papillomas of the oral cavity are common with a prevalence of 0.1 to 0.5%. Squamous papillomas are common in children and in adults between the ages 30 and 50 years. Approximately one half of these lesions are associated with HPV infection and are the oral equivalent of verruca vulgaris on the skin. The most common sites affected are the hard and soft palate, labial mucosa, tongue, and gingiva. Clinically they are soft pedunculated lesions and are usually single with a diameter of about 6 mm. Histologically they resemble verruca vulgaris. There is no malignant potential, and these lesions often regress spontaneously but can be removed by simple excision or cryosurgery. Focal epithelial hyperplasia is a condition where there are multiple oral papillomas induced by HPV serotypes 13 and 32. This usually affects children and adolescents and affects mainly the labial and buccal mucosa and tongue. Clinically there are multiple soft-rounded or flat swellings with a slight nodular surface. They are usually pink in color and range from 2 to 10 mm in diameter. Histologically they are more distinct than squamous papilloma. The condition has no malignant potential and regresses spontaneously. Granular cell tumors are rare and usually arise in the tongue. The lesion appears as a smooth sessile swelling 1 to 2 cm in diameter covered by normal epithelium. The lesion occurs between the ages of 40 and 60 and is more common in females. They are thought to be of Schwann cell origin. Histologically eosinophilic cells with abundant granular cytoplasm are seen. These cells extend into adjacent tissues merging with muscle cells. Characteristically many lesions show pseudoepitheliomatous hyperplasia of the overlying epithelium. The lesion stains strongly for S-100 protein and neurone specific enolase. They are benign and rarely recur after excision.

Salivary Gland Tumors
Malignant Salivary Gland Tumors
Minor salivary gland tumors can arise anywhere in the mucosa of the upper aerodigestive tract. They account for 9 to 23% of all salivary gland neoplasms with the most common sites being the palate (44–58%), lips (15–22%), and buccal mucosa (12–15%) (2). Approximately 40 to 50% of intraoral minor salivary gland tumors are malignant (3,4). The most common carcinoma is mucoepidermoid carcinoma (54%), polymorphous low-grade adenocarcinoma (17%), adenoid cystic carcinoma (15%), adenocarcinoma not otherwise specified (NOS) (5%), acinic cell carcinoma (4%), clear cell carcinoma NOS (2.4%), and carcinoma ex pleomorphic

adenoma (1.2%) (3). The most common site affected is the palate in 33% of cases (4). They appear as rounded masses with a smooth overlying mucosa (Fig. 11.4) and may be confused with more benign swellings, for example, torus palatinus on the palate (Fig. 11.5).

Benign Salivary Gland Tumors
Approximately 50 to 60% of intraoral minor salivary gland tumors are benign (3,4). Of the benign tumors pleomorphic adenoma is the most common (66%) followed by cystadenoma (11%), canalicular adenoma (10%), ductal papillomas (7.5%), basal cell adenoma (3.3%), and myoepithelioma (2.2%) (3).

Soft Tissue Tumors
Kaposi's Sarcoma
Kaposi's sarcoma (KS) is a locally aggressive vascular tumor most often found in immunocompromised patients due to human immunodeficiency virus (HIV) disease or transplants.

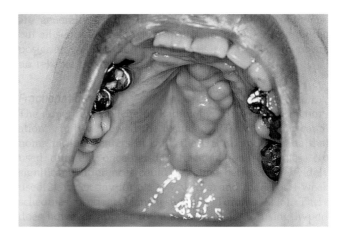

Figure 11.4 Pleomorphic adenoma arising from the minor salivary glands of the hard palate.

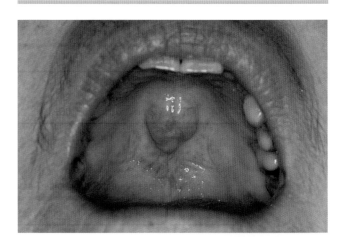

Figure 11.5 Torus palatinus of the hard palate.

The disease is caused by a complex interaction between human herpes virus 8 (HHV8) and immunologic and environmental factors. HHV8 is found in KS cells in all patients and appears to be contracted by oral exposure to infectious saliva. Although the majority of KS occur on the skin, mucosal membranes such as the oral mucosa can also be affected. Oral KS most frequently occurs on the palate followed by the gingiva and tongue. The lesion appears as a purplish nodule on the palate that may then ulcerate. Histologically the nodules consist of fascicles of spindle cells and numerous slit-like spaces containing red cells.

Lymphangioma

Lymphangioma is a benign cavernous/cystic lymphovascular lesion comprising dilated lymphatic channels. Most are congenital, and in the head and neck region the dorsal aspect of the anterior tongue is the most common site. They present as a painless swelling of the tongue with irregular nodularity. Macroscopically they form a multicystic spongy mass the cavities of which contain milky fluid. Histologically they have thin-walled dilated lymphatic vessels lined by flattened endothelium. Malignant transformation does not occur, and these lesions are best treated by surgical resection or injection with sclerosing agents.

Haematolymphoid Tumors

Non-Hodgkins lymphoma (NHL) accounts for 3.5% of all oral malignancies (5). It most commonly affects the palatine tonsils but can also occur in the oral cavity with the most common site being the palate followed by the gingiva and tongue. Patients present with an ulcer, swelling, pain, paraesthesia, or loose teeth. Most NHL of the oral cavity are diffuse large B cell lymphoma followed by mantle cell lymphoma, follicular lymphoma, and extranodal marginal zone B cell lymphomas of mucosa associated lymphoid tissue (MALT) type.

Mucosal Malignant Melanoma

Mucosal melanomas are particularly virulent tumors and are fortunately rare. Men are affected 3 times as commonly as women, and the palate (Fig. 11.6) and gingiva are the most common sites involved. Roughly one third of cases are preceded by melanosis, and therefore pigmented oral lesions should be carefully followed and biopsied if appropriate. Early diagnosis is often difficult, and the gross appearance can vary from a typically pigmented lesion to a nonpigmented, soft vascular tumor. Histological diagnosis of difficult cases may be aided by immunohistochemical demonstration of S100 protein.

Tumors of Bone

An exceptional degree of interdisciplinary cooperation is required between clinician, radiologist, and pathologist for diagnosis of bone tumors and tumor-like conditions. All of the tumors that affect bone elsewhere in the body can also occur in the facial skeleton. Imaging information should be made available to the pathologist as a given histological picture may be interpreted differently depending upon its location in the skeleton. Odontogenic tumors of the jaw are derived from the dental soft and hard tissues and may have a purely epithelial origin, a purely mesenchymal origin, or a mixture of both. The most important of these is the ameloblastoma (Fig. 11.7), which is an epithelial neoplasm. The most frequent site of affliction is the molar region of the mandible, and these tumors are locally aggressive, often producing extensive bone destruction.

Secondary Metastases

Metastases to soft tissues of the oral cavity are extremely rare (0.1% of all oral malignancy) and arise most commonly from melanomas, breast, lung, or kidney. Metastases to the jaw are more common (1% of all oral malignancy), involve the mandible 4 times as commonly as the maxilla, and arise most frequently (6) from adenocarcinoma of the breast, prostate, gastrointestinal tract, or hypernephroma of the kidney (Fig. 11.8).

Epithelial Precursor Lesions

Epithelial precursor lesions can be classified into leukoplakia (white plaques) and erythroplakia (red patch).

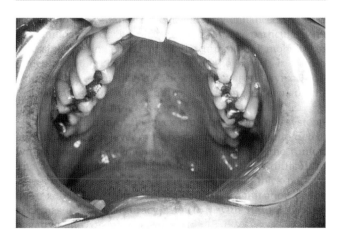

Figure 11.6 Malignant melanoma of the soft palate.

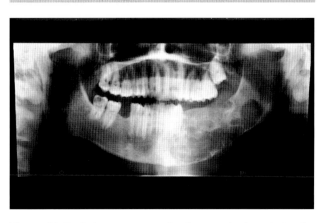

Figure 11.7 Orthopantomogram showing extensive bone destruction from an ameloblastoma of the right mandible.

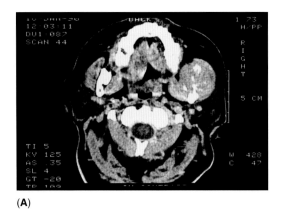

(A)

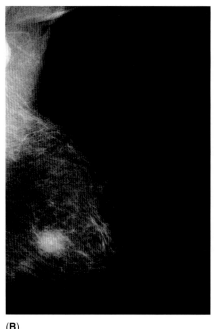

(B)

Figure 11.8 **(A)** Computed tomography scan demonstrates extensive osseous metastasis to the ascending ramus of the right mandible. **(B)** The primary tumor in the breast is clearly seen on mammography.

Leukoplakia is a "white patch or plaque that cannot be characterised clinically or pathologically as any other disease" (7). It is important to realize that the term has no histological meaning and is often loosely used to imply a premalignant condition. The prevalence of leukoplakia worldwide is about 2% and erythroplakia is 0.05%. Both conditions are associated with smoking and alcohol.

Leukoplakia

Clinical features. Clinically, leukoplakia can be subdivided into a homogeneous type (flat, thin, uniform white) (Fig. 11.9) and a nonhomogeneous type. In the nonhomogeneous type there is a white and red lesion (erythroleukoplakia). This may be either irregularly flat (speckled), nodular, or verrucous.

Homogeneous leukoplakia (Leukoplakia simplex) This is the most common variety, and lesions appear as homogeneous, sharply circumscribed, thickened whitish areas broken up by longitudinal fissures (Fig. 11.9). They are generally hyperorthokeratotic but can less frequently be hyperparakeratotic on histological examination. Dysplastic changes are seen in only 2 to 5% of patients. Excision, at least in part, may be necessary; after exclusion of risk factors such as smoking and tobacco use, these patients may be satisfactorily managed by follow-up at reasonable intervals along with maintenance of oral hygiene.

Nonhomogeneous leukoplakia Nonhomogeneous leukoplakia can be nodular, speckled, or verrucous. Nodular and speckled lesions are usually associated with severe epithelial dysplasia and candida infection. Common light microscopic features of these lesions include hyperkeratosis, acanthosis, parakeratosis, widening of rete pegs, dyskeratosis, and carcinoma in situ, which is a term used to signify

full thickness involvement of the mucosa by dysplasia. Verrucous leukoplakia has a warty surface and is often associated with dysplasia. This variety can develop into a squamous cell or verrucous carcinoma.

Histopathology

There are different classification schemes used for precursor lesions as shown in Table 11.2. In general, most clinicians and pathologists use the WHO 2005 classification scheme that classifies lesions according to the degree of dysplasia. The criteria used for diagnosing dysplasia is dependent upon architecture and cytological features and these are listed in Table 11.3.

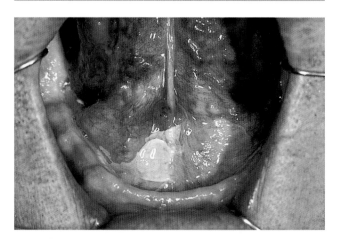

Figure 11.9 Homogenous leukoplakia of the anterior floor of mouth.

Table 11.2 Classification of Epithelial Precursor Lesions

2005 WHO Classification	Squamous intraepithelial neoplasia (SIN)	Ljubljana classification squamous intraepithelial lesions (SIL)
Squamous cell hyperplasia		Squamous cell hyperplasia
Mild dysplasia	SIN1	Basal/parabasal hyperplasia
Moderate dysplasia	SIN2	Atypical hyperplasia
Severe dysplasia	SIN3	Atypical hyperplasia
Carcinoma in situ	SIN3	Carcinoma in situ

Table 11.3 Criteria Used for Diagnosing Dysplasia

Architecture	Cytology
Irregular epithelial stratification	Abnormal variation in nuclear size (anisonucleosis)
Loss of polarity of basal cells	Abnormal variation in nuclear shape (nuclear pleomorphism)
Drop shaped rete ridges	Abnormal variation in cell size (anisocytosis)
Increased number of mitotic figures	Abnormal variation in cell shape (cellular pleomorphism)
Abnormally superficial mitoses	Increased nuclear-cytoplasmic ratio
Premature keratinization in single cells (dyskeratosis)	Increased nuclear size
Keratin pearls within rete pegs	Atypical mitotic figures
	Increased number and size of nucleoli
	Hyperchromasia

Hyperplasia. There is increased cell numbers either in the basal, parabasal cell layers, or in the spinous layer (acanthosis). There is no cellular atypia.

Dysplasia. Dysplasia is the term used when architecture and cytology are atypical. It is a spectrum classified into mild, moderate, severe, and finally carcinoma in situ.

Mild dysplasia: Architectural disturbance is limited to the lower third of the epithelium accompanied by cellular atypia.
Moderate dysplasia: Architectural disturbance extends to the lower two thirds of the epithelium accompanied by cellular atypia.
Severe dysplasia: Architectural disturbance extends greater than two thirds of the epithelium accompanied by cellular atypia.
Carcinoma in situ: Architectural disturbance extends to full thickness of the epithelium accompanied by pronounced cellular atypia, but changes are limited to layers superficial to the basement membrane. Atypical mitotic figures and abnormal superficial mitoses are common.

Malignant Transformation

Approximately 1% of leukoplakias undergo malignant transformation annually (8). This figure is much higher for nonhomogeneous leukoplakia. Vital staining using toluidine blue (9) or Lugol's iodine (10) may be useful diagnostic adjuncts, especially in high-risk patients and as a method of ruling out false-negative clinical impressions. Suspicious lesions must be biopsied and in the absence of dysplasia less than 5% of lesions will develop malignant features. The presence of dysplasia increases this to 15 to 30% (11).

The risk factors which carry a statistically significant risk of malignant transformation are

- Female gender
- Long duration of leukoplakia
- Location on the tongue or floor of mouth (12)
- Leukoplakia in nonsmokers
- Size greater than 2 cm (2,11)
- Nonhomogeneous type
- Presence of dysplasia

Of these factors, the presence of epithelial dysplasia in a nonhomogenous lesion is the most important.

Molecular Risk Markers for Transformation

Although grade of dysplasia may help to predict the risk of cancer, experienced pathologists vary widely in grading oral dysplasia. Furthermore it is difficult to distinguish between severe dysplasia and carcinoma in situ. Therefore the diagnosis and grading of dysplasia is often uncertain, which poses a dilemma for surgeons about how aggressively to treat these lesions. Molecular markers of risk may be more useful. Loss of heterozygosity (LOH) studies have shown a correlation with high-risk lesions. Several studies have shown that loss of chromosome regions containing known tumor suppressor genes (e.g., at locus 3p14 and 9p21) can determine cancer risk in oral dysplasia (13–15). If we stratify patients by LOH status, patients can have either a low (2%) versus high (50%) 5-year cancer risk. Recently it has been reported that toluidine blue staining is associated with the presence of LOH even when dysplasia is absent or minimal, suggesting toluidine blue as a means of identifying high-risk lesions (16).

There have been several recent reports documenting other possible molecular markers that may help in predicting the malignant transformation of leukoplakia lesions. These include the expression of a novel molecule podoplanin (17), suprabasal expression of p53 (18), presence of high-risk HPV 16 (19), immunohistochemistry pattern of cyclin D1, p27 and p63 (20), and the expression of cytokeratin 8 (21).

Management

In general a biopsy should be carried out to confirm the diagnosis and determine the degree of dysplasia. If possible the presence or absence of aneuploidy should be assessed. Most clinicians actively treat leukoplakia irrespective of the absence or presence of epithelial dysplasia by surgical excision. For patients with multiple lesions, surgical excision of all lesions may have too much morbidity, and in these patients treatment often consists of cessation of any etiological factors such as smoking and alcohol and close observation. In these patients, other therapies may be particularly useful. These include photodynamic therapy (22) and the use of chemopreventative agents (discussed in detail later). The use of toluidine blue (23,24), optical spectroscopy (25), direct fluorescence visualization (26,27), and chemiluminescence (28) in such patients may also prove useful in trying to predict which lesions are most likely to be malignant.

Erythroplakia

Erythroplakia is defined as a "bright red velvety patch that cannot be characterised clinically or pathologically as being caused by any other condition" (Fig. 11.10). Histologically erythroplakia shows at least some degree of dysplasia and often even carcinoma in situ. These lesions have a very high rate of aneuploidy (68%), and if present the majority go on to develop into cancer. As such all erythroplakia lesions should be treated aggressively by wide surgical excision.

Other Premalignant Lesions
Oral Lichen Planus

There is debate as to whether or not this is a premalignant lesion. If it is, the malignant transformation rate is extremely low and certainly less than 1%.

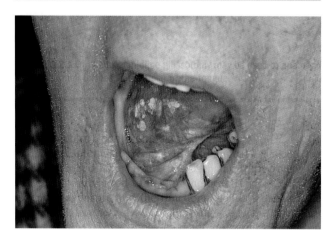

Figure 11.10   Erythroplakic patch on the lateral border of the tongue.

Oral Submucous Fibrosis

This condition is caused by the chewing of areca and betal quid. As such it is a condition confined to South-East Asia where this habit ensues. Clinically this condition is characterized by extreme sensitivity to spicy and hot foods, fibrosis and stiffening of the oral mucosa, and the development of trismus. Histologically there is fibrosis of the lamina propria with atrophy of the overlying epithelium. This atrophied epithelium predisposes to the development of SCC. The annual malignant transformation rate is approximately 0.5% (29).

EPIDEMIOLOGY

Worldwide there are an estimated 405,000 new cases of oral cancer diagnosed each year with two thirds occurring in developing countries. In the European Union there are an estimated 66,650 new cases each year. The countries with the highest rates are Sri Lanka, India, Pakistan, Bangladesh, Hungary, and France (30) (Fig. 11.11).

In Sri Lanka, India, Pakistan, and Bangladesh, oral cancer is the most common cancer in men and accounts for 30% of all new cancer cases each year. This is in comparison to 3% in the U.K. and 6% in France. The oral cavity ranks only 20th on the list of cancers in the U.K., and in 2005 there were 4926 new cases reported.

Geographical Variation in Oral Cancer Incidence in the U.K.

The incidence rates from oral cancer are significantly higher in Scotland (12.1 per 100,000) than in England (7.7. per 100,000) and Wales (10.0 per 100,000) (31). This correlates with the higher rates of tobacco and alcohol consumption in Scotland than in other parts of the U.K. Oral cancer mortality rates are also highest in Scotland reflecting their incidence rates.

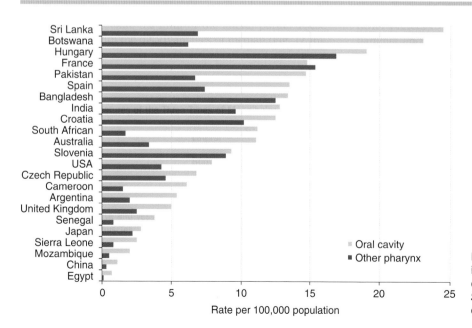

Figure 11.11   World age-standardized male incidence rates for oral cancers, selected countries of the world, 2002 estimates. *Source:* http://info.cancerresearchuk.org/ cancerstats/types/oral/incidence

Age and Sex Distribution

Incidence increases with age, and about 85% of cases in Britain occur after the fifth decade (Fig. 11.12), but in poorer countries the age range is much smaller, and oral cancer is seen in much younger people. The male:female ratio has decreased steadily over recent decades as the incidence rate in men has fallen more sharply relative to that in women.

Trends in Incidence and Mortality

In the U.K., incidence rates have shown a growing trend in recent decades, at 7 per 100,000 in males between 1975 and 1989 increasing to 10 per 100,000 in 2005, an increase of 41% since 1989 (Fig. 11.13). Female oral cancer rates have remained much lower than that of males, but the incidence trend is similar with an average increase of 2.7% each year

since 1989. When oral cancer rates are analyzed by age group, the rates have halved for men older than age 80, remained stable for men age 60 to 70 years, but increased markedly in men between age 40 and 60 years (32) (Fig. 11.14). For men between age 40 and 49 years, incidence has more than doubled from 3.6 to 9.2 per 100,000 and from 11.5 to 25.3 for men age 50 to 59 years (Fig. 11.15). Other European countries have also experienced an upward trend in younger birth cohorts of men (33), and this has been attributed to increasing levels of alcohol consumption (34). The role of smokeless tobacco has remained unresolved in the U.K., and there is no evidence that HIV disease has contributed to the rising incidence in young males (35). Although incidence has increased in the U.K., overall mortality remained fairly stable between 1971 and 2006 at around 3.5 and 1.4 per 100,000 for males and

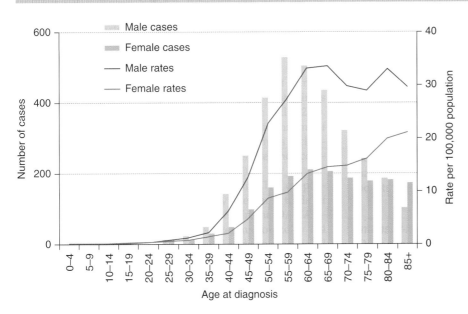

Figure 11.12 Numbers of new cases and age specific incidence rates, by sex, oral cancer, UK 2005. *Source*: http://info.cancerresearchuk.org/cancerstats/types/oral/incidence

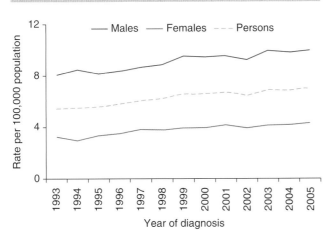

Figure 11.13 Incidence rates for oral cancer, by sex, in the UK from 1993-2005. *Source*: http://info.cancerresearchuk.org/cancerstats/types/oral/incidence

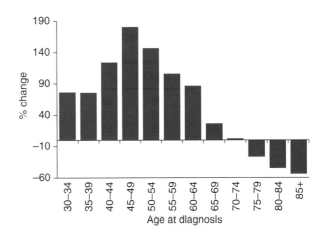

Figure 11.14 Percentage change in incidence rates for oral cancer in British men, 1975/6-2004/5. *Source*: http://info.cancerresearchuk.org/cancerstats/types/oral/incidence

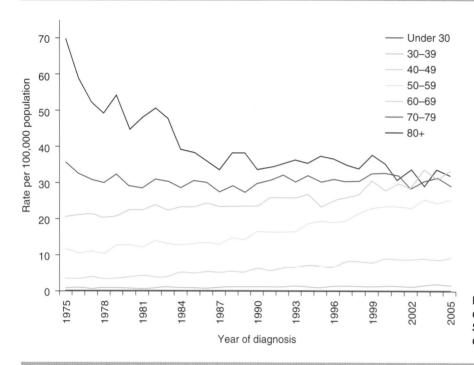

Figure 11.15 Age-specific incidence rates, oral cancer, males, Great Britain, 1975–2005. *Source:* http://info.cancerresearchuk.org/cancerstats/types/oral/incidence

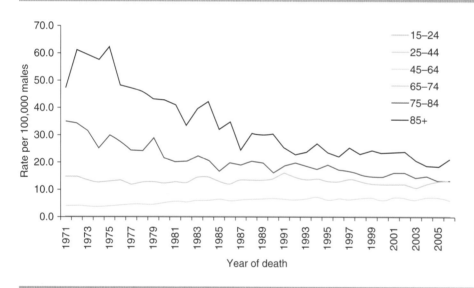

Figure 11.16 Oral cancer mortality rates, by age, males, UK, 1971–2006. *Source:* http://info.cancerresearchuk.org/cancer-stats/types/oral/incidence

females respectively (36). As with incidence trends, the mortality figures reflect the age-specific incidence trends with halving of the figures for men age 70 to 80 years, but a steady increase in mortality for men in their 40s, 50s, and 60s (Fig. 11.16).

ETIOLOGICAL FACTORS

The epidemiology of oral cancer reflects the importance of etiological factors: smoking and alcohol drinking are the major risk factors in Whites whereas betel nut and tobacco consumption have been associated with oral cancer in the Asian population.

Tobacco

Tobacco is the most important factor, and more than 90% of patients have a history of smoking. Tobacco contains many carcinogenic molecules such as polycyclic hydrocarbons and nitrosamines. A clear dose-response relationship has been demonstrated between tobacco exposure and oral cancer (37). As many as 34,000 of the 56,000 estimated annual cases of oral cancer in India are thought to be tobacco induced and are therefore potentially avoidable (38). Cigarette smoking, however, cannot be the sole etiological factor as only a small percentage of smokers develop oral cancer, and genetic predisposition must be taken into account. Although the precise molecular targets of tobacco have eluded conclusive identification thus far, there is proof that significant tobacco and alcohol use is associated with a high frequency of p53 mutations (39). Other genetic factors associated with increased risk include mutagen sensitivity (40), which reflects a defect in DNA repair seen in conditions like xeroderma pigmentosum, Fanconi anaemia, and ataxia telangiectasia.

Epidemiological studies from India have correlated the form and method of tobacco consumption to the site of involvement. "Bidi" smoking (Fig. 11.17) has been linked to cancer of the oral commissure and the tongue. "Reverse smoking" ("Chutta") (41) is a practice peculiar to parts of India and has been linked with an increase in the incidence of cancer of the hard palate. The habit of chewing "paan" has been linked to the increased risk of alveolobuccal cancer in the Indian subcontinent (Fig. 11.18) (42). Khaini (43) is a mixture of tobacco and lime that is retained in the inferior gingivolabial sulcus and leads to cancer in this site.

Alcohol

There is strong evidence that alcohol acts synergistically with tobacco (44), most probably because of a topical effect, and mucosal areas exposed to prolonged contact with alcohol are at increased risk. Others have proposed an independent effect (45), and American (46) as well as French (47) studies have demonstrated a positive correlation of alcohol to oral cancer. This link has not been proved in the U.K., probably because of the prohibition of unmatured, pot-stilled spirits containing toxic by-products (48). Alcohol may act as a solvent increasing the cellular permeability of tobacco carcinogens. Chronic alcohol use may upregulate enzymes of the cytochrome p450 system resulting in activation of protocarcinogens into carcinogens. Other possible mechanisms include the ability of alcohol to impair macrophage activity and reduce T lymphocyte numbers. Alcohol may also reduce the activity of DNA repair enzymes, resulting in increased chromosomal damage.

Dietary Factors

A diet deficient in vitamin A is thought to predispose to oral cancer while fruits and vegetables have been found to have a protective effect (49).

Chronic Irritation

Various epidemiological studies have implicated chronic irritation in carcinogenesis. Factors include poor dental hygiene (7), syphilis, chronic use of mouthwash (50), and marijuana smoking (51).

Viruses

The herpes simplex virus (HSV-1) has long been suspected but has never been identified within oral cavity carcinoma (52). Types 2, 11, and 16 of the human papilloma virus (53) have also been associated with oral cancer without conclusive proof.

Immunosuppression

Immunosuppression associated with kidney transplantation and bone marrow transplant has been implicated in the development of oral cancer (54). HIV-infected patients with acquired immunodeficiency syndrome are more prone to KS and NHL but squamous cancer can also occur (55).

Premalignant Lesion

As discussed above, premalignant lesions include nonhomogeneous leukoplakia, erythroplakia, and oral submucous fibrosis.

Genetic Factors

Genetic factors associated with increased risk include mutagen sensitivity (40), which reflects a defect in DNA repair seen in conditions like xeroderma pigmentosum, Fanconi anaemia, and ataxia telangiectasia.

THE BIOLOGY AND NATURAL HISTORY OF ORAL SQUAMOUS CELL CARCINOMA

Over four decades ago, Slaughter et al. (56) hypothesized the role of "field cancerization" in the etiology of oral cancer. Their theory was based on the premise that an inherent

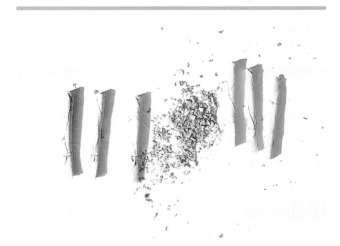

Figure 11.17 The "bidi" is made of tobacco rolled up in a dried temburni leaf and is the most common form of tobacco use in India.

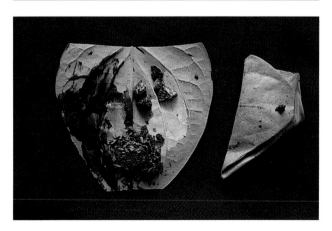

Figure 11.18 "Paan" is a quid of betel leaf (Piper betel) which contains areca nut, lime, other aromatic spices and may contain catechu and tobacco.

instability of the mucosa of the entire upper aerodigestive tract combined with repeated carcinogenic insults leads to an increased risk of developing multiple independent pre-malignant and malignant foci. Until recently this theory was only indirectly supported by the observation of the high incidence of second primary tumors in patients with oral cancer. With advances in our understanding of tumor biology and molecular biology, there is now evidence to support this hypothesis.

Oral carcinogenesis appears to evolve through a complex, multistage process involving biomolecular changes that precede premalignant lesions, which in turn precede invasive cancer. The exact sequence of events in human oral carcinogenesis has not yet been accurately mapped, and the following is only a synopsis of our current understanding of this complex process.

The genetic changes caused by exposure to carcinogens like tobacco and alcohol tend to accumulate over time in the entire mucosa exposed to this insult. Clonal malignant foci, however, develop only in specific sites where tumorigenesis is possible. The fundamental genetic events associated with carcinogenesis have not yet been established, but several nonrandom chromosomal alterations such as those in chromosomes 1, 3, 5, 7, 8, 9, 10, 11, 13, and 17 have been identified (57). The carcinogen-containing environment that initiated tumorigenesis also affects the adjacent tissue, and loss of heterozygosity and other chromosomal abnormalities have been demonstrated in this histologically normal tissue, lending support to the field cancerization theory (58).

The fundamental regulatory mechanism in carcinogenesis is thought to be the cellular balance between oncogenes and tumor suppressor genes. The proto-oncogenes stimulate cell growth and proliferation and are under negative control of the tumor suppressor genes, which prevent overgrowth. A cancer may therefore arise either from activation of a proto-oncogene or due to loss of a tumor suppressor gene. Uncontrolled cell growth can be caused by only a single mutation of an oncogene, but deletion or mutation of both alleles of a tumor suppressor gene is necessary for the same effect. Numerous genetic events are required to cause a cancer, but the most frequently observed molecular abnormality is mutation of the p53 tumor suppressor gene which is seen in 40 to 70% of malignant lesions (59) and 20% of premalignant lesions (60). Several other oncogenes and tumor suppressor genes have been studied, but no clear relationship has been demonstrated with phenotypic behavior or survival.

Once the cancer has developed, its phenotypic behavior is dependent on complex microenvironmental and biologic systems. The capability of a tumor to invade and metastasize depends on its production of degradative enzymes, for example, collagenase, plasminogen activators like urokinase, and cathepsin, as well as angiogenic factors, growth factors,

cytokines, receptors, cell-surface properties, and motility factors. The tumor milieu is also influenced by host factors such as stromal cells, nerve fibers, and tumor-associated and tumor-infiltrating lymphocytes.

The tumor then increases in size horizontally and vertically to invade adjacent and deep structures. It may present as a local mass, producing symptoms such as pain, airway obstruction, infection and hemorrhage, cranial nerve involvement secondary to invasion, or fungation with fistula formation. Later on in the course of the disease, there is invasion of the lymphatics leading to locoregional disease. Usually late in the sequence there may be disseminated metastasis. Death is most commonly related to the effects of locoregional disease either due to direct invasion of vital structures or large nodal masses producing catastrophic hemorrhage.

Site Distribution

The importance of the "cancer-prone crescent" has been known for several decades, and its significance is related to the postulate that most oral cancers should occur in mucosa where saliva pools due to gravity exposing it to salivary carcinogens (61). Moore and Catlin (62) reported a very interesting analysis of the site distribution of oral cancer in patients from two separate hospitals and showed that roughly 25% of lesions occurred in each of the two "alveolar-lingual areas" (corresponding to the posterior floor of mouth and adjacent lateral border of tongue), 25% in the anterior floor of mouth, and 25% in the rest of the mouth. The distribution of oral cancer in developing countries is, however, very different and may be explained by certain habits peculiar to that population, for example, betel quid chewing that contributes to the high incidence of buccal cancer in the Indian subcontinent (Table 11.4) (63).

Nodal Metastases

Lymphatic spread of the tumor from the oral cavity into the neck generally follows a step-wise, orderly, and predictable fashion. The lymph node basins of the neck have traditionally been described as named groups of nodes, but this had led to confusion in comparison of terminology. The Memorial Sloan-Kettering classification is a more precise system of describing the cervical nodes and is now well accepted (64). The patient with a clinically negative neck is at highest risk of metastasis to levels I through III, whereas about 15% of patients with an N+ neck are at risk of developing metastases at level IV in addition to the upper three levels (65). Skip metastases to level IV do occur, missing out levels II and III, and are more commonly associated with cancer of the anterior tongue. Metastases to level V are seen in only about 1% of patients with clinically palpable

Table 11.4 Site Distribution in Percentage of Total Cases of Oral Cancer

	Anterior tongue (%)	Floor of the mouth (%)	Buccal mocosa (%)	Alveolar ridges (%)	Hard palate (%)
United Kingdom	36	← 46 →			
USA (40)	36	35	10	16	3
France (41)	22	68	7	2	1
India (42)	22	4	43	18	3.5

nodes at other levels and are almost never seen as skip metastases. This understanding of the patterns of nodal metastasis from lesions of the oral cavity has practical implications in the design of neck dissection for patients with oral cancer, and these have been outlined elsewhere in this book.

The primary echelons of drainage from alveolar ridge cancers are levels I and II (Fig. 11.19), but about 6% of tumors will metastasize to level V. The probability of lymph node metastases is directly related to T stage (70% for T4 with an average of 30%) (66,67), but mandibular ridge cancers have been shown to metastasize more frequently than those of the maxillary ridge.

Tumors of the floor of mouth drain initially to the submental and submandibular nodes (Fig. 11.20) and 12 to 30% of early (T1–T2) lesions will have occult metastases depending upon the thickness of the lesion (68). The incidence of lymph node metastases in larger lesions (T3–T4) is between 47 and 53%. The floor of the mouth therefore is a high-risk area for cervical nodal metastases, and elective treatment of the neck should be considered in the initial management of selected patients.

Carcinoma of the oral tongue has the greatest propensity among all oral cancers for metastasis to the neck. The primary echelon of drainage is level II, but other levels may be also involved (Fig. 11.21). Depending upon the size of the primary tumor, as many as 15 to 75% of patients will have neck metastases (69,70), and about 25% of patients will have occult nodal metastases at presentation (63). The incidence of bilateral metastases is 25% whereas 3% of patients have

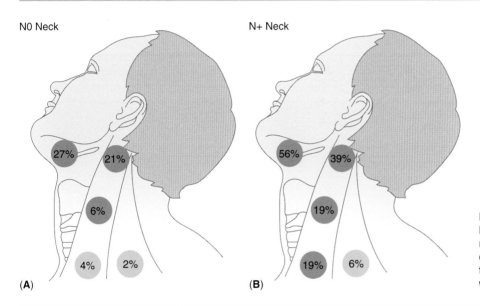

Figure 11.19 (A) Incidence of occult lymph node involvement in the clinically node negative patient with alveolar ridge cancer. (B) Incidence of lymph node metastasis in the clinically node-positive patient with alveolar ridge cancer.

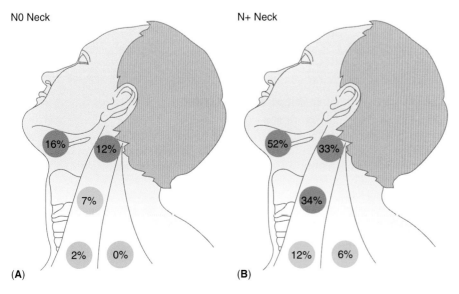

Figure 11.20 (A) Incidence of occult lymph node involvement in the clinically node-negative patient with cancer of the floor of mouth. (B) Incidence of lymph node metastasis in the clinically node-positive patient with cancer of the floor of mouth.

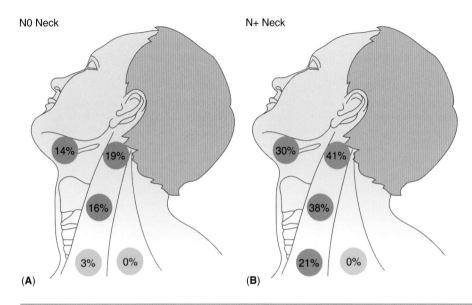

NO Neck   N+ Neck

(A)   (B)

Figure 11.21 **(A)** Incidence of occult lymph node involvement in the clinically node-negative patient with cancer of the oral tongue. **(B)** Incidence of lymph node metastasis in the clinically node-positive patient with cancer of the oral tongue.

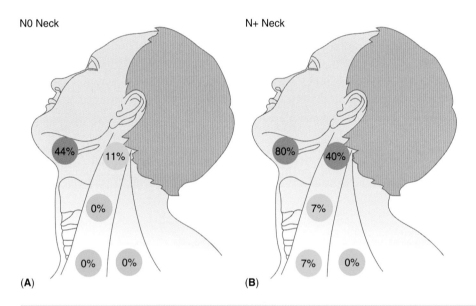

NO Neck   N+ Neck

(A)   (B)

Figure 11.22 **(A)** Incidence of occult lymph node involvement in the clinically node-negative patient with cancer of the buccal mucosa. **(B)** Incidence of lymph node metastasis in the clinically node-positive patient with cancer of the buccal mucosa.

only contralateral metastases, a pattern that is more common in tumors that approach or cross the midline. The depth of invasion and tumor thickness seem to be significant predictors of lymph node metastasis (63,71).

Only 10% of patients with buccal cancer have clinically significant neck nodes at presentation. The primary echelons are levels I and II (Fig. 11.22). Buccal cancer has a recognized risk for metastatic spread to the facial and prevascular facial lymph nodes. As such, careful attention to these lymph nodes should be carried out to ensure adequate removal during a neck dissection. Tumor thickness is a significant prognostic factor, and the 5-year survival has been shown to be significantly better in tumors less than 6 mm thick as compared to deeper tumors (72).

CLINICAL PRESENTATION
Symptoms
Despite the fact that the oral cavity is an easily accessible site for the patient and the physician, a surprisingly large number of oral tumors present late because of the painless and rather vague nature of the symptomatology. The relatively phlegmatic personality types associated with the major risk factors related to the disease may also contribute to the relatively advanced stage at presentation.

Tumors of the alveolar ridge commonly present with pain while chewing, but patients may present with intermittent bleeding and loose teeth, and edentulous patients may complain of ill-fitting dentures. The development of symptoms such as trismus and altered sensation or anesthesia of the lower teeth and lip from involvement of the mandibular canal and the inferior alveolar nerve signify locally advanced disease.

Lesions in the floor of mouth are typically painful, infiltrative lesions that extend to invade bone anteriorly, muscles of the floor of mouth deeply, or tongue posteriorly. Patients often complain of "food getting trapped under the tongue." Early spread to the alveolus and periosteum of the mandible is common; clinical fixation of the tumor to the mandible indicates periosteal involvement, and direct bone invasion may be present in a high number of cases.

Tumors of the oral tongue usually start as a small ulcer that gradually infiltrates the musculature of the tongue until its normal motility is lost. An early lesion may appear as a small granular excrescence, which may arouse suspicion only because of a subtle difference from surrounding normal mucosa or because of the patient's anxiety about the nature of the lesion. More advanced tumors present either as exophytic or ulcerative lesions, which are usually quite evident.

Endophytic infiltrative lesions, however, may be more difficult to recognize, and their extent may not be apparent until an adequate evaluation under a general anesthetic is carried out. Patients may be aware of a difficulty swallowing or speaking, which becomes even more pronounced when the tumor spreads to the floor of the mouth. Cancer of the tongue is generally painful even in its early stage, but lesions can be painless; this feature may contribute to a considerable delay in diagnosis. Any painful ulcer in the oral cavity that fails to heal within a week after a suspected irritant has been eliminated must be investigated by a biopsy. As the disease progresses the lesion may be the cause of an excruciating pain that may radiate to the neck or the ear. Cervical lymph node metastases occur early in the course of the disease, and an occasional patient may present with a lump in the neck.

Buccal mucosal cancer, like that of the gums, is more common in developing countries as a consequence of peculiar patterns of tobacco abuse among the population. Lesions may be papillary or erosive and are often located near the dental occlusal line where they are more likely to be traumatized. Leukoplakia of the surrounding mucosa may be a striking feature. Buccal cancers are more frequently exophytic than other oral cancers, but they rarely present as T1 tumors because pain is not a prominent symptom. The presence of trismus indicates extension into pterygoid musculature and signifies locally advanced disease.

Physical Examination

There should be a thorough examination of the lesion and the rest of the upper aerodigestive tract. Line drawings and photographic records of the tumor are extremely useful and provide a baseline for comparison on later occasions. A TNM-staged record at original examination is similarly essential and may incorporate information from further staging investigations.

Investigation

Radiological investigations including orthopantomogram, computed tomography and magnetic resonance imaging examination of the primary tumor and neck can provide valuable information, which must be used to stage the disease accurately. Imaging of bone may be necessary to detect involvement by the tumor or for planning surgical treatment and is discussed later in this chapter.

Most accessible lesions may be adequately biopsied in the clinic, but thorough examination under general anesthesia offers the optimal conditions for assessment of the depth of invasion, tumor biopsy, and palpation of neck nodes. The value of routine panendoscopy of all upper aerodigestive tract mucosa for assessment of second primary tumors is doubtful and should probably be reserved for investigation of symptoms in high-risk individuals. Biopsy may be achieved with a knife, punch biopsy forceps, trucut needle, or fine-needle aspiration. Each technique has its protagonists and each has its disadvantages extending from crush artefact to the potential risk of tumor seeding as a result of the biopsy technique. The clinician and the histologist are usually able to arrive at a protocol that suits their own and the patient's circumstances.

TNM Staging

The clinical staging of a particular tumor consists of staging the primary tumor (Table 11.5), the neck (Table 11.6), and assessment for distant metastases (Table 11.7). This information can then be assimilated and a TNM stage grouping for the tumor derived (Table 11.8) (73).

Although the TNM system is useful for comparing outcome after treatment with various modalities in tumors

Table 11.5 Staging of Primary Tumor (T)

TX	Primary tumor cannot be assessed
T0	No evidence of primary tumor
Tis	Carcinoma in situ
T1	Tumor 2 cm or less in greatest dimension
T2	Tumor more than 2 cm but not more than 4 cm in greatest dimension
T3	Tumor more than 4 cm in greatest dimension
T4 (lip)	Tumor invades adjacent structures e.g., through cortical bone, inferior alveolar nerve, floor of mouth, skin of face
T4 (oral cavity)	Tumor invades adjacent structures e.g., through cortical bone, into deep (extrinsic) muscle of tongue, maxillary sinus, skin. (Superficial erosion alone of bone/tooth socket by gingival primary is not sufficient to classify a tumor as T4)

Table 11.6 Staging of Regional Lymph Nodes (N)

NX	Regional lymph nodes cannot be assessed
N0	No regional lymph node metastasis
N1	Metastasis in a single ipsilateral lymph node, 3 cm or less in greatest dimension
N2a	Metastasis in a single ipsilateral lymph node more than 3 cm but not more than 6 cm in greatest dimension
N2b	Metastasis in multiple ipsilateral lymph nodes, none more than 6 cm in greatest dimension
N2c	Metastasis in bilateral or contralateral lymph nodes, none more than 6 cm in greatest dimension
N3	Metastasis in a lymph node more than 6 cm in greatest dimension

Note: Midline nodes are ipsilateral nodes.

Table 11.7 Staging of Distant Metastases (M)

MX	Presence of distant metastases cannot be assessed
M0	No distant metastases
M1	Distant metastases

Table 11.8 Stage Grouping of Oral Cancer

Stage I	T1N0M0
Stage II	T2N0M0
Stage III	T3N0M0
	T3N1M0
Stage IV	T1–3N2M0
	Any T, N3, M0
	Any T, Any N, M1

of similar severity, it is far from perfect as a prognostic indicator for individual patients. One of its major limitations is that it fails to take into consideration the prognostic implications of the third dimension or depth of invasion of the primary tumor. This aspect of tumor spread has been shown in various studies (63,66) to be a more reliable predictor of cervical nodal metastasis than the conventional T stage, especially for tumors of the tongue. However, until better prognosticators are available, the TNM system will continue to be the standard language of communication among clinicians treating oral and other cancers.

TREATMENT: GENERAL PRINCIPLES

Treatment of squamous carcinoma of the oral cavity is in general either by surgery or by radiation alone or in combination. Chemotherapy and new immunologically based treatment protocols are at the moment reserved for patients with what is considered to be incurable disease in normal terms or for those patients in whom conventional treatment has failed.

The choice of the best initial therapy for a particular patient must take into account a variety of interrelated factors (Fig. 11.23). As with most other cancers, only a very general policy of treatment selection can be outlined, and the management of each patient must be tailored individually.

The chronological age by itself should not be a deterrent to aggressive treatment. Rather, the risk of treatment should be assessed based on intercurrent conditions, cardiopulmonary status, and other factors. The patient's enthusiasm and acceptance of a particular plan of management also need to be taken into account. Treatment decisions may be influenced by the patient's lifestyle (i.e., unwillingness to give up smoking and alcohol) and by their occupation and socioeconomic status.

The team approach to treatment planning cannot be overemphasized, and a combined clinic with physicians, surgeons, radiotherapists, medical oncologists, nurses, dieticians, physiotherapists, and rehabilitation staff is of great importance. In addition to allowing time to collate all clinical and investigational data, the pretreatment phase allows discussion between doctor and patient and also with all those

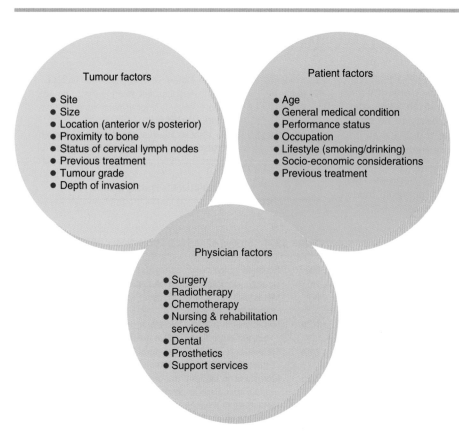

Figure 11.23 Factors determining the choice of initial treatment.

potentially involved in the future management of the patient including family, friends, and other healthcare professionals. The emotional and spiritual needs of the patient must also be given due weight in this phase. The diagnosis and treatment plan are now explained carefully and clearly to the patient in terms that he or she can understand. It is also important that the patient realizes the potential for failure of treatment and that management of complications of treatment may require staged procedures over a long period of time, so that informed consent can be obtained.

Cessation of smoking in the period leading up to treatment, especially major surgery, is important in minimizing complications. In addition, a prospective study (74) has shown the adverse prognostic effect of continued tobacco consumption and advice to stop smoking is essential from a prophylactic as well as from a therapeutic point of view.

For some patients, notably those with advanced disease or underlying medical conditions that militate against optimal treatment, nonstandard treatment regimens must be entertained; options including clinical trials, supportive treatment, or even of no treatment at all other than supportive or palliative care may be discussed.

As single modality treatment using either radiation or surgery offers comparable control rates for early lesions (T1–2), other factors including functional results, compliance of the patient, cost of treatment, and long-term sequelae must be considered. For more advanced lesions (stage III and IV), primary surgery followed by postoperative radiation therapy is generally accepted as standard treatment.

Surgical Management

Surgical excision is one of the two mainstays of locoregional treatment of oral cancer. It allows histopathological assessment of the clearance margins of the tumor together with further information regarding tumor spread and dynamics. Considerable controversy has been generated in recent years over the comparison of results of surgery with radiation, and it is important to choose the modality best suited to the individual patient.

A detailed description of operative procedures for cancer of the oral cavity is outside the scope of this chapter but some general principles are outlined below

Access to the Oral Cavity

A detailed and meticulous examination, often under anesthetic, must be undertaken before deciding the choice of surgical approach. Small, superficial, anteriorly located tumors can be easily resected per orally. Larger, infiltrative lesions, and those located more posteriorly will require more extensive surgical exposure using techniques such as cheek flaps or mandibulotomy. Some form of neck dissection is now regarded as mandatory except perhaps for the most superficial T1 lesion. This can be carried out either as an en bloc procedure or via a separate neck incision.

Transoral excision. Premalignant lesions and small, superficial tumors of the anterior floor of mouth, alveolus, and tongue may be resected through the open mouth (Fig. 11.24). The ability to use this approach also depends on how wide the patient's mouth can be opened under anesthetic as well as on other physical factors like the transverse diameter of the oral commissure and the size of the tongue. In general, one of the other more extensive approaches must be used if there is any doubt about the adequacy of surgical exposure. Laser vaporization may be used for superficial premalignant lesions, but all other lesions must be excised using palpation to achieve adequate resection margins.

Cheek flaps. Tumors of the posterior oral cavity are not easily accessible transorally, and a cheek flap may give more adequate exposure in appropriate cases. An upper cheek flap is raised using a median upper lip split and carrying the incision around the nose with the corresponding mucosal incision in the upper gingivobuccal sulcus. The lower cheek flap requires a midline lip split that continues over the chin into the neck. The flap is raised subplatysmally, but great care must be exercised not to strip the periosteum off the mandible. Accurate replacement of a cheek flap is facilitated by leaving a substantial mucosal cuff on the alveolar side. A midfacial degloving flap through bilateral gingivobuccal incisions is preferable in appropriate cases as this avoids midfacial scars. A visor flap can give access to both sides of the neck and avoids splitting the lip, but adequate mobilization results in division of both mental nerves with anesthesia of the lip.

Mandibulotomy. Larger tumors of the lateral border of the tongue or those involving or extending onto the floor of the mouth may occasionally be resected transorally with a separate neck dissection approach, but most require a lip-splitting mandibulotomy approach. Similarly, adequate surgical exposure of tumors located in the posterior oral cavity may be obtained using a mandibulotomy.

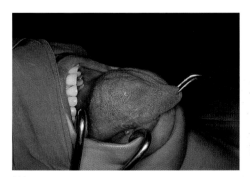
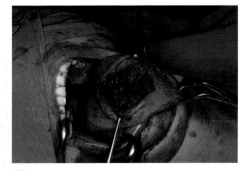

(A) (B)

Figure 11.24 Transoral excision of a tongue tumor: **(A)** preexcision **(B)** postexcision.

The technical aspects of mandibulotomy have been discussed in Chapter 13.

Management of the Mandible

Mechanism of invasion of the mandible. Tumors of the floor of the mouth, the ventral surface of the tongue, and the gingivobuccal sulcus spread along the mucosa and submucosa to the adjacent gingiva. The mechanism of invasion of these tumors into the mandible has been established (75,76), and we know that periosteum acts as a deterrent to mandibular invasion (77). Apart from the obvious implication of upstaging of the tumor with bony invasion, involvement of the mandible increases the risk of invasion of the inferior alveolar nerve within the mandibular canal and raises the possibility of perineural spread of the tumor toward the base of the skull. Figure 11.25 shows that in the dentate mandible tumor creeps up from the gingiva, through the dental socket into the cancellous bone. In contrast, the edentulous mandible offers much less resistance, and tumor invasion of cancellous bone occurs through the dental pores of the alveolar process (Fig. 11.26).

Assessment of bony invasion. Early cortical invasion of the mandible is extremely difficult to image radiographically even with modern technology. A number of radiological investigations are available: plain radiography, cephalometric orthognathic films, orthopantomogram (OPG), dental occlusal films, radionuclide bone scans, CT scans, MRI, and positron emission tomography (PET) scans. The accuracy of conventional radiography in detecting early invasion is limited by the fact that 30 to 50% mineral loss must occur before the changes are radiologically apparent. The OPG (Fig. 11.27) is currently the first-line investigation, but early invasion of the lingual cortex, especially in the region

of the mental symphysis, may not be evident and intraoral dental films are indicated in patients with anterior floor of mouth lesions. Although its accuracy in demonstrating bone invasion in edentulous patients has been reported (78), the accuracy of CT scanning in routine assessment of bony invasion is limited by artefacts produced by irregular dental sockets, other dental artefacts, and by patient motion. However, 1:1 reconstruction of axial images may be useful in fabricating templates for planning accurate bony microvascular reconstruction. Computerized tomography multiplanar reformation (CT/MPR or Dentascan) is a computer software technique that uses information from CT scan slices to generate true cross-sectional images and panoramic views of the mandible and maxilla (79). The oblique sagittal view on Dentascan reportedly allows accurate evaluation of buccal and lingual cortical bone margins

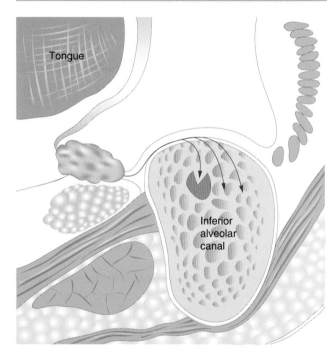

Figure 11.26 Route of mandibular invasion in the edentulous mandible.

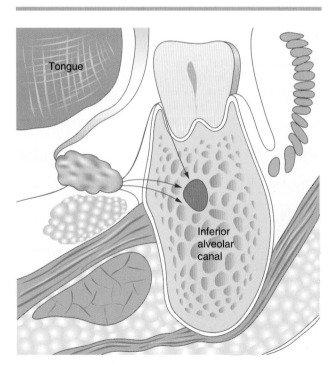

Figure 11.25 Route of mandibular invasion in the dentate mandible.

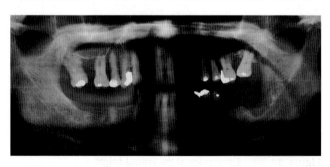

Figure 11.27 OPG showing gross invasion of the left mandible.

as well as clear visualization of the incisive and inferior alveolar canals (80). The role of MRI has also been investigated and reports indicate that though a negative study virtually excludes periosteal or cortical involvement, the overall usefulness of this investigation is hampered by the high rate of false-positive results in dental infections, previously irradiated mandibles, and in osteoradionecrosis (81). Bone scans, for example, ^{99m}Tc-labelled diphosphonate are not specific and suffer from a high rate of false-positive results due to infections and inflammatory processes (82). Overall, clinical evaluation has been shown to be reliable in assessment of early bony invasion (83), but radiological investigation must be ordered if any form of bone resection and reconstruction are planned.

Marginal resection of the mandible. The understanding of tumor invasion into mandible enables the use of marginal resection of bone (Table 11.9) based on the observation that the cortical part of the bone containing the mandibular canal lies inferior to the dental roots, remains relatively uninvolved in early stage disease, and can be safely spared.

In practical terms, however, the ability to perform a marginal mandibulectomy in a given patient depends upon the vertical height of the body of the mandible (Fig. 11.28). Resorption of the mandible with age results in recession of the alveolar process, and the mandibular canal with the inferior alveolar nerve is at increased risk of involvement in these patients. Marginal resection in edentulous patients is fraught with danger as the residual bone is very liable to iatrogenic or spontaneous fracture. The risk of fracture after marginal resection can be minimized by using smooth, rounded cuts

Table 11.9 Indications for Marginal Mandibulectomy

Primary tumor abutting against the mandible
Minimal involvement of the alveolar process
Minimal cortical erosion

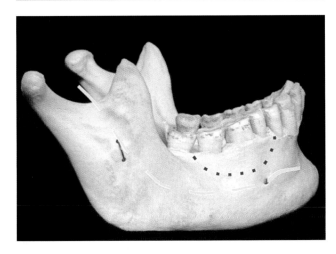

Figure 11.28 Significance of the vertical height of the mandible in relation to the mandibular canal.

because sharp angles tend to concentrate the forces of stress and increase the chances of fracture (Fig. 11.29).

Adequate tumor clearance in edentulous patients may necessitate a segmental mandibulectomy. Marginal mandibular resection is also best avoided in previously irradiated patients because of the more variable routes of tumor entry and multiple foci of tumor invasion coupled with the high risk of osteoradionecrosis. The indications for segmental resection are listed in Table 11.10, and resection of the normal uninvolved mandible to accomplish an en bloc resection can no longer be justified in view of the realization that there are no lymphatic channels passing through the mandible.

Management of the Neck

General principles. It is well known that although 60 to 70% of patients with early stage oral cancer will present with a clinically negative neck (N0), approximately 20 to

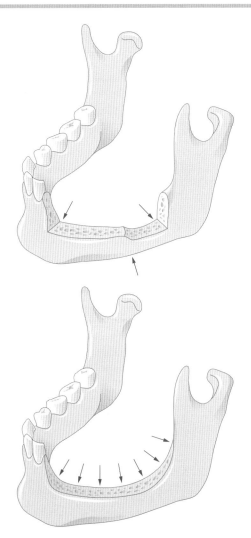

Figure 11.29 Sharp bony cuts in the mandible tend to concentrate the forces of stress and increase the chance of fracture after marginal resection. In contrast, a smooth, rounded resection distributes these forces more evenly and the residual mandible is therefore more resistant to fracture.

Table 11.10 Indications for Segmental Mandibulectomy

Invasion of the mandibular canal and inferior alveolar nerve
Gross invasion of the mandible
Primary mandibular osseous tumor
Metastatic tumor to the mandible

30% will have occult nodal metastasis if subjected to an elective neck dissection. Furthermore, about 30 to 50% of patients will eventually develop neck metastases during the course of their disease. It is also well recognized that metastasis to the cervical lymph nodes is the single most important prognostic factor in patients with head and neck cancer. The presence of a metastatic cervical node in a patient with oral cancer decreases the chance of cure by 50% when compared to those with similar primary tumors without nodal metastases (84). It therefore follows that management of the neck is a crucial and integral part of overall management of the patient with oral cancer. Primaries at certain subsites such as the oral tongue and the floor of the mouth are more liable to metastasize to the neck, and prophylactic treatment of the neck should be considered in their initial management. Tumors at other sites such as the hard palate, the upper alveolus, and the lips have a low rate of occult nodal metastasis and elective treatment of the neck may not be necessary in these patients (85). The risk of nodal metastasis is related to several factors (Table 11.11) and these must be taken into consideration in planning of neck treatment.

If a decision is taken to treat the neck, a neck dissection is carried out when the treatment of the primary is surgical, especially when the neck has to be accessed for reconstruction of the primary defect. If the primary is being treated with irradiation, the neck can be included in the treatment plan. Only very rarely do the primary tumor and the neck need to be treated using different modalities.

Selection of the type of neck dissection. As described earlier, metastasis to the neck from an oral primary generally occurs in an orderly and predictable manner, most often involving levels I through III. In a patient with a clinically N0, the risk of metastasis to levels IV and V is very small and a supraomohyoid neck dissection (SOHND) would therefore adequately address the neck in these patients. For similar patients with tongue primaries, inclusion of level IV in the dissection is probably justified in view of the higher incidence of skip metastases. When a SOHND is carried out, suspicious nodes are sent for frozen section analysis and if positive, the modified radical neck dissection is completed (i.e., levels IV and V are removed). A treatment policy combining SOHND with radiation therapy when indicated has resulted in failure rates of less than 10% in patients with clinically N0 necks (86,87). Although recognizing that each patient needs to be managed on an individual basis, our general policy of action if occult metastases are found on histopathological examination of the neck dissection specimen is outlined in Figure 11.30.

In patients with palpable cervical nodes, levels I to IV are at highest risk. The choice of neck dissection in these patients depends largely on the individual patient, but the general principle is that all five lymph node levels are dissected and the spinal accessory nerve is never sacrificed unless it is directly involved by tumor. The classical radical neck dissection is almost never indicated in the absence of direct infiltration of the relevant structures.

The classical radical neck dissection (RND) does, however, remain the gold standard against which the effectiveness of all other forms of neck dissection must be evaluated. When used alone, RND controls disease in the neck in more than 90% of N0 patients, but as many as 60% of patients with bulky neck disease will recur. The control rate for patients with a clinically positive neck improves to more than 80% if postoperative radiation therapy is added (88). For clinically N0 patients who are proven pathologically N0, failure rates of less than 10% have been reported (89,90). The 30% of patients who have pathologically proven occult metastases following SOHND develop neck recurrence in 10 to 24%, depending upon the number of positive nodes and the presence of extracapsular extension. The addition of postoperative radiation reduces the failure rate in these patients to 0 to 15%. The appropriate use of postoperative radiation therapy (Table 11.12) in combination with modified radical neck dissection has resulted in comparable control rates to RND for similar patients (89). With lesions approaching or crossing the midline, bilateral neck dissections are carried out.

Sentinel node biopsy. Sentinel node biopsy (SNB) is an experimental technique that is under active evaluation by prospective clinical trials and is only practiced in a few select centers. The sentinel lymph node is defined as the first echelon lymph node to which cancer spreads. The technique identifies patients with a positive neck, thus being able to

Table 11.11 Risk Factors for Nodal Metastasis in Patients with Oral Cancer

	High risk	Low risk
Subsite of the primary	Tongue and floor of mouth	Hard palate and lips
T stage	Advanced stage (T3–4)	Early stage (T1–2)
Depth of invasion	>8 mm	<2 mm
Histological grade	High grade	Low grade
Morphology of the primary tumor*	Infiltrative	Exophytic or verrucous Flat superficial
Other histopathological features*	Lymphatic permeation Vascular invasion Perineural invasion Invading front of tumor	Lymphocytic infiltration Pushing front of tumor

*These factors have not been shown to be statistically predictive of lymph node metastasis.

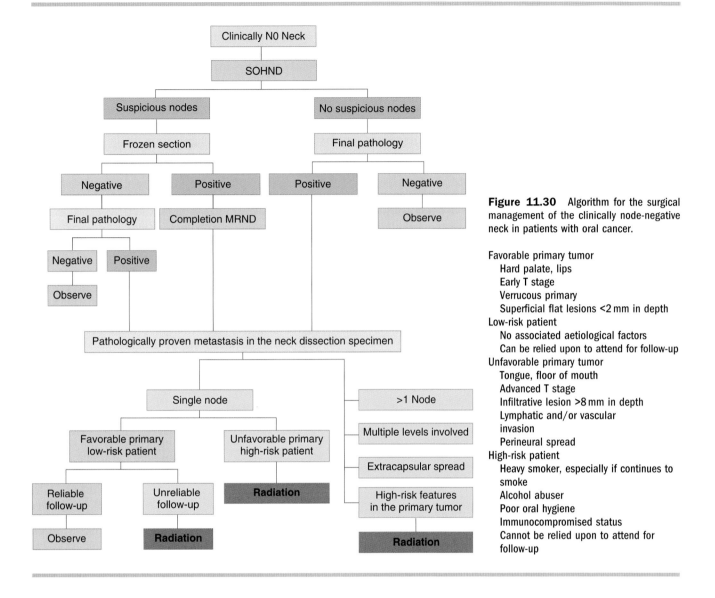

Figure 11.30 Algorithm for the surgical management of the clinically node-negative neck in patients with oral cancer.

Favorable primary tumor
    Hard palate, lips
    Early T stage
    Verrucous primary
    Superficial flat lesions <2 mm in depth
Low-risk patient
    No associated aetiological factors
    Can be relied upon to attend for follow-up
Unfavorable primary tumor
    Tongue, floor of mouth
    Advanced T stage
    Infiltrative lesion >8 mm in depth
    Lymphatic and/or vascular
    invasion
    Perineural spread
High-risk patient
    Heavy smoker, especially if continues to
    smoke
    Alcohol abuser
    Poor oral hygiene
    Immunocompromised status
    Cannot be relied upon to attend for
    follow-up

Table 11.12 Indications for Postoperative Radiation Therapy to the Neck

Features of the primary tumor
    Advanced T stage:
        Bulky tumor
        Involvement of bone, nerves or skin
    High histological grade
    Positive surgical resection margins
    Lymphatic permeation
    Vascular invasion
    Perineural spread

Features of the cervical lymph nodes
    Single pathologically involved node in high-risk patient and/or
        unfavorable primary tumor
    More than two pathologically involved nodes
    Involvement at more than one lymph node level in the neck
    Lymph node more than 3 cm in diameter (N2 or N3 stage)
    Presence of extracapsular spread
    Microscopic or gross residual disease in the neck

accurately stage patients as well as identify patients who require a neck dissection. The technique was first utilized for malignant melanoma and breast cancer and is now a widely accepted technique in these types of cancer. Identification of the sentinel node requires the use of preoperative lymphoscintigraphy using radioactive technetium and then blue dye injection (toluidine blue) at the time of surgery. The sentinel node is identified using a gamma probe and confirmed with the injection of blue dye at the time of biopsy. Pathology of the sentinel node requires hematoxylin and eosin staining and also immunohistochemistry. The node requires serial sectioning at 150 micron sections for accurate analysis. Melanoma and breast cancer are ideally suited to this technique because the primary tumor is easily palpated and visualized, making injection into the tumor relatively straight forward. The majority of oral cavity cancers are also easily visualized and are in general accessible to a direct injection. This has lead to the suggestion that the SNB technique may be useful in neck management for oral cavity cancer. Studies on the incidence of occult metastases in N0 necks have shown tumor spread in only 20% of patients (91). Therefore if neck dissection is carried out electively or as a staging procedure, a large majority of patients will have unnecessary surgery. The first report of this technique for SCC of the oral cavity was reported in 2001 by Shoaib et al. (92), where SNB was carried out prior to an elective neck dissection in patients with a clinically negative neck. A study by Ross et al. (93) reported on SNB on 57 clinically N0 necks in 48 patients and reported 15 (35%) were upstaged by SNB and 28 (65%) were staged SNB negative. With a mean follow-up of 18 months, only one patient developed regional neck disease after being staged negative on SNB. The overall sensitivity of the technique was 94%. A further multicenter trial reported upstaging in 42 of 135 patients (35%) (94). However, this technique is still experimental and should only be carried out in centers with the necessary expertise and the appropriate volume of cases, as it has been shown that centers who carry out this technique with fewer than 10 cases per year have a much lower sensitivity (95).

Reconstructive Surgery

The ultimate functional outcome of surgical treatment depends a great deal upon choosing the appropriate reconstructive procedure. Reconstruction of the head and neck and mandibular reconstruction are discussed in detail in this book.

Radiotherapy and Chemotherapy

Radical Radiotherapy

Radical radiotherapy is rarely used in the oral cavity due to morbidity associated with treatment and poorer results compared to surgery. If surgery is contraindicated due to medical comorbidity and high anesthetic risk, radiotherapy can be used as an alternative option. However, radiotherapy should not be used in the presence of bone invasion, as the chance of success is low, and even if the malignant cells are eradicated, the bone usually fails to regenerate, leading inevitably to troublesome osteoradionecrosis. The success rate of radiotherapy is appreciably higher if some or all of the dose is administered by brachytherapy, rather than by external beam alone (90,96). Long-term side effects of radiotherapy include xerostomia with increased risk of dental caries; this is much less of a problem after brachytherapy than external beam, because of the smaller volume of normal mucosa irradiated. Necrotic ulcers of the soft tissues occasionally occur, more commonly after brachytherapy.

Adjuvant Radiotherapy

Adjuvant radiotherapy is indicated for patients with clinical or pathological features that indicate a high risk of locogional recurrence. This includes patients with positive or close surgical margins, lymphovascular invasion, perineural invasion, pathological positive neck nodes, and extracapsular spread. Postoperative doses of 60 Gray or more result in good locoregional control (97,98).

Adjuvant Chemoradiotherapy

Administration of cisplatin chemotherapy concurrently with postoperative radiotherapy has been reported to improve locoregional control and survival versus radiotherapy alone in patients with extracapsular spread and/or positive surgical margins (99,100). However, concurrent chemoradiation is an extremely toxic treatment and should only be used judiciously at centers that are equipped to manage the intensive needs of these patients. In patients unsuitable for chemotherapy, concurrent administration of cetuximab with radiotherapy has also shown improved locoregional control in locally advanced oral cavity cancer (101). However even with this regime, cutaneous toxicity in the form of an acneiform rash has increasingly been observed (102). Recently there has been evidence that induction chemotherapy using docetaxel plus cisplatin and fluorouracil [Taxol, Platinum (TPF)] followed by concurrent chemoradiation can produce enhanced efficacy resulting in improved locoregional control and overall survival in patients with locally advanced unresectable SCC of the head and neck (103,104). Vermorken reported that the TPF group had a median overall survival of 18.8 months compared to 14.5 months in patients who received cisplatin and fluorouracil (PF), which equates to a 27% reduction in the risk of death. In patients with unresectable disease and also organ preservation patients, Posner reported a median survival of 71 months in the TPF group compared to 30 months in the PF group.

Osteoradionecrosis

Osteoradionecrosis is a serious sequel to treatment with radiation, and its management can be extremely challenging. The development of this complication can be largely prevented by a few simple precautions (Table 11.13). Diseased teeth within the treatment volume are the prime initiator of osteoradionecrosis, and almost all bone necrosis occurs in patients who were dentulous prior to radiotherapy. Risk factors include the size and location of the lesion, the volume of the mandible within the radiation field, dosage more than 65 Gy, and the health of the dentition. Three major pathological elements seem to be involved: periosteal and endosteal microangiopathy, primary or secondary osteomyelitis, and osteocyte damage (105).

The onset of osteonecrosis is heralded by intractable local pain and a high index of suspicion is essential to early diagnosis. This is, however, not easy, and the situation is often complicated by the need to exclude a local recurrence

Table 11.13 Prevention of Osteoradionecrosis

Preradiotherapy
   Avoid radiation therapy for tumors involving the mandible
   Extract poor-prognosis teeth prior to starting treatment
   Remove cysts and odontomes

Postradiotherapy
   Stress on maintenance of oral and dental hygiene through and
      after radiation therapy
   Avoid dental extraction, especially of multiple teeth after radiation
      therapy
   Removal of caries and extirpation of pulps
   Root canal therapy

Prevent tooth loss
   Fluoride gel and mouthwashes
   Chlorhexidine mouthwashes
   Limit radiation caries with dental splint coverage

of tumor. It is important to avoid traumatizing the suspicious area with multiple biopsies, which only serve to worsen the problem. Currently used radiological investigations are not very specific and PET scanning may prove more useful in differentiating viable tumor tissue in a previously irradiated mandible from the necrosis and inflammation associated with osteoradionecrosis (106).

Early and limited areas of osteoradionecrosis may be treated with conservative measures such as use of a Water Pik, debridement, long-term antibiotics, and only very rarely, hyperbaric oxygen. The use of systemic antibiotics remains controversial, but our policy is to use either a combination of metronidazole and a third-generation cephalosporin or long-term tetracycline, depending upon the extent and duration of bone exposure. For more extensive necrosis, the conservative approach requires protracted treatment with an often-disappointing outcome in terms of function and cosmesis. Selected patients with severe osteonecrosis may benefit from aggressive surgical excision of the necrotic mandible and immediate microvascular reconstruction (107).

Photodynamic Therapy

For oral dysplasia, carcinoma in situ, and early oral cancers, photodynamic therapy is an alternative modality of treatment. Photodynamic therapy involves the systemic administration of a photosensitizing agent to the patient. When the oral cavity lesion is illuminated with light, the photosensitizer is activated into a cytotoxic drug that then destroys the tissue illuminated. Thus, selective destruction of premalignant and malignant lesions can be achieved. The photosensitiser most commonly used is 5-aminolevulinic acid. As well as selectivity, the technique has other advantages in that it leaves little scarring and does not prevent the use of other treatments such as surgery or radiotherapy at a later date. The treatment can be repeated many times. The technique however is limited by the depth of cancers that can be treated because the technique relies on light application to the surface of the tumor. Therefore only superficial tumors can be treated in this way. The use of interstitial light-emitting probes may help to alleviate this problem, and this is currently under investigation for the palliative treatment of recurrent oral cancer. The other main problem with the technique is that patients remain sensitive to light for several weeks and have to avoid being exposed to sunlight by staying inside, wearing protective creams and glasses. Using this technique, cure rates of 94% can be achieved with early carcinomas of the oral cavity (108). Despite this, surgery still remains the mainstay for treatment in patients with solitary oral cavity cancers. Photodynamic therapy mainly has a role in patients who present with multiple primary tumors of the oral cavity where multiple excisions result in too much scarring and functional morbidity. Copper et al. (109) reported on 27 patients with 42 second or multiple primary head and neck tumors treated by photodynamic therapy and reported that 28 of 42 tumors were cured (67%) with cure rates for stage I or in situ disease being 85% versus 38% for stage II/III disease.

Chemoprevention of Oral Cancer

Premalignant lesions such as leukoplakia and erythroplakia can be removed surgically. However this often does not prevent cancer because the entire lining of the oral cavity is often precancerous due to field cancerization (69,110). In a study of 150 patients with dysplastic epithelium, Sudbo et al. reported patients with negative margins had a similar rate of oral cancer to those with positive margins; oral cancer developed in 32% of patients with negative margins and 30% patients with positive margins (111). Chemoprevention may therefore be a useful method of treating such patients.

Retinoids

The most extensively studied chemoprevention agents has been vitamin A analogues (retinoids). Vitamin A has an important role in epithelial differentiation by binding to retinoic acid receptors. High levels of retinoic acid metabolites can reverse epithelial dedifferentiation toward a normal phenotype, and therefore it was postulated that synthetic retinoids may have a role in reversing epithelial dysplasia. Indeed it has been shown that high levels of the drug isoretinoin (13-cis-retinoic acid [13cRA]) can reverse epithelial dysplasia and reduce the second primary tumor risk (112). Significant skin toxicity was found, and this limited its use for long-term prevention. Within 3 months of stopping, more than one half of the responders recurred or developed new lesions. Following this, a randomized trial of 3-month induction with high dose 13cRA followed by 9 months low dose versus placebo reported progression of only 8% in the cRA group versus 55% in the placebo group (113). There is some evidence that it reduces the risk of developing a second cancer in patients with a previous history of oral cancer, although this reduction in second primary tumor (SPT) disappears 3 years after stopping the retinoid (114).

COX-2 Inhibitors

Cyclooxygenases (COXs) are enzymes involved in the synthesis of prostaglandins from the fatty acid arachidonic acid. COX-1 is constitutively expressed in cells, whereas COX-2 is inducible by mitogens and is also highly expressed in many cancer types. COX-2 has been shown to be involved in several processes in carcinogenesis including apoptosis, angiogenesis, invasion, and immune response (115). COX-2 inhibitors may be useful in oral cancer prevention because it has been reported that it is overexpressed in high-risk oral dysplasia (116). In addition, there is a four-fold increased COX-2 expression in active smokers versus never smokers (117), and there is epidemiological evidence that the use of nonsteroidal anti-inflammatory drugs (NSAIDS) reduces head and neck cancer risk (118). Preclinical data has shown inhibition of COX-2 in the upper aerodigestive tract can be used for cancer prevention or treatment (119). However, disappointingly, a recent randomized, double-blind, placebo controlled trial of the COX-2 inhibitor ketorolac as an oral rinse found no effect on oral leukoplakia (120). Recently it has been shown that aneuploid oral dysplastic lesions, which are the lesions at greatest risk of cancer progression, have selective upregulation of COX2 (121). Therefore targeting these patients with COX-2 inhibition may be the way forward. Such targeting requires an assessment of aneuploidy in the patient's lesion to select the most appropriate patient. Such a trial is planned for the Nordic countries where classification of dysplastic lesions by ploidy status is standard practice.

Epidermal Growth Factor Receptor Inhibitors

Epidermal growth factor receptor (EGFR) overexpression occurs in 80 to 100% of premalignant and malignant lesions of the oral cavity (122,123). Activation of EGFR is by phosphorylation, which in turn activates signal transduction pathways (e.g., MAPK, Src, Pak1) leading to cell proliferation and invasion. Tobacco is able to induce phosphorylation of EGFR, and phosphorylated EGFR has been found in 50% of dysplastic oral lesions and 100% of carcinomas. This therefore suggests that EGFR inhibitors may be useful in the prevention of oral cancer. Recently it has been reported that COX-2 inhibitors and EGFR inhibitors can act in a synergistic way to inhibit growth in head and neck cell lines. As such, targeting a COX-2 inhibitor and an EGFR inhibitor in high-risk patients may have increased efficacy.

Other Chemoprevention Agents

It has been reported that oral administration of the antioxidant N-acetyl-L-cysteine reduced the frequency of DNA adducts, and abnormal micronuclei in oral mucosa in healthy smokers and oral dysplasia showed a clinical and histological response to lycopene, a naturally occurring carotenoid (124). The use of mouthwashes containing attenuated adenovirus (125,126) has been reported as have the use of gene therapy and vaccine therapy (127,128).

REHABILITATION AND FOLLOW-UP
Rehabilitation

Rehabilitation of the patient after treatment involves close cooperation with other health professionals including dieticians, speech therapists, dental surgeons, hygienists, and prosthodontists. In patients who have resection of tumors of the oral cavity, teeth and bone may be removed. Such patients require dental rehabilitation in the form of dentures or dental implants. Patients often have coexisting periodontal disease that accelerates if the patient receives radiotherapy. Such patients require dental care before and after radiotherapy. Dental extractions in irradiated mandibles should only be done in hospital by specialist dental surgeons due to the increased risk of osteoradionecrosis. This occurs in approximately 5% of patients who have radiation to the oral cavity (129). Surgery and radiotherapy to the oral cavity also have a major impact on speech and swallowing, particularly if large resections of the oral tongue are resected or if free flaps and pedicled myocutaneous flaps are required for reconstruction. These patients should be actively followed by speech and swallowing therapists to rehabilitate speech and also assess risk of aspiration. The use of modified barium swallow via videofluoroscopy can assess the risk for aspiration (130). Fiber optic endoscopic evaluation of swallowing is also being used more extensively to diagnose and rehabilitate dysphagia patients (131). Many of these patients will need percutaneous gastostomy (PEG) tubes to maintain nutrition in the immediate postoperative period, particularly if postoperative chemoradiation is planned. As such, careful monitoring of nutrition and patient weight should be carried out by a dietitian assigned to the head and neck team.

Follow-up

Patients who have been treated for oral cancer require a regular periodic examination on a graduated time scale dependent upon assessment of the state of the primary site, locoregional disease, and distant spread. The possibility of the occurrence of a second head and neck primary exists at a constant rate of about 4 to 7% of treated patients a year, and thorough examination and a high suspicion are synergistic activities. Although it is important for patients to stop abusing tobacco and alcohol, prevention strategies have not worked (132), and chemoprevention using agents such as retinoids have been under investigation (133). Routine chemoprevention cannot, however, be recommended just yet because of the doubtful value and low index of safety of currently available agents.

RESULTS OF TREATMENT
Alveolar Ridge and Retromolar Trigone Tumors

Surgery is the best option for patients with T1–2 lesions. Primary radiation is less feasible because the tendency of these tumors to invade through thin mucoperiosteum or tooth sockets, placing the patient at increased risk for osteoradionecrosis. A brachytherapy technique using iridium wires looped over the gum is available for superficial lesions (134) but is rarely used. Mucoperiosteal or minimal cortical invasion can be effectively managed by combining surgical excision of the lesion with a marginal mandibulectomy or partial maxillectomy, which can often be safely accomplished transorally (Fig. 11.31). Posteriorly located lesions may be better accessed using an appropriately planned upper or lower cheek flap. Edentulous patients with "pipestem" mandibles may however need segmental resection of their mandible for adequate tumor clearance. Elective neck dissection is carried out in most N0 cases en bloc with the primary or through a separate incision. More advanced tumors are best treated with combined modality treatment using surgery and radiation therapy. Surgery followed by postoperative radiation therapy is probably a better option compared to preoperative radiation, which is associated with a higher risk of osteoradionecrosis. Resection of the mandible and/or maxilla may be required, and functional outcome can be improved with osteomyocutaneous free tissue transfer (135) and osseointegrated implants as appropriate.

Surgery as the only modality of treatment has resulted in 5-year actuarial survival rates of 77% in early stage disease (stages I and II) (136). This figure drops sharply to 24% in patients with stage IV disease (137). Radical radiotherapy is best avoided for tumors of the alveolar ridge because of the likelihood of bone invasion, unless surgery is not possible for any reason. Early tumors of the retromolar trigone, on the other hand, tend to respond better to radiotherapy, there being no difference in survival rates between surgery and radiotherapy (138). Five-year survival rates of 88% for T1 and 69% for T2 tumors have been reported from a radical radiotherapy policy (139). Some radiotherapy failures result from perineural spread in the direction of the infratemporal fossa and so it is important to irradiate an adequate superior margin.

Floor of the Mouth

Equivalent control rates have been reported following surgery and radiation therapy for early tumors of the floor of mouth. Anterior and lateral floor of mouth lesions can be resected transorally (Fig. 11.32) and the defect closed using

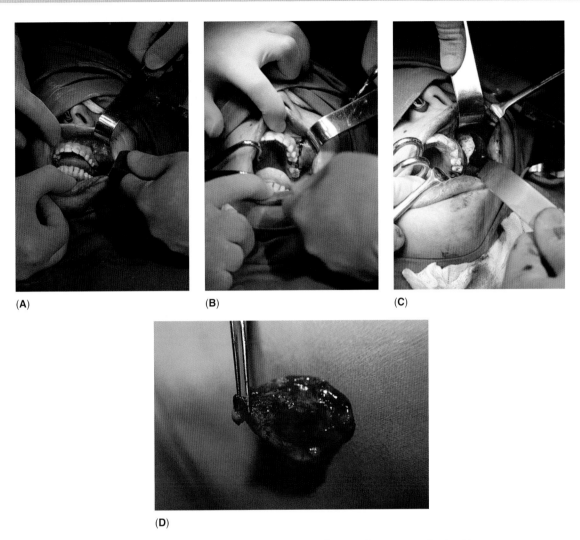

(A)   (B)   (C)

(D)

Figure 11.31 (A–D) Transoral excision with partial maxillectomy for an upper alveolar ridge cancer.

mucosal advancement or a skin graft. Superficial lesions can be excised with little postoperative morbidity. The submandibular gland ducts need to be carefully dissected and transplanted laterally while excising lesions of the anterior floor of mouth. Interstitial implants have also been used (140), but radiation therapy is contraindicated as the primary modality of treatment in lesions that abut against or are tethered to the mandible. The management of the clinically N0 neck is controversial; most authors recommend elective neck dissection, though some advocate neck dissection if the lesion is more than 4mm thick (66). Our practice is to carry out a supraomohyoid neck dissection and submit suspicious nodes for frozen section analysis with a view to a complete modified radical neck dissection if any node shows metastasis. Bilateral neck dissections are carried out for lesions approaching or crossing the midline. Locally advanced floor of mouth tumors are best treated using a combination of surgery and radiation therapy. Apart from the horizontal spread to involve mandibular bone, these lesions infiltrate the sublingual salivary gland and the space between the intrinsic tongue muscles and the genioglossus. Surgical excision of floor of mouth cancers may therefore include partial glossectomy, marginal or segmental

mandibulectomy, and reconstruction using skin grafts, pedicled flaps, or microvascular tissue transfer. Patients are subjected to elective or therapeutic neck dissection and lesions that approach or cross the midline may need bilateral neck dissection. As discussed previously, postoperative radiation therapy is an integral part of management when indicated.

The overall 5-year survival rates in patients with floor of mouth cancer reported in the literature are shown in Table 11.14. Early lesions (T1–T2) treated with surgery have a 10% local failure rate, whereas failure in the neck (40%) is a bigger concern in patients with larger lesions (T3–T4). Radiation therapy for stage I tumors has a 6% local failure rate, whereas 16% of stage II tumors will recur locally if treated with radiation alone (141). Locoregionally advanced tumors (stage III) are treated with a combination of surgery and radiation therapy achieving a 79% 5-year actuarial local control (142).

Oral Tongue
As with most other oral cancers, equivalent results have been reported with surgery and radiation therapy.

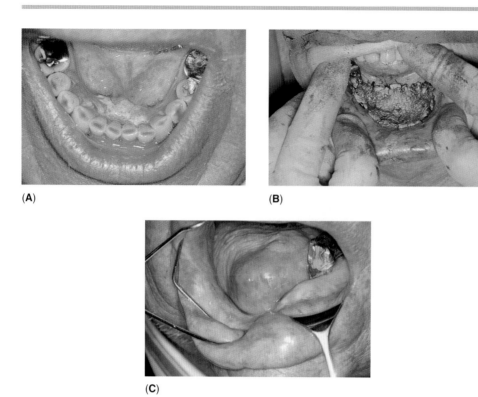

(A)

(B)

(C)

Figure 11.32 **(A–C)** Transoral excision and split skin graft for a cancer of the anterior floor of mouth.

Table 11.14 Overall 5-year Survival (%) in Patients with Cancer of the Floor of the Mouth

Series	No. of patients	Stage I	Stage II	Stage III	Stage IV
Harrold (91)	634	69	49	25	7
Panje et al. (92)	103	57	60	43	19
Nason et al. (93)	198	69	64	46	26
Shaha et al. (94)	320	88	80	66	32
Fu et al. (95)	153	83	71	43	10

192 Iridium (^{192}Ir) implants have been used successfully in the treatment of these tumors, and the functional results of radiation may be better than those after surgery, especially in the case of tumors on the dorsum and lateral border of the middle third. Lesions amenable to radiation include T1, and exophytic T2 and T3 lesions with minimal infiltration. Transoral excision of smaller tumors can often be safely accomplished, but surgical excision of larger T2 lesions with adequate margins most often results in a partial glossectomy. Reconstruction of the resultant defect using a free radial forearm flap gives good functional results and is our current treatment of choice.

The role of elective treatment of the clinically negative neck in the management of early tongue cancer continues to generate controversy, and there have been reports in the literature evaluating the predictive value of histological parameters such as the depth of tumor invasion (69,70). Despite the lack of conclusive survival benefit in two prospective trials (70,141) in early oral cavity cancer, there seems to be unanimity in opinion regarding the importance of elective treatment of the neck in early tongue cancer (143). Our practice of routine elective neck treatment for

early tongue lesions is based on our observation (144) that patients whose necks had not been treated had a statistically significant increase in the rate of neck failure. Although the difference in actuarial 5-year survival rates between those whose necks were treated electively and those who had no elective treatment was not statistically significant (75 vs. 65%; $p = 0.44$), there was a significant increase in risk for neck failure in the latter group (17% vs. 43%; $p = 0.025$). Multivariate analysis of another group of our cases treated by brachytherapy showed that elective neck irradiation was a statistically significant favorable prognostic factor (144); there was a similar finding in favor of elective neck dissection in a French study (145). Additionally, as many as 67% of our patients who failed in the neck succumbed to their disease, and it is our contention that the best chance for treatment of the neck is at initial presentation of the primary tumor.

Surgical excision of larger lesions may require a mandibulotomy or a lingual-releasing approach to gain access. Patients presenting with a clinically N0 neck should undergo a functional neck dissection whereas those with palpable nodes are treated with a modified or RND. Discontinuous resection of the primary has been shown to be oncologically safe, and we make no special effort to resect the neck nodes in continuity with the primary tumor.

The overall 5-year survival rates reported in the major series in the literature are listed in Table 11.15. Local control of the tumor using primary radiation can be achieved in 80 to 85% of patients with early lesions (T1–T2) and in 68% of patients with T3 lesions (146–150). Surgical excision gives local control in 85% of T1, 77% of T2, and only 50% of T3 lesions. Despite combined treatment with surgery and radiation therapy, only 35% of patients with advanced stage disease (stages III and IV) will survive 5 years, mainly as a result of recurrence in the neck.

Buccal Mucosa

As with other sites within the oral cavity, surgery and radiation therapy are equally effective in controlling T1 lesions. Smaller lesions can be excised transorally (Fig. 11.33) with minimal functional sequelae whereas larger lesions that approach the commissure are probably best managed by radiation. Exophytic or superficial lesions can be managed by radiation therapy, but infiltrative lesions are best managed by surgery. Patients with a clinically negative neck may be safely observed because, in contrast to other sites, less than 10% of patients fail in the neck.

Surgery combined with radiation therapy is the treatment of choice for more advanced tumor. Adequate exposure may be obtained by elevating a cheek flap. A full-thickness resection may be required if tumor invades into the buccal fat pad or the overlying skin. Other structures that need careful evaluation for invasion prior to surgery are the alveolar ridges and the mandible. Adequate clearance of tumor almost certainly necessitates resection of these structures, and preoperative planning of bony cuts facilitates reconstruction and rehabilitation. The surgical defect is reconstructed using pedicled myocutaneous flaps or free tissue transfer. An ipsilateral neck dissection is carried out in all patients with locally advanced tumors irrespective of nodal status. In addition to the obvious advantage in terms of regional control,

Table 11.15 Overall 5-year Survival (%) in Patients with Cancer of the Tongue

Series	No. of patients	Stage I	Stage II	Stage III	Stage IV
Callery et al. (102)	252	75	60	40	20
Decroix and Ghossein (103)	602	59	45	25	13
Wallner et al. (104)	424	68	50	33	20
Ildstad et al. (105)	122	48	48	18	26
O'Brien et al. (106)	97	73	62	–	–

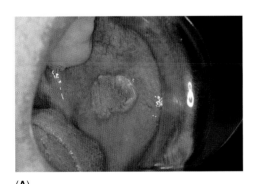

(A)

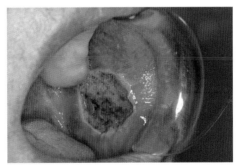

(B)

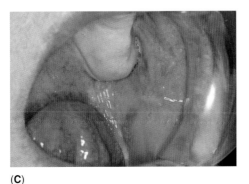

(C)

Figure 11.33 (A–C) Transoral laser excision of a carcinoma of the left buccal mucosa.

a modified neck dissection resecting the sternomastoid muscle may be essential if the pedicle of a myocutaneous flap has to be accommodated in that side of the neck.

Radiation therapy as a single modality offers limited control: 3-year disease-free survival is 85% for stage I, 63% for stage II, 41% for stage III, and only 14% for stage IV patients (151). Surgical excision as the only modality has slightly better results compared to radiation therapy: 5-year disease-free survival is 77% for stage I, 65% for stage II, 27% for stage III, and 18% for stage IV patients (152).

ORAL CANCER: THE WAY AHEAD

Although treatment results for patients with oral cancer have improved considerably over the last several decades, we have now reached a plateau in terms of survival because of the adverse effect of second and subsequent primary tumors in long-term survivors. Our focus must therefore be on prevention of oral cancer not only by better education but also by the use of novel targeted molecular therapies aimed at the epithelial precursor lesions that develop into oral cancer. Identification of high-risk lesions and targeting therapies to these patients with small molecule inhibitors will help to improve outcome. The use of global gene expression profiling using microarrays may also help us to identify molecular markers of invasion and metastases, thus allowing more effective therapeutic agents to be designed.

REFERENCES

1. Jovanovic A, Schulten EA, Kostense PJ et al. Tobacco and alcohol related to the anatomical site of oral squamous cell carcinoma. J Oral Pathol Med 1993; 22: 459–62.
2. Waldron CA, el Mofty SK, Gnepp DR. Tumors of the intraoral minor salivary glands: a demographic and histologic study of 426 cases. Oral Surg Oral Med Oral Pathol; 66: 323–33.
3. Buchner A, Merrell PW, Carpenter WM. Relative frequency of intra-oral minor salivary gland tumors: a study of 380 cases from northern California and comparison to reports from other parts of the world. J Oral Pathol Med 2007; 36: 207–14.
4. Pires FR, Pringle GA, de Almeida OP et al. Intra-oral minor salivary gland tumors: a clinicopathological study of 546 cases. Oral Oncol 2007; 43(5): 463–70.
5. Epstein JB, Epstein JD, Le ND et al. Characteristics of oral and paraoral malignant lymphoma: a population based review of 361 cases. Oral Surg Oral Med Oral Pathol Oral Radiol Endod 2001; 92: 519–25.
6. Meyer I, Shklar G. Malignant tumors metastatic to the mouth and jaws. Oral Surg 1965; 20: 350.
7. Axell T, Holmstrup P, Kramer IRH et al. International seminar on oral leukoplakia and associated lesions to tobacco habits. Community Dent Oral Epidemiol 1984; 12: 145.
8. Holmstrup P, Vedtofte P, Reibel J et al. Long term outcome of oral premalignant lesions. Oral Oncol 2006; 42: 461–74.
9. Warnakulasuriya KA, Johnson NW. Sensitivity and specificity of OraScan toluidine blue mouthrinse in the detection of oral cancer and precancer. J Oral Pathol Med 1996; 25: 97–103.
10. Epstein JB, Scully C, Spinelli J. Toluidine blue and Lugol's iodine application in the assessment of oral malignant disease and lesions at risk of malignancy. J Oral Pathol Med 1992; 21: 160–3.
11. Silverman S Jr, Gorsky M, Lozada F. Oral leukoplakia and malignant transformation: a follow-up study of 257 patients. Cancer 1984; 53: 563–8.
12. Kramer IR, El Labban N, Lee KW. The clinical features and risk of malignant transformation in sublingual keratosis. Br Dent J 1978; 144: 171–80.
13. Rosin MP, Cheng X, Poh C et al. Use of allelic loss to predict malignant risk for low grade oral epithelial dysplasia. Clin Cancer Res 2000; 6: 357–62.
14. Mao L. Can molecular assessment improve classification of head and neck premalignancy? Clin Cancer Res 2000; 6: 321–2.
15. Partridge M, Pateromichelakis S, Phillips E et al. A case-control study confirms that microsatellite assay can identify patients at risk of developing oral squamous cell carcinoma within a field of cancerization. Cancer Res 2000; 60: 3893–8.
16. Epstein JB, Zhang L, Poh C et al. Increased allelic loss in toluidine blue positive oral premalignant lesions. Oral Surg Oral Med Oral Pathol Oral Radiol Endod 2003; 95: 45–50.
17. Kawaguchi H, El-Nagger AK, Papadimitrakopoulou V et al. Podoplanin: a novel marker for oral cancer risk in patients with oral premalignancy. J Clin Oncol 2008; 26: 354–60.
18. Vora HH, Trivedi TI, Shukla SN et al. P53 expression in leukoplakia and carcinoma of the tongue. Int J Biol Markers 2006; 21: 74–80.
19. Luo CW, Roan CH, Liu CJ. Human papillomaviruses in oral squamous cell carcinoma and pre-cancerous lesions detected by PCR based gene-chip array. Int J Oral Maxillofac Surg 2007; 36: 153–8.
20. Kovesi G, Szende B. Prognostic value of cyclin D1, p27 and p63 in oral leukoplakia. J Oral Pathol Med 2006; 35: 274–7.
21. Gires O, Mack B, Rauch J et al. CK8 correlates with malignancy in leukoplakia and carcinomas of the head and neck. Biochem Biophys Res Commun 2006; 343: 252–9.
22. Kvaal SI, Warloe T. Photodynamic treatment of oral lesions. J Environ Pathol Toxicol Oncol 2007; 26: 127–33.
23. Gandolfo S, Pentenero M, Broccoletti R et al. Toluidine blue uptake in potentially malignant oral lesions in vivo: clinical and histological assessment. Oral Oncol 2006; 42: 89–95.
24. Zhang L, Williams M, Poh CF et al. Toluidine blue staining identifies high risk primary oral premalignant lesions with poor outcome. Cancer Res 2005; 65: 8017–21.
25. Sharwani A, Jerjes W, Salih V et al. Assessment of oral premalignancy using elastic scattering spectroscopy. Oral Oncol 2006; 42: 343–9.
26. Poh CF, Zhang L, Anderson DW et al. Fluorescence visualization detection of field alterations in tumor margins of oral cancer patients. Clin Cancer Res 2006; 12: 6716–22.
27. Westra WH, Sidransky D. Fluorescence visualization in oral neoplasia: shedding light on an old problem. Clin Cancer Res 2006; 12: 6594–7.
28. Epstein JB, Gorsky M, Lonky S et al. The efficacy of oral luminoscopy (ViziLite) in visualizing oral mucosal lesions. Spec Care Dentist 2006; 26: 171–4.
29. Murti PR, Bhonsle RB, Pindborg JJ et al. Malignant transformation rate in oral submucous fibrosis over a 17 year period. Community Dent Oral Epidemiol 1985; 13: 340–1.
30. GLOBOCAN 2002. Cancer incidence, mortality and prevalence Worldwide IARC. Cancer Base No.5 (computer program) version 2.0. Lyon IARC Press: 2004.
31. Kemp I. Atlas of cancer in Scotland 1975–1980. IARC scientific publications No.72. Scottish National Health Service. Information and Statistics division, Edinburgh, Great Britain: 1985.
32. Hindle I, Downer MC, Speight PM. The epidemiology of oral cancer. Br J Oral Maxillofac Surg 1996; 34: 471–6.
33. Boyle P, Macfarlane GJ, Scully C. Oral cancer: necessity for prevention strategies. Lancet 1993; 342: 1129.
34. Moller H. Changing incidence of cancer of the tongue, oral cavity and pharynx in Denmark. J Oral Pathol Med 1989; 18: 224–9.

35. Epstein JB, Scully C. Neoplastic disease in the head and neck of patients with AIDS. Int J Oral Maxillofac Surg 1992; 21: 219–26.

36. Office for National Statistics. Mortality statistics: cause, 2006–2008.

37. Spitz MR, Fueger JJ, Goepfert H et al. Squamous cell carcinoma of the upper aerodigestive tract: a case comparison analysis. Cancer 1988; 61: 203–8.

38. Jayant K, Notani PN. Epidemiology of oral cancer. In: Rao RS, Desai PB, eds. Oral cancer. Bombay, India: Tata Memorial Hospital, Professional Education Division, 1991.

39. Brennan JA, Boyle JO, Koch WM et al. Association between cigarette smoking and mutation of the p53 gene in squamous cell carcinoma of the head and neck. N Engl J Med 1995; 332: 712–17.

40. Schantz SP, Hsu TC. Head and neck cancer patients express increased clastogen-induced chromosome fragility. Head Neck 1989; 11: 337–43.

41. Reddy CRRM. Carcinoma of hard palate in relation to reverse smoking of chuttas. J Natl Cancer Inst 1974; 53: 615–19.

42. IARC Monographs on the evaluation of the carcinogenic risk of chemicals to the human. Tobacco habits other than smoking: betel-quid and areca nut chewing and some related nitrosamines. Lyon, France: International Agency for Research on Cancer, 1985.

43. Mehta FS, Gupta PC, Daftary DK et al. An epidemiologic study of oral cancer and precancerous conditions among 101761 villagers in Maharashtra, India. Int J Cancer 1972; 10: 134–41.

44. McCoy DG, Wynder EL. Etiological and preventive implications in alcohol carcinogenesis. Cancer Res 1979; 39: 2844–50.

45. Mashberg A, Garfinkel L, Harris S. Alcohol as a primary risk factor in oral squamous carcinoma. CA Cancer J Clin 1981; 31: 146–55.

46. Graham S, Dayal H, Rohrer T et al. Dentition, diet, tobacco, and alcohol in the epidemiology of oral cancer. J Natl Cancer Inst 1977; 59: 1611–18.

47. Szpirglas H. Alcohol et cancer buccaux. Actual Odontostomatol (Paris) 1976; 115: 448–54.

48. Binnie WH. Epidemiology and aetiology of oral cancer in Britain. Proc R Soc Med 1976; 69: 737–40.

49. McLaughlin JK, Gridley G, Block G et al. Dietary factors in oral and pharyngeal cancer. J Natl Cancer Inst 1988; 80: 1237–43.

50. Wynder EL, Kabat G, Rosenberg S et al. Oral cancer and mouthwash use. J Natl Cancer Inst 1983; 70: 255–60.

51. Donald PJ. Marijuana smoking – possible cause of head and neck cancer in young patients. Otolaryngol Head Neck Surg 1986; 94: 517–21.

52. Shillitoe EJ, Greenspan D, Greenspan JS et al. Immunoglobulin class of antibody to herpes simplex virus in patients with oral cancer. Cancer 1983; 51: 65–71.

53. Watts SL, Brewer EE, Fry TL. Human papillomavirus DNA types in squamous cell cancer of the head and neck. Oral Surg Oral Med Oral Pathol 1991; 7: 701–7.

54. Fortner JG, Shiu MH. Organ transplantation and cancer. Surg Clin North Am 1974; 54: 871–6.

55. Ficarra G, Eversole LE. HIV related tumors of the oral cavity. Crit Rev Oral Biol Med 1994; 5: 159–85.

56. Slaughter DP, Southwick HW, Smejkal W. "Field cancerization" in oral stratified squamous epithelium: clinical implications of multicentric origin. Cancer 1953; 6: 963.

57. Lester EP, Tharapel SA. Chromosome abnormalities in squamous carcinoma cell lines of head and neck origin. Presented at the Third International Head and Neck Oncology Research Conference, Las Vegas, 1990.

58. van der Riet P, Nawroz H, Hruban RH et al. Frequent loss of chromosome 9 p21–22 early in head and neck cancer progression. Cancer Res 1994; 54: 1156–8.

59. Brachman DG, Graves D, Vokes E et al. Occurrence of p53 gene deletions and human papilloma virus infection in human head and neck cancer. Cancer Res 1992; 53: 4832.

60. Boyle JO, Hakin J, Koch W et al. The incidence of p53 mutations increases with progression of head and neck cancer. Cancer Res 1993; 53: 4477–80.

61. Lederman M. The anatomy of oral cancer. J Laryngol Otol 1964; 78: 181.

62. Moore C, Catlin D. Anatomic origins and locations of oral cancer. Am J Surg 1967; 114: 510–13.

63. Ahmed F, Islam KM. Site of predilection of oral cancer and its correlation with chewing and smokings habits—a study of 103 cases. Bangladesh Med Res Counc Bull 1990; 16: 17–25.

64. Robbins KT, Medina JE, Wolfe GT et al. Standardizing neck dissection terminology. Arch Otolaryngol Head Neck Surg 1991; 117: 601–5.

65. Shah JP, Candela FC, Poddar AK. The patterns of cervical lymph node metastases from squamous carcinoma of the oral cavity. Cancer 1990; 66: 109–13.

66. Byers RM, Newman R, Russell N, Yue A. Results of treatment for squamous carcinoma of the lower gum. Cancer 1981; 47: 2236–8.

67. Willen R, Nathanson A. Squamous cell carcinoma of the gingiva. Acta Otolaryngol 1973; 75: 299–300.

68. Spiro RH, Huvos AG, Wong GY et al. Predictive value of tumor thickness in squamous carcinoma confined to the tongue and floor of the mouth. Am J Surg 1986; 152: 345–50.

69. Lindberg R. Distribution of cervical lymph node metastases from squamous cell carcinoma of the upper respiratory and digestive tracts. Cancer 1972; 29: 1446–9.

70. Strong EW. Carcinoma of the tongue. Otolaryngol Clin North Am 1979; 12: 107–13.

71. Fakih AR, Rao RS, Borges AM et al. Elective versus therapeutic neck dissection in early carcinoma of the oral tongue. Am J Surg 1989; 158: 309–13.

72. Urist MM, O'Brien CJ, Soong SJ et al. Squamous carcinoma of the buccal mucosa: analysis of prognostic factors. Am J Surg 1987; 154: 411–14.

73. Beahrs OH, Henson DE, Hutter RVP et al. Manual for staging of cancer, 4th ed. Philadelphia: JB Lippincott, 1992.

74. Bundgaard T, Bentzen SM, Wildt J. The prognostic effect of tobacco and alcohol consumption in intraoral squamous cell carcinoma. Eur J Cancer Oral Oncol 1994; 30B: 323–28.

75. McGregor AD, McDonald DG. Routes of entry of squamous cell carcinoma to the mandible. Head Neck Surg 1988; 10: 294–301.

76. McGregor AD. Patterns of spread of squamous cell carcinoma in the mandible. Head Neck 1989; 11: 457–61.

77. Marchetta FC, Sako K, Murphy JB. The periosteum of the mandible and intraoral carcinoma. Am J Surg 1971; 122: 711–13.

78. Huntley TA, Busmanis I, Desmond P et al. Mandibular invasion by squamous cell carcinoma: a computed tomography and histological study. Br J Oral Maxillofac Surg 1996; 34: 69–74.

79. King JM, Caldarelli DD, Petasnick JP. Dentascan—a new diagnostic method for evaluating mandibular and maxillary pathology. Laryngoscope 1992; 102: 379–87.

80. Yanagisawa K, Friedman CD, Vining EM et al. Dentascan imaging of the mandible and maxilla. Head Neck 1993; 15: 1–7.

81. Chung TS, Yousem DM, Seigerman HM et al. MR of mandibular invasion in patients with oral and oropharyngeal malignant neoplasms. Am J Neuroradiol 1994; 15: 1949–55.

82. Ahuja RB, Soutar DS, Moule B et al. Comparative study of technetium-99m bone scans and orthopantomography in determining mandible invasion in intraoral squamous cell carcinoma. Head Neck 1990; 12: 237–43.

83. Shaha AR. Preoperative evaluation of the mandible in patients with carcinoma of the floor of the mouth. Head Neck 1991; 13: 398–402.

84. Shah JP, Andersen PE. Evolving role of modifications in neck dissection for oral squamous carcinoma. Br J Oral Maxillofac Surg 1995; 33: 3–8.

85. Farr HW, Arthur K. Epidermoid carcinoma of the mouth and pharynx 1960–1964. J Laryngol Otol 1972; 86: 243–53.

86. Spiro JD, Spiro RH, Shah JP et al. Critical assessment of supraomohyoid neck dissection. Am J Surg 1988; 156: 286–89.

87. Mannii JJ, van den Hoogen FJA. Supraomohyoid neck dissection with frozen section biopsy as a staging procedure in the clinically node-negative neck in carcinoma of the oral cavity. Am J Surg 1991; 162: 373–6.

88. Tupchong L, Scott CB, Blitzer PH et al. Randomized study of preoperative versus postoperative radiation therapy in advanced head and neck carcinoma: long-term follow-up of RTOG study 73–03. Int J Radiat Oncol Biol Phys 1991; 20: 21–8.

89. Andersen PE, Spiro RH, Cambronero E et al. The role of comprehensive neck dissection with preservation of the spinal accessory nerve in the clinically positive neck. Am J Surg 1994; 168: 499–502.

90. Chu A, Fletcher GH. Incidence and cause of failure to control by irradiation the primary lesions in squamous cell carcinomas of the anterior two-thirds of the tongue and floor of mouth. Am J Roentgenol 1973; 117: 502–8.

91. Ferlito A, Shaha AR, Rinaldo A. The incidence of lymph node micrometastases in patients staged N0 in cancer of the oral cavity and oropharynx. Oral Oncol 2002; 38: 3–5.

92. Shoaib T, Soutar DS, MacDonald DG et al. The accuracy of head and neck carcinoma sentinel lymph node biopsy in the clinically N0 neck. Cancer 2001; 91: 2077–83.

93. Ross G, Shoaib T, Soutar DS et al. The use of sentinel node biopsy to upstage the clinically N0 neck in head and neck cancer. Arch Otolaryngol Head Neck Surg 2002; 128: 1287–91.

94. Ross GL, Soutar DS, MacDonald DG et al. Sentinel node biopsy in head and neck cancer: preliminary results of a multicenter trial. Ann Surg Oncol 2004; 11: 690–6.

95. Ross GL, Shoaib T, Soutar DS et al. The first international conference on sentinel node biopsy in mucosal head and neck cancer and adoption of a multicenter trial protocol. Ann Surg Oncol 2002; 9: 406–10.

96. Wallner PE, Hanks GE, Kramer S et al. Patterns of care study: analysis of outcome survey data: anterior two-thirds of tongue and floor of mouth. Am J Clin Oncol 1986; 9: 50–7.

97. Zelefsky MJ, Harrrison LB, Fass DE et al. Postoperative radiation therapy for squamous cell carcinomas of the oral cavity and oropharynx: impact of therapy on patients with positive surgical margins. Int J Radiat Oncol Biol Phys 1993; 25: 17–21.

98. Bartelink H, Breur K, Hart G et al. The value of postoperative radiotherapy as an adjunct to radical neck dissection. Cancer 1983; 52: 1008–13.

99. Bernier J, Domenge C, Ozsahin M et al. Postoperative irradiation with or without concomitant chemotherapy for locally advanced head and neck cancer. N Eng J Med 2004; 350: 1945–52.

100. Cooper JS, Pajak TF, Forastiere AA et al. Postoperative concurrent radiotherapy and chemotherapy for high risk squamous cell carcinoma of the head and neck. N Eng J Med 2004; 350: 1937–44.

101. Bonner JA, Harari PM, Giraly J et al. Radiotherapy plus cetuximab for squamous cell carcinoma of the head and neck. N Eng J Med 2006; 354: 567–78.

102. Budach W, Bolke E, Homey E. Severe cutaneous reaction with radiotherapy and cetuximab. N Eng J Med 2007; 357: 514–17.

103. Vermorken JB, Remenar E, van Herpen C et al. Cisplatin, fluorouracil and Docetaxel in unresectable head and neck cancer. N Eng J Med 2007; 356: 1695–704.

104. Posner MR, Hershock DM, Blajman CR et al. Cisplatin and fluorouracil alone or with docetaxel in head and neck cancer. N Eng J Med 2007; 356: 1705–15.

105. Archer DJ. Osteoradionecrosis and the dental surgeon. In: Bloom HJ, Hanham IWF, eds. Head and Neck Oncology. New York: Raven Press, 1986: 253–8.

106. Minn H, Aitasalo K, Happonen RP. Detection of cancer recurrence in irradiated mandible using positron emission tomography. Eur Arch Otorhinolaryngol 1993; 250: 312–15.

107. Shaha AR, Cordeiro PG, Hidalgo DA et al. Resection and immediate microvascular reconstruction in the management of osteoradionecrosis of the mandible. Head Neck 1997; 19: 406–11.

108. Biel MA. Photodynamic therapy treatment of early oral and laryngeal cancers. Photochem Photobiol 2007; 83: 1063–8.

109. Copper MP, Triesscheijn M, Tan IB et al. Photodynamic therapy in the treatment of multiple primary tumors in the head and neck, located to the oral cavity and oropharynx. Clin Otolaryngol 2007; 32: 185–9.

110. Braakhuis BJ, Tabor MP, Kummer JA et al. A genetic explanation of Slaughter's concept of field cancerization: evidence and clinical implications. Cancer Res 2003; 63: 1727–30.

111. Sudbo J, Lippman SM, Lee JJ et al. The influence of resection and aneuploidy on mortality in oral leukoplakia. N Eng J Med 2004; 350: 1405–13.

112. Hong WK, Endicott J, Itri LM et al. 13-cis-retinoic acid in the treatment of oral leukoplakia. N Engl J Med 1986; 315: 1501–5.

113. Lippman SM, Batsakis JG, Toth BB et al. Comparison of low dose isotretinoin with beta carotene to prevent oral carcinogenesis. N Eng J Med 1993; 328: 15–20.

114. Khuri FR, Lee JJ, Lippman SM et al. Randomised phase III trial of low-dose isotretinoin for prevention of second primary tumors in stage I and II head and neck cancer patients. J Natl Cancer Inst 2006; 98: 426–7.

115. Dannenberg AJ, Lippman SM, Mann JR et al. Cyclooxygenase-2 and epidermal growth factor receptor: Pharmacologic targets for chemoprevention. J Clin Oncol 2005; 23: 254–66.

116. Sudbo J et al. Cyclooxygenase-2 (COX-2) expression in high risk premalignant oral lesions. Oral Oncol 2003; 39: 497–505.

117. Moraitis D, Du B, De Lorenzo MS et al. Levels of COX-2 are increased in the oral mucosa of smokers. Evidence for the role of EGFR and its ligands. Cancer Res 2005; 65: 664–70.

118. Bosetti C, Talamini R, Franceshi S et al. Aspirin use and cancers of the upper aerodigestive tract. Br J Cancer 2003; 88: 672–4.

119. Altorki NK, Subbaramaiah K, Dannenberg AJ. COX-2 inhibition in upper aerodigestive tract tumors. Semin Oncol 2004; 31: 30–6.

120. Mulshine JL, Atkinson JC, Greer RO et al. Randomised, double blind, placebocontrolled phase IIB trial of the cyclooxygenase inhibitor ketorolac as an oral rinse in oropharyngeal leukoplakia. Clin Cancer Res 2004; 10: 1565–73.

121. Sudbo J, Soland TM, Ristmaki A et al. COX-2 is selectively up regulated in aneuploid oral leukoplakia: a rationle for targeted use of COX-2 inhibitors to prevent oral cancer. Cancer Epidemiol Biomarkers Prev.

122. Grandis JR, Tweardy DJ. Elevated levels of transforming growth factor alpha and epidermal growth factor receptor messenger RNA are early markers of carcinogenesis in head and neck cancer. Cancer Res 1993; 53: 3579–84.

123. Shin DM, Ro JY, Hong WK et al. Dysregulation of epidermal growth factor receptor expression in premalignantlesions during head and neck tumorogenesis. Cancer Res 1994; 54: 3153–9.

124. Singh M, Krishanappa R, Bagewadi A et al. Efficacy of oral lycopene in the treatment of oral leukoplakia. Oral Oncol 2004; 40: 591–6.

125. Rudin CM, Cohen EEW, Papadimitrakopoulou VA et al. An attenuated adenovirus, ONYX-015, as mouthwash therapy for premalignant oral dysplasia. J Clin Oncol 2003; 21: 4546–52.

126. Gaballah K, Hills A, Curiel D et al. Lysis of dysplastic but not normal oral keratinocytes and tissue engineered epithelia with conditionally replicating adenoviruses. Cancer Res 2007; 67: 7284–94.

127. Clayman GL, Lippman SM. Gene therapy in preventing cancer in patients with premalignant carcinoma of the oral cavity and pharynx. ClinicalTrials.gov Identifier:NCT00064103.

128. Strome SE. MAGE–A3/HPV 16 vaccine for squamous cell carcinoma of the head and neck. ClinicalTrials.gov Identifier:NCT00257738.

129. Jereczek-Fossam BA, Orecchia R, Radiotherapy induced mandibular bone complications. Cancer Treat Rev 2002; 28: 65–74.

130. Stenson KM, MacCracken E, List M et al. Swallowing function in patients with head and neck cancer prior to treatment. Arch Otolaryngol Head Neck Surg 2000; 126: 371–7.

131. Aviv JE, Wu CH, Hisao TY et al. Prospective randomised outcome study of endoscopy versus modified barium swallow in patients with dysphagia. Dysphagia after radiotherapy: endoscopic examination of swallowing in patients with nasopharyngeal carcinoma. Laryngoscope 2000; 110: 564–74.

132. COMMIT Research Group. Community intervention trial for smoking cessation (COMMIT): I. Cohort results from a four-year community intervention. Am J Public Health 1995; 85: 183–92.

133. Lippman SM, Hong WK. Retinoid chemoprevention of upper aerodigestive tract carcinogenesis. In: DeVita VT, Hellman S, Rosenberg SA, eds. Important advances in oncology. Philadelphia: Lippincott, 1992: 93–109.

134. Alcock CJ, Paine CH, Weatherburn H. Interstitial radiotherapy in treatment of superficial tumors of the lower alveolar ridge. Clin Radiol 1984; 35: 363–6.

135. Hidalgo DA. Aesthetic improvements in free-flap mandible reconstruction. Am Soc Plast Reconst Surg 1991; 88: 574–5.

136. Cady B, Catlin D. Epidermoid carcinoma of the gum: a 20-year survey. Cancer 1969; 23: 551–69.

137. Soo KC, Spiro RH, King W et al. Squamous carcinoma of the gingiva: an update. Am J Surg 1988; 156: 281–5.

138. Byers RM, Fields RS, Anderson B et al. Treatment of squamous carcinoma of the retromolar trigone. Am J Clin Oncol 1984; 7: 647–52.

139. Wang CC. Radiation therapy for head and neck neoplasms, 2nd ed. Chicago: Year Book Medical Publishers, 1990.

140. Mazeron J, Grimard L, Raynal M et al. Iridium-192 curietherapy for T1 and T2 epidermoid carcinomas of the floor of mouth. Int J Radiat Biol Phys 1990; 18: 1299–306.

141. Vandenbrouck C, Sancho GH, Chassagne D et al. Elective vs therapeutic neck dissection in epidermoid carcinoma of the oral cavity. Results of a randomized trial. Cancer 1980; 46: 386–90.

142. Dearnaley DP, Dardoufas C, A'Hern RP et al. Interstitial irradiation for carcinoma of the tongue and floor of mouth: Royal Marsden experience 1970–86. Radiother Oncol 1991; 21: 1883–92.

143. DeSanto LW, Johnson JT, Million RR. Controversies: cost-effective management of T1N0 carcinoma of the tongue. Head Neck 1996; 18: 573–76.

144. Yii NW, Patel SG, Rhys Evans PH et al. Management of the N0 neck in early cancer of the oral tongue. Clin Otolaryngol 1999; 24: 75–9.

145. Piedbois P, Mazeron JJ, Haddad E et al. Stage I–II squamous carcinoma of the oral cavity treated by iridium-192: is elective neck dissection indicated? Radiother Oncol 1991; 21: 100–6.

146. Callery CD, Spiro RH, Strong EW. Changing trends in the management of squamous carcinoma of the tongue. Am J Surg 1984; 148: 449–54.

147. Decroix Y, Ghossein NA. Experience of the Curie Institute in treatment of cancer of the mobile tongue: treatment policies and results. Cancer 1981; 47: 503–8.

148. Wallner PE, Hanks GE, Kramer S et al. Patterns of care study: analysis of outcome survey data–anterior two thirds of tongue and floor of mouth. Am J Clin Oncol 1986; 9: 50–7.

149. Ildstad ST, Bigelow ME, Remensnyder JP. Squamous cell carcinoma of the mobile tongue: Clinical behavior and results of current therapeutic modalities. Am J Surg 1983; 145: 443–9.

150. O'Brien CJ, Lahr CJ, Soong SJ et al. Surgical treatment of early stage carcinoma of the oral tongue-would adjuvant treatment be beneficial? Head Neck Surg 1986; 8: 401–8.

151. Nair M, Sankaranarayanan R, Padmanabhan TK. Evaluation of the role of radiation therapy in the management of carcinoma of the buccal mucosa. Cancer 1988; 61: 1326–31.

152. Bloom NO, Spiro RH. Carcinoma of the cheek mucosa: a retrospective analysis. Am J Surg 1980; 140: 556–9.

12

Tumors of the Oropharynx

Raghav C Dwivedi, Peter H Rhys Evans and Snehal G Patel

INTRODUCTION

Tumors of the oropharynx are relatively infrequent with an incidence of about 0.8 to 3.8 per 100,000 population per annum, but for head and neck tumors, this is the most common site for carcinomas of the pharynx. Functionally, the oropharynx is one the most critical sites in the upper aerodigestive tract because it is situated at the important bifurcation of the respiratory and digestive tract. Tumors at this site will affect swallowing, speech, and ultimately the airway; therefore, decisions about treatment are influenced not only by which is the optimal method of tumor ablation, but also by important functional considerations.

The oropharynx also includes important lymphatic structures in the base of tongue and tonsils that form part of Waldeyer's ring and, therefore, are a significant extranodal site for development of lymphomas, which have a quite different morphology and natural history to squamous cell carcinomas (SCCs) arising in this site.

Tumors may arise from any site within the oropharynx, but there is considerable variation in the type and behavior of tumors in these different sites even for SCC. It is therefore of practical importance to divide the oropharynx into the palatine arch and the oropharynx proper (Table 12.1) (1). In general, SCCs of the palatine arch tend to be less aggressive and metastasize later than those elsewhere in the oropharynx.

ANATOMICAL SUBSITES

The oropharynx is the middle part of the pharynx and is functionally unique in that it forms the common conduit for the upper respiratory and digestive tracts. Superiorly it communicates through the velopalatine isthmus with the nasopharynx, anterosuperiorly through the palatoglossal arch with the oral cavity, and inferiorly it continues as the hypopharynx with an anteroinferior opening into the larynx. Each of these orifices is surrounded by a complex independent sphincter mechanism that controls the integrity of the opening during respiration and deglutition. Under normal circumstances these sphincters are functionally synchronized by cortical and local neuromuscular reflex pathways, but these can be easily disrupted under pathological conditions causing serious functional complications.

The oropharynx extends from the level of the hard palate above to the hyoid bone below (Fig. 12.1). It is further subdivided into four main anatomical subsites for the purpose of tumor classification (Table 12.2).

Anterior Wall

This comprises the base or posterior third of the tongue bounded anteriorly by the V-shaped line of circumvallate papillae. These commence laterally adjacent to the base of the palatoglossal fold and come to an apex in the midline at the vestigial foramen caecum (Fig. 12.2). It extends caudally to include the valleculae at the junction of the base of the tongue with the lingual aspect of the epiglottis and the lateral pharyngoepiglottic and the midline glosseoepiglottic folds. The epiglottis itself is classified as part of the supraglottic larynx. Laterally it extends to the margins of the tongue.

The base of the tongue is mostly covered with aggregates of lymphoid tissue forming the lingual tonsil. Mucous glands open onto the surface and also into the crypts of the lingual tonsil. The bulk of the tongue base is formed by the interlacing network of intrinsic (vertical and transverse) and extrinsic (styloglossus, genioglossus, and hyoglossus) muscle bundles (Fig. 12.3). The attached part or root of the tongue also contains the important vascular and nerve pedicles on each side. The septum linguae is a strong midline connective tissue septum that effectively separates the deeper structures of the tongue base. Small tumors at this site however may invade both neurovascular bundles and thus compromise the function and viability of the whole tongue.

Vascular Supply

The base of the tongue has a rich vascular supply from the lingual artery, which is the third branch of the external carotid artery. Normally there is a good collateral circulation from the facial artery so that ligation of the origin of the lingual artery does not significantly reduce bleeding. Venous drainage is via the deep lingual vein that accompanies the hypoglossal nerve, "protecting" its superficial surface during dissection of the area.

Innervation

The afferent supply to the posterior part of the tongue is through the glossopharyngeal (IX) nerve except for a small area in the valleculae and adjacent part of the tongue mucosa, which is supplied by twigs from the superior laryngeal branch of the vagus (X). The glossopharyngeal nerve contains fibers of general sensation and of taste, the latter especially distributed to the circumvallate papillae. The acute pain on swallowing, eating, and talking associated with tumors of the tongue base, similar to glossopharyngeal

Table 12.1 Divisions of the Oropharynx

Palatine arch
    Soft palate and uvula
    Anterior faucial pillar

Oropharynx proper
    Lateral and posterior wall including the pharyngoepiglottic fold
    Base of tongue and vallecula
    Glossotonsillar sulcus
    Tonsillar fossa and posterior faucial pillar

Table 12.2 Anatomical Subsites of the Oropharynx

Anterior wall (glossoepiglottic area)
    Tongue posterior to the circumvallate papillae (base of tongue)
    Vallecula (but not the lingual surface of the epiglottis, which is now included in the larynx – suprahyoid epiglottis)

Latqeral wall
    Tonsil
    Tonsillar fossa and faucial pillars
    Glossotonsillar sulcus

Posterior wall

Superior wall
    Inferior surface of the soft palate
    Uvula

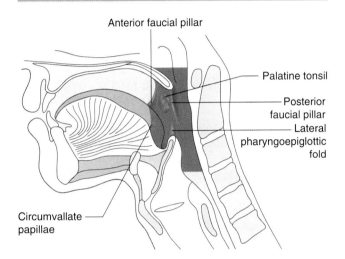

Figure 12.1 Surface anatomy of the oropharynx.

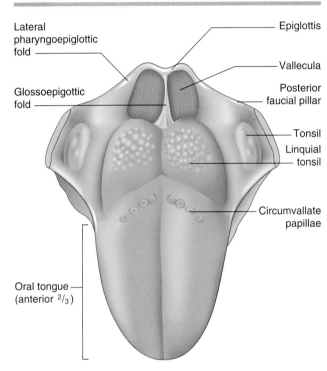

Figure 12.2 Dorsum of the tongue.

neuralgia, often radiating to the ear, is an important clinical sign even in the absence of mucosal abnormality, which must not be missed.

Motor innervation to the muscles of the tongue is via the hypoglossal (XII) nerve, which emerges between the internal jugular vein and internal carotid artery, descending to a point above the carotid bifurcation where it gives off the descendans hypoglossi branch of the ansa cervicalis. It curves forward on the surface of the internal and external carotid arteries adjacent to the deep aspect of the jugulodigastric lymph node. Here it can be invaded by metastatic tumor or may need to be resected if there is extracapsular spread (ECS).

Lymphatic Drainage

Lymphatics from the tongue posterior to the circumvallate papillae run downward towards the hyoid bone where they pierce the pharyngeal wall to enter the nodes of the upper deep cervical chain (level II). Tumors typically drain into the largest of these nodes (jugulodigastric), which lies on the lateral aspect of the internal jugular vein, just below the inferior border of the posterior belly of digastric muscle (Fig. 12.3). From here lymphatics normally drain sequentially to levels III, IV, and V although under pathological conditions or following surgery to the neck there may be retrograde spread to level I, the retropharyngeal nodes

or to the contralateral side of the neck. Tumors near the midline are more likely to exhibit bilateral spread.

Lateral Wall

This includes the tonsil, the tonsillar fossae, the faucial pillars, and more posteriorly the lateral pharyngeal wall, which merges into the posterior wall. The anterior boundary is the vertical fold of the palatoglossus muscle (anterior faucial pillar) which separates it from the oral cavity. The posterior faucial pillar is formed by the palatopharyngeus and deep to both muscles is the superior pharyngeal constrictor. Inferiorly the lateral wall includes the glossotonsillar sulcus, which separates it from the border of the tongue (Fig. 12.2).

The tonsil is the largest aggregation of lymphoid tissue in Waldeyer's ring. It is characterized by deep crypts in which SCCs may arise without causing obvious surface

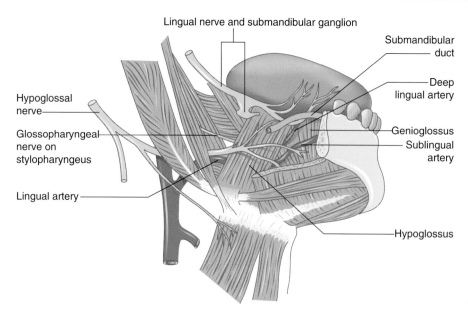

Figure 12.3   Innervation and musculature of the tongue.

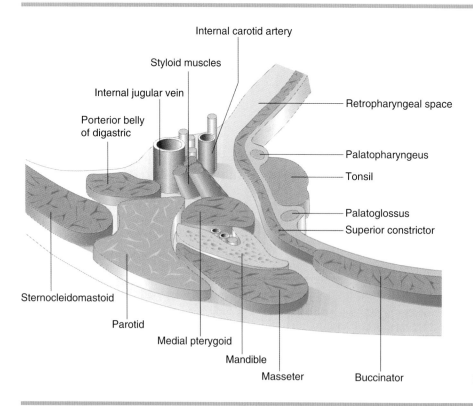

Figure 12.4   Deep relations of the tonsil.

ulceration. It has a distinct capsule that separates it from the superior constrictor and deep to that the contents of the parapharyngeal space (Fig. 12.4).

Vascular Supply

The tonsillar branch of the facial artery is the main supply with other branches from the lingual, the ascending palatine, and superiorly from the lesser palatine arteries. The tonsillar and other pharyngeal veins drain into a plexus situated on the posterior wall of the pharynx, which communicates above with the pterygoid plexus and below with the superior thyroid and lingual veins or directly into the facial or internal jugular (2). A separate ring-like submucosal pharyngeal plexus is situated around the entrance to the larynx and is particularly dense with veins 1 to 3 mm in diameter. It is arranged in two parts, one on the anterior and the other on the posterior wall of the pharynx, and is thought to be concerned with pressure adjustments accompanying swallowing (3). It accounts for the increased vascularity noticed in this area during pharyngeal resections.

Innervation

The sensory innervation of the tonsillar region is via the glossopharyngeal nerve that passes forward lateral to the stylopharyngeus and deep to the lower pole of the tonsil. Tumors arising in the depths of the tonsillar crypts may invade branches of this exquisitely sensitive nerve causing pain and otalgia before surface ulceration becomes apparent. Sensation from the upper part of the tonsil is through descending branches of the lesser palatine nerves coursing through the sphenopalatine ganglion from the facial (VII) nerve.

The pharyngeal plexus provides the motor and most of the sensory innervation to the pharynx from branches of the glossopharyngeal and vagus nerves. The former contributes only sensation to the plexus, but the vagus supplies sensory fibers as well as all the motor fibers including those joining from the internal ramus of the accessory (XI) nerve. Loss of the glossopharyngeal nerve either from tumor invasion or from surgery will therefore impair sensation and the swallow reflex, but good function is maintained unless there is additional loss of the vagus or its pharyngeal branches at the skull base.

Lymphatic Drainage

The oropharyngeal mucosa has a rich lymphatic network, especially the tonsils, which drain directly through the pharyngeal wall into the upper deep cervical (jugulodigastric) nodes. Large early metastatic deposits may present here; and because this node has a tendency to undergo cystic degeneration in the presence of SCC, it is often mistaken for a branchial cyst with serious consequences for the patient. In addition, fine-needle aspiration of the cystic fluid may often be acellular or nondiagnostic giving a false sense of security. It can never be said too often that in an adult, particularly where there is a history of smoking, an enlarged node that has been present for more than 1 month should be regarded as metastatic carcinoma until proved otherwise, irrespective of whether or not it has partly responded to antibiotics. Ultrasound-guided fine-needle aspiration cytology (FNAC) may help to take samples from the wall of the cyst rather than the fluid itself. From level II nodes drainage continues to levels III and IV.

Lymphatics from the upper lateral wall drain to the retropharyngeal nodes of which the only constant one is the node of Rouvier situated close to the skull base between the internal carotid artery and the lateral wall of the pharynx. Lymph from here drains into the deep cervical chain (levels II, III, and IV).

Posterior Wall

This extends superiorly from the level of the hard palate and Passavant's ridge down to the hyoid bone where the posterior pharyngeal wall is continuous with that of the hypopharynx. Laterally it curves forward to merge with the lateral wall. The mucosa is smooth and contains occasional small aggregates of lymphoid tissue. Deep to this are the overlapping posterior fibers of the superior and middle constrictor muscles that insert largely into each other in a midline pharyngeal raphe. The muscular wall with its thin covering of buccopharyngeal fascia is separated from the prevertebral fascia by an area of loose connective tissue forming the retropharyngeal space.

Vascular Supply

The arterial supply of the posterior wall is from branches of the ascending pharyngeal and superior thyroid arteries. The venous drainage is through the pharyngeal plexus previously described.

Innervation

Details of the motor and sensory distribution of the vagus and glossopharyngeal nerves to the pharyngeal wall are described above.

Lymphatic Drainage

The primary echelons of drainage are the retropharyngeal nodes and the nodes at levels II and III with midline lesions drain bilaterally.

Roof

The roof of the oropharynx is formed by the curved arch of the inferior surface of the soft palate and the uvula in the midline. There are numerous palatine glands opening onto the mucosa on the oral surface of the soft palate, and they are especially abundant over the uvula. The palatine aponeurosis forms the skeletal framework of the soft palate and is firmly attached anteriorly to the posterior margin of the hard palate. The tensor and levator veli palatine muscles fuse with each other in the midline raphe and are responsible for closing off the nasopharynx during speech and swallowing. The palatoglossus and palatopharyngeus control the sphincteric action of the faucial pillars.

Vascular Supply

The soft palate is supplied by the lesser palatine arteries, which are branches of the descending palatine from the maxillary artery. The venous drainage is mainly to the pharyngeal and pterygoid plexus.

Innervation

Sensory innervation from the soft palate is through fibers in the lesser palatine nerve via the pterygopalatine ganglion. All the muscles of the soft palate are supplied from the pharyngeal plexus from the vagus (X), with the exception of the tensor veli palatini, which is innervated by a branch from the mandibular nerve.

Lymphatic Drainage

Lymphatic drainage is mainly to the upper deep cervical nodes (level II).

HISTOLOGY

As with other sites in the upper aerodigestive tract, tumors may arise in the oropharynx from different epithelial elements, and three main histological types are well recognized:

1. SCC from the squamous epithelium
2. Lymphomas from the tonsils and lymphoid follicles in the base of the tongue
3. Salivary gland tumors from minor salivary glands concentrated in the soft palate, uvula and the capsule of the tonsil.

As seen in other head and neck regions, SCC is the most common type of cancer encountered in the oropharynx and accounts for almost 90% of all malignant neoplasms (4–6). Because of the higher concentration of lymphoid tissue in the oropharynx, non-Hodgkin's lymphomas tend to occur more frequently as compared to other sites in the head and neck. Salivary gland tumors and other rare tumors account for less than 5% of oropharyngeal malignancies.

Squamous Cell Carcinoma
Epidemiology
There is no consensus about the use of oral and oropharyngeal cancer demographic data (prevalence and incidence data) in the world literature. Many authors have quoted oral and oropharyngeal cancers rates collectively while describing oropharyngeal cancers. Also the term *pharyngeal cancer* is being used frequently as a synonym to describe oropharyngeal cancers. Our position is that the prevalence and behavior of oropharyngeal cancers is different from cancers of other subsites of the pharynx (nasopharynx and hypopharynx) and oral cavity and, hence, they should be reported separately (7).

There is very little concrete demographic data available on oropharyngeal cancers separately. However, oral and pharyngeal cancers collectively account for more than 400,000 new cases and nearly 200,000 deaths per year across the globe (8,9). The vast majority of these cases come from developing countries (66%–75%) (8,9).

In the western world, oropharyngeal carcinomas account for about 5% of all cancers (10), and approximately 10,000 new cases of oropharyngeal cancer are diagnosed in U.S.A. annually (11). In the U.K. more than 1,000 new cases of SCC of the oropharynx were registered in England and Wales in 2005 (12,13). According to an estimate, more than 10,000 new cases of oropharyngeal cancer will be diagnosed, and more than 2,000 patients will die of oropharyngeal cancer in U.S.A. in 2008 (14).

The incidence of oropharyngeal cancer varies considerably around the world, but in most series it ranks second or third in order of frequency of head and neck cancers and in general is not as common as laryngeal or oral cavity tumors (12,13,15). The global incidence rate among males is 3.8 per 100,000 population whereas in Europe worst affected is Western Europe with an overall incidence of 9.7. Central Europe, Southern Europe, and Northern Europe have comparatively low incidence rates with 5.4, 5.3, and 2.6 per 100,000 population per year, respectively (8). Some European countries have much higher incidence rates than global or European standards. Hungary (16.9), France especially Bas-Rhin and Doubs regions (15.4), Luxemburg (13.1), Slovakia (11.1), and Croatia (10.2) are among the highest incidence areas in the world. The reported incidence rates in U.K. and U.S.A. are 2.5 and 4.3, respectively (8). The

maximum number of oropharyngeal cancer patients are reported from South East Asia, especially India, which not surprisingly has both one of the highest incidence registering areas with 12.5 cases per 100,000 population per year and a very large population.

Reported incidence rates in females are less than 1.0 per 100,000 population in most areas of the world, whereas calculated global incidence is 0.8 per 100,000 people per year (8). Again the same geographical preponderance is seen in certain countries like France (2.5), Hungary (2.1), Luxemburg (1.8), India (1.8), and Croatia (1.0). The exact reason for this selectivity is not known, however it has been associated with different social, cultural, genetic, and environmental factors.

The disease is more common in males with the male/female ratio ranging between 2 and 5:1 (12–14) and is seen most frequently in the sixth and seventh decade in men and women (4,16,17). Some recent reports indicate toward an increasing trend of oral and oropharyngeal cancer among younger population around the globe (18,19).

Etiological Factors
Tobacco. Tobacco is the single most important etiologic factor responsible for SCC of the upper aerodigestive tract and other cancers in general. Tobacco contains more than 19 known carcinogens (collectively known as tar) and more than 4,000 chemicals, most of which have been identified as toxic, tumorigenic, and carcinogenic (20,21). Burning of tobacco releases methylchloranthrene, benzopyrine, benzanthracene, and other polycyclic aromatic hydrocarbons that reach the cellular surface of the epithelium in the smoke or dissolved in saliva. Arylhydrocarbon hydroxylation breakdown of these carcinogens produces carcinogenic epoxides which bind to DNA and RNA molecules, damaging them and initiating the process of cancer formation (22). N-nitroso compounds, well-known carcinogens found in tobacco smoke, play a major role in the malignant transformation of the upper aerodigestive tract mucous membrane (23).

It is observed that tobacco users have a high frequency of p53 mutation (24), which is a key feature of all cancers including oropharyngeal cancers. The process of development of the carcinoma depends on all possible determinants; like the type of tobacco used, the length and intensity of carcinogen exposure, type of vehicle used, response of the epithelium (production of mucous and ciliary paralysis), genetically determined arylhydrocarbon hydroxylase inducibility, use of fresh fruits (naturally occurring antioxidants), and other dietary factors (25).

Regional differences in the form and method of tobacco consumption are responsible for varied prevalence of oral and oropharyngeal cancers. In South Asian countries, especially India, oral and oropharyngeal cancers account for as many as 20 to 25% of all cancers (8). The use of Beedi (26) (crude form of cigarette with about 0.2 gms of tobacco wrapped in specific tree leaf) tobacco quid, Khaini (tobacco quid with slaked lime) betal quid or "paan" (arecanut and slaked lime wrapped in a betal leaf) chewing, paan masala (dry complex mixture of arecanut, catechu, flavoring agents), and gutka (dry complex mixture of arecanut, catechu, flavoring agents with tobacco) are the main culprits for this mammoth rate of oral-oropharyngeal cancers in the Indian subcontinent (22,27). It is observed that paan masala and gutka contain over 2,000 chemicals, many of which have been proved to be carcinogenic (28). Besides having direct irritating effect on the mucosa, betel quid chewing causes genomic instability (29). It is noted that it also interferes with cell-mediated immunity, which might play a role in the malignant transformation of the oral and oropharyngeal mucous membrane (30).

It is observed that smokers have a sixfold increase of developing oral cancers compared to nonsmokers (31). Similarly tobacco quid/betel quid chewing leads to a five- to sixfold increase in risk of developing oral cavity cancers (32,33). Quitting tobacco and stopping smoking reduces the risk of oral-oropharyngeal cancers and premalignant lesions; although it may take 10 to 20 years or more for a former smoker's risk to reduce to that of nonsmokers (34,35).

Alcohol. Alcohol is another well established risk factor for the development of oral and oropharyngeal cancers. The chronic consumption of alcohol is estimated to increase the risk of upper aerodigestive tract cancer by 2 to three-fold (36,37). It affects oncogenes at initiation and promotion stages of carcinogenesis, impairs the cell's ability to repair its DNA, and overexpresses certain oncogenes responsible for cancer formation.

Alcohol use has a synergistic effect with tobacco and is known to increase the risk of developing head and neck SCC (HNSCC) up to 20 to 120 times than of nonsmoker and nonalcoholic person (37,38). The nitrocarbon carcinogens in tobacco are relatively insoluble in normal saliva but are more soluble in alcohol and therefore are more readily absorbed into the surface epithelium (20). In normal cigarette smokers, the oropharyngeal site most commonly affected is within the capsule of the tonsil, but where additional alcohol consumption is an important factor, tumors also commonly arise in the glossotonsillar sulci and more posteriorly in the pharyngoepiglottic fold. Alcohol also dehydrates the cell wall and hence enhances the ability of tobacco carcinogens to permeate the local tissues; additionally it retards the body's natural defense mechanisms and depletes antioxidants that have a protective role in cancers (36). Some alcoholic beverages contain chemical impurities like N-nitrosodiethylamine and polycyclic aromatic hydrocarbons that are well-known carcinogens (39,40). As seen with smoking, incidence and severity of oral and oropharyngeal cancer is affected by quantity, quality, and duration of alcohol consumed (41,42).

Viruses. Human papilloma virus (HPV) belongs to the family of small double-stranded DNA viruses that infect the basal cells of squamous epithelium (43). At present the sequences for more than 320 types of HPV have already been identified, with several additional poorly characterized types described. The different types have been traditionally separated based on tropism for cutaneous and mucosal sites, as well as their association with malignancy (high, intermediate, and low risk) (44). Their role in causation of cervical carcinoma has been known for many decades, but their potential as a possible etiologic factor in HNSCCs has been established recently. Mucosal high-risk types HPV 16 and HPV 18 has been linked to the etiology of SCC of oral cavity and oropharynx. More than 90% of HPV positive oral cancers are HPV-16 positive (34), and the rate of positivity is even greater (95%) in oropharyngeal cancers (45). High-risk HPV 16 genome is found in 50% of

oropharyngeal tumors (46) and varies in geographical distribution (47).

Two oncogenic proteins of HPV 16, E6 and E7, can target two critical areas of the p53 and Rb tumor suppressor pathways and subsequently cause genomic instability through the deregulation of important cellular process, including DNA repair, cell cycle control, and apoptosis (48).

HPV infection is particularly associated with young, sexually active, nonsmoker males and may be responsible for changing trends of oral and oropharyngeal cancers toward younger nonsmoking population (19,38). Because risk factors for HPV infection include having a large number of sexual partners and first intercourse at a younger age, changing sexual practices in our society may increase the effect of HPV infection on the development of oral cancers and premalignant lesions, especially in younger adults (49). Oral sex practices have been recently associated with increased risk of developing oral and oropharyngeal cancers (50). There is strong evidence that HPV infection may be an independent risk factor for oral and oropharyngeal cancers (51). This finding is further supported by demonstration of HPV from cervical nodes of patients presenting with occult primary, confirming them to come from oropharynx (52).

Oropharyngeal cancer caused by HPV behaves differently from the other, more common variety that affects older age group. It is known to affect a younger nonsmoking nondrinking population that is sexually active. These patients often present with a neck node, respond well to radiation, and have a better prognosis than the other counterpart. It is because of these reasons some authors advocate to adopt different treatment paradigms in treating these cancer patients (46,53,54). These patients have been shown to have genetic predisposition as well (55).

It is now known that smoking, HPV infection, and chronic alcohol consumption has a synergistic effect in causation of upper aerodigestive tract SCCs (56).

Human immunodeficiency virus (HIV) also probably accelerates development of SCC in high-risk patients (20).

Genetic and familial factors. Cigarette smoking cannot be the sole etiological factor as only a small percentage of smokers will develop carcinoma. This suggests that tobacco-associated susceptibility to HNSCC is influenced by host factors as well (57). Several studies have suggested that risk for development of HNSCC is inherited, as individuals with a first-degree family member with cancer have a 2- to 14-fold increase in HNSCC (58,59). Accumulation of p53 in tumor cell nuclei predicts a significantly increased risk of death, independent of tumor grade, stage, and lymph node status (60).

Aberrant human leukocyte antigen (HLA) expression patterns, allelic polymorphism of HLA genes, and the major histocompatibility complex (MHC) class I chain related gene A, HLA-B*35, HLA-B*40 are found to be associated with oral squamous cell carcinomas (OSCC) patients (61). Preferential deletion of regions at chromosomes 2q21–24, 2q33–35, and 2q37.3 that contain several putative tumor suppressor genes such as LRP1B, CASP8, CASP10, BARD1, ILKAP, PPP1R7, and ING5 have been linked with oral and oropharyngeal SCC (62). Chromosome 18 may also be a possible site for a tumor suppressor gene deletion (63).

Single nucleotide polymorphisms of the DNMT3B promoter region, C46359T (–149C > T), –283T > C, and –579G > T might be a cancer-susceptible factor for several cancers including OSCC (64). The base excision repair system, which comprises the MUTYH, OGG1, and MTH1 genes and repairs mutations involving 8-oxoguanine, may have some role to play in the etiology of OSCC (65).

Epithelial adhesion molecule, a transmembrane glycoprotein involved in intercellular adhesion, is overexpressed by the majority of human epithelial carcinomas, including oral and oropharyngeal cancers and is significantly found associated with tumor size, regional lymph node metastasis, histological differentiation, and invasion pattern (66). Overexpression of vascular endothelial growth factor has been shown to be associated with angiogenic phenotypes and a poor prognosis (67).

Some other genetic factors associated with increased risk include abnormal induceability of cytochrome P450 (68–71) and mutagen sensitivity (72), which reflects a defect in DNA repair. Patients with xeroderma pigmentosum, Fanconi anaemia, and ataxia telangiectasia are known to have in risk of developing HNSCC.

Dietary factors. Approximately 15% of oral and oropharyngeal cancers can be attributed to dietary deficiencies or imbalances (22). Increase in risk has been reported to derive from high intake of foods that represent important source of calories, such as starchy foods, pulses, certain meats especially processed meat, charcoal grilled meat, pork, and eggs (73,74). Ingestion of salted meat has also been shown to be a risk factor in oral cavity and pharyngeal carcinoma (75).

Reactive oxygen species and reactive nitrogen species can function as initiators and promoters in carcinogenesis, whereas antioxidants provide protection against the cellular and molecular damage caused by them (76). Fruits and vegetables have naturally occurring antioxidants; similarly vitamin A and vitamin C also act as antioxidants and prevent from development of cancers (77). It has been shown that dietary deficiencies, particularly of vitamin A (and related carotenoids), vitamin C, vitamin E, iron, selenium, folate, and other trace elements, have been linked to increased risk of oral cancer (78–80).

Immunosuppression. Increased incidence of oral malignancy has been documented in chronic immunodeficiency states (81–84). Oral SCC has been reported in younger persons undergoing immunosuppression regimens following organ transplantation (85). However, the incidence of oral cancer is stated to be very low with no evidence of a particular preponderance in these patients (85,86). Although SCC of the oral cavity has been reported (87–89) in patients with HIV, there is no evidence that HIV disease has contributed to the rising incidence of oral cancer in the U.K., or elsewhere (90).

Occupation. Epidemiological evidence exists for an association between workers exposed to formaldehyde (91,92), electronics workers (93), textile workers (94), and an increased risk of oral and oropharyngeal cancer.

Other factors. Chronic irritants, poor dental hygiene (polymicrobial supragengival dental plaque) (95), candidiasis (96), diabetes (97), syphilis, and marijuana smoking (98,99)

have been identified as predisposing factors in upper aerodigestive tract carcinoma.

Precancer Precancerous lesions of the oropharynx include leukoplakia, erythroplakia, and mixed erythroleukoplakia (100); however, these do not have such significance in predisposition for oropharyngeal cancer as they do in SCC of the oral cavity. There is an accepted predisposition for cancer development in certain conditions such as submucous fibrosis (Fig. 12.5), which predisposes to tumors developing in the oropharynx particularly in the anterior palatoglossal fold and mucosal atrophy associated with iron deficiency anemia found in the Plummer–Vinson syndrome.

Site Distribution

The distribution of carcinomas at various sites in the oropharynx follows similar patterns to that seen in the oral cavity in that the sites most commonly affected are those in more prolonged contact with surface carcinogens (101–103). The crypts of the tonsils, the glossotonsillar sulci, and the tongue base are bathed in saliva to a greater extent than the soft palate or posterior pharyngeal wall and are thus more common sites where smoking and alcohol are etiological factors.

There is also considerable geographical variation in the incidence of SCC at different sites due to environmental and other etiological agents. The practice of "reverse smoking" (Chutta) in women in certain parts of India is associated with a higher incidence of carcinoma of the soft and hard palate (73,104). "Beedi" smoking in India also predisposes to development of tumors in the base of the tongue (26). In France and other Mediterranean countries there is a higher incidence of oropharyngeal tumors than in the U.K. because of differences in tobacco and alcohol consumption. In these regions carcinoma is more common in the glossotonsillar sulcus and on the pharyngoepiglottic fold.

The most common site for carcinoma in the oropharynx is the tonsil followed by the base of the tongue, and these two sites account for between 60 to 90% of cases (5) (Table 12.3). The soft palate and posterior wall are much

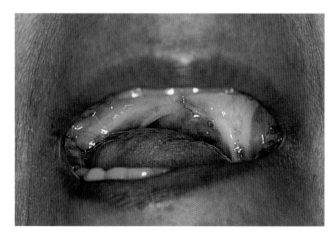

Figure 12.5   Oral submucous fibrosis, a condition that is associated with cancer developing in the anterior palatoglossal fold.

Table 12.3 Site Distribution in Oropharynx

Site	Sundaram et al. (2005) (106) Number	(%)	Selek et al. (2004) (107) Number	(%)	Johansen et al. (2000) (108) Number	(%)	Pradier et al. (1996) (105) Number	(%)	Mak-Kregar et al. (1995) (109) Number	(%)	Henk et al. (1992) (110) Number	(%)
Base of tongue	17	15.2	40	22.9	68	23.5	288	37.5	179	28	42	57
Tonsillar region	66	58.9	60	34.3	169	58.5	333	43.5	372	58.0	73	33
Soft palate and uvula	29[a]	25.9	55	31.4	33	11.4	119	15.5	62	10	8	6
Posterior pharyngeal wall	–	–	20	11.4	19	6.6	27	3.5	27	4.0	6	4
Total	112	100	175	100	289	100	767	100	650	100	129	100

[a]Includes soft palate, uvula and posterior pharyngeal wall.

less common, and those tumors occurring on the posterior wall almost invariably are situated low down near the junction with the hypopharynx at the level of the hyoid (105).

Nodal Metastases

The incidence of nodal metastases in oropharyngeal SCC is reported to vary from 12 to 85% (111,112). In majority of cases it is nearer to the higher values of spectrum (50%–85%) (113,114) (Table 12.4) and may be influenced by a number of potential tumor factors including grade of differentiation, site, and size of the tumor (115,116).

Despite numerous lymphatic pathways and cervical lymph nodes, the lymphatic spread of oropharyngeal cancers usually occurs in a predictable way (121) from superior to inferior, the upper deep cervical lymph nodes (level II) being the first echelon at risk (122). Retropharyngeal

adenopathy is relatively common (123) and usually associated with lymphadenopathy in other neck levels; isolated retropharyngeal adenopathy without involvement of other lymph nodes also occurs particularly in posterior oropharyngeal wall cancer (124). For midline structures the risk of bilateral node involvement is much greater with base-of-tongue tumors than soft palate or posterior pharyngeal wall (125) (Table 12.5), similarly tonsillar carcinoma is also more prone to bilateral disease than soft palate and posterior pharyngeal wall tumors (Table 12.5).

Grade does not seem to be an influential factor because metastases are just as common with poorly differentiated lesions as with well-differentiated tumors. Site, however, does influence the occurrence of nodal disease because of the richer distribution of lymphatics in the tongue base and tonsillar fossae (Table 12.5). Tumors in these two sites have a high risk of metastatic nodal disease at presentation (Table 12.5 and 12.6).

Table 12.4 Nodal Status Depending on Oropharyngeal Sites

Site	N0	%	N1	%	N2	%	N3	%	N+	%	Total	%
Base of tongue (117)	49	(14.7)	54	(16.2)	191	(57.4)	39	(11.7)	284	(85.3)	333	(100)
Tonsil including tonsillar pillars (118)	153	(30.4)	68	(13.5)	233	(46.3)	49	(9.8)	350	(69.6)	503	(100)
Soft palate and uvula (119)	73	(50.3)	24	(16.6)	38	(26.2)	10	(6.9)	72	(49.7)	145	(100)
Posterior pharyngeal wall (120)[a]	28	(55.0)	7	(13.7)	12	(23.6)	4	(7.8)	23	(45.0)	51	(100)

[a]Includes posterior hypopharyngeal wall also.

Table 12.5 Nodal Metastasis in Base-of-tongue Carcinoma (117)

	N0	N1	N2a	N2b	N2c	N2 Total	N3	N+
Number of patients	49	54	25	85	81	191	39	284
Percentage (%)	14.7	16.2	7.5	25.5	24.4	57.4	11.7	85.3

Table 12.6 Nodal Metastasis in Tonsillar Carcinomas (118)

	N0	N1	N2a	N2b	N2c	N2 Total	N3	N+
Number of patients	153	68	48	123	62	233	49	350
Percentage (%)	30.4	13.5	9.5	24.5	12.3	46.3	9.8	69.6

Table 12.7   Clinical Stage Wise Distribution of Tongue Base and Tonsil Carcinoma

	Base of tongue (127)						Tonsil (128)					
	N0	N1	N2	N3	N+ (%)	Total	N0	N1	N2	N3	N+ (%)	Total
T1	67	16	43	10	50.7	136	14	15	12	3	68.1	44
T2	34	10	30	1	54.6	75	38	26	19	8	58.2	91
T3	7	5	6	2	65	20	22	21	18	6	67.1	67
T4	9	3	15	4	71	31	35	29	26	18	67.6	108
Total	117	34	94	17	145	262	109	91	75	35	201	310
(%)	44.6	13.0	35.9	6.5	55.4	100	35.2	29.3	24.2	11.3	64.8	100

The T stage of oropharyngeal carcinoma is based on size, and as a group there does not appear to be any overall correlation between size and N stage because positive nodes are seen just as commonly with T_1 as with T_4 tumors (Table 12.7). This is probably related to the dominant sites of the tonsil and to a lesser extent the tongue base because of their rich lymphatic drainage (123,126). For posterior wall and soft palate the numbers are too small for analysis, but node metastases are generally not so commonly seen from smaller tumors at these sites.

Staging

The tumor node metastasis (TNM) classification of SCC has undergone several changes but the accepted joint International Union Against Cancer/American Joint Committee on Cancer (UICC/AJCC; 2002) (129) classification for oropharyngeal tumors is shown in Tables 12.8 to 12.11 with the following provisions:

1. The classification only applies to SCC.
2. There must be histological verification of the disease and the grade may range from well-differentiated to poorly differentiated or anaplastic carcinoma. Spindle cell or basal cell variants may be seen.
3. The extent and staging must include clinical, radiological, and endoscopic findings.

Distant metastases at presentation are rarely seen, but in large series with long follow-up, the frequency may range between 10 to 15%, which is high and stands only second to hypopharynx among all HNSCCs (130). The rate of

distant metastasis for HNSCC in general varies between 4 and 26% (131–133). Lung is the most common site to be involved (46–83%) followed by bones (20–34%) and liver (3–6%) (130,134,135).

Second Primary SCC

The frequent development of second primary/multiple primary tumors (Figs. 12.6 and 12.7) may well be explained by the "field cancerization theory" proposed by Slaughter et al. (136) in 1953 that was later on supported by other researchers (101–103,137). This theory proposes that tumors develop in a multifocal fashion within a field of tissue chronically exposed to carcinogens.

The development of a second primary SCC within the head and neck is thought to approximate 2% per patient-year of follow-up (138). This risk may translate to a lifetime incidence of second primary between 5 and 36% patients who survive their initial HNSCC (139,140). Most commonly, these figures include second primary malignancies developing at all sites, not only those within the head and neck. Approximately two thirds of these reported second primaries occur within the head and neck region (139). For primaries occurring outside of the head and neck, pharyngeal primary HNSCC is most closely linked with subsequent development of esophageal carcinoma (digestive axis) (141); however, careful search should also be made in whole upper aerodigestive tract including respiratory axis (142). Continued smoking and alcohol consumption

Table 12.8   Classification of Primary Tumor (UICC/AJCC) (129)

TX	Primary tumor cannot be assessed
Tis	Carcinoma in situ
T0	No evidence of primary tumor
T1	Tumor 2 cm or smaller in greatest dimension
T2	Tumor larger than 2 cm but 4 cm or smaller in greatest dimension
T3	Tumor larger than 4 cm in greatest dimension
T4a	Tumor invades the larynx, deep/extrinsic muscle of tongue, medial pterygoid, hard palate, or mandible
T4b	Tumor invades lateral pterygoid muscle, pterygoid plates, lateral nasopharynx, or skull base or encases carotid artery

Abbreviation: UICC/AJCC, International Union Against Cancer/American Joint Committee on Cancer.

Table 12.9   Classification of Cervical Nodes

NX	Regional lymph nodes cannot be assessed
N0	No regional lymph node metastasis
N1	Metastasis in a single ipsilateral lymph node, 3 cm or smaller in greatest dimension
N2	Metastasis in a single ipsilateral lymph node, larger than 3 cm but 6 cm or smaller in greatest dimension, or in multiple ipsilateral lymph nodes, 6 cm or smaller in greatest dimension, or in bilateral or contralateral lymph nodes, 6 cm or smaller in greatest dimension
N2a	Metastasis in a single ipsilateral lymph node larger than 3 cm but 6 cm or smaller in greatest dimension
N2b	Metastasis in multiple ipsilateral lymph nodes, 6 cm or smaller in greatest dimension
N2c	Metastasis in bilateral or contralateral lymph nodes, 6 cm or smaller in greatest dimension
N3	Metastasis in a lymph node larger than 6 cm in greatest dimension

Table 12.10 Classification of Metastatic Disease

MX	Distant metastasis cannot be assessed
M0	No distant metastasis
M1	Distant metastasis

Table 12.11 Stage Grouping

Stage 0	Tis, N0, M0
Stage I	T1, N0, M0
Stage II	T2, N0, M0
Stage III	T3, N0, M0
	T1, N1, M0
	T2, N1, M0
	T3, N1, M0
Stage IVA	T4a, N0, M0
	T4a, N1, M0
	T1, N2, M0
	T2, N2, M0
	T3, N2, M0
	T4a, N2, M0

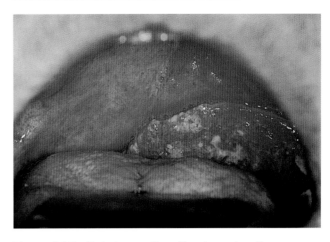

Figure 12.6 Patient presenting with a large ulcerating squamous carcinoma of the soft palate was also found on examination to have a synchronous asymptomatic squamous carcinoma of the floor of mouth (Fig. 12.7).

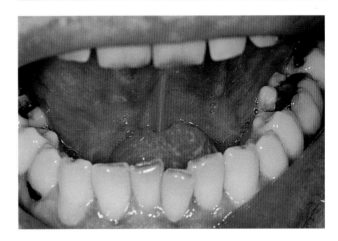

Figure 12.7 Patient with a synchronous asymptomatic squamous carcinoma of the floor of mouth (Fig. 12.6).

after treatment has been shown to have increased risk of development of second primary tumors within the aerodigestive tract (143,144).

Lymphoepithelioma

Otherwise known as undifferentiated carcinoma of nasopharyngeal type (UCNT) this variant of SCC is found most commonly, as its name implies, in the nasopharynx. It is however also found in the tonsil and base of tongue. The squamous component may be extremely undifferentiated, but the lymphoid element is composed of nonneoplastic lymphocytes that permeate widely throughout the tumor. Surface marker studies have shown these lymphoid cells to be reactive B cells, T helper, and T suppressor cells. Metastases are characterized by the presence of only the squamous element similar to the primary tumor and do not contain lymphocytes. The important clinical features of this tumor are its increased tendency to metastasize, similarity to nasopharyngeal UCNT, and also its extreme radiosensitivity.

Lymphoma

Due to the abundant lymphoid tissue in the oropharynx, non-Hodgkin's lymphoma occurs in this region as extranodal lymphatic disease. Also, adenopathies may be present at sites unusual for an untreated carcinoma, or the oropharyngeal lesion may be associated with another extranodal neck lymphoma localization (145). Non-Hodgkin's lymphoma accounts for about 8% of oropharyngeal tumors (146), the usual sites being the tonsil (5%) and base of tongue (3%), but more commonly presents in the head and neck as nodal metastases. The most common type of lymphoma presenting in the oropharynx is the B cell lymphoma that is a large cell lymphoma of high-grade malignancy. T cell lymphomas are rare in the oropharynx but do show a well-documented association with T lymphotrophic virus type 1 especially in Japan and the Caribbean countries (147).

The classification of lymphomas has undergone major modifications over the past 20 years, and a working formulation has been devised by the National Cancer Institute (148). A comprehensive review of lymphomas of the oropharynx and head and neck is given elsewhere (1).

Salivary Gland Tumors

Salivary gland tumors account for about 3 to 5% (149) of all tumors of the oropharynx, and the majority of such tumors arising from the minor salivary glands. In the soft palate, these are often benign pleomorphic adenomas, but in other oropharyngeal sites malignant tumors, such as mucoepidermoid and adenoid cystic carcinoma, predominate (150). Spiro has described a large series of minor salivary gland tumors, 3% of which affected the oropharynx, and almost all of them arose in the tonsillar fossa (149). The majority of these are adenoid cystic carcinomas, and they behave in a similar way to those arising in other sites within the head and neck in that they do have a propensity to spread along nerve sheaths in the perineural lymphatics with late metastases to lymph nodes, lung, and bone. Although the short-term prognosis for these tumors is very good with an 80% 5-year survival rate, eventually about 60 to 80% of patients die from or with metastatic disease.

Metastatic Disease

Metastases to the oropharynx from primaries outside the head and neck region are rare but are occasionally found (Fig. 12.8).

CLINICAL PRESENTATION

Symptoms

Diagnosis of oropharyngeal carcinoma in its early stages is uncommon, and more than two thirds of patients present in advanced stage (stage III or IV) (Table 12.12). Only 4 to 10% of patients are stage I at presentation, roughly 10 to 20% are stage II, and about 70% are stage III and IV (151). The reason for late presentation of disease is the vagueness of initial presenting symptoms such as soreness or discomfort in the throat particularly on swallowing and otalgia that are reported in about 38 and 6% of the patients, respectively (5). The most common presenting complaint

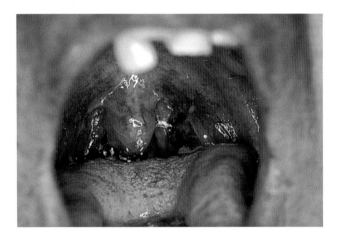

Figure 12.8 Metastatic malignant melanoma in the left tonsil from a primary located on skin of the back.

in oropharyngeal cancers is neck mass which is seen in approximately 57 to 79% of the cases (5). It can often be misdiagnosed as a branchial cyst when it lies in the jugulo-digastric region. Sometimes these nodes can rapidly enlarge due to hemorrhage or necrosis and are often tender. Other symptoms include a foreign-body sensation in the throat or altered voice with a "plum in the throat" quality. For more advanced tumors otalgia and throat pain become more pronounced and ulceration, necrosis and secondary infection may result in foul breath. There may also be progressive impairment of tongue movement affecting speech and swallowing.

Physical Examination

A full clinical examination of the upper aerodigestive tract and the neck including fiber-optic examination is essential. The extent of involvement is often misleading on inspection, and bimanual palpation of the tumor must be undertaken in all patients. The pharyngoglossoepiglottic folds and the posterior surface of the soft palate are blind spots that are not readily accessible to routine examination, and the importance of a thorough examination cannot be overemphasized. Anterior faucial pillar, soft palate, and tonsillar tumors may be visible with good lighting, but advanced lesions may be associated with trismus, which will make oral examination difficult. Surface appearance of SCCs is either ulcerative (Fig. 12.9) or exophytic (Fig. 12.10), although early lesions of the tonsil or tongue base arising in the lymphatic crypts may not be visible and may only be detectable on palpation under anesthetic or following tonsillectomy. In general the exophytic tumor spreads superficially and may be associated with other areas of leukoplakia in the oral cavity; the ulcerative type invades deeply. An adenocarcinoma may present as a smooth lobulated swelling without surface ulceration (Fig. 12.11), and a malignant lymphoma typically causes nodular enlargements in the tonsil or tongue base (Fig. 12.12).

Sensory and motor function should be assessed, particularly mobility of the tongue as well as fixation. A twelfth-nerve paralysis causes wasting of the ipsilateral tongue with deviation to the affected side on protrusion, but in the early stages fasciculations may be apparent. Palatal movement may be impaired by the tumor mass, but a palsy of the vagus nerve near the skull base will also cause weakness (and also a vocal cord palsy). Impaired sensation over the anterior chin distribution of the mental nerve and the lateral part of the tongue is an ominous sign indicating invasion of the inferior alveolar nerve or the lingual nerve in the infratemporal fossa.

Table 12.12 Overall Staging at Presentation

Reference	Stage I (%)	Stage II (%)	Stage III (%)	Stage IV (%)
Chen et al. (2007) (151)	7.7	11.9	21.5	59
Preuss et al. (2007) (10)	8.6	14.8	22.5	49.2
Kljajic et al. (2007) (152)	6	15	24	55
Hannisdal et al. (2003) (128)	4.5	12.2	27.4	55.8
Johansen et al. (2000) (108)	8	19	46	28
Woolger et al. (1999) (153)	7.5	37.5	22.5	32.5
Mak-Kregar et al. (1995) (109)	7	17	24	50

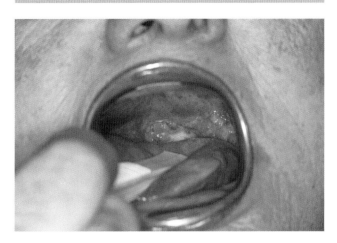

Figure 12.9 Squamous cell carcinoma of the soft palate (ulcerative type).

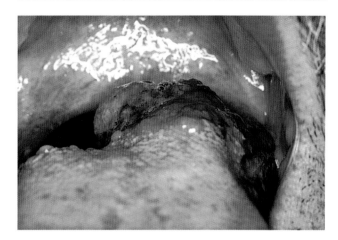

Figure 12.11 Adenocarcinoma of the base of the tongue.

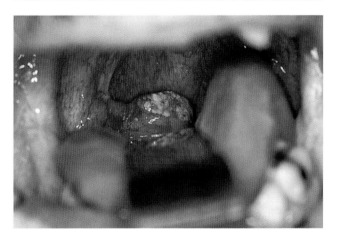

Figure 12.10 Squamous cell carcinoma of the right tonsil (exophytic type).

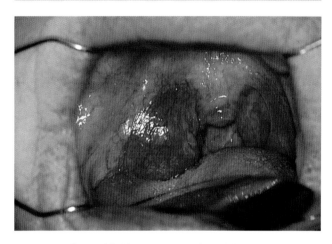

Figure 12.12 Lymphoma of the right tonsil.

Fiber-optic examination either with a rigid or flexible scope under local anesthetic has greatly enhanced the ease of examination of the pharynx and larynx, particularly in assessing the lower extent of the tumor and mobility of structures at or below the level of the hyoid. It is also valuable for estimating invasion of the nasopharynx. Indirect laryngoscopy with a mirror is no longer deemed sufficient for optimum assessment.

Examination of the neck must be carried out systematically, and each level must be carefully palpated to detect lymph node enlargement or deep invasion of the tumor. The deep cervical chain of nodes is particularly difficult to assess correctly especially if the patient has a thick neck or there is muscle spasm. At best, clinical examination of the neck has a 30% inaccuracy rate (154) with 10 to 30% false negative and/or false positive (155,156).

Nodal metastases from SCCs are typically hard and irregular and when small are generally mobile. As they enlarge, those in the deep cervical chain (levels II, III, and IV)

initially become attached to the structures in the carotid sheath and the overlying sternomastoid muscle with restriction of vertical mobility (Fig. 12.13), but later become attached to the deeper structures in the prevertebral region with absolute fixation. Cystic degeneration or necrosis in a metastatic jugulodigastric node may cause rapid enlargement and may initially be confused for a branchial cyst, with potential delay in proper diagnosis. Lymphomatous nodes have a firm and rubbery consistency and are generally larger and multiple with matting together of adjacent nodes.

INVESTIGATIONS
Fine-needle Aspiration Cytology
Any suspicious swelling or node in the neck should have FNAC at initial consultation, which should allow rapid differentiation between a branchial cyst, lymphoma, and SCC. Aspiration of cystic fluid from a necrotic metastatic node may give a false negative result and should be repeated

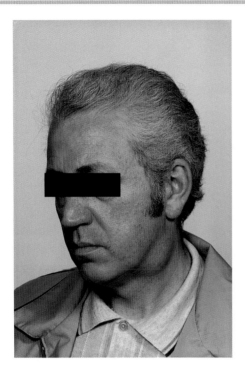

Figure 12.13 N3 metastasis from a T1 squamous cell carcinoma of the tonsil.

to sample the solid portion or wall of the cyst, if necessary under ultrasound guidance. In cases of lymphomas FNAC is usually inconclusive, mandating FNA biopsy/open biopsy.

Radiological Investigations

Orthopantomogram may be necessary

- to assess dentition prior to radiotherapy (RT)
- if a mandibulotomy is planned
- to show mandibular invasion.

Chest X-ray [Postero-anterior (PA) and lateral] is essential to rule out

- metastatic carcinoma
- synchronous bronchial primary
- coexisting acute or chronic pulmonary disease.

Suspicious lesions will need further investigation with chest computed tomography (CT) scan, lung function studies, or bronchoscopy. Some times CT guided FNAC/fine-needle aspiration biopsy may be required to establish the diagnosis.

CT and/or magnetic resonance imaging (MRI) of the head and neck are essential:

- For assessing the extent of the primary tumor and its relation to adjacent structures; an MRI is preferable to CT scan to show up small tongue base tumors and to assess the extent of soft tissue invasion (157).
- To assess any mandibular invasion, which is far better shown on CT scan (157).
- For accurate evaluation of the neck to assess the presence, the site, the size, and invasive potential of cervical

lymphadenopathy and in particular their relation to the carotid artery. Following RT treatment to the neck these examinations are less dependable in accurately assessing disease in the carotid sheath because of postradiotherapy fibrosis, which may be mistaken for tumor.

- To assess [clinically negative (N0) necks], particularly in obese patients, those with a thick neck or where there is spasm, and help identify possible nodes in the deep cervical chain or parapharyngeal space.
- To help distinguish between lymphoma and carcinomatous nodes.

The calculated sensitivity of CT and MRI for detecting lymph node metastases ranges from 36 to 94%, whereas specificity ranges between 5% and 98% (158).

Ultrasound Examination

Ultrasound examination of the neck to detect metastatic nodal disease is more sensitive than palpation and has a specificity of about 75%. The specificity is improved to more than 90% with the use of ultrasound-guided FNAC as compared with CT and MRI scans (approximately 80%) (159). This technique is very dependable in experienced hands but is not really practical in the routine head and neck clinic.

PET and PET CT

Positron emission tomography (PET) scanning is a useful imaging modality that is helpful in detecting neoplasms by demonstrating an increased concentration of radionucleotidelabeled tracer in neoplastic tissue (160). The most commonly used tracer is a glucose analog tagged with a positron-emitting isotope of fluorine: 2- [18F] fluoro-2-deoxy-d-glucose (FDG) (161,162). Malignant tumor cells are known to be metabolically more active than the cells within normal surrounding tissue. This metabolic hyperactivity is represented by increased tracer concentration on PET in the area of the tumor cells allowing for the use of FDG-PET imaging in the detection of head and neck cancers (163). It is important to note, however, that accumulation of FDG tracer can also occur in areas of infection, inflammation, and normal lymphoid tissue leading to potentially misleading PET scan results (164,165).

The sensitivity of FDG-PET in detecting cervical lymph node metastases of head and neck cancers varies between 67 and 96% whereas specificity ranges between 82 and 100% (166,167). These figures appear to be more impressive than other conventional imaging modalities in detecting nodal involvement (168–170). Because SCC of oropharynx has higher metastatic potential than SCC of other head and neck regions, it is important to determine the presence and extent of metastases from oropharyngel SCC at initial stage (164).

FDG-PET is also more accurate in detecting primary tumors in general as well as in patients with unknown primary neck metastases. Rusthoven et al (171) was found to be 88% sensitive, 75% specific, and 79 % accurate in detecting primary SCC of head neck region in a study involving 302 patients. However, they reported lower sensitivity rates for base-of-tongue cancers and lower specificity for tonsillar carcinomas (171). Sensitivity of FDG-PET in detecting occult primary varies between 25% and 50% (161,172).

Although FDG-PET has difficulty locating sites of abnormality relative to normal structures in functional images, the combination of FDG-PET and CT can overcome these limitations by fusing the anatomic data of CT with the functional data of FDG-PET (173,174). The combination of FDG-PET and CT has been reported to be more accurate than either alone in the detection and anatomic localization of head and neck cancers and thus may affect patient care and final outcome (175,176). PET has also shown to be of value in detecting recurrent HNSCC, including oropharyngeal cancers (177).

To summarize, potential clinical applications of FDG PET may be:

- to assess occult metastatic nodal disease, which is not amenable to detection by clinical examination or any other imaging modality.
- to assess occult distant metastatic disease in lung or bones or to rule out a possible granulomatous lesion in lung and prevent from unnecessary morbidity (172).
- to detect second primary carcinomas in head neck region or elsewhere (161).
- pretreatment staging (178); diagnosis may be upstaged in up to 20% patients, requiring gross alteration in treatment regimen especially from M0 to M1 (172).
- to find an unknown primary carcinoma (161).
- to detect primary HNSCC greater than 1 cm size (172).
- to detect recurrent disease (161,177).
- for treatment monitoring and evaluation of primarily treated patient (161,172).
- for proper intensity-modulated radiotherapy (IMRT) planning (161,179).
- as a prognostic marker in HNSCC (161).

Examination Under Anesthetic and Biopsy

A biopsy may be taken under local anesthetic in the clinic when appropriate, and this may suffice in elderly or infirm patients where there may be unacceptable risks with a general anesthetic. In all other patients a full examination of the upper aerodigestive tract under general anesthesia is essential:

- for biopsy of the primary
- to look for a possible synchronous primary
- to assess fixation of the primary, for example to the mandible
- for bimanual palpation, particularly lesions of the tongue base
- to assess involvement of the pre-epiglottic space, larynx and hypopharynx
- to assess the neck and perform FNAC if necessary
- to assess the airway and carry out tracheostomy if necessary
- for percutaneous endoscopic gastrostomy (PEG) insertion if nutritional support is required
- for dental extraction prior to treatment
- for bone marrow aspirate in cases of lymphoma.

Integrated Multidisciplinary Clinic

Full evaluation of the patient with all investigations should be discussed in a joint assessment (180,181) with

- head and neck surgeon
- radiologist

- pathologist
- radiotherapist
- medical oncologist
- reconstructive surgeon,
- dental oncologist
- speech therapist
- clinical nurse specialist
- dietician.

TREATMENT
General Principles

The goals of therapy are cure, organ preservation, attenuation of the morbidities associated with therapy, and improvement in quality of life (181). For those patients who achieve cure, second primary cancers pose a significant risk; therefore, prevention of second malignancies are goals of therapy in the treatment of patients with oropharyngeal cancers and HNSCC (182).

Curative treatment of oropharyngeal carcinoma is either by surgery or RT or a combination of both (7). As with other head and neck cancers, chemotherapy and newer forms of biological therapy or immunotherapy do not give consistent results and at the moment are reserved for patients with advanced or recurrent disease following conventional therapy. Early disease (T_{1-2}) is generally best treated by single modality, either RT or surgery with equivalent results (183). Radiation may be the preferred modality where the functional deficit will be great, such as the tongue base or tonsil (117,184). For advanced lesions (stage III and IV), combined therapy with radical surgery followed by postoperative radiotherapy (PORT) is generally accepted as giving the best chance of cure and still remains the gold standard (15,183). The most difficult dilemmas however in the treatment of oropharyngeal carcinoma concern the choice of optimal treatment for T_{3-4} tumors where radical surgery may well involve unacceptable loss of the larynx, tongue, or both, leading to swallowing and speech impairment. This ultimately results in decreased quality of life in many aspects, including nutrition, social functioning, and personal hygiene (185). In these instances, organ preservation using a combination of induction chemotherapy and radiation should be considered as an option (186–189).

The benefit of concomittent chemoradiotherapy compared with RT alone or induction chemotherapy followed by radiation (151) is now well established and has been shown to have improved outcome in patients with locally advanced disease that is surgically unrecectable (190,191). A trial has shown that chemotherapy (i.e., carboplatin plus fluorouracil) with RT provides better local control and improved 3-year actuarial overall survival (OS) and disease-free survival (DFS) than daily RT alone (186,187). In some situations curative treatment may not be applicable, and palliative therapy may be the only option.

In general, the choice for the individual patient will depend on a number of factors. The site and size of the primary tumor is one of the most important factors in determining treatment. Where cure rates for surgery and RT are similar, the choice is usually that which causes least functional disability (117,184). Deeply ulcerative lesions of the oropharynx are best treated with initial surgery followed by PORT as the results of salvage surgery in this setting are poor.

It is now commonly agreed that the single most important prognostic factor in oropharyngeal and other HNSCCs is the nodal status of the disease (113,192,193). The presence of nodal metastases in the neck at presentation reduces the prognosis by about 50% (194,195); and although radical RT may be effective in N0 and early N1 nodal disease, optimum treatment for N+ disease usually involves a combination of primary surgery with PORT (196).

Radiotherapy

RT has been the major treatment modality for the past 80 years, as it is only quite recently that improved reconstructive techniques have made a surgical approach possible. Despite surgical advances there is evidence that primary treatment by RT gives equal survival rates and a better quality of life than primary surgical treatment, especially in the case of soft palate and base-of-tongue tumors (118). Mostly RT is delivered solely by external beam techniques, but in some centers, especially in France, brachytherapy boosts are used. Because most cases of carcinoma of the oropharynx have in the past been treated by external beam, this disease has been the frequent subject of trials of new approaches in RT.

Patients should be counseled to stop smoking before beginning RT as smoking during treatment with RT has been shown to lower response rates and overall survival in these patients (197). Higher incidences (30–40%) of postirradiation hypothyroidism have been noted in patients who received external-beam radiation therapy (EBRT) to the entire thyroid gland or to the pituitary gland. Therefore thyroid function testing of patients should be considered prior to therapy and as part of posttreatment follow-up (198,199).

External Beam Radiotherapy

The results of external beam radiotherapy (EBRT) are best seen in large series from Canada, France, and the U.S.A. and show small but steady improvement in local tumor control and survival since the advent of supervoltage therapy. Mendenhall et al. (117) reported more than 90% local control rates (LCR) for early base-of-tongue tumors using EBRT alone, whereas LCR for advanced lesion varied between 53

and 82%. Similar results have been shown by some other researchers as well (Table 12.13). Charbonneau et al. (200) achieved nearly 90% LCRs for early tonsillar cancers treated with EBRT alone, whereas LCR for advanced tonsillar carcinoma varied between 60 and 72%. Similar results have been reported in some other studies also (Table 12.14).

There are few reports of results from the U.K. reflecting the relative rarity of the disease. A series of 144 patients was treated at the South Wales Radiotherapy Centre from the introduction of supervoltage RT in 1960 up to 1971 (204). They were treated according to the philosophy of the Christie Hospital in Manchester, namely irradiation of small, localized volumes over a 3-week period without elective nodal irradiation. A series of 127 patients treated at the Royal Marsden Hospital (RMH) from 1983 to 1991 (205) showed some improvement in survival (40 vs. 28% at 5 years) and local control (71 vs. 57% in radically irradiated patients), attributable to improvements in RT techniques and supportive care together with the use of elective nodal irradiation; the increase in survival was modest because of the influence of distant metastases and deaths from other causes.

Results of treatment of carcinoma of the soft palate are generally similar to those of the tonsillar carcinoma, but all series are relatively small. Carcinoma arising on the posterior wall of the oropharynx is so rare that there are no reliable treatment statistics.

Fractionation

The American College of Radiology "patterns of fractionation" study reviewed the results of RT for tonsillar carcinoma in nine centers in U.K., the U.S.A., and Canada that used different once-per-day fractionation schedules. No significant differences could be found between the widely used 2 Gy per day for 6½ to 7 weeks, and the 3- or 4-week schedules used at Manchester and Toronto (206). There does however appear to be an advantage to using hyperfractionation. A regime using twice daily fractions of 1.2 Gy to a total dose of 74 to 79 Gy was introduced at the University of Florida in 1978; retrospective comparison with daily fractionation revealed an improvement in local control for all sites and T stages, especially the more advanced (207).

Table 12.13 Local Control Rates for Carcinoma of Base of Tongue Treated with External Beam Radiation

Reference	Number of patients	T1 (%)	T2 (%)	T3 (%)	T4 (%)
Mendenhall et al. (2006) (117)	333	98	92	82	53
Brunin et al. (1999) (201)	216	93	66	45	18
Mak et al. (1995) (202)	54	100	96	67	NR

Abbreviation: NR, Not reported.

Table 12.14 Local Control Rates for Tonsillar Carcinoma Treated with External Beam Radiation

Reference	Number of patients	T1 (%)	T2 (%)	T3 (%)	T4(%)
Charbonneau et al. (2006) (200)	164	91	84	72	60
Mendenhall et al. (2006) (118)	503	88	84	78	61
Perez et al. (1998) (203)	154	76	63	59	33

A multicenter controlled trial conducted by the European organization for research and treatment of cancer (EORTC) compared 70 Gy given in daily fractions of 2 Gy with 80.5 Gy in twice daily fractions of 1.15 Gy, both over the same time of 7 weeks; the hyperfractionated arm gave a significantly higher LCR with no greater morbidity, but subgroup analysis showed that the advantage was confined to the T3 group (208).

There is also some evidence of the benefits of accelerated RT. The continuous hyperfractionated accelerated radiotherapy (CHART) regime showed equal local control with reduced late morbidity (209), whereas the EORTC trial of an accelerated hyperfractionated split-course regime led to a better local LCR but increased late morbidity (210). The concomitant boost technique introduced at the MD Anderson Hospital shows promising early results, but which are yet to be confirmed in a randomized trial (202). The Danish head and neck cancer study (DAHANCA)-7 trial compared five against six 2 Gy fractions per week, to the same total dose; six fractions per week gave a higher LCR, with increased early, but not late, morbidity (211).

Hypoxia

Hypoxia is a characteristic feature of all malignant tumors (212,213). It can render tumorous cells up to three times more resistant to radiation relative to aerobic cells (214). Hypoxia has been shown to be an important determinant of locoregional control (LRC) and OS in many tumors including head and neck cancers (215,216), and its presence compromises tumor control, DFS, and OS (217).

There is evidence of the oxygen effect in RT of oropharyngeal carcinoma, as demonstrated by the early trials of irradiation in high pressure oxygen (218). In the DAHANCA-5 trial of the hypoxic cell sensitizer nimorazole, 414 patients were randomized, of whom 187 had oropharyngeal carcinoma. The nimorazole group had a highly significantly better LCR and disease-free rate, but the oropharynx cases were not reported separately (219). The combination of nimorazole with six fractions per week in the DAHANCA-7 study appears to be the most effective regime yet studied, but it could not make a noticeable impact among clinicians. Currently newer hypoxia targeting agents like misonidazole,

pimonidazole, and hypoxic cell cytotoxin tirapazamine are under investigation and hope to offer some benefit in future (180,220).

Brachytherapy

Tumors at all sites in the oropharynx can be treated by interstitial implantation. Brachytherapists nowadays almost invariably use loops of plastic tubing, which are afterloaded with iridium-192 wire. The loops are inserted through either the lateral neck skin in the case of tonsillar and soft palate tumors (221) or the submental region in the case of base-of-tongue tumors (222). Brachytherapy can be used as monotherapy or as a combination therapy (boost) with equivalent success rates. A dose of 46 to 55 Gy is delivered by EBRT that is subsequently augmented (boosted) further by 18 to 36 Gy with the use of iridium-192 wires implanted in the tumor. This kind of brachytherapy boost is commonly known as low dose rate interstitial brachytherapy (223).

Recently a newer technique of high dose rate interstitial brachytherapy with EBRT has shown promising results with LCRs of around 90% in early and advanced disease (223,224).

Implantation of the oropharynx is technically difficult and therefore applicable only in centers treating a large number of cases where the expertise can be acquired. There is no added advantage in terms of LCR and OS with brachytherapy as compared to other techniques of radiation; it is no longer used in most of the centers except occasionally for a second primary tumor in a patient who has already received RT. Typical results of brachytherapy boosts are shown in Tables 12.15 and 12.16.

Intensity-modulated Radiotherapy

Over the past decade there have been rapid advances in RT techniques. Altered fractionation RT, specifically hyperfractionation and accelerated RT, have been associated with improved LRC and DFS in these patients (184,230) and in patients with head and neck cancers in general (231). IMRT has been shown to decrease the radiation dose to critical structures without compromising target dosimetry (232,233). Early reports with IMRT have shown improvements in

Table 12.15 Local Control Rates of Base-of-tongue Carcinoma by Combined External Beam and Brachytherapy

Reference	Number of patients	T1 (%)	T2 (%)	T3 (%)	T4 (%)
Gibbs et al. (2003) (225)	41	85	89	89	70
Harrison LB et al. (1998) (226)	68	87	93	82	100
Lusinchi et al. (1989) (227)	108	85	50	69	NR

Abbreviation: NR, not reported.

Table 12.16 Local Control Rates of Tonsillar Fossa Carcinoma by Combined External Beam and Brachytherapy

Reference	Number of patients	T1 (%)	T2 (%)	T3 (%)	T4 (%)
Pernot et al. (1994) (228)	361	89	85	67	NR
Puthawala et al. (1985) (229)	80	NR	NR	NR	NR

Abbreviation: NR, not reported.

toxicity, particularly xerostomia due to parotid gland sparing (234–237) and radiation-induced mucositis (220). This can be attributed to relatively low dose delivery (25–50 Gy) to potentially less involved areas and at the same time maintaining complete tumoricidal dose (70–75 Gy) to the gross tumor volume. IMRT with or without chemotherapy has been shown to achieve 88 to 98% local and LRC and has demonstrated 69 to 94% 5-year survival in oropharyngeal cancers (Table 12.17).

Among newer RT techniques, IMRT is associated with significantly reduced rates of skin and mucous membrane complications as compared to three-dimensional conformal radiotherapy or accelerated fractionation with concomitant boost technique. Only 6% of patients treated with IMRT had long-term xerostomia compared to 79% treated with other techniques. Reported local LCRs at 2 years for three-dimensional conformal radiotherapy are 81% and for concomitant boost technique are 82% which are much less than IMRT. This further support its continued use in the management of patients with locally advanced SCC of the oropharynx (171).

Concomitant Chemoradiation

Use of concomitant chemoradiotherapy (CRT) is based on a belief that chemotherapy synergistically acts with RT by inhibiting repair of DNA damage caused by RT, arresting cells in radiosensitive phases and possibly preventing regrowth between RT treatments. In addition it is thought that chemotherapy may treat radio-resistant tumor lineages such as hypoxic cells (244). The addition of concomitant chemotherapy to RT has been shown to be superior to RT alone for LRC and survival in head and neck SCC (245) (Table 12.18). A meta-analysis of 63 randomized prospective trials published between 1965 and 1993 showed an 8% absolute survival advantage in the subset of patients receiving concomitant chemotherapy and RT (190). Concomitant cisplatin-based chemotherapy has been shown to improve LRC and OS in patients with stage III to IV disease (246). Some more recent studies have shown concurrent chemoradiation to achieve good survival rates in early oropharyngeal tumors, but survival rates for advanced disease are reported to be poor which needs to be investigated further (247,248).

Nodal Irradiation

In view of the high incidence of occult metastases in the [clinically negative (N0) neck] elective nodal irradiation is widely advocated. In any case the first echelon lymph nodes are in the path of the radiation beams with most radiotherapeutic techniques. Tumors of the base of tongue, soft palate, and posterior wall are treated with lateral opposing beams, and the first echelon nodes (levels II and III) bilaterally are included. Well-lateralized T_{1-2} N0 tonsillar carcinomas rarely give rise to contralateral nodal metastases, so irradiation can be limited to the primary tumor and homolateral nodes with consequent reduction of subsequent xerostomia. Node-positive cases often have widespread subclinical nodal involvement, so elective irradiation of all node areas bilaterally is advisable (252).

In node-positive cases in which the primary tumor is treated by RT alone, the management of the neck is controversial. Some institutions use the policy of specifically targeting the gross neck disease with full tumoricidal dose of 70 Gy. Whereas others prefer to limit the radiation dose to the neck disease to 60 Gy when a neck dissection is planned to limit the potential morbidity in a radiated field.

Table 12.17 Clinical Outcomes with IMRT ± Chemotherapy for Oropharyngeal Cancers

Study	No of patients	Time point (years)	Local control (%)	Locoregional control (%)	Overall survival (%)
Hodge et al. (2007) (238)	52	3	NR	96	88
Garden et al. (2007) (239)	51	2	96	94	94
De Arruda et al. (2006) (240)	48	2	98	88	98
Mendenhall et al. (2006) (241)	64	2	NR	90	89
Milano et al. (2006) (242)	69	3	NR	94	69
Studer et al. (2006) (243)	53	2	88	93	87
Yao et al. (2005) (236)	56	3	NR	98	82

Abbreviations: IMRT, intensity-modulated radiotherapy; NR, not reported.

Table 12.18 Randomized Trials Comparing Outcome of Postoperative RT Versus Concomitant CRT

Reference	Arm	LRC (%)	DFS (%)	OS (%)
RTOG 9501	RT	71.3	29.1	37
Cooper et al. (2006) (249)	CRT	79.6	37.4	45.1
Bernier et al. (2004) (188)				
Cooper et al. (2004) (250)				
EORTC 22931	RT	69	36	40
Bernier et al. (2005) (251)	CRT	82	47	53
Bernier et al. (2004) (188)				

Abbreviations: RTOG, Radiation Therapy Oncology Group; EORTC, European Organization for Research and Treatment of Cancer; LRC, locoregional control; DFS, disease-free survival; OS, overall survival; RT, radiotherapy; CRT, chemo-radiotherapy

In these cases the only nodes that receive a full tumoricidal dose of 70 Gy are those in close proximity to the primary tumors and are treated incidentally (7). Undifferentiated carcinoma, especially of the nasopharyngeal type (253), is very radiosensitive, and LCRs by RT are high so that neck dissection is unnecessary. For other types of SCC many authorities recommend neck dissection, either before or after RT to the primary. However, size-for-size primary tumors and nodal metastases in the same patient tend to be equally radiosensitive (254), and RT failures at the primary site are as difficult to salvage surgically as nodal recurrences, in contrast to other head and neck sites such as the supraglottis. Therefore, in patients with small nodal metastases that become impalpable after RT there may be little or no gain from planned neck dissection. Peters et al. (255) reported only three isolated neck failures in a series of 62 node-positive patients managed by RT without planned neck dissection.

Postoperative Radiotherapy
The indications for PORT are the same as for other head and neck sites, namely large or infiltrating primary tumors, close or positive resection margins, multiple nodal involvement or ECS from a nodal metastasis (10,196,256). Postoperative radiotherapy has been shown to improve LRC rates and survival in patients with ECS (257). The RMH gives 60 Gy to the primary site and involved nodal areas, or 66 Gy to areas where gross residual tumor is suspected. Where there is unilateral nodal involvement the opposite side of the neck is irradiated electively to a dose of 50 Gy.

The British Association of Head & Neck Oncology (now has a consensus to give adjuvant RT to high recurrence risk patients with positive margins or ECS (258); however its use in intermediate recurrence risk patients may be associated with increased morbidity (259).

Surgical Management
Transoral Excision
Early tumors of the tonsil, faucial arches, and the soft palate may be adequately excised per orally. The resultant defect may be closed primarily, skin grafted or left to epithelialize. Larger tumors requiring bony resection, and more posteriorly located tumors, require more extensive access; and every effort must be made to carry out the surgical excision under direct vision. Selected, superficial early lesions, especially those involving the soft palate or posterior pharyngeal wall, may be resected using a transoral endoscopic laser (260) combined with discontinuous neck dissection as indicated (261). Steiner W et al. successfully used transoral laser microsurgery technique for early tongue base tumors. Tumors with deep infiltration of musculature (ulcerative rather than exophytic) or involving adjacent sites makes poor candidates for transoral laser microsurgery approach (262).

Transhyoid Pharyngotomy
This is a useful approach to small tumors of the base of the tongue even in the presence of limited involvement of the supraglottic larynx. The hyoid bone is transected or excised and the vallecula is entered blindly (Fig. 12.14). After resection of the tumor inferiorly from the neck, the resultant defect is closed primarily. Access is limited, and the technique must be used only in very selected patients to excise small lesions. Great care must be exercised to avoid damaging the lingual artery and the hypoglossal nerve if any tongue remnant is preserved on the side of the lesion. The advantage of this technique is that it maintains the integrity of the mandible and preserves the mobility of the tongue by preventing scarring in the anterior oral cavity (263). Larger tumors of the tonsil and base of the tongue may be excised using a combination of the transoral and transhyoid approaches (264).

Lateral Pharyngotomy
Small lesions of the posterior and lateral pharyngeal walls may be excised through a lateral pharyngotomy. The mucosa of the pyriform sinus is stripped off the medial surface of the thyroid ala that is retracted anteriorly. The superior laryngeal nerve is carefully preserved, and the pyriform sinus is entered in its superior aspect to gain access to the oropharynx. The superior extent of the mucosal incision is limited by the mandible, and this approach can be safely used in only selected instances.

Anterior Midline Glossotomy
Small, locally limited lesions of the base of the tongue may be resected via this approach. The tongue is bisected anteriorly in its relatively avascular midline to access the region of the base (Fig. 12.15). After adequate resection of the tumor, the defect is closed primarily, and the bisected halves of the anterior tongue are sutured back in layers. Although the functional outcome of this operation is excellent, it must be stressed that only very small lesions in selected patients are suitable. Larger tumors cannot be adequately excised without creating a substantial soft tissue defect with a tongue remnant of doubtful viability, and one of the other more extensive approaches must be used in these patients.

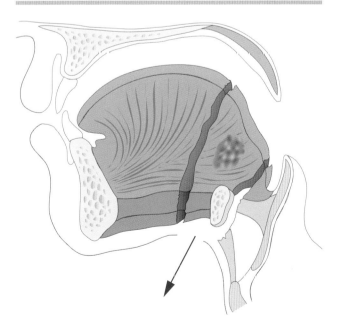

Figure 12.14 Transhyoid pharyngotomy.

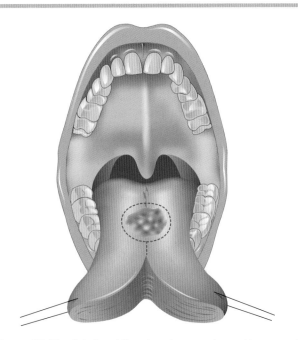

Figure 12.15 Anterior midline glossotomy may be used to approach selected, small lesions of the base of the tongue.

Mandibulotomy and Mandibular Swing

A mandibulotomy approach with paralingual extension, the so-called mandibular swing has been used effectively for resection of advanced tumors of the oropharynx (265). The extent of exposure and the functional consequences of the procedure depend a great deal on the site of the mandibular osteotomy. Three types of mandibulotomy have been described, and the relative advantages and disadvantages of each have been outlined in Table 12.19.

The paramedian mandibulotomy is designed to be anatomically less disruptive and results in lesser functional deficit postoperatively. It is also inherently more stable mechanically than a lateral osteotomy and, if RT becomes necessary, lies outside the limit of the lateral portal. These features along with the disadvantages of median (Fig. 12.16), and lateral mandibulotomy make the paramedian mandibulotomy the procedure of choice in access to the oropharynx (Tables 12.20 and 12.21).

The lower lip is split in the midline, and the gingivolabial sulcus is incised toward the side of the osteotomy leaving an adequate mucosal cuff to facilitate subsequent closure. The mandible is exposed by raising short cheek flaps bilaterally, dissecting in the plane above the periosteum and taking care to limit dissection to the point where the mental nerve exits the mental foramen. For a paramedian mandibulotomy, the osteotomy is sited between the lateral incisor and canine teeth. This is a natural area where the roots curve away from each other and are at minimal risk of exposure or direct injury. There is considerable debate in the literature about the shape of the osteotomy; notched (Fig. 12.17) or stair-step (Fig. 12.18) osteotomies tend to be preferred over a straight one (Fig. 12.19) because of their mechanical stability. Both these osteotomies are technically more demanding, and the mandible is more liable to fracture if the horizontal cut of the stair-step is sited too close to the inferior border of the bone. An oscillating power saw with the appropriate attachments is essential for accurate bony cuts. The mucosa and muscles of the floor of the mouth are now incised posteriorly right up to the anterior pillar of the soft palate, and this requires transection of the lingual nerve and the styloglossus muscle which cross the field. The mandible can then be swung out laterally to expose the oropharynx (Fig. 12.20).

Opinions regarding the type of fixation after mandibulotomy are divided, but no difference in stability and healing has been reported using either stainless steel wires or compression miniplates (266). The RMH prefers to use miniplates, and prelocalization of the plates across the osteotomy before the cuts are actually made that allow accurate approximation at the end of the procedure. Two plates are used across the osteotomy on the anterior surface, and one is contoured to fit the inferior edge of the mandible (Fig. 12.21).

There are conflicting reports in the literature about the incidence of nonunion and osteoradionecrosis after mandibulotomy in previously irradiated patients (267,268). The RMH prefers to avoid splitting the mandible in irradiated patients and relies on other approaches such as the floor

Table 12.19 Features of the Three Types of Mandibular Osteotomy

	Lateral	Median	Paramedian
Site of osteotomy	Body or angle of mandible	Midline	Between lateral incisor and canine
Exposure	Limited	Good	Good
Dental extraction	May be required	One central incisor	Not required
Inferior alveolar nerve and vessels	Have to be transected	Spared	Spared
Division of genial muscles	Not required	Inevitable	Not required. Only the mylohyoid needs division
Mechanical stability	Poor because of unequal pull of muscles on the two mandibular segments	Good	Good
Fixation of osteotomy	May require intermaxillary fixation	Compression miniplates or stainless steel wire	Compression miniplates or stainless steel wire
Postoperative radiation therapy	Osteotomy lies within the lateral portal. Increased risk of complications	Lies outside the lateral portal. Safe	Lies outside the lateral portal. Safe

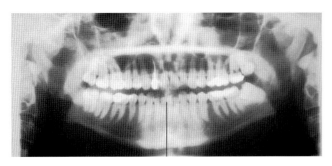

Figure 12.16 A median osteotomy.

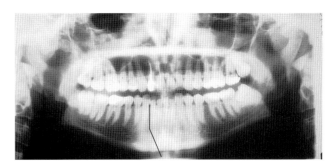

Figure 12.17 The notched paramedian osteotomy.

Table 12.20 Disadvantages of Lateral Mandibulotomy

- Provides limited exposure
- Inferior alveolar nerve has to be transected leading to denervation of all teeth distal to the osteotomy and the skin in the mental area
- Causes interruption of endosteal supply to the mandibular segment and distal teeth
- Unequal muscular pull on the mandibular segments causes stress at the site of osteotomy and this may necessitate intermaxillary fixation, which may interfere with postoperative oral hygiene.
- The mandibulotomy site lies directly within the lateral portal of radiation: may delay bony healing in radiated mandibles, and increase the risk of osteoradionecrosis if followed by postoperative radiation.

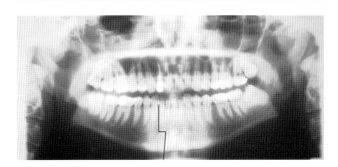

Figure 12.18 The horizontal cut of the step paramedian osteotomy must be carefully sited to avoid damaging the roots and at the same time must leave a reasonable thickness of bone on the inferior segment.

Table 12.21 Disadvantages of Median Mandibulotomy

- Requires extraction of one central incisor
- Division of the geniohyoid and genioglossus muscles, which arise from the genial tubercle interferes with normal mastication and swallowing

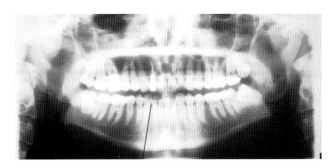

Figure 12.19 The straight paramedian osteotomy.

of mouth, transhyoid, or lateral pharyngotomy in these patients.

Floor-of-mouth (Lingual-releasing) Approach

This is an alternative to the more extensive mandibulotomy approach. It avoids splitting the mandible, especially in patients who have had previous irradiation and are at risk of nonunion or osteoradionecrosis.

It is usually combined with neck dissection, and the superior laryngeal nerve is carefully dissected and preserved. The glossopharyngeal and lingual nerves are then dissected and preserved if a partial glossectomy is planned, and part of the ipsilateral anterior tongue is to be preserved. Once the two nerves have been displaced downward, the muscles of the floor of mouth are ready for incision. The hyoid bone may have to be resected depending upon the extent of the disease. The mucosa of the floor of the mouth is then incised, leaving an adequate cuff on the alveolus (Fig. 12.22). The muscles of the floor of the mouth are divided, and branches of the lingual artery need ligation. The lingual nerve is divided posteriorly in the lateral floor of the mouth, and the tongue can then be drawn downward into the neck. Lesions requiring partial

excision of the tongue can often be excised by combining peroral excision with the floor-of-mouth approach. If a total glossectomy is planned, the opposite submandibular triangle is also dissected, and the floor of the mouth is incised all around the tongue. When the incision of the floor of mouth is complete, the tongue can be pulled through into the neck, and the tumor excised under direct vision. The RMH has found this approach very useful, especially in patients who have had previous irradiation. The surgical defect after total glossectomy (Fig. 12.23) is reconstructed using a free latissimus dorsi flap (Fig. 12.24) as it results in excellent vertical movement and thus

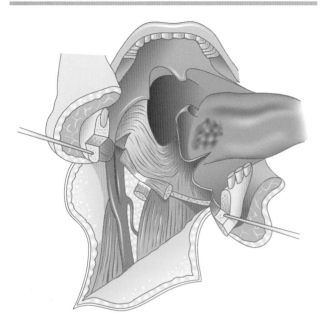

Figure 12.20 When the incision of the floor of the mouth is completed, the mandible can be swung out laterally to expose the tumour in the oropharynx.

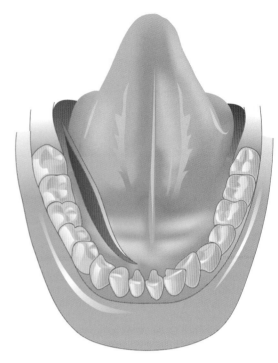

Figure 12.22 Incision of the mucosa of the floor of the mouth: leaving an adequate cuff on the alveolus facilitates subsequent closure.

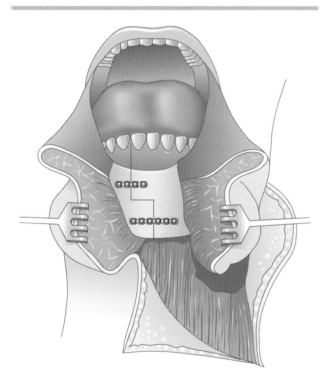

Figure 12.21 Miniplates are used to approximate the two halves of the mandible at the end of the procedure.

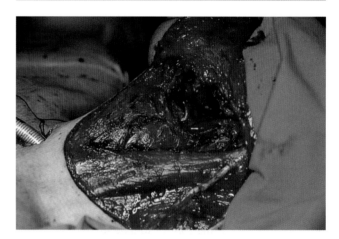

Figure 12.23 The surgical defect after total glossectomy using the floor of mouth lingual-releasing approach.

in closure is to place all the sutures approximating the inferior tip of the flap to the mucosa of the inferior edge of the defect, and then tying them transorally. The rest of the flap can be sutured in quite easily through the open mouth.

Resection of Soft Tissue

The importance of surgical margins cannot be overlooked in any oncosurgical procedure as it is one of the most important predictors of patient survival. Positive margins have shown to significantly decrease 5-year survival (38%)

provides far better functional mobility and velopharyngeal closure for swallowing and speech than a tethered pedicled myocutaneous or cutaneous flap. Although the surgical access using this approach is good, suturing in a myocutaneous flap may not always be easy. A useful technique

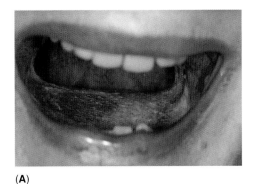

(A)

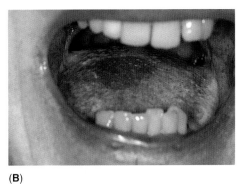

(B)

Figure 12.24 Free latissimus dorsi flap for reconstruction following total glossectomy showing excellent vertical movement that provides far better functional mobility and velopharyngeal closure for swallowing and speech than a tethered pedicled myocutaneous or cutaneous flap. **(A)** At rest; **(B)** on laryngeal elevation.

as compared to close margins (58%) and clear margins (69%). Also the risk of death from primary cancer increases up to 90% at 5 years with positive margins (269). Resection of the tumor along with an adequate cuff of normal surrounding tissue forms the basis of good oncologic surgery. Nowhere is this principle more difficult to follow than in the base of the tongue, mainly because of the difficulty in judging the extent of the tumor through the nodular surface of the organ. The tumor must be carefully palpated to ensure adequate margins as excision proceeds, but frozen section evaluation of the margins and the base of excision can minimize the chances of incomplete resection. Partial glossectomy may be oncologically adequate for limited tumors of the base of the tongue, but the anterior tongue can be salvaged only if the hypoglossal nerve and the blood supply via the lingual artery can be preserved on one side. Although a total glossectomy is a formidable procedure, it may be the only hope for survival in patients with locally advanced base-of-tongue tumors. Most patients requiring major glossectomy have conventionally been subjected to a total laryngectomy, either as a concomitant or subsequent procedure to prevent chronic aspiration (270). The functional results after glossectomy are as greatly influenced by the volume of tongue lost as by the mobility, sensitivity, and the shape of the tongue remnant. Significant advances in reconstructive surgery, prosthetics, and speech therapy have, however, greatly contributed in reducing the incidence of prophylactic total laryngectomy in patients with good performance status (271). Locally advanced tumors of the base of tongue involving adjacent sites require extended resections such as pharyngoglossectomy with complex reconstruction. The salient technical aspects of excision of particular tumors within the oropharynx have been discussed under the relevant subsites.

Management of the Neck

As with other sites within the head and neck, the management of the clinically negative neck depends on the risk of occult metastases, which in turn depends on size and location of primary tumor, perinural invasion, sex, and tumor thickness (272). Early lesions of the soft palate and the posterior pharyngeal wall are at low risk, and the clinically negative neck in these patients may be safely observed. In all other patients, elective treatment of the N0 neck must be considered. The type of treatment of the N0 neck depends largely upon the mode of treatment of the primary; if the primary is treated with RT, the neck is included in the fields; and if surgery is chosen for the primary, treatment of the neck is guided by the principles outlined in Figure 12.25. The uninvolved neck in well-lateralized lesions of the tonsil and tongue may be treated unilaterally, but both sides need treatment in lesions approaching or involving the midline.

The histology of the primary tumor obviously plays an important role in deciding treatment of positive neck nodes; UCNT and lymphomas are radiosensitive and do not require primary surgery. For all other well-lateralized primary lesions with an N+ neck, surgical treatment must include a comprehensive neck dissection including all five levels. A modified radical neck dissection is the procedure of choice, preserving as many normal structures as possible to minimize the postoperative functional deficit. A radical neck dissection should be necessary only if the relevant structures are directly infiltrated by nodal disease. Bilaterally involved nodes can be treated with simultaneous bilateral neck dissection.

The side with more advanced neck disease is dissected first aiming to preserve the internal jugular vein. At least one internal jugular vein must be preserved to minimize postoperative complications such as raised intracranial tension and mucosal edema. Preservation of the external jugular veins may help venous drainage and reduce edema of the skin flaps postoperatively. PORT is given for the usual indications, either due to adverse features of the primary or the neck nodes.

When the tumor is being treated with radical RT alone, a planned postradiotherapy neck dissection may be necessary for patients who have greater than N1 disease in the neck (273,274). Histopathological examination of the residual nodal tissue in such patients fails to demonstrate viable tumor in almost two thirds of patients (273–275). The RMH has recently modified its approach to local excision and frozen section analysis of the residual node, followed by neck dissection only if viable tumor cells are demonstrated.

Around 50% of patients with stage III and IV oropharyngeal carcinoma have involvement of the retropharyngeal nodes (276). Routine surgical procedures do not dissect these nodes, but virtually all of these patients with locoregionally advanced disease require PORT (277), and the retropharyngeal area can be easily included in the fields.

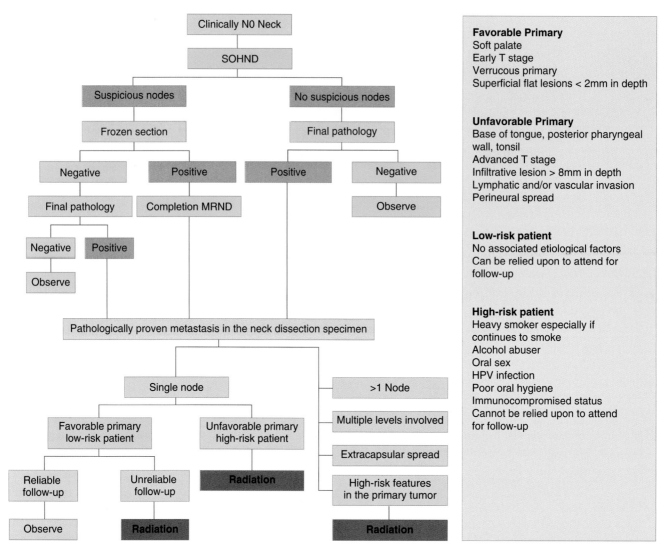

Figure 12.25   Algorithm for the surgical management of the clinically negative neck in patients with oropharyngeal carcinoma.

One of the advantages in treating the clinically negative neck with primary RT is that this policy includes the retropharyngeal nodes that are not usually included in neck dissection.

Those who favor elective neck dissection (END) for clinically negative (N0) neck advocate it to be the best way to assess occult nodal metastasis and helps in accurate pathological staging, which is most factor in predicting survival and disease-free interval (278). END also provides best information about extracapsular spread (153) and is the gold standard in assessing residual disease after treatment (7).

Management of Mandibular Involvement

Invasion of the mandible is less common in oropharyngeal carcinoma as compared to oral cancer, but as with oral tumors, there is a high degree of correlation between clinical and histopathological findings (279), and mandibular invasion influences the prognosis (280). Segmental resection of the mandible may be required in locally advanced oropharyngeal tumors, especially of the tonsil. Excellent

access to all sites within the oropharynx can be obtained using a mandibulotomy, and the uninvolved mandible should never be resected solely to gain access to the tumor. Marginal resection of the ascending ramus (Fig. 12.26) or inner table "rim resection" of the mandible (Fig. 12.27) may be carried out to obtain deep clearance in tumors of the tonsil or tongue base that abut against the periosteum of the body or ramus of the mandible.

Management of the Airway and the Larynx

Oropharyngeal tumors, by virtue of their location, can cause great difficulty in endotracheal intubation. This problem is compounded if the patient has trismus secondary to invasion of the pterygoid muscles. Fiber-optic endoscope-guided endotracheal intubation is an option, but in most instances it may be safer to perform a preliminary tracheostomy under local anesthetic. The temporary tracheostomy may then be used to protect the airway in the postoperative period, especially in patients who have had a total glossectomy with flap reconstruction. Decannulation of the tracheostomy

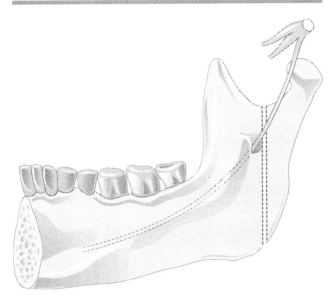

Figure 12.26 Marginal resection of the ascending ramus of the mandible for a posterior tonsullar tumour.

depends on a combination of factors including the efficacy of deglutition, the extent of aspiration, and the performance status of the patient. In selected patients who have had a limited excision of the base of the tongue with free radial forearm flap reconstruction, we have been able to avoid a tracheostomy by maintaining the patient on endotracheal tube ventilation overnight. The patient is extubated on the high-dependency unit after endoscopic evaluation of the tongue and the flap by the surgeon and the anesthetist. It is necessary to emphasize that this approach is used in very selected instances and requires a great deal of experience and judgment. It is always safer to perform a tracheostomy if there is any doubt whatsoever about the adequacy of the airway.

Tumors of the base of the tongue may break through the hyoepiglottic ligament and invade the preepiglottic space, or even the framework of the larynx. Depending upon the extent of involvement of the larynx, surgical excision of such lesions requires excision of the base of the tongue to be combined with either partial supraglottic or total laryngectomy. As a general rule, the performance status of the patient is a major factor when choosing between a partial and total laryngectomy; poor-risk patients will benefit from a total laryngectomy even when a supraglottic laryngectomy is technically feasible.

Reconstruction

Major soft tissue defects of the oropharynx can be broadly divided into those that require thin, pliable flaps for resurfacing and those that need bulkier myocutaneous flaps to provide volume. The posterior pharyngeal wall is an area that is best resurfaced using either a split skin graft or a free radial forearm flap. Substantial defects of the base of the tongue, tonsillar, and lateral pharyngeal walls need reconstruction with myocutaneous flaps such as the pectoralis major or the latissimus dorsi pedicled flaps. Although

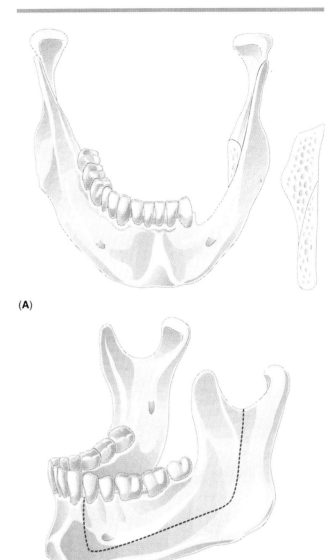

(A)

(B)

Figure 12.27 "Rim resection" of the mandible. **(A)** Inner cortical plate; **(B)** extended alveolar.

it is tempting to attempt primary closure of small defects of the base of the tongue, the best functional results are obtained by adequately replacing the volume of tongue lost, and an appropriately planned myocutaneous flap should be used to provide adequate bulk and shape to the tongue remnant. Partial circumference defects of the pharynx are reconstructed using pedicled myocutaneous flaps whereas circumferential defects are best restored by a gastric pull-up or microvascular jejunal transfer. Mandibular continuity may be restored after segmental resection, and these issues are discussed elsewhere in this book as are the individual reconstruction techniques.

Ancillary procedures such as laryngeal suspension and palatal augmentation may help improve functional results after major glossectomy (271). Swallowing after a total glossectomy suffers from a lack of the "oral phase" of swallowing. The "oral hold" phase is lost, and the bolus passes immediately to the oropharynx and then directly to the hypopharynx aided only by gravity. As a result, the material tends to pool in the pyriform sinuses and spills over into the larynx causing aspiration. A cricopharyngeal myotomy facilitates the passage of the bolus into the esophagus and prevents the "pharyngeal hold" phase of the swallowing sequence in glossectomized patients.

According to a recent study, cutaneous free flaps grafted to sites of field cancerization have been shown to develop severe epithelial dysplasia with concomitant deregulation of proliferation and increased p53 expression, raising the potential for malignant transformation (281). It therefore mandates careful examination of the local area in this group of patients posttreatment follow-up visits.

Role of Tube Feeding

Most patients with dysphagia and weight loss will have been on tube feeds preoperatively, and this must be continued into the postoperative period. Percutaneous endoscopic gastrostomy must be considered at the time of the operation if tube feeding is anticipated for more than 10 days postoperatively, for example, in patients who have had major glossectomy and reconstruction, and in those who have been planned for PORT.

Salvage Surgery and Management of Recurrences

Recurrence is a major problem in treating oropharyngeal and other HNSCC. Almost 40% of patients have recurrence following initial treatment. More than one half of these patients show a recurrent disease within 1 year and almost 99% within 5 years (282). This implies that if a patient did not show any recurrent disease up till 5 years posttreatment, he or she is virtually cured of the initial cancer.

Surgical salvage of recurrent tumors after RT is difficult because fibrosis makes palpation of the extent of the tumor inaccurate, and frozen section control of margins is extremely useful in this situation. Meticulous sharp dissection, avoidance of excessive diathermy charring, and careful hemostasis contribute to minimizing postoperative complications with healing. Patients who have required partial or total pharyngeal reconstruction commence feeds on around the tenth postoperative day. Early detection of recurrence after surgery, especially in the presence of a flap, is extremely difficult. A high index of suspicion based on symptoms such as localized pain is vital to timely diagnosis. The recurrence commonly involves the undersurface of the flap or the suture line, and although conventional imaging using CT or MRI may aid detection (283,284), but a PET scan appears to be the most useful investigation in this setting available currently (160,161).

SITE-SPECIFIC PRESENTATION, TREATMENT, AND RESULTS

Carcinoma of the Base of the Tongue

Tumors of the base of the tongue are diagnosed late, and as many as three fourths of patients present with stage III or IV disease (117). In addition, these tumors tend to infiltrate diffusely into the surrounding tissues, and regional nodal metastases are more common. Consequently, treatment is difficult, and the outcome, in terms of function and survival, is poor.

Lymph Node Metastases

The most commonly involved nodes are those at levels II and III, but level IV is more commonly involved than oral cavity tumors (Fig. 12.28). Bilateral lymphatic spread (Fig. 12.29) occurs in approximately one third of patients (117), the risk of nodal metastasis progressively increases from 51% for T_1 to 71% for T_4 lesions (127) (Tables 12.4, 12.5, and 12.7). As most tumors are treated with RT and do not undergo elective neck dissection, the actual risk of occult nodal metastases may be much higher than the reported figure of around 20%.

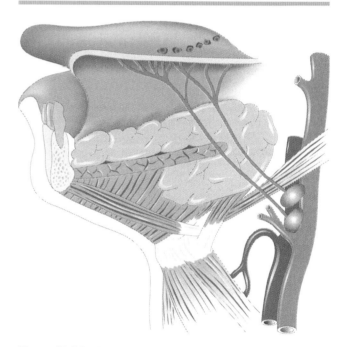

Figure 12.28   The base of the tongue drains lymph directly to level II nodes.

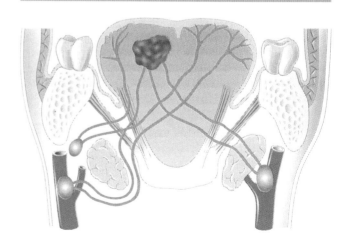

Figure 12.29   Cross-over lymphatics result in a high percentage of bilateral cervical nodal metastases.

Treatment of Early Disease

Surgery and RT give equivalent results in the treatment of early lesions of the base of the tongue (117). RT is generally favored because it causes lesser functional deficit (285,286). In view of the high propensity of these lesions to metastasize to the lymph nodes, elective treatment of the clinically negative neck is an integral part of the treatment. Dissection of the neck is recommended in patients who present with clinically involved nodes.

Early lesions can be approached either transorally, by a lateral pharyngotomy or through a combination of transoral and transhyoid approaches. Adequate resection of small unilateral lesions usually results in a defect that can be reconstructed with good functional outcome using a free radial forearm flap.

Treatment of Advanced Disease

RT may be used to treat most T_3 lesions in combination with neck dissection for palpable nodes. In view of the diffuse infiltration associated with advanced lesions, surgical resection results in positive margins in about one fourth of the cases (287). RT is generally offered to patients with negative necks, but salvage neck dissection can be performed in patients who have residual neck disease after a course of radical radiation (117).

Alternatively, a neck dissection can be carried out at the same time as the implants when the primary tumor is treated with brachytherapy. Some form of laryngeal resection may be required in locally advanced tumors of the base of the tongue as the hyoepiglottic ligament provides only a flimsy barrier to the preepiglottic space (Fig. 12.30).

Smaller lesions of the vallecula, which do not extend along the pharyngoepiglottic fold to involve the lateral pharyngeal wall, may be adequately encompassed by an extended supraglottic laryngectomy.

The major problem of combining glossectomy with laryngeal resection is the impairment of normal deglutition that results in chronic postoperative aspiration and pulmonary infection (288,289). The performance status of the patient must be taken into account when planning such a procedure, and a total laryngectomy may often be the only surgical option available to protect the airway. Induction chemotherapy with RT may be tried in appropriate patients in an effort to preserve the larynx, keeping the option of surgery for salvage of failures.

Results of Treatment

Early lesions of the base of the tongue can be controlled using surgery in approximately 85% of cases. As in many other upper aerodigestive tract tumors, the morphology of the tumor is a major determinant of outcome: exophytic tumors do much better than infiltrative, endophytic tumor. A retrospective functional evaluation has confirmed that RT provides a better posttreatment performance status than surgery for both early as well as advanced tumors (285,290). There are, however, no prospective randomized trials in literature comparing the oncologic and functional results of surgery alone with either radiation alone or combined treatment. The functional results of surgical treatment of base-of-tongue tumors as reported in the literature are listed in Table 12.22. Any attempt at comparison of these results is meaningless, as most reports are based on subjective evaluations, and the ones that have used objective parameters cannot be compared because of a lack of standardization.

Although most centers use a combined modality treatment policy when indicated, the results of surgery alone in the treatment of base-of-tongue tumors have been reported from the Mayo Clinic (294). A total of 55 patients, almost 75% with stage III or IV tumors, underwent complete surgical excision without pre- or postoperative chemotherapy or irradiation. Failure in the neck (44%) was the main cause of treatment failure with local recurrence in 22% and distant metastases in 13%. Surgical mortality was 4%, and the cause-specific survival at 5 years was 65%. Nisi et al. from Mayo Clinic achieved 82% LCRs, 59% LRC rates, and 51% OS rates in 79 patients treated with surgery with or without RT (289). Other authors have reported almost similar results (Table 12.23).

The results of RT are comparable to that of surgery. Mendenhall et al. reported 82% LCRs, 77% LRC, and 54% 5-year OS rates in his series of 333 patients. Similar results have been by other groups (Table 12.24).

Carcinoma of the Tonsil

Tumors of the tonsillar pillar tend to be more superficial than those of the tonsillar fossa that tend to present as bulky tumors. As they progress, these tumors spread to involve the adjacent structures. Tonsillar tumors present in stage III or IV in as many as 75% cases, mainly because symptoms like pain and dysphagia occur relatively late (4,301). Other symptoms include mass in the neck, weight loss, and if the pterygoid muscles are involved, trismus (Fig. 12.31). Lesions originating at the inferior pole of the tonsil may

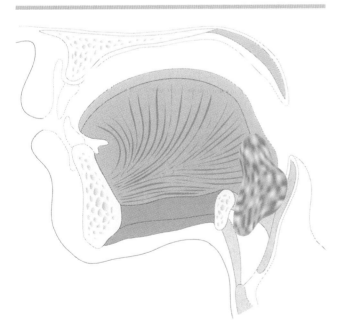

Figure 12.30 The pathways of invasion in tongue base tumours: the hyoepiglottic ligament offers little resistance to spread into the preepiglottic space.

Table 12.22 The Functional Results of Surgical Treatment of Base-of-tongue Tumors

Reference (No. of patients)	Survival	Total glossectomy	Mandibular resection	Impaired swallowing	"Useful" speech	Severe aspiration	Concomitant/ interval laryngectomy
Weber et al. (1990) (287)	51% at 2 years	27	?	56	92	11	0/8
Ruhl et al. (1997) (291)	41% at 5 years	54	?	?	?	?	?
Razack et al. (1983) (292)	20% at 5 years	45	49	69	84	37	40/13
Gehanno et al. (1992) (293)	65% at 1 year	80	?	49	39	?	?
Kraus et al. (1993) (288)	65% at 5 years	?	14	?	?	?	20

Table 12.23 Results of Surgical Treatment (With/Without Radiation) for Base-of-tongue Cancers

Reference	Number of patients	Follow-up (years)	Local control (%)	Locoregional control (%)	Overall survival (%)
Azizzadeh et al. (2002) (295)	28	5	NR	NR	80
Gourin et al. (2001) (296)	87	5	92	NR	49
Nisi et al. (1998) (289)	79	5	82	59	51
Machtay et al. (1997) (297)	17	3	77	68	46
Kraus et al. (1993) (288)	100	5	82	72	55
Thawley et al. (1983) (298)	101	5	74	57	45
Dupont et al. (1978) (299)	34	NR	NR	56	NR

Abbreviation: NR, Not reported.

Table 12.24 Results of Radiation Treatment for Base-of-tongue Cancers

Reference	Number of patients	Follow-up (years)	Local control (%)	Locoregional control (%)	Overall survival (%)
Mendenhall et al. (2006) (117)	333	5	82	77	54
Gibbs et al. (2003) (225)	41	5	82	NR	66
Brunin et al. (1999) (201)	216	5	50	45	27
Harrison et al. (1998) (226)	68	5	89	NR	87
Mak et al. (1995) (202)	54	5	85	76	59
Lusinchi et al. (1989) (227)	108	5	64	NR	26
Puthawala et al. (1988) (300)	70	5	NR	77	35

Abbreviation: NR, Not reported.

be visible only on endoscopic examination, and thorough bimanual palpation is necessary to establish their extent.

Lymph Node Metastases

Lymphatics from the tonsillar region drain into the jugulo-digastric nodes and also into the nodes of the submandibular and upper posterior triangles (153). Tumors involving the tonsillar pillars present with lymph node involvement less frequently as compared to tonsillar fossa tumors (4,301). Likewise, contralateral metastases are more common with tonsillar fossa tumors, and about 55% of patients present with advanced stage (N2–3) neck disease (117) (Tables 12.4, 12.6, and 12.7). Lesions of the posterior tonsillar pillar are more prone to metastasize to the spinal accessory and upper posterior triangle nodes.

Treatment of Early Lesions

Early lesions of the tonsillar region can be treated using a single-modality approach (15). If surgery is chosen as an option, transoral resection is generally possible, and every effort must be undertaken to ensure adequate margins.

In patients with limited mouth opening one of the other approaches described previously, such as lateral pharyngotomy or mandibulotomy, is to be preferred. Tumors abutting against the periosteum of the mandible may need marginal resection including the coronoid process (Fig. 12.26). A neck dissection is an integral part of treatment, even for patients with a clinically negative neck in view of the high risk of lymph node metastasis.

An early, asymptomatic lesion arising deep within a tonsillar crypt may present with a metastatic neck node, the so-called unknown primary. Optimal management of these patients must include a meticulous endoscopic evaluation of the entire upper aerodigestive tract, and if no lesion is obvious, an ipsilateral tonsillectomy is the only reliable method to detect a small, tonsillar crypt primary.

Equivalent results can be obtained using RT alone for the treatment of early tonsillar tumors (183). It offers excellent cure rates with a potentially better functional outcome (282). As with surgical management, elective treatment of the negative neck must be undertaken, and it is usually possible to avoid irradiating the contralateral neck for well-lateralized lesions.

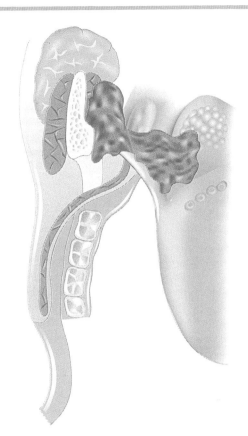

Figure 12.31 Trismus is an ominous clinical sign caused by invasion of tonsillar tumours into the pterygoid muscles.

Treatment of Advanced Lesions

Surgery combined with PORT has been conventionally used in the treatment of advanced (15,302) lesions, but radiation alone for the primary combined with neck dissection for involved nodes has been reported (228). A policy of radiation alone needs to be very selective as it has been shown that endophytic T_{3-4} lesions do not respond well to radiation and are best managed by surgery and PORT. Exophytic T_3 lesions, on the other hand, can be managed by EBRT with or without interstitial implants and a neck dissection for involved lymph nodes (300). Adequate surgical resection of advanced tonsillar tumors has conventionally required a mandibulectomy, the so-called tonsil commando operation (Fig. 12.32). Involvement of the inferior alveolar nerve is an ominous sign and is more common in elderly patients with edentulous mandibles. Conservation mandibular surgery is hazardous in patients with resorbed, edentulous mandibles; but for most other patients whose tumors do not directly invade the mandible, optimal functional results may be obtained using segmental resection combined with reconstruction and osseointegrated implants.

Results of Treatment

Although surgical resection alone is not commonly used for early tonsillar cancer, excellent control rates have been reported for such a policy (302,303). When the disease has spread to extend to the base of the tongue or lateral pharyngeal wall, the local recurrence rates for surgery alone tend to be unacceptable (304).

The results of treatment for more advanced lesions are uniformly poor. Most authors recommend surgery combined with PORT, although there are advocates of RT alone, reserving surgery for salvage. The results of both treatment approachs are nearly the same (55,305,306); however, complication are more commonly seen with surgical group as compared to organ preservation (117).

Some authors have shown a survival benefit for combination therapy in the treatment of advanced tonsillar carcinoma whereas others could not demonstrate any advantage in treating stage III and IV disease using a combined modality approach. While these studies were based on retrospective data, the Radiation Therapy Oncology Group 73–03 study (307) compared preoperative RT (50 Gy) plus surgery, surgery plus PORT (60 Gy), and RT alone (65–70 Gy) with surgery reserved for salvage in a prospective

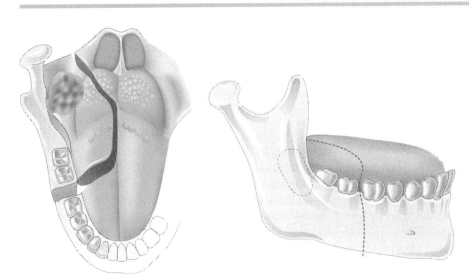

Figure 12.32 Composite resection of an advanced tonsillar tumor including the mandible: the "tonsil commando" operation.

randomized setting. No benefit could be demonstrated, either in terms of LRC or in survival, on comparison of results of the three methods of treatment. The study, however, did not stratify the patient population into subsites, and the conclusions cannot be reliably applied to any one site such as the tonsil.

CRT has clearly shown better LCR, LRC, and improved OS in advanced tonsillar carcinomas, as compared to RT alone (308,309). However, there still has not been a direct comparison between CRT and surgery alone.

Poulsen et al. reported 87% actuarial 5 year LRC and 57% overall 5-year survival with initial surgery and PORT as compared to 73 and 41%, respectively, with RT with/without CT (15). Shirazi et al. also reported 94% 4-year LCR, 87% LRC, and 71% 4-year OS with surgery and PORT as against 86, 92, and 48%, respectively, with organ preservation approach (303).

Analysis of our data from more than 300 oropharyngeal cancers patients treated at RMH in past two decades also shows OS benefits with primary surgery and PORT as compared to definitive RT alone. We currently prefer postoperative, rather than preoperative, RT for advanced lesions because it allows more reliable assessment of locoregional extent of the disease and surgical margins and is also associated with a lower rate of surgical complications. The choice of treatment and the sequence of therapy must

however be tailored to the individual patient with the aim to cure the disease with the least functional deficit. The results of surgery with or without radiation and RT alone are summarized in Tables 12.25 and 12.26.

Carcinoma of the Pharyngeal Wall

Tumors of the posterior pharyngeal wall tend to present late (4,301). Common symptoms at presentation include dysphagia, odynophagia, mass in the neck, weight loss, and bleeding. Tumors in this location tend to be more superficial and less bulky than those at other sites within the oropharynx, but they can be associated with extensive submucosal spread and "skip" areas. Most tumors originate at the junction between the oropharynx and the hypopharynx. The tumor may spread superiorly to the nasopharynx, inferiorly to the pyriform sinuses and hypopharynx, and posteriorly to infiltrate the prevertebral fascia.

Tumors of the posterior pharyngeal wall have a higher than usual rate of second primary tumors (37%) in one series (322), and the importance of a meticulous examination of the entire upper aerodigestive tract cannot be overemphasized in these patients.

Lymph Node Metastases

The primary echelons of drainage are the retropharyngeal nodes and the nodes at levels II and III (124). The incidence

Table 12.25 Results of Surgical Treatment (With/Without Radiation) for Tonsillar Carcinoma

Reference	Number of patients	Follow-up (years)	Local control (%)	Locoregional control (%)	Cause specific survival (%)
Laccourreye et al. (2005) (310)	166	5	82	NR	58 (OS)
Perez et al. (1998) (203)	230	5	68	NR	NR
Hicks et al. (1998) (302)	56	5	75	48	61
Foote et al. (1994) (311)	72	5	71	63	NR
Mizono et al. (1986) (312)	40	5	NR	73	NR
Gluckman et al. (1985) (313)	82	5	NR	NR	56
Rabuzzi et al. (1982) (314)	47	5	NR	NR	57
Givens et al. (1981) (315)	22	5	NR	NR	32
Schuller et al. (1979) (316)	20	5	NR	NR	20

Abbreviations: NR, not reported; OS, overall survival.

Table 12.26 Results of Radiation Treatment for Tonsillar Carcinoma

Reference	Number of patients	Follow-up (years)	Local control (%)	Locoregional control (%)	Cause specific survival (%)
Charbonneau et al. (2006) (200)	164	5	80	80	57 (OS)
Mendenhall et al. (2006) (118)	503	5	79	73	72 53 (OS)
Perez et al. (1998) (203)	154	5	56	NR	NR
Gwozdz et al. (1997) (317)	83	5	NR	NR	71 60 (OS)
Pernot et al. (1994) (228)	361	5	80	75	63 53 (OS)
Bataini et al. (1989) (318)	465	5	64	58	NR
Wong et al. (1989) (319)	150	5	75	77	70
Puthawala et al. (1985) (229)	80	5	84	75	NR
Garrett et al. (1985) (320)	372	5	NR	NR	54
Amornmarn et al. (1984) (321)	185	5	58	NR	42 30 (OS)

Abbreviations: NR, not reported; OS, overall survival.

of lymph node metastasis corresponds to the T stage and rises from 25% for T_1 lesions to more than 75% for T_4 tumors (323). As most of the tumors cross midline, bilateral cervical metastasis is common (124).

Treatment of Early Lesions

Transoral excision may be possible for small lesions in patients with good mouth opening when the lower limit of the tumor is well visible. For most other tumors, a transhyoid or lateral pharyngotomy approach can be used to resect the lesion. The avascular retropharyngeal space acts as a good plane of cleavage, and the tumor can usually be easily separated from the underlying prevertebral fascia, which is very rarely involved in early lesions. Alternative approaches like the median labiomandibular glossotomy and mandibular swing are more extensive and are usually reserved for more advanced lesions. Reconstruction of the defect commonly entails a split thickness skin graft or a free radial forearm flap. The functional results of surgery, even for small lesions, are far from optimal because of impairment of swallowing that results from denervation and resection of the pharyngeal musculature. Surgery is generally not extensive enough to encompass the retropharyngeal nodes and PORT to the neck may be indicated in high-risk patients.

Treatment of Advanced Lesions

Advanced tumors of the posterior pharyngeal wall are treated using surgery combined with PORT (324). An important issue in deciding resectability is involvement of the prevertebral fascia, encasement of carotid arteries, perineural spread, reteropharyngeal adenopathy, and overall patients' performance status (124). CT and MRI can detect advanced infiltration by obliteration of retropharyngeal fat plane, asymmetric enlargement of prevertebral muscles, thickening, and signal abnormality but are unreliable in cases of early involvement of the fascia, which is most often apparent only at operation (124,325,326). Resection of locally advanced pharyngeal wall tumors may at times require a total laryngopharyngectomy. However, larynx should be preserved whenever possible, as conservative surgery does not impair local control and survival in these patients (322,324). The resultant defect may be reconstructed using one of the various available options like tubed fasciocutaneous or myocutaneous flaps, gastric transposition, or microvascular free jejunal transfer. These operations have been discussed in detail elsewhere in this book; however, currently the free jejunal transfer is the procedure of choice for reconstructing circumferential pharyngeal defects as it allows early return to swallowing with the minimum of physiological disturbance. PORT is recommended in view of the high incidence of retropharyngeal node involvement and locoregional failure (124).

Results of Treatment

Tumor classification is often difficult because by the time they are detected, most lesions involve two separate anatomical regions, each having its own distinct classification; tumors of the oropharynx are also classified by size whereas those of the hypopharynx are classified by site of involvement. This, combined with the fact that these are rare tumors, makes comparison of treatment modalities difficult. RT alone has limited effectiveness in treatment mainly because of the technical difficulty in delivering adequate doses to tissue in such close proximity to the spinal cord (324), but also because these tumors are not very radiosensitive. The predominant feature of surgical treatment of these tumors is the high incidence of local failure that ranges between 40% (322) and 50% (324). The probability of local recurrence is directly related to stage (16% for stage I and 63% for stage IV) and salvage rates are only about 21 to 33% (324). Table 12.27 lists the results of treatment of posterior pharyngeal wall tumors reported in the literature.

Carcinoma of the Soft Palate

The anterior surface of the palate tends to be the most commonly involved (301), and the posterior surface is spared until the tumor is well advanced. Most lesions tend to be superficial initially (4) and start as leukoplakia or as raised lesions. Clinical diagnosis may be difficult in heavy smokers as leukoplakic areas on the palate are very common in this population. Also, delineation of the extent of a biopsy-proven lesion may be difficult because of the keratinization of the mucosa associated with heavy smoking. Common presenting symptoms include bleeding and a sore throat, but patients may complain of altered speech

Table 12.27 Results of Treatment of Posterior Pharyngeal Wall Carcinoma

References	No. of patients	Treatment	Follow-up (years)	Survival (%)
Yoshida et al. (2004) (120)	51	R	2	45
			5	31
Cooper et al. (2000) (327)	22	R	3	50
Spiro et al. (1990) (322)	78	S ± R	2	49
			5	32
Jaulerry et al. (1986) (328)	98	R	3	30
			5	14
Schwaab et al. (1983) (329)	24	C ± R	3	60
			5	25
Talton et al. (1981) (330)	35	S ± R	5	27
		R	5	35

Abbreviations: R, radiotherapy; S, surgery; C, chemotherapy.

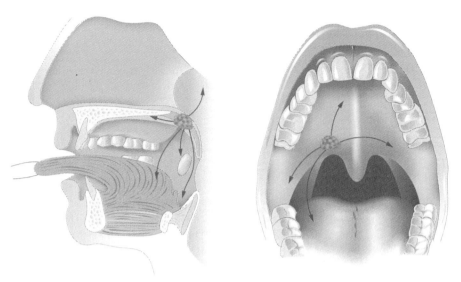

Figure 12.33 Pathways of local spread of tumors of the soft palate.

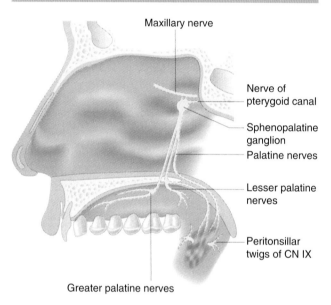

Figure 12.34 Involvement of the nerves of the palate results in pain, and the tumor may extend cranially along this path.

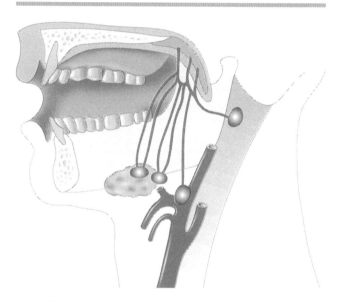

Figure 12.35 Lymphatic drainage of the soft palate.

or swallowing. As the tumor advances, it may spread to involve the tonsillar pillars, the base of the tongue, or the nasopharynx (Fig. 12.33). Involvement of the pharyngeal muscles results in pain as may extension along the palatine nerves (Fig. 12.34).

Lymph Node Metastases

Primary drainage is to the upper jugulodigastric and the retropharyngeal nodes (Fig. 12.35). About 30% of patients present with clinically positive neck nodes, but extension of the tumor to involve the tonsillar fossa increases this risk. Occult nodal metastases occur in 16% of patients, and about 15% of patients who have a midline primary lesion will have bilateral or contralateral neck metastases (124).

Treatment of Early Disease

The treatment of carcinoma of the soft palate is essentially by RT because surgical excision of all but the very small lesions results in unacceptable functional deficit such as nasal speech, regurgitation, and difficulty swallowing (119). Small primary tumors with clinically positive nodes can be treated with radical radiation to the primary and the neck, surgery being reserved for salvage of failures. Hyperfractionation is preferred over conventional fractionation owing to survival benefits (231).

Treatment of Advanced Disease

As with other sites, advanced tumors of the soft palate are also best managed using surgery combined with PORT.

Table 12.28 Results of Treatment for Carcinoma of the Soft Palate

References	No. of patients	Treatment	Follow-up (years)	Survival (%)
Chera et al. (2008) (119)	145	R	3.8	44
Mendini et al. (1997) (332)	24	R	3	81
Leemans et al. (1994) (333)	52	S, R, C, L	5	77
Keus et al. (1988) (334)	146	R	3	59
			5	40
Esche et al. (1988) (335)	43	I ± R	3	81
			5	37
Garrett et al. (1985) (320)	70	R	5	43

Abbreviations: R, external radiation; S, surgery; C, chemotherapy; L, laser resection; I, interstitial implant.

Table 12.29 Overall 5-year Survival (%) Depending on Sites in Oropharynx

Site	Sundaram et al. (2005) (106)	Johansen et al. (2000) (108)	Mark-Kregar et al. (1995) (109)
Base of tongue	15.2	36	33
Tonsillar region	58.9	31	42
Soft palate and uvula	21.4[a]	34	54
Posterior pharyngeal wall		13	32

[a]Includes soft palate, uvula, and posterior pharyngeal wall.

Local control rates for T_3 and T_4 tumors with continuous-course radiation are 45 and 25%, respectively, and the results of salvage surgery in these patients are poor (331). Some recent studies recommend CRT for advanced lesions ($\geq T_3$ or $\geq$ N2) (187,190).

Results of Treatment

Overall 5-year survival rates range between 52 to 61% for early disease (stage I and II) and 0 to 56% for advanced disease (stage III and IV) (119). The results of treatment reported in the literature are listed in Table 12.28.

FOLLOW UP AND REHABILITATION

Rehabilitation of patients who have had surgery for oropharyngeal tumors is often a prolonged and painstaking process. Apart from a great deal of patience, successful rehabilitation requires close co-operation between the surgeon, the speech therapist, the dietitian, the nursing staff, and the physiotherapist. Palatal augmentation prostheses and videofluoroscopy are useful adjuncts to rehabilitation. The time scale of posttreatment follow-up for these patients is identical to that for other head and neck patients, but it is vitally important to examine them thoroughly using palpation, fiber-optic endoscopy, and imaging as appropriate. The patients should be examined every month for the first posttreatment year, every 2 months for the second year, every 3 months for the third year, and every 6 months thereafter. It is essential to obtain a baseline follow-up CT/MRI three to six months after the end of therapy. Persisting or recurrent tissue asymmetry and/or increased tissue enhancement after therapy should be looked with suspicion for residual or recurrent tumor. Such findings needs further exploration, when no clinical correlate is apparent, it is safe to perform an additional nuclear imaging study or to obtain a follow up CT/MRI study about four months later. Recurrences under a flap reconstruction are notoriously difficult to detect, and in case of persisting or progressive tissue changes biopsy under anesthetic is required.

CONCLUSION

OS rates for different subsites of oropharynx differ considerably but remain constantly poor. Patients with posterior pharyngeal wall cancers have the least overall 5-year survival rates followed by base-of-tongue and soft palate cancers. Tonsillar carcinomas by far have the most favorable prognosis among this group, which however is still unsatisfactory (Table 12.29).

ACKNOWLEDGMENT

The authors would like to thank Dr. Ravi Chandra Dwivedi and Dr. Namita Kanwar from the Department of Internal Medicine, University of Mannitoba, Winnipeg, Canada, for their valuable contribution in completing the chapter.

REFERENCES

1. Rhys Evans PH. Tumours of the oropharynx and lymphomas of the head and neck. In: Kerr AG, ed. Scott-Brown's Otolaryngology, Vol. 5, 6th ed. London: Butterworth, 1997.
2. Hollinshead WH. In: Anatomy for Surgeons: Volume 1 The Head and Neck. 3rd ed. Philadelphia: Harper and Row, 1982; 336.
3. Batson OV. Veins of the pharynx. Arch Otolaryngol 1942; 36: 212.
4. Mendenhall WM, Riggs CE Jr, Cassisi NJ. Treatment of head and neck cancers. In: DeVita VT Jr, Hellman S, Rosenberg SA, 7th ed., Cancer: Principles and Practice of Oncology. Philadelphia: 2005: 662–732.

5. Ho T, Zahurak M, Koch WM. Prognostic significance of presentation-to-diagnosis interval in patients with oropharyngeal carcinoma. Arch Otolaryngol Head Neck Surg 2004; 130: 45–51.

6. Forastiere A, Koch W, Trotti A et al. Medical progress—head and neck cancer. New Engl J Med 2001; 345: 1890–1900.

7. Mau T, Oh Y, Bucci MK et al. Management of cervical metastases in advanced squamous cell carcinoma of the tonsillar fossa following radiotherapy. Arch Otolaryngol Head Neck Surg 2005; 131: 600–604.

8. Ferlay J, Bray F, Pisani P. Cancer Incidence, Mortality and Prevalence Worldwide. IARC Cancer Base 2004.

9. Robinson KL, Macfarlane GJ. Oropharyngeal cancer incidence and mortality in Scotland: are rates still increasing? Oral Oncology 2003; 39: 31–36.

10. Preuss SF, Dinh V, Klussmann JP et al. Outcome of multimodal treatment for oropharyngeal carcinoma: a single institution experience. Oral Oncol 2007; 43: 402–407.

11. Jemal A, Siegel R, Ward E et al. Cancer statistics, 2006. Ca-Cancer J Clin 2006; 56: 106–130.

12. Cancer incidence inn Wales. Cancer incidence in Wales. 2008.

13. Cancer statistics- registrations, England 2005. Series MB1 no 36, Office for National Statistics, 2008. Available on the National Statistics website: http://www.statistics.gov.uk/downloads/theme_health/MB1_36/MB1_No36_2005.pdf

14. Jemal A, Siegel R, Ward E et al. Cancer statistics, 2008. Ca-Cancer J Clin 2008; 58: 71–96.

15. Poulsen M, Porceddu SV, Kingsley PA et al. Locally advanced tonsillar squamous cell carcinoma: Treatment approach revisited. Laryngoscope 2007; 117: 45–50.

16. American Cancer Society. Cancer Facts and Figures 2004. Atlanta, GA: American Cancer Society, 2004.

17. Parkin DM, Bray F, Ferlay J et al. Estimating the world cancer burden: GLOBOCAN 2000. Int J Cancer 2001; 94: 153–6.

18. Conway DI, Stockton DL, Warnakulasuriya KA et al. Incidence of oral and oropharyngeal cancer in United Kingdom (1990–1999)—recent trends and regional variation. Oral Oncol 2006; 42: 586–92.

19. Shiboski CH, Schmidt BL, Jordan RC. Tongue and tonsil carcinoma—increasing trends in the US population ages 20–44 years. Cancer 2005; 103: 1843–9.

20. Singh B, Balwally AN, Shaha AR et al. Upper aerodigestive tract squamous cell carcinoma—the human immunodeficiency virus connection. Arch Otolaryngol-Head Neck Surg 1996; 122: 639–43.

21. Hoffmann D, Hoffmann I. Chemistry and Toxicology. In: Cigars, Smoking and Tobacco Control [Monograph]. National Institutes of Health, National Cancer Institute; 1998: 55–104.

22. Kapil U, Singh P. Nutritional risk factors in oral carcinoma. Pak J Nutrit 2004; 3: 366–70.

23. Patel BP, Rawal UM, Shah PM et al. Study of tobacco habits and alterations in enzymatic antioxidant system in oral cancer. Oncol 2005; 68: 511–9.

24. Lazarus P, Stern J, Zwiebel N et al. Relationship between p53 mutation incidence in oral cavity squamous cell carcinomas and patient tobacco use. Carcinogenesis 1996; 17: 733–9.

25. Reledi E, Kaaks R, Esteue J. Nutrition and laryngeal cancer. Cancer Causes Control 1996; 7: 147–56

26. Rahman M, Sakamoto J, Fukui T. Bidi smoking and oral cancer: A meta-analysis. Int J Cancer 2003; 106: 600–4.

27. Bedi R. Betel-quid and tobacco chewing among the United Kingdom's Bangladeshi community. Br J Cancer Suppl. 1996; Sep 29: 73–7.

28. Chaturvedi P, Chaturvedi U, Sanyal B. Prevalence of tobacco consumption in School children in rural India- an epidemic of tobaccogenic cancers looming ahead in the third world. J Cancer Educ 2002; 17: 6.

29. Zienolddiny S, Aguelon AM, Mironov N et al. Genomic instability in oral squamous cell carcinoma: relationship to betel-quid chewing. Oral Oncol 2004; 40: 298–303.

30. Chang MC, Chiang CP, Lin CL et al. Cell-mediated immunity and head and neck cancer: With special emphasis on betel quid chewing habit. Oral Oncol 2005; 41: 757–75

31. LaVecchia C, Tavani A, Franceschi S et al. Epidemiology and prevention of oral cancer. Oral Oncol 1997; 33: 302–12.

32. Balaram P, Sridhar H, Rajkumar T et al. Oral cancer in southern India: the influence of smoking, drinking, paan-chewing and oral hygiene. Int J Cancer 2002; 98: 440–5.

33. Dikshit RP, Kanhere S. Tobacco habits and risk of lung, oropharyngeal and oral cavity cancer: a population-based case-control study in Bhopal, India. Int J Epidemiol 2000; 29: 609–14.

34. Mayne S, Morse D, Winn D. Cancers of the oral cavity and pharynx. In: Schottenfeld D, Fraumeni J Jr, ed. Cancer Epidemiology and Prevention. New York: Oxford University Press; 2006: 647–96.

35. Cawson RA, Langdon JD, Eveson JW. Surgical Pathology of the Mouth and Jaws. Oxford: Butterworth and Heinemann, 1996; 204–8.

36. Seitz HK, Becker P. Alcohol metabolism and cancer risk. Alcohol Res Health 2007; 30: 38–41, 44–7.

37. Pelucchi C, Gallus S, Garavello W et al. Cancer risk associated with alcohol and tobacco use: focus on upper aerodigestive tract and liver. Alcohol Res Health 2006; 29: 193–8.

38. Laronde DM, Hislop TG, Elwood JM et al. Oral cancer: just the facts. J Can Dent Assoc 2008; 74: 269–72.

39. Klienjans JC, Monnen EJ, Dallinga JW. Polycyclic aromatic hydrocarbons in whiskey. Lancet 1996; 348: 1731.

40. Rogers MA, Vaughan TL, Davis S et al. Consumption of nitrate, nitrite and nitrosodimethylamine and the risk of upper aerodigestive tract cancer. Cancer Epidemiol Biomarkers Prev 1995; 4: 29–36.

41. Rodriguez T, Altieri A, Chatenoud L et al. Risk factors for oral and pharyngeal cancer in young adults. Oral Oncol 2004; 40: 207–13.

42. De Stefani E, Boffetta P, Oreggia F et al. Smoking patterns and cancer of the oral cavity and pharynx: a case-control study in Uruguay. Oral Oncol 1998; 34: 340–6.

43. Chang SS, Califano J. Current status of biomarkers in head and neck cancer. J Surg Oncol 2008; 97: 640–3.

44. zurHausen H. Papillomavirus infections—a major cause of human cancers. Biochimica et Biophysica Acta-Reviews on Cancer 1996; 1288: F55–F78.

45. Kreimer AR, Clifford GM, Boyle P et al. Human papillomavirus types in head and neck squamous cell carcinomas worldwide: A systematic review. Cancer Epidemiol Biomarkers Prev 2005; 14: 467–75.

46. Fakhry C, Gillison ML. Clinical implications of human papillomavirus in head and neck cancers. J Clin Oncol 2006; 24: 2606–11.

47. Herrero R, Castellsague X, Pawlita M et al. Human papillomavirus and oral cancer: The international agency for research on cancer multicenter study. J Natl Cancer Inst 2003; 95: 1772–83.

48. Dahlstrom KR, Little JA, Zafereo ME et al. Squamous cell carcinoma of the head and neck in never smoker-never drinkers: a descriptive epidemiologic study. Head Neck 2008; 30: 75–84.

49. D'Souza G, Kreimer AR, Viscidi R et al. Case-control study of human papillomavirus and oropharyngeal cancer. New Engl J Med 2007; 356: 1944–56.

50. Johns Hopkins Medical Institutions (2007, May 10). Oral Sex Increases Risk of Throat Cancer. ScienceDaily. Retrieved March 12, 2009, from http://www.sciencedaily.com/releases/2007/05/070509210142.htm

51. Rose Ragin CC, Taioli E. Second primary head and neck tumor risk in patients with cervical cancer—SEER data analysis. Head Neck 2008; 30: 58–66.

52. Begum S, Gillison ML, Ansari-Lari MA et al. Detection of human papillomavirus in cervical lymph nodes: A highly effective strategy for localizing site of tumor origin. Clin Cancer Res 2003; 9: 6469–75.

53. Forastiere AA. Chemotherapy in the treatment of locally advanced head and neck cancer. J Surg Oncol 2008; 97: 701–7.

54. Cmelak AJ, Li S, Goldwasser MA et al. Phase II trial of chemoradiation for organ preservation in resectable stage III or IV squamous cell carcinomas of the larynx or oropharynx: results of Eastern Cooperative Oncology Group Study E2399. J Clin Oncol 2007; 25: 3971–7.

55. Jones AS, Fenton JE, Husband DJ. The treatment of squamous cell carcinoma of the tonsil with neck node metastases. Head Neck 2003; 25: 24–31.

56. Smith EM, Ritchie JM, Summersgill KF et al. Human papillomavirus in oral exfoliated cells and risk of head and neck cancer. J Natl Cancer Instit 2004; 96: 449–55.

57. Llewellyn CD, Johnson NW, Warnakulasuriya KA. Risk factors for squamous cell carcinoma of the oral cavity in young people—a comprehensive literature review. Oral Oncol 2001; 37: 401–18.

58. Ho T, Wei QY, Sturgis EM. Epidemiology of carcinogen metabolism genes and risk of squamous cell carcinoma of the head and neck. Head Neck 2007; 29: 682–99.

59. Lynch HT, Fusaro RM, Lynch J. Hereditary cancer in adults. Cancer Detect Prev 1995; 19: 219–33.

60. Caminero MJ, Nunez F, Suarez C et al. Detection of p53 protein in oropharyngeal carcinoma—prognostic implications. Arch Otolaryngol-Head Neck Surg 1996; 122: 769–72.

61. Reinders J, Rozemuller EH, Otten HG et al. HLA and MICA associations with head and neck squamous cell carcinoma. Oral Oncol 2007; 43: 232–40.

62. Cengiz B, Gunduz M, Nagatsuka H et al. Fine deletion mapping of chromosome 2q21-37 shows three preferentially deleted regions in oral cancer. Oral Oncol 2007; 43: 241–7.

63. Rowley H, Jones AS, Field JK. Chromosome-18—a possible site for a tumor-suppressor gene deletion in squamous-cell carcinoma of the head and neck. Clinical Otolaryngol 1995; 20: 266–71.

64. Chang KP, Hao SP, Liu CT et al. Promoter polymorphisms of DNMT3B and the risk of head and neck squamous cell carcinoma in Taiwan: a case-control study. Oral Oncol 2007; 43. 345–51.

65. Gorgens H, Muller A, Kruger S et al. Analysis of the base excision repair genes MTH1, OGG1 and MUTYH in patients with squamous oral carcinomas. Oral Oncol 2007; 43: 791–5.

66. Bagan JV, Scully C. Recent advances in oral oncology 2007: Epidemiology, aetiopathogenesis, diagnosis and prognostication. Oral Oncol 2008; 44: 103–8.

67. Masuda M, Ruan HY, Ito A et al. Signal transducers and activators of transcription 3 up-regulates vascular endothelial growth factor production and tumor angiogenesis in head and neck squamous cell carcinoma. Oral Oncol 2007; 43: 785–90.

68. Scully C, Field JK, Tanzawa H. Genetic aberrations in oral or head and neck squamous cell carcinoma (SCCHN): 1. Carcinogen metabolism, DNA repair and cell cycle control. Oral Oncol 2000; 36: 256–63.

69. Katoh T, Kaneko S, Kohshi K et al. Genetic polymorphisms of tobacco- and alcohol-related metabolizing enzymes and oral cavity cancer. Int J Cancer 1999; 83: 606–9.

70. Sato M, Sato T, Izumo T et al. Genetic polymorphism of drug-metabolizing enzymes and susceptibility to oral cancer. Carcinogenesis 1999; 20: 1927–31.

71. Tanimoto K, Hayashi S, Yoshiga K et al. Polymorphisms of the CYP1A1 and GSTM1 gene involved in oral squamous cell carcinoma in association with a cigarette dose. Oral Oncol 1999; 35: 191–6.

72. Brennan JA, Boyle JO, Koch WM et al. Association between cigarette-smoking and mutation of the p53 gene in squamous-cell carcinoma of the head and neck. New Engl J Med 1995; 332: 712–17.

73. Gupta PC, Hebert JR, Bhonsle RB et al. Influence of dietary factors on oral precancerous lesions in a population-based case-control study in Kerala, India. Cancer 1999; 85: 1885–93.

74. Franceschi S, Bidoli E, Baron AE et al. Nutrition and cancer of the oral cavity and pharynx in North-East Italy. Int J Cancer 1991; 47: 20–5.

75. Destefani E, Oreggia F, Ronco A et al. Salted meat consumption as a risk factor for cancer of the oral cavity and pharynx—a case-control study from Uruguay. Cancer Epidemiol Biomarkers Prev 1994; 3: 381–5.

76. Rasheed MH, Beevi SS, Geetha A. Enhanced lipid peroxidation and nitric oxide products with deranged antioxidant status in patients with head and neck squamous cell carcinoma. Oral Oncol 2007; 43: 333–8.

77. World Cancer Research Fund International and American Institute for Cancer Research. Mouth, pharynx, and larynx. Food, nutrition, physical activity and the prevention of cancer: a global perspective. Washington, DC: AICR, 2007.

78. Key T, Schatzkin A, Willett WC et al. Diet, nutrition and the prevention of cancer. Public Health Nutr 2004; 7: 187–200.

79. Bosetti C, Gallus S, Trichopoulou A et al. Influence of the Mediterranean diet on the risk of cancers of the upper aerodigestive tract. Cancer Epidemiol Biomarkers Prev 2003; 12: 1091–4.

80. Pelucchi C, Talamini R, Negri E et al. Folate intake and risk of oral and pharyngeal cancer. Ann Oncol 2003; 14: 1677–81.

81. Quon H, Hershock D, Feldman M et al. Cancer of the head and neck. In: Abeloff M, Armitage J, Niederhuber J et al., 3rd ed. Clinical Oncology. Orlando, USA: Churchill Livingstone: An imprint of Elsevier; 2004: 1499–500.

82. Bhatia S, Louie AD, Bhatia R et al. Solid cancers after bone marrow transplantation. J Clin Oncol 2001; 19: 464–71.

83. Curtis RE, Rowlings PA, Deeg HJ et al. Solid cancers after bone marrow transplantation. New Engl J Med 1997; 336: 897–904.

84. Streilein JW. Immunogenetic factors in skin-cancer. New Eng J Med 1991; 325: 884–7.

85. Varga E, Tyldesley WR. Carcinoma arising in cyclosporine-induced gingival hyperplasia. Br Dent J 1991; 171: 26–7.

86. Thomas DW, Seddon SV, Shepherd JP. Systemic immunosuppression and oral malignancy—a report of a case and review of the literature. Br J Oral Maxillofac Surg 1993; 31: 391–3.

87. Roland JT Jr, Rothstein SG, Mittal KR et al. Squamous-cell carcinoma in HIV-positive patients under age-45. Laryngoscope 1993; 103: 509–11.

88. Greenspan JS, Greenspan D, Lennette ET et al. Replication of Epstein-Barr Virus within the epithelial-cells of oral hairy leukoplankia, an AIDS-associated lesion. New Engl J Med 1985; 313: 1564–71.

89. Silverman S, Migliorati CA, Lozadanur F et al. Oral findings in people with or at high-risk for AIDS—a study of 375 homosexual males. J Am Dental Assoc 1986; 112: 187–92.

90. Epstein JB, Scully C. Neoplastic disease in the head and neck of patients with AIDS. Int J Oral Maxillofac Surg 1992; 21: 219–26.

91. Blair A, Stewart P, Oberg M et al. Mortality among industrial-workers exposed to formaldehyde. J Natl Cancer Instit 1986; 76: 1071–84.

92. Dubrow R, Wegman DH. Cancer and occupation in Massachusetts—a death certificate study. Am J Ind Med 1984; 6: 207–30.

93. Vagero D, Olin R. Incidence of cancer in the electronics industry—using the new "Swedish-Cancer-Environment" registry as a screening instrument. Br J Ind Med 1983; 40: 188–92.

94. Moulin JJ, Mur JM, Wild P et al. oral cavity and laryngeal cancers among man-made mineral fiber production workers. Scandinavian J Work Environ Health 1986; 12: 27–31.

95. Bloching M, Reich W, Schubert J et al. The influence of oral hygiene on salivary quality in the Ames test, as a marker for genotoxic effects. Oral Oncol 2007; 43: 933–9.

96. Rautemaa R, Hietanen J, Niissalo S et al. Oral and oesophageal squamous cell carcinoma—a complication or component of autoimmune polyendocrinopathy-candidiasis-ectodermal dystrophy (APECED, APS-I). Oral Oncol 2007; 43: 607–13.

97. Goutzanis L, Vairaktaris E, Yapijakis C et al. Diabetes may increase risk for oral cancer through the insulin receptor substrate-1 and focal adhesion kinase pathway. Oral Oncol 2007; 43: 165–73.

98. Hashibe M, Ford DE, Zhang ZF. Marijuana smoking and head and neck cancer. J Clin Pharmacol 2002; 42: 103S–107S.

99. Lingen M, Sturgis EM, Kies MS. Squamous cell carcinoma of the head and neck in nonsmokers: clinical and biologic characteristics and implications for management. Curr Opin Oncol 2001; 13: 176–82.

100. Neville BW, Day TA. Oral cancer and precancerous lesions. Ca-Cancer J Clin 2002; 52: 195–215.

101. Ha PK, Califano JA. The molecular biology of mucosal field cancerization of the head and neck. Crit Rev Oral Biol Med 2003; 14: 363–9.

102. Braakhuis BJM, Tabor MP, Leemans CR et al. Second primary tumors and field cancerization in oral and oropharyngeal cancer: molecular techniques provide new insights and definitions. Head Neck 2002; 24: 198–206.

103. Tabor MP, Brakenhoff RH, Ruijter-Schippers HJ et al. Multiple head and neck tumors frequently originate from a single preneoplastic lesion. Am J Pathol 2002; 161: 1051–60.

104. Pedapenki RM. Epidemiological study of reverse smoking (chutta) and the prevalence of carcinoma palate in North Coastal Andhra Pradesh, India. UICC World Cancer Congress 2006, July 10th 2006 Washington DC, USA.

105. Pradier RN, Califano L. Cancer of the oropharynx. In: Shah J, Johnson, eds. Proceedings of the 4(th) International Conference on Head and Neck Cancer. 1996.

106. Sundaram K, Schwartz J, Har-El G et al. Carcinoma of the oropharynx: factors affecting outcome. Laryngoscope 2005; 115: 1536–42.

107. Selek U, Garden AS, Morrison WH et al. Radiation therapy for early-stage carcinoma of the oropharynx. Int J Radiat Oncol Biol Phys 2004; 59: 743–51.

108. Johansen LV, Grau C, Overgaard J. Squamous cell carcinoma of the oropharynx—an analysis of treatment results in 289 consecutive patients. Acta Oncologica 2000; 39: 985–94.

109. Mak-Kregar S, Hilgers FJ, Levendag PC et al. A nationwide study of the epidemiology, treatment and survival of oropharyngeal carcinoma in The Netherlands. Eur Arch Otorhinolaryngol 1995; 252: 133–8.

110. Henk JM. Treatment of oral-cancer by interstitial irradiation using Ir-192. Br J Oral Maxillofac Surg 1992; 30: 355–9.

111. Krabbe CA, Dijkstra PU, Pruim J et al. FDG PET in oral and oropharyngeal cancer. Value for confirmation of N0 neck and detection of occult metastases. Oral Oncol 2008; 44: 31–6.

112. Lee SY, Lim YC, Song MH et al. Level llb lymph node metastasis in elective neck dissection of oropharyngeal squamous cell carcinoma. Oral Oncol 2006; 42: 1017–21.

113. Vartanian JG, Pontes E, Agra IM et al. Distribution of metastatic lymph nodes in oropharyngeal carcinoma and its implications for the elective treatment of the neck. Arch Otolaryngol-Head Neck Surg 2003; 129: 729–32.

114. Jose J, Coatesworth AP, Johnston C et al. Cervical node metastases in oropharyngeal squamous cell carcinoma: prospective analysis of prevalence and distribution. J Laryngol Otol 2002; 116: 925–8.

115. Pimenta Amaral TM, Da Silva Freire AR, Carvalho AL et al. Predictive factors of occult metastasis and prognosis of clinical stages I and II squamous cell carcinoma of the tongue and floor of the mouth. Oral Oncol 2004; 40: 780–6.

116. O-charoenrat P, Pillai G, Patel S et al. Tumour thickness predicts cervical nodal metastases and survival in early oral tongue cancer. Oral Oncol 2003; 39: 386–90.

117. Mendenhall WM, Morris CG, Amdur RJ et al. Definitive radiotherapy for squamous cell carcinoma of the base of tongue. Am J Clin Oncol 2006; 29: 32–9.

118. Mendenhall WM, Morris CG, Amdur RJ et al. Definitive radiotherapy for tonsillar squamous cell carcinoma. Am J Clin Oncol 2006; 29: 290–7.

119. Chera BS, Amdur RJ, Hinerman RW et al. Definitive radiation therapy for squamous cell carcinoma of the soft palate. Head Neck 2008; 30: 1114–9.

120. Yoshida K, Inoue T, Inoue T et al. Treatment results of radiotherapy with or without surgery for posterior pharyngeal wall cancer of oropharynx and hypopharynx: prognostic value of tumor extension. Radiat Med 2004; 22: 30–6.

121. Stoeckli SJ. Sentinel node biopsy for oral and oropharyngeal squamous cell carcinoma of the head and neck. Laryngoscope 2007; 117: 1539–51.

122. Vikram B, Strong EW, Shah JP et al. Failure in the neck following multimodality treatment for advanced head and neck-cancer. Head Neck Surg 1984; 6: 724–9.

123. Werner JA, Dunne AA, Myers JN. Functional anatomy of the lymphatic drainage system of the upper aerodigestive tract and its role in metastasis of squamous cell carcinoma. Head Neck 2003; 25: 322–32.

124. Hermans R. Oropharyngeal cancer. Cancer Imaging 2005; 5: S52–S57.

125. Lindberg RD. Distribution of cervical lymph node metastases from squamous cell carcinoma of the upper respiratory and digestive tracts. Cancer 1972; 29: 1446–9.

126. Doweck I, Robbins KT, Mendenhall WM et al. Neck level-specific nodal metastases in oropharyngeal cancer: is there a role for selective neck dissection after definitive radiation therapy? Head Neck 2003; 25: 960–7.

127. Sessions DG, Lenox J, Spector GJ et al. Analysis of treatment results for base of tongue cancer. Laryngoscope 2003; 113: 1252–61.

128. Hannisdal K, Boysen M, Evensen JF. Different prognostic indices in 310 patients with tonsillar carcinomas. Head Neck 2003; 25: 123–31.

129. Sobin LH, Wittekind CH. TNM classification for malignant tumors. UICC, International Union Against Cancer, 6th ed. New York: Wiley-Liss; 2002.

130. Garavello W, Ciardo A, Spreafico R et al. Risk factors for distant metastases in head and neck squamous cell carcinoma. Arch Otolaryngol-Head Neck Surg 2006; 132: 762–6.

131. Leon X, Quer M, Orus C et al. Distant metastases in head and neck cancer patients who achieved locoregional control. Head Neck 2000; 22: 680–6.

132. Alvi A, Johnson JT. Development of distant metastasis after treatment of advanced-stage head and neck cancer. Head Neck 1997; 19: 500–5.

133. Troell RJ, Terris DJ. Detection of metastases from head and neck cancers. Laryngoscope 1995; 105: 247–50.

134. Kowalski LP, Carvalho AL, Priante AV et al. Predictive factors for distant metastasis from oral and oropharyngeal squamous cell carcinoma. Oral Oncol 2005; 41: 534–41.

135. Al-Othman MO, Morris CG, Hinerman RW et al. Distant metastases after definitive radiotherapy for squamous cell carcinoma of the head and neck. Head Neck 2003; 25: 629–33.

136. Slaughter DP, Southwick HW, Smejkal LW. Field cancerization in oral stratified squamous epithelium; clinical implications of multicentric origin. Cancer 1953; 6: 963–8.

137. Braakhuis BJ, Tabor MP, Kummer JA et al. A genetic explanation of Slaughter's concept of field cancerization: evidence and clinical implications. Cancer Res 2003; 63: 1727–30.

138. Bhattacharyya N, Nayak VK. Survival outcomes for second primary head and neck cancer; A matched analysis. Otolaryngol-Head Neck Surg 2005; 132: 63–8.

139. Vaamonde P, Martin C, Del Rio M et al. Second primary malignancies in patients with cancer of the head and neck. Otolaryngol-Head Neck Surg 2003; 129: 65–70.

140. Ota Y, Aoki T, Karakida K et al. Simultaneous treatment of multiple primary cancers of the oral cavity and other sites. Tokai J Exp Clin Med 2000; 25: 165–71.

141. Leon X, Quer M, Diez S et al. Second neoplasm in patients with head and neck cancer. Head Neck 1999; 21: 204–10.

142. Pharynx (including base of tongue, soft palate and uvula). In: Greene FL, Balch CM, Page DL et al. eds. American Joint Committee on Cancer. AJCC Cancer Staging Manual, 6th ed. New York: Springer, 2002: 31–46.

143. Do KA, Johnson MM, Doherty DA et al. Second primary tumors in patients with upper aerodigestive tract cancers: joint effects of smoking and alcohol (United States). Cancer Causes Control 2003; 14: 131–8.

144. Khuri FR, Kim ES, Lee JJ et al. The impact of smoking status, disease stage, and index tumor site on second primary tumor incidence and tumor recurrence in the head and neck retinoid chemoprevention trial. Cancer Epidemiol Biomarkers Prev 2001; 10: 823–9.

145. Hermans R. Extranodal lymphoma-neck Cancer Imaging 2004.

146. Stell PM, Nash JRG. Tumours of the oropharynx. In: Kerr AG, ed. Scott-Brown's Otolaryngology, Vol. 5. London: Butterworth, 1997.

147. Million R.R. The lymphomatous diseases. In: Textbook of Radiotherapy. Philadelphia: Lea and Febiger, 1980.

148. Rosenberg S, Berard C, Brown B Jr. et al. National Cancer Institute sponsored study of classifications of non-Hodgkin's lymphomas: summary and description of a working formulation for clinical usage. The Non-Hodgkin's Lymphoma Pathologic Classification Project. Cancer 1982; 49: 2112–35.

149. Spiro RH, Koss LG, Hajdu SI et al. Tumors of minor salivary origin. A clinicopathologic study of 492 cases. Cancer 1973; 31: 117–29.

150. Watkinson JC, Gaze MN, Wilson JA. Stell & Maran's Head & Neck Surgery. Oxford: Butterworth Heinemann, 2000.

151. Chen AY, Schrag N, Hao YP et al. Changes in treatment of advanced oropharyngeal cancer, 1985–2001. Laryngoscope 2007; 117: 16–21.

152. Kljajic V, Jovic R, Canji K et al. [Surgical techniques and outcomes in the treatment of malignant tongue base tumors]. Med Pregl 2007; 60: 49–53.

153. Woolgar JA. Histological distribution of cervical lymph node metastases from intraoral oropharyngeal squamous cell carcinomas. Br J Oral Maxillofac Surg 1999; 37: 175–80.

154. Shoaib T, Soutar DS, MacDonald DG et al. The accuracy of head and neck carcinoma sentinel lymph node biopsy in the clinically N0 neck. Cancer 2001; 91: 2077–83.

155. Kowalski LP, Carvalho AL. Feasibility of supraomohyoid neck dissection in N1 and N2a oral cancer patients. Head Neck 2002; 24: 921–4.

156. Ali S, Tiwari RM, Snow GB. False-positive and false-negative neck nodes. Head Neck Surg 1985; 8: 78–82.

157. Weber AL, Romo L, Hashmi S. Malignant tumors of the oral cavity and oropharynx: clinical, pathologic, and radiologic evaluation. Neuroimaging Clin N Am 2003; 13: 443–64.

158. Lin DT, Cohen SM, Coppit GL et al. Squamous cell carcinoma of the oropharynx and hypopharynx. Otolaryngol Clin N Am 2005; 38: 59–74.

159. Castelijns JA, van den Brekel MW. Imaging of lymphadenopathy in the neck. Eur Radiol 2002; 12: 727–38.

160. McGuirt WF, Greven K, Williams D et al. PET scanning in head and neck oncology: A review. Head Neck 1998; 20: 208–15.

161. Wong RJ. Current status of FDG-PET for head and neck cancer. J Surg Oncol 2008; 97: 649–52.

162. Nolop KB, Rhodes CG, Brudin LH et al. Glucose-utilization in vivo by human pulmonary neoplasms. Cancer 1987; 60: 2682–9.

163. Braams JW, Pruim J, Kole AC et al. Detection of unknown primary head and neck tumors by positron emission tomography. Int J Oral Maxillofac Surg 1997; 26: 112–5.

164. Kim MR, Roh JL, Kim JS et al. Utility of F-18-fluorodeoxyglucose positron emission tomography in the preoperative staging of squamous cell carcinoma of the oropharynx. Eur J Surg Oncol 2007; 33: 633–8.

165. Paulus P, Sambon A, Vivegnis D et al. ^{18}FDG-PET for the assessment of primary head and neck tumors: clinical, computed tomography, and histopathological correlation in 38 patients. Laryngoscope 1998; 108: 1578–83.

166. Ng SH, Yen TC, Chang JTC et al. Prospective study of [F-18] fluorodeoxyglucose positron emission tomography and computed tomography and magnetic resonance imaging in oral cavity squamous cell carcinoma with palpably negative neck. J Clin Oncol 2006; 24: 4371–76.

167. Ng SH, Yen TC, Liao CT et al. F-18-FDG PET and CT/MRI in oral cavity squamous cell carcinoma: a prospective study of 124 patients with histologic correlation. J Nucl Med 2005 46: 1136–43.

168. Schoder H, Carlson DL, Kraus DH et al. F-18-FDG PET/CT for detecting nodal metastases in patients with oral cancer staged N0 by clinical examination and CT/MRI. J Nucl Med 2006; 47: 755–62.

169. Schmid DT, Stoeckli SJ, Bandhauer F et al. Impact of positron emission tomography on the initial staging and therapy in locoregional advanced squamous cell carcinoma of the head and neck. Laryngoscope 2003; 113: 888–91.

170. Kunkel M, Forster GJ, Reichert TE et al. Detection of recurrent oral squamous cell carcinoma by [F-18]-2-fluorodeoxyglucose-positron emission tomography—implications for prognosis and patient management. Cancer 2003; 98: 2257–65.

171. Rusthoven KE, Raben D, Ballonoff A et al. Effect of radiation techniques in treatment of oropharynx cancer. Laryngoscope 2008; 118: 635–9.

172. Shah GV, Wesolowski JR, Ansari SA et al. New directions in head and neck imaging. J Surg Oncol 2008; 97: 644–8.

173. Nakamoto Y, Tatsumi M, Hammoud D et al. Normal FDG distribution patterns in the head and neck: PET/CT evaluation. Radiology 2005; 234: 879–85.

174. Townsend DW, Carney JPJ, Yap JT et al. PET/CT today and tomorrow. J Nucl Med 2004; 45: 4S–14S.

175. Branstetter BF, Blodgett TM, Zimmer LA et al. Head and neck malignancy: is PET/CT more accurate than PET or CT alone? Radiology 2005; 235: 580–6.

176. Schoder H, Yeung HWD, Conen M et al. Head and neck cancer: Clinical usefulness and accuracy of PET/CT image fusion. Radiology 2004; 231: 65–72.

177. Wong RJ, Lin DT, Schoder H et al. Diagnostic and prognostic value of [F-18]fluorodeoxyglucose positron emission tomography for recurrent head and neck squamous cell carcinoma. J Clin Oncol 2002; 20: 4199–208.

178. Hitchcock YJ, Bentz BG, Sharma PK et al. Planned neck dissection after definitive radiotherapy or chemoradiation for base of tongue cancers. Otolaryngol-Head Neck Surg 2007; 137: 422–7.

179. Newbold KL, Partridge M, Cook G et al. Evaluation of the role of 18FDG-PET/CT in radiotherapy target definition in patients with head and neck cancer. Acta Oncol 2008; 47: 1229–36.

180. Peters LJ. Changes in radiotherapeutic management of head and neck cancer: A 30-year perspective. Int J Radiat Oncol Biol Phys 2007; 69: S8–S11.

181. Yao M, Epstein JB, Modi BJ et al. Current surgical treatment of squamous cell carcinoma of the head and neck. Oral Oncol 2007; 43: 213–3.

182. Vokes EE, Weichselbaum RR, Lippman SM. Head and neck-cancer—reply. New Engl J Med 1993; 328: 1784.

183. Parsons JT, Mendenhall WM, Stringer SP et al. Squamous cell carcinoma of the oropharynx—surgery, radiation therapy, or both. Cancer 2002; 94: 2967–80.

184. Fu KK, Pajak TF, Trotti A et al. A Radiation Therapy Oncology Group (RTOG) phase III randomized study to compare hyperfractionation and two variants of accelerated fractionation to standard fractionation radiotherapy for head and neck squamous cell carcinomas: first report of RTOG 9003. Int J Radiat Oncol Biol Phys 2000; 48: 7–16.

185. Gillison ML, Forastiere AA. Larynx preservation in head and neck cancers—a discussion of the National Comprehensive Cancer Network practice guidelines. Hematology-Oncology Clinics N Am 1999; 13: 699–718.

186. Semrau R, Mueller RP, Stuetzer H et al. Efficacy of intensified hyperfractionated and accelerated radiotherapy and concurrent chemotherapy with carboplatin and 5-fluorouracil: updated results of a randomized multicentric trial in advanced head-and-neck cancer. Int J Radiat Oncol Biol Phys 2006; 64: 1308–16.

187. Denis F, Garaud P, Bardet E et al. Final results of the 94-01 French Head and Neck Oncology and Radiotherapy Group randomized trial comparing radiotherapy alone with concomitant radiochemotherapy in advanced-stage oropharynx carcinoma. J Clin Oncol 2004; 22: 69–76.

188. Bernier J, Domenge C, Ozsahin M et al. Postoperative irradiation with or without concomitant chemotherapy for locally advanced head and neck cancer. New Engl J Med 2004; 350: 1945–52.

189. Olmi P, Crispino S, Fallai C et al. Locoregionally advanced carcinoma of the oropharynx: conventional radiotherapy vs. accelerated hyperfractionated radiotherapy vs. concomitant radiotherapy and chemotherapy—a multicenter randomized trial. Int J Radiat Oncol Biol Phys 2003; 55: 78–92.

190. Pignon JP, Bourhis J, Domenge C et al. Chemotherapy added to locoregional treatment for head and neck squamous-cell carcinoma: three meta-analyses of updated individual data. Lancet 2000; 355: 949–55.

191. Brizel DM, Albers ME, Fisher SR et al. Hyperfractionated irradiation with or without concurrent chemotherapy for locally advanced head and neck cancer. New Engl J Med 1998; 338: 1798–804.

192. Layland MK, Sessions DG, Lenox J. The influence of lymph node metastasis in the treatment of squamous cell carcinoma of the oral cavity, oropharynx, larynx, and hypopharynx: N0 versus N+. Laryngoscope 2005; 115: 629–39.

193. Leemans CR, Tiwari R, Nauta JJP et al. Regional lymph-node involvement and its significance in the development of distant metastases in head and neck-carcinoma. Cancer 1993; 71: 452–6.

194. Audet N, Beasley NJ, MacMillan C et al. Lymphatic vessel density, nodal metastases, and prognosis in patients with head and neck cancer. Arch Otolaryngol-Head Neck Surg 2005; 131: 1065–70.

195. Shah JP, Andersen PE. Evolving role of modifications in neck dissection for oral squamous carcinoma. Br J Oral Maxillofac Surg 1995; 33: 3–8.

196. Leemans CR, Tiwari R, Vanderwaal I et al. The efficacy of comprehensive neck dissection with or without postoperative radiotherapy in nodal metastases of squamous-cell carcinoma of the upper respiratory and digestive tracts. Laryngoscope 1990; 100: 1194–8.

197. Browman GP, Wong G, Hodson I et al. Influence of cigarette-smoking on the efficacy of radiation-therapy in head and neck-cancer. New Engl J Med 1993; 328: 159–63.

198. Constine LS. What else dont we know about the late effects of radiation in patients treated for head and neck-cancer. Int J Radiat Oncol Biol Phys 1995; 31: 427–9.

199. Turner SL, Tiver KW, Boyages SC. Thyroid dysfunction following radiotherapy for head and neck cancer. Int J Radiat Oncol Biol Phys 1995; 31: 279–83.

200. Charbonneau N, Gelinas M, del Vecchio P et al. Primary radiotherapy for tonsillar carcinoma: a good alternative to a surgical approach. J Otolaryngol 2006; 35: 227–34.

201. Brunin F, Mosseri V, Jaulerry C et al. Cancer of the base of the tongue: Past and future. Head Neck 1999; 21: 751–9.

202. Mak AC, Morrison WH, Garden AS et al. Base-of-tongue carcinoma—treatment results using concomitant boost radiotherapy. Int J Radiat Oncol Biol Phys 1995; 33: 289–96.

203. Perez CA, Patel MM, Chao KSC et al. Carcinoma of the tonsillar fossa: prognostic factors and long-term therapy outcome. Int J Radiat Oncol Biol Phys 1998; 42: 1077–84.

204. Henk JM. Results of radiotherapy for carcinoma of oropharynx. Clin Otolaryngol 1978; 3: 137–43.

205. Henk JM. Treatment of oral-cancer by interstitial irradiation using Ir-192. Br J Oral Maxillofac Surg 1992; 30: 355–9.

206. Withers HR, Peters LJ, Taylor JMG et al. Local-control of carcinoma of the tonsil by radiation-therapy—an analysis of patterns of fractionation in 9 institutions. Int J Radiat Oncol Biol Phys 1995; 33: 549–62.

207. Fein DA, Lee WR, Amos WR et al. Oropharyngeal carcinoma treated with radiotherapy: a 30-year experience. Int J Radiat Oncol Biol Phys 1996; 34: 289–96.

208. Horiot JC, Le FR, N'Guyen T et al. Hyperfractionated compared with conventional radiotherapy in oropharyngeal carcinoma: an EORTC randomized trial. Eur J Cancer 1990; 26: 779–80.

209. Dische S, Saunders M, Barrett A et al. A randomised multicentre trial of CHART versus conventional radiotherapy in head and neck cancer. Radiother Oncol 1997; 44: 123–36.

210. Horiot JC, Bontemps P. An overview of the EORTC accelerated and hyperfractionated radiotherapy trials in head and neck cancer. Radiother Oncol 1996; 40: S30.

211. Overgaard J, Saad Hansen H, Sapra W. Conventional radiotherapy as the primary treatment of squamous-cell carcinoma of the head and neck. A randomized multicentre study of 5 versus 6 fractions per week: preliminary report from the DAHANCA 6 and 7 trial. Radiother Oncol 1996; 40: S31.

212. Isa AY, Ward TH, West CM et al. Hypoxia in head and neck cancer. Br J Radiol 2006; 79: 791–8.

213. Terris DJ. Head and neck cancer: the importance of oxygen. Laryngoscope 2000; 110: 697–707.

214. Gray LH, Conger AD, Ebert M et al. The concentration of oxygen dissolved in tissues at the time of irradiation as a factor in radiotherapy. Br J Radiol 1953; 26: 638–48.

215. Tatum JL, Kelloff GJ, Gillies RJ et al. Hypoxia: importance in tumor biology, noninvasive measurement by imaging, and value of its measurement in the management of cancer therapy. Int J Radiat Biol 2006; 82: 699–757.

216. Nordsmark M, Bentzen SM, Rudat V et al. Prognostic value of tumor oxygenation in 397 head and neck tumors after primary radiation therapy. An international multi-center study. Radiother Oncol 2005; 77: 18–24.

217. Nordsmark M, Overgaard J. Tumor hypoxia is independent of hemoglobin and prognostic for locoregional tumor control after primary radiotherapy in advanced head and neck cancer. Acta Oncol 2004; 43: 396–403.

218. Henk JM. Late results of a trial of hyperbaric-oxygen and radiotherapy in head and neck-cancer—a rationale for hypoxic cell sensitizers. Int J Radiat Oncol Biol Phys 1986; 12: 1339–41.

219. Overgaard J, Hansen HS, Overgaard M et al. A randomized double-blind phase III study of nimorazole as a hypoxic radiosensitizer of primary radiotherapy in supraglottic larynx and pharynx carcinoma, results of the Danish Head and Neck Cancer Study (DAHANCA) protocol 5-85. Radiother Oncol 1998; 46: 135–46.

220. Lee NY, Mechalakos JG, Nehmeh S et al. Fluorine-18-labeled fluoromisonidazole positron emission and computed tomography-guided intensity-modulated radiotherapy for head and neck cancer: a feasibility study. Int J Radiat Oncol Biol Phys 2008; 70: 2–13.

221. Pernot M, Malissard L, Taghian A et al. Velotonsillar squamous cell carcinoma: 277 cases treated by combined external irradiation and brachytherapy—results according to extension, localization, and dose rate. Int J Radiat Oncol Biol Phys 1992; 23: 715–23.

222. Harrison LB, Zelefsky MJ, Sessions RB et al. Base-of-tongue cancer treated with external beam irradiation plus brachytherapy—oncologic and functional outcome. Radiology 1992; 184: 267–70.

223. Nose T, Koizumi M, Nishiyama K. High-dose-rate interstitial brachytherapy for oropharyngeal carcinoma: results of 83 lesions in 82 patients. Int J Radiat Oncol Biol Phys 2004; 59: 983–91.

224. Rudoltz MS, Perkins RS, Luthmann RW et al. High-dose-rate brachytherapy for primary carcinomas of the oral cavity and oropharynx. Laryngoscope 1999; 109: 1967–73.

225. Gibbs IC, Le QT, Shah RD et al. Long-term outcomes after external beam irradiation and brachytherapy boost for base-of-tongue cancers. Int J Radiat Oncol Biol Phys 2003; 57: 489–94.

226. Harrison LB, Lee HJ, Pfister DG et al. Long term results of primary radiotherapy with/without neck dissection for squamous cell cancer of the base of tongue. Head Neck 1998; 20: 668–73.

227. Lusinchi A, Eskandari J, Son Y et al. External irradiation plus curie therapy boost in 108 base of tongue carcinomas. Int J Radiat Oncol Biol Phys 1989; 17: 1191–7.

228. Pernot M, Malissard L, Hoffstetter S et al. Influence of tumoral, radiobiological, and general factors on local-control and survival of a series of 361 tumors of the velotonsillar area treated by exclusive irradiation (external-beam irradiation plus brachytherapy or brachytherapy alone). Int J Radiat Oncol Biol Phys 1994; 30: 1051–7.

229. Puthawala AA, Syed AMN, Eads DL et al. Limited external irradiation and interstitial ir-192 implant in the treatment of squamous-cell carcinoma of the tonsillar region. Int J Radiat Oncol Biol Phys1985; 11: 1595–602.

230. Overgaard J, Hansen HS, Specht L et al. Five compared with six fractions per week of conventional radiotherapy of squamous-cell carcinoma of head and neck: DAHANCA 6&7 randomised controlled trial. Lancet 2003; 362: 933–40.

231. Bourhis J, Overgaard J, Audry H et al. Hyperfractionated or accelerated radiotherapy in head and neck cancer: a meta-analysis. Lancet 2006; 368: 843–54.

232. Garden AS, Morrison WH, Rosenthal DI et al. Target coverage for head and neck cancers treated with IMRT: review of clinical experiences. Sem Radiat Oncol 2004; 14: 103–9.

233. Cozzi L, Fogliata A, Bolsi A et al. Three-dimensional conformal vs. intensity-modulated radiotherapy in head-and-neck cancer patients: comparative analysis of dosimetric and technical parameters. Int J Radiat Oncol Biol Phys 2004; 58: 617–24.

234. Li Y, Taylor JMG, Ten Haken RK, Eisbruch A. The impact of dose on parotid salivary recovery in head and neck cancer patients treated with radiation therapy. Int J Radiat Oncol Biol Phys 2007; 67: 660–9.

235. Lee NY, de Arruda FF, Puri DR et al. A comparison of intensity-modulated radiation therapy and concomitant boost radiotherapy in the setting of concurrent chemotherapy for locally advanced oropharyngeal carcinoma. Int J Radiat Oncol Biol Phys 2006; 66: 966–74.

236. Yao M, Dornfeld KJ, Buatti JM et al. Intensity-modulated radiation treatment for head-and-neck squamous cell carcinoma—The University of Iowa experience. Int J Radiat Oncol Biol Phys2005; 63: 410–21.

237. Chao KSC, Ozyigit G, Blanco AI et al. Intensity-modulated radiation therapy for oropharyngeal carcinoma: impact of tumor volume. Int J Radiat Oncol Biol Phys 2004; 59: 43–50.

238. Hodge CW, Bentzen SM, Wong G et al. Are we influencing outcome in oropharynx cancer with intensity modulated radiotherapy? An inter-era comparison. Int J Radiat Oncol Biol Phys 2007; 69: 1032–41.

239. Garden AS, Morrison WH, Wong PF et al. Disease-control rates following intensity-modulated radiation therapy for small primary oropharyngeal carcinoma. Int J Radiat Oncol Biol Phys 2007; 67: 438–44.

240. de Arruda FF, Puri DR, Zhung J et al. Intensity-modulated radiation therapy for the treatment of oropharyngeal carcinoma: the Memorial Sloan-Kettering Cancer Center experience. Int J Radiat Oncol Biol Phys 2006; 64: 363–73.

241. Mendenhall WM, Amdur RJ, Palta JR. Intensity-modulated radiotherapy in the standard management of head and neck cancer: promises and pitfalls. J Clin Oncol 2006; 24: 2618–23.

242. Milano MT, Vokes EE, Kao J et al. Intensity-modulated radiation therapy in advanced head and neck patients treated with intensive chemoradiotherapy: preliminary experience and future directions. Int J Oncol 2006; 28: 1141–51.

243. Studer G, Huguenin PU, Davis JB et al. IMRT using simultaneously integrated boost (SIB) in head and neck cancer patients. Radiat Oncol 2006; 1: 7.

244. Lamont EB, Vokes EE. Chemotherapy in the management of squamous-cell carcinoma of the head and neck. Lancet Oncol 2001; 2: 261–9.

245. Denis F, Garaud P, Manceau A et al. Prognostic value of the number of involved nodes after neck dissection in oropharyngeal and oral cavity carcinoma. Cancer Radiother 2001; 5: 12–22.

246. Adelstein DJ, Li Y, Adams GL et al. Intergroup phase III comparison of standard radiation therapy and two schedules of concurrent chemoradiotherapy in patients with unresectable squamous cell head and neck cancer. J Clin Oncol 2003; 21: 92–8.

247. Nguyen NP, Vos P, Smith HJ et al. Concurrent chemoradiation for locally advanced oropharyngeal cancer. Am J Otolaryngol 2007; 28: 3–8.

248. Machtay M, Rosenthal DI, Hershock D et al. Organ preservation therapy using induction plus concurrent chemoradiation for advanced resectable oropharyngeal carcinoma: a University of Pennsylvania phase II trial. J Clin Oncol 2002; 20: 3964–71.

249. Cooper JS, Pajak TF, Forastiere AA et al. Long-term survival results of a phase III intergroup trial (RTOG 95-01) of surgery followed by radiotherapy vs. radiochemotherapy for resectable high risk squamous cell carcinoma of the head and neck. Int J Radiat Oncol Biol Phys 2006; 66: S14–S15.

250. Cooper JS, Pajak TF, Forastiere AA et al. Postoperative concurrent radiotherapy and chemotherapy for high-risk squamous-cell carcinoma of the head and neck. New Engl J Med 2004; 350: 1937–44.

251. Bernier J, Cooper JS, Pajak TF et al. Defining risk levels in locally advanced head and neck cancers: a comparative analysis of concurrent postoperative radiation plus chemotherapy trials of the EORTC (#22931) and RTOG (#9501). Head and Neck-Journal for the Sciences and Specialties of the Head and Neck 2005; 27: 843–50.

252. Fletcher GH. Elective irradiation of subclinical disease in cancers of head and neck. Cancer 1972; 29: 1450–54.

253. Klijanienko J, Micheau C, Azli N et al. undifferentiated carcinoma of nasopharyngeal type of tonsil. Arch Otolaryngo-Head Neck Surg 1989; 115: 731–4.

254. Henk JM. Radiosensitivity of lymph node metastases. Proc R Soc Med 1975; 68: 85–6.

255. Peters LJ, Weber RS, Morrison WH et al. Neck surgery in patients with primary oropharyngeal cancer treated by radiotherapy. Head Neck 1996; 18: 552–9.

256. Huang DT, Johnson CR, Schmidtullrich R, Grimes M. Postoperative radiotherapy in head and neck-carcinoma with extracapsular lymph-node extension and or positive resection margins—a comparative-study. Int J Radiat Oncol Biol Phys 1992; 23: 737–42.

257. Clark J, Li W, Smith G et al. Outcome of treatment for advanced cervical metastatic squamous cell carcinoma. Head Neck 2005; 27: 87–94.

258. Blackburn TK, Bakhtawar S, Brown JS et al. A questionnaire survey of current UK practice for adjuvant radiotherapy following surgery for oral and oropharyngeal squamous cell carcinoma. Oral Oncol 2007; 43: 143–9.

259. Brown JS, Blackburn TK, Woolgar JA et al. A comparison of outcomes for patients with oral squamous cell carcinoma at intermediate risk of recurrence treated by surgery alone or with post-operative radiotherapy. Oral Oncol 2007; 43: 764–73.

260. Rhys Evans PH, Frame JW, Brandrick J. A review of carbon dioxide laser surgery in the oral cavity and pharynx. J Laryngol Otol 1986; 100: 69–77.

261. Eckel HE, Volling P, Pototschnig C et al. Transoral laser resection with staged discontinuous neck dissection for oral cavity and oropharynx squamous cell carcinoma. Laryngoscope 1995; 105: 53–60.

262. Steiner W, Fierek O, Ambrosch P, Hommerich CP, Kron M. Transoral laser microsurgery for squamous cell carcinoma of the base of the tongue. Arch Otolaryngol Head Neck Surg 2003; 129: 36–43.

263. Zeitels SM, Vaughan CW, Ruh S. Suprahyoid pharyngotomy for oropharynx cancer including the tongue base. Arch Otolaryngol Head Neck Surg 1991; 117: 757–60.

264. Civantos F, Wenig BL. Transhyoid resection of tongue base and tonsil tumors. Otolaryngol Head Neck Surg 1994; 111: 59–62.

265. Spiro RH, Gerold FP, Shah JP et al. Mandibulotomy approach to oropharyngeal tumors. Am J Surg 1985; 150: 466–9.

266. Shah JP, Kumaraswamy SV, Kulkarni V. Comparative-evaluation of fixation methods after mandibulotomy for oropharyngeal tumors. Am J Surg 1993; 166: 431–4.

267. Dubner S, Spiro RH. Median mandibulotomy—a critical-assessment. Head and Neck-Journal for the Sciences and Specialties of the Head and Neck 1991; 13: 389–93.

268. Altman K, Bailey BMW. Non-union of mandibulotomy sites following irradiation for squamous cell carcinoma of the oral cavity. Br J Oral Maxillofac Surg 1996; 34: 62–5.

269. Binahmed A, Nason RW, Abdoh AA. The clinical significance of the positive surgical margin in oral cancer. Oral Oncol 2007; 43: 780–4.

270. Krespi YP, Sisson GA. Reconstruction after total or subtotal glossectomy. Am J Surg 1983; 146: 488–92.

271. Weber RS, Ohlms L, Bowman J et al. Functional results after total or near total glossectomy with laryngeal preservation. Arch Otolaryngol-Head Neck Surg 1991; 117: 512–15.

272. Capote A, Escorial V, Munoz-Guerra MF et al. Elective neck dissection in early-stage oral squamous cell carcinoma—does it influence recurrence and survival? Head Neck 2007; 29: 3–11.

273. Wang SJ, Wang MB, Yip H et al. Combined radiotherapy with planned neck dissection for small head and neck cancers with advanced cervical metastases. Laryngoscope 2000; 110: 1794–7.

274. Roy S, Tibesar RJ, Daly K et al. Role of planned neck dissection for advanced metastatic disease in tongue base or tonsil squamous cell carcinoma treated with radiotherapy. Head Neck 2002; 24: 474–81.

275. Boyd TS, Harari PM, Tannehill SP et al. Planned postradiotherapy neck dissection in patients with advanced head and neck cancer. Head Neck 1998; 20: 132–7.

276. Hasegawa Y, Matsuura H. Retropharyngeal node dissection in cancer of the oropharynx and hypopharynx. Head Neck 1994; 16: 173–80.

277. Duvvuri U, Simental AA, D'Angelo G et al. Elective neck dissection and survival in patients with squamous cell carcinoma of the oral cavity and oropharynx. Laryngoscope 2004; 114: 2228–34.

278. Greenberg JS, El Naggar AK, Mo V et al. Disparity in pathologic and clinical lymph node staging in oral tongue carcinoma—implications for therapeutic decision making. Cancer 2003; 98: 508–15.

279. Jones AS, England J, Hamilton J et al. Mandibular invasion in patients with oral and oropharyngeal squamous carcinoma. Clin Otolaryngol 1997; 22: 239–45.

280. Patel RS, Dirven R, Clark JR et al. The prognostic impact of extent of bone invasion and extent of bone resection in oral carcinoma. Laryngoscope 2008; 118: 780–5.

281. Robinson CM, Prime SS, Paterson IC, Guest PG, Eveson JW. Expression of Ki-67 and p53 in cutaneous free flaps used to reconstruct soft tissue defects following resection of oral squamous cell carcinoma. Oral Oncol 2007; 43: 263–71.

282. Mendenhall WM, Amdur RJ, Stringer SP et al. Radiation therapy for squamous cell carcinoma of the tonsillar region: a preferred alternative to surgery? J Clin Oncol 2000; 18: 2219–25.

283. Hudgins PA, Burson JG, Gussack GS et al. CT and MR appearance of recurrent malignant head and neck neoplasms after resection and flap reconstruction. Am J Neuroradiol 1994; 15: 1689–94.

284. Velazquez RA, McGuff S, Sycamore D et al. The role of computed tomographic scans in the management of the N-positive neck in head and neck squamous cell carcinoma after chemoradiotherapy. Arch Otolaryngol-Head Neck Surg 2004; 130: 74–7.

285. Malone JP, Stephens JA, Grecula JC et al. Disease control, survival, and functional outcome after multimodal treatment for advanced-stage tongue base cancer. Head Neck 2004; 26: 561–72.

286. Friedlander P, Caruana S, Singh B et al. Functional status after primary surgical therapy for squamous cell carcinoma of the base of the tongue. Head Neck 2002; 24: 111–14.

287. Weber RS, Gidley P, Morrison WH et al. Treatment selection for carcinoma of the base of the tongue. Am J Surg 1990; 160: 415–19.

288. Kraus DH, Vastola AP, Huvos AG et al. Surgical management of squamous cell carcinoma of the base of the tongue. Am J Surg 1993; 166: 384–8.

289. Nisi KW, Foote RL, Bonner JA et al. Adjuvant radiotherapy for squamous cell carcinoma of the tongue base: improved local-regional disease control compared with surgery alone. Int J Radiat Oncol Biol Phys 1998; 41: 371–7.

290. Harrison LB, Zelefsky MJ, Armstrong JG et al. Performance status after treatment for squamous-cell cancer of the base

of tongue—a comparison of primary radiation-therapy versus primary surgery. Int J Radiat Oncol Biol Phys1994; 30: 953–7.

291. Ruhl CM, Gleich LL, Gluckman JL. Survival, function, and quality of life after total glossectomy. Laryngoscope 1997; 107: 1316–21.

292. Razack MS, Sako K, Bakamjian VY et al. Total glossectomy. Am J Surg 1983; 146: 509–11.

293. Gehanno P, Guedon C, Barry B et al. Advanced-carcinoma of the tongue—total glossectomy without total laryngectomy—review of 80 cases. Laryngoscope 1992; 102: 1369–71.

294. Foote RL, Olsen KD, Davis DL et al. Base of tongue carcinoma—patterns of failure and predictors of recurrence after surgery alone. Head Neck 1993; 15: 300–7.

295. Azizzadeh B, Enayati P, Chhetri D et al. Long-term survival outcome in transhyoid resection of base of tongue squamous cell carcinoma. Arch Otolaryngol Head Neck Surg 2002; 128: 1067–70.

296. Gourin CG, Johnson JT. Surgical treatment of squamous cell carcinoma of the base of tongue. Head Neck 2001; 23: 653–60.

297. Machtay M, Perch S, Markiewicz D et al. Combined surgery and postoperative radiotherapy for carcinoma of the base of tongue: analysis of treatment outcome and prognostic value of margin status. Head Neck 1997; 19: 494–9.

298. Thawley SE, Simpson JR, Perez CA et al. Preoperative irradiation and surgery for carcinoma of the base of the tongue. Ann Otol Rhinol Laryngol 1983; 92: 485–90.

299. Dupont JB, Guillamondegui OM, Jesse RH. Surgical treatment of advanced carcinomas of base of tongue. Am J Surg 1978; 136: 501–3.

300. Puthawala AA, Syed AMN, Eads DL et al. Limited external beam and interstitial Ir-192 irradiation in the treatment of carcinoma of the base of the tongue—a 10 year experience. Int J Radiat Oncol Biol Phys 1988; 14: 839–48.

301. Hu KS, Harrison LB, Culliney B. Head and neck cancer: a multidisciplinary approach. In: Harrison LB, Sessions RB, Hong WK, eds. Philadelphia: Lippincott Williams & Wilkins, 2004: 306–51.

302. Hicks WL Jr, Kuriakose MA, Loree TR et al. Surgery versus radiation therapy as single-modality treatment of tonsillar fossa carcinoma: the Roswell Park Cancer Institute experience (1971-1991). Laryngoscope 1998; 108: 1014–9.

303. Shirazi HA, Sivanandan R, Goode R et al. Advanced-staged tonsillar squamous carcinoma: organ preservation versus surgical management of the primary site. Head Neck 2006; 28: 587–94.

304. Tong D, Laramore GE, Griffin TW et al. Carcinoma of the tonsillar region—results of external irradiation. Cancer 1982; 49: 2009–14.

305. Soo KC, Tan EH, Wee J et al. Surgery and adjuvant radiotherapy vs concurrent chemoradiotherapy in stage III/IV nonmetastatic squamous cell head and neck cancer: a randomised comparison. Br J Cancer 2005; 93: 279–86.

306. Gillespie MB, Brodsky MB, Day TA et al. Laryngeal penetration and aspiration during swallowing after the treatment of advanced oropharyngeal cancer. Arch Otolaryngol-Head Neck Surg 2005; 131: 615–19.

307. Kramer S, Gelber RD, Snow JB et al. Combined radiation-therapy and surgery in the management of advanced head and neck-cancer—final report of Study 73–03 of the Radiation Therapy Oncology Group. Head Neck Surg 1987; 10: 19–30.

308. Browman GP, Hodson DI, Mackenzie RJ et al. Choosing a concomitant chemotherapy and radiotherapy regimen for squamous cell head and neck cancer: a systematic review of the published literature with subgroup analysis. Head Neck 2001; 23: 579–89.

309. Mendenhall WM, Riggs CE, Amdur RJ et al. Altered fractionation and/or adjuvant chemotherapy in definitive irradiation of squamous cell carcinoma of the head and neck. Laryngoscope 2003; 113: 546–51.

310. Laccourreye O, Hans S, Menard M et al. Transoral lateral oropharyngectomy for squamous cell carcinoma of the tonsillar region: II. An analysis of the incidence, related variables, and consequences of local recurrence. Arch Otolaryngol Head Neck Surg 2005; 131: 592–9.

311. Foote RL, Schild SE, Thompson WM et al. Tonsil cancer—patterns of failure after surgery alone and surgery combined with postoperative radiation-therapy. Cancer 1994; 73: 2638–47.

312. Mizono GS, Diaz RF, Fu KK et al. Carcinoma of the tonsillar region. Laryngoscope 1986; 96: 240–4.

313. Gluckman JL, Black RJ, Crissman JD. Cancer of the oropharynx. Otolaryngol Clin N Am 1985; 18: 451–9.

314. Rabuzzi DD, Mickler AS, Chung CT et al. Treatment results of combined high-dose preoperative radiotherapy and surgery for oropharyngeal cancer. Laryngoscope 1982; 92: 989–92.

315. Givens CD, Johns ME, Cantrell RW. Carcinoma of the Tonsil—analysis of 162 cases. Arch Otolaryngol-Head Neck Surg 1981; 107: 730–4.

316. Schuller DE, McGuirt WF, Krause CJ et al. Increased survival with surgery alone vs combined therapy. Laryngoscope 1979; 89: 582–94.

317. Gwozdz JT, Morrison WH, Garden AS et al. Concomitant boost radiotherapy for squamous carcinoma of the tonsillar fossa. Int J Radiat Oncol Biol Phys 1997; 39: 127–35.

318. Bataini JP, Asselain B, Jaulerry C et al. A multivariate primary tumor-control analysis in 465 patients treated by radical radiotherapy for cancer of the tonsillar region—clinical and treatment parameters as prognostic factors. Radiother Oncol 1989; 14: 265–77.

319. Wong CS, Ang KK, Fletcher GH et al. Definitive radiotherapy for squamous-cell carcinoma of the tonsillar fossa. Int J Radiat Oncol Biol Phys 1989; 16: 657–62.

320. Garrett PG, Beale FA, Cummings BJ et al. Carcinoma of the Tonsil—the effect of dose-time-volume factors on local-control. Int J Radiat Oncol Biol Phys 1985; 11: 703–6.

321. Amornmarn R, Prempree T, Jaiwatana J et al. Radiation management of carcinoma of the tonsillar region. Cancer 1984; 54: 1293–9.

322. Spiro RH, Kelly J, Vega AL et al. Squamous carcinoma of the posterior pharyngeal wall. Am J Surg 1990; 160: 420–3.

323. Guillamondegui OM, Meoz R, Jesse RH. Surgical treatment of squamous cell carcinoma of the pharyngeal walls. Am J Surg 1978; 136: 474–6.

324. Julieron M, Kolb F, Schwaab G et al. Surgical management of posterior pharyngeal wall carcinomas: functional and oncologic results. Head Neck 2001; 23: 80–6.

325. Hsu WC, Loevner LA, Karpati R et al. Accuracy of magnetic resonance imaging in predicting absence of fixation of head and neck cancer to the prevertebral space. Head Neck 2005; 27: 95–100.

326. Loevner LA, Ott IL, Yousem DM et al. Neoplastic fixation to the prevertebral compartment by squamous cell carcinoma of the head and neck. Am J Roentgenol 1998; 170: 1389–94.

327. Cooper RA, Slevin NJ, Carrington BM et al. Radiotherapy for carcinoma of the posterior pharyngeal wall. Int J Oncol 2000; 16: 611–15.

328. Jaulerry C, Brunin F, Rodriguez J et al. [Carcinomas of the posterior pharyngeal wall. Experience of the Institut Curie. Analysis of the results of radiotherapy]. Ann Otolaryngol Chir Cervicofac 1986; 103: 559–63.

329. Schwaab G, Vandenbrouck C, Luboinski B et al. Posterior pharyngeal wall carcinomas treated by primary surgery. J Eur de Radiother 1983; 4: 175–9.

330. Talton BM, Elkon D, Kim JA et al. Cancer of the posterior hypopharyngeal wall. Int J Radiat Oncol Biol Phys 1981; 7: 597–9.

331. Amdur RJ, Mendenhall WM, Parsons JT et al. Carcinoma of the soft palate treated with irradiation—analysis of results and complications. Radiother Oncol 1987; 9: 185–94.

332. Medini E, Medini A, Gapany M et al. External beam radiation therapy for squamous cell carcinoma of the soft palate. Int J Radiat Oncol Biol Phys1997; 38: 507–11.

333. Leemans CR, Engelbrecht WJ, Tiwari R et al. Carcinoma of the soft palate and anterior tonsillar pillar. Laryngoscope 1994; 104: 1477–81.

334. Keus RB, Pontvert D, Brunin F, Jaulerry C, Bataini JP. Results of irradiation in squamous-cell carcinoma of the soft palate and uvula. Radiother Oncol 1988; 11: 311–17.

335. Esche BA, Haie CM, Gerbaulet AP et al. Interstitial and external radiotherapy in carcinoma of the soft palate and uvula. Int J Radiat Oncol Biol Phys 1988; 15: 619–25.

13

Tumors of the Hypopharynx

David P Goldstein, J John Kim, Patrick J Gullane and Paul Q Montgomery

INTRODUCTION

Hypopharyngeal tumors have one of the poorest survival rates of any head and neck site and are associated with significant morbidity. Early symptoms are often vague, and most patients are diagnosed at a late stage when the tumor is locally advanced and nodal metastases are frequently present. Progressive dysphagia over several months prior to diagnosis may reduce the patient to a poor physical state with a correspondingly increased risk of morbidity and mortality following treatment. The larynx is frequently involved, although in the early stages of the disease hoarseness is not a common symptom. Primary total laryngectomy with partial or total pharyngectomy is associated with a profound alteration in quality of life. However, advances in reconstructive surgery and voice rehabilitation has allowed for more extensive surgery with reduced morbidity and better functional outcomes. Some patients will require adjuvant radiotherapy (RT) with or without chemotherapy.

Because of the poorer prognosis of hypopharyngeal cancers, even early-stage cancers are often treated with aggressive organ preservation strategies. Altered radiation dose-fractionation schedules or combined modality treatment with radiation and concurrent chemotherapy has offered a rational basis to avoid laryngectomy with improvements in control rates and survival compared to standard once-daily RT. Primary RT is associated with a risk of chronic dysphagia because of postradiation fibrosis. For those patients who recur after primary RT, salvage surgery is associated with an increased risk of complications and may not be feasible. The complex management of these tumors exemplifies the essential need for a multidisciplinary team approach.

SURGICAL ANATOMY

The hypopharynx is the part of the pharynx that extends from the level of the hyoid cartilage superiorly to the lower border of the cricoid cartilage. It is divided into three subsites: the piriform fossae, the postcricoid region, and the posterior pharyngeal wall (Fig. 13.1) (1,2).

Piriform Fossa
Relations
Each piriform fossa is analogous to an inverted pyramid with a base (superior), medial and lateral walls and an apex (inferior) (1–4). The base is formed by the hypopharyngeal aspect of the lateral pharyngoepiglottic and adjacent aryepiglottic folds. The apex is at the confluence of the medial and lateral walls at the entrance of the cervical esophagus at or just below the inferior border of the cricopharyngeus muscle. The medial wall of the hypopharynx includes the lateral surface of the aryepiglottic fold, the arytenoid and cricoid cartilages, and is related to the paraglottic space, the laryngeal ventricle, saccule, and the intrinsic muscles of the larynx. A distinction is made by some authors (5,6) between the superior aspect of the medial wall (aryepiglottic fold: part of the epilarynx) and the inferior aspect (the piriform fossa proper), as the prognosis of squamous cell carcinomas (SCCs) in the former site is better. The lateral wall of the piriform fossa is formed by the inferior constrictor (thyropharyngeus and cricopharyngeus muscles), and deep to this the internal branches of the superior laryngeal neurovascular bundle, the hyoid, thyrohyoid membrane and thyroid ala. A descriptive distinction is also made between the upper "membranous" and lower "cartilaginous" piriform fossa, that part of the lateral wall mucosa that is, respectively, adjacent to the thyrohyoid membrane and the cartilaginous thyroid ala (7).

Innervation
Sensation is via the glossopharyngeal and vagal cranial nerves through the pharyngeal plexus. Lesions within the piriform fossa may cause a sensation medial to the sternomastoid muscle and lateral to the thyroid ala. The common origin of Arnold's nerve to the external auditory canal and the internal branch of the superior laryngeal nerve from the vagus results in the phenomenon of referred otalgia associated with invasive piriform lesions (8). Motor innervation is via the pharyngeal plexus and the recurrent laryngeal nerve from the vagus.

Lymphatic Drainage
Lymphatic channels draining the piriform fossa pierce the thyrohyoid membrane (with associated nodes at the lateral margin of the thyrohyoid muscle) to follow the superior laryngeal artery where they drain into three main lymph node groups: the subdigastric nodes, the lateral jugular nodes, and the jugular nodes below the common facial vein. Pathological studies suggest that midjugular nodes (level III) drain twice the lymphatic flow as the upper (level II) or lower jugular nodes (level IV) (9). Hasegawa and Matsuura (10) noted the significance of retropharyngeal nodes in the lymphatic drainage of the piriform fossa in advanced carcinoma (Fig. 13.2).

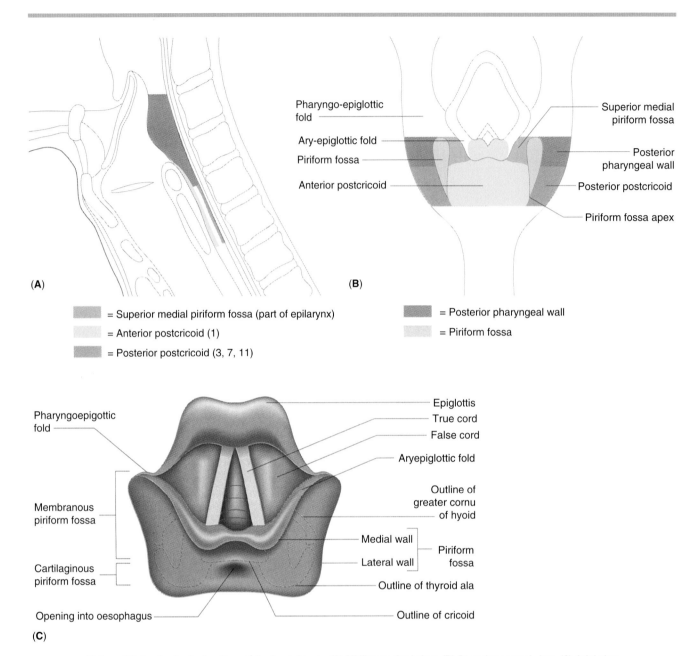

Figure 13.1 Anatomical regions of the hypopharynx. **(A)** Midline sagittal view. **(B)** Posterior coronal view. **(C)** Axial view.

Postcricoid

The postcricoid area is the anterior (laryngeal) surface extending from the superior aspect of the arytenoid cartilages to the inferior border of the cricoid cartilage. Silver (3), Ogura et al. (11), and Million and Cassisi (7) also included the opposing posterior pharyngeal mucosal surface enclosed by cricopharyngeus, thus regarding this subsite as a circumferential surface.

Relations

Deep to the mucosa are the arytenoids, the cricoarytenoid joints, the cricoid and the interarytenoid and posterior cricoarytenoid muscles. Inferiorly, any tumor growth on the anterior (laryngeal) surface below the cricoid, toward the esophagus, brings the tumor into direct relationship with the trachealis muscle and recurrent laryngeal nerves.

Innervation

Sensation is through the glossopharyngeal and vagus nerves via the pharyngeal plexus (8). Lesions produce a globus sensation, prior to true dysphagia, at the level of the suprasternal notch.

Lymphatic Drainage

The postcricoid mucosa may drain directly through the muscular layer to local lymph nodes or pass submucosally

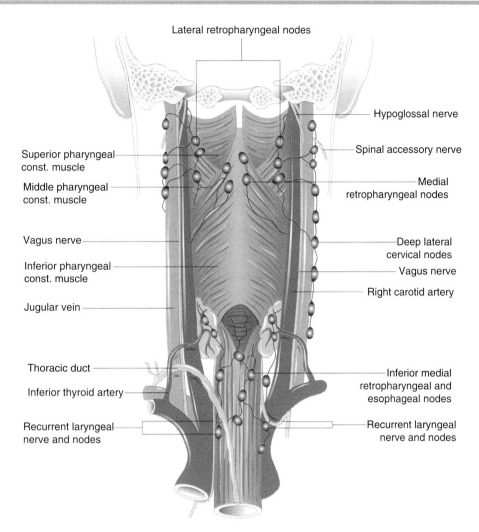

Lateral retropharyngeal nodes

Superior pharyngeal
const. muscle

Middle pharyngeal
const. muscle

Vagus nerve

Inferior pharyngeal
const. muscle

Jugular vein

Thoracic duct

Inferior thyroid artery

Recurrent laryngeal
nerve and nodes

Hypoglossal nerve

Spinal accessory nerve

Medial
retropharyngeal nodes

Deep lateral
cervical nodes

Vagus nerve

Right carotid artery

Inferior medial
retropharyngeal and
esophageal nodes

Recurrent laryngeal
nerve and nodes

Figure 13.2 Lymphatic drainage of the hypopharynx viewed posteriorly.

then pierce the muscular layer. Thus midline flow is not only bilateral (12), but also submucosal; and this has surgical implications as to the extent of resection. The lymphatics drain to the nodes associated with the recurrent laryngeal nerve in the paratracheal and esophageal grooves (Fig. 13.2) and then to level IV, or to ascend with the lymphatic drainage of the piriform fossa (levels II and III), or to drain down into the superior mediastinum (8).

Posterior Pharyngeal Wall

The posterior wall of the hypopharynx extends from the horizontal level of the floor of the vallecula to the inferior border of the cricoid (1), and laterally it merges into the piriform fossa (Fig. 13.1). In the International Union Against Cancer (UICC) definition (1) it is implicit that the term *posterior pharyngeal wall* includes the lateral walls of the hypopharynx. It is difficult to define precisely and has a maximum anteroposterior extent of 2 cm (7). Pure lateral pharyngeal wall lesions are correspondingly very rare [7% of oro- and hypopharyngeal tumors (13)]. The deep relations of the lateral wall are significantly different to those

of the posterior wall. Local control, recurrence, and survival between the two areas is similar for T1/2/3 growths (14) but T4 lesions of the posterior pharyngeal wall have a much poorer local control than those of the lateral pharyngeal wall (29 vs. 68%) (15).

Relations
The deep relation of the lateral aspect of the posterior pharyngeal wall is the lateral pharyngeal space containing the carotid sheath whereas that of the posterior aspect of the posterior pharyngeal wall is the prevertebral fascia and muscles.

Innervation
This is from the glossopharyngeal and vagus nerves via the pharyngeal plexus, the superior and recurrent laryngeal nerves (8).

Lymphatic Drainage
The posterior pharyngeal wall lymphatics may drain bilaterally, passing to the lateral retropharyngeal nodes or the

internal jugular nodes (levels II and III) (9,16). Hasegawa and Matsuura (10) and Ballantyne (17) highlighted the significance of the retropharyngeal nodes in the lymphatic drainage of the posterior pharyngeal wall in advanced carcinoma.

HISTOLOGY

The vast majority of hypopharyngeal malignancies are SCCs, accounting for more than 95% of cases (18–20). The majority of the remaining malignancies are adenocarcinomas. Occasionally other tumor types such as sarcomas, lymphomas, and melanomas have been reported.

EPIDEMIOLOGY

Hypopharyngeal carcinomas account for less than 10% of all SCCs of the upper aerodigestive tract (3). The reported incidence rates varies worldwide, with Northern France exhibiting one of the highest incidence rates (21) of 14.8 per 100,000 per annum, accounting for 18% of all upper aerodigestive tract (UADT) lesions (Table 13.1). In North America the overall reported incidence rate is 1 per 100,000 per year (19). In North America and France hypopharyngeal carcinomas most commonly arise in the piriform fossa, whereas postcricoid lesions appear more commonly in Northern Europe (Table 13.2).

The mean age at presentation of hypopharyngeal tumors is approximately 60 years. Piriform fossa and posterior pharyngeal wall lesions demonstrate the typical male predominance: for piriform fossa lesions this sex difference is marked in North America [approximately 5–20 males to 1 female (22–24)] and extreme in France with ratios of nearly 50:1 (6,25). Postcricoid lesions, unlike all other sites, show a consistent moderate female preponderance (approximately 1.5:1 female/male ratio) (12,26–29).

ETIOLOGY

As with all head and neck SCCs there is a significant association with alcohol and smoking, which also act synergistically. Postcricoid carcinoma is associated with previous radiation exposure; variously reported in 4 to 7% of cases (12,26,30) and sideropenic dysphagia (12,27,28) also known as Plummer–Vinson or Patterson Brown-Kelly syndrome. The syndrome, which tends to occur in females aged 30 to 50 without a history of tobacco and alcohol use, is characterized by dysphagia, associated weight loss and iron-deficiency anemia (31). Today the syndrome is rare in regions with improved nutrition and fortification of food with vitamins and iron. Radiation exposure has also been implicated in posterior pharyngeal wall carcinomas (32). Although human papilloma virus has been implicated in oropharyngeal carcinoma, its role in the carcinogensis of hypopharyngeal cancer is less well defined. Rates of detection range from 19 to 29% (33–35).

STAGING SYSTEMS

As with other carcinomas of the upper aerodigestive tract, hypopharyngeal carcinomas are staged using the system adopted by the UICC/American Joint Committee on Caner (AJCC) (1) (Table 13.3). The sixth and latest edition (1,36) subdivides T4 lesions into T4a and T4b based on their resectability.

Piriform Fossa
The UICC/AJCC (1) system, as applied to the piriform fossa, is generally accepted by most centers as the reporting system of choice in its ability to reflect the natural history and prognoses of lesions at this subsite. Bataini (6) excludes the superior part of the piriform aspect of the aryepiglottic fold, which he regards as part of the epilarynx, where tumors have a better prognosis. Other systems have been used (6,11) in an attempt to reflect the natural history/prognosis of the disease. It is worth noting that a tumor may progress from a T1 to T4 without intermediate T stages depending on its position and direction of spread (see below).

Postcricoid
Prior to 1997 the UICC/AJCC system attracted criticism as tumor length was not included. This was a significant omission as tumor length relates to the degree of invasion through the muscle coat to the adventitia, circumferential spread, and into the thyroid gland (37). Other staging systems therefore evolved to address this issue (11,28), and in 1997 the UICC/AJC system was amended to include length.

Posterior Pharyngeal Wall
As with postcricoid lesions the pre-1997 UICC/AJC system was criticized as the size of the lesions was not taken into

Table 13.1 Incidence of Hypopharyngeal Carcinoma per 100 000 per Year

Sweden (21)	0.84
USA (8)	1
Canada (22)	0.75
UK (23)	0.7
France (20)	14.8

Table 13.2 Distribution by Site of Hypopharyngeal Carcinoma

Site	France (6)	Canada (22)	USA (24)	Brazil (25)	Belgium (26)	UK (27)	Finland (28)
Piriform fossa (%)	90	85	59	97	89	60	52
Posterior pharyngeal wall (%)	7	8	35	3	9	5	18
Postcricoid (%)	3	7	6	–	2	35	30

Table 13.3 Staging System for Hypopharyngeal Tumours (1)

T1   One subsite of the hypopharynx and 2 cm or less in greatest dimension

T2   More than one subsite of the hypopharynx or an adjacent site, or measures more than 2 cm but not more than 4 cm in greatest dimension, without fixation of hemilarynx

T3   Tumor measures more than 4 cm in greatest dimension, or with fixation of hemilarynx

T4a Tumor invades thyroid/cricoid cartilage, hyoid bone, thyroid gland, esophagus, or central compartment soft tissue, which includes prelaryngeal strap muscles and subcutaneous fat

T4b Tumor invades prevertebral fascia, encases carotid artery, or involves mediastinal structures

NX   Regional lymph nodes cannot be assessed

N0   No regional lymph node metastasis

N1   Metastasis in a single ipsilateral lymph node, 3 cm or less in greatest dimension

N2a Metastasis in a single ipsilateral lymph node more than 3 cm but not more than 6 cm in greatest dimension

N2b Metastasis in multiple ipsilateral lymph nodes, none more than 6 cm in greatest dimension

N2c Metastasis in bilateral or contralateral lymph nodes, none more than 6 cm in greatest dimension

N3   Metastasis in a lymph node more than 6 cm in greatest dimension

Stage grouping

Stage 0: Tis, N0, M0
Stage I: T1, N0, M0
Stage II: T2, N0, M0
Stage III: T1, 2 or 3, N1, M0 or T3, N0, M0
Stage IVA: T1, 2 or 3, N2, M0, or
T4a, N0, 1 or 2, M0
Stage IVB: T4b, Any N, M0, or
Any T, N3, M0
Stage IVC: Any T, Any N, M1

Note: midline nodes are considered ipsilateral nodes.

Table 13.4 Symptoms of Hypopharyngeal Carcinoma

Symptoms	Piriform fossa (26) (%)	Postcricoid (12,33) (%)		Posterior wall (42) (%)
Dysphagia	41	99	90	46
Odynophagia	18	–	18	60
Otalgia	9	–	9	14
Hoarseness	31	20	15	11
Neck lump	–	–	7	14
Weight loss	–	54	–	–
Dyspnoea	1	–	–	–

nodal metastases, and up to 75% of patients have pathologically involved nodes on presentation of which at least 10% are bilateral (41,42).

Postcricoid

Rapid onset of dysphagia is common with 50% of patients having symptoms for fewer than 3 months (28). Other symptoms such as voice change are common because of the proximity of the larynx. Large retropharyngeal nodes may produce occipital and nape of the neck pain radiating to the retrorbital area (Table 13.4) (8).

Posterior Pharyngeal Wall

Dysphagia and sore throat are common symptoms, but the primary complaint of a neck mass has been reported in 18% of cases; 10% are asymptomatic and found incidentally (43). As with postcricoid lesions large retropharyngeal nodes may produce occipital and nape of the neck pain radiating to the retrorbital area (Table 13.4) (8).

NATURAL HISTORY: CLINICOPATHOLOGICAL FEATURES
Piriform Fossa
Primary Tumor

Piriform fossa lesions behave in a similar manner to transglottic rather than supraglottic laryngeal tumors (26). The appearance is usually classified as either exophytic or endophytic with the former having generally a better prognosis. Tani et al. (44) reported 20% of tumors predominantly medial, 35% lateral, and 45% involving both walls (Fig.13.3). The majority of lesions (>80%) present late (Table 13.5) with vocal cord immobility and/or cartilage invasion.

Lateral and apical extension is associated with invasion of cartilage (22) and submucosal spread may be beyond 10 mm (45). Superiorly, the base of the tongue is at risk if extension is beyond the lateral pharyngoepiglottic fold into the vallecula (22).

Cervical esophageal involvement is seen less commonly than with primary postcricoid tumors, but apical spread is an ominous sign as it is associated with a high probability of invasion of the thyroid and cricoid cartilages (22). Involvement of the tracheo-esophageal groove and cricopharyngeus occurs by deep extension after postcricoid involvement (3).

Medial invasion is via the paraglottic space into the larynx (Fig. 13.4) and thence through the cricothyroid

account. T1 lesions would not only include the smallest invasive lesion but also a massive lesion completely occupying the posterior pharyngeal wall and thus many clinicians used the size-based UICC (1) oropharyngeal system. Another consideration was that posterior pharyngeal wall carcinomas often arise at the junction of the oro- and hypopharynx creating a dilemma as to which UICC (1) system should be used. Pene et al. (38) and Schwaab et al. (39) suggested a compromise classification for all posterior pharyngeal wall carcinomas. The 1997 UICC/AJC classification was updated to include site and size criteria to answer these issues.

NATURAL HISTORY: SYMPTOMS
Piriform Fossa

Unilateral sore throat and dysphagia are common symptoms of intraluminal growth although their onset may be late. As these symptoms become more severe they are associated with weight loss. Otalgia is associated with invasion through the pharyngeal wall and hoarseness from involvement of laryngeal musculature (Table 13.4) (40). The profuse lymphatic drainage from the piriform fossa results in early

membrane to involve the lower border of the thyroid and upper border of the cricoid cartilage (22). Olofssen and Van Nostrand (26) noted invasion of the laryngeal muscles in 42% of cases with spread to the false cord in 16%, preepiglottic invasion in 5% and tracheal invasion in 5%. Tani et al. (44) found that tumors originating on the medial wall,

which had extended to the posterior pharyngeal wall or postcricoid region, had all extended into the laryngeal structures.

Tumors of the lateral wall are associated with cartilaginous involvement in 55%, predominantly the posterior border of the thyroid cartilage (22), and invasion of the thyroid gland in 11% (26). Superficially tumors may spread onto the posterior pharyngeal wall. Tumors on the lateral wall may penetrate through the pharyngeal wall into the neck without necessarily causing vocal cord fixation, so T1/2 lesions may progress directly to a T4 lesion without a T3 stage (44).

Tani et al. (44) reported normal vocal cord mobility in 20% of cases, partial mobility in 10%, and fixed cord in 70% of cases and found that fixation of the cords was strongly associated with intrinsic laryngeal muscle invasion. Involvement of the arytenoid cartilage or cricoarytenoid joint occurred in only 30% of cases, and all of these had significant invasion of the intrinsic laryngeal muscles. Tani suggested that in medially based tumors a T1 lesion may progress to a T3 lesion due to involvement of the intrinsic laryngeal muscles without passing through the T2 stage (44).

Kirchner also found that limitation of vocal cord mobility or fixation was due to invasion of the posterior cricoarytenoid or interarytenoid muscles (46). Olofsson and Van Nostrand (26) noted that in cases of vocal cord fixation, 42% showed invasion of the intrinsic laryngeal muscles and invasion of the cricoarytenoid joint in 16%. Perineural invasion of the recurrent laryngeal nerve is quite common but is unlikely to be the primary cause of vocal cord fixation (26).

Kirchner highlighted the problem of understaging with 47% of clinical T3 lesions having cartilage invasion (Fig. 13.5) (22) mainly associated with apical and lateral surface extension. None of the T1 or T2 tumors had histological involvement of cartilage. Tani et al. (44) pointed out that cartilage involvement was more likely to be contact

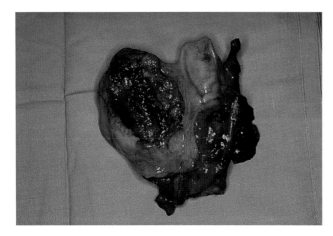

Figure 13.3 Piriform fossa tumour involving medial and lateral walls.

Table 13.5 Percentage T Stage Distribution at Presentation

T stage	Kirchner (AJC 1973) (29)	El Badawi et al. (AJC 1977) (45)
T1	5	5
T2	4	12
T3	91	38
T4	–	45

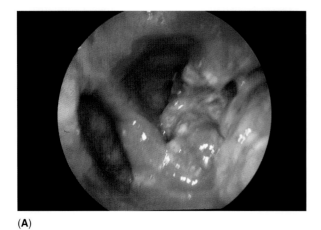

(A)

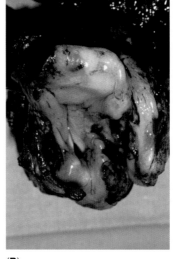

(B)

Figure 13.4 **(A)** Advanced carcinoma of the right piriform fossa with extension to the larynx (courtesy of JP Shah, Mosby). **(B)** Piriform fossa tumour invading medially into the larynx.

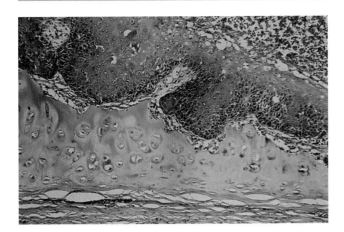

Figure 13.5 Laryngeal cartilage invasion by tumour.

Table 13.6 Analysis of Cartilage Involvement in Piriform Fossa Lesions (44)

Cartilage	'Involvement' (%)	Contact(%)	Invasion(%)
Thyroid	90	60	30
Cricoid	45	40	5
Arytenoid	50	All	None

Table 13.7 Stage Groupings (1988 AJC) at Presentation for Piriform Fossa Lesions

Stage	Bataini et al. (6) (%)	El Badawi et al. (45) (%)
I	3	6
II	4	22
III	50	38
IV	43	34

rather than invasion (Table 13.6) and concluded that the arytenoid cartilage diverts spread either anteromedially to the thyroarytenoid muscle or posteromedially towards the cricoarytenoid joint (seldom invading it) and thence to the postcricoid laryngeal muscles.

Olofssen and Van Nostrand (26) found 42% of pharyngolaryngectomy specimens had thyroid lamina invasion with half of these extending beyond the larynx, 58% involving one or more laryngeal cartilages, and epiglottic invasion occurring in 5%.

Regional Metastasis

Neck metastasis at presentation is common, and the majority of piriform fossa lesions are stage III to IV, reflecting a large primary tumor and a high propensity for nodal metastasis (Table 13.7).

Kirchner (22) reported an incidence of 57%, Harrison (45) 65%, Million and Cassisi (41) 75%, and Olofssen 63% (26). In those who had no palpable disease and who had an elective neck dissection, 60% had micrometastases (22,42).

Table 13.8 Correlation of Clinical with Pathological Nodal State (29)

	pN+ve (%)	pN-ve (%)
cN+ve	72	28
cN-ve	60	40

Table 13.9 Patterns of Histologically Proven Cervical Node Metastases Related to Clinical Nodal Status (16)

Lymph node region	cN-ve (%)	cN+ve (%)
I	0	6
II	15	72
III	8	72
IV	0	47
V	0	8

In patients who had palpable neck disease (cN+ve) there was a significant false positive rate of 28% (Table 13.8) (22).

Levels II and III are mainly at risk of micrometastases in cN-negative necks (16), but in cN-positive patients the pattern of nodal spread suggests that all levels were at significant risk of metastasis (Table 13.9). Involvement of levels I or V is unlikely without simultaneous nodes in levels II, III, and IV being present. Patients classified as cN1 were in fact pN2b in 75% of cases (i.e., more than one node involved).

Retropharyngeal node involvement has been found in 56% of patients with T2/3 lesions (10) and bilateral and contralateral nodal disease has been reported in 3 to 30% (10,47,48) associated with advancing T stage but not with tumor differentiation (22). Involvement of paratracheal nodes is much lower in hypopharyngeal tumors (8.3%) than with cervical esophageal carcinoma (71%) (49).

Second Primaries

Approximately 6% of patients develop second primaries (50).

Postcricoid

Primary Tumor

Small tumors are unusual (Fig. 13.6), and macroscopic mucosal spread at presentation is often extensive (Tables 13.10–13.13) with involvement of the piriform fossa and/or the posterior pharyngeal wall in 20 to 50% of cases. Willatt et al. (37) found 35% had a longitudinal macroscopic extension of over 5 cm. Tumors greater than 5 cm in length were associated with circumferential involvement of the hypopharynx and invasion of the thyroid.

The extent of submucosal spread beyond the macroscopic tumor edge is of critical importance as it influences the RT fields, the extent of resection, and the mode of reconstruction. Davidge-Pitts and Mannel (51) found submucosal spread 5 to 10 mm above the superior macroscopic extent of the tumor. Inferiorly the average macroscopic extension into the cervical esophagus was 10 mm with a further 6 to 30 mm (average 15 mm) of submucosal spread. In Harrison's series (52) submucosal spread was found 5 mm inferiorly and 10 mm superior to the macroscopic margin.

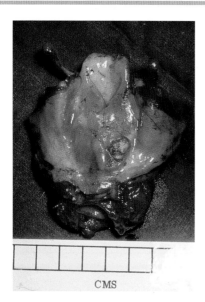

Figure 13.6 Small postcricoid carcinoma.

Table 13.10 T Stage Presentation for Postcricoid Carcinoma

T stage	Stell et al. (12) (%)	Farrington et al. (33) (%)	Tandon et al. (34) (%)	Olofsson and Van Nostrand (21) (%)
T1	32	8	0	27
T2	62	26	17	49
T3	6	24	39	19
T4	–	43	43	5

Vocal cord immobility or hemilaryngeal fixation in postcricoid carcinoma is due to direct spread into the paraglottic space or to involvement of the recurrent laryngeal nerve. It is a late feature and may be associated with laryngeal cartilage invasion in 26% of patients (37).

Olofsson and Van Nostrand (26) found that 43% of postcricoid tumors at laryngectomy had invasion of the cricoid cartilage and 14% had involvement of the trachea and thyroid gland.

Regional Metastasis
The incidence of cervical node involvement in postcricoid tumors is in the region of 33 to 52% (12,45) of which one fourth may be bilateral or fixed (Tables 13.11 and 13.12).

Table 13.11 Nodal Status in Postcricoid Carcinoma

Nodel status	Stell et al. (12) (%)	Pingree et al. (53) (%)	Tandon et al. (34) (%)	Harrison (46) (%)
N0	67	65	74	48
N+	33	35	26	52

Table 13.12 Incidence of Nodal Involvement as Related to T Stage

T stage	Stell et al. (12) (%)	Farrington et al. (33) (%)	Tandon et al. (34) (%)
T1	34	6	0
T2	38	17	25
T3	50	38	11
T4	–	50	40

Unrecognized spread to paratracheal and lower deep cervical nodes may result in stomal and tracheal recurrence (45). Hasegawa and Matsuura (10) noted that retropharyngeal nodes were involved in 75% of patients with advanced (stage III–IV) postcricoid primaries.

Node involvement is associated with a 50% incidence of vocal cord paralysis, and 40% of patients will have tumors larger than 5 cm (23). Like piriform fossa tumors the majority of postcricoid lesions are stage III to IV at presentation (Table 13.13).

Distant Metastases and Second Primaries
Distant metastases from postcricoid carcinomas are rare at presentation with an incidence of between 0 and 2% (12,26, 28,37). The 2% incidence of second primaries (12,50) is less than for piriform fossa tumors (6%).

Patient Status
Patients with postcricoid cancer may be unsuitable for radical therapy not only due to very advanced disease but also due to severe weight loss secondary to dysphagia and/or concomitant disease, which precludes radical treatment. Jones et al. (53) found 25% unsuitable for any treatment, and Stell et al. (12) noted that in the 30% who had no treatment, one half were unsuitable because of poor general health.

Posterior Pharyngeal Wall
Primary Tumor
The commonest site of origin is at the oro-hypopharyngeal junction (38,39): 80% are ulcerative/infiltrative (38,39) and

Table 13.13 Stage Grouping Presentation of Postcricoid Lesions

Stage	Stell et al. (12) (%)	Farrington et al. (33) (%)	Pingree et al. (53) (%)	Tandon et al. (34) (%)	Olofsson and Van Nostrand (21) (%)
I	21	7		0	21
II	37	21	{15.5}	13	36
III	22	23		39	25
IV	20	49	{77.6}	48	18

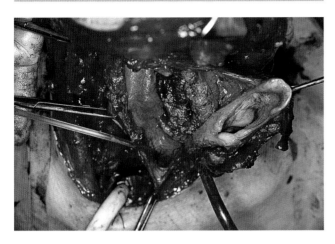

Figure 13.7 Posterior hypopharyngeal wall tumour.

Table 13.14 T Stage Presentation of Posterior Hypopharyngeal Wall Tumours [Site-Based (%)]

T stage	Spiro et al. (43)	Pene et al. (38)	Teichgraeber and McConnel (55)
T1	14	7	10
T2	48	15	26
T3	23	78	30
T4	15	–	33

20% are nodular (with a better prognosis). The majority (64%) of tumors (Fig. 13.7) are larger than 4 cm at presentation, whereas 8% are under 2 cm, 14% are 2 to 3 cm and 14% are 3 to 4 cm (38).

More than 85% of tumors (using the site-dependent T system) are T2–4 lesions (Table 13.14) and, in addition, 38 to 78% are associated with cord fixation (38,43,54).

Once through the pharyngeal wall these tumors may involve the prevertebral fascia, which acts as a barrier to spread, and laterally through the parapharyngeal space to involve structures of the carotid sheath (7). These extensions are rare at presentation but are common with recurrent disease following primary RT.

Regional Metastasis

The first echelon of nodes to be involved in posterior hypopharyngeal wall tumors are levels II, III, and retropharyngeal (32). Candela's study of elective and therapeutic neck dissections also showed that once the neck was clinically positive all nodal levels were pathologically involved at a significant rate with 20%, 84%, 72%, 40% and 21% in levels I, II, III, IV, and V, respectively (16). It was also noted that involvement of the submandibular (I) or posterior triangles (V) did not occur without cN-positive nodes in II, III, and IV. Three fourths of clinically N1 necks had multiple histologically involved nodes involved (pN2), and thus levels I and V were at significant risk. Retropharyngeal node involvement is in the region of 42% (17), rising to 67% with stage III to IV disease (10).

Table 13.15 Posterior Hypopharyngeal Wall Staging at Presentation (%)

Stage	Spiro et al. (43)	Jones and Stell (36)	Teichgraeber and McConnel (55)*
I	9	26	6
II	37	16	23
III	29	26	16
IV	25	32	55

*Orohypopharyngeal (using an unspecified TNM system in 1985).

Overall, the incidence of nodal disease is between 35 and 45% and is associated with increasing T stage with the incidence of nodal disease being 33%, 10 to 12%, 40 to 77%, and 50 to 80% at T1, T2, T3 and T4, respectively (32,43,54).

Stage Grouping

As with other hypopharyngeal carcinomas, very few cases present as stage I, and two thirds of patients have stages III or IV disease (Table 13.15) (32,43,54).

Distant Metastasis and Second Primaries

Distant metastases are seen more frequently on presentation (3–10%) than with postcricoid lesions (38,54). There is often a history (37%) of previous malignancy of the upper aerodigestive tract (50% laryngeal, 33% oral), and 10% may be found incidentally as part of a diagnostic work-up for another primary (43). Teichgraeber et al. (54) reported 20% with metachronous and 3% synchronous second carcinomas with two thirds of metachronous carcinomas occurring in the upper aerodigestive tract.

INVESTIGATIONS

The diagnostic work-up and clinical staging of a patient with a suspected hypopharyngeal malignancy involves a history and physical examination followed by imaging and panendoscopy with biopsy. Endoscopic examination (panendoscopy) under general anesthetic is essential to determine the mucosal extent of the tumor, involvement of adjacent structures, presence of deep fixation, and to investigate the possibility of a second primary malignancy. Flexible esophagoscopy should be considered over rigid techniques in patients with postcricoid lesions or cervical esophageal involvement to reduce the risk of perforation, particularly if one wants to assess the distal extent of the tumor. Biopsy of the primary tumor has traditionally been carried out at the time of panendoscopy. With the introduction of the trans-nasal esophagoscope with a biopsy port, biopsies of laryngeal and hypopharyngeal tumors are potentially possible under local anesthetic in the clinic setting. In the presence of palpable nodal disease, a fine needle aspiration may be obtained to confirm suspicion of a metastatic node.

Imaging should include computed tomography (CT), and/or magnetic resonance imaging (MRI), of the neck and superior mediastinum to assess local extension and cervical, paratracheal, retropharyngeal, and mediastinal nodal disease. Imaging will upstage a significant proportion of patients (55). CT and MRI are complementary examinations and should ideally be performed. CT scanning is particularly valuable in assessing invasion of the thyroid and cricoid cartilages, as well as assessing adenopathy. MRI has better soft tissue definition and the potential to detect occult submucosal disease, invasion of the intrinsic laryngeal musculature or paraglottic space, and spread along the superior neurovascular pedicle (56,57). The search for distant metastasis with a chest CT is important for accurate clinical staging and treatment planning. Functional imaging with fusion positron emission tomography (PET) combined with CT (PET/CT) is becoming increasingly recognized as an additional staging tool. It has been shown to assist in assessment of the extent of the primary tumor, as well as assessment of second primaries, distant metastases, and extent of cervical adenopathy. However, it is limited by cost, availability, and the false positive rates resulting from inflammation and other confounding factors.

TREATMENT – GENERAL COMMENTS

Hypopharyngeal carcinoma has the poorest survival rate of all squamous cell cancers of the upper aerodigestive tract. Overall 5-year survival rates rarely exceed 35% regardless of the treatment approach used (19,58–60). Population-based databases have investigated the survival rate in patients with hypopharynx cancer. Using the United States Surveillance Epidemiology and End Results (SEER) cancer registry Carvalho et al. reported a 5-year survival rate of 33%, and Hoffman et al. reported a disease specific survival rate of 31.4% (19,58). Wahlberg et al. reported an overall survival rate of only 15% for all patients with hypopharyngeal cancer in the Swedish Cancer Registry treated between 1960 and 1989 (61).

Given the poor survival as well as the potential effects treatment may have on speech and swallowing, the management of hypopharyngeal carcinoma remains one of the most challenging and controversial areas in head and neck oncology. There is potential conflict among organ (larynx) preservation, optimum quality of life, and survival. Overall, the goal is to provide single-modality treatment where possible, with multimodality treatment reserved for patients where there is additive survival benefit from the additional modality.

Management is therefore a complex assessment of tumor factors (i.e., the response of the tumor to treatment modalities), patient factors (i.e., the wishes of the patient, his or her ability to attend follow-up, and physical and psychological health), and physician factors (i.e., the ability of the physician to deliver effectively the treatment modality of choice).

Tumor Factors

Larger and deeply infiltrating tumors are less likely to be controlled with RT because of high "tumor load" and an associated higher proportion of hypoxic radioresistant cells. Tumors with true invasion of cartilage, rather than just "contact" are also less likely to be cured with RT. The presence of neck metastases is a poor prognostic factor, particularly multiple nodes, nodes greater than 3cm, extranodal

extension, and metastases to level IV. Persistent or recurrent tumor in the neck after RT is difficult to diagnose, and salvage surgery rarely succeeds. Based on the high likelihood of overt and occult nodal metastases at presentation management of the neck should be performed in almost all patients, even the clinically negative neck.

Patient Factors

It is of paramount importance that the patient is given balanced information concerning the benefits and risks of the treatment options available. This includes information not only on survival but also the expected and potential short- and long-term sequalae of treatment. Hypopharynx cancer patients are often debilitated by a period of progressive dysphagia and weight loss and are thus often poor candidates for aggressive surgical and nonsurgical treatment protocols. It is important to consider, at a very early stage, some form of hyperalimentation irrespective of the choice of treatment to avoid the debilitating effects of weight loss alone. In a proportion of patients whose tumor persists or recurs after radical RT, long-term survival can still be achieved by salvage surgery. Successful salvage surgery can only be achieved with meticulous follow-up and early diagnosis. Where regular visits are not feasible or the patient's attendance unpredictable, conservation surgery or RT alone may not be the optimum primary treatment choice.

Physician Factors

The multidisciplinary team dealing with the patient must not only have an appreciation of the best treatment choice but also must know their ability to deliver the treatment modality of choice with acceptable levels of morbidity, peri-operative mortality and survival. Referral to another center may be appropriate.

Ablative Surgery
Early Stage Tumors

Only select patients with early stage (T1/T2) tumors are suitable for surgery without the need for total laryngectomy, many of which will still require postoperative radiation therapy (PORT) with or without concurrent chemotherapy. Partial hypopharyngeal surgery with laryngeal preservation can be performed through open approaches or transoral laser endoscopic excision (TOL). Tumors most amenable to either of these conservation surgical approaches are T1/T2 piriform sinus tumors and small posterior pharyngeal wall tumors. Although TOL surgery has advantages over open approaches in terms of reduced fistula rates, avoidance of reconstruction, and shorter hospitals stays, there are no well-designed studies comparing the two.

Locally Advanced Tumors

As most hypopharyngeal tumors are locally advanced at presentation total laryngectomy with partial or total pharyngectomy is often the only curative primary surgical approach. Total laryngectomy with partial pharyngectomy is required when the larynx is significantly involved precluding partial laryngeal surgery and the disease is limited to the piriform sinus. Circumferential laryngopharyngectomy is required when clear margins cannot be achieved with a partial pharyngectomy. Primary surgery with laryngeal sacrifice is indicated in patients with (1) advanced disease with extensive destruction of the thyroid cartilage and extension into the surrounding soft tissues, (2) patients with extensive disease recurrence following nonsurgical modalities, and (3) advanced disease that is unlikely to be controlled with good functional outcomes with radiation or chemoradiation. In patients with disease extension below the cervical esophagus, esophagectomy should be combined with total laryngopharyngectomy. Thyroid gland invasion with piriform sinus cancers has been noted to occur in up to 30% of specimens (62–64). Thyroidectomy with parathyroid gland preservation should be performed in all patients undergoing surgical management of piriform sinus cancers due to the frequent invasion of the thyroid gland (65).

Reconstructive Surgery

Factors to consider in deciding on the appropriate reconstructive option include the extent of the defect, the patient's body habitus and co-morbidities, history of prior radiation or chemoradiation, and the surgeon's experience. The goals of reconstruction are to restore the patient's ability to eat, rehabilitate the voice, and prevent significant peri-operative complications. In cases of partial surgery the reconstructive options depend upon the site of the tumor.

Reconstruction following partial surgery depends upon whether open approaches or TOL is used, as well as the size and location of the defect. Following transoral laser surgery Steiner et al. (66) reported little morbidity after allowing the defect to heal by secondary intention. With open approaches defects in the lateral aspect of the piriform sinus with preservation of the larynx can be closed primarily if the defect is small or reconstructed with a regional flap or free tissue transfer. A thin pliable cutaneous flap is often preferred in this situation, making reconstruction with either a radial forearm flap or anterolateral thigh flap the preferred modality for reconstruction.

Resections of the medial wall of the piriform fossa combined with total laryngectomy may be closed primarily provided that there is a residual pharyngeal circumference of at least 6 to 7cm. In the majority of cases there is insufficient remaining mucosa to close primarily without a significant risk of stricture and therefore requires reconstruction with either a regional or free flap (Fig. 13.8). Regional flaps, such as the pectoralis major or latissmus dorsi flap, are highly dependable (67). Both flaps provide an additional layer of vascularized muscle to cover the anastomosis and great vessels, which is especially important in salvage surgery following radiation or chemoradiation. The major drawback of the pectoralis major muscle flap is the donor site defect created on the chest, as well as the risk of distal flap necrosis and associated fistula in 13 to 68% of cases (67). The other option is reconstruction with a fasciocutaneous free flap, such as the radial forearm flap and anterolateral thigh flap. In centers with extensive microvascular experience, free tissue transfer has a lower rate of partial flap necrosis and avoids the donor site defect in the chest.

In cases of a total laryngopharyngectomy the resultant defect is typically a circumferential pharyngeal defect requiring a "tubed" reconstruction (Fig.13.9) (68). In cases where the cervical esophagus is involved requiring an esophagectomy the only option available is transposed abdominal viscera, the most common of which is the gastric pull-up. In centers with extensive experience the mortality rate is reduced but still not insignificant, with an average complication and mortality rate of 37 and 16%, respectively (69). In the total laryngopharyngectomy without cervical esophagus resection a number of potential reconstructive options exist. Regional flaps such as the pectoralis major and latissmus dorsi myocutaneous flaps should be avoided as they are usually difficult to tube due to the bulk of the subcutaneous tissue and the muscle, and are at risk of distal flap necrosis and associated fistula (67).

Free flaps have become the best option for reconstructing the total laryngopharyngectomy defect. Enteric and fasciocutaneous free flaps have been frequently used. With free jejunal flaps the rates of stricture tend to be low, large segments of jejunum can be harvested to span large defects, and the lumen caliber closely matches that of the esophagus. The drawbacks to the jejunal flap are the requirement for a laparatomy in centers not experienced in the laparoscopic harvest technique and the "wet" speech quality when rehabilitated with at tracheo-esophageal puncture (TEP) prosthesis (70–71). Another option for an enteric flap is the tubed gastro-omental free flap (72–73). The potential advantages of this flap over free jejunum include improved swallowing and TEP speech due to lack of peristalsis and wet speech quality. As well, a large amount of omentum can be harvested to drape over the vessels, microvascular anastomosis, and pharyngeal reconstruction. This is particularly valuable in patients requiring salvage laryngopharyngectomy following chemoradiation failure. When total laryngopharyngectomy is performed in the primary setting or as salvage following standard radiation alone fasciocutaneous flaps are ideal for reconstruction. The anterolateral thigh flap and radial forearm flap are the most commonly used flaps. In thin patients these flaps are thin, pliable, and easily tubed. Compared with free jejunal flaps fasciocutaneous flaps appear to have superior TEP speech, lower free flap failure rates, and avoidance of a laparatomy. Although stricture rates were initially reported to be higher in fasciocutaneous flaps, the use of salivary bypass tube appears to reduce the stricture rate (74–76).

Radiation

RT has a role in the primary management of hypopharyngeal cancers, as well as in the postoperative setting. Indications for RT are similar to those of other head and neck SCCs. RT also plays a role in palliation of pain and bleeding. Organ preservation strategies with primary RT have become the mainstay of treatment in patients with hypopharyngeal cancer. Radiation may be used as single modality therapy or in conjunction with concurrent chemotherapy. In early-stage tumors, control and survival rates appear to be similar to surgery based on observational data (77–79). Control rates with RT for early-stage tumors decreases as tumor burden increases (i.e., greater than 2.5cm, or bulky tumors) or those that extend to the piriform fossa apex (79–82). Altered fractionation techniques with accelerated and/or

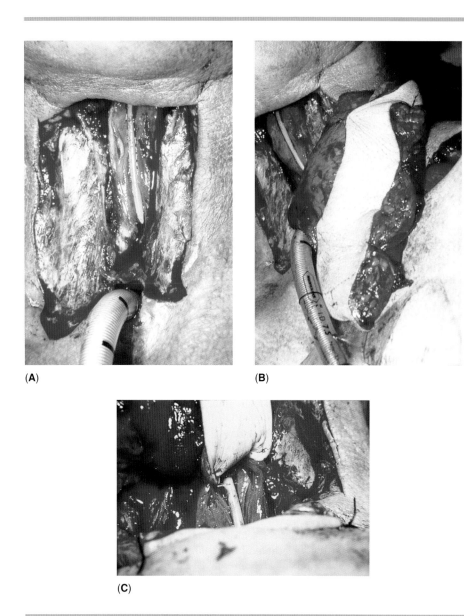

(A)

(B)

(C)

Figure 13.8 **(A)** Hypopharyngeal defect following subtotal pharyngolaryngectomy, leaving posterior strip of mucosa. **(B)** Latissimus dorsi flap raised. **(C)** Flap being sutured into position.

hyperfractionated RT have resulted in improved local control rates in these high-risk early-stage tumors (78,79, 83–84), and in locally advanced carcinomas (85). Accelerated fractionation reduces the overall treatment time as a strategy to overcome tumor clonogenic repopulation (86). Hyperfractionation is a radiation dose-escalation strategy using multiple small fractions per day over conventional treatment times to allow greater normal tissue recovery that occurs in the interval between fractions (86). To improve control and survival rates in advanced stage lesions (stage III or IV) chemotherapy has been added concurrently with various RT schedules (87).

Neck control following RT, either with standard or altered fractionation, appears to decrease with increasing nodal size (88–90). Less than two thirds of lymph nodes greater than 3 cm are controlled with standard RT alone at doses less than 70 Gy (91). Although it is commonly accepted that early metastatic neck disease (N1) can be effectively

treated with single modality therapy, controversy exists regarding the optimal treatment of advanced neck disease (N2 and N3). Patients with neck disease that incompletely responds to RT tend to have a high likelihood of residual disease and should undergo neck dissection. For patients with N2 or N3 disease that completely responds to RT, some advocate serial observation and surgical salvage for recurrent neck disease, whereas others advocate planned PORT neck dissection. An observation approach is based on the low probability of isolated recurrence and the fact that many patients will undergo a neck dissection to benefit a few. A planned neck dissection approach is based on the observation that neck dissection reduces the regional failure rate and may improve cause-specific survival. However, there exists no randomized control trials addressing this issue and the introduction of functional imaging with PET/CT may help differentiate between residual fibrosis and persistent disease.

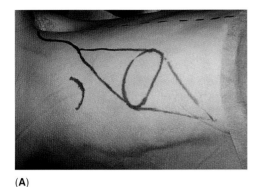

(A)

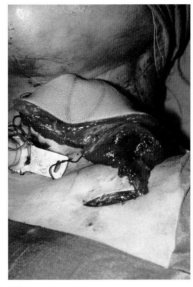

(B)

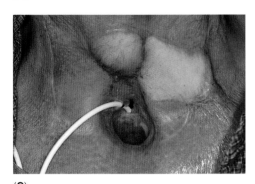

(C)

Figure 13.9 (A) Latissimus dorsi flap used for circumferential reconstruction of the hypopharynx and anterior neck skin defect. (B) Flap raised. (C) Six months postoperation (note large tracheo-oesophageal fistula tract requiring subsequent closure with a sternomastoid flap).

Along with advances in altered fractionation schedules and chemoradiation, there have also been significant advances in the delivery of RT over the past two decades. Conformal RT allows the delivery of high doses of radiation to be shaped around the tumor target while limiting dose to critical normal tissues. Examples of conformal RT include three-dimensional conformal radiotherapy (3D-CRT), intensity modulated radiation therapy (IMRT), and tomotherapy.

Chemotherapy

Chemotherapy initially had its role in the palliative treatment of patients with incurable disease. Over the past decade chemotherapy given concurrently with RT has had an increasing role in the primary management of stage III and IV hypopharynx cancers. Compared with single modality radiation and induction chemotherapy regimens, the addition of chemotherapy in advanced-stage tumors has resulted in improved control and survival rates while allowing preservation of the larynx. Cisplatin is the most active chemotherapeutic agent (83,87,92). A meta-analysis by Pignon et al. on concurrent chemoradiation noted an absolute survival benefit at 5 years of 8% (87). Chemotherapy has also been used concurrently with PORT in patients with high-risk pathologic features of recurrence. A meta-analysis of four trials comparing postoperative concurrent chemoradiation compared with RT alone for patients with high risk of recurrence (stage III or IV cancers, or high-risk pathologic features) showed improved locoregional control rates and survival in favor of concurrent chemoradiation (93). The addition of chemotherapy in either

the primary or adjuvant setting is associated with increases in acute and long-term toxicity (87). Two recent studies have demonstrated the benefit of two versus three neoadjuvant chemotherapeutic agents (91,94). The benefit of induction chemotherapy in patients receiving concurrent chemotherapy is unknown. Although induction chemotherapy followed by RT in nonresponders failed to show any significant improvement in control rates or survival in a meta-analysis, current ongoing studies evaluating outcomes with induction chemotherapy with cisplatin followed by concurrent chemoradiation in responders are being performed (95).

Molecular Targeted Therapy

Molecular targeted therapies exert their anticancer effect against specific protein or pathways that are over expressed or abnormally activated in malignant cells. The epidermal growth factor receptor (EGFR) which is frequently overexpressed in head and neck squamous cell carcinoma (HNSCC) is the main receptor/pathway targeted with either monoclonal antibodies or small molecule tyrosine kinase inhibitors (96–98). In phase II trials of patients with recurrent and/or metastatic disease EGFR inhibitors given with chemotherapy (platinum agents) showed response rates in the range of 4 to 13% and disease control rates in the range of 40 to 50% (99–102). Cetuximab, a monoclonal antibody against EGFR, has been the most successful in clinical development (96). Bonner et al. published their landmark randomized trial comparing RT only to RT plus cetuximab in patients with newly diagnosed HNSCC (103). The mean overall survival was improved by 20 months and progression free survival of 5 months in the RT plus cetuximab arm. As well the median duration of locoregional control was also improved in the combined modality arm. Toxicities were comparable between the two arms with the exception of a skin rash occurring in the cetuximab arm. The study is limited by the fact that the regimen was not compared to concurrent chemoradiation, the current regimen for treating advanced stage HNSCC. As well, there was heterogeneity of radiation regimens used. Although the exact role of molecular targeted therapy in the treatment of HNSCC is yet to be determined, current trials with different molecular targeted genes and as different combined therapy protocols are ongoing.

TREATMENT – SUBSITE SPECIFIC: PIRIFORM FOSSA
Primary Tumor

Early-stage tumors (T1–T2, N0 or N1) of the piriform fossa can be effectively managed with either RT or surgery. Organ preservation strategies are the mainstay of treatment for advanced tumors (T3–T4 or any T with N2 or N3 disease) with surgery reserved for salvage. However, preservation of function should be the goal rather than just preservation of the organ. Primary surgery should be considered in advanced cases with extensive tumor burden, or in cases where preservation of function will not be possible with nonsurgical modalities.

Radiotherapy

For T1 and "low-risk" T2 lesions without nodal metastases, the proposed benefit of RT is better speech and swallowing outcomes compared with surgery, although evidence to support this is lacking. In patients with more advanced local disease, consideration should be given to radical irradiation of the primary and neck using altered fractionated RT or concurrent chemoradiation.

Standard radiation dose-fractionation schedules deliver 70 Gy in 35 daily fractions over 7 weeks to the primary tumor. Tissues at risk for subclinical microscopic spread typically receive 50 Gy in 25 daily fractions over 5 weeks. Concurrent chemotherapy is delivered with standard doses of radiation whereas altered fractionated RT typically employs multiple nonstandard doses of radiation per day. RT targets are defined by the International Commission on Radiation Units and Measurements (104). Regions of gross and microscopic disease are encompassed by clinical target volumes (CTV). An additional margin is required to account for day-to-day variation of treatment set-up, patient movement and organ movement (e.g., swallowing, breathing). The CTV and additional margin are encompassed by the planning target volume (PTV). Patients are immobilized in head and neck immobilization devices to limit day-to-day set-up variation and movement during treatment.

Conventional RT techniques are typically field based with radiation portals delineated to encompass the PTV and a build-up of the radiation dose at the edge of the radiation beam (penumbra). Conventional external beam RT is delivered with photons and electrons. Conformal RT techniques such IMRT requires state-of-the-art CT-based planning software and radiation treatment units. Unlike conventional RT, the beam intensity across each IMRT treatment field is varied in a complex manner that enables shaping of the radiation dose. The advantage of IMRT compared to conventional techniques is the ability to shape the radiation dose conformally around the PTV. Additionally, the dose gradient between the radiation target and normal tissue can be made very steep if they are in close proximity to each other. This enables the dose to be limited to normal tissues such as parotids and uninvolved pharynx with the potential benefit of avoiding permanent xerostomia and dysphagia, respectively.

A large randomized study conducted by the Radiation Therapy Oncology Group demonstrated improved locoregional control with altered fractionation in locally advanced HNSCCs (105). Similarly, two Danish studies, Danish head and neck cancer group (DAHANCA) 6 and 7, showed improved local control using a simple accelerated fractionation scheme by delivering six daily fractions per week compared to the usual five fractions per week, thus shortening overall treatment time by 7 days (106). At the Princess Margaret Hospital, 64 Gy is delivered to the primary in forty 1.6 Gy twice-daily fractions over 4 weeks (107). The benefit of altered fractionation may be greater for the primary tumor than for the neck (92). Trials to date have reported results using conventional RT. Whether the use of conformal RT techniques may improve neck control outcomes is unknown.

Surgery

As most tumors are advanced at presentation the mainstay of surgical treatment is total laryngectomy with partial or total pharyngectomy with reconstruction of the pharyngeal defect and voice restoration. For the rare early (T1/T2) lesion in young healthy individual with good respiratory function, transoral endoscopic laser surgery or open partial surgical approaches should be considered. It must be recognized that PORT is frequently still required, and patients will be subjected to the toxicities of two modalities. For open partial laryngeal surgery, various approaches have been described for piriform sinus tumors including the lateral pharyngotomy approach, and numerous combinations of open partial laryngectomy and pharyngectomy. Stringent criteria exist when determining candidacy for any of these operations and are listed in Table 13.16. These criteria are highly selective for early tumors of the upper lateral wall of the piriform fossa provided that the patient's cardio-respiratory function is good.

Transoral CO_2 laser microsurgery as described by Steiner et al. (66,108–110) has the advantage of not precluding further endoscopic resection, conventional partial, or radical resections or RT. Nodal disease is managed with a unilateral or bilateral neck dissection for cN-negative and cN-positive disease. Adjuvant postoperative therapy with either radiation alone or concurrent chemoradiotherapy is based on pathologic findings. Whichever surgical approach

Table 13.16 Indications for Partial/Conservation Surgery (56,57)

The true cords and arytenoids must be freely mobile and free of gross tumour involvement
No involvement of the apex of the piriform sinus
No thyroid cartilage invasion
No postcricoid involvement

is chosen margin determination must take into account the propensity for hypopharynx cancers to exhibit skip lesions and submucosal extension, particularly in the salvage situation. As well, TOL excision and open partial surgery of the hypopharynx should be performed only in centers with the appropriate expertise.

Regional Disease
Radiotherapy
Treatment of the neck is indicated for almost all SCCs of the hypopharynx regardless of stage. In the clinically and radiographically negative neck management is still indicated given the high rate of micrometastases at presentation (111–112). The neck should be managed with the same principles used to treat the primary tumor. In patients with piriform sinus cancer and a clinically negative neck undergoing RT, elective irradiation of levels II, III, IV, and V is advisable. The retropharyngeal nodal regions are included in node-negative patients. In node-positive patients the entire lymphatic drainage of the neck must be treated including the contralateral deep cervical chain, which is involved in about 15% of cases (48).

Radiation dose-fractionation schedules used for the primary tumor are also used for the neck with the exception of the possible use of an intermediate gross disease dose range to treat small nodes in the lower neck in an attempt to limit the risk of radiation-induced brachioplexopathy.

Surgery
If a primary surgical approach is chosen for management of hypopharynx cancer, the neck needs to be managed whether clinically negative or positive. In the clinically negative neck the ipsilateral nodal basins at risk are managed with a selective neck dissection (levels II, III, and IV). Level I and V metastases are rarely involved and therefore not routinely dissected in the cN0 neck. In patients with clinically positive nodes a comprehensive neck dissection incorporating levels I through V should be performed. Bilateral neck dissections should be performed for advanced primary tumors and those involving the medial wall of the piriform sinus. As well, clearance of the paratracheal nodes (level VI) in piriform sinus tumors is required. These nodes are particularly at risk in patients with piriform sinus tumors involving the apex (113–114). PORT with or without chemotherapy is considered in patients with multiple positive nodes or evidence of extracapsular extension.

TREATMENT – SUBSITE SPECIFIC: POSTCRICOID
General Comments
As with all patients with a resectable head and neck cancer a fundamental management decision has to be made between primary surgery and PORT versus primary RT (with salvage surgery). The advantage of primary surgery in postcricoid carcinoma is immediate restitution of swallow and reasonable cure rates, but the disadvantages are loss of the larynx and the morbidity and mortality associated with resection and reconstruction.

The option of no treatment results in a rapid and unpleasant demise of the patient with 50% dead at 6 weeks, 90% at 4 months, and 100% at 9 months (28). The results

of palliative RT, however, are only marginally better with 50% dead at 5 months, 90% dead at 12 months, and none surviving 4 years (28).

Primary Tumor
Radiotherapy
Postcricoid tumors are often large and infiltrate down the cervical esophagus. Often, the inferior extent of the tumor is poorly visualized on diagnostic imaging and planning CT scans. The surgical description is critical to the accurate delineation of the gross disease and CTV highlighting the importance of a multidisciplinary approach to this cancer. Involvement of the cervical esophagus may necessitate a large CTV and hence, a large PTV that is difficult to irradiate with conventional techniques if the volume extends into the upper mediastinum. These lesions are optimally treated with conformal RT. Patients with cervical esophageal involvement are at significant risk for dysphagia given the volume of pharynx and esophagus that must be irradiated. The same dose-fractionation principles used for piriform fossa tumors apply to postcricoid lesions.

Surgery
The aim of surgery is to eradicate the cancer with the minimum morbidity and mortality. This will result in a circumferential defect with the loss of the larynx. Minimal oncological clearance of the inferior margin requires resection at least 3 cm beyond the macroscopic extent thus resulting in a total laryngo-pharygectomy. If the resection involves the cervical esophagus extending below the thoracic inlet the entire esophagus is removed in continuity thus resulting in a total laryngo-pharyngoesophagectomy. Postcricoid tumors are less amenable to transoral laser surgery because of the proximity of the laryngeal muscles, arytenoids, and recurrent laryngeal nerves (63).

Involvement of the tracheo-esophageal groove/ posterior tracheal wall is also an important consideration. It is often difficult to dissect low in the neck and care must be taken to avoid tearing the trachealis muscle as this can rapidly dissect toward the carina with associated ventilatory difficulties (3). Extensive tracheal resection may require a low suprasternal tracheostomy or even a manubrial resection.

Regional Disease
Radiotherapy
The superior mediastinum and the upper cervical nodes may be involved (level II), and RT should cover levels II, III, IV, paratracheal, and retropharyngeal areas as well as level V if there is palpable disease.

Surgery
In N0 necks levels II, III, IV, paratracheal, and retropharyngeal are cleared on both sides because of bilateral lymphatic drainage. If there is palpable disease at levels II, III, or IV, level V should also be dissected as well as the superior mediastinum if there is radiological or palpable disease in this area using, if necessary, an upper sternotomy approach (115).

TREATMENT – SUBSITE SPECIFIC: POSTERIOR PHARYNGEAL WALL

Primary Tumor

Radiotherapy

Similar to postcricoid tumors, delineation of posterior pharyngeal tumors may be difficult, and these patients are also at significant risk for dysphagia. Additionally, meticulous RT planning is required as the PTV is often in close proximity to the spinal cord, a critical normal tissue. Full thickness tumor infiltration of the posterior wall may often result in a large necrotic ulcer on the prevertebral fascia and anterior spinal ligament. This is frequently painful and due to the poor vascularity in this area may take a long time to heal.

Surgery

The size of the lesion dictates the extent of the resection and reconstruction (Table 13.17), but the most important

Table 13.17   Methods of Resection and Reconstruction (43)

Resection	Percentage
Transoral local resection	12
Transhyoid/anterior pharyngotomy	12
Lateral pharyngotomy	11
Median labiomandibular glossotomy	11
Mandibular swing, paralingual extension	11
Pharyngo-oesophagectomy	2
Pharyngolaryngectomy	16
Pharyngolaryngo-oesophagectomy	21
Circumferential pharyngectomy	5
Reconstruction (by site staging)	
T1 Split skin graft	100
T2 Split skin graft	29
Deltopectoral flap	29
Pectoralis major flap	21
Gastric transfer	7
Radial forearm free flap	14
T3 Deltopectoral flap	20
Pectoralis major flap	20
Gastric transfer	60
T4 Gastric transfer	100

functional consideration is whether the larynx is removed or retained. The age and health status of the patient must also be taken into consideration. Early stage (T1/T2) lesions of the posterior pharyngeal wall are amenable to TOL excision. After resection the defect is allowed to heal by secondary intention. Early-stage lesions of the upper posterior pharyngeal wall may also be approached via a transhyoid approach that involves dividing the suprahyoid musculature and depressing the hyoid bone or resecting the central portion. This approach has limited exposure. Better exposure can be achieved through a lateral pharyngotomy. To minimize the risk of postoperative complications several points of surgical technique are important:

1. The posterior margin of the thyroid cartilage may be removed to improve access.
2. The main postoperative risk is from aspiration because of loss of sensation and muscular activity on the posterior pharyngeal wall. Identification and preservation of the internal and external branches of the superior laryngeal nerve is therefore essential.
3. A small defect may be left to granulate and epithelialize or may be covered with a split skin graft (Fig. 13.10A). Larger resections extending onto the lateral pharyngeal wall in very selected cases may be suitable for reconstruction with a free radial forearm flap (Fig. 13.10B). In our experience more bulky flaps do not give a satisfactory functional result.
4. Temporary tracheostomy and insertion of a percutaneous gastrostomy tube (PEG) are required to minimize the risk of aspiration but even so, rehabilitation may be prolonged.
5. Postoperative problems of healing and aspiration are much more likely in salvage surgery following previous irradiation.

Regional Disease

Radiotherapy

In node-positive and -negative patients, a radical dose is given to the primary and any gross nodes and elective irradiation of node levels II, III, IV, V bilaterally and retropharyngeal nodes.

Nodal metastases are often bilateral and primarily involve levels II, III, and retropharyngeal nodes. If surgery for the primary is the treatment of choice with a cN-negative

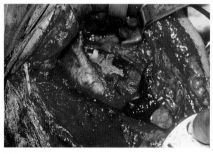

(A)

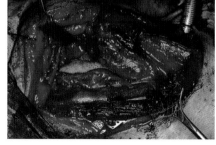

(B)

Figure 13.10   (A) Skin graft for defect on posterior pharyngeal wall. (B) Radial forearm free flap for defect on posterior pharyngeal wall extending on to the lateral pharyngeal wall.

neck a bilateral selective dissection of levels II, III, IV, and retropharyngeal nodes is advisable with a modified radical neck dissection where the neck is clinically involved.

TREATMENT RESULTS: GENERAL COMMENTS

There are few randomized controlled trials on the management of hypopharyngeal tumors with most of the literature on this subject being observational and poorly controlled. Most of the literature comprises observational studies that are limited by small patient numbers, changes in staging systems over time, lack of uniform treatment approaches, inclusion of different subsites, and comparisons to historical controls. RT regimes and surgical techniques have also changed radically over time making comparisons difficult between different institutions and over time. Dosages have been increased above 60 Gy, altered fractionation techniques have improved control rates, and image-guided RT and conformal and IMRT have been developed. Protocols combining RT and chemotherapy have been adopted as well. Similarly, surgical management of hypopharyngeal cancers has also changed with the introduction of transoral laser surgery and advances in microvascular reconstructive surgery. Microvascular surgery has allowed surgeons to perform more aggressive ablative surgery particularly in the salvage situation. Given the limitations in the literature comparing nonsurgical to surgical methods one needs to interpret the literature with caution. There also exists a paucity of data on the "quality of life" consequences of each treatment modality.

TREATMENT RESULTS: PIRIFORM FOSSA
Primary Radiotherapy

Million and Cassisi (116) reviewed the policy of radical irradiation for carcinoma of the piriform fossa between 1964 and 1978 and reported that RT gave high levels of local control for early (Tl and T2) lesions, but more advanced lesions were associated with significantly lower survival (Tables 13.18 and 13.19). Failure of T1 lesions was

mainly due to apical involvement in laterally originating lesions with 100% control with RT for anteriorly and medially originating lesions and 63% control for laterally originating lesions. Apical involvement is a poor prognostic sign due to the high probability of early cartilaginous involvement and understaging.

Million and Cassisi (116) recommended that T1 and favorable T2/3 lesions (i.e., no apical involvement) should be treated with primary RT and salvage surgery. Unfavorable T2/3 lesions (with apical involvement) may be managed with a policy of either (1) primary surgery with postoperative RT or (2) primary RT to a level of 50 Gy provided that if the response is poor (e.g., failure of return of vocal cord mobility) early salvage surgery should be advised. They also recommended T4 lesions require primary surgery with postoperative RT.

From the same institution Mendenhall et al. (117) in 1987 reviewed all stages of piriform fossa lesions treated with RT and salvage surgery from 1964 to 1984. It was again noted that local control for T1–3 lesions was good, but there was no success with T4 lesions [ultimate local control was 89%, 90%, 60% and 0% for T1, T2, T3 and T4, respectively (117)]. The determinate survival was also proportionately reduced in stage III to IV disease with 5-year determinate survival at 100% for stages I and II and 62% and 45% for stages III and IV, respectively.

Bataini et al. (6) reported a series of 434 piriform fossa carcinomas (excluding the epilarynx as these had a 15% better overall survival) treated with primary RT and salvage surgery at the Institute Curie using the 1972 UICC staging system in which T3 lesions in 1972 are equivalent to T3/4 lesions using the 1997 system (Table 13.20). The cause-specific survival was twice the absolute survival indicating the high level of intercurrent disease and second primaries. In T1/2 lesions local control was significantly better if the dose level was greater than or equal to 65 Gy (65%) as compared with less than 65 Gy (36%). T3 lesions showed no dose-related improvement between 50 Gy and 75 Gy.

Mendenhall et al. (118) also compared RT alone or followed by neck dissection for T1/2 lesions. The 5-year rates of local control and ultimate local control were 88 and 94% for stage I and 79 and 91% for stage ll disease. When grouped for stage the cause-specific survival was 100% for I and II, 83% for III, and 51% for IV. He concluded that comparison with available data from series using conservation surgery showed similar rates of local control and survival but less risk of fatal and nonfatal complications.

Rabbani et al. recently reported on 123 patients with T1 to T2 piriform sinus SCC treated primarily with RT

Table 13.18 Ultimate Local Control with Primary Irradiation (58)

T stage	Local control (%)
T1	79
T2	90
T3	50
T4	14

Table 13.19 Survival with Radiation in Relation to Stage (70)

Stage	Determinate survival	
	2 years (%)	5 years (%)
I/II	83	66
III	73	43
IV	55	11
Overall	64	32

Table 13.20 Survival as Related to T Stage (6)

T Stage	Determinate survival	
	2 years (%)	5 years (%)
T1	56	49
T2	62	48
T3	52	39
Overall	54	41

between 1964 and 2003. The 5-year local control rate, overall survival, and cause-specific survival was 85%, 35%, and 61%, respectively. The overall local control rate with a functioning larynx was 83% (119).

Primary Surgery
Conservation Surgery

Conservation of the larynx with primary surgery is achievable in a proportion of carefully selected early lesions. In 1980, Ogura et al. (120) found that partial laryngopharyngectomy and low-dose preoperative radiation in selected cases resulted in a 59% 3-year actuarial survival with 52% of patients treated by conservation surgery. Barton (121) found the 5-year determinate survival was 55% when treating 22 selected cases of early piriform fossa carcinoma with partial laryngopharyngectomy. Czaja and Gluckman, however, noted that the rare hypopharyngeal lesions, which were amenable to partial pharyngectomy, had a local recurrence rate of 44%. This high recurrence rate was thought to be due to submucosal disease and "skip lesions," and they suggested that limited resection for early hypopharyngeal lesions was ill advised (122). Plouin-Goudin et al. reported on 34 patients with piriform sinus cancer treated with partial surgery of which 66% received PORT. The 5-year local control rate with a functional larynx of 80%, overall survival rate of 50%, and cause-specific survival of 65%. The majority of patients (31 of 34) were T1 or T2 tumors (123). Holsinger et al. reported on 30 patients with T1 and T2 piriform sinus cancer managed with lateral pharyngectomy and primary closure and PORT. The 5-year local control rate was 80%, and the survival rate was 23% (124).

Steiner (66,108–110) has pioneered the use of transoral laser microsurgery for piriform sinus cancer with the goal of achieving complete locoregional tumor resection with laryngopharyngeal function preservation. The group consisted of 70% of patients with stage III to IV disease (previously untreated). With a median follow-up of 104 months the reported results were that four patients required a temporary tracheostomy and none had a laryngectomy. The 5-year crude survival was 64% (83% adjusted survival rate) with 17% dying of the hypopharyngeal cancer, 10% of second primarie, and 10% of intercurrent diseases. In 2001 Steiner et al. reported their results on 129 patients with piriform sinus cancer of all local stages managed with TOL surgery. With a median follow up was 44 months the local control rate was 87% and the 5-year overall survival rate for patients with stage I to II disease was 71% and for stage III to IV disease was 47%.

Radical Surgery

El Badawi et al. (125) at MD Anderson found that primary surgery and PORT for predominantly T3/4 lesions gave an actuarial survival at 2 and 5 years of 55% and 40%. Primary surgery and RT as compared to RT alone halved locoregional recurrence rates.

Surgery Compared with Radiotherapy

In the 1987 series from the Institute Gustave-Roussy, Van den Brouck et al. (25) reports two groups treated with primary surgery or RT. The RT group had a greater proportion of T2 tumors with the primary surgery group having

Table 13.21   T Stage Distribution of Two Treatment Modalities (32)

T stage	Radiotherapy (%)	Surgery (%)
T1	13	14
T2	26	3
T3	54	78
T4	8	5

Table 13.22   Survival and Locoregional Recurrence Rates Related to Treatment Modality (32)

	Overall survival (%)		Locoregional recurrence (%)
	3 years	5 years	
Radiotherapy	25	14	44
Surgery	48	33	17.5

more T3 lesions (Table 13.21). The overall survival was higher with surgery compared with RT even though the lesions treated with RT were generally earlier. Locoregional recurrence was also much higher in the RT group (Table 13.22). This paper (25) suggests that survival is higher with surgery compared to RT for advanced disease and that locoregional recurrence is much higher with RT alone. They conclude that the strategy of primary surgery followed by PORT appeared to be the better course.

The piriform fossa is the only hypopharyngeal subsite that has had treatment outcomes, comparing primary surgery with primary RT investigated using a randomized trial; the European organisation for research and treatment of cancer (EORTC) Organ Preservation Study (126). The trial was designed to investigate the effect of chemoselection followed by RT in T2-4, N0-2ab (and operable N3) piriform fossa lesions, in which the control was radical surgery and PORT. Chemoresponders were treated with radical RT and salvage surgery if necessary or possible. Nonresponders were assumed to be relatively radioinsensitive and had immediate surgery followed by PORT. These patients were compared with the control arm where all patients were treated with primary radical surgery and PORT. The results showed that survival in the chemoselection arm was better at 3 years (57% vs. 43%) than in those undergoing surgery but the 5-year survival remained similar (30% vs. 35%). This may be due to later appearance of distant metastases in the chemotherapy group leading to a better 3-year survival, but this effect does not last long enough to affect the 5-year survival (127). Survivors in the chemoselection arm had a 50% chance of retaining a functioning larynx at 3 years and at 5 years. All the survivors in the primary surgical arm had undergone total laryngectomy. Those patients who had a complete response to chemotherapy had a 64% and 58% chance of retaining a functioning larynx at 3 and 5 years, respectively. None of the T4 lesions in the chemoselection had a complete response, and therefore all had primary surgery. The relapse pattern was equal in both arms with respect to local and locoregional failures. This latter aspect is unusual as most other reports indicate poorer locoregional control with RT alone and may be attributable to the chemotherapy. Thirty-six percent of patients in the surgery arm developed distant metastases as compared with 25% in the chemoselection arm.

Forastiere (128) and Stockwell (129) comment that this trial should be viewed as an alternative therapy for the informed patient desiring voice preservation and mandates enrolment in investigational protocols, if feasible. Forastiere states that it is too soon to adopt this as a new standard and also advises caution because the functional and productive quality of life of patients treated by chemotherapy and RT treatment programs is not established (128).

In 1999 Lefebvre (127,130) commented that preservation regimes have not jeopardized survival and have allowed preservation of the larynx. In addition meta-analysis of this study, the French Groupe d'Etude des Tumeurs de la Tete et du Cou (GETTEC) study [a study similar to the Veterans Affairs (VA) study but including T3 larynx disease] and the VA study showed no significant difference in survival but a laryngeal preservation rate of 53%. The analysis by subgroups of patients may vary positively and negatively according to anatomical subsite, biological profiles, and tumor extension. This method of selection may be only one of many strategies used to detect those patients who are suitable for either laryngeal preservation or ablation as the best treatment for them. He concludes that surgery remains, in some cases, the best solution and suggests that a larynx-preserving approach cannot be considered as a standard and remains in the field of clinical research.

TREATMENT RESULTS: POSTCRICOID
General Comments
There are no randomized controlled trials, and therefore one can draw only very limited conclusions.

Primary Radiotherapy and Salvage Surgery
In a large series from the U.K., treated with RT (96% of cases) and salvage surgery Farrington et al. (28) reported a cause-specific 5-year survival in the radically treated group of 22% (Table 13.23). Survival decreased significantly with lesions more than 2 cm in length and for tumors over 4 cm the survival at 5 years was less than 5% (Table 13.24). In addition vocal cord palsy was a very poor prognostic feature (Table 13.25) irrespective of the treatment modality.

Primary Surgery and Salvage Surgery
Harrison and Thompson (30) reported a series of 101 gastric transpositions (including 45% salvage operation after failed RT). The lesions were predominantly postcricoid (66%) in origin (19% piriform fossa, 9% cervical esophagus, 4% larynx, 1% posterior pharynx, and 1% thyroid). The survival rates (68%, 65%, 63%, and 58% at 1, 2, 3 and 5 years, respectively) were high despite the fact that almost half of the patients were treated for recurrent disease following previous RT. This report clearly demonstrates that one of the fundamental issues about complex radical head and neck surgery is that it should only be carried out by an experienced surgical team and not on an occasional basis. The excellent results in this series, even for recurrent cases, reflect the low hospital mortality rate of 11%, which in the latter part of the study fell to 6%. Overall results showed that two thirds of patients survived the first year, with 58% having a 5-year survival.

Table 13.23 Primary Radiotherapy: Cause-Specific Survival (33)

T stage	Cause-specific survival by year (%)				
	1	2	3	4	5
T1 (<2 cm)	80	70	55	50	50
T2 (2–4 cm)	55	40	25	20	20
T3 (>4 cm)	30	20	10	5	3
T4	25	10	5	5	3

Table 13.24 Tumour Length Correlated to Actuarial Survival (33)

Tumour length (cm)	Actuarial survival by year (%)		
	1	2	5
<5	60	40	30
>5	30	23	20

Table 13.25 Vocal Palsy Correlated to Actuarial Survival (33)

	Actuarial survival by year (%)		
	1	2	5
Vocal cord palsy	15	10	0
No vocal cord palsy	45	45	35

Following irradiation Farrington et al. (28) found a recurrence rate of 75% of whom only 10% were thought to be suitable for salvage surgery with 25% success (i.e., one twelfth of recurrences are successfully salvaged) (53). The cause-specific survival at 5 years was 22% (20% as a result of successful RT and an additional 2% with salvage). This compares with a 58% 5-year actuarial survival where surgery is advocated (30).

Primary Radiotherapy Compared with Primary Surgery
Axon et al. (130) compared the effect of surgery or RT in treating postcricoid carcinoma and recommended that surgery was a better method of improving survival especially in patients with no nodal disease. In this series, however, the surgical group consisted of 69% stage III to IV whereas the RT arm had 71% stage I to II. In addition, 28% of patients in the surgical arm had had previous RT. There was a 14% peri-operative mortality, an average stay of 22 days, 17% incidence of gastric reflux, and 5% requiring repeated dilation. The RT group had minimal complications with 20% undergoing salvage surgery. The 5-year survival figures for surgery versus RT were 45% and 23% irrespective of nodal status, 63% and 25% without nodes, and 10% and 0% with nodes.

Stell et al (12). reported a series of postcricoid carcinomas where early lesions (stage I to II) were treated with RT, but more advanced tumors and patients with nodal involvement were treated with primary surgery using either flap or viscus repair. The 5-year survival for the surgical group repaired with a flap was 32% with RT being approximately 22%. The additional 10% overall survival advantage for those patients treated with primary surgery, and a flap repair occurred despite the fact that the lesions in this group were more advanced (Table 13.26).

In a subsequent paper Stell et al. (131) reported a 38% 5-year survival in patients treated with primary RT and also in a group treated surgically and reconstructed with a flap. (Those with a visceral repair had only a 10% 5-year survival). The RT group included T1 and small T2 lesions with a vertical length not greater than 5 cm and with no cervical nodes. Those in the surgery group included tumors greater than 5 cm in length and/or had cervical nodes or had radiorecurrent disease. It was concluded that early lesions should be treated with primary RT and surgery used for larger or recurrent tumors, but again the problem with this report is that the groups are noncomparable.

Management of Regional Disease

As at other sites nodal disease correlates with poor survival (Table 13.27) and advanced cases respond better to a combination of surgery and RT.

TREATMENT RESULTS: POSTERIOR PHARYNGEAL WALL
General Comments

There are again no randomized controlled trials, and the literature is sparse with all published series being very small. Most report the combined results of treatment of carcinomas of the posterior walls of the hypopharynx and the oropharynx, and consequently it is impossible to compare the outcomes of different methods of treatment with any certainty.

Primary Radiotherapy

In one of the very few reports of a series of posterior hypopharyngeal wall carcinomas treated by radical RT Talton et al. (132) reported overall crude and cause-specific survival of 36 to 39% (Table 13.28) with nodal disease diminishing survival. Recurrence was seen in 79% of cases, but RT was recommended as the treatment of choice. Meoz-Mendez et al. (133) reported the results of radical RT at the MD Anderson Hospital for the posterior pharyngeal wall including hypopharynx and oropharynx with recurrence at the primary site associated with increasing T stage. Local failure was 9%, 27%, 39%, and 63% for stages T1, T2, T3, and T4, respectively.

Table 13.26 Crude Survival (12)

	Crude survival by year (%)				
	1	2	3	4	5
Early (T1/2 N0): R/T	50	40	32	25	22
Advanced: surgery + flap	63	46	40	35	32
Advanced: surgery + viscus	10	5	5	5	5

Table 13.27 Nodal Disease and Survival (%) (12)

	Survival by year (%)				
Nodal disease	1	2	3	4	5
N0	35	28	27	27	24
N1	30	20	12	5	3
N2	15	0	0	0	0
N3	22	12	0	0	0

Table 13.28 Survival Related to T Stage (77)

	Crude 5-year survival (%)		Determinate 5-year survival (%)	
T stage	N−ve	N+ve	N−ve	N+ve
T1	43	20	50	n/c
T2	50	0	50	n/c
T3/4	0	0	n/c	n/c
Overall	36	10	39	14

n/c = no comment.

Pene et al. (38) reported a group of oro- and hypopharyngeal malignancies predominantly treated with RT. Lesions over 4 cm had a worse prognosis than smaller tumors. The degree of lymph node involvement did not appear to affect survival. Seventy-five percent of patients died of local disease. The overall 5-year (crude) survival was 3%, and local control was achieved in 69% of lesions under 4 cm and 10% in larger tumors.

Fein et al. (15) from the University of Florida found the results of RT were no worse than surgery. At 2 years, local control was 100%, 76%, 51%, and 25% for stages T1, T2, T3, and T4, respectively. However 11% developed RT complications with one patient dying after developing quadriplegia secondary to a peridural abscess, and 2% developed severe soft tissue necrosis of the posterior pharyngeal wall.

Son and Kacinski (134) reported the use of combination brachytherapy and external beam RT in sequence for 14 pharyngeal wall cancers. For hypopharyngeal cancers local control was obtained in 80% of cases with an average follow-up of 3 years, and the actuarial survival rate for oro- and hypopharyngeal wall tumors was 82% at 2 and 5 years.

Primary Surgery

In a series of 78 patients with oro- and hypopharyngeal lesions, with surgery as the main treatment modality (76%) to the primary site and neck, Spiro et al. (43) found that the overall 2- and 5-year actuarial survival was 49% and 32%. For lesions confined to the posterior pharyngeal wall the overall 2- and 5-year actuarial survival was 58% and 34%. For stage I to II disease the overall 2- and 5-year actuarial survival was four times better than stage IV disease. In the N0 neck the overall 2- and 5-year actuarial survival was 61% and 41%. Local recurrence occurred in 41% of patients, regional failure in 21%, and distant metastasis in 9%.

In Pene et al.'s series (38) primary surgery with postoperative RT was employed in only 7% of cases, in earlier lesions (mainly T1/2) with minimal nodal disease and fitter/younger patients giving a crude 5-year survival of 30%. Their recommendation of surgical treatment for the rare early lesions to reduce the risk of local recurrence was borne out by a subsequent publication (39). Pene concluded that primary surgery with postoperative RT is indicated in tumors confined to the mucosa of the posterior pharyngeal wall without invasion of the lateral wall or adjacent structures. They also comment that at first presentation the extent of the disease frequently indicates the use of RT only.

Primary Surgery Compared to Primary Radiotherapy

In the Liverpool series, Jones and Stell (32) found no difference in survival between primary surgery and primary RT when treatment was adjusted for stage with a 5-year stage I survival of 45 to 50%. There were no 5-year survivors for stage II, III, and IV disease. Marks et al. (13) reported preoperative RT and surgery for oro- and hypopharyngeal lesions versus RT and salvage surgery. The two groups were age, sex, and tumor stage comparable. In the primary surgery group there was a 20% survival advantage at 5 years (Table 13.29), but a higher complication rate (11% major and 89% lesser vs. 5% major and 48% lesser). They recommended surgical intervention with pre- or postoperative RT as the primary modality of treatment.

TREATMENT RESULTS: CONCLUSION

Hypopharyngeal cancer provides one of the clearest examples in the management of head and neck tumors where referral to an experienced multidisciplinary team is essential for optimum survival and quality of life for the patient. It is a rare disease and should not be treated on an occasional basis. A careful balanced view should be given between the obvious potential benefits of larynx-preserving RT and conservation surgery, which may be appropriate in early selected lesions, and the survival advantage of chemoradiation or radical surgery for more advanced tumors. The management of these cases should be undertaken by an experienced multidisciplinary team.

From the above review it is evident that there is a need for high-quality trials to justify not only the introduction of new therapies but also to support present practice. It would be ideal, where possible, for most patients to be entered into trials.

Whatever choice is thought by the multidisciplinary team to be the "best" for the patient, it is essential that the patient is given a balanced view of all options and his or her wishes being of paramount importance.

Table 13.29 Survival with Primary Surgery or Radiotherapy (13)

	Actuarial survival by year (%)			
	1	2	3	5
Preoperative radiotherapy and surgery	70	40	30	25
Radiotherapy	50	30	15	5

REFERENCES

1. Sobin LH, Wittekind Ch, eds. TNM classification of malignant tumours, 6th ed. UICC/AJC. New York: John Wiley, 2002.
2. Beahrs OH, Henson DE, Hutter RVP et al., eds. Manual for Staging of Cancer; American Joint Committee on Cancer, 3rd edn. New York: JB Lippincott, 1988.
3. Silver CE. Surgery for Cancer of the Larynx and Related Structures, 2nd edn. Philadelphia: WB Saunders, 1996.
4. Warwick R, Williams PL, eds. Gray's Anatomy, 35th edn. London: Longman, 1978.
5. Lefebvre JL, Castelain B, De La Torre JC et al. Lymph node invasion in hypopharyngeal and lateral epilarynx carcinoma: a prognostic factor. Head Neck Surg 1987; 10: 14–18.
6. Bataini P, Brugere J, Bemier J et al. Results of radiotherapeutic treatment of carcinoma of the pyriform sinus: experience of the Institut Curie. Int J Radiat Oncol Biol Phys 1982; 8: 1277–86.
7. Million RR, Cassisi NJ, eds. Management of Head and Neck Cancer: A Multidisciplinary Approach. Philadelphia: JB Lippincott, 1994.
8. Myers EN, Suen JY. Cancer of the hypopharynx and cervical esophagus. In: Cancer of the Head and Neck, 3rd edn. Philadelphia: WB Saunders, 1996; 423–38.
9. Haagensen CD, Feind CR, Herter FP et al. In: The Lymphatics in Cancer. Philadelphia: WB Saunders, 1972; 171.
10. Hasegawa Y, Matsuura H. Retropharyngeal node dissection in cancer of the oropharynx and hypopharynx. Head Neck 1994; 16: 173–80.
11. Ogura JH, Sessions DG, Spector G et al. Long term therapeutic results: cancer of the larynx and hypopharynx. Preliminary report. Laryngoscope 1974; 85: 1746–61.
12. Stell PM, Carden EA, Hibbert J et al. Post cricoid carcinoma. Clin Oncol 1978; 4: 215–26.
13. Marks JE, Smith PG, Sessions DG. Pharyngeal wall cancer: a reappraisal after comparison of treatment methods. Arch Otolaryolol 1985; 111: 79–85.
14. Barzan L, Barra S, Franchin G et al. Squamous cell carcinoma of the posterior pharyngeal wall: characteristics compared with the lateral wall. J Laryngol Otol 1995; 109: 120–5.
15. Fein DA, Mendenhall WM, Parsons JT et al. Pharyngeal wall carcinoma treated with radiotherapy: impact of treatment technique and fractionation. Int J Radiat Oncol Biol Phys 1993; 26: 751–7.
16. Candela FC, Kothari K, Shah JP. Patterns of cervical node metastases from squamous carcinoma of the oropharynx and hypopharynx. Head Neck 1990; 12: 197–203.
17. Ballantyne AJ. Principles of surgical management of cancer of the pharyngeal walls. Cancer 1967; 20: 663–7.
18. Menvielle G, Luce D, Goldberg P et al. Smoking, alcohol drinking and cancer risk for various sites of the larynx and hypopharynx. A case-control study in France. Eur J Cancer Prev 2004; 13: 165–72.
19. Parkin DM, Ferlay J, Raymond L, Young J. Cancer Incidence in Five Continents. Lyon, France: International Agency for Research on Cancer, 1997.
20. Hoffman HT, Karnell LH, Shah JP et al. Hypopharyngeal cancer patient care evaluation. Laryngoscope 1997; 107: 1005–17.
21. Adenis L, Lefebvre JL, Cambier L. Registre des cancers des voies aerodigestives superieures des departements du Nord et du Pas-de-Calais 1984–1986. Bull Cancer Paris 1988; 75: 745–50.
22. Kirchner JA. Pyriform sinus cancer: a clinical and laboratory study. Ann Otolaryngol 1975; 84: 793–803.
23. Eisbach KJ, Krause CJ. Carcinoma of the pyriform sinus. A comparison of treatment modalities. Laryngoscope 1977; 87: 1904–10.

24. Driscoll WG, Nagorsky MJ, Cantrell RW et al. Carcinoma of the piriform sinus: analysis of 102 cases. Laryngoscope 1983; 93: 556–60.

25. Van den Brouck C, Eschwege F, De La Rochefordiere A et al. Squamous cell carcinoma of the pyriform sinus: a retrospective study of 351 cases treated at the Institut Gustave-Roussy. Head Neck Surg 1987; 10: 4–13.

26. Olofsson J, Van Nostrand AWP. Growth and spread of laryngeal and hypopharyngeal carcinoma with reflections on the effect of preoperative irradiation: 139 cases studied by whole organ serial sectioning. Acta Otolaryngol Suppl 1973; 308: 1–84.

27. Kajanti M, Mantyla M. Carcinoma of the hypopharynx. Acta Oncol 1990; 29: 903–7.

28. Farrington WT, Weighill JS, Jones PH. Post-cricoid carcinoma (ten-year retrospective study). J Laryngol Otol 1986; 100: 79–84.

29. Tandon DA, Bahadur S, Chatterji TK et al. Carcinoma of the hypopharynx: results of combined therapy. Indian J Cancer 1991; 28: 131–8.

30. Harrison DFN, Thompson AE. Pharyngolaryngoesophagectomy with pharyngogastric anastamosis for cancer of the hypopharynx: review of 101 operations. Head Neck Surg 1986; 8: 418–28.

31. Jones PH, Farrington WT, Weighill JS. Surgical salvage in postcricoid cancer. J Laryngol Otol 1986; 100: 85–95.

32. Jones AS, Stell PM. Squamous cell carcinoma of the posterior pharyngeal wall. Clin Otolaryngol 1991; 16: 462–5.

33. Mineta H, Ogino T, Amano HM et al. Human papilloma virus (HPV) type 16 and 18 detected in head and neck squamous cell carcinoma. Anticancer Res 1998; 18: 4765–8.

34. Rodrigo JP, Alvarez I, Martinez JA et al. Relationship of human papillomavirus to ploidy in squamous cell carcinomas of the head and neck. Otolaryngol Head Neck Surg 1999; 121: 318–22.

35. Rodrigo JP, Gonzalez MV, Lazo PS et al. Genetic alterations in squamous cell carcinomas of the hypopharynx with correlations to clinicopathological features. Oral Oncol 2002; 38: 357–63.

36. Greene F, Page DL, Fleming I et al. AJCC cancer staging manual. New York: Springer-Verlag, 1997: 220.

37. Willatt DJ, Jackson SR, McCormick MS et al. Vocal cord paralysis and tumour length in staging postcricoid cancer. Eur J Surg Oncol 1987; 13: 131–7.

38. Pene F, Avedian V, Eschwege F et al. A retrospective study of 131 cases of carcinoma of the posterior pharyngeal wall. Cancer 1978; 42: 2490–3.

39. Schwaab G, Vandenbrouck C, Luboinski B et al. Les carcinomas de la paroi posterieure du pharynx traites par chirurgie premiere. J Eur Radiother 1983; 4: 175–9.

40. Van den Bogaert W, Ostyn F, Van der Schueren E. Hypopharyngeal cancer: results of treatment with radiotherapy alone and combinations of surgery and radiotherapy. Radiother Oncol 1985; 3: 311–18.

41. Million RR, Cassisi NJ, eds. In: Management of Head and Neck Cancer: A Multidisciplinary Approach. Philadelphia: JB Lippincott, 1984.

42. Ogura JH, Biller BF, Wette R. Elective neck dissection for pharyngeal and laryngeal cancers: an evaluation. Ann Otol Rhinol Laryngol 1971; 80: 646–53.

43. Spiro RH, Kelly J, Vega AL et al. Squamous carcinoma of the posterior pharyngeal wall. Am J Surg 1990; 160: 420–3.

44. Tani M, Amatsu M. Discrepancies between clinical and histopathologic diagnosis in T3 pyriform sinus cancer Laryngoscope 1987; 97: 93–6.

45. Harrison DFN. Pathology of hypopharyngeal cancer in relation to surgical management. J Laryngol Otol 1970; 84: 349–66.

46. Stell PM. Cancer of the hypopharynx. J R Coll Surg Edinb 1973; 18: 20–30.

47. Kirchner JA. One hundred laryngeal cancers studied by serial section. Ann Otol Rhinol Laryngol 1969; 78: 689–709.

48. Lindberg R. Distribution of cervical lymph node metastases from squamous cell carcinoma of the upper respiratory and digestive tracts. Cancer 1972; 29: 1446–9.

49. Weber RS, Marvel J, Smith P et al. Paratracheal lymph node dissection for carcinoma of the larynx, hypopharynx and cervical oesophagus. Otolaryngol Head Neck Surg 1993; 108: 11–7.

50. Dalley VM. Cancer of the laryngopharynx. J Laryngol Otol 1968; 82: 407–20.

51. Davidge-Pitts KJ, Mannel A. Pharyngolaryngectomy with extrathoracic esophagectomy. Head Neck Surg 1983; 6: 571–4.

52. Harrison DFN. Malignant disease of the hypopharynx: surgical pathology of hypopharyngeal neoplasms. J Laryngol Otol 1971; 85: 1215–18.

53. Jones PH, Farrington WT, Weighill JS. Surgical salvage in postcricoid cancer. J Laryngol Otol 1986; 100: 85–95.

54. Teichgraeber JF, McConnel FMS. Treatment of posterior pharyngeal wall carcinoma. Otolaryngol Head Neck Surg 1979; 94: 287–90.

55. Muir C, Weiland L. Upper aerodigestive tract cancers. Cancer 1995; 75: 147–53.

56. Million RR, Cassisi NJ, Mancuso AA. Hypopharynx: Pharyngeal walls, pyriform sinus, postcricoid pharynx. In: Million RR CN, ed. Management of Head and Neck Cancer. Philadelphia: JB Lippincott Company, 1994: 505–32.

57. Wenig BL, Ziffra KL, Mafee MF et al. MR imaging of squamous cell carcinoma of the larynx and hypopharynx. Otolaryngol Clin North Am 1995; 28: 609–19.

58. Carpenter RJ, De Santo LW. Cancer of the hypopharynx. Surg Clinics N Am 1977; 57: 723–35.

59. Kirchner JA. Pyriform sinus cancer: a clinical and laboratory study. Ann Otol Rhinol Laryngol 1975; 84: 793–803.

60. Steiner W, Ambrosch P, Hess CF et al. Organ preservation by transoral laser microsurgery in piriform sinus carcinoma. Otolaryngol Head Neck Surg 2001; 124: 58–67.

61. Wahlberg PC, Andersson KE, Biorklund AT et al. Carcinoma of the hypopharynx: analysis of incidence and survival in Sweden over a 30-year period. Head Neck 1998; 20: 714–19.

62. Van den Bogaert W, Ostyn F, Lemkens P et al. Are postoperative complications more frequent and more serious after irradiation for laryngeal and hypopharyngeal cancer? Radiother Oncol 1984; 2: 31–6.

63. Olofsson J, van Nostrand AW. Growth and spread of laryngeal and hypopharyngeal carcinoma with reflections on the effect of preoperative irradiation. 139 cases studied by whole organ serial sectioning. Acta Otolaryngol Suppl 1973; 308: 1–84.

64. Wei WI. The dilemma of treating hypopharyngeal carcinoma: more or less: Hayes Martin Lecture. Arch Otolaryngol Head Neck Surg 2002; 128: 229–32.

65. Adams GL. Malignant tumors of the larynx and hypopharynx. In: Cummings CW, Harker LA, Krause CJ et al., eds. Otolaryngology Head and Neck Surgery. St. Louis, MO: Mosby, 1998: 2130–75.

66. Steiner W, Stenglein C, Fietkau R et al. Therapy of hypopharyngeal cancer. Part IV: Long-term results of transoral laser microsurgery of hypopharyngeal cancer. HNO 1994; 42: 147–56.

67. Spriano G, Pellini R, Roselli R. Pectoralis major myocutaneous flap for hypopharyngeal reconstruction. Plast Reconstr Surg 2002; 110: 1408–13; discussion 1408–13.

68. Lam KH, Ho CM, Lau WF et al. Immediate reconstruction of pharyngoesophageal defects. Arch Otolaryngol Head Neck Surg 115: 608–12.

69. Wei WI, Lam LK, Yuen PW et al. Current status of pharyngolaryngo-esophagectomy and pharyngogastric anastomosis. Head Neck 1998; 20: 240–4.

70. Reece GP, Bengtson BP, Schusterman MA. Reconstruction of the pharynx and cervical esophagus using free jejunal transfer. Clin Plast Surg 1994; 21: 125–36.

71. Mendelsohn M, Morris M, Gallagher R. A comparative study of speech after total laryngectomy and total laryngopharyngectomy. Arch Otolaryngol Head Neck Surg 1993; 119: 508–10.

72. Genden EM, Kaufman MR, Katz B et al. Tubed gastroomental free flap for pharyngoesophageal reconstruction. Arch Otolaryngol Head Neck Surg 2001; 127: 847–53.

73. Righini CA, Bettega G, Lequeux T et al. Use of tubed gastroomental free flap for hypopharynx and cervical esophagus reconstruction after total laryngo-pharyngectomy. Eur Arch Otorhinolaryngol 2005; 262: 362–7.

74. Takato T, Harii K, Ebihara S et al. Oral and pharyngeal reconstruction using the free forearm flap. Arch Otolaryngol Head Neck Surg 1987; 113: 873–9.

75. Nakatsuka T, Harii K, Asato H et al. Comparative evaluation in pharyngo-oesophageal reconstruction: radial forearm flap compared with jejunal flap. A 10-year experience. Scand J Plast Reconstr Surg Hand Surg 1998; 32: 307–10.

76. Anthony JP, Singer MI, Deschler DG et al. Long-term functional results after pharyngoesophageal reconstruction with the radial forearm free flap. Am J Surg 1994; 168: 441–5.

77. Pfister DG, Kenneth Hu, Lefebvre JL. Cancer of the hypopharynx and cervical esophagus. In: Harrison LB SR, Hong WK, eds. Head and Neck Cancer: A Multidisciplinary Approach. Philadelphia: Lippincott, 2004: 406–43.

78. Garden AS, Morrison WH, Clayman GL et al. Early squamous cell carcinoma of the hypopharynx: outcomes of treatment with radiation alone to the primary disease. Head Neck 1996; 18: 317–22.

79. Amdur RJ, Mendenhall WM, Stringer SP et al. Organ preservation with radiotherapy for T1-T2 carcinoma of the pyriform sinus. Head Neck 2001; 23: 353–62.

80. Robson A. Evidence-based management of hypopharyngeal cancer. Clin Otolaryngol 2002; 27: 413–20.

81. Pameijer FA, Mancuso AA, Mendenhall WM et al. Evaluation of pretreatment computed tomography as a predictor of local control in T1/T2 pyriform sinus carcinoma treated with definitive radiotherapy. Head Neck 1998; 20: 159–68.

82. Mendenhall WM, Parsons JT, Devine JW et al. Squamous cell carcinoma of the pyriform sinus treated with surgery and/or radiotherapy. Head Neck Surg 1987; 10: 88–92.

83. Rosenthal DI, Ang KK. Altered radiation therapy fractionation, chemoradiation, and patient selection for the treatment of head and neck squamous carcinoma. Semin Radiat Oncol 2004; 14: 153–66.

84. Wang CC, Blitzer PH, Suit HD. Twice-a-day radiation therapy for cancer of the head and neck. Cancer 1985; 55: 2100–4.

85. Bourhis J, Overgaard J, Audry H et al. Hyperfractionated or accelerated radiotherapy in head and neck cancer: a meta-analysis. Lancet 2006; 368: 843–54.

86. Withers, HR. Biologic basis for altered fractionation schemes. Cancer 1985; 55: 2086–95.

87. Pignon JP, Bourhis J, Domenge C et al. Chemotherapy added to locoregional treatment for head and neck squamous-cell carcinoma: three meta-analyses of updated individual data. MACH-NC Collaborative Group. Meta-Analysis of Chemotherapy on Head and Neck Cancer. Lancet 2000; 355: 949–55.

88. Chan AW, Ancukiewicz M, Carballo N et al. The role of postradiotherapy neck dissection in supraglottic carcinoma. Int J Radiat Oncol Biol Phys 2001; 50: 367–75.

89. Clayman GL, Johnson CJ 2nd, Morrison W et al. The role of neck dissection after chemoradiotherapy for oropharyngeal

cancer with advanced nodal disease. Arch Otolaryngol Head Neck Surg 2001; 127: 135–9.

90. Peters LJ, Weber RS, Morrison WH et al. Neck surgery in patients with primary oropharyngeal cancer treated by radiotherapy. Head Neck 1996; 18: 552–9.

91. Bernier J, Bataini JP. Regional outcome in oropharyngeal and pharyngolaryngeal cancer treated with high dose per fraction radiotherapy: analysis of neck disease response in 1646 cases. Radiother Oncol 1986; 6: 87–103.

92. Cohen EE, Lingen MW, Vokes EE. The expanding role of systemic therapy in head and neck cancer. J Clin Oncol 2004; 22: 1743–52.

93. Winquist E, Oliver T, Gilbert R. Cancer Care Ontario Head and Neck Group Guidelines. The Role of Post-operative Chemoradiotherapy for Squamous Cell Carcinoma of the Head and Neck: Cancer Care Ontario Program in Evidence Based Medicine, Toronto Ontario Canada: 2004. http://www.cancercare.on.ca/toolbox/qualityguidelines/diseasesite/head-neck-ebs/

94. Posner MR, Hershock DM, Blajman CR et al. Cisplatin and fluorouracil alone or with docetaxel in head and neck cancer. New Engl J Med 2007; 357: 1705–15.

95. Altundag O, Gullu I, Altundag K et al. Induction chemotherapy with cisplatin and 5-fluorouracil followed by chemoradiotherapy or radiotherapy alone in the treatment of locoregionally advanced resectable cancers of the larynx and hypopharynx: results of a single-centre study of 45 patients. Head Neck 2005; 27: 15–21.

96. Kim S, Grandis JR, Rinaldo A et al. Emerging perspectives in epidermal growth factor receptor targeting in head and neck cancer. Head Neck 2008: 30: 667–74.

97. Hamakawa H, Nakashiro K, Sumida T et al. Basic evidence of molecular targeted therapy for oral cancer and salivary gland cancer. Head Neck 2008; 30: 800–9.

98. He Y, Zeng Q, Drenning SD et al. Inhibition of human squamous cell carcinoma growth in vivo by epidermal growth factor receptor antisense RNA transcribed from the U6 promoter. J Natl Cancer Inst 1998; 90: 1080–7.

99. Baselga J, Trigo JM, Bourhis J et al. Phase II multicenter study of the antiepidermal growth factor receptor monoclonal antibody cetuximab in combination with platinum-based chemotherapy in patients with platinum-refractory metastatic and/or recurrent squamous cell carcinoma of the head and neck. J Clin Oncol 2005; 23: 5568–77.

100. Cohen EE, Rosen F, Stadler WM et al. Phase II trial of ZD1839 in recurrent or metastatic squamous cell carcinoma of the head and neck. J Clin Oncol 2003; 21: 1980–7.

101. Herbst RS, Arquette M, Shin DM et al. Phase II multicenter study of the epidermal growth factor receptor antibody cetuximab and cisplatin for recurrent and refractory squamous cell carcinoma of the head and neck. J Clin Oncol 2005; 23: 5578–87.

102. Soulieres D, Senzer NN, Vokes EE et al. Multicenter phase II study of erlotinib, an oral epidermal growth factor receptor tyrosine kinase inhibitor, in patients with recurrent or metastatic squamous cell cancer of the head and neck. J Clin Oncol 2004; 22: 77–85.

103. Bonner JA, Harari P Giralt J et al. Radiotherapy plus cetuximab for squamous cell carcinoma of the head and neck. N Engl J Med 2006; 354: 567–78.

104. International Commission on Radiation Units and Measurements. ICRU Report 62: Prescribing, recording, and reporting photon beam therapy (supplement to ICRU Report 50). Bethesda, MD, 1999.

105. Fu KK, Pajak TF, Trotti A et al. A Radiation Therapy Oncology Group (RTOG) phase III randomized study to compare hyperfractionation and two variants of accelerated fractionation to standard fractionation radiotherapy for head and neck squamous cell carcinomas: first report of RTOG 9003. Int J Radiat Oncol Biol Phys 2000; 48: 7–16.

106. Overgaard J, Hansen HS, Specht L et al. Five compared with six fractions per week of conventional radiotherapy of squamous-cell carcinoma of head and neck: DAHANCA 6 and 7 randomised controlled trial. Lancet 2000; 362: 933–40.

107. Waldron J, Warde P, Irish J et al. A dose escalation study of hyperfractionated accelerated radiation delivered with integrated neck surgery (HARDWINS) for the management of advanced head and neck cancer. Radiother Oncol 2008; 87: 173–80.

108. Steiner W. Therapy of hypopharyngeal cancer. Part III: the concept of minimally invasive therapy of cancers of the upper aerodigestive tract with special reference to hypopharyngeal cancer and trans-oral laser microsurgery. HNO 1994; 42: 104–12.

109. Steiner W. Therapy of hypopharyngeal cancer. Part V: Discussion of long-term results of transoral laser microsurgery of hypopharyngeal cancer. HNO 1994; 42: 157–65.

110. Ambrosch P, Brinck U, Fischer G et al. Special aspects of histopathological diagnosis in laser microsurgery of cancers of the upper aerodigestive tract. Laryngorhinootologie 1994; 73: 78–83.

111. Ho CM, Lam KH, Wei WI et al. Squamous cell carcinoma of the hypopharynx–analysis of treatment results. Head Neck 1993; 15: 405–12.

112. Buckley JG, MacLennan K. Cervical node metastases in laryngeal and hypopharyngeal cancer: a prospective analysis of prevalence and distribution. Head Neck 2000; 22: 380–5.

113. Peters LJ, Goepfert H, Ang KK et al. Evaluation of the dose for postoperative radiation therapy of head and neck cancer: first report of a prospective randomized trial. Int J Radiat Oncol Biol Phys 1993; 26: 3–11.

114. Clayman GL, Weber RS, Guillamondegui O et al. Laryngeal preservation for advanced laryngeal and hypopharyngeal cancers. Arch Otolaryngol Head Neck Surg 1995; 121: 219–23.

115. Ladas G, Rhys Evans PH, Goldstraw P. Anterior cervical transsternal approach for the resection of benign tumours at the thoracic inlet. Ann Thorac Surg 1999; 67: 785–9.

116. Million RR, Cassisi NJ. Radical irradiation for carcinoma of the pyriform sinus. Laryngoscope 1981; 91: 439–50.

117. Mendenhall WM, Parsons JT, Cassisi NJ et al. Squamous cell carcinoma of the pyriform sinus treated with radical radiation therapy. Radiother Oncol 1987; 9: 201–8.

118. Mendenhall WM, Parsons JT, Stringer SP et al. Radiotherapy alone or combined with neck dissection for T1–T2 carcinoma of the pyriform sinus: an alternative to conservation surgery. Int J Radiat Oncol Biol Phys 1993; 27: 1017–27.

119. Rabbani A, Amdur RJ, Mancuso AA et al. Definitive radiotherapy for T1–T2 squamous cell carcinoma of pyriform sinus. Int J Radiat Oncol Biol Phys 2008; 72: 351–5.

120. Ogura JH, Marks JE, Freeman RB. Results of conservation surgery for cancers of the supraglottis and pyriform sinus. Laryngoscope 1980; 90: 591–600.

121. Barton RT. Surgical treatment of carcinoma of the pyriform sinus. Arch Otolaryngol 1973; 97: 337–9.

122. Czaja J, Gluckman JL. Surgical management of early-stage hypopharyngeal carcinoma. Ann Otol Rhinol Laryngol 1997; 106: 909–13.

123. Plouin-Gaudon I, Lengelé B, Desuter G et al. Conservation laryngeal surgery for selected pyriform sinus cancer. Eur J Surg Oncol 2004; 30: 1123–30.

124. Holsinger FC, Motamed M, Garcia D et al. Resection of selected invasive squamous cell carcinoma of the pyriform sinus by means of the lateral pharyngotomy approach: the partial lateral pharyngectomy. Head Neck 2006; 28: 705–11.

125. El Badawi SA, Goepfert H, Fletcher GH et al. Squamous cell carcinoma of the pyriform sinus. Laryngoscope 1982; 92: 357–64.

126. Lefebvre JL, Chevalier D, Luboinski B et al. Larynx preservation in pyriform sinus cancer: preliminary results of a European Organization for Research and Treatment of Cancer phase III trial. J Natl Cancer Inst 1996; 88: 890–9.

127. Lefebvre JL. What is the role of primary surgery in the treatment of laryngeal and hypopharyngeal cancer: Hayes Martin Lecture. Arch Otolaryngol Head Neck Surg 2000; 126: 285–8.

128. Forastiere A. Another look at induction chemotherapy for organ preservation in patients with head and neck cancer. J Natl Cancer Instit 1996; 88: 855–6.

129. Stockwell S. EORTC Trial: larynx preservation does not jeopardize survival in hypopharyngeal cancer. Oncol Times 1996; 8: 11–2.

130. Axon PR, Woolford TJ, Hargreaves P et al. A comparison of surgery and radiotherapy in the management of postcarcinoma. Clin Otolaryngol 1997; 22: 370–4.

131. Stell PM, Rarnadan MF, Dalby JE et al. Management of postcricoid carcinoma. Clin Otolaryngol 1982; 7: 145–52.

132. Talton BM, Elkon D, Kim JA. Cancer of the posterior hypopharyngeal wall. Int J Radiat Oncol Biol Phys 1981; 7: 597–9.

133. Meoz-Mendez RT, Fletcher GH, Guillamondegui OM et al. Analysis of the results of irradiation in the treatment of squamous cell carcinomas of the pharyngeal walls. Int J Radiat Oncol Biol Phys 1978; 4: 579–85.

134. Son YH, Kacinski BM. Therapeutic concepts of brachytherapy/megavoltage in sequence for pharyngeal wall cancers. Results of integrated dose therapy. Cancer 1987; 59: 1268–73.

14

Tumors of the Larynx

Patrick Sheahan, Ian Ganly, Peter H Rhys Evans and Snehal G Patel

INTRODUCTION

Impairment of laryngeal function from disease and/or its treatment results in gross disturbances in breathing, speech, and swallowing with profound impact on the patient's lifestyle and self-esteem.

The successful management of laryngeal cancer is dependent as much upon individualizing the plan of management to suit the particular patient and his or her expectations, as on close co-operation among members of a head and neck multidisciplinary team.

ANATOMY

The larynx is divided into three distinct regions based on topographical landmarks (Fig. 14.1). The supraglottis comprises the epiglottis, the false cords, the ventricles, the aryepiglottic folds, and the arytenoids. The glottis includes the true vocal cords, and the anterior and posterior commissures. The subglottis begins 10mm below the level of the free margin of the vocal cords and extends to the inferior edge of the cricoid cartilage.

In Europe, especially France, the larynx is also described as being divisible into an "epilarynx" (or the "marginal zone") and an "endolarynx." This distinction is based on the similar natural history of tumors of the epilaryngeal region and those arising in the adjacent hypopharynx. The epilarynx consists of the free border and posterior surface of the suprahyoid epiglottis (anterior epilarynx), and the aryepiglottic fold (lateral epilarynx), the arytenoids and interarytenoid incisure (posterior epilarynx); whereas the "endolarynx" consists of the infrahyoid supraglottis (infrahyoid epiglottis, false cords and venticles), glottis, and subglottis.

Fibroelastic Membrane

An understanding of the fibroelastic membrane of the larynx is key to understanding the internal structure of the larynx. The upper part of the fibroelastic membrane is also known as the quadrangular membrane. This runs on each side from the lateral border of the epiglottis to the anterolateral surface of the arytenoid cartilage. The free upper border is concave and forms the aryepiglottic fold. The free lower border is convex and forms the vestibular ligament (false vocal cords). The lower part of the fibroelastic membrane is also known as the conus elasticus, the triangular membrane, or the cricovocal membrane. It arises from the whole of the superior border of the cricoid cartilage, anterior to the facets for the arytenoid cartilages. The anterior (median) part of the membrane is thick and runs to the inferior border of the thyroid cartilage to form the cricothyroid ligament. The lateral part of the membrane is thin and ascends within the thyroid cartilage, to be attached anteriorly to the inner surface of the thyroid cartilage in the region of anterior commissure (AC), and posteriorly to the vocal process of the arytenoid cartilage. Between these two points, the membrane thus forms a free upper border. This upper free border constitutes the vocal ligament.

The AC is a clinical concept used to describe the anterior part of the glottis. There is no universally agreed anatomic definition. Several important structures converge in the region of the AC. These include the vocal ligaments (upper free edges of the conus elasticus), the thyroepiglottic ligament, which is a strong fibrous band connecting the apex of the epiglottis to the inner surface of the thyroid cartilage, and the AC tendon (Broyle's ligament). The latter structure lies beneath the mucosa, extending from the inner margin of the thyroid notch to the insertion of the vocal ligaments. It serves as a perichondrium for the inner aspect of the thyroid cartilage in this area. These structures constitute a thick, poorly vascularized, gland-free region that resists the spread of tumor. Beneath the AC tendon, the thyroid cartilage has no inner perichondrium; here (in Guerrier's so-called plane zero), the mucosa is next to the thyroid cartilage. Tumor can easily invade the thyroid cartilage in this location (1). Caudal to the glottic plane, tumor may invade the anterior subglottic wedge, between the AC and the cricoid cartilage, and from here it may invade the cricothyroid ligament.

Laryngeal Spaces

The concept of laryngeal spaces is vital to understanding the growth and spread of laryngeal cancer and, therefore, to the understanding of the principles of conservation laryngeal surgery.

The preepiglottic space (of Boyer) is a funnel-shaped space bounded anteriorly by the upper part of the thyroid cartilage and thyrohyoid membrane down to the insertion of the thyroepiglottic ligament; superiorly by the hyoepiglottic ligament, and posteriorly by the epiglottis and the quadrangular membrane (Fig. 14.2). It is continuous laterally with the paraglottic space and contains adipose and areolar tissue along with lymphatic channels. Tumors in an infrahyoid location at the base of the epiglottis tend to

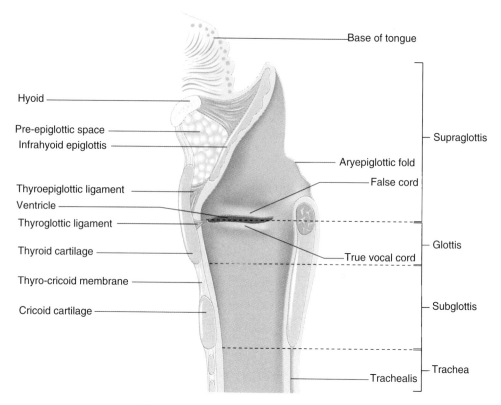

Figure 14.1 Anatomical divisions of the larynx.

spread into the preepiglottic space and have a poorer prognosis than those located in the suprahyoid epiglottis.

The paraglottic space is bound anterolaterally by the thyroid cartilage, inferomedially by the cricovocal (triangular) membrane, superomedially by the ventricle and quadrangular membrane, and posteriorly by the pyriform sinus mucosa. It contains the thyroarytenoid and vocalis muscles surrounded by the paramycium that separates these muscles from the adipose tissue of the posterior projection of the preepiglottic space. This space is therefore in continuity with the preepiglottic space and also the paralaryngeal tissues of the neck through the lateral cricothyroid space. The latter is an important route for the extralaryngeal spread of cancer.

Vocal Cords

The true vocal cords consist of five layers: (1) epithelium, (2) superficial layer of lamina propria, (3) intermediate layer of lamina propria, (4) deep layer of lamina propria, and (5) vocalis muscle. The superficial layer of lamina propria immediately underneath the epithelium consists of loose fibrous tissue and is named Reinke's space. This space is almost devoid of blood vessels and lymphatics and thus affords resistance to the spread of early glottic cancers. Together with the epithelium, this layer forms the cover of the vocal cords. The intermediate and deep layers of the lamina propria consist of elastic and collagenous fibers that form the vocal ligament. Together with the vocalis muscle, these layers form the body of the vocal cords.

Lymphatic Drainage

As with the arterial and venous supply, the glottis constitutes a watershed that divides the larynx into two units that have a distinct embryological derivation (2,3). The supraglottic larynx is drained by lymphatics that run with the superior thyroid artery and drain into deep cervical nodes at Level II. The vocal cords and their subepithelial spaces are largely devoid of lymphatics, which explains the relative rarity of cervical nodal metastases in glottic cancer. The subepithelial lymphatic vessels, which are densely concentrated in the region of the arytenoids, thin out progressively anteriorly and are sparsest in the anterior third of the cords (4). The subglottis has a superficial lymphatic plexus that drains into three main pedicles: one anterior and two posterior. The anterior pedicle pierces the cricothyroid membrane and drains into the prelaryngeal *or* Delphian node that in turn drains into the pretracheal and supraclavicular nodes. The paired posterolateral pedicles pierce the cricotracheal membrane to drain into the paratracheal and other superior mediastinal nodes.

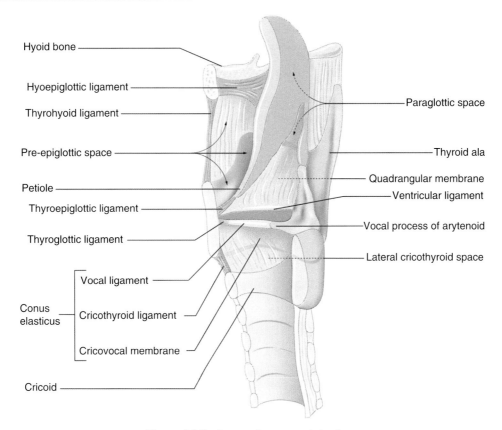

Figure 14.2 Laryngeal spaces and structures.

Labels on figure:
Hyoid bone
Hyoepiglottic ligament
Thyrohyoid ligament
Pre-epiglottic space
Petiole
Thyroepiglottic ligament
Thyroglottic ligament
Vocal ligament
Conus elasticus — Cricothyroid ligament
Cricovocal membrane
Cricoid
Paraglottic space
Thyroid ala
Quadrangular membrane
Ventricular ligament
Vocal process of arytenoid
Lateral cricothyroid space

Surgical Applications of Laryngeal Anatomy

The structure of the larynx and the arrangement of its membranes and cartilages (Fig. 14.3) play an important role in the way laryngeal tumors spread:

1. The conus elasticus resists the inferior spread of glottic tumors, and therefore subglottic extension is a relatively late and ominous manifestation.
2. Tumors involving the AC frequently invade the adjacent thyroid cartilage as the internal perichondrium is deficient at this site. Similarly, the external perichondrium is thinner near the midline and thickens laterally.
3. The paraglottic space containing the vocalis muscle is deficient laterally at the lateral cricothyroid space through which glottic tumors can spread into the neck. Some glottic cancers may be understaged as clinical evaluation of this extension is difficult. The paraglottic space also communicates with the preepiglottic space, and glottic cancer may extend into the supraglottic larynx through this route.
4. Epiglottic carcinoma can spread directly into the preepiglottic space through dehiscences in the epiglottic cartilage, thus this space must be resected completely during a supraglottic laryngectomy (Fig. 14.4).

HISTOLOGICAL VARIANTS

The histology of the tumor has an impact on the management of the patient and the eventual outcome (5) (Table 14.1).

Although the vast majority of primary tumors of the larynx are squamous cell carcinomas, a variety of other pathological types can occur.

Squamous cell carcinomas (Fig. 14.5) comprise 85 to 90% of all laryngeal neoplasms. The majority of vocal cord carcinomas are well to moderately differentiated and almost always arise anteriorly from the epithelium of the membranous part of the glottis. The inferior arcuate line, which is the boundary separating the squamous and columnar epithelium, is a common site of origin.

Verrucous carcinomas (Fig. 14.6) are a highly differentiated variant of squamous cell carcinoma (SCC) that constitute about 1 to 4% of laryngeal neoplasms and about 1 to 2% of vocal cord tumors. Their importance lies in the fact that they present diagnostic difficulties to the clinician and the pathologist, as the lesion that appears clinically malignant may only show histologically benign features. Human papillomavirus DNA sequences have been found in the tumor and in the adjacent normal tissue, pointing to a possible etiological link (6). The tumor is locally invasive but has very little tendency to metastasize. The surface of the tumor shows characteristic papillary fronds with prominent hyperkeratosis. In 10% of patients, hybrid tumors are present that show areas of classical SCC alongside verrucous carcinoma (7).

Spindle Cell Carcinoma

Most laryngeal tumors that have been previously classified as laryngeal sarcomas are now thought to be a biphasic

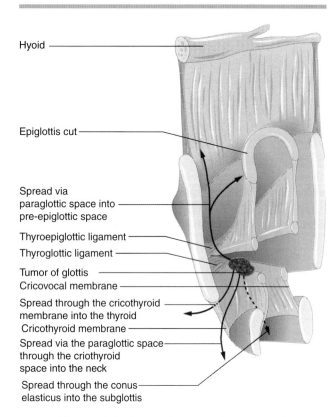

Hyoid

Epiglottis cut

Spread via paraglottic space into pre-epiglottic space

Thyroepiglottic ligament

Thyroglottic ligament

Tumor of glottis

Cricovocal membrane

Spread through the cricothyroid membrane into the thyroid

Cricothyroid membrane

Spread via the paraglottic space through the criothyroid space into the neck

Spread through the conus elasticus into the subglottis

Figure 14.3 Laryngeal spaces and tumor spread.

variant of squamous cell carcinoma with a predominant pseudosarcomatous component. The incidence of these spindle cell carcinomas is difficult to assess reliably because of differences in histological interpretation. These tumors most commonly arise in the vocal cords especially in the region of the AC.

Basaloid Squamous Cell Carcinoma

This is a biologically aggressive biphasic variant of SCC with a high propensity to regional and distant metastases (the latter may be seen even in the absence of cervical nodes) (8).

Neuroendocrine Tumors

Atypical carcinoid tumor is the most frequent neuroendocrine tumor of the larynx and has been mistaken for laryngeal paragangliomas. The vast majority (90%) occur in the supraglottis, and some are associated with the carcinoid syndrome (9). Cervical nodal metastasis is seen in 43% cases, distant metastases in 45%, and painful skin or subcutaneous metastases in 22% of patients. Surgical excision must be preceded by detailed metastatic workup. Elevated calcitonin levels are considered specific markers and may be used to monitor therapy (10).

Small cell neuroendocrine tumors ("oat cell" carcinoma) are rare but extremely aggressive. They account for only 0.5% of all laryngeal neoplasms, but almost 75% of patients die of widespread metastases. They are most commonly seen in males who are in their fifth or sixth

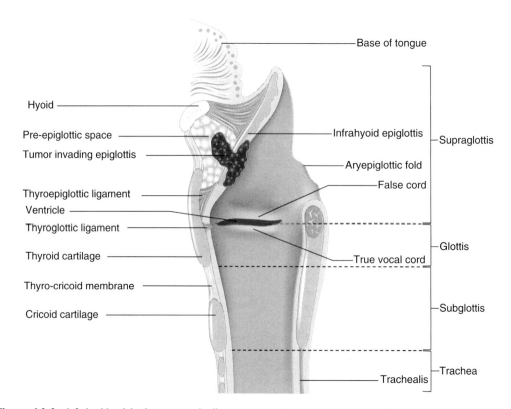

Base of tongue

Hyoid

Pre-epiglottic space

Tumor invading epiglottis

Thyroepiglottic ligament

Ventricle

Thyroglottic ligament

Thyroid cartilage

Thyro-cricoid membrane

Cricoid cartilage

Infrahyoid epiglottis

Aryepiglottic fold

False cord

True vocal cord

Trachealis

Supraglottis

Glottis

Subglottis

Trachea

Figure 14.4 Infrahyoid epiglottic tumors gain direct access to the preepiglottic space through epiglottic dehiscenses.

Table 14.1 Histological Type and Survival

Histological type	5-year survival rate (%)	10-year survival rate (%)
Verrucous squamous cell carcinoma	95	
Chondrosarcoma	90	
Mucoepidermoid carcinoma	80	
Squamous cell carcinoma	68	
Spindle cell carcinoma	68	
Atypical carcinoid	48	
Melanoma	20	
Basaloid squamous cell carcinoma	17.5	
Small cell neuroendocrine carcinoma	5	

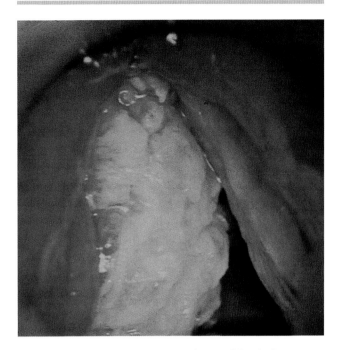

Figure 14.6 Verrucous carcinoma of the glottis.

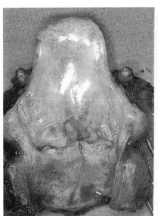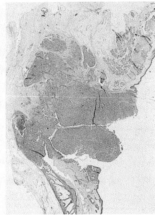

Figure 14.5 Squamous cell carcinoma of the vocal cord.

decade of life and who have been heavy smokers. Cervical nodal metastasis is seen in half of all patients, and distant spread most commonly involves the liver, lungs, bone, and bone marrow. A detailed metastatic work-up, including computed tomography (CT) scans of the lung and brain, bone and brain scintigraphy, and bone marrow aspiration biopsy is mandatory at diagnosis. The tumor is associated with various paraneoplastic syndromes, and the work-up must encompass this possibility.

Mucosal Melanomas

Primary melanoma of the larynx is extremely rare (11). It is commonly a tumor of elderly male Whites, and the majority are found in the supraglottis. Histological diagnosis of difficult cases may be aided by immunohistochemical demonstration of S100 protein and by electron microscopy. The differential diagnosis includes metastasis to the larynx from a cutaneous primary that must be ruled out before treatment commences. The incidence of lymphatic metastasis is low, and elective neck dissection is not routinely indicated.

Other Tumor Types

Adenoid cystic carcinoma is an uncommon tumor that is unusual in many ways. It affects males and females almost

equally, and approximately two thirds of tumors occur in the subglottis, often as a smooth submucosal mass (12). The tumor has a high tendency to recur locally and to metastasize to the lungs in the absence of cervical nodal metastases.

Mucoepidermoid carcinomas are rare tumors that may metastasize to the neck and the lungs. The histological grade of the tumor determines survival: 5-year survival in low-grade tumors is 90 to 100% whereas that for high-grade tumors is 50% (13).

Sarcomas of the larynx are uncommon, and chondrosarcoma (Fig. 14.7) is the most common mesenchymal malignancy. It most commonly involves the cricoid cartilage with the thyroid cartilage, the arytenoids and the epiglottis being more rarely affected. Chondrosarcomas are slow-growing tumors with a high potential for local recurrence. Lymphatic and distant metastases are rare.

Lymphomas of the larynx are predominantly of the B cell variety.

THE EPIDEMIOLOGY OF LARYNGEAL CANCER

Tumors of the larynx constitute about 3.5% of all new malignancies diagnosed annually worldwide. They cause about 200,000 deaths that is about 1% of all deaths from cancer (14). SCC of the larynx has, over the years, been the most frequent malignant tumor of the upper aerodigestive tract in Europe, but recent increases in the incidence of oral and oropharyngeal cancer have narrowed the gap.

Worldwide Distribution

The incidence of laryngeal cancer generally ranges from 2.5 to 17.2 per 100,000 per year. The highest incidence of

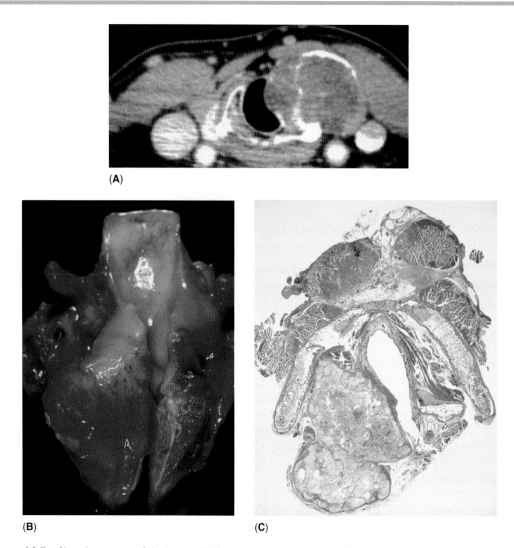

Figure 14.7 Chrondrosarcoma of the larynyx. **(A)** Computed tomography (CT); **(B)** Resected larynx; **(C)** Histological section.

laryngeal carcinoma has been reported from the Basque Country, Spain (20.4), and the lowest incidence for men from Qidong, China (0.1) (15). The incidence and mortality of laryngeal cancer has declined in Europe since the 1990s (16). European countries with the highest incidence in males include Spain (9.9), Croatia (9.5), France (9.3), and Lithuania (9.0) (16). Other areas of high incidence include Southern Brazil (15.1), Uruguay, Northern Thailand (18.4), and western Asia. Overall, laryngeal cancer constituted only 3% of the total number of new cases of cancer recorded in the European community (EC) in 1990 (17).

In the UK, the age-standardized (world population) incidence rate of laryngeal cancer in 2005 was 5.3 per 100,000 for men and 1.0 per 100,000 for women (16) (Fig. 14.8). Within the British Isles, Scotland and Ireland have higher incidence rates as compared to England and Wales.

Age and Sex Distribution

Larynx cancer is rarely diagnosed in people younger than 40, but incidence rises steeply thereafter peaking in people aged 75 to 84 years (Fig. 14.9). Most cases (72%) occur in people older than age 60. Women being affected at a younger age than males (18). The male/female ratio shows marked geographical variation, being 4:1 in Scotland, and 49:1 in Spain (16). In most developed countries, previously high male/female ratios have steadily declined, due to a relatively greater decrease in smoking prevalence in men compared to females (19). In patients younger than 35 years, the incidence in males and females is equal (20). Another difference among the sexes is that supraglottic carcinomas are relatively more frequent in women; according to one study 64% of laryngeal carcinomas were supraglottic in women against 46% in men (21).

Site Distribution

The pattern of distribution of SCC within the larynx appears to be related to the type of carcinogenic insult. In the UK and the USA, the vast majority of laryngeal cancers may be related to smoking tobacco; therefore, the vocal cords are the most commonly affected. In contrast, the supraglottis, which is more exposed to other carcinogenic influences such as alcohol, is more frequently involved in countries like France that have a relatively higher per capita consumption (Table 14.2). The distribution of laryngeal cancers in many countries appears to be changing over the last two decades, with a relative increase in the proportion of glottic cancers. In Spain, the incidence of supraglottic cancers has decreased, and the incidence of laryngeal cancers has increased, since the 1980s (22).

Etiological Factors

SCC of the larynx is a preventable disease resulting from an interplay of numerous etiological factors such as chronic consumption of tobacco and/or alcohol, environmental

carcinogens, socioeconomic status, occupational hazards, dietary factors, and genetic susceptibility.

Tobacco

Smoking is, without doubt, the major risk factor for laryngeal cancer. Tobacco smoke contains more than 30 different carcinogenic agents such as polycyclic aromatic hydrocarbons and nitrosamines. Nicotine from tobacco is not carcinogenic by itself but burning releases the tar that contains numerous carcinogens, notably methylcholanthrene, benzopyrene, and benzanthracene. These carcinogens reach the epithelial cellular surface in the tobacco smoke or dissolved in saliva. They are then broken down by cellular enzymes like arylhydrocarbon hydroxylase into epoxides that bind to DNA and RNA and cause genetic damage that can result in cancer. A dose-dependent increase in risk of laryngeal cancers, both of the supraglottis and glottis, has been demonstrated by several case-control studies (27–32). Patients smoking more than 40 cigarettes a day are 13 times more likely to die of laryngeal cancer than nonsmokers (33). Smoking nonfilter cigarettes (34) and/or black (air-cured) tobacco (35) has been linked to higher risk due to the higher exposure to carcinogens. The Heidelberg case-control study estimated a ninefold increase in the tobacco-associated relative risk in heavy smokers independent of

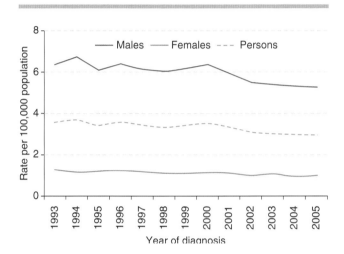

Figure 14.8 Age-standardized (European) incidence rates, laryngeal cancer, by sex, UK 1993–2005. *Source*: http://info.cancerresearchuk. org/cancerstats/types/larynx/incidence

Table 14.2 Site Distribution in Percentage of Total Cases of Laryngeal Cancer (Data Shown in Percentages)

	Supraglottis	Glottis	Subglottis
UK (23)	27	69	4
USA (24)	31	56	1
India (25)	71	28.6	0.2
France (26)	60	30	
Spain (22)	45	55	

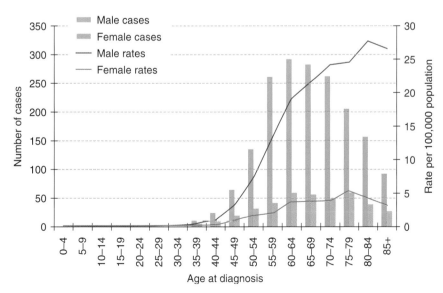

Figure 14.9 Numbers of new cases and agespecific incidence rates, by sex, laryngeal cancer, UK, 2005. *Source*: http://info.cancerresearchuk. org/cancerstats/types/larynx/incidence

alcohol consumption (36). The role of passive or "second-hand" smoking in cancer of the larynx is not clear. Apart from the etiological role of tobacco smoking, its importance in prognosis of patients who develop laryngeal cancer is also relevant. It has been shown that patients who survive 3 years or more after treatment of laryngeal cancer and who continue to smoke, are 7 times more likely to develop a second primary cancer.

Alcohol

Recent epidemiological studies have provided definitive evidence that alcohol consumption is an independent risk factor for laryngeal cancer. The risk increases with the amount of alcohol consumed (28,37). A twofold risk has been estimated in drinkers of 50 g of alcohol per day, and a fourfold risk in drinkers of 100 g of alcohol daily (37,38). A study from Italy suggested that wine drinking is associated with a greater risk than either beer or spirits (39). Within the larynx, the risks of cancer from heavy alcohol consumption are greater for the supraglottis than for the glottis (32,38).

In conjunction with chronic tobacco use, the risk due to alcohol multiplies several fold (28,29,32). Alcohol is presumed to act as a cocarcinogen and acts locally as well as systemically through various mechanisms at different stages during initiation and promotion. Carcinogenesis is also influenced by the malnutrition and depletion of protective vitamins and minerals that accompany chronic alcoholism (40).

Diet

Multicenter case-control studies from Europe have shown that a high and diverse intake of fruit, vegetables, vegetable oil, fish, and low intake of butter and preserved meats are associated with reduced risk of laryngeal cancers after adjustment for risk factors such as alcohol, tobacco, socio-economic status, and nutrition (41,42). A high intake of vitamins C and E, riboflavine, iron, zinc, and selenium, and a high polyunsaturated/saturated fatty acid ratio in diet were also found to have a protective effect. The micro-nutrients act as antioxidants and/or inducers of differentiation and are thought to inhibit carcinogenesis at different stages. Therefore, foods like fruit, salad, and vegetables may have a protective effect against the risk of laryngeal cancer.

Socioeconomic Status

Laryngeal cancer has been associated with lower social class due to poor health care, smoking, drinking, dietary habits, and exposure to environmental and occupational carcinogens. This association has also been demonstrated in the southwest of England where the incidence of laryngeal carcinoma has shown a gradual increase with increasing deprivation (43). The Heidelberg case-contol study (44) showed an increased independent relative risk for people of low educational standard and unskilled workers.

The impact of air pollution has resulted in a two- to three- fold increase in the risk for laryngeal cancer in heavily industrialized cities as compared to rural populations (45). In developing countries, indoor air pollution by emission products of fossil fuel single stoves is a major risk factor (46).

Burning lignite, hard coal, oil, or wood in these stoves causes an emission of high concentrations of carcinogenic combustion products such as polycyclic hydrocarbons into the indoor air, and their use in confined spaces increases the risk many fold.

Viruses

Human papillomavirus (HPV) is a DNA virus that has recently been recognized as an important etiological factor in SCC of the oropharynx (47,48). However the role of HPV in laryngeal cancers remains controversial. HPV is well established as the cause of recurrent respiratory papillomatosis. The HPV subtypes most commonly associated with recurrent respiratory papillomatosis are types 6 and 11 (49). Rarely, malignant transformation of laryngeal or pulmonary papillomas, many years after initial treatment, has been reported. Such an occurrence would appear to be more likely in patients whose papillomas had been treated with irradiation (50–52).

The prevalence of HPV in laryngeal cancer specimens has been reported to be between 4.4 and 58%. It is likely that much of this variation is explained by different detection methods or small numbers of patients included (44,47). Studies with large numbers of subjects using polymerase chain reaction (PCR) techniques for HPV detection have generally reported prevalence rates for HPV of between 4.4 and 25% (37,53–55). The most common subtype of HPV in larynx cancer is type 16 (54). The prevalence of HPV in larynx cancer would appear to be significantly less than that seen in oropharyngeal cancer (47,54).

Thus, though there is some evidence to suggest a possible relationship between HPV and some laryngeal cancers, the evidence is certainly less convincing than that for tonsillar or other oropharyngeal carcinomas.

Occupation

Blue-collar workers exposed to asbestos (31), metal dusts, diesel fumes (31), sulphuric acid mists, tar products, and other inorganic and organic agents may have an increased risk of laryngeal cancer (56). Though the carcinogenic effect of these agents may be important independently, the high incidence of tobacco and alcohol consumption in this social group must be taken into consideration. A high risk for wood-related occupations such as furniture making and woodworking has been reported in a case-control study from Spain (57).

Genetic Susceptibility

It has been hypothesized that genetic polymorphisms in enzymes such as glutathione S-transferase, which is involved in the detoxification of several tobacco smoke-derived carcinogens, and alcohol dehydrogenase (ADH), which converts ethanol to acetylaldehyde, a potential carcinogen, may modulate susceptibility to smoking and alcohol-induced laryngeal cancers. A number of studies have shown an increased risk of laryngeal cancer in the GSTM1 null genotype, particularly among light-to-medium smokers (58–61). It has been reported that certain genetic variants of the alcohol dehydrogenase may have a protective effect against laryngeal and other head and neck cancers, whereas other variants are associated with a higher risk, particularly among moderate drinkers (62,63); however, this remains controversial (64). Indirect evidence of a genetic predisposition to laryngeal cancer is also provided by studies on familial laryngeal cancer and in patients with the Lynch syndrome (65) and Bloom's syndrome (66).

Ionizing Radiation

The use of ionizing radiation in the treatment of benign conditions such as thyrotoxicosis, tuberculosis, and skin conditions has been associated with development of laryngeal carcinoma and sarcoma (67). Radiation-induced sarcoma may also follow treatment of laryngeal cancer with radiation therapy (68,69).

Leukoplakia and Erythroleukoplakia

These are considered under Precancerous Lesions.

Chronic Esophagogastric Reflux Disease

Chronic esophagogastric reflux disease has been linked to laryngeal cancer (70). However, after adjustment for alcoholism, Nilsson reported no significantly increased risk of larynx cancer in patients with reflux (71).

PRECANCEROUS LESIONS

Leukoplakia is a descriptive clinical term for a white patch on the mucosa and has no histologic or prognostic significance. It usually occurs on the true vocal cords and is often bilateral (72). Examination of most laryngeal leukoplakic patches reveals *keratosis*, a histological term used to describe complete replacement of superficial epithelial cells by keratin filaments with dissolution of the nuclei. Laryngeal keratosis is only a superficially visible manifestation of an underlying pathological process that can range from simple hyperplasia to invasive SCC. **Erythroplakia** is a descriptive term for a red patch on the mucosa and is considered to be a higher risk finding than simple leukoplakia.

The rate of malignant transformation of leukoplakic lesions depends mainly on the degree of dysplasia present. Clinical signs of high risk include erythroplakia, surface granularity, increased keratin thickness, increased size, recurrence after conservative excision, and long duration. Five histological parameters have been described as reliable indicators of malignant potential: abnormal mitotic figures, mitotic activity, stromal inflammation, maturation level, and nuclear pleomorphism (73).

At least two dozen classification schemes for laryngeal dysplasia have been proposed. Of these, the most commonly used are the World Health Organisation (WHO) classification; the Squamous Intraepithelial Neoplasia (SIN) classification, and the Ljubljana classification.

The WHO classifies premalignant lesions of the larynx into the following categories: (1) squamous cell hyperplasia (increased cell numbers); (2) mild dysplasia (architectural disturbance limited to lower third of the epithelium, with mild cytological atypia); (3) moderate dysplasia (architectural disturbance extending into the middle third of the epithelium, with more marked nuclear abnormalities); (4) severe dysplasia (architectural disturbance in greater than two thirds of the epithelium with marked cytological atypia); and (5) carcinoma in situ (full thickness architectural abnormalities with no evidence of invasion). The SIN has three categories: SIN 1 (corresponding to mild dysplasia); SIN 2 (corresponding to moderate dysplasia); and SIN 3 (including severe dysplasia and carcinoma in situ. Both of these have the same high risk of developing invasive carcinoma and are grouped together). The Ljubljana classification has four categories: simple hyperplasia (which is considered not to be premalignant); abnormal hyperplasia (which is considered to be a precursor to premalignant lesions); atypical hyperplasia ("risky" for malignancy); and carcinoma in situ (malignant but without invasion) (74,75).

Dysplasia is reported in 35 to 54% of cases of leukoplakia (76–81) (Table 14.3). The overall risk of malignant change is between 3.8 and 8.2%, and is higher in patients with more severe dysplasia (76–81) (Table 14.3). The incidence of recurrent dysplasia after excision is also dependent on the severity of dysplasia (Table 14.3). In addition, though only 7.8% of patients with mild dysplasia are reported to develop more severe dysplasia, up to 55% of patients with moderate dysplasia are reported to develop severe dysplasia or carcinoma in situ (81).

Management of patients with leukoplakic lesions generally involves microlaryngoscopy in the operating room and excision biopsy of the lesion. Further follow-up will be dictated by histological findings. Patients with no evidence of dysplasia are at low risk of developing cancer and so may be followed up routinely after 6 months. Patients with severe dysplasia or carcinoma in situ may warrant repeat operative microlaryngoscopy with biopsy of any suspicious lesions within 6 weeks.

THE NATURAL HISTORY OF LARYNGEAL CANCER
The Primary
Supraglottic Carcinoma

Although there are no doubts about the distinct embryological origin of the supraglottis, no actual anatomical barrier has been found in the body of the ventricle to support the traditional division of the larynx into the supraglottic, glottis, and subglottic areas (82,83). Tumors of the supraglottis generally tend to spread in an upward direction, an observation that has been verified by isotope injection studies (84). When the isotope is injected into the false vocal fold, it fills up the paraglottic space laterally and then spreads into the preepiglottic space and the aryepiglottic folds superiorly. Inferior spread into the deep

Table 14.3 Incidence of Dysplasia in Leukoplakic Lesions, Recurrence after Excision, and Risk of Malignant Transformation

	No dysplasia (%)	Mild/ moderate dysplasia (%)	Severe dysplasia (%)
Incidence (76–81)	46–65	18–73	10–15
Recurrence of dysplasia after excision (76,78)	12.5	7–17	15–28
Risk of malignant transformation (76–81)	3.0–4.2	5.8–11.9	9.4–40

aspect of the vocal fold via the paraglottic space is seen only after a large volume of isotope has been injected. Tumors of the infrahyoid epiglottis spread anteriorly into the preepiglottic space. The perichondrium of the epiglottis and the thyroepiglottic ligament act as the first barriers to anterior spread. Once this barrier is breached, the tumor enters the preepiglottic space through fenestrations in the epiglottic cartilage. Within the space, the tumor grows with a "pushing" margin, and therefore invasion of the hyoid bone is rare. Preservation of the hyoid bone during supraglottic laryngectomy is therefore safe in most patients and may decrease postoperative problems with swallowing. Tumors that are restricted to above the ventricle almost never invade the thyroid cartilage, and its outer perichondrium can be safely preserved during supraglottic laryngectomy. Inferior spread in the region of the AC is limited by the AC tendon and the "x-space," which is a completely avascular triangular zone at the upper anterior end of the vocal cords separating the supraglottis from the glottis.

Tumors of the "marginal zone," which is the suprahyoid epiglottis and the aryepiglottic folds, behave much more aggressively and are significantly more prone to lymphatic metastases. Once the tumor breaks through the quadrangular membrane to invade the adjacent medial wall of the pyriform sinus, it has ready access to the rich lymphatic supply of the vallecula or tongue base.

Glottic Carcinoma

Cancers of the glottis are contained locally in the early stage by four major barriers: the vocal ligament, the AC, the thyroglottic ligament, and the conus elasticus.

The thyroglottic ligament is that part of the conus elasticus that fans out from the anterior free border (the anterior vocal ligament) in an anterior and lateral direction thus covering the superior surface of the vocalis muscle to attach to the medial aspect of the thyroid lamina with the vocalis muscle. Its importance is that it acts as a barrier to tumor spread of anteriorly sited vocal cord cancers.

Tumors of the free margin of the true vocal cords. These are initially confined to the underlying Reinke's space by the vocal ligament. The tumor often spreads on the mucosal surface to involve the entire length of the cord, but once it breaches the vocal ligament and infiltrates the underlying thyroarytenoid (vocalis) muscle, vocal cord mobility is affected.

Tumors of the anterior commissure. These lie in close anatomical proximity to the thyroid cartilage, and an important clinical decision in their management is assessment of cartilage invasion. Tumor cells have been shown growing along collagen bundles of the AC tendon that provides them access to the thyroid cartilage (85). As this area is deficient in perichondrium at the site of attachment of the AC tendon, subclinical invasion by the tumor is likely. On laryngeal serial sections, however, thyroid cartilage invasion has been shown only in tumors that extend upward at the AC to involve the base of the epiglottis. Clinical evaluation of cancers involving this site should, therefore, be supplemented by imaging in an effort to determine early cartilage invasion.

Cancer of the middle and posterior true cords. These tend to spread laterally. After the barrier of the Reinke's space is overcome, superior spread into the ventricle is hampered by the thyroglottic ligament that is an extension of the vocal ligament along floor of the ventricle. Lateral spread into the thyroarytenoid muscle produces vocal cord fixation. The conus elasticus resists inferior spread, but once through it, the tumor can spread laterally into the paraglottic space or it may be deflected medially into the submucosa of the subglottis. Invasion of the paraglottic space may also occur by tumor spread along the superior surface of the vocal cord upward and laterally into the ventricle, above the thyroglottic ligament. From the paraglottic space, the tumor spreads inferiorly and may breach the cricothyroid membrane to invade the thyroid gland and soft tissues of the neck. The inner perichondrium of the cartilage and the thyroid cartilage itself are effective barriers to tumor spread. Transglottic tumors and glottic cancers with more than 1 cm of subglottic extension are most likely to invade into the thyroid cartilage. Areas of ossification are at highest risk of invasion due to the better vascularity and biochemical changes associated with bone formation. The inferior rim of the thyroid cartilage and the superior rim of the cricoid cartilage are areas of early ossification that border the cricothyroid space. These ossified rims of the cricothyroid space are at increased risk of involvement as tumor spreads from the paraglottic space into the neck through the cricothyroid membrane.

Subglottic Carcinoma

Primary tumors of the subglottis are rare, and not much is known about the pathology and pathways of their spread. These tumors can extend submucosally in a superior direction through the conus elasticus to produce vocal cord fixation. The hypopharynx and esophagus may be involved by posterior spread beneath the cricoid cartilage, and subepithelial spread along the mucous glands may allow spread to the cricothyroid membrane and cricoid cartilage (86).

Lymphatic Nodal Metastases

As with other sites within the head and neck, cervical lymphatic metastasis in cancer of the larynx is the single most important determinant of prognosis. Although there are no doubts about the importance of treating palpable cervical nodes, considerable controversy exists in the literature regarding management of the clinically negative neck.

Supraglottic Carcinoma

Cancers of the supraglottic larynx are significantly more likely to present with cervical nodal metastasis compared to other laryngeal subsites. The incidence of occult metastasis in supraglottic carcinoma ranges from 20 to 50% depending on the T stage of the primary. The overall rate of nodal metastasis is also related to the T stage (Table 14.4).

The primary echelons of nodal drainage are levels II, III, and IV (Table 14.5). In the clinically negative neck, micrometastases are found in 37% of patients with levels II and III most frequently involved. Occult metastases at levels I and V were found on pathological examination in only 6 and 1%, respectively (87). The patients who had occult metastases at levels I and V, respectively, had metastases at other levels. Surgical treatment of the clinically N0 or N1 neck may, therefore, safely include levels II, III, and IV whereas levels I and V need be dissected only for higher

Table 14.4 The Overall (Occult and Clinical) Incidence of Lymphatic Metastasis in Supraglottic Carcinoma

Stage of the primary tumour	Incidence (%)
T1	5–25
T2	30–70
T3–T4	60–80

Table 14.5 The Levels of Nodal Involvement in Supraglottic Cancer (61)

Level of nodal involvement	Clinically N0 neck (%)	Clinically N+ neck (%)	
		Immediate RND*	Subsequent RND*
I	6	5	11
II	18	62	63
III	18	53	68
IV	9	31	37
V	1	0	6

*Radical neck dissection.

Table 14.6 The Incidence of Lymphatic Metastasis in Supraglottic Carcinoma According to Subsite (89)

	"Marginal zone"	Infrahyoid epiglottis
Clinically N+ at presentation	48–57%	32–41%
Occult metastases	20–38%	14–16%

neck stages and for T4 primaries. For patients presenting with clinically obvious nodes, the incidence of involvement of levels I and V is up to 11 and 6%, respectively. Level V is almost never involved in the absence of nodal disease at other levels whereas level I involvement is generally associated with adverse features of the primary tumor such as extralaryngeal spread, either into the soft tissues of the neck or the base of the tongue, or high grade.

Within the supraglottis, tumors of the "marginal zone" that includes the suprahyoid epiglottis and the aryepiglottic folds have a greater propensity to neck metastases compared to those of the infrahyoid epiglottis (Table 14.6).

Of note, carcinomas of the supraglottis, particularly those arising in the epiglottis, have a high propensity for contralateral (39%)/bilateral cervical metastases (88).

Glottic Carcinoma

The risk of lymphatic metastases from carcinoma of the true vocal cords is relatively lower than that for supraglottic carcinoma. Because most early glottic cancers are treated using radiation therapy, the incidence of occult cervical metastasis has been reported only for surgically treated higher stage primaries, and ranges from 10% for T3 to 29% for T4 tumors (90). The overall rate of metastasis is less than 5% for T1, 5 to 10% for T2, 10 to 20% for T3, and 25 to 40% for T4 tumors (91,92). The primary echelons of drainage are levels II, III and IV (Table 14.7). As with other laryngeal tumors, isolated involvement of levels I and V is uncommon. Tumors of the vocal cords rarely metastasize bilaterally or into the contralateral neck except in the

Table 14.7 The Levels of Nodal Involvement in Glottic Cancer (61)

Level of nodal involvement	Clinically N0 neck (%)	Clinically N+ neck (%)	
		Immediate RND*	Subsequent RND*
I	0	15	6
II	21	54	38
III	29	61	75
IV	7	15	28
V	7	8	0

*Radical neck dissection.

presence of extensive supra- or subglottic involvement or invasion of the thyroid cartilage.

In a study of 92 whole-organ laryngeal sections, about 9% revealed involvement of the Delphian or cricothyroid lymph node, and involvement seemed to be dependent more on the anatomic location of the primary tumor rather than its size (93). Most tumors that metastasize to the Delphian node lie in an anterior location. Tumors that involve the conus elasticus, subglottis, or cricoid cartilage anteriorly are at high risk of involving the Delphian node that, in turn, is associated with an increased risk of paratracheal node involvement and stomal recurrence. Although a positive Delphian node may be not be relevant to the technique of total laryngectomy, it is an important consideration in the planning and performance of partial laryngeal surgery. The probability of total laryngectomy is much greater in these patients compared to other similar-sized tumors. It is generally agreed that involvement of the Delphian node is associated with a poor outcome (94).

Subglottic Carcinoma

The overall incidence of lymphatic metastasis from primary subglottic carcinoma is less than 20%. The incidence of paratracheal node involvement is, however, much higher at 50 to 65% (95,96). Mediastinal nodes may be involved in a high percentage of cases, with one series reporting an incidence of 46% (97). These statistics underscore the importance of treating the paratracheal nodes in management of subglottic cancers.

Distant Metastases

The lung is the most commonly affected systemic site followed by the mediastinum, bone, and liver. About 15% of patients with supraglottic cancers and 3% with glottic cancers will develop distant metastases within 2 years of diagnosis (98). The development of distant metastases is generally preceded by locoregional failure, but one study has reported that 11% of supraglottic and 7% of glottic carcinomas developed distant metastases in the absence of local failure or neck recurrence (99).

SCC of the larynx is characterized by the relatively high incidence of second primary tumors. Most of these develop in the lungs and are more likely after supraglottic rather than glottic primaries. The incidence of second primary tumors increases linearly with time; 11 to 19% of patients develop second primary tumors within 5 years of treatment that increases to 30% at 10 years (100). The value of routine chest radiography during follow-up is debatable. In a study of 556 patients with laryngeal carcinoma, yearly chest radiographs detected lung cancer in 12.4% of patients. Sixty-eight percent patients were asymptomatic at diagnosis, but their survival averaged only 10 months against 4 months for the symptomatic patients (101).

STAGING

The use of the most recent version of the International Union Against Cancer/American Joint Committee on Cancer (UICC/AJC) rules for staging is mandatory (Tables 14.8–14.11). However, the tumor-nodes-metastases (TNM) system (and associated stage grouping) is far from perfect as a prognostic indicator for individual patients. For instance, stage III includes patients with T3N0 as well as those with T1–3N1 tumors. The prognostic impact of positive lymph nodes is well recognized and must be considered in planning treatment. The staging system gives no consideration to the biological behavior of the primary tumor; an exophytic T1 tumor of the free edge of the vocal cord behaves

Table 14.8 T Staging of Supraglottic Tumors

Tx	Primary tumor cannot be assessed
T0	No evidence of primary tumor
T1	Tumor limited to one subsite of supraglottis with normal vocal cord mobility
T2	Tumor invades mucosa of more than one adjacent subsite of supraglottis or glottis or region outside supraglottis (e.g., base of tongue, vallecula, medial wall of pyriform sinus) without fixation of the larynx
T3	Tumor limited to larynx with vocal cord fixation and/or invades any of the following: postcricoid area, preepiglottic tissues, paraglottic space, and/or minor thyroid cartilage erosion (e.g., inner cortex).
T4a	Tumor invades through thyroid cartilage and/or invades tissues beyond the larynx (e.g., trachea, soft tissues of the neck including deep extrinsic muscle of the tongue, strap muscles, thyroid, or oesophagus).
T4b	Tumor invades prevertebral space or encases carotid artery or invades mediastinal structures.

Table 14.9 T Staging of Glottic Tumors

Tx	Primary tumor cannot be assessed
T0	No evidence of primary tumor
Tis	Carcinoma in situ
T1	Tumor limited to vocal cord(s) with normal mobility (may involve anterior or posterior commissures) T1a Tumor limited to one vocal cord T1b Tumor involves both vocal cords
T2	Tumor extends to supraglottis and/or subglottis and/or with impaired vocal cord mobility T2a normal vocal cord mobility T2b impaired vocal cord mobility
T3	Tumor limited to larynx with vocal cord fixation and/or invades paraglottic space and/or minor thyroid cartilage erosion (e.g., inner cortex).
T4a	Tumor invades through thyroid cartilage and/or invades tissues beyond the larynx (e.g., trachea, soft tissues of the neck including deep extrinsic muscle of the tongue, strap muscles, thyroid, or esophagus).
T4b	Tumor invades prevertebral space or encases carotid artery or invades mediastinal structures.

Table 14.10 T Staging of Subglottic Tumors

Tx	Primary tumor cannot be assessed
T0	No evidence of primary tumor
Tis	Carcinoma in situ
T1	Tumor limited to subglottis
T2	Tumor extends to vocal cord(s) with normal or impaired mobility
T3	Tumor limited to larynx with vocal cord fixation
T4	Tumor invades cricoid or thyroid cartilage and/or invades tissues beyond the larynx (e.g., trachea, soft tissues of the neck including deep extrinsic muscle of the tongue, strap muscles, thyroid, or esophagus).
T4b	Tumor invades prevertebral space or encases carotid artery or invades mediastinal structures.

Table 14.11 TNM Stage Grouping for Laryngeal Tumors

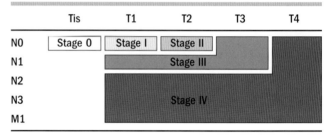

very differently from a similarly staged superficial tumor that extends across the AC to involve both the cords. The TNM system is, however, the most widely accepted staging system and does provide a means of comparison of treatment methods and results.

CLINICAL PRESENTATION
Symptoms

The common symptoms of laryngeal cancer are hoarseness, sore throat, dysphagia, and odynophagia. Hoarseness is an early symptom of glottic cancer but may be seen later in advanced supraglottic or subglottic tumors signifying spread to the vocal cord, arytenoid or cricoarytenoid joint. Paraglottic spread can occur submucosally from these sites to produce hoarseness without any mucosal irregularity. Sore throat and dysphagia are more commonly associated with supraglottic tumors, and odynophagia signifies involvement of the hypopharynx or tongue base. Referred otalgia generally indicates base of tongue involvement but may also be seen in tumors that have extended into the neck through cartilage. Ulceration and bleeding from exophytic tumors may present as hemoptysis. Dyspnoea and stridor occur with bulky supraglottic tumors or in the presence of vocal cord fixation. A neck mass almost always indicates lymphatic metastasis but may result from direct extension of the tumor into the soft tissues of the neck.

Physical Examination and Investigation

Clinical examination is limited by the fact that certain areas of the larynx are inaccessible to visualization and palpation, and involvement of these structures has an important bearing on staging as well as management. Information from radiologic imaging and operative endoscopy must be utilized in conjunction with physical findings to document an accurate pretreatment TNM staged record.

Supraglottic tumors are frequently understaged because the preepiglottic and paraglottic spaces cannot be assessed clinically. Infrahyoid tumors of the epiglottis are especially prone to invade the preepiglottic space. A study found invasion of the preepiglottic space in 89% of infrahyoid tumors as against none in suprahyoid tumors (102). CT and magnetic resonance imaging (MRI) can detect invasion of the preepiglottic space. Signs of preepiglottic space invasion include loss of normal fat density and absent visualization of the superior extent of the lateral cricoarytenoid muscle (103). Radiographic assessment is also useful to assess subglottic extension and the status of the laryngeal ventricle in glottic primaries. Although CT and MRI are excellent for assessing subglottic extension, coronal MR reconstruction may be better at delineating ventricular and paraglottic submucosal spread. MRI may also be superior at differentiating thyroarytenoid muscle invasion from involvement of the cricoarytenoid joint as the cause of vocal cord fixation (104). The value of CT in detecting cartilage invasion is doubtful because of the inconsistent mineralization patterns. If the sclerotic appearance of the cartilage is taken as a radiologic marker, only 46% of patients actually show histologic features of cartilage invasion (105). Another study found microscopic invasion of the thyroid cartilage in as many as 50% of clinically and radiologically staged T3 tumors of the glottis (106). Table 14.12 shows the radiological and clinical criteria that may be used to predict an increased risk of cartilage invasion in glottic cancers.

Positron emission tomography using fluorine-labeled deoxyglucose may be useful in detecting recurrent tumor after primary treatment (108). In addition, high pretreatment standardized uptake value (SUVs) have been associated with a poorer prognosis, particularly among patients who are not surgically treated (109).

The role of routine esophagoscopy in asymptomatic patients is controversial. The incidence of synchronous esophageal primaries in patients with head and neck cancer is about 1 to 2%, and retrospective studies have not demonstrated any survival advantage for patients whose tumors were discovered using routine oesophagoscopy (110). Esophagoscopy is therefore recommended only to investigate symptoms such as difficulty swallowing.

TREATMENT
General Principles
Treatment of the patient with laryngeal cancer, as for patients suffering from other cancers, must provide the best chance for cure while minimizing potential adverse effects on the normal laryngeal functions of phonation, protection of the airway, and breathing. The psychosocial effects of loss of normal laryngeal function can be crippling, and optimal treatment planning must be individually tailored based on a variety of interrelated factors. The patient's age, occupation, ability to read and write, general health and co-morbid conditions, lifestyle issues such as refusal to stop smoking, distance from the hospital, and family status need to be taken into account while planning treatment. The patient's opinion and preference for a particular treatment should be factored into the process of decision making (Table 14.13).

Although the chronological age by itself is not a deterrent to aggressive treatment, the risk of treatment

Table 14.12 Radiologic and Clinical Predictors of Cartilage Invasion in Glottic Cancer (106)

	Risk %
Paraglottic spread	74
Extensive cartilage ossification	73
Extensive involvement of anterior commissure	67
Tumor >2 cm	66
Vocal cord fixation	54

Table 14.13 Considerations in Choice of Treatment for Patients with Laryngeal Cancer

Tumor factors	Site
	Volume
	Extent
	Status of neck
	Presence of distant metastases
Patient factors	Pulmonary status
	Medical comorbidity
	Alcohol dependency
	Other cancers
	Occupation/professional voice use
	Expectations
	Literacy, intelligence, and motivation
	Preferences
Other factors	Social support
	Distance from hospital
	Availability of facilities and resources for radiotherapy, conservation laryngeal surgery, speech therapy, etc.

associated with intercurrent conditions and the cardiopulmonary status generally prevalent in this population may modify treatment approaches considerably. Patients who are technically amenable to conservation laryngeal surgery may be unsuitable due to medical conditions such as chronic obstructive pulmonary disease or congestive heart failure. The pretreatment phase must be utilized to reinforce lifestyle issues such as cessation of smoking and alcohol abuse. In addition to joint treatment planning by the surgical, radiation, and medical oncology teams, multidisciplinary input from speech therapists, physiotherapists, nutritionists, and psychological and social support services is invaluable to achieving a favorable outcome. Patients planned for total laryngectomy may benefit from meeting others who have tolerated the procedure well, and where available, the services of laryngectomee clubs must be utilized routinely.

Treatment Options
In general, the primary tumor can be treated by one of the following techniques: (1) transoral laser surgery (endoscopic resection); (2) open partial laryngectomy; (3) primary radiotherapy alone; (4) primary combined chemoradiotherapy; and (5) total laryngectomy.

Transoral Laser Surgery
Transoral laser surgery was initially proposed as a treatment for small glottic tumors. However, it has gained popularity

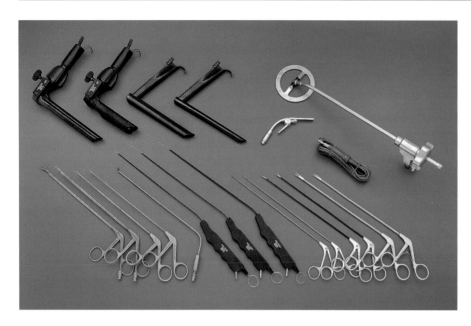

Figure 14.10 Instruments for transoral endoscopic laser resection. Courtesy of Karl Storz GMBH & Co.

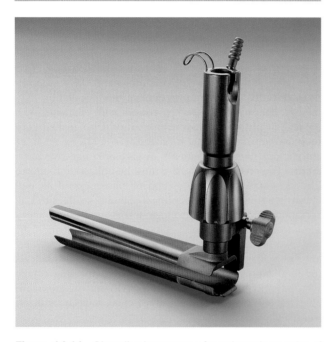

Figure 14.11 Distending laryngoscope for endoscopic resection of supraglottic tumors and tumors of the pyriform sinus. Courtesy of Karl Storz GMBH & Co.

in the treatment of supraglottic and moderately advanced laryngeal cancers. Typically, a double-cuff endotracheal tube is used, with the cuffs inflated with saline. The laryngeal structures are exposed using large laryngoscopes, including adjustable bivalved laryngoscopes. Surgery is generally performed using a CO_2 laser coupled to an

operating microscope, and manipulated using a micromanipulator. The use of 0°, 30°, and 70° laryngeal telescopes and fiber-optic laser delivery systems may also be helpful. Microlaryngeal instruments with electrocautery and suction are essential for the success of the technique (Figs. 14.10 and 14.11).

The technique relies on removal of cancer in a systematic, blockwise method, resulting in several resection specimens. This requires cutting through cancerous tissue, which of course is against the principles of conventional oncologic surgery. However with microscopic laser surgery it is possible to see the structure of the cut surface of the tumor, allowing exposure of the superficial and deep extension of the tumor more precisely and allowing one to differentiate between malignant and nonmalignant structure (Fig. 14.12). This way the surgeon can individually adjust the safety margin. Using this technique, smaller tumors may often be excised en-bloc as a single specimen. On the other hand, larger tumors require piecemeal removal.

When performed by experienced surgeons, transoral laser surgery offers a number of advantages over conventional treatment techniques:

1. The oncologic results are excellent, with ultimate local control, laryngectomy-free survival, and overall survival rates being comparable to those achieved by either open surgery or radiotherapy (Tables 14.17, 14.20, and 14.24).
2. Disruption of laryngeal function is minimal. This is because unlike open surgery transoral surgery avoids disruption of the cartilaginous framework of the larynx, and of the surrounding strap musculature. In addition, the sensory innervation through the superior laryngeal nerve is preserved. Thus, tracheostomies are generally avoided, and the need for temporary feeding tubes is minimized.

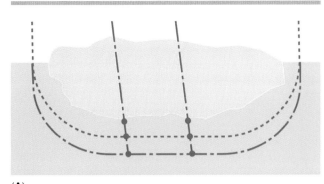

(A)

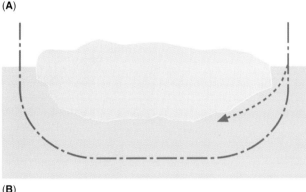

(B)

Figure 14.12 Blockwise resection of tumors by laser microsurgery **(A)** as opposed to en-bloc resection **(B)**. Courtesy of Georg Thieme Verlag.

3. It leaves open all treatment options for patients who develop local recurrence or second primary tumors, including transoral laser reexcision, open partial laryngectomy, or radiotherapy.
4. It may be performed expeditiously in a single sitting, at low cost, unlike radiotherapy which generally requires 6 to 7 weeks of treatment.

To perform transoral laser surgery, good access to the larynx is necessary. Factors that impede laryngeal access, including stiffness of the neck, anterior position of the larynx, and prominent upper teeth, may render transoral laser surgery difficult or even impossible. Access to the larynx may be particularly difficult in patients who have undergone previous neck radiotherapy or chemoradiotherapy.

Reported complications of transoral laser surgery include hemorrhage (2.6–8%) (111–116), pneumonia (0–11.5%) (112,113,117–119), cervical emphysema (1%) (113), perichondritis (0.7%) (113), laryngeal synechiae (0–8.3%) (111,120), and airway ignition (0.3%) (113). Complications after transoral laser surgery are more common with more extensive tumors (113), less experienced surgeons (113), and patients with diabetes (113). The incidence of tracheostomies reported in patients undergoing transoral laser surgery is 0 to 3.8% (111–115,119,120).

In patients who also require neck dissection, it has been recommended that this is performed in a delayed fashion (10–15 days after the transoral surgery) to minimize the risk of airway swelling and hence the need for a tracheostomy (121).

Open Partial Laryngectomy

When considering a patient for conservation laryngeal surgery, the following general principles should be considered:

1. The patient must be able to tolerate a general anesthetic.
2. The patient should not have any medical problems that may impair wound healing, for example, transplantation patients or patients with diabetes mellitus.
3. The patient should have good pulmonary function to tolerate the postoperative course, which commonly involves a period of aspiration. Vertical hemilaryngectomy typically causes little impact on swallowing function, whereas supraglottic laryngectomy results in dysphagia and aspiration. A percutaneous gastrostomy tube may be required for patients with a significant prolonged period of aspiration.
4. The patient should play an active role in speech and swallowing rehabilitation.
5. Any patient undergoing partial laryngectomy should be informed of the complexities of salvage conservation procedures and must give consent for total laryngectomy. Any patient who cannot do this is not a good candidate for conservation laryngeal surgery. Careful preoperative planning will reduce the incidence of conversion to total laryngectomy. Various types of partial laryngectomy have been described, depending on the site and extension of the tumor.

Conservation surgery for glottic laryngeal cancer. The possible surgical options include vertical partial laryngectomy and supracricoid partial laryngectomy with cricohyoidoepiglottopexy (CHEP).

Vertical partial laryngectomy This procedure may be a lateral or an anterolateral vertical partial laryngectomy. The technique involves vertical cuts through the laryngeal cartilage (Fig. 14.13). The majority of the ipsilateral thyroid cartilage, true vocal cord, portions of the subglottic mucosa, and false cord are removed. The extent of resection depends on the preoperative and intraoperative assessment of tumor extent. The strap muscles are closed over the residual perichondrium to form a pseudocord. A tracheostomy is generally required for 3 to 7 days. If the AC is involved, a frontolateral partial laryngectomy can be done. Contraindications include subglottic extension to the level of the cricoid cartilage, extensive preepiglottic space invasion, postcricoid or crico-arytenoid joint invasion, or invasion through the thyroid cartilage.

Supracricoid partial laryngectomy with CHEP This operation involves resection of both true cords, both false cords, the entire thyroid cartilage, paraglottic spaces bilaterally, and a maximum of one arytenoid. Reconstruction is done using the epiglottis, hyoid bone, cricoid cartilage, and tongue. A temporary tracheostomy and feeding tube is required. This procedure is mainly used for T1b glottic carcinomas with AC involvement, selected T2, and T3 glottic carcinomas.

Conservation surgery for supraglottic laryngeal cancer Surgical treatment of tumors of the supraglottic larynx creates a significant physiologic disturbance in the act of

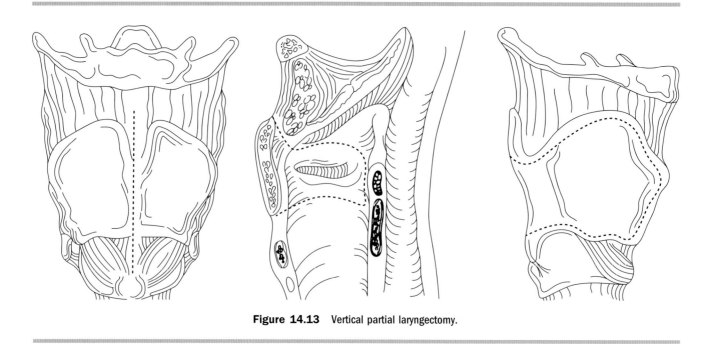

Figure 14.13   Vertical partial laryngectomy.

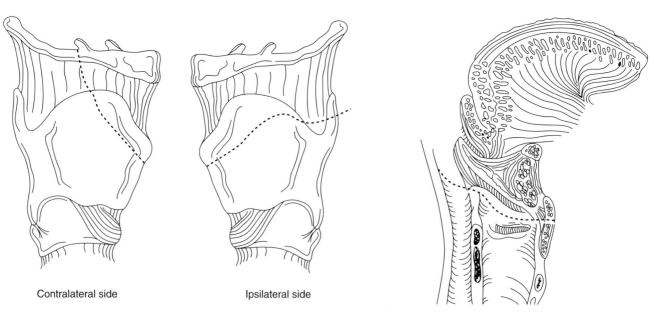

Contralateral side   Ipsilateral side

Figure 14.14   Horizontal supraglottic partial laryngectomy.

deglutition. Almost every patient aspirates to a varying degree following surgery. Most patients handle this with little difficulty and can handle most types of foods without significant pulmonary complications. However patients with a poor pulmonary reserve, advanced stage of emphysema, and those of advanced age are poor candidates for conservation surgery. The conservative open surgical options available for supraglottic cancers include the supraglottic horizontal partial laryngectomy and the supracricoid laryngectomy with cricohyoidopexy.

Horizontal supraglottic partial laryngectomy In this procedure, the epiglottis, hyoid bone, preepiglottic space, thyrohyoid membrane, upper half of the thyroid cartilage, and the supraglottic mucosa are removed (Fig. 14.14).The vallecula is transected superiorly, the ventricles inferiorly, and the aryepiglottic folds laterally. The vocal cords and paraglottic space are preserved. This operation is used for tumors of the supraglottis with a clear margin from the AC of at least 5 mm, and with normal vocal cord mobility. Closure is by approximating the base of tongue to the lower half of the thyroid cartilage and closing the posterior false cord mucosa to the medial pyriform sinus mucosa. A temporary tracheostomy is required. Bilateral selective neck dissection is carried out at the same time. In this procedure it is important to identify and preserve the internal and external branches of the superior laryngeal nerve. The tongue base sutures are placed in the midline and 1cm off to avoid damage to the hypoglossal nerves and lingual arteries. Contra-indications to supraglottic laryngectomy are given in Table 14.22.

Supracricoid partial laryngectomy with cricohyoidopexy (CHP)
This operation is suitable for supraglottic carcinomas not amenable to supraglottic laryngectomy due to either

1. Glottic level involvement through the AC or ventricle
2. Preepiglottic space invasion
3. Decreased cord mobility
4. Limited thyroid cartilage invasion.

Lesions that may be suited to CHP are not rare especially because between 20 and 54% of tumors involve the paraglottic space. This operation involves resection of both true cords, both false cords, the entire thyroid cartilage, both paraglottic spaces bilaterally, and a maximum of one arytenoid, thyrohyoid membrane, and epiglottis. Reconstruction is done using the hyoid bone, cricoid cartilage, and tongue. A temporary tracheostomy and feeding tube are required. Contraindications to supracricoid partial laryngectomy with CHP are given in Table 14.23.

In properly selected patients, open partial laryngectomies offer excellent local control rates. However, the surgery involves considerable disruption of laryngeal framework and surrounding strap musculature; consequently, it leads to considerable functional disturbance in most. Temporary tracheostomy tubes and feeding tubes are usually required. In most patients, swallowing function returns to near normal within a few weeks, allowing tubes to be removed (122). After open supraglottic laryngectomy, a mean time to removal of nasogastric tubes of 17 to 19 days, and a mean time to removal of tracheostomy tubes of 35 days has been reported (117,118). After supracricoid laryngectomy, mean times of 15 to 16 days and 19 to 30 days respectively are reported (122–124). However, many patients will continue to experience silent aspiration (117). For this reason, candidates for partial laryngectomy must have adequate pulmonary reserve to tolerate this chronic, low-grade aspiration. The incidence of aspiration pneumonia after partial laryngectomy is generally reported to be between 0 and 13.5% (88,117,118). The reported incidence of long-term tracheostomy tubes in large series of supraglottic or supracricoid laryngectomies is 0 to 15% (88,117,118,122,123, 125,126). The reported incidence of total laryngectomy for intractable aspiration is 0.5 to 9% (88,122,124–126).

Primary Radiotherapy
Among patients with early laryngeal cancers, primary radiotherapy offers excellent local control and cure rates. For more advanced cancers, the local control rate of radiotherapy alone is not as good as that of surgery; however, when surgical salvages are taken into account, survival outcomes are generally considered to be equivalent (127). Large tumor volume (128), cartilage involvement, vocal

cord fixation, AC involvement (127–132), T4 stage (133), and transglottic tumors have been reported to predict a poorer response to radiotherapy.

The main advantage of radiotherapy is that it preserves the structure of the larynx, hence functional disturbance should be minimized. However, preservation of structure does not necessarily equate with preservation of function. In the case of early larynx cancers, functional outcomes after radiotherapy are generally very favorable. With larger tumors, more significant functional disturbances may be seen.

Disadvantages of primary radiotherapy include the following:

1. Once patients have received radiotherapy, they usually cannot be reirradiated. Thus, radiotherapy is not available as a treatment option in the case of local recurrence or second primary tumor.
2. In a considerable number of patients with early glottic carcinoma, the primary tumor is completely removed with the diagnostic biopsy. Thus a policy of primary radiotherapy may result in overtreatment for a significant number of patients (134).
3. The start of radiotherapy may be significantly delayed by such factors as access to radiotherapy facilities, dental extractions, and treatment planning. Furthermore, the duration of radiotherapy is typically 6 to 7 weeks, with completion of the treatment schedule highly dependent on patient compliance
4. Postradiotherapy edema and fibrosis makes monitoring for the early signs of recurrent tumor very difficult.
5. Local control is not as good as surgery for advanced tumors.
6. In some patients who fail radiotherapy, the only feasible salvage option is total laryngectomy.

Late complications of radiotherapy include severe edema necessitating permanent trachestomy (1.5–2%) (133,135), chondronecrosis necessitating total laryngectomy (1–2%) (128,133,135), permanent inability to swallow necessitating a gastrostomy tube (1–2%) (133,135), hypothyroidism, spinal cord injury (<1%) (133), and fatal carotid blow-out (133).

Primary Chemoradiotherapy
Combined chemotherapy and radiotherapy may be administered to patients with advanced laryngeal cancer in a sequential or concurrent fashion. Concurrent chemoradiation appears to show better local control than sequential radiation, but with increased toxicity (136). Chemoradiotherapy offers the opportunity for larynx preservation in patients with advanced laryngeal cancers that are unlikely to respond to radiotherapy alone (137), and has thus had a major impact on the contemporary management of laryngeal cancer.

The disadvantages of chemoradiotherapy are as follows:

1. Increased early and late toxicity compared to radiotherapy alone, particularly with concurrent chemoradiation (136). Because of this, elderly patients or patients with medical comorbidity may not tolerate the treatment.
2. There is a high incidence of long-term functional sequelae, including swallowing problems, aspiration,

feeding tube and/or tracheostomy tube dependence, and weight loss (104,107,138–143).

3. Monitoring for the earliest signs of recurrence may be extremely difficult.
4. For patients who fail chemoradiation, the only realistic salvage option is total laryngectomy.

Chemoradiotherapy is discussed in more detail in the section on Advanced Laryngeal Cancer.

Total Laryngectomy

In the past, total laryngectomy has been considered the treatment of choice for advanced laryngeal cancers. Total laryngectomy is associated with excellent local control (144–148).The major disadvantages of total laryngectomy are the significant functional and psychological problems (Tables 14.14 and 14.15).

Nowadays, total laryngectomy as first-line treatment is generally reserved for patients with very advanced tumors, with cartilage destruction, and/or extralaryngeal extension. Most other patients with tumors that are not suitable for conservation surgery undergo either radiotherapy alone or combined chemoradiotherapy as first-line treatment, in an effort to preserve the larynx. Total laryngectomy is reserved for salvage of radiotherapy and chemoradiotherapy failures. This approach has allowed for laryngeal preservation in a large number of patients without adversely affecting survival (137). However, one disadvantage of this approach is the increased incidence of pharyngocutaneous fistulae and other complications that are seen after total laryngectomy in patients who have previously been treated with radiotherapy or chemoradiotherapy (149).

Table 14.14   Functional Effects of Total Laryngectomy

Loss of larynx	Loss of normal speech
Loss of glottic closure and ability to raise intrathoracic pressure	Loss of airway protective mechanism
	Less effective cough
	Inability to strain
	Difficulty lifting heavy objects
Loss of nasal airflow	Impaired olfaction and taste
	Rhinitis
	Tendency to develop airway crusts
Presence of stoma	Body image issues
	Inability to swim and need for water precautions
	Need to protect stoma from wind-blown sand/dust

Table 14.15   Patient Factors Affecting Outcome of Total Laryngectomy

Motivation	Success of speech rehabilitation strongly depends on motivation
Literacy	Ability to communicate in writing
Manual dexterity	Ability to clean stoma and use tracheo-esophageal prosthesis
Parkinson's disease	Handwriting may be illegible
Visual acuity	Ability to care for stoma and write
Family/social support	Provide motivation and support

Choice of Treatment by Tumor Status and Results
Severe Dysplasia/Carcinoma In Situ (CIS)

The management of severe dysplasia and carcinoma in situ (CIS) is considered together as both of these lesions have the same high propensity to invasive cancer (150). In fact, both of these lesions are categorized together as "carcinoma in situ" in the Ljubljana classification (74).

CIS continues to carry significant morbidity and even mortality. In patients who progress to invasive cancer, total laryngectomy rates of between 13.5 and 82% have been reported (80,81,151,152). The optimum management of CIS is controversial: on the one hand, treatment should be adequate to minimize morbidity and mortality from recurrence and progression to invasive carcinomas. On the other hand, treatment should not unnecessarily sacrifice function or cause undue morbidity.

One of the issues with CIS is that recurrences frequently represent new disease developing in dysplastic epithelium rather than recurrences of the original lesion (151). Many patients will thus ultimately need retreatment, the options for which may be complicated by the initial treatment.

Radiotherapy has been shown to be effective in preventing progression to invasive cancer, and in achieving local control in patients with CIS. Stenersen (153) and Hintz (148) compared rates of invasive carcinoma in patients treated with irradiation with observed patients. The observed rates in irradiated patients were 19 to 28%, and those in observed patients were 46 to 63%.

Among recent large series of patients undergoing radiotherapy for CIS, 5-year control rates of 88 to 98% (154,155), 5-year local control rates with laryngeal preservation of 88 to 98% (154), and 5-year ultimate local control rates of 100% have been reported (154). Le reported a 10-year local control rate of 79%, and a 10-year laryngeal preservation rates of 85% (152).

Proponents of radiation therapy cite posttreatment voice quality as its major advantage. However, though radiotherapy may cure individual lesions, it provides no assurance that another lesion will not develop in an already diseased and unstable mucosa.

The alternative to radiotherapy is surgical treatment. This may take the form of either vocal cord stripping or transoral laser resection of individual lesions. Nowadays, transoral laser surgery is generally preferred as it causes less vocal sequelae than vocal cord stripping. One of the major advantages of surgical treatment over radiotherapy is that it can be easily repeated, and radiotherapy is still a treatment option for recurrences or new primary lesions arising elsewhere in the unstable mucosa.

The control rates of surgical treatment are similar to those seen with radiotherapy, with reported 5-year local control rates of between 85 and 95% (156–158). Ultimate local control rates, after repeat excisions or radiotherapy, are generally excellent. In most cases, excision of the diseased mucosa via subepithelial cordectomy, passing through Reinke's space, is performed. In selected patients, Damm recommended performing subligamental cordectomy to obtain adequate excision (158).

Vocal outcomes after transoral laser surgery for early glottic lesions are generally excellent. However, many patients with CIS have a history of multiple previous biopsies, often alongside a history of chronic laryngitis secondary to smoking. Thus, many of these patients will have extensive scarring in Reinke's space, particularly those who have previously undergone traditional stripping surgeries.

In general, radiation therapy is recommended for patients with

- recurrence after one or more procedures
- lesions that recur relatively soon after excision
- patients whose voice quality is critical to their livelihood, for example, professional singers, etc.
- poor operative risk
- patients who are unlikely to attend for regular follow-up
- lesions that are not easily accessible to surgical treatment, for example, AC lesions.

Patients must be encouraged to stop smoking, and treatment must be followed up by regular follow-up.

Early Glottic Cancer (T1/2, N0)

Management of the primary. Early stage (T1/2, N0) carcinoma of the vocal cords may be effectively treated with either endoscopic resection or primary irradiation. Both of these treatment options offer excellent local control and survival (Tables 14.16 and 14.17), although some authors have reported surgery to have slightly better local control and laryngeal preservation rates than radiotherapy (127,159,160). Thus, the choice of treatment should strive to optimize functional outcomes.

Radiotherapy and transoral resection may have adverse effects on speech. The effect of radiotherapy on the vocal cords is to cause submucosal fibrosis, leading to stiffness and derangement of the mucosal wave. This results in a harsh, "raspy" voice. Compared to controls, patients treated with radiotherapy for early glottic cancer show significant perturbations in jitter, shimmer, and maximum phonation time (161,162). However, overall, long-term vocal outcomes after radiotherapy for early vocal cord cancers are generally very good (163).

In the case of transoral resection, vocal outcomes depend to a large extent on the extent of resection (164–166). This in turn depends on the depth of invasion of the tumor, as assessed by visual examination and palpation at the time of endoscopy (120). The European Laryngological Society has classified cordectomies into five types: type I (subepithelial), type II (subligamental), type III (transmuscular), type IV (total), and type V (extended) (167). After type III cordectomy, many patients develop a fibrous "neocord" that allows for good speech (168). With more extensive resections, other compensatory patterns (false cordal, or arytenoideus hyperadduction types) are seen (168), correlating with poorer voice outcomes (164,165,168). In the long-term, most patients with T1a tumors will eventually experience a satisfactory vocal outcome (164,166).

There continues to be lack of consensus regarding whether vocal outcomes are better after either transoral surgery or radiotherapy for treatment of early glottic carcinoma. Several authors have reported a better outcome for radiotherapy on objective (169) and subjective measures (170,171). Peeters reported better Voice Handicap Index scores in patients with T1a tumors treated with transoral surgery. However, in this series, patients were selected for either radiotherapy or transoral laser resection on the basis of videostroboscopic findings (172,189). Other studies found no difference for T1a tumors (173–178,190–195).

Transoral resection may have an advantage for small lesions as it allows complete tumor removal with excellent functional outcomes, and without the side effects of radiotherapy (165). The best functional results are likely to be obtained in tumors with an intact mucosal wave on videostroboscopy (172). Transoral resection also avoids the

Table 14.16 Results of Treatment of T1/2 N0 Glottic Cancer with Primary Radiation Therapy

	Initial local control (%)	Ultimate local control (%)	Larynx preservation (%)	Disease-specific survival (%)	Overall survival (%)
T1	82–95 (128,130,132, 181–184)	91–98 (128,182–184)	85–96 (128,160, 181,185)	95–99 (130,160,181, 183–185)	69–84 (128,130, 132,160,184)
T2	68–78 (182,186–188)	92–94 (182,187)	74–82 (185–187)	86–92 (185–188)	59–69 (187,188)
T2a	80 (181)		82 (181)	95 (181)	
T2b	72 (181)		76 (181)	90 (181)	
T3	60–63 (189,190)	86 (189)		58–78 (185,189)	35–54 (189,190)

Table 14.17 Results of Treatment of T1/2 N0 Glottic Cancer with Transoral Laser Resection

	Initial local control (%)	Ultimate local control with laser alone (%)	Larynx preservation (%)	Disease-specific survival (%)	Overall survival (%)
T1	86–96 (156, 191–194)	87–95	97–100 (160)	97–100 99[a] (160)	75–98[a] (160)
T2	100 (156,192)	91–100	100		
T1/2	88–100 (120,156, 195–197)	84–100	90–96	97–98	87–93

[a]3-year survival.

risk of overtreatment in cases where the entire tumor is removed by the initial biopsy (179,196). In such cases, the surgical specimen will be negative, and the patient can be safely followed. The cost of transoral laser resection has also been reported to be lower than that of radiotherapy (180,197).

Involvement of the AC in patients with early glottic cancer would appear to be a worrisome sign. Such cases may show early invasion of the petiole of the epiglottis, the thyroid cartilage, cricothyroid membrane, and the anterior subglottic wedge, which is missed by endoscopic examination. Imaging studies (CT and/or MRI) (1,198) and the use of the 70° endoscope (199) may be useful in diagnosing AC involvement. AC involvement has been reported to affect local control but not survival after transoral resection (197,200). Other authors did not find AC involvement to have a significant impact on local control (120,191). However, patients in some of these institutions with deep AC involvement were treated with supracricoid laryngectomy (120). AC involvement has also been reported to lead to an increased local recurrence rate after radiotherapy (127–132).

When performing transoral surgery in cases with AC involvement, it is important to carry the extent of resection down to the underlying thyroid cartilage and cricothyroid membrane. Frequently, the anterior parts of the false vocal cords and infrahyoid epiglottis will also need to be removed to get adequate access. However, although excellent local control rates have been reported for endoscopic surgery, the extent of resection required may lead to a suboptimal voice outcome. This is particularly true in cases where removal of large portions of both vocal cords is necessary; in such cases, the resultant phonatory gap may lead to a persistent breathy voice. Furthermore, synechiae and webbing of the AC is common in patients undergoing bilateral anterior vocal cord resections.

Another option for early glottic cancer with AC involvement is open resection, either by means of a frontolateral partial laryngectomy, or supracricoid laryngectomy. Excellent local control rates of 95 to 98%, and laryngeal

preservation rates of 100% have been reported for early glottic lesions with AC invasion after supracricoid laryngectomy (201,202). However, supracricoid laryngectomy is associated with a much more pronounced early disturbance in function than either radiotherapy or endoscopic resection.

Besides AC involvement, other factors that have been reported to lead to a worse outcome after transoral resection of early glottic carcinoma are T2 versus T1 stage (203), vocalis muscle infiltration (120,156), and subglottic involvement (120). Positive surgical margins (196) have also been reported to lead to poorer local control, although Steiner reported that there was no difference in ultimate outcome between patients with initially negative margins, and those with initially positive margins whose re-resection specimens showed no residual tumor (204). Some authors elect to closely follow patients with positive margins, performing re-resection only in patients in whom recurrence later develops (191).

The probability of second tumors in patients with early glottic cancers has been estimated to be 13% at 10 years, and 23 to 26% at 20 years (130,188). The mortality of these second tumors is greater than that from laryngeal cancer in patients with T1 tumors (130).

Management of the neck. The overall incidence of nodal metastasis in glottic cancer is low and is directly related to the volume of the primary tumor. For T1 and T2 glottic cancers the risk of nodal metastasis is negligible, and therefore elective treatment of the neck with surgery or radiation is not generally necessary.

Early supraglottic cancer

Management of the primary. Compared to glottic carcinomas, cancers of the supraglottis tend to be more advanced at presentation. Thus early lesions (T1/2) are less commonly seen. Treatment options for such cases include primary radiotherapy, transoral laser resection, and open supraglottic laryngectomy.

Local control and survival rates are shown in Tables 14.18, 14.19, and 14.20. When primary radiotherapy

Table 14.18 Results of Treatment of T1/2 N0 Supraglottic Cancer with Radiation Alone

	Initial local control (%)	Ultimate local control (%)	Larynx preservation (%)	Disease-specific survival (%)	Overall survival (%)
T1	92–100 (133,135,213,214)	96–100 (133,135,214)	94–100 (133,135,214)	100 (214)	
T2	81–86 (133,135,213,214)	76–93 (133,135,214)	80–86 (133,135,214)	100 (214)	
T3	56–76 (133,135,213,215)	80–88 (133,135)	68–72 (133,135)		
T4	43–62 (133,135,213,215)	51–76 (133,135)	43–68 (133,135)		

Table 14.19 Results of Treatment of Supraglottic Squamous Cell Carcinoma with Open Supraglottic Laryngectomy

	Initial local control (%)	Ultimate local control (%)	Larynx preservation (%)	Disease-specific survival (%)	Overall survival (%)
T1	99–100 (125,207)			93 (207)	
T2	91 (125,207)			91 (207)	
T1/2	84–90 (88,206)	88 (206)	80 (206)	49–78 (88,206)	52–89 (88,126,206)
T3	92 (125,207)			100 (207)	

Table 14.20 Results of Treatment of T1/2 N0 supraglottic Cancer with Transoral Laser Resection without Radiation

	Initial local control (%)	Ultimate local control (%)	Larynx preservation (%)	Disease-specific survival (%)	Overall survival (%)
T1 (111,112,210,216)	82–100	93–100	89	97	91
T2 (111,112,210,216)	63–89	75–97	85	94	88

is compared to open supraglottic laryngectomy, the initial local control rates are somewhat lower for primary radiotherapy, especially in the case of T2 lesions (205,206). However, when the effect of surgical salvage is added to the results, ultimate local control rates and survival are comparable (206). The advantage of primary radiotherapy with surgical salvage of failures is that it provides the opportunity to preserve laryngeal function without compromising ultimate control rates. Many patients who fail radiotherapy may still be candidates for conservation surgery as salvage. However, in others, total laryngectomy is the only salvage option.

Local control rates in excess of 90% are reported for early supraglottic cancer after open supraglottic laryngectomy (125,207,208,211,212) (Table 14.19). However, open supraglottic laryngectomy has a high immediate postoperative morbidity, with most patients requiring trachestomy and feeding tubes, and having a prolonged recovery of swallowing function. Aspiration may lead to pneumonia in patients without adequate pulmonary function. On the other hand, among appropriately selected patients, long-term functional outcomes are generally reported to be very good, and are comparable to those seen after radiotherapy (206).

Impressive local control rates are also reported for transoral laser resection (Table 14.20). The oncologic outcomes are reported to be comparable to those of open supraglottic laryngectomy (209). The major advantage of transoral laser surgery over open surgery is that functional sequelae are minimized, owing to less disruption of normal structures. Thus, tracheostomies are generally avoided, rehabilitation of swallowing is faster, and hospital stay is shorter.

The functional outcomes of open versus endoscopic supraglottic laryngectomy have been compared in two studies. Both of these studies reported a significantly lower incidence of tracheostomy tubes, and a faster time to removal of nasogastric tubes, in patients treated with transoral surgery. There was no difference in medium- or long-term subjective swallowing scores, indicating that patients undergoing open supraglottic laryngectomy eventually achieve acceptable swallowing outcomes (117,118). However, a significantly higher incidence of videofluoroscopic abnormalities was seen at long-term follow-up in patients undergoing open surgery, suggesting ongoing silent aspiration (117).

Management of the neck. Patients with supraglottic carcinoma have a high incidence of cervical metastases. The risk of occult metastases in early supraglottic cancer with a clinically N0 neck ranges from 15 to 28% (206,207,210,214). Thus, treatment planning should also take into consideration

elective treatment of the neck. Patients undergoing primary radiotherapy should receive elective neck irradiation, whereas those undergoing open surgery should undergo simultaneous unilateral or bilateral neck dissection. Patients undergoing transoral resection should also undergo elective neck dissection. Some authors have recommended delaying this for 10 to 15 days to minimize the risk of airway swelling or pharyngocutaneous fistulae after extensive resections (121). An alternative for patients undergoing transoral resection is to undergo planned postoperative radiotherapy that also includes the neck. This has been reported to yield regional control rates of 96% in patients with clinical N0 (cN0) necks (211,215).

Among patients undergoing open or transoral supraglottic laryngectomy, the indications for postoperative radiotherapy are pathological evidence of nodal metastases; and close or positive surgical margins, which are reported in 21 to 23% of open supraglottic laryngectomy specimens (88,125,207). Routine postoperative radiotherapy in cases with N0 necks and negative margins is not indicated (212,216).

Moderately Advanced (T3) Laryngeal Cancer (Glottic and Supraglottic)

Glottic tumors are classified as T3 when there is a fixed vocal cord indicating invasion of the paraglottic space. In contrast, supraglottic tumors may be classified as T3 if the vocal cord is fixed but also if there is invasion of the preepiglottic space with normal vocal cord mobility. In general, vocal cord fixation portends poorer local control rates and poorer outcome. The choice of treatment modality for the T3 cancers of the larynx is therefore dependent on the subsite (glottis vs. supraglottis) and the fixation of the cord. As well as tumor factors, patient factors such as age, pulmonary status, swallowing dysfunction, and other medical comorbidity needs to be taken into account.

Management of the primary. Treatment options for the T3 larynx include (1) radiotherapy alone, (2) combined chemoradiotherapy, (3) open partial laryngectomy, (4) transoral laser resection, and (5) total laryngectomy.

Radiotherapy The main advantage of radiotherapy alone over open surgical approaches is that it allows the opportunity for preservation of a functioning larynx in a large proportion of patients, while avoiding the immediate morbidity of open partial laryngeal surgery. The disadvantage is that local control rates after radiotherapy alone for more advanced laryngeal cancers tend to be poorer than those seen after surgery (Tables 14.16, 14.18, 14.21, and 14.24). Certain features, such as increased T stage (133),

Table 14.21   Results of Treatment of Supraglottic Squamous Cell Carcinoma with Open Supraglottic Laryngectomy

Author	N	Site	T Stage	Treatment	Adjuvant RT	LC (%)	LP (%)	DSS (%)	OS (%)
Bron (207)	75	Supraglottis	T1–3	Supraglottic laryngectomy	25	92.5	98.5	92	75
Sevilla (125)	267	Supraglottis	T1–4	Supraglottic laryngectomy	125	71	85	72	
Maurizi (126)	163	Supraglottis	T1–4	Supraglottic laryngectomy	25				86
Dufour (237)	118	Glottis and supraglottis	T3	Supracricoid laryngectomy	24 (20)	91	90		
Gallo (123)	253	Glottis and supraglottis	T1–4	Supracricoid laryngectomy	10	92.5			79
Laudadio (124)	206	Glottis and supraglottis	T1–4	Supracricoid laryngectomy	36 (17.5)	93	97	88	81
Lima (238)	43	Glottis	T3–4	Supracricoid laryngectomy	14 (33)	85	84	78	
Laccourreye (202)	60	Glottis and supraglottis	T3–4	Supracricoid laryngectomy		92	92		73

Abbreviations: N, Number of patients; RT, radiotherapy; LC, local control; LP, laryngeal preservation; DSS, disease-specific survival; OS, overall survival.

greater tumor volume (128,189,213), presence of vocal cord fixation (182,213), and subglottic extension (186) have been associated with poorer local control. In addition, posttreatment edema and fibrosis may make detection of recurrence difficult.

Among patients who fail initial radiotherapy, salvage surgery is successful in 45 to 68% (133,135,188). Thus, ultimate local control rates and survival outcomes are generally equivalent in patients treated by either primary surgery or radiotherapy. However, though some patients with moderately advanced cancer may be candidates for conservation surgery after failed radiotherapy, for many others, the only feasible salvage option is total laryngectomy (217). Thus, laryngeal preservation rates for T3 tumors treated with primary radiotherapy drop to 68 to 72% (133,135), which is less than that reported for T3 cancers treated by conservation laryngeal surgery.

Chemoradiotherapy Chemoradiotherapy has been shown to produce superior local control rates to radiotherapy alone (137). However, it is associated with significant acute toxicity, as well as significant long-term functional problems. The use of chemoradiation is considered further in the section on advanced laryngeal cancer.

Conservation surgery T3 glottic cancers can be treated by vertical partial laryngectomy or by supracricoid partial laryngectomy with CHEP. With vertical partial laryngectomy, local recurrence rates range from 11–46% (218–220). In contrast, supracricoid laryngectomy with CHEP has a lower local recurrence rate of 10% (221). The consistently low recurrence rate is mainly due to the complete resection of the entire thyroid cartilage and bilateral paraglottic spaces.

T3 supraglottic cancers can be treated by supraglottic horizontal partial laryngectomy or supracricoid laryngectomy with CHP. For horizontal partial laryngectomy, high local recurrence of 75% has been reported for T3 tumors. Therefore horizontal supraglottic laryngectomy should be considered with extreme caution in T3 lesions (207, 222–226). The criteria for patient selection for supraglottic laryngectomy are shown in Table 14.22. In contrast, supracricoid laryngectomy with CHP has much better local control rates and outcome. Laccourreye (227) has reported no local recurrences of supraglottic carcinomas treated this way in 68 patients (T1–1, T2–40, T3–26, T4–1) over a fol-

Table 14.22   Contraindications to Supraglottic Laryngectomy

Extension to glottis or floor of ventricle
Invasion of petiole of epiglottis or anterior commissure
Paraglottic space involvement
Interarytenoid invasion
Vocal cord fixation
Extension to apex of piriform sinus
Bilateral fixed nodes requiring bilateral radical neck dissection
Impaired tongue base mobility
Inadequate pulmonary reserve

Source: From Ref. 239.

low-up period of 18 months. Chevalier and Piquet (228) reported a local recurrence rate of 3.3%. In tumors with pre-epiglottic space invasion, Laccourreye (229) reported a local control of 94% in 19 patients with a 5-year follow up period. The reason for such good results is due to the en-bloc resection of bilateral paraglottic spaces, preepiglottic space, and thyroid cartilage.

Therefore for glottic and supraglottic T3 cancers, the supracricoid laryngectomy gives superior results to traditional open partial laryngectomy operations of vertical laryngectomy and horizontal laryngectomy. It also results in excellent laryngeal preservation rates in appropriately selected patients with moderately advanced tumors. The local control rates approach those for total laryngectomy in patients with similarly staged disease. The downside is the immediate postoperative morbidity, such as the need for tracheostomy and feeding tubes, delayed recovery of swallowing function, and aspiration, which is present in nearly every patient. Long-term functional outcomes are generally acceptable, with most patients being decannulated (91–100%) and regaining normal swallowing function (81–99%) within 1 to 3 months of surgery (122,124,126, 230,231). However, most series report a small proportion of patients who eventually require total laryngectomy for intractable aspiration (88,122,124–126).

Careful patient selection is crucial in patients with moderately advanced disease. Most patients will continue to experience some degree of ongoing aspiration; thus it is critical that they have adequate pulmonary reserve to tolerate this. Careful assessment should also be made of the anatomic extent of the tumor. Patients with transglottic tumors who are not suitable for supraglottic laryngectomy may be candidates for supracricoid laryngectomy. Patient selection criteria for supracricoid laryngectomy are shown in Table 14.23. Laccourreye reported that the use of neo-adjuvant chemotherapy allowed for remobilization of fixed crico-arytenoid joints, thus allowing many patients to undergo supracricoid laryngectomy (202).

Transoral laser resection Several recent reports have detailed the use of transoral laser surgery for moderately advanced laryngeal carcinomas (Table 14.24). In expert hands, impressive oncologic outcomes are reported. In a series of 50 patients with pathological T3 (pT3) supraglottic carcinoma, Ambrosch reported a 5-year local control rate of 86%, a 5-year ultimate local control rate of 91%, and a 5-year recurrence-free survival rate of 71% (232). For glottic carcinoma Ambrosch reported a local control rate of 68%, larynx preservation rate of 86% and recurrence-free survival of 62%. A multi-institution review of 117 patients with stage III or stage IV glottic or supraglottic carcinomas undergoing transoral laser surgery at centers in Germany and the USA reported a 5-year local control rate of 74%, a 5-year laryngeal preservation rate of 86%, and a 5-year disease-free survival of 58% (114). In a direct comparison between 26 patients undergoing open supraglottic laryngectomy and 26 patients undergoing transoral resection (15 in each group with T3 primary tumors), Cabanillas reported equivalent oncologic outcomes in both groups (209).

Transoral laser surgery in moderately advanced laryngeal cancers is technically demanding, however, compared to open surgery, functional outcomes of endoscopic surgery are excellent. Positive resection margins are associated with increased risk of local recurrence, thus such patients should undergo either re-resection or postoperative radiotherapy. Many of the local recurrences seen after endoscopic surgery can be treated with further endoscopic resection, thus ultimate local control and laryngectomy-free survival rates are excellent. Of note, extensive spread into the preepiglottic space is considered by some authors to be a contra-indication to transoral resection (111,209).

Total laryngectomy Patients with T3 glottic and supraglottic cancer can be effectively treated with total laryngectomy and bilateral neck dissection with excellent recurrence-free survival and overall survival that is comparable to or superior to other forms of treatment. For glottic carcinoma many patients can be managed by surgery alone without postoperative radiotherapy provided margins are clear and there are no positive neck nodes after bilateral selective neck dissection. Disease-specific survival rates of 60 to 80% are reported (90,145,233–235). With T3 supraglottic cancer management is by total laryngectomy, bilateral neck dissection followed by adjuvant postoperative radiotherapy. The addition of postoperative radiotherapy (PORT) has improved locoregional control rates and disease-specific survival in supraglottic cancer with reported figures of 60 to 90% (214,236).

Management of the neck. Many patients with moderately advanced laryngeal cancer will also have established cervical metastases. Patients undergoing primary surgical treatment should have a neck dissection performed at the time of the surgery, or possibly some days later in the case of transoral surgery. Bilateral selective neck dissections (levels II–IV) should be carried out due to the high incidence of occult metastasis especially for supraglottic primaries. For small-volume glottic T_3 cancers an ipsilateral selective neck dissection can be done. For clinically positive neck disease a modified radical neck dissection is recommended. Postoperative radiotherapy should be administered according to pathological findings (multiple nodes,

Table 14.23 Contra-Indications to Supracricoid Laryngectomy with Cricohyoidopexy

Arytenoid cartilage fixation
Subglottic extension >10 mm anteriorly, or >5 mm laterally, or reaching cricoid cartilage
Major preepiglottic space invasion
Hyoid bone invasion
Cricoid cartilage invasion
Outer thyroid perichondrium invasion or extralaryngeal spread
Inadequate pulmonary reserve

Source: From Ref. 240.

Table 14.24 Transoral Resection of Advanced Laryngeal Cancers

Author	N	Site	Stage	Postoperative RT (%)	Local control (%)	Larynx preservation (%)	Survival
Hinni (114)	117	Glottis and supraglottis	11 T2, 73 T3, 33 T4	34	82[a] (74)	92[a] (86)	68% 2-yr DFS 75% 2-yr OS
Motta (111)	18	Supraglottis	T3	0	77	94	81
Iro (210)	48	Supraglottis	15 T3, 33 T4	45	84		
Ambrosch (232)	167	Glottis	97 T2b 70 T3		74 68	87 86	62% DFS
Ambrosch (232)	50	Supraglottis	T3	26	86	96	71% DFS
Cabanillas (209)	24	Supraglottis	3 T1, 8 T2, 15 T3	23	67	86	80% DSS

[a]2-year rate (5-year estimate in parentheses).
Abbreviations: N, number of patients; RT, radiotherapy; DFS, disease-free survival; OS, overall survival; DSS, disease-specific survival.

pN2+ disease, or extracapsular spread). Among patients undergoing nonsurgical treatment, the options are as follows: (1) up-front neck dissection, followed by definitive radiotherapy to primary site and neck; (2) primary radiotherapy to the primary site and neck, with a delayed neck dissection in patients who do not show a complete response in the neck; or (3) primary combined chemoradiotherapy (see section on advanced laryngeal cancer).

Advanced Laryngeal Cancer

Advanced laryngeal cancers with invasion of cartilage, demonstrating extralaryngeal spread, or with spread to the postcricoid region, or to the apex of the piriform sinus, are generally not suitable for conservation surgery. The choice of treatment in such cases is between primary total laryngectomy, primary radiotherapy, or primary combined chemoradiotherapy. In general invasion of cartilage is a contraindication to organ preservation radiotherapy or chemoradiotherapy. These cases are best treated with primary total laryngectomy.

Total laryngectomy. Total laryngectomy is an effective treatment for advanced laryngeal cancer but has the disadvantage of loss of the larynx, with the attendant functional and psychosocial problems. PORT is typically administered to patients who are able to tolerate it. This appears to improve locoregional control, however, there is no evidence that this improves survival (241). Among patients with advanced laryngeal cancers, local control rates in excess of 85 to 90% have been reported (90,144–147). In these patients, the status of the neck generally has a greater impact on survival (133). Patients with N+ necks undergoing total laryngectomy should undergo concomitant neck dissection. Among patients with N0 necks for whom PORT is planned regardless, it is reasonable not to perform neck dissection, and to treat both sides of the neck with radiation. Regional control rates depend on N stage. Many patients (15–25%) will ultimately succumb to a second primary tumor. The incidence of distant metastases in patients undergoing surgical treatment for advanced laryngeal cancer is 7% (145,146).

In patients with primary glottic SCC with significant (>15 mm) subglottic spread, or with primary subglottic SCC, there is a high incidence of paratracheal lymph node metastases, and extralaryngeal spread into the ipsilateral thyroid lobe (242,243). Thus, surgery in these patients should include ipsilateral thyroid lobectomy and clearance of pretracheal and paratracheal nodes.

Larynx preservation therapy for advanced laryngeal cancer. Larynx preservation therapies for advanced laryngeal cancer include radiotherapy, sequential chemoradiotherapy, and concurrent chemoradiation. In these patients, surgery to the larynx and neck is reserved for salvage for persistent or recurrent disease. Salvage surgery for the larynx is by total laryngectomy.

Primary radiotherapy Until the 1980s, the only alternative approach to total laryngectomy in patients with advanced laryngeal cancer was radical radiotherapy, reserving surgery for patients who fail this treatment. Using this protocol, typical local control rates of 56 to 76% for T3 tumors (133,135,213,215), and 43 to 57% for T4 tumors were reported (133,135,213,215). Unfortunately, monitoring these patients for the earliest signs of recurrence is hindered by postradiotherapy edema and fibrosis. However, thanks to the anatomic compartmentalization of the larynx, for most patients the recurrence is still contained within the larynx, and suitable for salvage total laryngectomy. Roughly 66% of patients with laryngeal cancer who fail radiotherapy are suitable for salvage surgery (133), which is successful in 45–68% (133,135,188). Thus, 41 to 45% of patients failing radiotherapy ultimately achieve local control (133,135).

The use of primary radiotherapy thus affords the opportunity for a large number of patients to retain a functional larynx. However, the benefits of this treatment protocol would appear to be limited to a subset of patients with moderately advanced primary cancers as discussed previously. Radiation alone appears to be much less effective in tumors with T4 stage (133,135), evidence of thyroid cartilage destruction, and extralaryngeal spread of tumor. Only 20% of patients with initial T4 tumors are successfully salvaged by total laryngectomy if they fail primary radiation therapy (135). Thus, primary total laryngectomy is likely to be a better option in such patients.

Primary chemoradiation In the 1980s, in an effort to improve the results of nonsurgical treatment, the use of induction chemotherapy followed by radical radiotherapy was investigated. Since then, two randomized controlled trials comparing total laryngectomy with chemoradiation have been published. In 1991 the Department of Veterans Affairs Laryngeal Cancer Study Group (VALCSG) published its landmark trial (137) comparing conventional treatment (surgery with postoperative radiation) to induction chemotherapy followed by radiation therapy in patients with advanced laryngeal cancer. Two-year survival in each arm was equal at 68%, but as much as 64% of patients in the chemoradiation arm retained a functional larynx. This study was regarded as showing that a treatment strategy involving sequential chemoradiotherapy for advanced laryngeal cancer may be effective in preserving the larynx in a high proportion of patients without compromising overall survival.

In contrast, in 1998, the French Groupe d'Etude de Tumeurs de Tete Et du Cou (GETTEC) group published the results of a prospective randomized study comparing total laryngectomy to three cycles of induction chemotherapy followed by radiotherapy if there was a better than 80% clinical response, or total laryngectomy in other cases. Unlike the VALCSG study, all patients in the GETTEC study had primary tumors staged T3 or higher. The authors reported significantly better locoregional control and disease-free survival in the total laryngectomy group. The major drawback of this study was that CT was not routinely performed to assess tumor extension and response, however, this weakness in no way invalidates the findings of this study (244).

In 2003, Forastiere published the results of the Radiation Therapy Oncology Group (91–11) study comparing radiation alone, sequential chemoradiotherapy, and concurrent chemoradiotherapy in patients with advanced laryngeal cancer. Overall survival rates were similar in all three groups. However, at 2 years, a significantly higher percentage of patients undergoing concurrent chemoradiotherapy had an intact larynx (88%) than did patients undergoing sequential chemoradiotherapy (75%) or radiotherapy alone

(70%). Patients undergoing concurrent chemoradiotherapy also had significantly better local control (78% vs. 61% vs. 56%, respectively). The major disadvantage of chemoradiotherapy regimes compared to radiotherapy alone was the significantly increased incidence of severe toxic effects during and after treatment (136).

A notable criticism of the VALCSG and Radiation Therapy Oncology Group 91-11 studies was that many tumors were considered "advanced" on the basis of advanced nodal status, not because of primary stage. Thus, there were many patients with mobile vocal cords included in these trials who may have been candidates for conservation laryngeal surgery. Despite this, these trials have demonstrated the feasibility of nonsurgical approaches to advanced laryngeal cancer.

The development of chemoradiotherapy protocols has thus afforded the opportunity for larynx preservation in patients whose only surgical option would have been total laryngectomy. However, although concurrent chemoradiation is now considered first-line treatment in many institutions for patients with advanced laryngeal cancer, it is clear that there still exists a subset of patients who do not respond so well. Such patients, which include those with tumor invasion of laryngeal cartilage, or extension of tumor outside the larynx, would thus be better served with up-front total laryngectomy.

It is well established that the response of tumors to induction chemotherapy is predictive of the tumor response to radiotherapy or chemoradiotherapy. In an effort to identify those tumors which are likely to be cured by nonsurgical treatment, there has been much recent interest in protocols consisting of induction chemotherapy, with patients showing complete response proceeding to concurrent chemoradiation, and nonresponders proceeding to total laryngectomy (245,246). With such regimes, impressive 3-year (85%) and 5-year (68%) overall survival and laryngeal preservation rates have been reported (245,246). Induction chemotherapy has also been described to select patients for treatment with radiotherapy alone (complete responders) as opposed to concurrent chemoradiotherapy (all others) (247).

Serious concerns persist regarding the function of the preserved larynx after concurrent chemoradiotherapy, particularly with respect to airway protection and swallowing (138–140). A high requirement for tracheostomy and feeding tubes is reported (104,141). In a series of 29 patients treated with chemoradiotherapy who underwent prospective evaluation of swallow function with videofluoroscopy and esophagogram, Eisbruch reported an incidence of aspiration which increased from 14% pretreatment, to 65% in the early posttreatment period, and 62% in the late (6–12 months) posttreatment period. Six patients developed pneumonia requiring hospitalization (142). Nguyen reported an incidence of aspiration of 54% in chemoradiotherapy patients, compared to 33% in radiotherapy alone patients (140), while Langmerman reported trace aspiration in 56%, and frank aspiration in 33%, of patients with larynx cancer treated with chemoradiotherapy (143). Aspiration in these patients is typically silent, with no symptoms of coughing or choking (142,143). Swallowing disorders persist 12 months after completion of chemoradiotherapy (104,139), in contrast to patients treated with radiotherapy alone (139). Even 2 years or more after treatment, a high proportion of patients still have aspiration and are dependent on tracheostomy tubes (107). Pretreatment vocal cord fixation has been reported to be a strong predictor of poor functional outcome (141).

Patients treated with chemoradiotherapy also show abnormalities of voice (248). However, compared to patients undergoing total laryngectomy, patients treated with chemoradiotherapy are reported to have better speech function (249,250). Fung also reported swallowing function to be comparable between total laryngectomy and chemoradiotherapy patients (249).

Recently, several investigators have attempted to compare quality of life in patients treated with either total laryngectomy and PORT or combined chemoradiotherapy. Hanna found no difference in overall quality of life (251), whereas Boscolo-Rizzo reported a better global quality of life score in nonsurgical patients (252). In both studies, surgical patients had poorer scores for physical, social, and role functioning, and more problems with pain and sensory disturbance, whereas chemoradiotherapy patients had more problems with dry mouth and sticky saliva (251,252).

Newer approaches, using biological therapy with tyrosine kinase inhibitors (gefitnib and erlotinib) and monoclonal antibodies directed against epidermal growth factor receptor (cetuximab) may allow for comparable efficacy when combined with radiation as conventional concurrent chemoradiotherapy, but with less toxicity. The combination of cetuximab and radiotherapy has been shown to have a survival benefit over radiotherapy alone (253).

Subglottic Carcinoma

Primary SCC of the subglottis is rare, comprising less than 2% of laryngeal carcinomas (254–256). Far more common is subglottic spread of glottic SCC, or transglottic spread of supraglottic SCC via the paraglottic space (243). Unlike SCC arising on the vocal cords which produce symptoms early, primary subglottic SCC produces symptoms late, and so is usually advanced at presentation (159,254,257). Diagnosis may be missed if careful examination of the subglottis is not performed. Swelling of the vocal cord, with reduced mobility, but with intact vocal cord mucosa, may be the only endoscopic sign of a subglottic carcinoma which has spread superiorly to the level of glottis. Because most cases are advanced presentation, total laryngectomy is the only surgical option in most (96). Partial laryngectomy may be feasible in select cases (96).

Subglottic SCC is associated with a much higher incidence of lymphatic metastases than glottic SCC. Typically, spread occurs first to paratracheal nodes (243). Extralaryngeal spread and distant metastases are common (257).

The prognosis of subglottic SCC is generally regarded to be very poor. Paisley reported local control rates with radiation alone of 56%, with ultimate local control rates after salvage surgery of 81% (258). On the other hand, others reported dismal control rates with radiation alone, and found combined surgery and radiotherapy to be associated with a significantly better outcome (154). After primary surgical treatment, disease-specific survival rates of up to 70% (96) have been reported. Overall survival rates after 3 to 5 years are reported to be between 25 and 58% (254,257,258).

Recurrent Laryngeal Cancer

Assessment and diagnosis. One of the disadvantages of treatment of head and neck cancer with radiotherapy or chemoradiotherapy is that the diagnosis of recurrent disease is often difficult to make, and by the time recurrence is diagnosed, the tumor is unresectable. In addition, salvage surgery is more difficult than primary surgery, owing to fibrosis and scarring of tissue planes. Postoperative complications, such as pharyngocutaneous fistulae, are reported to be more common after salvage laryngectomies than in primary laryngectomies (149).

In the case of the larynx, postradiotherapy edema of the supraglottis impairs visualization of the rest of the larynx. In particular, the laryngeal ventricle, AC, and subglottic region may be difficult to examine. Fibrosis of the soft tissues of the neck leading to stiffness of the neck and tongue base can also increase the difficulty of operative endoscopy. Recurrences may frequently develop in a multicentric fashion beneath an intact mucosa (259). The distinction between recurrent cancer and chondronecrosis can be very difficult using standard imaging (CT and MRI) modalities (260,261). Finally, the histological diagnosis of recurrence may also be difficult owing to the effects or radiation in the surrounding tissues, and false negative biopsies are common.

Traditional teaching has been that patients showing persistent laryngeal edema more than 6 months after completion of radiotherapy should undergo direct laryngoscopy with biopsy of suspicious areas. In the era of chemoradiotherapy, this protocol needs to be tempered to take into account the significant risk of chondronecrosis of the larynx that may be precipitated by large biopsies. Thus, in the absence of lesions that are clearly suspicious of recurrence, restraint should be exercised in taking biopsies of the chemo-irradiated larynx. The advent of positron emission tomography scanning may be useful in detecting areas that are considered to be at high risk of harboring recurrent disease, although false positives and negatives may occur.

On the other hand, the anatomic position and compartmentalization of the larynx mean that, uniquely among head and neck cancers, laryngeal cancer recurrences tend to remain localized within the larynx, and thus it is usually possible to achieve complete clearance by salvage total laryngectomy. Thus, in contrast to other head and neck cancers, the results of salvage surgery are acceptable.

Recurrence after radiotherapy.

Salvage conservation surgery by transoral laser surgery In patients who develop recurrence after undergoing radiotherapy alone for less advanced disease, it is frequently possible to perform larynx-sparing salvage surgery. This may be either by transoral resection or open partial laryngectomy. In properly selected patients, such an approach does not appear to lead to any compromise of oncologic outcomes (217,262–264).

Local control rates for transoral laser resection of recurrences after radiotherapy range from 65 to 81% (263, 265,266). Subsequent total laryngectomy is required in 6 to 30% (263,265). Five-year disease-specific survival rates of 86 to 95% have been reported (262,263). To perform adequate transoral resection, adequate visualization of the tumor is necessary. This may be difficult in irradiated patients due to laryngeal edema, and stiffness of the neck, and tongue base. The distinction between tumor and normal tissue in the irradiated larynx may also be difficult. Frozen sections should always be sent in such cases, with all margins subsequently confirmed by permanent section.

Recurrence at the AC after radiotherapy presents a particular problem. This is due to difficulties with exposure, the tangential viewing angle in this location, difficulties distinguishing between tumor and nontumor tissue in an irradiated field, and the high incidence of thyroid cartilage involvement reported in these cases (267). A high recurrence rate compared to cases without AC involvement is reported (267,268). Steiner reported no significant difference in ultimate local control in patients with and without AC involvement, however, the laryngectomy rate was higher in patients with AC involvement. He advocated taking wider margins, including a part of the thyroid cartilage (263).

Salvage conservation surgery by open partial laryngectomy In patients who are not suitable for transoral resection, good results may be achieved by salvage open partial laryngectomy. Careful radiologic and endoscopic assessment of the recurrent tumor is critical to good patient selection, and this may be difficult for the reasons given above. Excellent oncologic outcomes have been reported in appropriately selected patients (217,231). Functional outcomes are also reported to be acceptable. Length of hospitalization and tracheostomy tube dependence after supracricoid laryngectomy are reported to be higher in patients treated with initial radiotherapy, however, long-term functional outcomes are equivalent (122,230).

Salvage surgery by total laryngectomy In many patients with recurrent laryngeal cancer after radiotherapy, the only viable salvage option is total laryngectomy (264). The salvage rate for total laryngectomy in such cases is generally reported to be between 45 and 68% (133,135,188).

Recurrence after chemoradiation.

After failed chemoradiotherapy, laryngeal conservation surgery is seldom feasible. For most of these patients, the only salvage option is total laryngectomy. A significantly higher incidence of complications such as pharygocutaneous fistulas after salvage laryngectomy compared to primary laryngectomy has been reported (149,269). When performing total laryngectomy on these patients, careful assessment should be made of the quality of the remaining tissues of the trachea and pharynx prior to performing tracheo-esophageal puncture. If the quality of the tissues is dubious, a secondary tracheo-esophageal puncture may be advisable. In addition, reinstitution of oral feeding should be delayed to ensure full healing has occurred. The use of pectoralis major flaps to prevent pharyngo-cutaneous fistulae has been advocated.

Recurrence after total laryngectomy.

Local recurrence after total laryngectomy usually takes the form of stomal recurrence.

Stomal recurrence is most commonly related to paratracheal nodal metastases (147,270). Other suggested risk factors for stomal recurrence include pre-operative tracheostomy (147,270–272), (unrecognized) subglottic extension of tumor (271–273), and unrecognized second primary tumor in the esophagus. When performing total laryngectomy for patients with glottic, subglottic, or transglottic cancers, care should be taken to ensure an adequate inferior margin of resection. In patients who have had a previous tracheostomy, complete excision of the tracheostomy tract, with an adequate margin of normal trachea below the tracheostomy should be performed (270,272). Pretracheal and paratracheal nodal clearance, as well as ipsilateral thyroid lobectomy, should be performed to reduce the risk of stomal recurrence (243,270,272).

Reirradiation using intensity modulated radiotherapy, with or without chemotherapy, is an option in selected patients with recurrent laryngeal cancer postsurgery and radiotherapy. Patients who underwent primary radiotherapy with intensity modulated radiotherapy for early laryngeal cancers may be good candidates as the original radiotherapy fields in many cases will have been small, and most of the irradiated tissue may have been removed during the course of subsequent surgery. The rate of toxicity is high in patients undergoing reirradiation (274–276). Serious late complications such as fatal carotid rupture and osteoradionecrosis are also commonly reported (276). Although the absolute number of serious late complications in most series would appear to be within acceptable limits, it should be borne in mind that the number of patients at risk for late complications is small, so that the true rate of serious complications in survivors is even higher. Overall 2-year survival rates in the region of 15 to 58% have been reported in patients receiving reirradiation for recurrent head and neck cancers of all sites (274,276,277). In patients undergoing salvage surgery postradiotherapy who are planned for reirradiation, the use of free flaps for surgical reconstruction has been advocated to facilitate wound healing (278).

FOLLOW-UP AND REHABILITATION

Rehabilitation of the patient after treatment involves close co-operation with other health professionals including the speech therapist, dietician, and nursing staff. The follow-up schedule must incorporate appropriate evaluation of the patient by these members of the treating team at regular intervals. In addition to a thorough examination of the head and neck region, a yearly chest radiograph may be useful, although its value in improving outcome of second primary lung cancer remains unproven.

The rehabilitation of speech and swallowing in postlaryngectomy patients is discussed elsewhere in this book.

FUTURE DIRECTIONS
Chemotherapy Alone
Laccourreye reported that patients with glottic carcinoma staged T1-4 who show a complete response to platinum-based induction chemotherapy regimen may be treated with chemotherapy alone. Patients with glottic primaries were reported to have a 5-year local control rate of 65.7%, a 5-year ultimate local control of 100%, a 5-year laryngeal preservation rate of 100%, and a 5-year neck control rate of 90% (279). Other authors have also reported a high survival in patients who had a complete response to induction chemotherapy who proceeded to treatment with chemotherapy alone (280).

Molecular Markers of Chemoradiation Response
Chemoradiation using newer agents may result in an improvement in survival in addition to the already proven benefit of laryngeal organ preservation. However, it is more important to identify patients who will respond best to chemoradiation so that patients who will not respond can be treated with primary surgery and avoid the unnecessary toxicity of chemoradiation. There seems to be some promise in markers such as p53 overexpression, p105 labeling, S-phase fraction labeling, and potential doubling time (281–283). An in vitro histoculture drug sensitivity has demonstrated the ability to predict which patients may respond favorably to chemotherapy (284), but much study will be required before these tests come into routine clinical practice. A recent study by Ganly et al. (285) reported that mdm2 and ErbB2 may be useful markers of chemoradiation response.

Gene Therapy
Viral vectors have been used to transfer the p53 tumor suppressor gene into SCC of the human lung (286) and several centers are investigating the application of gene therapy in head and neck cancer.

Laryngeal Transplantation
The role of laryngeal transplantation has been explored for quite some time now, and interest in the subject has been renewed mainly because microvascular reconstruction is now an everyday routine in head and neck surgery. Parallel to the advances in microsurgical technique, improvements in immunosuppressive agents have now made laryngeal transplantation look more feasible. However, the major technical problem in achieving successful functional outcome remains reinnervation of the transplanted organ. Various techniques have been tried and the use of growth factors has not improved success. The possibility of using gene therapy to aid, and possibly guide, nerve regeneration needs to be explored. Apart from the difficulty in reinnervating the transplanted larynx, there are numerous other technical issues that are unresolved. The central question is the wisdom of immunosuppressing patients who are already at risk of developing subsequent malignant tumors. In summary, future research and developments need to focus not only on understanding the basic mechanisms of the disease and how to prevent it, but efforts must also be made to help those who have been unfortunate to develop the disease and suffer its consequences.

REFERENCES

1. Bradley PJ, Rinaldo A, Suarez C et al. Primary treatment of the anterior vocal commissure squamous carcinoma. Eur Arch Otorhinolaryngol 2006; 263: 879–88.
2. Pressman JJ, Dowdy A, Libby R et al. Further studies upon the submucosal compartments and lymphatics by the injection of dyes and radioisotopes. Ann Otol Rhino Laryngol 1956; 65: 963.
3. Welsh LW, Welsh JJ, Rizzo TA Jr. Laryngeal spaces and lymphatics: current anatomic concepts. Ann Otol Rhinol Laryngol 1983; 105: 19–31.
4. Werner JA, Schunke M, Rudert H et al. Description and clinical importance of the lymphatics of the vocal fold. Otolaryngol Head Neck Surg 1990; 102: 13–9.

5. Ferlito A, Rinaldo A, Devaney KO et al. Impact of phenotype on treatment and prognosis of laryngeal malignancies. J Laryngol Otol 1998; 112: 710–14.

6. Fliss DM, Noble Topham SE, McLachlin M et al. Laryngeal verrucous carcinoma: a clinicopathologic study and detection of human papillomavirus using polymerase chain reaction. Laryngoscope 1994; 104: 146–52.

7. Orvidas LJ, Olsen KD, Lewis JE et al. Verrucous carcinoma of the larynx: a review of 53 patients. Head Neck 1998; 20: 197–203.

8. Ferlito A, Altavilla G, Rinaldo A et al. Basaloid squamous cell carcinoma of the larynx and hypopharynx. a clinicopathological study of 15 new cases with review of the literature. Ann Otol Rhinol Laryngol 1997; 106: 1024–35.

9. Overholt SM, Donovan DT, Schwartz MR et al. Neuroendocrine neoplasms of the larynx. Laryngoscope 1995; 105: 789–94.

10. Batsakis JG, El-Naggar AK, Luna MA. Neuroendocrine tumours of the larynx. Ann Otol Rhinol Laryngol 1992; 101: 710–14.

11. Wenig BM. Laryngeal mucosal malignant melanoma. A clinicopathologic, immunohistochemical, and ultrastructural study of four patients and a review of the literature. Cancer 1995; 75: 1568–77.

12. Batsakis JG, Luna MA, El-Naggar AK. Nonsquamous carcinomas of the larynx. Ann Otol Rhinol Laryngol 1992; 101: 1024–6.

13. Hyams VJ, Heffner DK. Laryngeal pathology. In: Tucker HM, ed. The Larynx, 2nd ed. New York: Thieme, 1993; 35–80.

14. Cantrell RW. The current status of laryngeal cancer. In: Inouye T, Fukuda H, Sato T, Hinohara T, eds. Recent Advances in Bronchesophagology. Amsterdam: Excerpta Medica, 1990; 3–12.

15. Parkin DM, Muir CS, Whelan S et al., eds. Cancer Incidence in Five Continents (Vol. VI. IARC Scientific Publication No. 120). Lyon, France: World Health Organization, International Agency for Research on Cancer, 1992.

16. Karim-Kos HE et al. Recent trends of cancer in Europe: A combined approach of incidence, survival and mortality for 17 cancer sites since the 1990s. Eur J Cancer, 2008; 44: 1345–89.

17. Esteve J, Kricker A, Ferlay J et al., eds. Facts and Figures of Cancer in the European Community. Lyon, France: World Health Organization, International Agency for Research on Cancer Commission of the European Communities, 1993.

18. Maier H, Tisch M. Epidemiology of laryngeal cancer. In: Kleinsasser O, Glanz H, Olofsson J, eds. Advances in Laryngology in Europe. Amsterdam: Elsevier Science B.V., 1997; 129–33.

19. Wunsch Filho V. The epidemiology of laryngeal cancer in Brazil. Sao Paulo Med J 2004; 122: 188–94.

20. Schottenfeld S. Alcohol as a co-factor in the etiology of cancer. Cancer 1979; 43: 1962–6.

21. Wynder EL, Covey LS, Mabuchi K et al. Environmental factors in cancer of the larynx: a second look. Cancer 1976; 38: 1591–601.

22. Tamarit Conejeros JM et al. [Supraglottic and glottic carcinomas. Study of the incidence in the last 31 years]. Acta Otorrinolaringol Esp 2007; 58: 449–53.

23. Data from the Royal Marsden Hospital Head and Neck Cancer Database. Personal communication with Roger A'hern, Department of Computing and Statistics, Royal Marsden Hospital, London, September 1998.

24. Shah JP, Karnell LH, Hoffman HT et al. Patterns of care for cancer of the larynx in the United States. Arch Otolaryngol Head Neck Surgery 1997; 123: 475–83.

25. Desai PB, Rao RS, Dinshaw KA et al. Hospital Cancer Registry Annual Report 1993. Bombay, India: Tata Memorial Hospital 1993.

26. Robin PE, Powell J, Holme GM et al. Incidence. In: Robin PE, ed. Cancer of the Larynx (Clinical Cancer Monographs, vol. 2). New York: Stockton Press, 1989; 64–5.

27. Polesel J, Talamini R, La Vecchia C et al. Tobacco smoking and the risk of upper aero-digestive tract cancers: a reanalysis of case-control studies using spline models. Int J Cancer 2008; 122: 2398–402.

28. Talamini R, Bosetti C, La Vecchia C et al. Combined effect of tobacco and alcohol on laryngeal cancer risk: a case-control study. Cancer Causes Control 2002; 13: 957–64.

29. Hashibe M, Boffetta P, Zaridze D et al. Contribution of tobacco and alcohol to the high rates of squamous cell carcinoma of the supraglottis and glottis in Central Europe. Am J Epidemiol 2007; 165: 814–20.

30. Menvielle G, Luce D, Goldberg P et al. Smoking, alcohol drinking and cancer risk for various sites of the larynx and hypopharynx. A case-control study in France. Eur J Cancer Prev 2004; 13: 165–72.

31. Muscat JE, Wynder EL. Tobacco, alcohol, asbestos, and occupational risk factors for laryngeal cancer. Cancer 1992; 69: 2244–51.

32. Tuyns AJ, Esteve J, Raymond L et al. Cancer of the larynx/hypopharynx, tobacco and alcohol: IARC international case-control study in Turin and Varese (Italy), Zaragoza and Navarra (Spain), Geneva (Switzerland) and Calvados (France). Int J Cancer 1988; 41: 483–91.

33. Hoffman D, Melkian A, Adams JD et al. New aspects of tobacco carcinogenesis. Carcinogenesis 1985; 8: 239–56.

34. Maier H, Dietz A, Gewelke U et al. Tobacco and alcohol and the risk of head and neck cancer. Clin Invest 1992; 70: 320–7.

35. Sancho-Garnier J, Theobald S. Black (air-cured) and blond (flue-cured) tobacco and cancer risk: pharynx and larynx cancer. Eur J Cancer 1993; 29A: 273–6.

36. Maier H, Tisch M. Epidemiology of laryngeal cancer: results of the Heidelberg case-control study. Acta Otolaryngol Suppl (Stockh) 1997; 527: 160–4.

37. Koskinen WJ, Brondbo K, Mellin Dahlstrand H et al. Alcohol, smoking and human papillomavirus in laryngeal carcinoma: a Nordic prospective multicenter study. J Cancer Res Clin Oncol 2007; 133: 673–8.

38. La Vecchia C, Zhang ZF, Altieri A. Alcohol and laryngeal cancer: an update. Eur J Cancer Prev 2008; 17: 116–24.

39. Garavello W et al. Type of alcoholic beverage and the risk of laryngeal cancer. Eur J Cancer Prev 2006; 15: 69–73.

40. Brugere J, Guenel P, Leclerc A et al. Differential effects of tobacco and alcohol in cancer of the larynx, pharynx and mouth. Cancer 1986; 57: 391–5.

41. Garavello W, Lucenteforte E, Bosetti C et al. Diet diversity and the risk of laryngeal cancer: a case-control study from Italy and Switzerland. Oral Oncol 2009; 45: 85–9.

42. Esteve J, Riboli E, Pequignot G et al. Diet and cancers of the larynx and hypopharynx: The IARC multi-center study in southwestern Europe. Cancer Causes Control 1996; 7: 240–52.

43. Thorne P, Etherington D, Birchall MA. Head and neck cancer in the South West of England: Influence of socio-economic status on incidence and second primary tumours. Eur J Surg Oncol 1997; 23: 503–8.

44. Torrente MC, Ojeda JM. Exploring the relation between human papilloma virus and larynx cancer. Acta Otolaryngol 2007; 127: 900–6.

45. Doll R. The epidemiology of cancer. Cancer 1980; 45: 2475–85.

46. World Health Statistics Annual 1983. Geneva, Switzerland: World Health Organisation, 1983.

47. Hobbs CG, Sterne JA, Bailey M et al. Human papillomavirus and head and neck cancer: A systematic review and meta-analysis. Clin Otolaryngol 2006; 31: 259–66.

48. Klussmann JP, Weissenborn SJ, Wieland U et al. Prevalence, distribution, and viral load of human papillomavirus 16 DNA in tonsillar carcinomas. Cancer 2001; 92: 2875–84.

49. Rabah R, Lancaster WD, Thomas R et al. Human papillomavirus-11-associated recurrent respiratory papillomatosis is more aggressive than human papillomavirus-6-associated disease. Pediatr Dev Pathol 2001; 4: 68–72.

50. Klozar J, Taudy M, Betka J et al. Laryngeal papilloma—precancerous condition? Acta Otolaryngol Suppl 1997; 527: 100–2.

51. Lindeberg H, Elbrond O. Malignant tumours in patients with a history of multiple laryngeal papillomas: the significance of irradiation. Clin Otolaryngol Allied Sci 1991; 16: 149–51.

52. Gerein V, Rastorquev E, Gerein J et al. Incidence, age at onset, and potential reasons of malignant transformation in recurrent respiratory papillomatosis patients: 20 years experience. Otolaryngol Head Neck Surg 2005; 132: 392–4.

53. Gorgoulis VG, Zachataros P, Kotsinas A et al. Human papilloma virus (HPV) is possibly involved in laryngeal but not in lung carcinogenesis. Hum Pathol 1999; 30: 274–83.

54. Kreimer AR, Clifford GM, Boyle P et al. Human papillomavirus types in head and neck squamous cell carcinomas worldwide: a systematic review. Cancer Epidemiol Biomarkers Prev 2005; 14: 467–75.

55. Smith EM, Summersqill KF, Allen J et al. Human papillomavirus and risk of laryngeal cancer. Ann Otol Rhinol Laryngol 2000; 109: 1069–76.

56. Elwood JM, Pearson JCG, Skippen DH et al. Alcohol, smoking, social and occupational factors in the etiology of cancer of the oral cavity, pharynx and larynx. Int J Cancer 1984; 34: 603–12.

57. Pollan M, Lopez Abente G. Wood-related occupations and laryngeal cancer. Cancer Detect Prev 1995; 19: 250–7.

58. Peters ES, McClean MD, Marsit CJ et al. Glutathione S-transferase polymorphisms and the synergy of alcohol and tobacco in oral, pharyngeal, and laryngeal carcinoma. Cancer Epidemiol Biomarkers Prev 2006; 15: 2196–202.

59. Acar H, Ozturk K, Muslumanoglu MH et al. Relation of glutathione S-transferase genotypes (GSTM1 and GSTT1) to laryngeal squamous cell carcinoma risk. Cancer Genet Cytogenet 2006; 169: 89–93.

60. Bardakci F, Canbay E, Degerli N et al. Relationship of tobacco smoking with GSTM1 gene polymorphism in laryngeal cancer. J Cell Mol Med 2003; **7**: 307–12.

61. Jourenkova N, Reinikainen M, Bouchardy C et al. Larynx cancer risk in relation to glutathione S-transferase M1 and T1 genotypes and tobacco smoking. Cancer Epidemiol Biomarkers Prev 1998; **7**: 19–23.

62. Hashibe M, McKay JD, Curado MP et al. Multiple ADH genes are associated with upper aerodigestive cancers. Nat Genet 2008; 40: 707–9.

63. Nishimoto IN, Pinheiro NA, Rogatto SR et al. Alcohol dehydrogenase 3 genotype as a risk factor for upper aerodigestive tract cancers. Arch Otolaryngol Head Neck Surg 2004; 130: 78–82.

64. Olshan AF, Weissler MC, Watson MA et al. Risk of head and neck cancer and the alcohol dehydrogenase 3 genotype. Carcinogenesis 2001; 22: 57–61.

65. Lynch HT, Kriegler M, Christiansen TA et al. Laryngeal carcinoma in a Lynch syndrome II kindred. Cancer 1988; 62: 1007–13.

66. Berkower AS, Biller JF. Head and neck cancer associated with Bloom's syndrome. Laryngoscope 1988; 98: 746–9.

67. Baker DC, Weismann B. Postirradiation carcinoma of the larynx. Ann Otol 1971; 80: 631–7.

68. van der Laan BFAM, Baris G, Gregor R Th et al. Radiation-induced tumors of the head and neck. J Otol Laryngol 1995; 109: 346–9.

69. Glaubiger DL, Casler JD, Garrett WL et al. Chondrosarcoma of the larynx after radiation treatment for vocal cord cancer. Cancer 1991; 68: 1828–31.

70. Morrison MD. Is chronic gastroesophageal reflux a causative factor in glottic carcinoma? Otolaryngol Head Neck Surg 1988; 99: 370–3.

71. Nilsson M, Chow WH, Lindblad M et al. No association between gastroesophageal reflux and cancers of the larynx and pharynx. Cancer Epidemiol Biomarkers Prev 2005; 14: 1194–7.

72. Bouquot JE, Gnepp DR. Laryngeal precancer: a review of the literature, commentary, and comparison with oral leukoplakia. Head Neck 1991; 13: 488–97.

73. Blackwell KE, Fu YS, Calcaterra TC. Laryngeal dysplasia. A clinicopathologic study. Cancer 1995; 15: 457–63.

74. Hellquist H, Cardesa A, Gale N et al. Criteria for grading in the Ljubljana classification of epithelial hyperplastic laryngeal lesions. A study by members of the Working Group on Epithelial Hyperplastic Laryngeal Lesions of the European Society of Pathology. Histopathology 1999; 34: 226–33.

75. Gale N, Kambic V, Michaels L et al. The Ljubljana classification: a practical strategy for the diagnosis of laryngeal precancerous lesions. Adv Anat Pathol 2000; **7**: 240–51.

76. Gallo A, de Vincentiis M, Della Rocca C et al. Evolution of precancerous laryngeal lesions: a clinicopathologic study with long-term follow-up on 259 patients. Head Neck 2001; 23: 42–7.

77. Isenberg JS, Crozier DL, Dailey SH. Institutional and comprehensive review of laryngeal leukoplakia. Ann Otol Rhinol Laryngol 2008; 117: 74–9.

78. Motta G, Esposito C, Motta S et al. [Microlaryngoscopy treatment of laryngeal dysplasia with CO2 laser]. Acta Otorhinolaryngol Ital 2001; 21: 32–43.

79. Ricci G, Molini E, Faralli M et al. Retrospective study on precancerous laryngeal lesions: Long-term follow-up. Acta Otorhinolaryngol Ital 2003; 23: 362–7.

80. Sllamniku B, Bauer W, Painter C et al. The transformation of laryngeal keratosis into invasive carcinoma. Am J Otolaryngol 1989; 10: 42–54.

81. Hojslet PE, Nielsen VM, Palvio D. Premalignant lesions of the larynx. A follow-up study. Acta Otolaryngol 1989; 107: 150–5.

82. Kirchner JA, Carter D. Intralaryngeal barriers to the spread of cancer. Acta Otolaryngol (Stockh) 1987; 103: 503–13.

83. Kirchner JA. Glottic-supraglottic barrier: Fact or fantasy? Ann Otol Rhinol Laryngol 1997; 106: 700–4.

84. Welsh LW, Welsh JJ, Rizzo TA. Internal anatomy of the larynx and the spread of cancer. Ann Otol Rhinol Laryngol 1989; 98: 228–34.

85. Yeager VL, Archer CR. Anatomical routes for cancer invasion of laryngeal cartilages. Laryngoscope 1982; 92: 449–52.

86. Bridger GP, Nassar VH. Carcinoma in situ involving the laryngeal mucous glands. Arch Otolaryngol 1971; 94: 389–400.

87. Candela FC, Shah J, Jacques DP et al. Patterns of cervical node metastases from squamous carcinoma of the larynx. Arch Otolaryngol Head Neck Surg 1990; 116: 432–5.

88. Prades JM, Simon PG, Timoshenko AP et al. Extended and standard supraglottic laryngectomies: a review of 110 patients. Eur Arch Otorhinolaryngol 2005; 262: 947–52.

89. Marks JE, Breaux S, Smith PG et al. The need for elective irradiation of occult lymphatic metastases from cancers of the larynx and pyriform sinus. Head Neck 1985; 8: 3–8.

90. Johnson JT, Myers EN, Hao SP et al. Outcome of open surgical therapy for glottic carcinoma. Ann Otol Rhinol Laryngol 1993; 102: 752–5.

91. Daly CJ, Strong EW. Carcinoma of the glottic larynx. Am J Surg 1975; 130: 489–92.

92. Jesse RH. The evaluation and treatment of patients with extensive squamous cancer of the vocal cords. Laryngoscope 1975; 85: 1424–9.

93. Thaler ER, Montone K, Tucker J et al. Delphian lymph node in laryngeal carcinoma: A whole organ study. Laryngoscope 1997; 332–4.

94. Olsen K, DeSanto LW, Pearson BW. Positive Delphian lymph node: clinical significance in laryngeal cancer. Laryngoscope 1987; 97: 1033–7.

95. Harrison DF. The pathology and management of subglottic cancer. Ann Otol Rhinol Laryngol 1971; 80: 6–12.

96. Shaha AR, Shah JP. Carcinoma of the subglottic larynx. Am J Surg 1982; 144: 456–8.

97. Lamprecht J, Lamprecht A, Kurten-Rothes R. Mediastinal involvement in cancers of the subglottis. Laryngol Rhinol Otol (Stuttg) 1987; 66: 88–90.

98. Merino OR, Lindberg RD, Fletcher GH. An analysis of distant metastases from squamous cell carcinoma of the upper respiratory and digestive tracts. Cancer 1977; 40: 145–51.

99. Johnson JT. Carcinoma of the larynx: selective approach to the management of cervical lymphatics. Ear Nose Throat J 1994; 73: 303–5.

100. Rovirosa A, Beullmunt J, Lopez A et al. The incidence of second neoplasms in advanced laryngeal cancer. Impact on survival. Med Clin (Barc) 1994; 102: 121–4.

101. Engelen AM, Stalpers LJ, Manni JJ et al. Yearly chest radiography in the early detection of lung cancer following laryngeal cancer. Eur Arch Otorhinolaryngol 1992; 249: 364–9.

102. Zeitels SM, Vaughan CW. Preepiglottic space invasion in "early" epiglottic cancer. Ann Otol Rhinol Laryngol 1991; 100: 789–92.

103. Mancuso AA. Evaluation and staging of laryngeal and hypopharyngeal cancer by computed tomography and magnetic resonance imaging. In: Silver, ed. Laryngeal Cancer. New York: Thieme, 1991.

104. Dworkin JP, Hill SL, Stachler RJ et al. Swallowing function outcomes following nonsurgical therapy for advanced-stage laryngeal carcinoma. Dysphagia 2006; 21: 66–74.

105. Munoz A, Ramos A, Ferrando J et al. Laryngeal carcinoma: sclerotic appearance of the cricoid and arytenoid cartilage – CT-pathologic correlation. Radiology 1993; 189: 433–7.

106. Nakayama M, Brandenburg JH. Clinical underestimation of laryngeal cancer. Predictive indicators. Arch Otolaryngol Head Neck Surg 1993; 119: 950–7.

107. Nguyen NP, Moltz CC, Frank C et al. Long-term aspiration following treatment for head and neck cancer. Oncology 2008; 74: 25–30.

108. Oe A, Kawabe J, Torii K et al. Detection of local residual tumor after laryngeal cancer treatment using FDG-PET. Ann Nucl Med 2007; 21: 9–13.

109. Roh JL, Pae KH, Choi SH et al. 2-[18F]-Fluoro-2-deoxy-D-glucose positron emission tomography as guidance for primary treatment in patients with advanced-stage resectable squamous cell carcinoma of the larynx and hypopharynx. Eur J Surg Oncol 2007; 33: 790–5.

110. Atabek U, Mohit-Tabatabai MA, Rush BF et al. Impact of esophageal screening in patients with head and neck cancer. Am Surg 1990; 56: 289–92.

111. Motta G, Esposito E, Testa D et al. CO2 laser treatment of supraglottic cancer. Head Neck 2004; 26: 442–6.

112. Ambrosch P, Kron M, Steiner W. Carbon dioxide laser microsurgery for early supraglottic carcinoma. Ann Otol Rhinol Laryngol 1998; 107: 680–8.

113. Vilaseca-Gonzalez I, Bernal Sprekelsen M, Blanch Alejandro JL et al. Complications in transoral CO2 laser surgery for carcinoma of the larynx and hypopharynx. Head Neck 2003; 25: 382–8.

114. Hinni ML, Salassa J, Grant DG et al. Transoral laser microsurgery for advanced laryngeal cancer. Arch Otolaryngol Head Neck Surg 2007; 133: 1198–204.

115. Preuss SF, Cramer K, Klussman JP et al. Transoral laser surgery for laryngeal cancer: Outcome, complications and prognostic factors in 275 patients. Eur J Surg Oncol 2009; 35: 235–40.

116. Grant DG, Salassa J, Hinni ML et al. Transoral laser microsurgery for carcinoma of the supraglottic larynx. Otolaryngol Head Neck Surg 2007; 136: 900–6.

117. Peretti G, Piazza C, Cattaneo A et al. Comparison of functional outcomes after endoscopic versus open-neck supraglottic laryngectomies. Ann Otol Rhinol Laryngol 2006; 115: 827–32.

118. Cabanillas R, Rodrigo JP, Llorente JL et al. Functional outcomes of transoral laser surgery of supraglottic carcinoma compared with a transcervical approach. Head Neck 2004; 26: 653–9.

119. Bernal-Sprekelsen M, Vilaseca-Gonzalez I, Blanch-Alejandro JL. Predictive values for aspiration after endoscopic laser resections of malignant tumors of the hypopharynx and larynx. Head Neck 2004; 26: 103–10.

120. Mortuaire G, Francois J, Wiel E et al. Local recurrence after CO2 laser cordectomy for early glottic carcinoma. Laryngoscope 2006; 116: 101–5.

121. Ambrosch P, Kron M, Pradier O et al. Efficacy of selective neck dissection: A review of 503 cases of elective and therapeutic treatment of the neck in squamous cell carcinoma of the upper aerodigestive tract. Otolaryngol Head Neck Surg 2001; 124: 180–7.

122. Pellini R, Manciocco V, Spriano G. Functional outcome of supracricoid partial laryngectomy with cricohyoidopexy: radiation failure vs previously untreated cases. Arch Otolaryngol Head Neck Surg 2006; 132: 1221–5.

123. Gallo A, Manciocco V, Simonelli M et al. Supracricoid partial laryngectomy in the treatment of laryngeal cancer: Univariate and multivariate analysis of prognostic factors. Arch Otolaryngol Head Neck Surg 2005; 131: 620–5.

124. Laudadio P, Presutti L, Dall'olio D et al. Supracricoid laryngectomies: long-term oncological and functional results. Acta Otolaryngol 2006; 126: 640–9.

125. Sevilla MA, Rodrigo JP, Llorente JL et al. Supraglottic laryngectomy: analysis of 267 cases. Eur Arch Otorhinolaryngol 2008; 265: 11–6.

126. Maurizi M, Paludetti G, Galli J et al. Oncological and functional outcome of conservative surgery for primary supraglottic cancer. Eur Arch Otorhinolaryngol 1999; 256: 283–90.

127. Bron LP, Soldati D, Zouhair A et al. Treatment of early stage squamous cell carcinoma of the glottic larynx: endoscopic surgery or cricohyoidoepiglottopexy versus radiotherapy. Head Neck 2001; 23: 823–9.

128. Reddy SP, Hong RL, Nagda S et al. Effect of tumor bulk on local control and survival of patients with T1 glottic cancer: a 30-year experience. Int J Radiat Oncol Biol Phys 2007; 69: 1389–94.

129. Marshak G, Brenner B, Shvero J et al. Prognostic factors for local control of early glottic cancer: The Rabin Medical Center retrospective study on 207 patients. Int J Radiat Oncol Biol Phys 1999; 43: 1009–13.

130. Cellai E, Frata P, Magrini SM et al. Radical radiotherapy for early glottic cancer: Results in a series of 1087 patients from two Italian radiation oncology centers. I. The case of T1N0 disease. Int J Radiat Oncol Biol Phys 2005; 63: 1378–86.

131. Chen MF, Chang JT, Tsang NM et al. Radiotherapy of early-stage glottic cancer: analysis of factors affecting prognosis. Ann Otol Rhinol Laryngol 2003; 112: 904–11.

132. Jin J, Liao Z, Gao L et al. Analysis of prognostic factors for T(1)N(0)M(0) glottic cancer treated with definitive radiotherapy alone: Experience of the cancer hospital of Peking Union Medical College and the Chinese Academy Of Medical Sciences. Int J Radiat Oncol Biol Phys 2002; 54: 471–8.

133. Hinerman RW, Mendenhall WM, Amdur RJ et al. Carcinoma of the supraglottic larynx: treatment results with radiotherapy alone or with planned neck dissection. Head Neck 2002; 24: 456–67.

134. Ambrosch P. The role of laser microsurgery in the treatment of laryngeal cancer. Curr Opin Otolaryngol Head Neck Surg 2007; 15: 82–8.

135. Nakfoor BM, Spiro IJ, Wang CC et al. Results of accelerated radiotherapy for supraglottic carcinoma: a Massachusetts General Hospital and Massachusetts Eye and Ear Infirmary experience. Head Neck 1998; 20: 379–84.

136. Forastiere AA, Goepfert H, Maor M et al. Concurrent chemotherapy and radiotherapy for organ preservation in advanced laryngeal cancer. New Engl J Med 2003; 349: 2091–8.

137. Induction chemotherapy plus radiation compared with surgery plus radiation in patients with advanced laryngeal cancer. The Department of Veterans Affairs Laryngeal Cancer Study Group. N Engl J Med 1991; 324: 1685–90.

138. Rieger JM, Zalmanowitz JG, Wolfaardt JF. Functional outcomes after organ preservation treatment in head and neck cancer: a critical review of the literature. Int J Oral Maxillofac Surg 2006; 35: 581–7.

139. Logemann JA, Pauloski BR, Rademaker AW et al. Swallowing disorders in the first year after radiation and chemoradiation. Head Neck 2008; 30: 148–58.

140. Nguyen NP, Moltz CC, Frank C et al. Aspiration rate following nonsurgical therapy for laryngeal cancer. ORL J Otorhinolaryngol Relat Spec 2007; 69: 116–20.

141. Staton J, Robbins KT, Newman L et al. Factors predictive of poor functional outcome after chemoradiation for advanced laryngeal cancer. Otolaryngol Head Neck Surg 2002; 127: 43–7.

142. Eisbruch A, Lyden T, Bradford CR et al. Objective assessment of swallowing dysfunction and aspiration after radiation concurrent with chemotherapy for head-and-neck cancer. Int J Radiat Oncol Biol Phys 2002; 53: 23–8.

143. Langerman A, Maccracken E, Kasza K et al. Aspiration in chemoradiated patients with head and neck cancer. Arch Otolaryngol Head Neck Surg 2007; 133: 1289–95.

144. DeSanto LW. Cancer of the supraglottic larynx: a review of 260 patients. Otolaryngol Head Neck Surg 1985; 93: 705–11.

145. Razack MS et al. Management of advanced glottic carcinomas. Am J Surg 1989; 158: 318–20.

146. Ampil FL et al. Total laryngectomy and postoperative radiotherapy for T4 laryngeal cancer: A 14-year review. Am J Otolaryngol 2004; 25: 88–93.

147. Imauchi Y et al. Stomal recurrence after total laryngectomy for squamous cell carcinoma of the larynx. Otolaryngol Head Neck Surg 2002; 126: 63–6.

148. Hintz BL et al. A "watchful waiting" policy for in situ carcinoma of the vocal cords. Arch Otolaryngol, 1981; 107: 746–51.

149. Ganly I, Patel S, Matsuo J et al. Postoperative complications of salvage total laryngectomy. Cancer 2005; 103: 2073–81.

150. Sadri M, McMahon J, Parker A. Management of laryngeal dysplasia: a review. Eur Arch Otorhinolaryngol 2006; 263: 843–52.

151. Pene F, Fletcher GH. Results in irradiation of the in situ carcinomas of the vocal cords. Cancer 1976; 37: 2586–90.

152. Le QT, Takamiya R, Shu HK et al. Treatment results of carcinoma in situ of the glottis: An analysis of 82 cases. Arch Otolaryngol Head Neck Surg 2000; 126: 1305–12.

153. Stenersen TC, Hoel PS, Boysen M. Carcinoma in situ of the larynx: an evaluation of its natural clinical course. Clin Otolaryngol Allied Sci 1991; 16: 358–63.

154. Garcia-Serra A, Hinerman RW, Amdur RJ et al. Radiotherapy for carcinoma in situ of the true vocal cords. Head Neck 2002; 24: 390–4.

155. Spayne JA, Warde P, O'Sullivan B et al. Carcinoma-in-situ of the glottic larynx: results of treatment with radiation therapy. Int J Radiat Oncol Biol Phys 2001; 49: 1235–8.

156. Peretti G, Nicolai P, Redaelli De Zinis LO et al. Endoscopic CO2 laser excision for tis, T1, and T2 glottic carcinomas: cure rate and prognostic factors. Otolaryngol Head Neck Surg 2000; 123: 124–31.

157. Pradhan SA, Pai PS, Neeli SI et al. Transoral laser surgery for early glottic cancers. Arch Otolaryngol Head Neck Surg 2003; 129: 623–5.

158. Damm M, Sittel C, Streppel M et al. Transoral CO2 laser for surgical management of glottic carcinoma in situ. Laryngoscope 2000; 110: 1215–21.

159. Sjögren EV, Langeveld TP, Baatenburg de Jong RJ. Clinical outcome of T1 glottic carcinoma since the introduction of endoscopic CO(2) laser surgery as treatment option. Head Neck 2008; 30: 1167–74.

160. Thurnher D, Erovic BM, Frommlet F et al. Challenging a dogma—surgery yields superior long-term results for T1a squamous cell carcinoma of the glottic larynx compared to radiotherapy. Eur J Surg Oncol 2008; 34: 692–8.

161. Kazi R, Venkitaraman R, Johnson C et al. Prospective, longitudinal electroglottographic study of voice recovery following accelerated hypofractionated radiotherapy for T1/T2 larynx cancer. Radiother Oncol 2008; 87: 230–6.

162. Rovirosa A, Ascaso C, Abellana R et al. Acoustic voice analysis in different phonetic contexts after larynx radiotherapy for T1 vocal cord carcinoma. Clin Transl Oncol 2008; 10: 168–74.

163. Verdonck-de Leeuw IM, Keus RB, Hilgers FJ et al. Consequences of voice impairment in daily life for patients following radiotherapy for early glottic cancer: voice quality, vocal function, and vocal performance. Int J Radiat Oncol Biol Phys 1999; 44: 1071–8.

164. Vilaseca I, Huerta P, Blanch JL et al. Voice quality after CO2 laser cordectomy—what can we really expect? Head Neck 2008; 30: 43–49.

165. Ledda GP, Grover N, Pundir V et al. Functional outcomes after CO2 laser treatment of early glottic carcinoma. Laryngoscope 2006; 116: 1007–11.

166. Knott PD, Milstein CF, Hicks DM et al. Vocal outcomes after laser resection of early-stage glottic cancer with adjuvant cryotherapy. Arch Otolaryngol Head Neck Surg 2006; 132: 1226–30.

167. Remacle M Eckel HE, Antonelli A et al. Endoscopic cordectomy. A proposal for a classification by the Working Committee, European Laryngological Society. Eur Arch Otorhinolaryngol 2000; 257: 227–31.

168. Policarpo M, Aluffi P, Brovelli F et al. Oncological and functional results of CO2 laser cordectomy. Acta Otorhinolaryngol Ital 2004; 24: 267–74.

169. Krengli M, Policarpo M, Manfredda I et al. Voice quality after treatment for T1a glottic carcinoma—radiotherapy versus laser cordectomy. Acta Oncol 2004; 43: 284–9.

170. Rydell R, Schalén L, Fex S et al. Voice evaluation before and after laser excision vs. radiotherapy of T1A glottic carcinoma. Acta Otolaryngol 1995; 115: 560–5.

171. Nunez Batalla F, Caminero Cueva MJ, Senaris-Gonzales B et al. Voice quality after endoscopic laser surgery and radiotherapy for early glottic cancer: objective measurements emphasizing the voice handicap index. Eur Arch Otorhinolaryngol 2008; 265: 543–8.

172. Peeters AJ, van Gogh CD, Goor KM et al. Health status and voice outcome after treatment for T1a glottic carcinoma. Eur Arch Otorhinolaryngol 2004; 261: 534–40.

173. Cohen SM, Garrett CG, Dupont WD et al. Voice-related quality of life in T1 glottic cancer: irradiation versus endoscopic excision. Ann Otol Rhinol Laryngol 2006; 115: 581–6.

174. Wedman J, Heimdal JH, Elstad I et al. Voice results in patients with T1a glottic cancer treated by radiotherapy or endoscopic measures. Eur Arch Otorhinolaryngol 2002; 259: 547–50.

175. Loughran S, Calder N, MacGregor FB et al. Quality of life and voice following endoscopic resection or radiotherapy for early glottic cancer. Clin Otolaryngol 2005; 30: 42–7.

176. McGuirt WF, Blalock D, Koufman JA et al. Comparative voice results after laser resection or irradiation of T1 vocal cord carcinoma. Arch Otolaryngol Head Neck Surg 1994; 120: 951–5.

177. Delsupehe KG, Zink I, Lejaegere M et al. Voice quality after narrow-margin laser cordectomy compared with laryngeal irradiation. Otolaryngol Head Neck Surg 1999; 121: 528–33.

178. Tamura E, Kitahara S, Ogura M et al. Voice quality after laser surgery or radiotherapy for T1a glottic carcinoma. Laryngoscope 2003; 113: 910–4.

179. Ansarin M, Zabrodsky M, Bianchi L et al. Endoscopic CO2 laser surgery for early glottic cancer in patients who are candidates for radiotherapy: results of a prospective nonrandomized study. Head Neck 2006; 28: 121–5.

180. Goor KM, Peeters AJ, Mahieu HF et al. Cordectomy by CO2 laser or radiotherapy for small T1a glottic carcinomas: costs, local control, survival, quality of life, and voice quality. Head Neck 2007; 29: 128–36.

181. Mendenhall WM, Amdur RJ, Morris CG et al. T1-T2N0 squamous cell carcinoma of the glottic larynx treated with radiation therapy. J Clin Oncol 2001; 19: 4029–36.

182. Pellitteri PK, Kennedy TL, Vrabec DP et al. Radiotherapy. The mainstay in the treatment of early glottic carcinoma. Arch Otolaryngol Head Neck Surg 1991; 117: 297–301.

183. Small Jr W, Mittal BB, Brand WN et al. Results of radiation therapy in early glottic carcinoma: multivariate analysis of prognostic and radiation therapy variables. Radiology 1992; 183: 789–94.

184. Spector JG, Sessions DG, Chao KS et al. Stage I (T1 N0 M0) squamous cell carcinoma of the laryngeal glottis: therapeutic results and voice preservation. Head Neck 1999; 21: 707–17.

185. Jorgensen K, Godballe C, Hansen O et al. Cancer of the larynx—treatment results after primary radiotherapy with salvage surgery in a series of 1005 patients. Acta Oncol 2002; 41: 69–76.

186. Dagan R, Morris CG, Bennett JA et al. Prognostic significance of paraglottic space invasion in T2N0 glottic carcinoma. Am J Clin Oncol 2007; 30: 186–90.

187. Howell-Burke D, Peters LJ, Goepfert H et al. T2 glottic cancer. Recurrence, salvage, and survival after definitive radiotherapy. Arch Otolaryngol Head Neck Surg 1990; 116: 830–5.

188. Frata P, Cellai E, Magrini SM et al. Radical radiotherapy for early glottic cancer: results in a series of 1087 patients from two Italian radiation oncology centers. II. The case of T2N0 disease. Int J Radiat Oncol Biol Phys 2005; 63: 1387–94.

189. Mendenhall WM, Parsons JT, Mancuso AA et al. Definitive radiotherapy for T3 squamous cell carcinoma of the glottic larynx. J Clin Oncol 1997; 15: 2394–402.

190. Kowalski LP, Batista MB, Santos CR et al. Prognostic factors in T3, N0-1 glottic and transglottic carcinoma. A multifactorial study of 221 cases treated by surgery or radiotherapy. Arch Otolaryngol Head Neck Surg 1996; 122: 77–82.

191. Hartl DM, de Monès E, Hans S et al. Treatment of early-stage glottic cancer by transoral laser resection. Ann Otol Rhinol Laryngol 2007; 116: 832–6.

192. Ledda GP, Puxeddu R. Carbon dioxide laser microsurgery for early glottic carcinoma. Otolaryngol Head Neck Surg 2006; 134: 911–5.

193. Bocciolini C, Presutti L, Laudadio P. Oncological outcome after CO2 laser cordectomy for early-stage glottic carcinoma. Acta Otorhinolaryngol Ital 2005; 25: 86–93.

194. Gallo A, de Vincentiis M, Manciocco V et al. CO2 laser cordectomy for early-stage glottic carcinoma: A long-term follow-up of 156 cases. Laryngoscope, 2002; 112: 370–4.

195. Moreau P. Treatment of laryngeal carcinomas by laser endoscopic microsurgery. Laryngoscope 2000; 110: 1000–6.

196. Crespo AN, Chone CT, Gripp FM et al. Role of margin status in recurrence after CO2 laser endoscopic resection of early glottic cancer. Acta Otolaryngol 2006; 126: 306–10.

197. Chone CT, Yonehara E, Martins JE et al. Importance of anterior commissure in recurrence of early glottic cancer after laser endoscopic resection. Arch Otolaryngol Head Neck Surg 2007; 133: 882–7.

198. Barbosa MM, Araujo VJ Jr, Boasquevisque E et al. Anterior vocal commissure invasion in laryngeal carcinoma diagnosis. Laryngoscope 2005; 115: 724–30.

199. Eryilmaz A, Akmansu H, Topcu E et al. The role of 70-degree telescopic examination during direct laryngoscopic evaluation of laryngeal cancers. Eur Arch Otorhinolaryngol 2004; 261: 267–9.

200. Steiner W, Ambrosch P, Rodel RM et al. Impact of anterior commissure involvement on local control of early glottic carcinoma treated by laser microresection. Laryngoscope 2004; 114: 1485–91.

201. Laccourreye O, Laccourreye L, Garcia D et al. Vertical partial laryngectomy versus supracricoid partial laryngectomy for selected carcinomas of the true vocal cord classified as T2N0. Ann Otol Rhinol Laryngol 2000; 109: 965–71.

202. Laccourreye O, Muscattello L, Laccourreye L et al. Supracricoid partial laryngectomy with cricohyoidoepiglottopexy for "early" glottic carcinoma classified as T1-T2N0 invading the anterior commissure. Am J Otolaryngol 1997; 18: 385–90.

203. Motta G, Esposito E, Motta S et al. CO(2) laser surgery in the treatment of glottic cancer. Head Neck 2005; 27: 566–73, discussion 573–4.

204. Jäckel MC, Ambrosch P, Martin A et al. Impact of re-resection for inadequate margins on the prognosis of upper aerodigestive tract cancer treated by laser microsurgery. Laryngoscope 2007; 117: 350–6.

205. Robbins KT, Davidson W, Peters LJ et al. Conservation surgery for T2 and T3 carcinomas of the supraglottic larynx. Arch Otolaryngol Head Neck Surg 1988; 114: 421–6.

206. Orus C, Leon X, Vega M et al. Initial treatment of the early stages (I, II) of supraglottic squamous cell carcinoma: partial laryngectomy versus radiotherapy. Eur Arch Otorhinolaryngol 2000; 257: 512–6.

207. Bron LP, Soldati D, Monod ML et al. Horizontal partial laryngectomy for supraglottic squamous cell carcinoma. Eur Arch Otorhinolaryngol 2005; 262: 302–6.

208. Suarez C, Rodrigo JP, Herranz J et al. Supraglottic laryngectomy with or without postoperative radiotherapy in supraglottic carcinomas. Ann Otol Rhinol Laryngol 1995; 104: 358–63.

209. Cabanillas R, Rodrigo JP, Llorente JL et al. Oncologic outcomes of transoral laser surgery of supraglottic carcinoma compared with a transcervical approach. Head Neck 2008; 30: 750–5.

210. Iro H, Waldfahrer F, Altendorf-Hofman A et al. Transoral laser surgery of supraglottic cancer: follow-up of 141 patients. Arch Otolaryngol Head Neck Surg 1998; 124: 1245–50.

211. Davis RK, Kristokovich MD, Galloway EB et al. Endoscopic supraglottic laryngectomy with postoperative irradiation. Ann Otol Rhinol Laryngol 2004; 113: 132–8.

212. Esposito E, Motta S, Motta G. Exclusive surgery versus postoperative radiotherapy for supraglottic cancer. ORL J Otorhinolaryngol Relat Spec 2002; 64: 213–8.

213. Mendenhall WM, Parsons JT, Mancuso AA et al. Radiotherapy for squamous cell carcinoma of the supraglottic larynx: An alternative to surgery. Head Neck 1996; 18: 24–35.

214. Weems DH, Mendenhall WM, Parsons JT et al. Squamous cell carcinoma of the supraglottic larynx treated with surgery and/or radiation therapy. Int J Radiat Oncol Biol Phys 1987; 13: 1483–7.

215. Harwood AR, Beale FA, Cummings BJ et al. Supraglottic laryngeal carcinoma: an analysis of dose-time-volume factors in 410 patients. Int J Radiat Oncol Biol Phys 1983; 9: 311–9.

216. Eckel H. Endoscopic laser resection of supraglottic carcinoma. Otolaryngol Head Neck Surg 1997; 117: 681–7.

217. Ganly I, Patel S, Matsuo J et al. Results of surgical salvage after failure of definitive radiation therapy for early-stage squamous cell carcinoma of the glottic larynx. Arch Otolaryngol Head Neck Surg 2006; 132: 59–66.

218. Biller HF, Lawson W. Partial laryngectomy for vocal cord cancer with marked limitation or fixation of the vocal cord. Laryngoscope 1986; 96: 61.

219. Kessler DJ, Trapp TK, Calcaterra TC. The treatment of T3 glottic carcinoma with vertical partial laryngectomy. Arch Otolaryngol Head Neck Surg 1987; 113: 1196.

220. Mendenhall WM, Million RR, Sharkey DE et al. Stage T3 squamous cell carcinoma of the glottic larynx treated with surgery and/or radiation therapy. Int J Radiat Oncol Biol Phys 1984; 10: 357.

221. Laccourreye O, Salzer SJ, Brasnu D et al. Glottic carcinoma with a fixed true vocal cord: outcome after neoadjuvant chemotherapy and supracricoid partial laryngectomy with cricohyoidoepiglottopexy. Otolaryngol Head Neck Surg 1996; 114: 400.

222. Burstein FD, Calcaterra TC. Supraglottic laryngectomy: Series report and analysis of results. Laryngoscope 1985; 95: 833.

223. Coate HL, DeSanto LW, Devine KD et al. Carcinoma of the supraglottic larynx. A review of 221 cases. Arch Otolaryngol 1976; 102: 686.

224. Lee NK, Goepfert H, Wendt CD. Supraglottic laryngectomy for immediate stage cancer: UT MD Anderson Cancer Center experience with combined therapy. Laryngoscope 1990; 100: 831.

225. Som ML. Conservation surgery for carcinoma of the supraglottis. London: University of London, 1969.

226. Spaulding CA, Constable WC, Levine PA et al. Partial laryngectomy and radiotherapy for supraglottic cancer: a conservative approach. Ann Otol Rhinol Laryngol 1988; 98: 125.

227. Laccourreye H, Laccourreye O, Weinstein G et al. Supracricoid laryngectomy with cricohyoidopexy: a partial laryngeal procedure for selected supraglottic and transglottic carcinomas. Laryngoscope 1990; 100: 735.

228. Chevalier D, Piquet JJ. Subtotal laryngectomy with cricohyoidopexy for supraglottic carcinoma: Review of 61 cases. Am J Surg 1994; 168: 472.

229. Laccourreye O, Brasnu D, Merite-Drancy A et al. Cricohyoidopexy in selected infrahyoid epiglottic carcinomas presenting with pathological preepiglottic space invasion. Arch Otolaryngol Head Neck Surg 1993; 119: 881.

230. Lewin JS, Hutcheson KA, Barringer DA et al. Functional analysis of swallowing outcomes after supracricoid partial laryngectomy. Head Neck 2008; 30: 559–66.

231. Pellini R, Pichi B, Ruscito P et al. Supracricoid partial laryngectomies after radiation failure: a multi-institutional series. Head Neck 2008; 30: 372–9.

232. Ambrosch P, Rodel R, Kron M et al. Transoral laser microsurgery for cancer of the larynx. A retrospective analysis of 657 patients. Onkologie 2001; **7**: 505–12.

233. Ogura JH, Sessions DG, Spector GJ. Analysis of surgical therapy for epidermoid carcinoma of the laryngeal glottis. Laryngoscope 1975; 85: 1522–30.

234. Leroux-Robert JL. A statistical study of 620 laryngeal carcinomas of the glottic region personally operated upon more than 5 years ago Laryngoscope 1975; 85: 1440–66.

235. De Santo LW. T3 glottic cancer. Options and consequences of the options. Laryngoscope 1984; 94: 1311–15.

236. Goepfert H, Jesse RH, Fletcher GH et al. Optimal treatment for technically resectable squamous cell carcinoma of the supraglottic larynx. Laryngoscope 1975; 85: 14–32.

237. Dufour X, Hans S, De Mones E et al. Local control after supracricoid partial laryngectomy for "advanced" endolaryngeal squamous cell carcinoma classified as T3. Arch Otolaryngol Head Neck Surg 2004; 130: 1092–99.

238. Lima RA, Freitas EQ, Dias FL et al. Supracricoid laryngectomy with cricohyoidoepiglottopexy for advanced glottic cancer. Head Neck 2006; 28: 481–6.

239. Rinaldo A, Ferlito A. Open supraglottic laryngectomy. Acta Otolaryngol 2004; 124: 768–71.

240. Brasnu D. Supracricoid partial laryngectomy with cricohyoidopexy in the management of laryngeal carcinoma. World J Surg 2003; 27: 817–23.

241. Ampil FL, Nathan CO, Lian TS et al. Total laryngectomy and T3-T4 laryngeal cancer without other adverse histopathology. Otolaryngol Head Neck Surg 2007; 136: 296–300.

242. Plaat RE, de Bree R, Kuik DJ et al. Prognostic importance of paratracheal lymph node metastases. Laryngoscope 2005; 115: 894–8.

243. Chiesa F, Tradati N, Calabrese L et al. Surgical treatment of laryngeal carcinoma with subglottis involvement. Oncol Rep 2001; 8: 137–40.

244. Richard JM, Sancho-Garnier H, Pessey JJ et al. Randomized trial of induction chemotherapy in larynx carcinoma. Oral Oncol 1998; 34: 224–8.

245. Urba S, Wolf G, Eisbruch A et al. Single-cycle induction chemotherapy selects patients with advanced laryngeal cancer for combined chemoradiation: a new treatment paradigm. J Clin Oncol 2006; 24: 593–8.

246. Majem M, Mesia R, Mañós M et al. Does induction chemotherapy still have a role in larynx preservation strategies? The experience of Institut Catala d'Oncologia in stage III larynx carcinoma. Laryngoscope 2006; 116: 1651–6.

247. Altundag O, Gallu I, Altundag K et al. Induction chemotherapy with cisplatin and 5-fluorouracil followed by chemoradiotherapy or radiotherapy alone in the treatment of locoregionally advanced resectable cancers of the larynx and hypopharynx: results of single-center study of 45 patients. Head Neck 2005; 27: 15–21.

248. Meleca RJ, Dworkin JP, Kewson DT et al. Functional outcomes following nonsurgical treatment for advanced-stage laryngeal carcinoma. Laryngoscope 2003; 113: 720–8.

249. Fung K, Lyden TH, Lee J et al. Voice and swallowing outcomes of an organ-preservation trial for advanced laryngeal cancer. Int J Radiat Oncol Biol Phys 2005; 63: 1395–9.

250. Kazi R, Venkitaraman R, Johnson C et al. Electroglottographic comparison of voice outcomes in patients with advanced laryngopharyngeal cancer treated by chemoradiotherapy or total laryngectomy. Int J Radiat Oncol Biol Phys 2008; 70: 344–52.

251. Hanna E, Sherman A, Cash D et al. Quality of life for patients following total laryngectomy vs chemoradiation for laryngeal preservation. Arch Otolaryngol Head Neck Surg 2004; 130: 875–9.

252. Boscolo-Rizzo P, Maronato F, Marchiori C et al. Long-term quality of life after total laryngectomy and postoperative radiotherapy versus concurrent chemoradiotherapy for laryngeal preservation. Laryngoscope 2008; 118: 300–6.

253. Bonner JA, Harari PM, Giralt J et al. Radiotherapy plus cetuximab for squamous-cell carcinoma of the head and neck. N Engl J Med 2006; 354: 567–78.

254. Dahm JD, Sessions DG, Paniello RC et al. Primary subglottic cancer. Laryngoscope 1998; 108: 741–6.

255. Santoro R, Turelli M, Polli G. Primary carcinoma of the subglottic larynx. Eur Arch Otorhinolaryngol 2000; 257: 548–51.

256. Sessions DG, Ogura JH, Fried MP. Carcinoma of the subglottic area. Laryngoscope 1975; 85: 1417–23.

257. Garas J, McGuirt WF Sr. Squamous cell carcinoma of the subglottis. Am J Otolaryngol 2006; 27: 1–4.

258. Paisley S, Warde PR, O'Sullivan B et al. Results of radiotherapy for primary subglottic squamous cell carcinoma. Int J Radiat Oncol Biol Phys 2002; 52: 1245–50.

259. Zbaren P, Nuyens M, Curshmann J et al. Histologic characteristics and tumor spread of recurrent glottic carcinoma: analysis on whole-organ sections and comparison with tumor spread of primary glottic carcinomas. Head Neck 2007; 29: 26–32.

260. Zbaren P, Caversaccio M, Thoeny HC et al. Radionecrosis or tumor recurrence after radiation of laryngeal and hypopharyngeal carcinomas. Otolaryngol Head Neck Surg 2006; 135: 838–43.

261. Zbaren P, Christe A, Caversaccio MD et al. Pretherapeutic staging of recurrent laryngeal carcinoma: clinical findings and imaging studies compared with histopathology. Otolaryngol Head Neck Surg 2007; 137: 487–91.

262. Piazza C, Peretti G, Cattaneo A et al. Salvage surgery after radiotherapy for laryngeal cancer. From endoscopic resections to open-neck partial and total laryngectomies. Arch Otolaryngol Head Neck Surg 2007; 133: 1037–43.

263. Steiner W, Vogt P, Ambrosch P et al. Transoral carbon dioxide laser microsurgery for recurrent glottic carcinoma after radiotherapy. Head Neck 2004; 26: 477–84.

264. Holsinger FC, Funk E, Roberts DB et al. Conservation laryngeal surgery versus total laryngectomy for radiation failure in laryngeal cancer. Head Neck 2006; 28: 779–84.

265. Ansarin M, Planicka M, Rotundo S et al. Endoscopic carbon dioxide laser surgery for glottic cancer recurrence after radiotherapy: oncological results. Arch Otolaryngol Head Neck Surg 2007; 133: 1193–7.

266. Puxeddu R, Piazza C, Mensi MC et al. Carbon dioxide laser salvage surgery after radiotherapy failure in T1 and T2 glottic carcinoma. Otolaryngol Head Neck Surg 2004; 130: 84–8.

267. Casiano RR, Cooper JD, Lundy DS et al. Laser cordectomy for T1 glottic carcinoma: a 10-year experience and videostroboscopic findings. Otolaryngol Head Neck Surg 1991; 104: 831–7.

268. de Gier HH, Knegt PP, de Boer MF et al. CO2-laser treatment of recurrent glottic carcinoma. Head Neck 2001; 23: 177–80.

269. Galli J, De Corso E, Volante M et al. Postlaryngectomy pharyngocutaneous fistula: Incidence, predisposing factors, and therapy. Otolaryngol Head Neck Surg 2005; 133: 689–94.

270. Amatsu M, Makino K, Kinishi M. Stomal recurrence—etiologic factors and prevention. Auris Nasus Larynx 1985; 12: 103–10.

271. Zbaren P, Greiner R, Kengelbacher M. Stoma recurrence after laryngectomy: an analysis of risk factors. Otolaryngol Head Neck Surg 1996; 114: 569–75.

272. Leon X, Quer M, Burgues J et al. Prevention of stomal recurrence. Head Neck 1996; 18: 54–9.

273. Petrovic Z, Djordjevic V. Stomal recurrence after primary total laryngectomy. Clin Otolaryngol Allied Sci 2004; 29: 270–3.

274. Sulman EP, Schwartz DL, Le TT et al. IMRT reirradiation of head and neck cancer- disease control and morbidity outcomes. Int J Radiat Oncol Biol Phys 2009; 73: 399–409.

275. Goldstein DP, Karnell LH, Yao M et al. Outcomes following reirradiation of patients with head and neck cancer. Head Neck 2008; 30: 765–70.

276. Langer CJ, Harris J, Horwitz EM et al. Phase II study of low-dose paclitaxel and cisplatin in combination with split-course concomitant twice-daily reirradiation in recurrent squamous cell carcinoma of the head and neck: Results of Radiation Therapy Oncology Group Protocol 9911. J Clin Oncol 2007; 25: 4800–5.

277. Spencer SA, Harris J, Wheeler RH et al. Final report of RTOG 9610, a multi-institutional trial of reirradiation and chemotherapy for unresectable recurrent squamous cell carcinoma of the head and neck. Head Neck 2008; 30: 281–8.

278. Cohn AB, Lang PO, Agarwal JP et al. Free-flap reconstruction in the doubly irradiated patient population. Plast Reconstr Surg 2008; 122: 125–32.

279. Laccourreye O, Veivers D, Hans S et al. Chemotherapy alone with curative intent in patients with invasive squamous cell carcinoma of the pharyngolarynx classified as T1–T4N0M0 complete clinical responders. Cancer 2001; 92: 1504–11.

280. Bonfils P, Trotoux J, Bassot V. Chemotherapy alone in laryngeal squamous cell carcinoma. J Laryngol Otol 2007; 121: 143–8.

281. Truelson JM, Fisher SG, Beals TE et al. DNA content and histologic growth pattern correlate with prognosis in patients with advanced squamous carcinoma of the larynx. Department of Veterans Affairs Cooperative Laryngeal Cancer Study Group. Cancer 1992; 70: 56–62.

282. Corvo R, Giaretti W, Sanguineti G et al. In vivo cell kinetics in head and neck squamous cell carcinomas predicts local control and helps guide radiotherapy regimen. J Clin Oncol 1995; 13: 1843–50.

283. Fu KK, Hammond E, Pajak TF et al. Flow cytometric quantification of the proliferation-associated nuclear antigen p105 and DNA content in advanced head and neck cancer: results of RTOG 91-08. Int J Radiat Oncol Biol Phys 1994; 29: 661–71.

284. Robbins KT, Connors KM, Storniolo AM. Sponge-gel-supported histoculture drug-response assay for head and neck cancer: correlations with clinical response to cisplatin. Arch Otolaryngol Head Neck Surg 1994; 120: 288–92.

285. Ganly I, Talbot S, Carlson D et al. Identification of angiogenesis/metastases genes predicting chemoradiotherapy response in patients with laryngopharyngeal carcinoma. J Clin Oncol 2007; 25: 1369–76.

286. Roth JA, Nguyen D, Lawrence DD et al. Retrovirus-mediated wild-type p53 gene transfer to tumors of patients with lung cancer. Nature Med 1996; 2: 985–91.

15

Management of the Neck

Ian Ganly, Hin Ngan Tay, Snehal G Patel, Ashok Shaha and Jatin P Shah

INTRODUCTION

The prognostic significance of cervical lymph node status in squamous cell carcinoma (SCC) of the upper aerodigestive tract is well recognized. Metastases to regional lymph nodes reduce 5-year survival rates to nearly one-half that of patients with disease confined to the primary site (1). Appropriate management of the neck is therefore critical in planning treatment for patients with SCC of the upper aerodigestive tract.

The management of metastases to regional cervical lymph nodes outlined in this chapter includes an overview of the relevant anatomy of the neck, a brief discussion of the biological mechanisms of lymphatic metastases, diagnostic evaluation, disease staging, and treatment principles. The major focus of this discussion will be on lymphatic metastases from SCC, but a brief mention will be made regarding other malignancies of the head and neck, such as those of the salivary glands or thyroid, and cutaneous melanoma.

THE ANATOMY AND BIOLOGY OF CERVICAL LYMPHATIC METASTASES

It has been estimated that about 300 of the 800 lymph nodes in the human body are located in the head and neck region. To standardize reporting and facilitate communication, the American Head and Neck Society (AHNS), in co-operation with the Committee for Head and Neck Surgery and Oncology of the American Academy of Otolaryngology-Head and Neck Surgery has made recommendations for classification of lymph node anatomy and neck dissections (2). Cervical lymph nodes are categorized into five nodal levels, and additionally levels VI and VII encompassing central compartment and superior mediastinal nodes, as illustrated in Figures 15.1 and 15.2. Levels I, II, and V are further subdivided into sublevels A and B. Table 15.1 lists the clinical and surgical landmarks used to describe these levels. This classification system is constantly being reevaluated and updated, with the current update in 2008 (3).

Other cervical lymph node groups relevant to patterns of nodal metastasis but lacking a standardized nodal level classification include lymph nodes of the retropharyngeal, facial, intraparotid, preauricular, postauricular, and suboccipital regions.

The Biology of Lymphatic Metastasis

Despite the continuing advances in our knowledge regarding the molecular mechanisms involved in primary carcinogenesis, many questions persist as to how malignant cells metastasize to regional lymphatics. The frustration in our inability to delineate fully these molecular events is further compounded when considering the prognostic significance of nodal metastases in head and neck squamous cell carcinoma (HNSCC).

Molecular Events in Carcinogenesis and Nodal Metastasis

The development of malignant tumors at the primary site appears to be the result of multiple accumulated genetic alterations (4). These genetic mutations must occur in the correct number and sequence for cancer to develop, a progression of genetic events first described by Fearon and Vogelstein for colorectal tumorigenesis (5). A genetic progression model for head and neck cancer has been established demonstrating the multiple steps involved in the expansion and migration of clonally related preneoplastic cells (6).

Once a primary malignancy progresses from carcinoma in situ to a microinvasive carcinoma to an invasive carcinoma extending into the surrounding stroma, the probability increases for metastasis to regional lymphatics. The primary processes involved in the complex cascade of invasion include changes in adhesion between cells, proteolytic degradation of the extracellular matrix, cellular migration, and angiogenesis (7–9). This cascade has yet to be completely characterized, but our present understanding is summarized by the following molecular events: cell–cell adhesion between tumor cells decreases as adhesion between tumor cells and the extracellular matrix increases (Fig. 15.3). Matrix metalloproteases (MMPs) provide enzymatic degradation of the basement membrane, giving way to cellular motility and migration, further assisted by neovascularization. Endothelial cell ligands continue this cascade, facilitating the passage of tumor cells to and from the circulation. This cascade highlights the complex interaction between the lymphatic and hematogenous patterns of circulation, underscoring the importance of considering the two systems as interrelated, and not distinct entities, in the mechanism of metastasis.

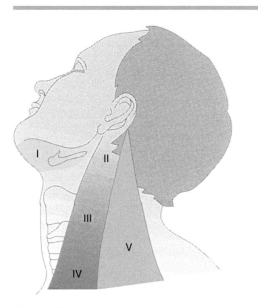

Figure 15.1   Lateral view of the neck to demonstrate the boundaries of lymph node levels I–V.

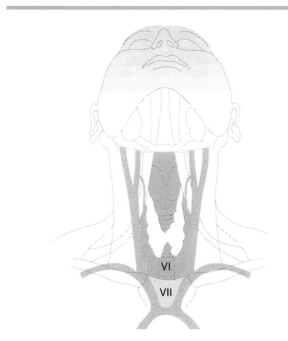

Figure 15.2   Regional lymph node levels of the anterior neck and superior mediastinum.

Patterns of Cervical Lymphatic Flow

Prior to the understanding of these molecular processes, Ugo Fisch used contrast cervical lymphography to characterize the pathways of circulation through the lymphatics in the neck (10). It was noted that following retroauricular injection of contrast, the cervical lymphatic network filled in an orderly sequence. Lymph nodes in the region

Table 15.1   Clinical and Surgical Landmarks for Description of Node Levels

Node level	Clinical landmarks	Surgical landmarks
Level I	Submental and submandibular triangles	Lower border of the body of the mandible superiorly, posterior belly of the diagastric muscle posteriorly, and hyoid bone inferiorly
Level II	Upper jugular lymph nodes	Base of skull superiorly, posterior belly of diagastric muscle anteriorly, posterior border of the sternocleidomastoid muscle posteriorly, and hyoid bone inferiorly
Level III	Middle jugular lymph nodes	Hyoid bone superiorly, lateral limit of the sternohyoid muscle anteriorly, the posterior border of sternocleidomastoid muscle posteriorly, and cricothyroid membrane inferiorly
Level IV	Lower jugular lymph nodes	Cricothyroid membrane superiorly, lateral limit of the sternohyoid muscle anteriorly, posterior border of the sternocleidomastoid muscle posteriorly, and clavicle inferiorly
Level V	Posterior triangle lymph nodes	Posterior border of sternocleidomastoid muscle anteriorly, anterior border of the trapezius muscle posteriorly, and clavicle inferiorly
Level VI	Anterior compartment of the neck	Hyoid bone superiorly, suprasternal notch inferiorly, and medial border of the carotid sheath on either side of the neck laterally
Level VII	Superior mediastinal lymph nodes	Suprasternal notch superiorly

of the upper lateral neck termed the "junctional area" by Fisch filled with contrast first. Direct connections from the "junctional area" then filled separately to the jugular nodes, to the supraclavicular nodes, and to the nodes along the spinal accessory nerve (SAN) in the lower posterior triangle. Radiation therapy with conventional X-rays and with cobalt-60 was found to markedly decrease the caliber and number of lymph vessels, as well as the size and the number of cervical lymph nodes. These postradiation changes resulted in disturbance in the normal filling of the cervical lymphatic system, with the main route of lymph flow directed toward the jugular chain. Following radical neck dissection (RND), Fisch noted that collateral lymphatic circulation developed through one of two mechanisms. Collateral circulation developed either by submental diversion through preexisting lymphatic channels (following unilateral neck dissection), or by retrograde flow to the subcutaneous and dermal lymphatic network of the neck (following bilateral neck dissection or unilateral neck dissection with postoperative radiation therapy [PORT]).

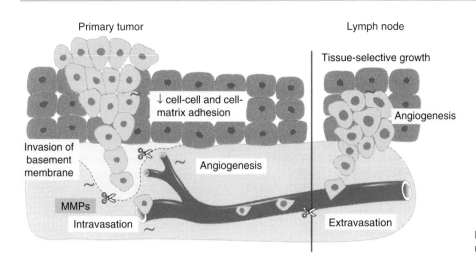

Figure 15.3 Cascade of events leading up to lymphatic metastases.

Immunological Aspects of Nodal Metastasis and Lymphadenectomy

A subject not often broached in the literature of managing cervical nodal metastases concerns the immunological implications involved in nodal metastasis and in lymph node removal. Previous studies have shown a hierarchical immunomodulatory relationship between the primary tumor and its draining lymphatics in HNSCC (11,12). These studies demonstrate that natural killer cell activity of lymph nodes positive for metastatic HNSCC was significantly diminished compared to uninvolved lymph nodes, and that interleukin-2 (IL-2)-activated cytotoxicity of lymph nodes closer to the primary tumor was depressed compared to lymph nodes further away from the primary site. These studies suggest that an immunosuppressive effect of the primary tumor on lymph nodes in close proximity to it and has been attributed to a change in the cytokine milieu. IL-10 produced by T-helper (Th2) cells suppress IL-12 and 18 mediated T helper 1 (Th1) antitumor activity (13). Inhibition of host immune responses in this manner has been proposed to play a role in perpetuating the spread of metastatic foci throughout cervical lymphatics.

The clinical significance of the immunity of regional lymphatics in HNSCC has been debated. In a double-blinded retrospective study, Berlinger et al. determined that an absence of histological signs of lymph node immunologic activity on light microscopy negatively affected 5-year survival rates in patients with SCC of the larynx, pharynx, and oral cavity (14). Gilmore and his colleagues however concluded in a double-blinded retrospective analysis of RND specimens that immunologic activity in lymph nodes by light microscopy did not correlate with survival outcome in patients with SCC of the larynx (15). A criticism applicable to both these reports is that neither study controlled for preoperative radiotherapy, which is known to affect cervical lymphatic drainage. Studying patients with oral cavity SCC undergoing elective neck dissection (END), Cernea et al. found that certain lymph node reactivity patterns on light microscopy (e.g., sinus histiocytosis) were more likely to predict local, regional, or distant recurrence than others (e.g., presence of germinal centers) in patients with N0 necks (16).

In light of the immunosuppressive mechanisms involved in HNSCC metastatic to cervical lymph nodes, attempts have been made to stimulate lymphokine-activated killer cells using regional injection of recombinant IL-2 (17). Although augmented cytotoxic effects of natural killer cells have been observed in vivo, immunotherapy remains an experimental modality requiring further study in the treatment of HNSCC.

Another immunological question relevant to nodal metastases from HNSCC concerns the effect of neck dissection on host immunity. Using skin homografts in immunocompetent cancer patients, Griffiths found that removal of regional lymph nodes in the head and neck, axilla, and groin did not significantly alter host immunity (18). Collateral lymphatic circulation was reestablished, and the remaining immune cells were observed to compensate for those lymph nodes that had been removed. Thus, regional lymphadenectomy did not inhibit local host response against homografts in this study.

Patterns of Cervical Lymphatic Metastasis

Characteristics of the primary tumor influencing nodal metastasis. Various characteristics of the primary tumor may influence the frequency of cervical nodal metastases. Such characteristics include site of origin, size, T stage, location, and histomorphologic presentation. As illustrated in Table 15.2, certain primary sites have an increased predilection to metastasize to cervical lymph nodes. For example, in the oral cavity, cancers of the floor of mouth and tongue are more likely to present with regional lymph node metastases than those arising from the hard palate. Increasing size or advanced T stage of the primary tumor also increases the risk for nodal metastases. The anatomic location of the primary tumor is also important. As a general rule, the risk for lymph node metastasis increases for tumors located more posteriorly, for example, oropharyngeal cancers are at higher risk than most oral cavity tumors. Similarly, within the laryngopharynx, the risk for nodal metastases increases centrifugally: glottic primaries are at lowest risk, whereas pyriform fossa and other

Table 15.2 The Incidence of Cervical Lymph Node Metastasis by Site of the Primary Tumor in Previously Untreated Patients. (Percentages are Approximate and are Based on a Review of the Literature)

Site	Clinically abnormal nodes at presentation (%)	Incidence of occult nodal metastases (%)	Regional failure with observation of the neck (%)
Oral cavity			
Oral tongue	35–55	25–30	25–35
Floor of mouth	25–35	15–25	20–30
Gum and hard palate	15–25	5–15	10–15
Buccal mucosa	15–25	10–20	10–15
Oropharynx			
Tonsillar fossa	40–50	45–55	?*
Base of the tongue	40–50	40–50	?*
Soft palate	25–30	30–35	35–40*
Pharyngeal wall	35–45	35–45	?*
Nasopharynx	60–70	?†	?*
Hypopharynx	60–70	65–70	?*
Larynx			
Supraglottic	35–45	25–35	25–30
Glottic	<5	<5	<5
Major salivary glands	15–20	5–10	10–15
Differentiated thyroid carcinoma	35–40	60–65	20–25

*Percentages not known or unreliable as most patients receive radiation therapy to the neck during initial treatment.
†Percentages not known as initial treatment is largely non-surgical.

Table 15.3 Distribution of Cervical Lymph Node Metastases from Squamous Cell Carcinoma of the Upper Aerodigestive Tract in N0 Patients (24)

Lymph node level	Oral cavity (%)	Oropharynx (%)	Hypopharynx (%)	Larynx (%)
I	58	7	0	14
II	51	80	75	52
III	26	60	75	55
IV	9	27	0	24
V	2	7	0	7

These patterns of cervical lymph node metastasis described above are not exclusive of other nodal levels but rather predict those first echelon nodes at highest risk for initial involvement, based on the location of the primary tumor in the head and neck. As illustrated in Table 15.3, tumors arising in the oral cavity are more likely to present with nodal metastases at levels I, II, and III. Initial involvement of level IV is much less common, and metastases at level V on presentation are even more infrequent. A topic of ongoing debate in the literature however concerns the concept of "skip metastases," or metastases to inferior cervical nodes at levels III or IV in the absence of demonstrable involvement at levels I and II (24). However, the likelihood of failure at level IV following supraomohyoid neck dissection (SOHND) (encompassing levels I through III) for oral cavity cancer is low (25). The reported failure rate at level IV in the absence of nodal involvement of levels I through III following SOHND is approximately 5% (26,27).

The orderly and predictable pattern of metastases no longer remains reliable once lymphatic drainage is altered following surgery or radiation. As described above, alterations in normal lymphatic architecture may result in nodal metastases presenting at unexpected sites so that selective neck dissections (SNDs) in these settings are inadequate for staging and treatment.

CLINICAL EVALUATION OF NODAL METASTASES
History and Physical Examination

When evaluating a patient with a neck mass suspicious for cervical nodal metastases, one cannot overemphasize the need for a systematic, comprehensive medical history and physical examination of the head and neck. Salient features of the history and physical examination are summarized in Table 15.4.

Should the primary tumor prove elusive during the physical exam, particular attention must be directed to sites of the head and the neck where a primary lesion may remain occult, for example, the tonsil and the base of tongue. The fiber-optic laryngoscope has proven invaluable in the office setting in examining and photographically documenting the nasopharynx, laryngopharynx, and pyriform sinuses.

Diagnostic Imaging

Errors may occur in the clinical assessment of regional lymph nodes by palpation alone (28), especially in patients

hypopharyngeal tumors metastasize quite frequently. Histomorphologic characteristics of the primary tumor that increase the risk of nodal metastasis include an endophytic, rather than exophytic, appearance, poorer degree of differentiation, and increased depth of invasion. Some of these factors have a site specific influence, e.g., Spiro and colleagues found that the risk of cervical metastasis approached 40% in patients with primary tumors of the floor of mouth and oral tongue that were greater than 2 mm in thickness (19). Other groups have established different cut-off criteria ranging between 2 and 6 mm pathologically or radiologically that have shown a similar trend (20). Other histologic factors predisposing to a higher rate of lymphatic metastases include lymphatic and vascular invasion by tumor, and perineural infiltration (21).

Predictable patterns of nodal metastasis. Appropriate management of cervical lymph nodes is based on the orderly and predictable spread of regional metastases based on the primary site (22,23). Lymph nodes at highest risk for metastasis from carcinoma of the oral cavity are located at levels I, II, and III. Carcinoma of the nasopharynx often presents initially with lymph node metastases situated in the posterior triangle at level V or the superior deep jugular nodes at level II. Cancers of the oropharynx, hypopharynx, and larynx tend to spread first to lymph nodes at levels II, III, and IV. Nodal metastases from thyroid carcinoma typically present in the central compartment, at levels VI and VII, before extending to either or both lateral necks.

Table 15.4 Salient Features in the History and Physical Examination of a Patient Presenting with a Cervical Nodal Mass

Clinical history	
	Otalgia (possibly referred)
	Epistaxis
	Trismus
	Dysphagia
	Odynophagia
	Dysarthria
	Globus sensation
	Hoarseness
	Dyspnea
	Hemoptysis
	Weight loss or other constitutional symptoms
Past medical history	
	Previous history of malignancy
	Previous history of radiation exposure
Social history	
	Tobacco use
	Alcohol use
	Occupational exposures, including sun exposure
Family history	
	Family history of malignancy
Physical examination	
	Overview of functional status and nourishment
	Comprehensive examination of the skin of the scalp, face and neck
	Otoscopy
	Anterior rhinoscopy
	Test symmetry of the somatosensory function of the lower divisions of the trigeminal nerve (V2 and V3)
	Test maximal interincisal (or interalveolar, if edentulous) distance
	Assess dentition
	Assess voluntary movement of the tongue
	Bimanual palpation of oral cavity and oropharynx
	Indirect mirror laryngoscopy or fiberoptic nasopharyngolaryngoscopy
	Bimanual palpation of thyroid gland
	Bimanual palpation of all cervical lymph node levels

with a short, stout neck, in patients with fibrotic changes secondary to previous radiotherapy, and in patients with metastatic lymph nodes at sites typically inaccessible by routine physical examination, such as the parapharyngeal space (29). In the presence of adequate clinical suspicion, imaging is also helpful in excluding other histologies, such as carotid body tumors or schwannomas, and can guide the clinician to the appropriate path along the diagnostic algorithm. Imaging modalities currently available in routine clinical practice include ultrasonography, computed tomography (CT), and magnetic resonance imaging (MRI) scans, and positron emission tomography (PET) scans. Other modalities, such as single photon emission computer tomography (SPECT) scans are currently under evaluation and presently have little application in clinical practice.

Relevant imaging should be undertaken prior to manipulation of the primary tumor or neck nodes, to maximize the information obtained from these studies. Inflammation and obliteration of tissue planes from a recent biopsy may not only create difficulty in interpreting anatomic relations but also cause artifacts on functional imaging studies, such as PET scans.

Computed Tomography and Magnetic Resonance Imaging

There is no substitute for a systematic, comprehensive examination of the neck; however, imaging studies provide valuable supplemental information of regional lymph node status. The sensitivity of CT and MRI for accurately detecting nodal metastases has been reported as 84 and 92%, respectively (30). Although the presence of metastatic involvement of a lymph node is a histologic, not a radiologic diagnosis, there are characteristic changes apparent on CT and MRI suggestive of metastatic SCC, including enhancement, poorly circumscribed margins, central necrosis, and nodal size in excess of 1 cm in diameter. Lymphoma of the head and neck typically presents radiographically as solid, homogeneous lymph nodes that are isointense with muscle.

Despite the advantages afforded by these imaging modalities, limitations of CT and MRI include difficulty differentiating reactive soft tissue inflammation or postradiotherapy fibrosis from residual or recurrent carcinoma. Furthermore, cervical lymph node size does not always correlate with the presence of tumor involvement. Although larger metastatic lymph nodes indicate greater tumor volume, a small lymph node less than 1 cm in diameter may still harbor foci of tumor cells. Conversely, lymph node size greater than 1 cm in diameter does not automatically herald metastatic cancer, because reactive lymphadenopathy following infection, inflammation, or surgical intervention may result in lymph nodes of such size. Another disadvantage of CT is that scatter artifact from dental fillings may result in poor image resolution.

Ultrasonography

Ultrasonography is a useful diagnostic imaging modality, which has been reported to be extremely sensitive in accurately characterizing cervical lymph nodes metastatic for SCC (31–33). On ultrasound, grey-scale sonography helps to assess nodal morphology including size, shape, internal architecture (loss of hilar architecture, necrosis, and calcification). Power Doppler ultrasonography assesses the vascular pattern of the lymph node. Grey-scale and Doppler ultrasonography are used to identify malignant nodes (34). Ultrasonography has advanced to such an extent now that the sensitivity and specificity of this technique is equivalent to that of CT and MRI. In a recent study by Yoon et al. (35) the sensitivity, specificity, and accuracy of ultrasound was 78, 98.5, and 94.8% versus 77, 99, and 95%, respectively, for CT and MRI imaging in 67 patients with head and neck cancer. Advantages of ultrasonography include its relative low cost, easy on-screen nodal measurement, low patient burden, and facility for guided fine-needle aspiration (FNA) (36). The use of FNA combined with ultrasound further increase the sensitivity and specificity of this technique making it a very powerful imaging modality for the assessment of malignant cervical lymph nodes. As such the use of serial ultrasound and FNA is used in many

European centers now for the conservative management of the clinically negative neck rather than END (34,37). The technique however is dependent of the experience of the ultrasonographer (38). In addition to evaluation of the neck in SCC, ultrasound is excellent for the evaluation of thyroid nodules (39) and for evaluation of the neck for paratracheal and lateral neck nodes in thyroid cancer (40). Indeed, this is the investigation of choice for neck node evaluation in thyroid cancer.

Positron Emission Tomography

PET scanning is a functional imaging modality that measures the metabolic rate of tissue using radioisotopes and is based on the principle that malignant tumors have higher metabolic rates compared to normal tissues. Glucose metabolism can be characterized following the administration of radiolabeled FDG. Although [18]FDG-PET imaging lacks the anatomic detail afforded by CT or MRI scans, it relies on metabolic activity from glucose transport, rather than gross lymph node size, to indicate metastatic foci. Sites of increased metabolic activity are reflected on PET scans by higher SUV_{BW}. Such a physiologic study aims to reduce the false negative rate of CT and MRI by identifying metastatic lymph nodes smaller than 1 cm. However, like these conventional imaging techniques, [18]FDG-PET is prone to the false-positive tendency of suggesting erroneously that reactive lymphadenopathy may be metastatic cancer.

PET and the evaluation of the N+neck. Evaluation of [18]FDG-PET for accurately identifying nodal metastases demonstrates results comparable to those of CT or MRI. Kau et al. found the sensitivity and specificity of [18]FDG-PET to be 87 and 94%, respectively, compared to 65 and 47%, respectively, for CT, and 88 and 41%, respectively, for MRI in patients with HNSCC metastatic to cervical lymph nodes (41). Prospective comparison of [18]FDG-PET with CT, MRI, and ultrasound demonstrated superior sensitivity and specificity of [18]FDG-PET for detecting cervical lymph node metastases from HNSCC (39). Other reports have suggested that [18]FDG-PET is particularly useful when the findings on conventional CT imaging are equivocal for nodal metastases (42). The lower limit in terms of resolution of [18]FDG-PET for detection of abnormal lymph nodes has not been clearly delineated, but accurate identification of metastatic SCC in cervical lymph nodes less than 5 mm in diameter has been reported (43). It is now possible to carry out PET/CT and fuse the CT image with the functional information from the PET scan. This fusion of functional information from [18]FDG-PET with the anatomic resolution of CT has allowed us an unprecedented level of appreciation and confidence of the location and activity of nodes at diagnosis or posttreatment (44–46).

PET and the evaluation of the N0 neck. Some authors have suggested that the indications for [18]FDG-PET may extend beyond the N+ neck and may also include patients without clinically apparent nodal metastases on presentation (N0 neck). Patients whose primary tumor is in a high-risk location for occult regional metastatic disease may be appropriate candidates for evaluation by [18]FDG-PET (47). However, a recent meta-analysis by Kyzas et al. (48)

showed the sensitivity was only 50% whereas specificity was 87%. This low sensitivity in conjunction with the greater expense of [18]FDG-PET may prohibit its routine use in this setting (49). The low yield associated with [18]FDG-PET in identifying intrathoracic second primaries or metastases from HNSCC not otherwise apparent on routine work-up also suggests that routine inclusion of the thorax in imaging a patient otherwise without pulmonary symptoms is not justified (50).

PET and the unknown primary. [18]FDG-PET may be of benefit in patients with cervical nodal metastases from an unknown primary (Fig. 15.4). Some studies have suggested a beneficial contribution of [18]FDG-PET in elucidating the primary tumor (51), whereas other reports have concluded that it did not significantly improve detection of the primary tumor and was hindered by false positive results (52).

PET and the detection of residual or recurrent neck disease. An area where [18]FDG-PET seems particularly beneficial is the detection of recurrent HNSCC following radiation therapy (53). Tumor cells should theoretically possess greater metabolic activity and express increased levels of glucose transporters, compared to edematous, scarred, or most normal tissues (54). Furthermore, clinical response to concurrent radiation therapy and chemotherapy for HNSCC is mirrored by a decrease in tumor hypermetabolism on serial [18]FDG-PET scans before, during, and after therapy (55).

In the N+ neck treated by concurrent chemoradiation, treatment response is determined clinically and by imaging utilizing CT scan and PET scan. Although the optimal time point for imaging the neck following completion of treatment continues to generate debate, in the absence of an

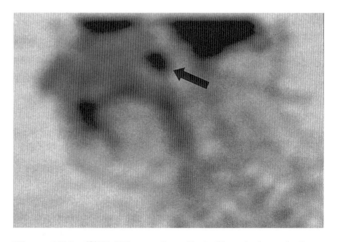

Figure 15.4 [18]FDG-PET scan of a patient with an 'unknown' primary showing intense activity in the nasopharynx. Nasopharyngoscopy had failed to reveal any mucosal abnormality and the patient was returned to the operating room for repeat examination and biopsy based on the PET findings. Histopathologic examination of the nasopharyngeal biopsy specimen confirmed the presence of squamous carcinoma.

extenuating reason, evaluation should generally be done approximately 3 months postcompletion of chemoradiation to avoid false positive scans because the effect of radiation on lymph node shrinkage continues for several weeks after completion of treatment.

PET and its use in thyroid cancer. For differentiated thyroid carcinoma, whole-body [18]FDG-PET imaging has been shown to be a useful tool for detecting recurrent and/ or metastatic disease in patients who present with serially rising thyroglobulin levels but negative 131 Iodine (^{131}I) and [201]T1 scans following total thyroidectomy (56). However it is in the evaluation of Hürthle cell carcinoma and poorly differentiated thyroid variants that PET has a specific role. These tumors are not iodine avid, and therefore the detection of lymph node or distant metastatic disease cannot be assessed accurately by radioactive iodine (RAI) imaging. These tumors are metabolically very active and therefore exhibit high [18]FDG uptake which means they are well imaged on [18]FDG-PET scan.

Prognostic role of SUV$_{BW}$. Previous studies have found no correlation between SUV$_{BW}$ and histologic grade of tumor in nodal metastases from HNSCC, possibly due to the heterogeneity of tumor cell clones or differential expression of glucose metabolism induced by oncogenic alteration (39).

Newer technologies. In light of the high cost associated with [18]FDG-PET, SPECT scans, using [18]FDG and [201]T1, have been evaluated as less expensive modalities. Unfortunately, the resolution of SPECT scanners is currently inferior to PET scanners (50).

Endoscopy

Endoscopic examination of the upper aerodigestive tract under anesthesia allows thorough inspection of the primary tumor as well as evaluation for second primary tumors, with the ability to biopsy suspicious sites. The oropharynx, hypopharynx, larynx, and esophagus should be examined in a systematic fashion through direct laryngoscopy and esophagoscopy.

Histologic Diagnosis

The diagnosis of metastatic cancer is made histologically, and so pathologic confirmation should be obtained for clinically and radiologically suspicious nodes.

Fine-needle Aspiration

FNA is an accurate, reliable procedure with minimal morbidity and may be performed in an outpatient setting, allowing for quick cytologic interpretation of suspicious neck masses. A diagnosis of metastatic epidermoid carcinoma may be distinguished from other malignant conditions, such as lymphoma, adenocarcinoma, or thyroid carcinoma. In addition, benign conditions, such as tuberculosis, chronic lymphadenitis, and hyperplastic lymph nodes, may be ruled out (57). Sensitivity and specificity of FNA of masses of the head and neck have been reported as 97 and 96%, respectively (58). Immunohistochemical staining for markers such as thyroglobulin, calcitonin, cytokeratin, and mucin

may be performed on the cellular aspirate to classify the histology if necessary.

Masses at sites in the head and neck inaccessible on routine examination (e.g., retropharyngeal lymph nodes) may be sampled under image guidance using CT, MRI, or ultrasonography (59–61).

An important caveat to remember regarding FNA concerns misinterpretation of cytologic results. A finding of epithelial cells in the presence of clear or straw-colored fluid on aspiration is occasionally misinterpreted as branchial cleft carcinoma, rather than cystic degeneration of a metastatic lymph node which is the more likely diagnosis in an adult. Metastases from SCC of certain sites, such as the tonsil or base of tongue, and from well-differentiated thyroid carcinomas are often cystic and therefore more likely to such misinterpretation. True branchial cleft carcinoma is an extremely rare condition, with few cases in the literature that satisfy all criteria originally proposed by Martin et al. (62,63). Repeat FNA, using image guidance if appropriate, should be considered following an initial non-diagnostic FNA. A metastatic lymph node with a necrotic center may occasionally yield a nondiagnostic specimen because of cellular debris in the hypoxic core, with viable tumor cells undetected at the periphery of the lymph node. Availability of immediate cytological stains and evaluation of the specimen under the microscope improves the diagnostic yield rate of FNA and obviates repeated outpatient visits and the associated delays in diagnosis.

Core-needle Biopsy

Should a repeat fine-needle biopsy performed for an initial nondiagnostic specimen fail to yield a diagnosis, one may consider a core-needle biopsy of the neck mass. The larger caliber of the needle generally provides an adequate specimen for cytologic and histologic evaluation. Core biopsy is typically not necessary for metastatic HNSCC, because a properly executed FNA should easily elucidate this diagnosis. It may, however, be useful in selected instances such as when malignant lymphoma is suspected or in the case of poorly differentiated or undifferentiated small-cell carcinomas where a tissue core may provide architectural information and sufficient tissue for immunohistochemistry (64–66). Extreme caution should be exercised when performing a core biopsy on a mass in the vicinity of the great vessels of the neck. In this situation, image guided core biopsies, with ultrasound or CT scan improves the level of safety.

Open Biopsy

The prognostic impact of open biopsy of a metastatic neck node during the work-up of a patient with SCC of the head and neck remains controversial. Unfortunately, data from retrospective reviews (67–70) that have shown "no adverse impact on overall outcome" are quoted to justify the practice. Ill-planned biopsy incisions create unwarranted difficulties with surgical planning during the definitive surgical operation. If the patient needs a subsequent neck dissection, it may need resection of structures that would ordinarily be spared, to fully excise contaminated tissue planes and scar from the previous open biopsy. In addition, therapy may be delayed if the patient develops wound complications from the biopsy, and there have been anecdotal reports of fungation of the tumor through the biopsy site. An open biopsy of a suspicious neck node should therefore be discouraged in most instances.

Open neck node biopsy does have a role in selected instances, particularly when the FNA suggests lymphoma. In such circumstances, the open neck node biopsy should be planned in such a manner that the incision scar be excised with the surgical specimen should biopsy results demonstrate SCC, necessitating subsequent neck dissection. At the time of open biopsy, communication with the pathologist is critical to facilitate the correct diagnosis. If lymphoma is the suspected diagnosis, the cervical nodal specimen should be transported to the pathology lab fresh (not fixed in formalin) to allow proper tissue typing. If mycobacterial infection is the suspected diagnosis, the microbiology lab should be contacted ahead of time to determine whether special handling or media is necessary.

Histopathologic Diagnosis

An important consideration in the accurate detection of nodal metastases concerns the sensitivity of routine histopathologic examination of nodal specimens. Intraoperative labeling of cervical nodal levels with tags may facilitate orientation for accurate pathologic reporting, but this practice is not widely utilized. Surgical pathology departments at different institutions may have different policies regarding the routine sampling of neck dissection specimens to evaluate for metastatic lymph nodes. Standard sectioning techniques result in microscopic examination of only a small portion of the nodal contents excised. Serial microscopic sectioning of all lymph nodes would improve the sensitivity of detection over traditional hematoxylin and eosin (H&E) staining, but at significant expense of time and manpower. Furthermore, the prognostic significance of such micrometastases from HNSCC detected by serial sectioning is not known (71). To improve on detection for occult nodal metastases, different immunohistochemical markers, such as proliferating cell nuclear antigen, MIB-1, E-cadherin, and c-myc, have been investigated for HNSCC (72,73). Likewise, immunohistochemistry for S-100 has been studied as a predictive marker of occult nodal metastases from malignant melanoma (74). Further study however is necessary to determine the prognostic significance of these immunohistochemical markers.

For cutaneous melanoma, standard techniques now include serial sectioning and immunostaining for S100, HMB-45, and Melan-A (75). In addition, the reverse transcriptase-polymerase chain reaction (RT-PCR) assay has been utilized as a sensitive technique to detect submicroscopic lymph node metastases (76). Shivers et al. have reported a significant difference in disease-free survival and overall survival between pathologically negative, RT-PCR positive and pathologically negative, RT-PCR negative patient groups undergoing lymphatic mapping and sentinel lymph node biopsy for malignant melanoma (77). Although the ability to detect metastasis at the cellular, and even molecular level exists, the prognostic significance of these findings remains to be determined. The Sunbelt Melanoma Trial, a multi-institutional, prospective randomized trial involving 79 centers in the U.S.A. and Canada has accrued more than 3,600 patients and may eventually answer this question, although the primary objective of the trial is a comparison of adjuvant interferon therapy against nodal dissection alone. One arm on this study consists of RT-PCR positive but histology-negative patients (78), and it will be interesting to compare their prognosis with the rest of the patients. A concern with the use of highly sensitive molecular markers is the potential for high false positive rate. Specificity of RT-PCR can be improved by using multiple markers, for example, tyrosinase and MART-1 and requiring more than 1 to be considered positive or using quantitative RT-PCR (79).

Molecular diagnosis in HNSCC has lagged behind melanoma, but more studies utilizing RT-PCR for different markers including the cytokeratin 5 or 14 and E48 have shown promise. The pemphigus vulgaris antigen has been reported 100% accurate in distinguishing between benign and malignant nodes (80). This may be useful for intraoperative staging with sentinel lymph node biopsy, as quantitative RT-PCR can be performed within 30 minutes, with a much higher sensitivity and specificity compared to frozen section.

Diagnosis of the Unknown Primary

The work-up of SCC metastatic to a cervical lymph node with an unknown primary represents a diagnostic challenge. Careful evaluation of the head and neck for an undetected primary tumor is critical (81). Location of the metastatic lymph node may suggest the primary site (82). Although primary malignancies for cervical metastases in the lateral neck often arise from the oral cavity or oropharynx, SCC more inferiorly in the neck at the supraclavicular region may herald primary lesions at the hypopharynx or cervical esophagus.

Supraclavicular metastases may also arise from an infraclavicular primary, such as carcinoma of the lung, breast, or stomach. The skin of the head and neck should be thoroughly examined to rule out cutaneous malignancy, which may not have been brought to light during the history taking, particularly if treated in the distant past. Sites of potential occult primaries should be carefully evaluated, including the nasopharynx, base of tongue, and pyriform sinuses. The benefit of fiber-optic nasopharyngolaryngoscopy in the office setting may be illustrated by a series of three reports from Memorial Sloan-Kettering Cancer Center (83–85). The most recent study found that the proportion of patients in whom occult primary tumors were subsequently identified dropped with each subsequent report from 31 to 15 to 12%. This decrease was largely attributed to improvements in technology that facilitated the identification of small primary tumors on initial evaluation.

With histologic diagnosis of SCC, attempts to identify the primary tumor should include direct laryngoscopy and esophagoscopy in the operating room. Bronchoscopy with bronchial washings has been advocated in the work-up of an unknown primary. Although controversial, the yield from routine bronchoscopy in the absence of clinical symptoms or signs and without abnormalities on chest X-ray may be low. Also controversial is the manner in which biopsies to determine the primary site should be performed. Rather than "blind" biopsies sampling tissues from various sites in the upper aerodigestive tract, biopsies directed by areas of suspicion based on preoperative clinical evaluation may be a more suitable approach. Some authors have

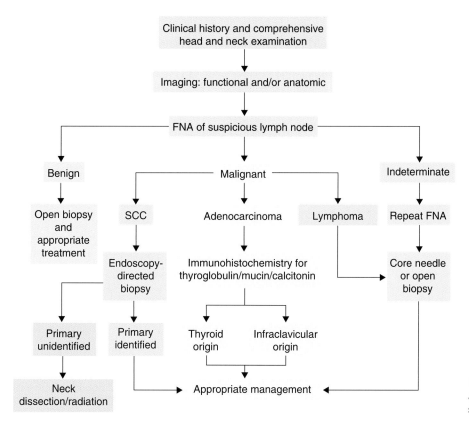

Figure 15.5 Algorithm for the work-up for a metastatic cervical lymph node with a suspected unknown primary.

advocated routine tonsillectomy to rule out microscopic tumor, especially within the tonsillar crypts (86,87). Although this is justifiable in level II and III nodal metastasis, especially when they are cystic, there is no consensus as to the validity of tonsillectomy in metastasis to other nodal stations. A similar controversy exists regarding unilateral versus bilateral tonsillectomy.

Good visualization with office endoscopy and widespread availability of imaging including CT, MRI, and PET scans have improved the detection rate of previously difficult to identify tumors, but should the primary tumor continue to be elusive, the pathologist may be requested to perform immunohistochemical stains on the cytologic aspirate. This is especially indicated where the cytology is not consistent with run-of-the-mill SCC. Thyroglobulin, thyroid transcription factor-1, PAX-8, or calcitonin stain may be requested if the diagnosis of thyroid malignancy is suspected. Epstein–Barr virus (EBV), viral capsid antigen, and early antigen IgA titers or Epstein–Barr virus DNA may be requested if nasopharyngeal carcinoma is suspected. For less differentiated tumors, immunohistochemical stains become even more important to guide localization efforts, for example, S100 for melanoma, CEA, and calcitonin for medullary thyroid cancer, thyroid transcription factor-1 for thyroid and lung cancer, cytokeratins for SCC and CD20, CD34 for lymphomas. An algorithm for the approach to a metastatic cervical lymph node with an unknown primary is depicted in Figure 15.5.

STAGING AND PROGNOSIS

The staging system of regional metastases to cervical lymph nodes established by the American Joint Committee on Cancer (AJCC) is outlined in Tables 15.5, 15.6, and 15.7 (88,89).

Characteristics of Nodal Metastases Influencing Outcome

The presence of cervical lymph node metastases results in decreased survival rates compared to those free of nodal metastases. However, various characteristics of the involved cervical lymph nodes can themselves impact on outcome. The current TNM staging system takes some of these into account, such as size, laterality, and number of involved lymph nodes. For example, the clinical stage of the neck at presentation has been shown by multivariate analysis to be an important predictor of disease specific and overall survival outcome irrespective of T stage in cancer of the larynx (90). It has also been shown to be an independent predictor of distant failure in cancer of the larynx (91). Matsuo et al reported that patients with cN3 disease at presentation had a 7.5-fold increased risk of distant failure compared to patients with cN0 disease. Extracapsular spread (ECS) of carcinoma in cervical lymph nodes, which is probably the single-most important predictor of poor prognosis has not been included in the TNM staging system. ECS has been associated with increased rates of regional

Table 15.5 Staging System of Regional Lymph Nodes (N Stage) for Squamous Cell Carcinoma of the Upper Aerodigestive Tract Excluding Nasopharynx

Nx	Regional lymph nodes cannot be assessed
N0	No regional lymph node metastasis
N1	Metastasis in a single ipsilateral lymph node, 3 cm or less in greatest dimension
N2a	Metastasis in a single ipsilateral lymph node more than 3 cm but not more than 6 cm in greatest dimension
N2b	Metastasis in multiple ipsilateral lymph nodes, none more than 6 cm in greatest dimension
N2c	Metastasis in bilateral or contralateral lymph nodes, none more than 6 cm in greatest dimension
N3	Metastasis in a lymph node more than 6 cm in greatest dimension

Table 15.6 Staging System of Regional Lymph Nodes (N Stage) for Squamous Cell Carcinoma of the Nasopharynx

Nx	Regional lymph nodes cannot be assessed
N0	No regional lymph node metastasis
N1	Unilateral metastasis in lymph node(s) 6 cm or less in greatest dimension, above the supraclavicular fossa
N2	Bilateral metastasis in lymph node(s) 6 cm or less in greatest dimension, above the supraclavicular fossa
N3a	Metastasis in a lymph node greater
N3b	Metastatic lymph node extension to the supraclavicular fossa

Table 15.7 Staging System of Regional Lymph Nodes (N Stage) for Thyroid Carcinoma. Regional Lymph Nodes are the Cervical and Upper Mediastinal Lymph Nodes

Nx	Regional lymph nodes cannot be assessed
N0	No regional lymph node metastasis
N1	Regional lymph node metastasis
N1a	Metastasis in ipsilateral cervical lymph node(s)
N1b	Metastasis in bilateral, midline, or contralateral cervical or mediastinal lymph node(s)

nodal recurrence (92), as well as significantly decreased survival rates (93). Multivariate analysis has demonstrated that ECS is an independent predictor of survival (94). The location of metastatic disease within the neck is also of prognostic value; as a general rule, the incidence of distant metastasis increases with, and prognosis worsens with, more inferiorly located cervical metastases (95,96).

PRINCIPLES OF TREATMENT

Despite the shortcomings of the current AJCC staging system, N staging of cervical metastases from HNSCC is useful in guiding treatment planning. Early stage (N1) regional lymph node metastases may be treated equally well with surgery or radiation therapy, with the treatment modality usually in keeping with that of the primary tumor. For more advanced cervical metastases (N2 or N3),

management is by combined therapy with surgery and PORT. Alternatively the neck and primary can be treated with concurrent chemoradiation with salvage neck dissection for residual disease. Management of the N0 neck is a subject fraught with considerable controversy. Details of the treatment strategies applicable to the clinically N+ neck and the N0 neck follow later in this chapter.

Surgery

Traditional surgical management of cervical nodal metastases entails comprehensive neck dissection with or without preservation of certain anatomic structures, such as the spinal accessory nerve (SAN), internal jugular vein (IJV), and the sternocleidomastoid muscle (SCM) when technically and oncologically feasible. There has been a continuing trend towards more selective procedures, sparing not only the XI, IJV, and SCM, but also lymph node groups thought to be at low risk for metastases.

History of Neck Dissection

Early attempts to resect cervical lymph nodes were met with pessimism. In the mid-nineteenth century, Chelius wrote "Once the growth in the mouth has spread to the submaxillary gland complete removal of the disease is impossible" (97). Towards the end of the nineteenth century however innovative surgical approaches incorporated regional lymph nodes during resection of tumors of the oral cavity. In 1880, Kocher described excising upper cervical lymph nodes at the time of resection of a cancer of the tongue (98). In 1906, Crile was the first to describe a systematic, comprehensive approach to dissect cervical lymph nodes, including removal of the SCM, IJV, and SAN (99). This procedure was popularized by Martin and colleagues, who described in 1951 the indications and technique of the so-called radical neck dissection (100).

Classification of Neck Dissections

The system of classifying neck dissections is undergoing continuous evolution. The Committee for Neck Dissection Classification of the American Head and Neck Society continues to publish its recommendations, which are widely adopted in head and neck literature. A brief description of the traditional and current classification is included here. Neck dissection is classified into comprehensive neck dissection, which is carried out for clinically positive neck disease, and SND, which is generally carried out for clinically negative neck disease.

Comprehensive neck dissection. This refers to procedures that remove cervical lymph nodes from levels I to V. They can be subclassified into RND, modified RND (MRND), and extended RND.

Radical neck dissection The classical RND is the gold standard of lymphadenectomy for clinically apparent lymphatic metastases and consists of surgical clearing of nodal lymphatics from all five levels of the neck. Included in the specimen with the cervical lymphatics are the SCM, SAN, IJV, submandibular gland, and tail of the parotid. Functional morbidity associated with RND arises primarily from sacrifice of one or more of the following

Table 15.8 Classification of Neck Dissections

Comprehensive neck dissection
    Classical radical neck dissection (RND)
    Type I modified radical neck dissection (MRND I)
    Type II modified radical neck dissection (MRND II)
    Type III modified radical neck dissection (MRND III)
    Extended radical neck dissection (ERND)

Selective neck dissection
    Supraomohyoid neck dissection (SOHND)
    Lateral neck dissection (LND)
    Posterolateral neck dissection (PLND)

structures: the SAN, the SCM, and the IJV. Sacrifice of the SAN results in loss of innervation to the trapezius muscle. The patient is unable to abduct the arm fully and suffers from chronic pain and stiffness of the shoulder. Destabilization of the shoulder results in a "winged scapula" deformity and increases the risk for sternoclavicular subluxation (101). Resection of the SCM gives the appearance of platysmal banding and removes a layer of cover for the carotid artery, potentially important in the irradiated neck. Sacrifice of the IJV may result in significant facial edema and possibly neurovascular compromise, particularly following bilateral RND and laryngopharyngectomy that disrupts collateral drainage into Batson's prevertebral venous plexus. In light of the functional morbidity and cosmetic deformity associated with RND, modifications to the procedure have been described. A classification scheme previously described to standardize nomenclature of the different types of neck dissection is listed in Table 15.8 (102).

Modified radical neck dissection MRNDs still encompass levels I to V but one or more nonlymphatic structures are preserved, either the SAN, the IJV, or the SCM. They are classified into types I, II, and III. Traditionally, Type I MRND selectively preserves the SAN and Type III modified neck dissection (functional neck dissection) preserves the SAN, SCM, and IJV. There is some variability about the Type II MRND where some describe preservation of SCM and SAN and others the IJV and SAN (103,104). The latest AHNS nomenclature is clearly useful in such situations, where the surgery is designated, for example, MRND with preservation of SCM and SAN.

Extended radical neck dissection Extended RND is also included in the category of comprehensive neck dissection. It may include nodal groups such as retropharyngeal or parapharyngeal lymph nodes or nonlymphatic structures not typically removed during the dissection, such as the carotid artery or hypoglossal nerve.

Selective neck dissection. In contrast to comprehensive neck dissections, procedures in this category selectively remove cervical lymph node groups at certain levels, while preserving the SAN, SCM, and IJV. This neck dissection is traditionally for the clinically negative neck. SND includes procedures such as supraomohyoid, extended supraomohyoid, lateral, and posterolateral. SOHND removes lymph nodes at levels I, II, and III and is usually carried out for cancers of the oral cavity and floor of mouth. Extended SOHND removes lymph nodes at levels I, II, III, and IV

and is usually carried out for cancer of the oral tongue due to the recognized incidence of skip metastases to level IV. Lateral neck dissection (jugular neck dissection) removes lymph nodes at levels II, III, and IV and is carried out for cancers of the oropharynx, larynx, and hypopharynx. Posterolateral neck dissection removes lymph nodes at levels II through V, as well as suboccipital nodes and postauricular nodes and is usually carried out for cancer of the skin where the primary is in the posterolateral region of the scalp. Current terminology is more cumbersome but allows less room for misinterpretation, for example, SND (sublevels IIA, IIB, III, and V). This method of reporting should be encouraged.

Nodal Yields in Neck Dissection

An area for which there is no easy answer concerns the impact of nodal count following neck dissection. Retrospective analyses that have quantified nodal counts exenterated in neck dissection illustrate the variation of nodal yields among different surgeons (105–109). These studies demonstrate that the mean number of lymph nodes harvested during RND has ranged from 22 to 39 nodes. Certainly, the technical expertise of the surgeon performing the neck dissection and the meticulousness of the pathologist examining the specimen affect the absolute number of the nodal yield. As described above, more sensitive detection techniques, such as serial sectioning or PCR, may further increase the number of pathologically positive lymph nodes over conventional H&E evaluation. There are no good data correlating the number of lymph nodes harvested during neck dissection and outcome regarding regional recurrence or survival. The absence of such data to suggest what constitutes an adequate neck dissection is particularly important in light of the increasing acceptance of more selective procedures. The absence of standardized nomenclature characterizing the minimum number of cervical lymph nodes resected to qualify a procedure as a neck dissection is evident in the fifth edition of the *AJCC Cancer Staging Manual*, indicating that "a selective neck dissection will ordinarily include six or more lymph nodes and a radical or modified radical neck dissection will ordinarily include 10 or more lymph nodes" (90). These small numbers suggested could result in a wide variety of surgical procedures yielding markedly different numbers of nodes harvested, and yet these procedures would all be grouped under the general heading of "neck dissection."

Radiation Therapy

Radiation therapy may be carried out as primary modality therapy for the neck for the clinically negative neck or the neck with N1 disease. Neck dissection, with or without adjuvant irradiation, is the preferred treatment for large cervical metastases (110). Heterogeneity among radiosensitivity may be due to several factors, including tumor volume, intrinsic cellular radiosensitivity, clonogen density, and hypoxia (111). In light of this heterogeneity, molecular markers to predict radiosensitivity have been investigated, including Ki-67 immunohistochemistry (112), as well as assays for p53 mutation, or *bcl*-2 expression (113). The prognostic significance of such molecular markers has yet to be determined.

Definitive Radiation Therapy for N0 and N1 Disease

Definitive radiotherapy shares comparable results with surgical treatment for N0 and N1 neck disease. SCC arising from certain subsites in the head and neck is particularly radiosensitive, such as the nasopharynx and lymphoepithelial carcinoma of the tonsil. Even advanced cervical metastases from these primary tumors respond well to definitive radiotherapy, reserving planned neck dissection for residual disease. Although a variety of different fractionation schemes may be employed, definitive radiotherapy generally delivers 60 to 70 Gy through a shrinking field technique over 6 to 7.5 weeks. In many major centers, intensity modulated radiation therapy (IMRT) has become the modality of choice for radiation treatment. The ability to configure the treatment volume tightly while sparing critical structures has significantly improved with the use of computer-aided reverse planning. This should maintain or increase the control rate while decreasing morbidity.

Adjuvant Radiation Therapy Post Neck Dissection for N2 and N3 Disease

Advanced cervical lymphatic metastases (N2 or N3) from most sites of the head and neck can be managed by a combination of neck dissection and radiation therapy. Early reports combining neck dissection and preoperative radiation therapy demonstrated reduction in regional recurrence, particularly for advanced nodal disease (114). The final report of study 73-03 of the Radiation Therapy Oncology Group did not demonstrate a statistically significant difference in survival between preoperative versus PORT for advanced HNSCC, although locoregional control was improved in the patients receiving PORT (115). The standard timing of radiation therapy when combined with neck dissection is currently in an adjuvant setting. The advantages of delivering radiation therapy after surgery include the ability to deliver a greater dose of radiation in the postoperative setting (usually 60–70 Gy over 6–7 weeks), than preoperatively (typically 45 Gy over 4–5 weeks); and the additional information gleaned during neck dissection to plan for appropriate portals of radiation therapy, based on the surgical extent of tumor. Potential disadvantages associated with PORT include possible contamination of tissue planes with tumor during surgical manipulation, or delayed wound healing from complications following neck dissection may delay the administration of radiation therapy. The ideal time to initiate PORT has been recommended as between 4 and 6 weeks following surgery, in light of the risk for increased locoregional failure (116). Indications for adjuvant radiotherapy include

- metastatic lymph node size greater than 3 cm
- multiple positive nodes
- extracapsular lymph node extension
- microscopic or gross residual disease
- adverse features of the primary tumor such as positive surgical margins, vascular and lymphatic invasion, or perineural infiltration.

Adjuvant radiation therapy has been shown to improve locoregional control and survival in the presence of ECS or positive resection margins following surgery (117).

PORT however should not be construed as a panacea for an inadequate operation. Surgical clips placed intraoperatively are useful to mark the extent of gross residual disease or suspected microscopic disease if adjuvant radiation therapy is planned, to facilitate planning. This is especially important in IMRT where more attention will be directed at the critical treatment areas.

The decision to employ PORT for HNSCC metastatic to cervical lymph nodes with an unknown primary mirrors that for nodal metastases from a known primary source. N1 disease without extracapsular extension can be managed by neck dissection alone (118), whereas more advanced nodal disease requires PORT to both sides of the neck, as well as to putative mucosal sites in the pharyngeal axis, particularly in the presence of extracapsular extension (119).

Brachytherapy

Treatment options for patients with nodal recurrence or gross persistent disease following previous irradiation to the neck include neck dissection with intraoperative radiation therapy, where a single dose of high-intensity external beam radiotherapy is employed, or neck dissection with brachytherapy. As illustrated in Figure 15.6, [121]I-Dexon mesh or afterloading catheters with [191]Ir wires may be used for brachytherapy. Care must be taken to protect the carotid artery when brachytherapy is employed. Either pedicled muscle flaps or vascularized free flaps are suitable tissue coverage to minimize the risk of flap necrosis and wound dehiscence with attendant risk of carotid exposure and subsequent blowout, when employing brachytherapy for gross residual or recurrent nodal disease.

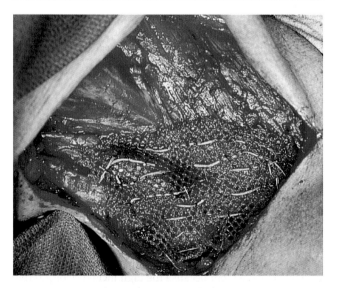

Figure 15.6 This patient had a regional recurrence following previous neck dissection and postoperative radiation therapy for a squamous carcinoma of the tonsil. The recurrent tumor was excised leaving gross residual disease in the region of the carotid bifurcation. A [121]I-Dexon mesh was sutured in place to deliver brachytherapy to the residual tumor.

Chemoradiation Therapy

Adjuvant Chemoradiation Post Neck Dissection for N2 and N3 Disease

Two recent multicenter randomized controlled trials, one conducted by the Radiation Oncology Therapy Group (RTOG) (120) and another conducted by the European Organization for Research and Treatment of Cancer (EORTC) (121) have established the superiority of concurrent chemoradiation over radiation alone as adjuvant treatment post-surgery in high-risk or locally advanced head and neck cancers. The RTOG study results which were based on 416 patients, showed a 10% improvement (82 vs. 72%) in locoregional control, with a longer disease-free survival, but no significant difference in overall survival. Locoregional failure rates were 29% in the radiation arm and 16% in the chemoradiation arm. In the EORTC study, 5-year progression-free survival (36 vs. 47%) and overall survival (40 vs. 53%) were significantly improved with the addition of concurrent chemotherapy, which consisted of cisplatin on days 1, 22, and 43 of radiation. Locoregional relapses were 31 and 18%. Patients recruited into both studies exhibited high-risk characteristics including multiple nodal metastasis, extracapsular nodal disease, microscopically involved mucosal margins, perineural invasion, and vascular tumour emboli. The incidence of grade 3 or 4 toxicity in the RTOG study was 77 as opposed to 34% for radiation alone, which makes it important that only patients with high-risk characteristics warrant this morbid treatment.

Definitive Chemoradiation for Advanced N2/N3 Neck Disease with Planned or Salvage Neck Dissection

Concurrent chemotherapy and radiation therapy has been demonstrated to provide improved disease control and survival rates over sequential chemoradiation or radiation therapy alone, when utilized in an organ preservation approach for advanced SCC of the head and neck (122–125). However, despite the improved benefit of concurrent chemoradiation, an area for which very little data exists, is the optimal management of nodal metastases in a concurrent approach. Because of the paucity of data, a number of controversies persist regarding the optimal treatment of the neck in concurrent chemoradiation.

Planned neck dissection postchemoradiation. Patients with N2 and N3 neck disease may be managed by planned neck dissection 6 to 8 weeks after completion of chemoradiation. This policy is carried out irrespective of the response to chemoradiation, that is, even if there has been a complete response to treatment, a neck dissection is still carried out. This policy has the advantage of carrying out the neck dissection before the onset of fibrosis has occurred and therefore makes the neck dissection technically similar in complexity to a prechemoradiation neck dissection.

There are several reports in the literature that advocate this management because the high incidence of positive nodes found at pathology even in necks which had no clinical or radiological signs of residual cancer. Lavertu and colleagues reported on 53 patients with stage III and IV head and neck cancer with N2 or N3 disease (126). All patients with N2 or N3 disease were planned to undergo neck dissection 4 to 6 weeks following concurrent chemoradiation. For patients demonstrating less than a complete response in the neck after concurrent chemoradiation, 47% of nodal specimens were found to have tumor. However, in patients with a complete response in the neck after concurrent therapy, 22% of these complete responders were found to have the presence of tumor in the nodal specimens. Moreover, this pathologic positivity was demonstrated to negatively impact on disease-specific survival. In light of this degree of pathological positivity in complete responders (greater than 20%), these authors concluded that all patients presenting with N2 or N3 disease should undergo planned neck dissection. Furthermore, they demonstrated a lower rate of nodal recurrence following neck dissection, and the inability to salvage nodal failure in patients who had not undergone neck dissection. Other studies (127,128) have reported an incidence of residual occult metastases of 28 and 29%, respectively. Moreover, Gourin et al. reported that these occult metastases were PET negative. Brizel et al. (129) also reported that the disease-specific survival was improved in patients who had neck dissection compared to those who did not (75 vs. 53%, $p = 0.04$).

Despite this evidence, other authors have reported very low incidence of regional recurrence in patients managed by observation followed by a complete response in the neck to chemoradiotherapy (CTRT). A recent study by Corry et al. (130) reported on 102 patients with N2/3 neck disease with a complete response clinically and radiologically at 12 weeks postchemoradiation where no planned neck dissection was done. With a median follow up of 4.3 years, no patient had neck recurrence. Lau et al. (131) reported that in patients with complete response postchemoradiation with N2/3 neck disease treated by observation, the 2-year locoregional recurrence-free survival was 95%. However Zelefsky et al. (132) reported on 65 patients who had a complete response to CTRT managed by neck observation. With a median follow-up of 9 years, there was a 10 to 15% incidence of neck recurrence. Patients who had a complete response to induction chemotherapy were less likely to recur raising the suggestion that response to induction chemotherapy could be used as the indicator to who should have a planned neck dissection.

The type of neck dissection most commonly reported for planned neck dissection is either the radical or MRND. However, there is some evidence that a SND 3 to 6 weeks post-CTRT is an alternative (133). This study reported a pathological positive incidence of 22% in 70 neck dissections on 58 patients with a similar regional recurrence rate to MRND.

Salvage neck dissection post chemoradiation. An alternative approach is to carry out neck dissection only if there is clinical or radiological evidence of neck disease after completion of chemoradiation. This approach is wholly dependent on the ability to assess the response to chemoradiation. This is an area fraught with controversy. For example,

1. What is the best imaging technique to use?
2. When is the most appropriate time to assess response?
3. Is needle biopsy necessary to confirm disease before carrying out neck dissection?
4. What type of neck dissection should be done?

Imaging for residual disease Clinical evaluation of response is unreliable because induration and erythema, combined with fibrosis and edema, obscure accurate assessment. Anatomic-based diagnostic imaging, such as CT, MRI, and ultrasonography, may also be difficult to interpret for the same reasons. However, more recently there have been several reports that suggest [18]FDG-PET scanning is particularly beneficial in this scenario. [18]FDG-PET scanning has been shown to correlate with clinical response to concurrent chemoradiation before, during, and after therapy (56). A recent study from MSKCC involving 65 patients with 84 hemi-necks established the utility of [18]FDG PET/CT for excluding residual locoregional disease with a high negative predictive value (134).

Time to assess response to treatment It is important not to assess response to treatment too early because the biological effect of chemoradiation continues for several weeks after the cessation of treatment. In addition there can be residual inflammation and infection following chemoradiation. Both of these factors can result in false positive results on PET/CT scanning if carried out too early following completion of treatment. It is now our policy to assess response to chemoradiation by PET/CT approximately 12 weeks posttreatment. An algorithm for neck management by PET/CT evaluation is shown in Figure 15.7. If the PET/CT is positive and suggests residual disease then patients are offered neck dissection. If PET/CT is negative then one may observe patients with no lymph node or if lymph nodes <1 cm are present on structural imaging; in patients with nodes >1 cm the decision to observe or carry out neck dissection is an individual decision because the radiologically or clinically evident node may have viable tumor that is too small to be detected on PET scan or the entire node may indeed contain nonviable

tumor. The use of ultrasound-guided biopsy may help in this situation, but the decision for surgical intervention versus continued observation is generally based on the clinician's perception of risk in each individual situation.

Need for biopsy confirmation before neck dissection Biopsy specimens either by FNA or core-needle biopsy may be falsely negative due to sampling artifact that miss focally dispersed residual tumor. Ghosting of dead cells with residual squamous architecture may give false positive results. It is now generally accepted that should the PET/CT scan be positive with a residual lymph node >1 cm then a neck dissection should be done without biopsy. In the situation where there is anatomical evidence of disease but a negative PET, biopsy under ultrasound control may be useful to confirm no evidence of viable tumor but may be confounded by the limitations as described above.

Type of neck dissection Most authors advocate RND or MRND for salvage postchemoradiation. This is because aberrant lymphatic pathways develop during radiation and may result in unpredictable lymphatic spread making SND less ideal. However, neck dissection carried out at 12 weeks postchemoradiation is technically more difficult due to the onset of fibrosis from treatment. As such, this can result in increased morbidity in terms of shoulder dysfunction, wound complications (135), and quality of life (136) compared to neck dissection carried out without chemoradiation. In addition, pathological examination of specimens often fails to show evidence of disease outside of the nodes positive on the initial CT scan. This has led many surgeons to question the need to carry out comprehensive neck dissection in this situation, and there are now several reports describing the use of selective or superselective (removal of two or fewer contiguous neck levels) (137)

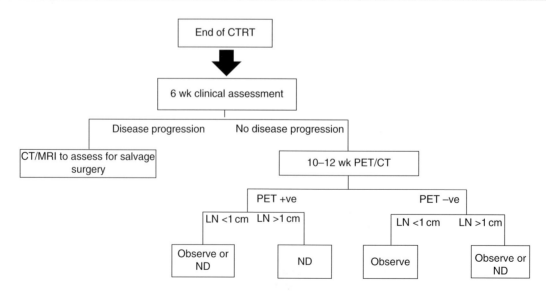

Figure 15.7 Algorithm for use of combined PET/CT in evaluation of patients with HNSCC after definitive chemoradiotherapy. *Abbreviations*: LN, lymph node; ND, neck dissection; ECE, extracapsular extension; CTRT, chemoradiotherapy; PET, positron emission tomography; CT, computed tomography; HNSCC, head and neck squamous cell carcinoma.

neck dissection to treat residual disease with no increase in regional recurrence. Sandhu et al. (138) recently reported on 48 salvage neck dissections carried out on 42 patients approximately 8 weeks after chemoradiation. The pathological positivity was 26%. The positive nodes were always confined to the clinically documented area of residual disease and in 50% of cases were only microscopic in nature. They concluded that comprehensive neck dissection was excessive, and that neck dissection should be confined to the area of clinically evident disease. However there are no randomized trials comparing regional recurrence rates for comprehensive and SND for residual disease postchemoradiation.

MANAGEMENT OF CERVICAL METASTASES FROM SQUAMOUS CELL CARCINOMA OF THE HEAD AND NECK
Management of the Clinically Positive Neck
N1 Neck Disease
As previously mentioned, early-stage (N1) regional lymph node metastases may be treated equally well with surgery or radiation therapy, with the treatment modality usually in keeping with that of the primary tumor.

N2 and N3 Neck Disease
Surgery and postoperative radiotherapy. For more advanced cervical metastases (N2 or N3), combined therapy with surgery and PORT can be done. Neck dissection is by comprehensive neck dissection which may be radical or modified radical type I. Some advocate the use of modified radical type II or III, but there is evidence that regional recurrence is greater in the type III neck dissection for SCC (139). For low-volume disease it may be possible to carry out a more SND providing PORT is given. Pathology reviews of nodal status in RNDs have demonstrated that for low-volume neck disease, some nodal stations are at low risk, for example, in N1 to N2a disease in oral cancer, 0.6% involved level IV, and none level V (140). Several studies have found no difference in locoregional control rate between SND and MRND, both with adjuvant radiation (141–143). Although no level 1 evidence exists, SND appears to be adequate in low-volume nodal disease with no extracapsular extension, provided adjuvant radiation is planned (144). For large-volume neck disease and in the presence of extranodal extension, comprehensive neck dissection is still the gold standard treatment.

CTRT and salvage neck dissection. If the primary and neck are treated by concurrent chemoradiation, neck dissection may be reserved for salvage as discussed above. The neck dissection is usually comprehensive, but there is recent evidence suggesting that selective and superselective neck dissections can be done without any negative impact on regional recurrence rates. One exception to this trend for conservative surgery has been nasopharyngeal carcinoma. Because the seminal study of patterns of nodal metastasis and analysis of nodal involvement in neck dissection specimens by Wei et al., which showed a 88% positive rate and 35% ECS with adherence to posterior triangle structures, RND has been the treatment of choice for N2 or N3 disease without complete response after chemoradiation (145).

Locally Advanced Neck Disease
Special mention should be made with regard to advanced nodal metastases encasing the carotid. Although carotid artery resection has been reported by some authors, the risk of locoregional failure is substantial because of the high likelihood of leaving residual disease at other sites such as the skull base, pharynx, or prevertebral region. In addition, the risk of neurological sequelae from carotid manipulation generally precludes the practice of carotid resection for advanced HNSCC. Balloon test occlusion demonstrating adequate collateral circulation has been suggested to avoid neurovascular complications from carotid resection. However, neurological injury may still arise from three mechanisms, namely, cholesterol emboli from atherosclerotic plaques during carotid manipulation, antegrade propagation of the clot in the distal stump of the carotid, or hypotension during the peri-operative period causing the perfusion pressure in the contralateral circulation to become insufficient. Furthermore, reconstruction of the carotid from saphenous vein or synthetic materials risks catastrophic hemorrhage from carotid rupture in the event of regional recurrence or postoperative infection.

Management of the Clinically Negative Neck
An issue of ongoing controversy concerns the management of the neck in patients without clinical evidence of regional nodal metastases (the N0 neck). Lymphatic metastases occur in a predictable fashion through sequential spread. Although previous surgery or irradiation may result in aberrant lymphatic drainage, there are well-established first echelon lymph nodes at highest risk for metastases depending on the primary site of cancer. Pathologic evidence of micrometastases has been observed on gross section in up to 33% of END specimens. More sensitive detection methods such as serial sectioning or PCR may result in an even higher prevalence. Primary tumors in different locations within the head and neck region have variable propensity for lymph node metastasis, so what constitutes the ideal approach to the N0 neck? Is the best approach observation or treatment? If treatment is chosen, is END or elective neck irradiation the optimal modality?

In light of the tumor characteristics influencing the propensity for nodal metastases, it has been suggested that if the probability of metastases to cervical lymph nodes exceeds 20%, then treatment of the neck is warranted (146). The need for appropriate management of the clinically negative neck has been demonstrated by the fact that patients whose clinically negative necks are observed tend to fail with regionally advanced disease that is difficult to salvage (147).

Elective Neck Dissection
It has been reported that there is no survival advantage offered by END when compared to observation (148). However, as previously mentioned, when observation is used for the neck at risk for metastasis, patients tend to fail with advanced nodal disease, even with close follow-up (146). END has been shown to be improve locoregional control and may therefore positively affect the quality of the patient's survival (149).

One criticism of END has focused on potential complications from the procedure. In light of the morbidity associated with the RND, there has been the trend toward selective, rather than comprehensive neck dissection, based on the predictable pattern of cervical lymph node metastases. Suarez described in 1963 that the SCM, IJV, and SAN may be preserved during neck dissection without compromising sound oncologic principles (150). Bocca popularized this technique as the "functional" neck dissection (151). SND has been demonstrated to be an oncologically sound procedure, providing effective treatment for the N0 neck (110). The specific levels to be dissected is based on an understanding of embryology and anatomy of the location of the primary, together with anatomic and pathologic studies of its pattern of nodal metastasis. Decision on the necessity for nodal dissection and its extent should not be arbitrary.

Oral cavity. SND (levels I to III), or SOHND has been recommended for N0 patients with primary SCCs of the oral cavity (24,152). Other reports have extended the indication for SND (levels I to III) for primary tumors in the oral cavity to include not only N0 necks, but also N1 necks without evidence of ECS (28,153). This latter proposition is a controversial subject that has not been resolved. For primary tumors of the oral tongue there is the potential for "skip metastases," or metastases to inferior cervical nodes at levels III or IV in the absence of demonstrable involvement at levels I and II (25,26). Oral tongue cancers should therefore have SND removing levels I to IV (extended SOHND). Meticulous care should be exercised in the region of level IV to prevent inadvertent injury either to the thoracic duct on the left side of the neck or to the main lymphatic duct on the right side of the neck. There is controversy as to whether removal of lymph nodes in level IIB is necessary in elective SOHND because dissection of this region can result in shoulder dysfunction due to traction or devascularization of the SAN. However in a study of 102 patients with oral cancer undergoing SOHND, Olofsson et al. (154) recently reported that there is an incidence of 7.3% positive nodes in level IIB for oral cancer in general and 12% for tongue cancer. However, no randomized controlled trial has been done to examine this issue.

Oropharynx. For the N0 neck with a primary arising in the oropharynx, the risk for level IV spread is higher compared to those arising from the oral cavity, whereas the risk for level I spread is correspondingly lower. Thus, an SND (levels II to IV) has been advocated for N0 necks with an oropharyngeal primary (24).

For primary tumors of the oral cavity or oropharynx, the risk of level V involvement has been shown to be minimal when only one level is involved, unless level IV is the involved level, or unless multiple levels are involved (155). Level V therefore is not routinely included in the selective lymphadenectomy of N0 necks for primaries of the oral cavity or oropharynx.

Larynx and hypopharynx. The lymphatic drainage pattern of the larynx has been well studied, and it has long been understood that the supraglottis, glottis, and subglottis have different drainage patterns, consistent with embryological development and therefore differing risk for nodal metastases depending on the site of the primary tumor. The supraglottis is rich in lymphatics that drain bilaterally into the jugular chain of nodes, leading to a concomitantly high risk of bilateral nodal metastasis. The subglottis is also lymphatic rich, but it drains through the cricothyroid membrane into the prelaryngeal or Delphian node, which derives its name from its ability to forewarn the surgeon of the presence of laryngeal cancer. The glottis which is the watershed of these two embryologically distinct segments has only sparse lymphatics that typically drain to the jugular chain unless there is subglottic extension. END for the larynx therefore usually entails bilateral SND (levels II to IV) for the supraglottic and glottis and, if there is subglottic involvement, level VI too. It may be possible to spare dissection of level IIB as Coskun et al. (156) reported that of 113 SND for N0 laryngeal cancer, none of the specimens contained cancer in level IIB. More recently Ferlito recommends limiting dissection to levels IIA and III for supraglottic and glottic primaries, citing a metastatic rate of 1.4% to level IIB and 3.4% to level IV (157).

Paranasal sinuses. Tumors of the paranasal sinuses do not typically require nodal dissection due to a low risk of nodal metastasis.

Ear canal and scalp. Squamous cancers in the ear canal and temporo-parietal scalp require superficial parotidectomy in addition to SND (levels II to V), previously known as posterolateral neck dissection to remove the first echelon of nodes, which are intraparotid.

Sentinel Node Mapping for Mucosal Squamous Cell Carcinoma of the Head and Neck

In the era of more SNDs, the utility of sentinel lymph node biopsy (SLNB), which is clinically useful for treatment of cutaneous melanoma, has been investigated for primaries of the oral cavity (158). SLNB is an experimental technique that is under active evaluation by prospective clinical trials and is only practiced in a few select centers. The sentinel lymph node is defined as the first echelon lymph node to which cancer spreads. The advantage of the technique is that it allows focused examination of the lymph nodes at highest risk for metastases, so that neck dissection is performed only in patients with a positive node, and the rest can be spared the morbidity of the operation. The technique was first utilized for malignant melanoma and breast cancer and is now a widely accepted technique in these types of cancer. Identification of the sentinel node requires the use of preoperative lymphoscintigraphy using radioactive technetium and then blue dye injection (toluidine blue) at the time of surgery. The sentinel node is identified using a gamma probe and confirmed with the injection of blue dye at the time of biopsy. Pathology of the sentinel node requires H&E staining and also immunohistochemistry. The node requires serial sectioning at 150 micron sections for accurate analysis. Melanoma and breast cancer are ideally suited to this technique because the primary tumor is easily palpated and visualized making injection into the tumor relatively straightforward. The majority of oral cavity cancers are also easily visualized and are in general accessible to a direct injection. This has led to the suggestion that the SLNB technique may be useful in neck management for oral cavity cancer. The first report of this technique for SCC of the oral cavity was reported in 2001 by Shoaib et al. (159) where SLNB was carried out prior to an END in patients with a clinically negative neck. A report by Ross et al. (160) examined SLNB in 57 clinically N0 necks in 48 patients and reported 15 (35%) were upstaged by SNB and 28 (65%) were staged SNB negative. With a mean follow up of 18 months only one patient developed regional neck disease after being staged negative on SNB. The overall sensitivity of the technique was 94%. A further multicenter trial reported upstaging in 42 of 135 patients (35%) (161). However this technique is still experimental and should only be carried out in centers with the necessary expertise and the appropriate volume of cases as it has been shown that centers who carry out this technique with fewer than 10 cases per year have a much lower sensitivity (162). Technical problems of "shine through," where the radioactivity level in the primary site potentially obscures the sentinel node, has been mitigated by the concurrent use of lymphoscintigraphy, blue dye injection, and the 10% rule using the gamma probe. Many studies have shown SLNB to be as effective as SND for staging of the neck (163–165). In reality however, the difference between SLNB and SND (levels I, IIA, and III) may not be significant in terms of extent of surgery and morbidity, especially if deeper nodes from level IIA need to be removed.

Trials of SLNB in T_1 and T_2 laryngeal and oropharyngeal tumors have yielded promising results, with sensitivity ranging between 93 and 97%. Injections are performed under general anesthesia, and resection of the primary tumor is performed prior to SLNB. An interval of 15 to 20 minutes is required for the tracer to reach the sentinel nodes. Compared to oral cavity tumors, the advantage of SLNB in the larynx and oropharynx is even more debatable. The nodal station most frequently involved in these cases is level IIA, and SND (IIA and III) is neither more morbid nor appreciably more extensive than excision of a deep level IIA node.

The role of SLNB in T_3 and T_4 HNSCC is controversial. There is a higher rate of failure in these cases, sometimes attributed to obstruction of lymphatic flow caused by tumor and redirecting of flow to neighboring nodes, resulting in false negative biopsies. In the setting of neo-adjuvant chemoradiation, the alteration in lymphatic drainage becomes unpredictable, and it is suggested that fused functional/anatomic imaging be employed instead, to avoid an unpleasant surprise during SLNB (166).

Elective Neck Irradiation

The theoretical advantages of treating the N0 neck with surgical lymphadenectomy include pathologic staging information, preparation of donor and recipient vessels for microvascular reconstruction, and avoidance of the morbidity associated with radiotherapy. However, elective neck irradiation has been shown to provide lymph node failure rates of less than 5% when the primary lesion has been adequately controlled (167,168). In fact, no significant differences in regional recurrence have been demonstrated following treatment with elective neck irradiation, compared to END (169).

The modality chosen to address the clinically negative neck may be largely influenced by philosophy of the treating physician and by the treatment planned for the primary tumor. Nevertheless, as a general rule, the treatment modality for the primary tumor is used concurrently to address occult metastases in the clinically negative neck if the risk is appreciable.

MANAGEMENT OF NECK METASTASES FROM AN UNKNOWN PRIMARY

The detailed evaluation of the patient with cervical metastases from an unknown primary has been discussed above. The management of the neck in these patients traditionally is by neck dissection followed by radiotherapy to possible primary sites. Even patients with N1 disease from an unknown primary benefit from neck dissection because the additional pathologic information that becomes available may help plan further treatment. However, metastatic lymph nodes at level IV are not recommended for neck dissection if the primary site is believed to lie below the level of the clavicles, unless the patient complains of compressive symptoms. Data from Memorial Sloan-Kettering have compared institutional outcome data from patients treated for cervical metastases with an unknown primary from the years of 1977 and 1990 to those treated from 1965 to 1976. In the cohort of patients treated from 1977 to 1990, control of the treated neck had improved from 50 to 74%, presumably from the addition of adjuvant radiation therapy following neck dissection. Five-year survival (45%) however had not significantly improved. The standard type of neck dissection employed for cervical metastases with an occult primary involves comprehensive neck dissection, with or without preservation of the SAN. More recently concurrent chemoradiation has been utilized in the treatment of patients with an unknown primary. It is most commonly utilized where there is evidence of ECS in the neck dissection specimen. Patients are treated with chemoradiation to the neck and to all possible primary sites. It is also possible that concurrent chemoradiation could be used as the primary modality treating the neck and possible primary sites and then carrying out planned neck dissection or salvage neck dissection posttreatment. There is however a shortage of evidence in the literature that advocate this approach (170) and as such is not to be recommended at present for the unknown primary.

MANAGEMENT OF CERVICAL METASTASES FROM SALIVARY NEOPLASMS

Occult cervical metastases are uncommon in cancers of the major salivary glands (171,172). Armstrong et al. reported an incidence of occult metastases of 12% in 407 patients who were clinically node negative. Significant risk factors for occult nodal metastases from cancers of the major salivary glands include primary tumor size greater than 4 cm in size (20 vs. 4%), and high tumor grade (49 vs. 2%) (170). END should therefore be done in patients with high-grade malignancies and T_3/T_4 tumors. SND for parotid cancer should encompass levels I, II, III, and IV (170). Alternatively, if it is anticipated that PORT will be given to the primary site then the ipsilateral neck can be treated by radiotherapy at the same time rather than by neck dissection.

For clinically apparent nodal metastases, patients should be treated by superficial parotidectomy, comprehensive neck dissection, followed by PORT. Klussman et al. (173)

reported that on multivariate analysis, lymph node involvement of level I was an independent predictor for poorer disease-specific survival.

The benefit of adjuvant radiotherapy has been demonstrated in a matched-pair analysis of patients receiving combined surgery and PORT compared to patients treated with surgery only (174). Five-year determinate survival for the combined therapy group was improved compared to the group undergoing surgery only (48.9 vs. 18.7%), and locoregional control was improved as well (69.1 vs. 40.2%). The benefit of PORT was especially pronounced in patients with high-stage and high-grade primary tumors.

Fast neutron radiotherapy is available at select institutions and has been suggested as effective treatment for locally advanced adenoid cystic carcinoma of the head and neck (175). However, its role in the management of nodal disease remains undefined.

MANAGEMENT OF CERVICAL METASTASES FROM THYROID CARCINOMA
Well-differentiated Thyroid Cancer

The first echelon lymph nodes for thyroid cancer are the central lymph node compartment (level VI) lymph nodes. These are bound by the hyoid bone superiorly, sternal notch inferiorly, and the carotid arteries laterally. Subdivisions are the pretracheal, paratracheal, precricoid (Delphian), and supramediastinal nodes. From the central compartment, metastatic spread is to the lateral compartment nodes, most commonly levels II to IV and less commonly to level V, level I, and retropharyngeal lymph nodes. However skip metastases to the lateral nodes can occur in 2 to 19% of cases bypassing the central nodes. This may suggest a direct route of spread from the thyroid to the lateral compartment or alternatively failure to identify micrometastases in the central compartment lymph nodes.

In patients with a clinically negative neck, the incidence of occult micrometastases ranges from 30 to 70% (176–178). The incidence depends on the size of the primary (26% in tumors <1 cm and 66% in tumors >1 cm). Machens et al. reported the central nodes and lateral nodes were involved in 29% each whereas Wada et al. (179) reported 61% for the central compartment and 40% for the lateral compartment. Mirallie (180) reported that the paratracheal nodes were the most common site involved (50%). Shaha reported on 1,038 patients at memorial sloan-kettering cancer center (MSKCC) and reported 56% of patients had a clinically positive neck at the initial evaluation (181). Given the fact that lymph node metastases are so common it may seem somewhat surprising that thyroid cancer has a 93 to 98% 10-year survival rate (182). There remains controversy about the impact of nodal metastasis on survival. Several studies suggest there is no decrease in survival in the presence of nodal disease, especially in the younger population of patients younger than age 45 years (183,184). Other studies report a reduced survival (185–187). Nodal size greater than 3 cm and ECS are poor prognostic signs (188). The management of the neck therefore is a controversial subject.

Ultrasound is excellent for the evaluation of thyroid nodules (40) and for evaluation of the neck for paratracheal and lateral neck nodes in thyroid cancer (41). Indeed, this is the investigation of choice for neck node evaluation in thyroid cancer.

Surgery

Elective treatment of the neck. Due to the high incidence of occult metastases, many have recommended elective treatment of the central compartment lymph nodes. In a case control study of 195 patients having central compartment neck dissection, the 10-year survival was greater in the group having neck dissection compared to those who did not (98.4 vs. 89–92%) (189). Lee et al. (190) suggested that only the ipsilateral central compartment need be dissected for tumors less than 2 cm; posttreatment thyroglobulin levels for patients having ipsilateral versus complete central compartment were equivalent. Other authors suggest that adjuvant RAI therapy may be an alternative treatment (191) because central compartment dissection is associated with a high incidence of temporary and permanent hypoparathyroidism as well as increasing the risk of damage to the recurrent laryngeal nerves. As such, dissection of the central compartment should only be done if any nodes appear enlarged or suspicious.

Treatment of the clinically negative lateral neck remains a controversial topic. Even though occult metastases are seen in up to 40% of patients (177) studies have shown that in patients having a lateral neck dissection and those that do not the regional recurrence rates were equivalent, suggesting that routine RAI therapy is sufficient to treat occult metastatic disease (177,192). Elective treatment of the lateral neck is therefore not standard practice.

Treatment of the clinically positive neck. Clinically apparent nodal metastases in the central compartment from differentiated thyroid cancer are treated with central compartment neck dissection. If nodes are present in the lateral compartment then a lateral neck dissection should also be carried out. Patients who have positive lateral nodes but no nodes in the central compartment clinically, that is, skip metastases, are treated with a combined lateral and central neck dissection; a recent study by Khafif et al. (193) reported that in patients with positive nodes in the lateral neck compartment 84% of these patients will also have positive nodes in the central compartment. The main debate is over what type of lateral neck dissection should be carried out. Several studies have shown that multiple neck levels are involved when the lateral neck is clinically positive (194–196). This is an argument against "berry picking" or superselective neck dissection as this may lead to a higher rate of missed disease and recurrent operations. It is recommended that a MRND type III be carried out for the positive neck. In the Kupferman et al. study of 44 neck dissections in 39 patients, all patients had levels II to V dissected; the incidence of metastases was 52% in level II, 57% in level III, 41% in level IV, and 21% in level V. Roh et al. reported 76% level IV and 70% level IIA and III nodes were involved, 17% of level IIb, 4% in level I, 16% in the infraaccessory compartment of level V, but 0% in the supraaccessory nerve compartment of level V. These authors therefore recommended dissection of levels II to V including level IIb but sparing the supraaccessory compartment of level V. In contrast however, a study by Turanli (197) comparing MRND type III to SND (levels II–IV) showed no differences in disease-free survival, overall survival, or local recurrence at 80 months follow-up.

Adjuvant Radioactive Iodine

Patients with bulky nodal disease are at increased risk for distant metastases, especially to the lung. RAI therapy after total thyroidectomy and appropriate neck dissection is recommended in this situation. RAI dosimetry 4 to 6 weeks after surgery is used to identify any residual thyroid tissue, followed by RAI ablative treatment. RAI treatment requires a hypothyroid state to elevate the patient's serum thyroid stimulating hormone (TSH) for optimal concentration of iodine. Traditionally, this hypothyroid state has been effected by cessation of supplemental thyroxine for 4 to 6 weeks prior to RAI dosimetry and treatment. Patients often complain of debilitating symptoms of hypothyroidism, including fatigue and difficulty with concentration. In light of these unpleasant side effects associated with several weeks of symptomatic hypothyroidism, a relatively recent advance has been the use of recombinant human TSH to elevate the patient's serum TSH to increase RAI uptake. Recombinant human TSH allows for elevated serum TSH without the debilitating symptoms of clinical hypothyroidism. Further studies are necessary however before recombinant human TSH supplants the traditional hypothyroid approach as standard therapy for RAI.

Poorly Differentiated Thyroid Cancer

Management of the clinically positive neck should involve central compartment neck dissection and a comprehensive type III neck dissection if the lateral nodes are positive. As previously mentioned, poorly differentiated tumors and thyroid cancer in older patients do not concentrate RAI effectively, and these patients may have to be treated either with external beam radiation or high-dose RAI on an empiric basis. External beam radiotherapy is not typically utilized for differentiated thyroid cancer and is usually reserved for bulky gross residual or recurrent disease and for anaplastic thyroid cancer.

MANAGEMENT OF CERVICAL METASTASES FROM MELANOMA

Clinically Negative Neck

Selective Neck Dissection

Regional nodal metastases are relatively rare in thin cutaneous melanomas (less than 1 mm in thickness) of the head and neck region, and END is therefore not recommended. Thicker lesions (greater than 4 mm) are associated with a high incidence of distant metastases and therefore END is unlikely to affect survival in this population. The role of END in patients with intermediate thickness (1.0–4 mm thick) melanomas continues to be debated, as only about 15% of patients will have histologically demonstrable metastatic nodes so that the remaining 85% may be considered to have undergone an unnecessary procedure. Four randomized trials (198–201) and a large, retrospective study (202) in patients with intermediate thickness melanomas have failed to demonstrate any improvement in survival following END.

Sentinel Lymph Node Biopsy (SLNB)

SLNB for cutaneous head and neck melanoma has the potential to avoid the morbidity of routine elective nodal dissections while accurately and pathologically staging the regional nodes at risk for micrometastases. The usefulness and reliability of the technique has been well described in numerous publications since it was first reported in 1990 (203). In our experience, a negative SLNB correctly predicted regional nodal control in 47/48 (98%) patients but missed one of the five (20%) patients who had regional lymphatic disease. The 2-year disease-specific survival for SLN-negative patients was 93% compared to 50% for SLN-positive patients (p = NS) (204). SLN mapping is a reliable indicator of the status of the draining lymphatic basins but patients with negative SLN(s) will need to be observed for longer periods to understand the true implications of the procedure. If patients are SLN positive they can be managed by either neck dissection or by systemic therapy with immunomodulating agents such as interferon, interleukin, or vaccine-based therapy. However there is no evidence to suggest that neck dissection in patients who are SLN positive improves overall survival compared to patients who are SLN negative (205). Whether or not to carry out a neck dissection in patients who are SLN positive is therefore an individual decision between surgeon and patient.

Clinically Positive Neck

Clinically apparent regional lymphatic spread to the parotid gland or to cervical lymph nodes should be managed with superficial parotidectomy and comprehensive neck dissection, with likely adjuvant radiation therapy. Originally believed to be a radioresistant tumor, cutaneous melanoma has a radiation response different from that of SCC, demonstrating effective tumor cell death at a higher dose per fraction than that of SCC. As a result, hypofractionation schemes utilizing large-dose fractions have been employed. Adjuvant hypofractionated radiotherapy has been shown to improve 5-year actuarial locoregional control rates for patients with stage II and III disease (206).

COMPLICATIONS OF TREATMENT

Surgery

Complications Following Primary Neck Dissection

Sacrifice of the SAN, SCM, and IJV during RND results in functional morbidity and cosmetic deformity described earlier in the chapter.

Air embolism refers to inadvertent entry of air into the cervical venous system and may occur following laceration of the internal jugular vein. Clinical signs include a precipitous drop in systolic blood pressure, cardiac output, and oxygen saturation, and an audible "to-and-fro" murmur. Further operating should cease immediately, and the following steps instituted: nitrous inhalation anesthesia should be terminated and the patient ventilated with 100% oxygen; the patient should be positioned in the left lateral decubitus position to trap the air embolus in the right atrium; aspiration of the air embolus may then be performed through cardiac puncture or central venous catheterization.

Chylous fistulae may be prevented by meticulous identification and ligation of the thoracic duct prior to division. The terminal branches of the thoracic duct on the left neck are at risk for inadvertent injury during dissection of lymph nodes at level IV. Intraoperative chylous leaks may be recognized by the extravasation of milky fluid at the lower neck, particularly with increased intrathoracic pressure by the Valsalva maneuver. Recognition of chylous fistulae intraoperatively should be treated immediately with suture ligatures or hemoclips. Postoperative chylous fistulae manifest with marked increase in output of milky fluid in suction drains. Conservative management of postoperative chylous fistulae includes cessation of wall suction, with drains on self-suction only, pressure dressings, and low-fat nutritional support. Failure of conservative measures warrants return to the operating room for surgical intervention.

Complications Following Salvage Neck Dissection Post Radiation and Chemoradiation

It is well known that wound healing can be significantly affected by radiotherapy and possibly also by chemotherapy. Wound healing is divided into three stages: the first stage is inflammation, the second stage is the proliferative stage where fibroblasts predominate producing collagen and capillary formation occurs, and the third stage is the maturation stage where disorganized collagen fibrils cross link and increase the tensile strength of the wound. Radiotherapy impairs the proliferative stage of wound healing by impairing the ability of the fibroblasts to produce collagen and by impairing new capillary formation. Irradiated tissue exhibits hypoxia due to occlusion of small blood vessels from endarteritis. The maturation stage is also impaired by reduced collagen cross linking. There seems to be an additive effect to impairment of wound healing when chemotherapy is added with increased obliterative endarteritis (207). As such wound complications following radiotherapy and CTRT are increased and have been reported to be as high as 45% (136). A study by Newman et al. (208) on age, TNM stage, and comorbidity matched patients showed surgical complication rates of 35% in the CTRT group versus 12% in the control group for patients having neck surgery.

Nonsurgical Treatment

In addition to side effects of mucositis and xerostomia, major complications of external beam radiotherapy for SCC of the oral cavity and oropharynx include osteoradionecrosis, pathologic fracture, or ulceration of mucous membranes (209). The risk of osteoradionecrosis necessitates comprehensive dental care prior to the initiation of radiotherapy (210).

Complications associated with RAI therapy following total thyroidectomy for differentiated thyroid cancer include self-limited parotitis. High cumulative doses of RAI have been associated with bone-marrow depression and pulmonary fibrosis.

CONCLUSION

The prognostic significance of cervical metastases from HNSCC necessitates sound management of clinically apparent nodal metastases, as well as thorough screening for detection of occult regional spread. Adequate treatment

planning requires recognition of the relevant anatomy as well as ongoing study into our understanding of the biological mechanisms involved. Further study is necessary to complement our armamentarium particularly in managing advanced cervical metastases, where locoregional control rates remain suboptimal.

REFERENCES

1. Shah JP. Cancer of the upper aerodigestive tract. In: Alfonso AE, Gardner B, eds. The Practice of Cancer Surgery. New York: Appleton-Century-Crofts, 1982.
2. Robbins KT, Clayman G, Levine PA et al. Neck dissection classification update: revisions proposed by the American Head and Neck Society and the American Academy of Otolaryngology-Head and Neck Surgery. Arch Otolaryngol Head Neck Surg 2002; 128: 751–8.
3. Robbins KT, Shaha AR, Medina JE et al. Consensus statement on the classification and terminology of neck dissection. Arch Otolaryngol Head Neck Surg 2008; 134: 536–8.
4. Knudson AG Jr. Hereditary cancer, oncogenes, and antioncogenes. Cancer Res 1985; 45: 1437–43.
5. Fearon ER, Vogelstein B. A genetic model for colorectal tumorigenesis. Cell 1990; 61: 759–67.
6. Califano J, van der RP, Westra W et al. Genetic progression model for head and neck cancer: implications for field cancerization. Cancer Res 1996; 56: 2488–92.
7. Liotta LA. Tumor invasion and metastases: role of the extracellular matrix: Rhoads Memorial Award lecture. Cancer Res 1986; 46: 1–7.
8. Petruzzelli GJ, Benefield J, Yong S. Mechanism of lymph node metastases: current concepts. Otolaryngol Clin North Am 1998; 31: 585–99.
9. Charoenrat P, Modjtahedi H, Rhys-Evans P et al. Epidermal growth factor-like ligands differentially up-regulate matrix metalloproteinase 9 in head and neck squamous carcinoma cells. Cancer Res 2000; 60: 1121–8.
10. Fisch UP. Cervical lymph flow in man following radiation and surgery. Trans Am Acad Ophthalmol Otolaryngol 1965; 69: 846–68.
11. Mickel RA, Kessler DJ, Taylor JM et al. Natural killer cell cytotoxicity in the peripheral blood, cervical lymph nodes, and tumor of head and neck cancer patients. Cancer Res 1988; 48: 5017–22.
12. Wang MB, Lichtenstein A, Mickel RA. Hierarchical immunosuppression of regional lymph nodes in patients with head and neck squamous cell carcinoma. Otolaryngol Head Neck Surg 1991; 105: 517–27.
13. Strauss L, Bergmann C, Szczepanski M et al. A unique subset of CD4+CD25highFoxp3+ T cells secreting interleukin-10 and transforming growth factor-beta1 mediates suppression in the tumor microenvironment. Clin Cancer Res 2007; 13: 4345–54.
14. Berlinger NT, Tsakraklides V, Pollak K et al. Prognostic significance of lymph node histology in patients with squamous cell carcinoma of the larynx, pharynx, or oral cavity. Laryngoscope 1976; 86: 792–803.
15. Gilmore BB, Repola DA, Batsakis JG. Carcinoma of the larynx: lymph node reaction patterns. Laryngoscope 1978; 88: 1333–8.
16. Cernea C, Montenegro F, Castro I et al. Prognostic significance of lymph node reactivity in the control of pathologic negative node squamous cell carcinomas of the oral cavity. Am J Surg 1997; 174: 548–51.
17. Rivoltini L, Gambacorti-Passerini C, Squadrelli-Saraceno M et al. In vivo interleukin 2–induced activation of lymphokine-activated killer cells and tumor cytotoxic T-cells in cervical

lymph nodes of patients with head and neck tumors. Cancer Res 1990; 50: 5551–7.

18. Griffiths CO Jr. Radical neck dissection. Should it be performed with excision of the primary tumor in the presence of clinically uninvolved regional lymph nodes? Effects of regional lymphadenectomy on immunity to simulated new growths in man. Am J Surg 1968; 116: 559–70.

19. Spiro RH, Huvos AG, Wong GY et al. Predictive value of tumor thickness in squamous carcinoma confined to the tongue and floor of the mouth. Am J Surg 1986; 152: 345–50.

20. Bilde AA, von Buchwald CC, Therkildsen MHMH et al. Need for intensive histopathologic analysis to determine lymph node metastases when using sentinel node biopsy in oral cancer. Laryngoscope 2008; 118: 408–14.

21. Kowalski LP, Medina JE. Nodal metastases: predictive factors. Otolaryngol Clin North Am 1998; 31: 621–37.

22. Lindberg R. Distribution of cervical lymph node metastases from squamous cell carcinoma of the upper respiratory and digestive tracts. Cancer 1972; 29: 1446–9.

23. Shah JP. Patterns of cervical lymph node metastasis from squamous carcinomas of the upper aerodigestive tract. Am J Surg 1990; 160: 405–9.

24. Byers RM, Weber RS, Andrews T et al. Frequency and therapeutic implications of 'skip metastases' in the neck from squamous carcinoma of the oral tongue [see comments]. Head Neck 1997; 19: 14–19.

25. O'Brien CJ, Traynor SJ, McNeil E et al. The use of clinical criteria alone in the management of the clinically negative neck among patients with squamous cell carcinoma of the oral cavity and oropharynx. Arch Otolaryngol Head Neck Surg 2000; 126: 360–5.

26. Spiro RH, Morgan GJ, Strong EW et al. Supraomohyoid neck dissection. Am J Surg 1996; 172: 650–3.

27. Medina JE, Byers RM. Supraomohyoid neck dissection: rationale, indications, and surgical technique. Head Neck 1989; 11: 111–22.

28. Woolgar JA. Pathology of the N0 neck. Br J Oral Maxillofac Surg 1999; 37: 205–9.

29. Shah JP. Cervical lymph node metastases: diagnostic, therapeutic, and prognostic implications. Oncology 1990; 4: 61–9.

30. Hillsamer PJ, Schuller DE, McGhee RB Jr et al. Improving diagnostic accuracy of cervical metastases with computed tomography and magnetic resonance imaging [see comments]. Arch Otolaryngol Head Neck Surg 1990; 116: 1297–301.

31. Baatenburg De Jong RJ, Rongen RJ, Lameris JS et al. Metastatic neck disease. Palpation vs ultrasound examination. Arch Otolaryngol Head Neck Surg 1989; 115: 689–90.

32. Castelijns JA, van den Brekel MW. Imaging of lymphadenopathy in the neck. Eur Radiol 2002; 12: 727–38.

33. van den Brekel MW, Castelijns JA. What the clinician wants to know: surgical perspective and ultrasound for lymph node imaging of the neck. Cancer Imaging 2005; 23(Spec No A): S41–9.

34. Ahuja AT, Ying M, Ho SY et al. Ultrasound of malignant cervical lymph nodes. Cancer Imaging 2008; 25: 48–56.

35. Yoon DY, Hwang HS, Chang SK et al. CT, MR, US 18F-FDG PET/CT and their combined use for the assessment of cervical lymph node metastases in squamous cell carcinoma of the head and neck. Eur Radiol 2009; 19: 634–42.

36. van den Brekel MW, Castelijns JA, Snow GB. Diagnostic evaluation of the neck. Otolaryngol Clin North Am 1998; 31: 601–20.

37. Richards PS, Peacock TF. The role of ultrasound in the detection of cervical lymph node metastases in clinically N0 squamous cell carcinoma of the head and neck. Cancer Imaging 2007; 19: 167–78.

38. Adams S, Baum RP, Stuckensen T et al. Prospective comparison of 18F-FDG PET with conventional imaging modalities (CT, MRI, US) in lymph node staging of head and neck cancer. Eur J Nucl Med 1998; 25: 1255–60.

39. Fish SA, Langer JE, Mandel SJ. Sonographic imaging of thyroid nodules and cervical lymph nodes. Endocrinol Metab Clin North Am 2008; 37: 401–17.

40. Langer JE, Mandel SJ. Sonographic imaging of cervical lymph nodes in patients with thyroid cancer. Neuroimaging Clin N Am 2008; 18: 479–89.

41. Kau RJ, Alexiou C, Laubenbacher C et al. Lymph node detection of head and neck squamous cell carcinomas by positron emission tomography with fluorodeoxyglucose F 18 in a routine clinical setting. Arch Otolaryngol Head Neck Surg 1999; 125: 1322–8.

42. McGuirt WF, Williams DW III, Keyes JW Jr et al. A comparative diagnostic study of head and neck nodal metastases using positron emission tomography. Laryngoscope 1995; 105: 373–5.

43. Bailet JW, Abemayor E, Jabour BA et al. Positron emission tomography: a new, precise imaging modality for detection of primary head and neck tumors and assessment of cervical adenopathy. Laryngoscope 1992; 102: 281–8.

44. Fakhry NN, Lussato DD, Jacob TT et al. Comparison between PET and PET/CT in recurrent head and neck cancer and clinical implications. Eur Arch Oto Rhino Laryngol 2007; 264: 531–8.

45. Branstetter BFIV, Blodgett TM, Zimmer LA et al. Head and neck malignancy: is PET/CT more accurate than PET or CT alone? Radiol 2005; 235: 580–6.

46. Schoder H, Yeung HWD, Gonen M et al. Head and neck cancer: clinical usefulness and accuracy of PET/CT image fusion. Radiol 2004; 231: 65–72.

47. Myers LL, Wax MK, Nabi H et al. Positron emission tomography in the evaluation of the N0 neck. Laryngoscope 1998; 108: 232–6.

48. Kyzas PA, Evangelou E, Denaxa-Kyza D et al. 18F-fluorodeoxyglucose positron emission tomography to evaluate cervical node metastases in patients with head and neck squamous cell carcinoma: a meta-analysis. J Natl Cancer Inst 2008; 100: 712–20.

49. McGuirt WF, Greven K, Williams D III et al. PET scanning in head and neck oncology: a review. Head Neck 1998; 20: 208–15.

50. Keyes JW Jr, Chen MY, Watson NE Jr et al. FDG PET evaluation of head and neck cancer: value of imaging the thorax. Head Neck 2000; 22: 105–10.

51. Jungehulsing M, Scheidhauer K, Damm M et al. 2[F]-fluoro-2-deoxy-D-glucose positron emission tomography is a sensitive tool for the detection of occult primary cancer (carcinoma of unknown primary syndrome) with head and neck lymph node manifestation. Otolaryngol Head Neck Surg 2000; 123: 294–301.

52. Greven KM, Keyes JW Jr, Williams DW III et al. Occult primary tumors of the head and neck: lack of benefit from positron emission tomography imaging with 2 [F18]fluoro-2-deoxy-D-glucose. Cancer 1999; 86: 114–8.

53. Bailet JW, Sercarz JA, Abemayor E et al. The use of positron emission tomography for early detection of recurrent head and neck squamous cell carcinoma in postradiotherapy patients. Laryngoscope 1995; 105: 135–9.

54. Farber LA, Benard F, Machtay M et al. Detection of recurrent head and neck squamous cell carcinomas after radiation therapy with 2-18F-fluoro-2-deoxy-D-glucose positron emission tomography. Laryngoscope 1999; 109: 970–5.

55. Berlangieri SU, Brizel DM, Scher RL et al. Pilot study of positron emission tomography in patients with advanced head and neck cancer receiving radiotherapy and chemotherapy. Head Neck 1994; 16: 340–6.

56. Muros MA, Llamas-Elvira JM, Ramirez-Navarro AT et al. Utility of fluorine-18–fluorodeoxyglucose positron emission tomography in differentiated thyroid carcinoma with negative radioiodine scans and elevated serum thyroglobulin levels. Am J Surg 2000; 179: 457–61.

57. Shaha A, Webber C, Marti J. Fine-needle aspiration in the diagnosis of cervical lymphadenopathy. Am J Surg 1986; 152: 420–3.

58. Peters BR, Schnadig VJ, Quinn FB Jr et al. Interobserver variability in the interpretation of fine-needle aspiration biopsy of head and neck masses. Arch Otolaryngol Head Neck Surg 1989; 115: 1438–42.

59. Robbins KT, vanSonnenberg E, Casola G et al. Image-guided needle biopsy of inaccessible head and neck lesions. Arch Otolaryngol Head Neck Surg 1990; 116: 957–61.

60. Davis SP, Anand VK, Dhillon G. Magnetic resonance navigation for head and neck lesions. Laryngoscope 1999; 109: 862–7.

61. Baatenburg De Jong RJ, Knegt P et al. Reduction of the number of neck treatments in patients with head and neck cancer. Cancer 1993; 71: 2312–18.

62. Martin H, Morfit HM, Ehrlich H. The case of branchiogenic cancer (malignant branchioma). Ann Surg 1950; 132: 867–87.

63. Singh B, Balwally AN, Sundaram K et al. Branchial cleft cyst carcinoma: myth or reality? Ann Otol Rhinol Laryngol 1998; 107: 519–24.

64. Pfeiffer J, Kayser G, Technau-Ihling K et al. Ultrasound guided core needle biopsy in the diagnosis of head and neck masses: indications, technique and results. Head Neck 2007; 29: 1033–40.

65. Nyquist GG, Tom WD, Mui S. Automatic core needle biopsy: a diagnostic option for head and neck masses. Arch Otolaryngol Head Neck Surg 2008; 134: 184–9.

66. Carbone A, Ferlito A, Devaney K et al. Ultrasound guided core needle biopsy: is it effective in the diagnosis of suspected lymphomas presenting in the head and neck? J Surg Oncol 2008; 98: 4–5.

67. Mack Y, Parsons JT, Mendenhall WM et al. Squamous cell carcinoma of the head and neck: management after excisional biopsy of a solitary metastatic neck node. Int J Radiat Oncol Biol Phys 1993; 25: 619–22.

68. Ellis ER, Mendenhall WM, Rao PV et al. Incisional or excisional neck-node biopsy before definitive radiotherapy, alone or followed by neck dissection. Head Neck 1991; 13: 177–83.

69. Parsons JT, Million RR, Cassisi NJ. The influence of excisional or incisional biopsy of metastatic neck nodes on the management of head and neck cancer. Int J Radiat Oncol Biol Phys 1985; 11: 1447–54.

70. Robbins KT, Cole R, Marvel J et al. The violated neck: cervical node biopsy prior to definitive treatment. Otolaryngol Head Neck Surg 1986; 94: 605–10.

71. Ambrosch P, Brinck U. Detection of nodal micrometastases in head and neck cancer by serial sectioning and immunostaining. Oncology 1996; 10: 1221–6.

72. Franchi A, Gallo O, Boddi V et al. Prediction of occult neck metastases in laryngeal carcinoma: role of proliferating cell nuclear antigen, MIB-1, and E-cadherin immunohistochemical determination. Clin Cancer Res 1996; 2: 1801–8.

73. Gapany M, Pavelic ZP, Kelley DJ et al. Immunohistochemical detection of c-myc protein in head and neck tumors. Arch Otolaryngol Head Neck Surg 1994; 120: 255–9.

74. Cochran AJ, Wen DR, Morton DL. Occult tumor cells in the lymph nodes of patients with pathological stage I malignant melanoma. An immunohistological study. Am J Surg Pathol 1988; 12: 612–18.

75. Cochran AJ, Roberts A, Wen DR et al. Update on lymphatic mapping and sentinel node biopsy in the management of

patients with melanocytic tumours. Pathology 2004; 36: 478–84.

76. Wang X, Heller R, VanVoorhis N et al. Detection of submicroscopic lymph node metastases with polymerase chain reaction in patients with malignant melanoma. Ann Surg 1994; 220: 768–74.

77. Shivers SC, Wang X, Li W et al. Molecular staging of malignant melanoma: correlation with clinical outcome. JAMA 1998; 280: 1410–15.

78. McMasters KM, Noyes RD, Reintgen DS et al. Lessons learned from the Sunbelt Melanoma Trial. J Surg Oncol 2004; 86: 212–23.

79. Reintgen D, Pendas S, Jakub J et al. National trials involving lymphatic mapping for melanoma: the Multicenter Selective Lymphadenectomy Trial, the Sunbelt Melanoma Trial, and the Florida Melanoma Trial. Semin Oncol 2004; 31: 363–73.

80. Ferris RL, Xi L, Raja S et al. Molecular staging of cervical lymph nodes in squamous cell carcinoma of the head and neck. Cancer Res 2005; 65: 2147–56.

81. Shaha AR. The unknown primary. In: Lucente FE, ed. AAO-HNS Instruction Courses. St Louis, MO: Mosby-Year Book, 1995; 199–204.

82. Johnson JT, Newman RK. The anatomic location of neck metastasis from occult squamous cell carcinoma. Otolaryngol Head Neck Surg 1981; 89: 54–8.

83. Barrie JR, Knapper WH, Strong EW. Cervical nodal metastases of unknown origin. Am J Surg 1970; 120: 466–70.

84. Spiro RH, DeRose G, Strong EW. Cervical node metastasis of occult origin. Am J Surg 1983; 146: 441–6.

85. Davidson BJ, Spiro RH, Patel S et al. Cervical metastases of occult origin: the impact of combined modality therapy. Am J Surg 1994; 168: 395–9.

86. Randall DA, Johnstone PA, Foss RD et al. Tonsillectomy in diagnosis of the unknown primary tumor of the head and neck. Otolaryngol Head Neck Surg 2000; 122: 52–5.

87. Koch WM, Bhatti N, Williams MF et al. Oncologic rationale for bilateral tonsillectomy in head and neck squamous cell carcinoma of unknown primary source. Otolaryngol Head Neck Surg 2001; 124: 331–3.

88. American Joint Committee on Cancer. AJCC Cancer Staging Manual, 6th ed. Philadelphia: Lippincott Raven Publishers, 2002.

89. American Joint Committee on Cancer. AJCC Cancer Staging Manual, 5th ed. New York: Lippincott-Raven, 1997.

90. Hinerman RW, Mendenhall WM, Amdur RJ et al. Carcinoma of the supraglottic larynx: treatment results with radiotherapy alone or with planned neck dissection. Head Neck 2002; 24: 456–7.

91. Matsuo JM, Patel SG, Singh B et al. Clinical nodal stage is an independently significant predictor of distant failure in patients with squamous cell carcinoma of the larynx. Ann Surg. 2003; 238: 412–21; discussion 421–2.

92. Snow GB, Annyas AA, van Slooten EA et al. Prognostic factors of neck node metastasis. Clin Otolaryngol 1982; 7: 185–92.

93. Johnson JT, Barnes EL, Myers EN et al. The extracapsular spread of tumors in cervical node metastasis. Arch Otolaryngol 1981; 107: 725–9.

94. Noguchi M, Kido Y, Kubota H et al. Prognostic factors and relative risk for survival in N1–3 oral squamous cell carcinoma: a multivariate analysis using Cox's hazard model. Br J Oral Maxillofac Surg 1999; 37: 433–7.

95. Glanz H, Popella C. Intrinsic weakness of the N/pN classification and proposal of a new pN classification. Presented at the 5th International Conference on Head and Neck Cancer, San Francisco, July 2000.

96. Kowalski LP, Bagietto R, Lara JR et al. Prognostic significance of the distribution of neck node metastasis from oral carcinoma. Head Neck 2000; 22: 207–14.

97. Chelius JM. A System of Surgery. Philadelphia: Lea and Blanchard, 1847.

98. Kocher ET. Uber radicalheilung des Krebses. Deutsche Chir 1880; 13: 134–66.

99. Crile GW. Excision of cancer of the head and neck with special reference to the plan of dissection based on one hundred and thirty-two operations. JAMA 1906; 47: 1780–6.

100. Martin H, DelValle B, Ehrlich H et al. Neck dissection. Cancer 1951; 4: 441–99.

101. Schuller DE, Reiches NA, Hamaker RC et al. Analysis of disability resulting from treatment including radical neck dissection or modified neck dissection. Head Neck Surg 1983; 6: 551–8.

102. Robbins KT, Medina JE, Wolfe GT et al. Standardizing neck dissection terminology. Official report of the Academy's Committee for Head and Neck Surgery and Oncology [see comments]. Arch Otolaryngol Head Neck Surg 1991; 117: 601–5.

103. Robbins KT. Classification of neck dissection: current concepts and future considerations. Otolaryngol Clin North Am 1998; 31: 639–55.

104. Medina JE. A rational classification of neck dissections. Otolaryngol Head Neck Surg 1989; 100: 169–76.

105. Agrama MT, Reiter D, Topham AK et al. Node counts in neck dissection: are they useful in outcomes research? Otolaryngol Head Neck Surg 2001; 124: 433–5.

106. Bhattacharyya N. The effects of more conservative neck dissections and radiotherapy on nodal yields from the neck. Arch Otolaryngol Head Neck Surg 1998; 124: 412–16.

107. Busaba NY, Fabian RL. Extent of lymphadenectomy achieved by various modifications of neck dissection: a pathologic analysis. Laryngoscope 1999; 109: 212–15.

108. Friedman M, Lim JW, Dickey W et al. Quantification of lymph nodes in selective neck dissection. Laryngoscope 1999; 109: 368–70.

109. Shah JP, Candela FC, Poddar AK. The patterns of cervical lymph node metastases from squamous carcinoma of the oral cavity. Cancer 1990; 66: 109–13.

110. Wang CC. Radiation therapy in the management of oral malignant disease. Otolaryngol Clin North Am 1979; 12: 73–80.

111. Bentzen SM, Thames HD. Tumor volume and local control probability: clinical data and radiobiological interpretations. Int J Radiat Oncol Biol Phys 1996; 36: 247–51.

112. Mothersill C, Seymour CB, O'Brien A et al. Proliferation of normal and malignant human epithelial cells post irradiation. Acta Oncol 1991; 30: 851–8.

113. Ravi D, Ramadas K, Mathew BS et al. Apoptosis, angiogenesis and proliferation: trifunctional measure of tumour response to radiotherapy for oral cancer. Oral Oncol 2001; 37: 164–71.

114. Strong EW. Preoperative radiation and radical neck dissection. Surg Clin North Am 1969; 49: 271–6.

115. Kramer S, Gelber RD, Snow JB et al. Combined radiation therapy and surgery in the management of advanced head and neck cancer: final report of study 73-03 of the Radiation Therapy Oncology Group. Head Neck Surg 1987; 10: 19–30.

116. Vikram B, Strong EW, Shah JP et al. Failure in the neck following multimodality treatment for advanced head and neck cancer. Head Neck Surg 1984; 6: 724–9.

117. Huang DT, Johnson CR, Schmidt-Ullrich R et al. Postoperative radiotherapy in head and neck carcinoma with extracapsular lymph node extension and/or positive resection margins: a comparative study. Int J Radiat Oncol Biol Phys 1992; 23: 737–42.

118. Coster JR, Foote RL, Olsen KD et al. Cervical nodal metastasis of squamous cell carcinoma of unknown origin: indications for withholding radiation therapy. Int J Radiat Oncol Biol Phys 1992; 23: 743–9.

119. Colletier PJ, Garden AS, Morrison WH et al. Postoperative radiation for squamous cell carcinoma metastatic to cervical lymph nodes from an unknown primary site: outcomes and patterns of failure. Head Neck 1998; 20: 674–81.

120. Cooper JS, Pajak TF, Forastiere AA et al. Postoperative concurrent radiotherapy and chemotherapy for high-risk squamous-cell carcinoma of the head and neck. N Engl J Med 2004; 350: 1937–44.

121. Bernier J, Domenge C, Ozsahin M et al. Postoperative irradiation with or without concomitant chemotherapy for locally advanced head and neck cancer. N Engl J Med 2004; 350: 1945–52.

122. Adelstein DJ, Saxton JP, Lavertu P et al. A phase III randomized trial comparing concurrent chemotherapy and radiotherapy with radiotherapy alone in resectable stage III and IV squamous cell head and neck cancer: preliminary results. Head Neck 1997; 19: 567–75.

123. Calais G, Alfonsi M, Bardet E et al. Randomized trial of radiation therapy versus concomitant chemotherapy and radiation therapy for advanced-stage oropharynx carcinoma. J Natl Cancer Inst 1999; 91: 2081–6.

124. Al Sarraf M, LeBlanc M, Giri PG et al. Chemoradiotherapy versus radiotherapy in patients with advanced nasopharyngeal cancer: phase III randomized Intergroup study 0099. J Clin Oncol 1998; 16: 1310–17.

125. Taylor SG, Murthy AK, Vannetzel JM et al. Randomized comparison of neoadjuvant cisplatin and fluorouracil infusion followed by radiation versus concomitant treatment in advanced head and neck cancer. J Clin Oncol 1994; 12: 385–95.

126. Lavertu P, Adelstein DJ, Saxton JP et al. Management of the neck in a randomized trial comparing concurrent chemotherapy and radiotherapy with radiotherapy alone in resectable stage III and IV squamous cell head and neck cancer. Head Neck 1997; 19: 559–66.

127. Sewall GK, Palazzi-Churas KL, Richards GM et al. Planned postradiotherapy neck dissection: rationale and clinical outcomes. Laryngoscope 2007; 117: 121–8.

128. Gourin CG, Williams HT, Seabolt WN et al. Utility of positron emission tomography-computed tomography in identification of residual nodal disease after chemoradiation for advanced head and neck cancer. Laryngoscope 2006; 116: 705–10.

129. Brizel DM, Prosnitz RG, Hunter S et al. Necessity for adjuvant neck dissection in setting of concurrent chemoradiation for advanced head and neck cancer. Int J Radiat Oncol Biol Phys 2004; 58: 1418–23.

130. Corry J, Peters L, Fisher R et al. N2-N3 neck nodal control without planned neck dissection for clinical/radiologic complete responders – results of Trans Tasman Radiation Oncology Group Study 98.02. Head Neck 2008; 30: 737–42.

131. Lau H, Phan T, Mackinnon J et al. Absence of planned neck dissection for the N2-N3 neck after chemoradiation for locally advanced squamous cell carcinoma of the head and neck. Arch Otolaryngol Head Neck 2008; 134: 257–61.

132. Rengan R, Pfister DG, Lee NY et al. Long term neck control rates after complete response to chemoradiation in patients with advanced head and neck cancer. Am J Clin Oncol 2008; 31: 465–9.

133. Mukhija V, Gupta S, Jacobson AS et al. Selective neck dissection following adjuvant therapy for advanced head and neck cancer. Head Neck 2009; 31: 183–8.

134. Ong SC, Schöder H, Lee NY et al. Clinical utility of 18F-FDG PET/CT in assessing the neck after concurrent chemoradiotherapy for locoregional advanced head and neck cancer. J Nucl Med 2008; 49: 532–40.

135. Lavertu P, Bonafede JP, Adelstein DJ et al. Comparison of surgical complications after organ preservation therapy in patients with stage III and IV squamous cell head and neck cancer. Arch Otolaryngol Head Neck Surg 1998; 124: 401–6.

136. Donatelli-Lassig AA, Duffy SA, Fowler KE et al. The effect of neck dissection on quality of life after chemoradiation. Otolaryngol Head Neck Surg 2008; 139: 511–18.

137. Robbins KT, Shannon K, Vieira F. Superselective neck dissection after chemoradiation: feasibility based on clinical and pathologic comparisons. Arch Otolaryngol Head Neck 2007; 133: 486–9.

138. Sandhu A, Rao N, Giri S et al. Role and extent of neck dissection for persistent nodal disease following chemoradiation for locally advanced head and neck cancer: how much is enough. Acta Oncol 2008; 47: 948–53.

139. Bocca E, Pignatato O, Oldini C et al. Functional neck dissection: an evaluation and review of 843 cases. Laryngoscope 1984; 94: 942–5.

140. Kowalski L. Feasibility of supraomohyoid neck dissection in N1 and N2a oral cancer patients. Head Neck 2002; 24: 921–4.

141. Traynor S. Selective neck dissection and the management of the node-positive neck. Am J Surg 1996; 172: 654–7.

142. Pellitteri PK, Robbins KT, Neuman T. Expanded application of selective neck dissection with regard to nodal status. Head Neck 1997; 19: 260–5.

143. Chepeha D. Selective neck dissection for the treatment of neck metastasis from squamous cell carcinoma of the head and neck. Laryngoscope 2002; 112: 434–8.

144. Gourin CG. Is selective neck dissection adequate treatment for node-positive disease? Arch Otolaryngol Head Neck Surg 2004; 130: 1431–4.

145. Wei WI, Lam KH, Ho CM et al. Efficacy of radical neck dissection for the control of cervical metastasis after radiotherapy for nasopharyngeal carcinoma. Am J Surg 1990; 160: 439–42.

146. Weiss MH, Harrison LB, Isaacs RS. Use of decision analysis in planning a management strategy for the stage N0 neck. Arch Otolaryngol Head Neck Surg 1994; 120: 699–702.

147. Andersen PE, Cambronero E, Shaha AR et al. The extent of neck disease after regional failure during observation of the N0 neck. Am J Surg 1996; 172: 689–91.

148. Vandenbrouck C, Sancho-Garnier H, Chassagne D et al. Elective versus therapeutic radical neck dissection in epidermoid carcinoma of the oral cavity: results of a randomized clinical trial. Cancer 1980; 46: 386–90.

149. Hughes CJ, Gallo O, Spiro RH et al. Management of occult neck metastasis in oral cavity squamous carcinoma. Am J Surg 1993; 166: 380–3.

150. Suarez O. El problema se las metastasis linfticas y alejadas del cancer de laringe e hipofaringe. Rev Otorhinolaryngol 1963; 23: 83–9.

151. Bocca E, Pignataro O. A conservation technique in radical neck dissection. Ann Otol Rhinol Laryngol 1967; 76: 975–87.

152. Spiro JD, Spiro RH, Shah JP et al. Critical assessment of supraomohyoid neck dissection. Am J Surg 1988; 156: 286–9.

153. Byers RM. Modified neck dissection. A study of 967 cases from 1970 to 1980. Am J Surg 1985; 150: 414–21.

154. Elsheikh MN, Rinaldo A, Ferlito A et al. Elective supraomohyoid neck dissection for oral cavity squamous cell carcinoma: is dissection of sublevel IIB necessary. Oral Oncol 2008; 44: 216–19.

155. Davidson BJ, Kulkarny V, Delacure MD et al. Posterior triangle metastases of squamous cell carcinoma of the upper aerodigestive tract. Am J Surg 1993; 166: 395–8.

156. Coskun HH, Erisen L, Basut O. Selective neck dissection for clinically N0 neck in laryngeal cancer: is dissection of

157. Ferlito A, Silver CE, Rinaldo A. Selective neck dissection (IIA, III): a rational replacement for complete functional neck dissection in patients with N0 supraglottic and glottic squamous carcinoma. Laryngoscope 2008; 118: 676–9.

158. Koch WM, Choti MA, Civelek AC et al. Gamma probe-directed biopsy of the sentinel node in oral squamous cell carcinoma. Arch Otolaryngol Head Neck Surg 1998; 124: 455–9.

159. Shoaib T, Soutar DS, MacDonald DG et al. The accuracy of head and neck carcinoma sentinel lymph node biopsy in the clinically N0 neck. Cancer 2001; 91: 2077–83.

160. Ross G, Shoaib T, Soutar DS et al. The use of sentinel node biopsy to upstage the clinically N0 neck in head and neck cancer. Arch Otolaryngol Head Neck Surg 2002; 128: 1287–91.

161. Ross GL, Soutar DS, MacDonald DG et al. Sentinel node biopsy in head and neck cancer: preliminary results of a multicenter trial. Ann Surg Oncol 2004; 11: 690–6.

162. Ross GL, Shoaib T, Soutar DS et al. The first international conference on sentinel node biopsy in mucosal head and neck cancer and adoption of a multicenter trial protocol. Ann Surg Oncol 2002; 9: 406–10.

163. Pitman KT, Johnson JT, Brown ML et al. Sentinel lymph node biopsy in head and neck squamous cell carcinoma. Laryngoscope 2002; 112: 2101–13.

164. Côté V, Kost K, Payne RJ et al. Sentinel lymph node biopsy in squamous cell carcinoma of the head and neck: where we stand now, and where we are going. J Otolaryngol 2007; 36: 344–9.

165. Alex JC. The application of sentinel node radiolocalization to solid tumors of the head and neck: a 10-year experience. Laryngoscope 2004; 114: 2–19.

166. Wagner AA, Kermer CC, Zettinig GG et al. Validity of sentinel lymph node (SLN) detection following adjuvant radiochemotherapy (RCT) in head and neck squamous cell carcinoma (HNSCC). Technol Cancer Res Treat 2007; 6: 655–60.

167. Rabuzzi DD, Chung CT, Sagerman RH. Prophylactic neck irradiation. Arch Otolaryngol 1980; 106: 454–5.

168. Mendenhall WM, Million RR, Cassisi NJ. Elective neck irradiation in squamous-cell carcinoma of the head and neck. Head Neck Surg 1980; 3: 15–20.

169. Weissler MC, Weigel MT, Rosenman JG et al. Treatment of the clinically negative neck in advanced cancer of the head and neck. Arch Otolaryngol Head Neck Surg 1989; 115: 691–4.

170. Argiris A, Smoth SM, Stenson K et al. Concurrent chemoradiotherapy for N2 and N3 squamous cell carcinoma of the head and neck from an occult primary. Ann Oncol 2003; 14: 1306–11.

171. McGuirt WF. Management of occult metastatic disease from salivary gland neoplasms. Arch Otolaryngol Head Neck Surg 1989; 115: 322–5.

172. Armstrong JG, Harrison LB, Thaler HT et al. The indications for elective treatment of the neck in cancer of the major salivary glands. Cancer 1992; 69: 615–9.

173. Klussman JP, Ponert T, Mueller RP et al. Patterns of lymph node spread and its influence on outcome in resectable parotid cancer. Eur J Surg Oncol 2008; 34: 932–7.

174. Armstrong JG, Harrison LB, Spiro RH et al. Malignant tumors of major salivary gland origin. A matched-pair analysis of the role of combined surgery and postoperative radiotherapy. Arch Otolaryngol Head Neck Surg 1990; 116: 290–3.

175. Douglas JG, Laramore GE, Austin-Seymour M et al. Treatment of locally advanced adenoid cystic carcinoma of the

head and neck with neutron radiotherapy. Int J Radiat Oncol Biol Phys 2000; 46: 551–7.

176. Qubain SW, Nakano S, Baba M et al. Distribution of lymph node micrometastaes in pN0 well differentiated thyroid carcinoma. Surgery 2002; 13: 249–56.

177. Attie JN, Khafif RA, Steckler RM. Elective neck dissection in papillary carcinoma of the thyroid. Am J Surg 1971; 122: 464–71.

178. Machens A, Hinze R, Thomusch O et al. Pattern of nodal metastases for primary and reoperative thyroid cancer. World J Surg 2002; 26: 22–8.

179. Wada N, Duh QY, Sugino K et al. Lymph nodemetastasis from 259 papillary thyroid microcarcinomas: frequency, pattern of occurrence and recurrence, and optimal strategy for neck dissection. Ann Surg 2003; 237: 399–407.

180. Mirallie E, Vissset J, Sagan C et al. Localisation of cervica node metastases of papillary thyroid carcinoma. World J Surg 1999; 23: 970–3.

181. Shaha AR, Shah JP, Loree TR. Risk group stratification and prognostic factors in papillary carcinoma of thyroid. Ann Surg Oncol 1996; 3: 534–8.

182. Hundahl SA, Fleming ID, Fremgen AM et al. A National Cancer Data Base report on 53,856 cases of thyroid carcinoma treated in the US, 1985–1995. Cancer 1998; 83: 2638–48.

183. Hughes CJ, Shaha AR, Shah JP et al. Impact of lymph node metastasis in differentiated thyroid carcinoma of the thyroid: a matched pair analysis. Head Neck 1996; 18: 127–32.

184. Sato N, Oyamatsu M, Koyama Y et al. Do the level of nodal disease according to the TNM classification and the number of involved cervical nodes reflect prognosis in patients with differentiated carcinoma of the throid gland? J Surg Oncol 1998; 69: 151–5.

185. Scheumann GF, Gimm O, Wegener G et al. Prognostic significance and surgical management of locoregional lymph node metastases in papillary thyroid cancer. World J Surg 1994; 18: 559–67.

186. Lundgren CI, Hall P, Dickman PW et al. Clinically significant prognostic factors for differentiated thyroid carcinoma: a population based, nested case control study. Cancer 2006; 106: 524–31.

187. Sugitani I, Yanagisawa A, Shimizu A et al. Clinicopathplogic and immunohistochemical studies of papillary thyroid microcarcinoma presenting with cervical lymphadenopathy. World J Surg 1998; 22: 731–7.

188. Kitajiri S, Hiraumi H, Hirose T et al. The presence of large lymph node metastasis as a prognostic factor of papillary thyroic carcinoma. Auris Nasus Larynx 2003; 30: 169–74.

189. Tisell LE, Nilsson B, Molne J et al. Improved survival of patients with papillary thyroid carcinoma after surgical microdissection. World J Surg 1996; 20: 854–7.

190. Lee YS, Kim SW, Kim SW et al. Extent of routine central lymph node dissection with small papillary thyroid carcinoma. World J Surg 2007; 31: 1954–9.

191. Cooper DS, Doherty GM, Haugen BR, et al. Management guidelines for patients with thyroid nodules and differentiated thyroid cancer. Thyroid 2006; 16: 109–42.

192. Ito Y, Jikuzono T, Higashiyama T et al. Clinical significance of lymph node metastasis of papillary thyroid carcinoma located in one lobe. World J Surgery 2006; 30: 1821–8.

193. Khafif A, Ben-Yosef R, Abergel A et al. Elective paratracheal neck dissection for lateral metastases from papillary carcinoma of the thyroid: is it indicated? Head Neck 2008; 30: 306–10.

194. Pingpank JF Jr, Sasson AR, Hanlon AL et al. Tumor above the spinal accessory nerve in papillary thyroid cancer that involves lateral neck nodes: a common occurrence. Arch Otolaryngol Head Neck Surg 2002; 128: 1275–8.

195. Kupferman ME, Patterson M, Mandel SJ et al. Patterns of lateral neck metastasis in papillary thyroid carcinoma. Arch Otolaryngol Head Neck Surg 2004; 130: 857–60.

196. Roh JL, Kim JM, Park CI. Lateral cervical lymph node metastases from papillary thyroid carcinoma: pattern of nodal metastases and optimal strategy for neck dissection. Ann Surg Oncol 2007; 15: 1177–82.

197. Turanli S. Is the type of dissection in lateral neck metastasis for differentiated thyroid carcinoma important? Otolaryngol Head Neck Surg 2007; 136: 957–60.

198. Balch CM, Soong SJ, Bartolucci AA et al. Efficacy of an elective regional lymph node dissection of 1 to 4mm thick melanomas for patients 60 years of age and younger. Ann Surg 1996; 224: 255–63.

199. Balch CM, Cascinelli N, Sim FH et al. Elective lymph node dissection: results of prospective randomized surgical trials. In: Balch CM, ed., Cutaneous Oncology. St. Louis, MO: Quality Medical Publishing, 1998: 209–26.

200. Sim FH, Taylor WF, Ivins JC et al. A prospective randomized study of the efficacy of routine elective lymphadenectomy in management of malignant melanoma. Preliminary results. Cancer 1978; 41: 948–56.

201. Veronesi U, Adamus J, Bandiera DC et al. Inefficacy of immediate node dissection in stage 1 melanoma of the limbs. N Engl J Med 1977; 297: 627–30.

202. Coates AS, Ingvar CI, Petersen-Schaefer K et al. Elective lymph node dissection in patients with primary melanoma of the trunk and limbs treated at the Sydney Melanoma unit from 1960 to 1991. J Am Coll Surg 1995; 180: 402–9.

203. Morton DL, Cagle LA, Wong JH et al. Intraoperative lymphatic mapping and selective lymphadenectomy: technical details of a new procedure for clinical stage I melanoma. Presented at the Annual Meeting of the Society of Surgical Oncology, Washington DC, 1990.

204. Patel SG, Coit DG, Shaha AR et al. Sentinel lymph node biopsy for cutaneous head and neck melanomas. Arch Otolaryngol Head Neck Surg. 2002; 128: 285–91.

205. Tanis PJ, Nieweg OE, van den Brekel MW et al. Dilemma of clinically node negative head and neck melanoma: outcome of watch and wait policy, elective lymph node dissection, and sentinel node biopsy-a systematic review. Head Neck 2008; 30: 380–9.

206. Ang KK, Peters LJ, Weber RS et al. Postoperative radiotherapy for cutaneous melanoma of the head and neck region. Int J Radiat Oncol Biol Phys 1994; 30: 795–8.

207. Drake DB, Oishi SN. Wound healing considerations in chemotherapy and radiation therapy. Clin Plast Surg 1995; 22: 31–7.

208. Newman JP, Terris DJ, Pinto HA et al. Surgical morbidity of neck dissection after chemoradiotherapy in advanced head and neck cancer. Ann Otol Rhinol Laryngol 1997; 106: 117–22.

209. Larson DL, Lindberg RD, Lane E et al. Major complications of radiotherapy in cancer of the oral cavity and oropharynx. A 10 year retrospective study. Am J Surg 1983; 146: 531–6.

210. Marx RE, Johnson RP. Studies in the radiobiology of osteoradionecrosis and their clinical significance. Oral Surg Oral Med Oral Pathol 1987; 64: 379–90.

16

Tumors of the Upper Jaw and Anterior Skull Base

Valerie J Lund

SELECTED ANATOMY

The maxillary and anterior ethmoidal sinuses arise as out-pouchings from the lateral nasal wall at an early stage of fetal development. At birth small maxillary, ethmoid, and sphenoid sinuses are present. The sphenoid may be regarded as embryologically arising from a posterior ethmoidal cell whereas the frontal sinuses do not begin to develop until some months after birth and should be regarded developmentally as deriving from the anterior ethmoidal system.

The maxillary, frontal, and anterior ethmoidal cells drain into the middle meatus. This area together with the middle turbinate, which overlies it, is a frequent site for deposition of carcinogenic particulate matter. The posterior ethmoids drain into the superior meatus whereas the sphenoid sinus drains most posterosuperiorly into the sphenoethmoidal recess.

All the paranasal sinuses have an intimate relationship with the orbit from which they are divided by relatively thin and sometimes dehiscent bone; for example the lamina papyracea, the infraorbital canal; whereas the frontal and ethmoidal sinuses together with the superior nasal cavity are directly related to the anterior cranial fossa (Fig. 16.1). Similarly diseases of the sphenoid may spread into the cavernous sinus and middle cranial fossa (and involve the internal carotid artery). Thus, although the lymphatic drainage of the sinuses and nasal cavity is poor, disease may spread directly into adjacent structures with catastrophic results.

CLASSIFICATION
Site

The late presentation of patients often makes it difficult to distinguish the exact origin of sinonasal malignancy. The maxillary sinus is regarded as the most common site, but lesions often arise within the middle meatus, involving the ethmoids, nasal cavity, and maxillary antrum from an early stage of the disease. The ICD code 160, which also includes the middle ear, does not separate individual paranasal sinuses though primary malignancy of the frontal and sphenoid sinuses is extremely rare.

Histology

The sinonasal region suffers from the greatest histological diversity in the body and every tumor type, both benign and malignant can be encountered (Table 16.1).

Nonetheless, squamous cell carcinoma (SCC) is the commonest malignancy, as in the rest of the aerodigestive tract and epithelial tumors predominate overall.

Accurate histological diagnosis can prove difficult because of the rarity and diversity of these tumors. The term *anaplastic* should be treated with caution as when immunohistochemistry is performed these tumors may prove to be poorly differentiated SCC, an olfactory neuroblastoma, malignant melanoma, or lymphoma.

Metastatic spread, the sine qua non of malignancy, is infrequently encountered as patients more often die of local disease before secondary spread is manifest. By contrast the concept of a benign tumor must be reevaluated in this area due to the proximity of vital structures.

NATURAL HISTORY
General Considerations
Presentation

From the maxilla the tumor may spread into the nasal cavity producing nasal obstruction and discharge that may be blood stained. Involvement of the infraorbital canal may produce pain and paraesthesia in the distribution of the infraorbital nerve, extension into the soft tissues of the cheek, or spread into the orbit (Fig. 16.2). This may produce displacement of the globe with proptosis, diplopia, epiphora, and chemosis; infiltration of the orbital structures leads to fixation of the globe and visual loss. Extension through the maxillary floor may occur through the dental roots to produce loosening of the teeth and/or a malignant oroantral fistula or erosion of the hard palate producing a mass or ulceration. Posterior extension into the pterygoid and infratemporal fossa may produce pain and trismus (Fig. 16.3).

Spread from the ethmoid sinuses will involve the nasal cavity on one or both sides and the orbit with symptoms as before. Superior extension into the anterior cranial fossa is generally silent and not associated with headache, cerebrospinal fluid (CSF) leaks, or meningitis (Fig. 16.4).

The middle cranial fossa may also be extensively involved at presentation either from the anterior cranial fossa or via the orbital apex (Fig. 16.5). Specific cranial nerve palsies may also result from involvement of the cavernous sinus (either via the orbital apex or sphenoid sinus) or from tumor spread through the foramen ovale.

Tumors of the nasal cavity in addition to symptoms of blockage, discharge, and occasionally bleeding may obstruct the Eustachian tube producing a serous otitis media, spread around the maxillary spine to affect the hard palate

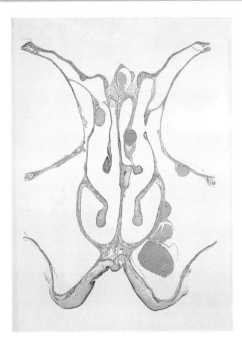

Figure 16.1 A coronal section from midfacial block (haematoxylin and eosin) showing proximity of orbit and anterior cranial fossa to nasal cavity and paranasal sinuses.

Table 16.1 Histological Range of Sinonasal Malignancy

Epithelial	
Epidermoid/ Squamous	Carcinoma (spindle cell, verrucous, transitional)
Nonepidermoid	Adenocarcinoma
	Adenoid cystic carcinoma
	Mucoepidermoid carcinoma
	Acinic cell carcinoma
	Metastases
Neuroectodermal	Malignant melanoma
	Olfactory neuroblastoma
	Neuroendocrine carcinoma
	Sinonasal undifferentiated carcinoma (SNUC)
	Peripheral neuroectodermal tumor/extraosseous
	Ewings sarcoma
	Mesenchymal
Vascular	Angiosarcoma
	Kaposi's sarcoma
	Hemagiopericytoma
Muscular	Leiomyosarcoma
	Rhabdomyosarcoma
	Chondrosarcoma (and mesenchymal)
Osseous	Osteosarcoma
Lymphoreticular	Burkitt's lymphoma
	Non-Hodgkin's lymphoma
	Extramedullary plasmacytoma
	T/NK lymphoma
	Fibrosarcoma
	Liposarcoma
	Malignant fibrous histiocytoma
	Alveolar soft part sarcoma

Abbreviation: T/NK, T cell/Natural Killer.

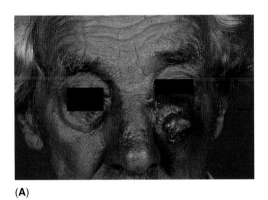

(A)

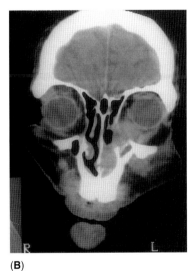

(B)

Figure 16.2 (A) Clinical photograph of patient with squamous cell carcinoma of the left maxilla extending into the orbit and facial soft tissues. (B) Coronal CT scan showing anterior extent of disease.

and anteriorly infiltrate, erode and/or splay the nasal bones to produce a mass in the region of the glabella (Fig. 16.6).

Risk Factors and Associations

A number of occupations have been linked with the development of sinonasal malignancy. In 1968 Acheson et al. (1) observed a high frequency of adenocarcinoma of the ethmoids in the woodworkers of the High Wycombe area in the U.K., which has been subsequently confirmed from many other parts of the world. The association is with hardwood dust exposure, for example, mahogany where fine dust of no more than 5 μm diameter is deposited in the middle meatus (2,3). The relative risk for a woodworker developing adenocarcinoma is 70 times that of a nonwoodworker.

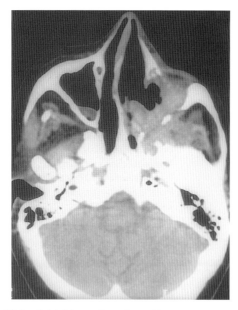

Figure 16.3   Axial CT scan in patient with recurrent squamous cell carcinoma showing infiltration of pterygoid and infratemporal regions.

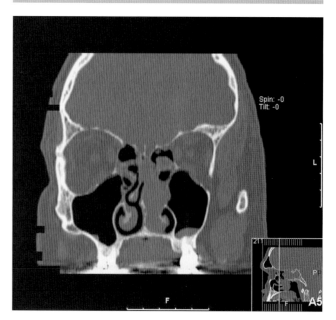

Figure 16.4   Coronal computed tomography showing extension of olfactory neuroblastoma up to skull base with early erosion of cribriform niche.

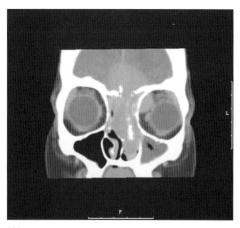

(A)

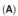

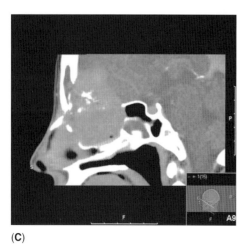

(C)

(B)

Figure 16.5   Computed tomography with contrast **(A)** coronal, **(B)** axial, and **(C)** sagittal view of an extensive sinonasal undifferentiated carcinoma.

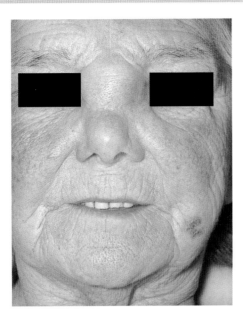

Figure 16.6 Clinical photograph showing infiltration of glabellar region by adenocarcinoma.

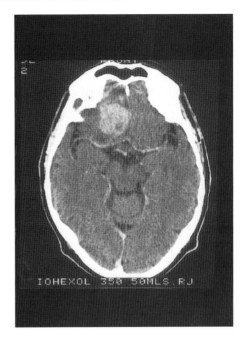

Figure 16.7 Axial CT scan of brain showing secondary deposit in frontal lobe of squamous cell carcinoma.

Adenocarcinoma has also been associated with the manufacture of chrome pigment, isopropyl alcohol, textiles, clothing, leather, and shoes though many patients with adenocarcinoma have no predisposing factors (4).

SCC has been linked with nickel refining, exposure to soft wood dust, and historically with radium dial painting and mustard gas manufacture (5). Cigarette smoking and alcohol have less impact in this area than elsewhere in the head and neck.

Incidence

Sinonasal malignancy is rare, constituting approximately 3% of head and neck cancer (excluding tumors of the external nose). Global figures suggest an incidence of fewer than 1 per 100,000 people per year in most countries though occupational factors may produce regional differences.

Sex Ratio

The male/female ratio for sinonasal malignancy is approximately 2:1 except where occupational factors impact.

Age Range

In our own cohort of nearly 800 cases of sinonasal malignancy, the age range is 5 to 88 years with the majority presenting between 50 and 69.

Pathophysiology/Modes of Spread

Sinonasal malignancy impacts most dramatically by local spread into the adjacent structures such as the orbit, skull base, cheek, oral cavity, nasopharynx, pterygoid, and infratemporal fossae.

Lymphatic Spread

The relatively poor lymphatic drainage of the nose and paranasal sinuses means that cervical lymphadenopathy is

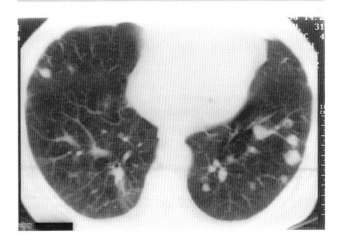

Figure 16.8 Axial CT scan of lung showing multiple deposits from squamous cell carcinoma of the antroethmoid.

relatively uncommon at presentation and is generally less than 10% during the course of the disease depending on the histology. The submandibular and jugulodigastric nodes are most frequently affected, particularly from SCC of the vestibule and columella where the cervical lymphadenopathy may be bilateral.

Hematological Spread

Hematological spread to bone, brain, lung, liver, and skin is also uncommon, generally occurring in the later stages of malignancies (Figs. 16.7–16.9). Adenoid cystic carcinoma is well known for its ability to spread along perineural

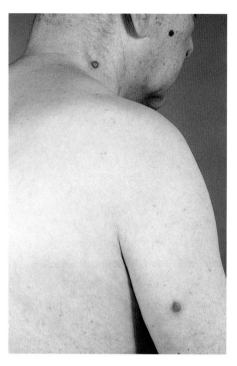

Figure 16.9 Clinical photograph showing skin metastases on neck and upper arm from poorly differentiated squamous cell carcinoma.

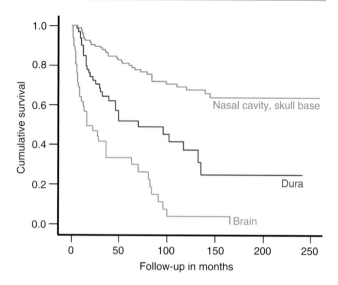

Figure 16.10 Actuarial survival Kaplan Meier curve in 308 craniofacial patients showing effect on prognosis of involvement of skull base alone, dura, and frontal lobes. *Source*: From Ref. 6.

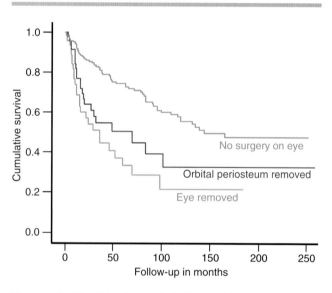

Figure 16.11 Actuarial survival Kaplan Meier curve in 308 craniofacial patients showing effect on prognosis of orbital involvement. *Source*: From Ref. 6.

lymphatics but may also embolize along adjacent cranial nerves and not infrequently metastases to the lungs.

Prognostic Factors

There have been a number of papers considering factors that influence prognosis. In general these relate to the extent of disease and histology. A multivariate analysis of 308 patients undergoing craniofacial resection of which 259 were for malignant tumors primarily of the ethmoid and nasal cavity demonstrated infiltration of the brain (as opposed to tumor onto dura) followed by infiltration of the orbit as the worst prognostic factors (6) (Figs. 16.10 and 16.11). The extent of orbital involvement has been classified because of its prognostic significance (7–9). From the maxilla, extensions into the pterygoid and infratemporal fossae offer the worst outcome (10) whereas invasion of the sphenoid was independently identified as significant in 100 tumors affecting the anterior skull base (8). In addition male sex, increasing age, and use of radiotherapy independently predicted poorer survival in a multi-institutional review of 783 cases of cancer of the nasal cavity, of which nearly half were squamous cell (11).

Tumors of the columella and nasal vestibule also have a poor survival largely due to bilateral lymphatic spread to the submandibular and jugulodigastric nodes at an early stage of disease. Generally lymphatic involvement signifies poor prognosis (9,11–13).

Similarly, although rare, secondary deposits in the bone, brain, lung, and liver invariably herald a rapid demise with the exception of adenoid cystic carcinoma where patients may survive up to 7 or 8 years with widespread pulmonary metastases.

Results of Treatment/Survival

Sinonasal malignancy is rare, and the different pathologies behave in very different ways. Consequently it is rather difficult to give an overall view of survival as this will depend upon the composition and size of the cohort and its length of follow-up. Indeed the concept of "benign" is arguably irrelevant in an area where any progressive disease, for example, an extracranial meningioma may result in bilateral blindness and the death of a patient even without the capability of metastatic spread.

In the cohort of 308 patients undergoing craniofacial resection, the overall actuarial survival for the whole group was 65% at 5 years, 47% at 10 years, and 41% at 15 years (6). The actuarial disease-free survival for malignant tumors was 59% at 5 years, dropping to 40 and 33% at 10 and 15 years, respectively. This group consisted of 259 individuals, comprising 22 different pathologies. Adenocarcinoma constituted the largest group (62) followed by olfactory neuroblastoma (54), SCC (34), and chondrosarcoma (24). For benign tumors, actuarial disease-free survival was 92% at 5, 82% at 10, and 76% at 15 years (Fig. 16.12). This group included 18 different pathologies, of which nine cases were meningioma (6). Local recurrence usually occurred within the first 2 years, which should be considered to be residual disease though in some individuals disease reappeared many years later, up to 14 years after surgery in one case of olfactory neuroblastoma. Thirty patients are known to have died with metastatic disease with or without evidence of local recurrence. The most common sites were bone (nine cases: brain; eight cases; and cervical lymph nodes: seven cases).

By contrast an increasing number of malignant tumors are being managed surgically by an endoscopic approach, either alone or in combination with a craniotomy. There are now a number of series in the literature though the numbers, varied histologies, and length of follow-up make direct comparison with craniofacial data difficult (14–16). Nonetheless an increasing body of experience suggests that with careful patient selection comparable results can be obtained, with minimal morbidity and early combination with additional medical oncology therapies (Table 16.2). In a personal series of 70 patients all managed with an entirely endoscopic resection with intention to cure and all with a mean follow-up in excess of 12 months (range 12–144 months), 54 are alive and well, 8 alive with recurrence, 5 dead of disease, and 3 dead of intercurrent disease. This includes a wide range of histopathologies, including 18 adenocarcinomas, 17 olfactory neuroblastomas, and 13 malignant melanomas. Three patients have been converted to craniofacial at approximately one year, emphasizing the need for careful long-term follow-up.

Orbital involvement is an important prognostic predictor of recurrence-free, disease-specific, and overall survival. Most studies suggest that orbital preservation as opposed to orbital clearance or exenteration (including eyelids) does not result in significant differences in local recurrence or actuarial survival. The eye may be preserved with resection of the periorbita as long as the tumor can be completely dissected away from the orbital fat (17). Malposition and malfunction of the eye, however, frequently result when patients have not had adequate rigid reconstruction of the orbital floor, particularly if they receive postoperative radiotherapy and require reconstruction. In 308 patients undergoing craniofacial resection (6), 53 had primary orbital clearance, 5 subsequent clearance, 50 had orbital preservation with resection of periosteum, of whom a further 5 had the eye removed at a later date. Thus 20.5% of this cohort lost an eye, but there was no statistical difference between those who had the eye removed at the time of the craniofacial and those who only had resection of orbital periosteum.

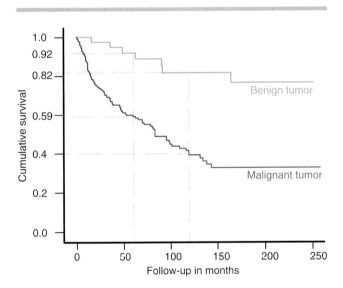

Figure 16.12 Actuarial survival Kaplan Meier curve in 308 craniofacial patients showing benign versus malignant tumors. *Source*: From Ref. 6.

CONSIDERATION BY HISTOLOGY/SUBSITE
Squamous Cell Carcinoma of the Maxillary Sinus
Presentation
The tumor must break out of the maxillary sinus to present with symptoms related to the adjacent nasal cavity, orbit, cheek, or pterygopalatine fossa. The most frequent symptoms at first onset are cheek swelling (29%), nasal obstruction (28%), and epistaxis (20%), and there is a reported average delay of 3 to 6 months before final diagnosis (18).

Table 16.2 Endoscopic Resection for Sinonasal Malignancy in the Literature

Author	Histology	n	Mean Follow-up in Months	Survival
Stammberger (16)	Olfactory neuroblastoma	6	57	100% 1 CFR
Goffart (15)	mixed	66	26	66%
Roh (67)	mixed	13	26	86% DFS
Shlpchandler (67)	SCC	7	31	91%
Poetker (67)	mixed	16	17	recurrence rate v
Bockmuhl (67)	adeno, SCC, ON	29	65	78% 5-year survival
Castelnuova (67)	mixed	18	25	61% @ 19.8 months
Lund (14)	mixed	49	35	88% overall, 68% DFS

Abbreviations: CFR, craniofacial resection; DFS, disease-free survival; SCC, squamous cell carcinoma; ON, olfactory neuroblastoma.

Risk Factors and Associations

An association has been described with soft wood exposure, but it is interesting that in Japan where maxillary sinus carcinoma has an unusually high incidence, there appeared to be little relationship with their traditional woodworking industry (19). Radium dial painting and mustard gas production manifested a high risk with exposure as short as 6 months but are no longer considered a source. Workers in the sintering and roasting processes in the nickel industry also had a risk that increases with age and duration of exposure (20). Nickel and chromium are found as traces in homemade snuff, which is used in South Africa by the indigenous black population who have been shown in the past to have a high incidence of antroethmoidal cancer (21). Exposure to irradiation and the radiological contrast agent thorium dioxide have also been shown to be carcinogenic (22) though the relationship with smoking and chronic infection is small if any. The incidence of advanced malignant transformation of inverted papilloma has been greatly overestimated in the literature, largely due to incorrect diagnosis of the initial material. The true incidence of SCC arising de novo in inverted papilloma is probably of the order of 1 to 2% (23).

Incidence

SCC is the most common of sinonasal histologies, comprising more than 60% of most series, though this will vary depending upon the interests of the unit concerned. An incidence of 1/100,000 population per year is quoted for the U.K., but 2.6/100,000 for men in Japan, Nigeria, and Jamaica.

Sex Ratio and Age Range

The sex ratio for SCC is 1.7:1 male/female, whereas the age range is 19 to 90 years, with an average of 60 years.

Pathophysiology/Modes of Spread

The tumor makes use of areas of natural weakness such as the inferior orbital fissure or ethmoid labyrinth, and early diagnosis with the tumor still confined within the maxilla is rare. Dura and orbital periosteum will resist disease for some time, but once breached, there is rapid infiltration of the brain and orbit. Extension into the nasopharynx is occasionally associated with spread up the Eustachian tubes, with tumor presenting in the middle ear cavity. Cervical lymphadenopathy is present in approximately 10% of patients at initial presentation. Distant metastases are uncommon at presentation though may be found at autopsy in the lungs, liver, and bone.

Prognostic Factors

Some authors have tried to link prognosis to the degree of differentiation. However, local spread into the orbital structures, frontal lobes, and pterygopalatine fossa and the presence of systemic metastases are of much greater prognostic significance.

Several subgroups of SCC have been described. Verrucous carcinoma is a slow-growing SCC that is locally aggressive but rarely metastasizes. Anaplastic carcinoma may be a poorly differentiated SCC but must be differentiated from other small-cell tumors such as olfactory neuroblastoma and lymphoma. Sinonasal undifferentiated SCC is now recognized as a specific and aggressive entity. Spindle cell carcinoma or carcinosarcoma should be regarded as an aggressive SCC. Transitional or cylindric cell carcinoma should be regarded as a poorly differentiated nonkeratinizing SCC.

Results of Treatment/Survival

Combined radiotherapy and surgery have remained the gold standard with 5-year survival rates of between 35 and 48% (24–26). Most recurrences occur within 2 years, and local recurrence is the prime cause of death. Radiotherapy may be given before or after surgery, and the surgery varies from partial maxillectomy to total or radical maxillectomy with orbital clearance or craniofacial resection.

Results in excess of 50% have been claimed for topical 5-fluorouracil applied via a palatal fenestration and combined with repeated debulking in Japan and Holland (27,28) though results have not been reported from other departments.

Adenocarcinoma
Presentation

Nasal obstruction, discharge, unilateral epistaxis, pain, epiphora, and other orbital symptoms are common (Fig. 16.13), and occasionally adenocarcinoma presents as a midline glabellar mass with involvement of the frontal bone (Fig. 16.6).

Risk Factors and Associations

As discussed previously there has been observed a high frequency of adenocarcinoma of the ethmoids in the woodworkers. The association is with hardwood dust exposure, for example, mahogany where fine dust of no more than 5 μm diameter is deposited in the middle meatus (2,3). The relative risk for a woodworker developing adenocarcinoma is 70 times that of nonwoodworkers. Adenocarcinoma has also been associated with the manufacture of chrome pigment, isopropyl alcohol, textiles, clothing, leather, and

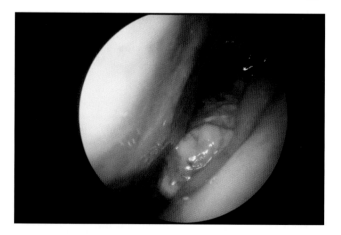

Figure 16.13 Endoscopic view of adenocarcinoma in left middle meatus.

shoes though many patients with adenocarcinoma have no predisposing factors (4).

Incidence, Sex Ratio, and Age Range

There is an incidence of 4 to 12% of sinonasal malignancies (29). The sex ratio is 4:1 male/female, and increasing to 11:1 in the older age group, which reflects longer previous carcinogenic exposure. There is an age range of 9 to 90 years, with an average of 50 to 60 years with higher grade tumors presenting in slightly older patients (30).

Pathophysiology/Modes of Spread

The tumor generally arises within the middle meatus spreading into the orbit, to the contralateral ethmoid, and through the anterior skull base at an early stage. The nasopharynx may be involved by spread from the spheno-ethmoidal recess. Cervical metastases are clinically palpable in 2 to 3% of cases at presentation.

Prognostic Factors

Improved prognosis is said to occur with low-grade adeno-carcinomas (30) though this is not always observed clinically Sex, age, site, size, histological type, and the presence of cervical metastases have also been cited as prognostic factors. The worst prognostic factor in our own group of 60 patients is frontal lobe infiltration with no survivors beyond 12 months.

Results of Treatment/Survival

Craniofacial resection (usually combined with radiotherapy) offers optimum long-term survival. In the past the majority of cases were managed by a radical maxillectomy or extended lateral rhinotomy frequently with sacrifice of the eye. The advent of the combined craniofacial approach has enabled an oncologic clearance with access to the anterior cranial fossa and orbit is of particular advantage in the management of ethmoidal adenocarcinoma. In a cohort of 62 patients treated by craniofacial resection, actuarial survival at 5 years was 58%, 40% at 10 years, and 33% at 15 years (6). Of our craniofacial patients who died, 50% had local disease, but a similar number developed distant metastases to lung, bone, and brain, which may be the result of improved local control afforded by the craniofa-cial resection, as distant metastases are rarely reported in noncraniofacial cohorts (Fig. 16.14).

Endoscopic resection is being used in increasing numbers of selected cases, usually combined with post-operative radiotherapy though the numbers and follow-up preclude definitive survival figures at present (14–16).

Adenoid Cystic Carcinoma
Presentation

Adenoid cystic carcinoma presents as nasal obstruction, rhinorrhoea, and epistaxis. Facial pain, tingling, and paraes-thesia occur affecting the infraorbital division of the tri-geminal nerve. Orbital involvement includes proptosis and diplopia. A palpable mass may be found in the medial canthal region or on hard palate.

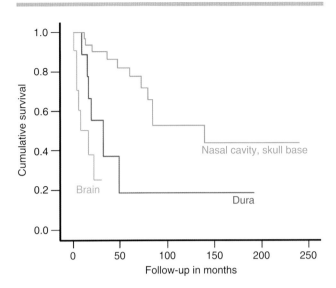

Figure 16.14 Actuarial survival Kaplan Meier curve for patients with adenocarcinoma treated with craniofacial resection. *Source*: From Ref. 6.

Incidence, Sex Ratio, and Age Range

Adenoid cystic carcinoma has an incidence of 1.3% of all sinonasal tumors (30). The sex ratio is 2:1 male/female and the age ranges between 12 and 84 years with the majority occurring in the fourth to sixth decades.

Pathophysiology/Modes of Spread

The maxilla and hard palate are the most common sites in the sinonasal region with spread to involve the orbit and nasolacrimal region in up to two thirds of cases (31). Early spread occurs by perineural infiltration along cranial nerves, and there is frequent hematogenous dissemination particularly to lungs. As a consequence local "recurrence" is the rule rather than the exception, and complete local excision is rarely possible. However, pulmonary metastases do not necessarily imply a rapid demise with patients living up to 7 or 8 years. By contrast, cervical lymphadenopathy is relatively rare. The true incidence of systemic metastases varies from 20 to 50%, which may manifest up to 15 to 22 years after initial presentation. Consequently, 5-year survival figures are rendered meaningless.

Prognostic Factors

There is no agreement on the prognostic importance of size, site, patient age, symptoms, or histological classifica-tion. However, of the three histological types—tubular, cribriform and solid—solid may be the more aggressive. Although two thirds of patients are alive in most series at 5 years, this falls to 10% or less at 20 years, suggesting that the majority of patients will die of the disease if followed for long enough (20).

Results of Treatment/Survival

Radical primary surgery combined with radiotherapy is rarely curative but will reduce the number and speed of local recurrence. As complete extirpation of all adjacent cranial nerves is impracticable, the patient should be offered the most radical operation, which also combines an acceptable morbidity, for example, a craniofacial resection or total maxillectomy with or without orbital clearance or in the case of a localized lesion on the palate, a subtotal maxillectomy preserving the orbital floor. Neck dissection is rarely indicated.

In a cohort of 19 patients undergoing craniofacial resection 5-year actuarial survival was 61 and 31% at 10 and 15 years, respectively (6).

Pulmonary metastases have been managed by wedge resection or lobectomy in selected cases, and the presence of pulmonary metastases does not preclude local surgery. Chemotherapy has no part to play either for cure or palliation. Carbamazepine may be used to control the associated neuralgia from perineural involvement.

Olfactory Neuroblastoma

Presentation

Olfactory neuroblastoma has a nonspecific presentation: nasal obstruction, epistaxis, and hyposmia. The tumor is generally slow growing with 24% of patients having symptoms for longer than 1 year (32).

Risk Factors and Associations

Experimental work with the Syrian hamster has produced olfactory neuroblastoma-type tumors with diethylnitrosamine (33).

Incidence, Sex Ratio, and Age Range

Approximately 5% of all sinonasal tumors are olfactory neuroblastomas with a slight male preponderance. A bimodal age distribution is seen with peaks in the second and third decades and later in the sixth and seventh decades (32).

Pathophysiology/Modes of Spread

The tumor arises almost exclusively in the superior nasal cavity corresponding to the anatomical distribution of the olfactory epithelium (Fig. 16.15). Early spread occurs along olfactory fibrils to involve the olfactory bulbs and tracts as confirmed by craniofacial resection (34).

Prognostic Factors

The natural history of this malignancy is variable and unpredictable. The anatomical location may make wide field resection on occasions impossible. The tumor can offer a range of local aggression, and the possibility of cervical lymphadenopathy and blood dissemination. The incidence of cervical metastases has been quoted at between 5 to 100% (mean 23%) in the literature and affects significantly prognosis (35). Extent of disease has been classified into stages I to III (36), but prognosis does not correlate with histological appearances (37).

Results of Treatment/Survival

The natural site of occurrence of the tumor makes it ideal for craniofacial resection. Several studies have demonstrated improved survival with craniofacial resection and radiotherapy as compared to extracranial resection and

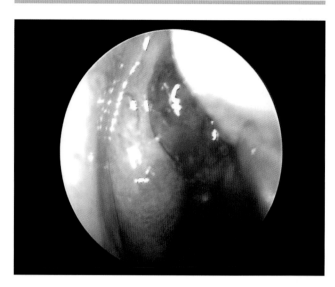

Figure 16.15 Endoscopic view of olfactory neuroblastoma in left nasal cavity.

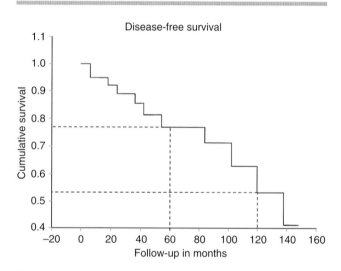

Figure 16.16 Actuarial survival Kaplan Meier curve in patients with olfactory neuroblastoma treated with craniofacial resection. *Source:* From Ref. 32.

radiotherapy. Most recent studies have suggested that craniofacial resection without radiotherapy for stages I and II produces satisfactory results (Fig. 16.16) (38,39). In a cohort of 56 patients treated by craniofacial resection (with radiotherapy for stage III disease) the 5-year actuarial survival rate was 74%, 50% at 10 years, and 40% at 15 years (6). In an earlier study of 42 patients with olfactory neuroblastoma who had undergone craniofacial resection, local recurrence overall was 17%. However, if they had received combined treatment with radiotherapy, this was only 4%, whereas if no radiotherapy had been given due to the limited nature of the tumor, that is, no involvement of the olfactory tracts and bulbs, the recurrence rate was 28% (32). It should also be noted that local recurrence may occur after a 14-year disease-free interval and can appear in the contralateral orbit or seeded at some distance on the dura. Therefore all patients are advised to undergo additional radiotherapy that is often combined with adjuvant chemotherapy (cyclophosamide, vincristine, cis-platinum, and 5-fluorouracil). This has also been advocated for extensive local disease and/or secondary spread (40). Again endoscopic resection is being offered for early tumors that involve the upper nasal cavity and skull base without macroscopic spread into the anterior cranial cavity but always in combination with radiotherapy (14,41).

Malignant Melanoma
Presentation
Unilateral nasal obstruction (46%), epistaxis (19%), a combination of the two (23%), or a visible mass (6%) are the common findings (42). Lesions on the palate produce a lump that often ulcerates and bleeds.

Risk Factors and Associations
Melanocytes are derivations of neural crest and are found throughout the nasal and oral mucosa. Experimental studies have suggested that exposure to formaldehyde may increase cutaneous melanoma, and in a cohort of 50 surviving patients, three had had extensive exposure to formaldehyde (43).

Incidence
Between 15 and 20% of all malignant melanomas arise in the head and neck, but the vast majority of these are cutaneous and only 0.5 to 2% affect the mucous membranes, and of these, the majority occur in the oral cavity. Malignant melanoma affecting the nasal cavity accounts for less than 1% of all malignant melanomas and 3% of all sinonasal neoplasia in our own cohort.

Sex Ratio and Age Range
The ratio of men to women is roughly equal with a slight male preponderance. The age ranges from 16 to 90 years with the majority presenting in the sixth to seventh decades, maximally between 60 and 69 years.

Pathophysiology/Modes of Spread
The most common site of origin is from the lateral wall particularly from the inferior and middle turbinates followed by the nasal septum. The tumor spreads along mucosal planes, is capable of producing satellite lesions, but tends not to destroy adjacent cartilage or bone extensively in the early stages.

Between 10 and 18% of patients will present with cervical lymphadenopathy and 4% with lung metastases. Local recurrence, cervical lymphadenopathy, and metastatic disease can occur at any time with systemic metastases in the lung, liver, brain, and skin usually present at the time of death from disease.

Prognostic Factor
The patients live in an interesting immunological balance with the tumor that may be upset by other factors such as a viral infection. Thus some patients succumb very rapidly to overwhelming disease whereas others may live for long periods of time with local or even systemic disease that may be resected many times.

The age, sex, degree of pigmentation, and mitotic activity do not directly correlate with prognosis, and unlike skin melanoma, correlation of depth of invasion and junction activity with outcome does not apply to mucosal disease.

Results of Treatment/Survival
The surgical approach of choice has been the lateral rhinotomy, which is a quick procedure in elderly patients with a low morbidity, offering good access to the common sites of origin of the disease. The incisions for a midfacial degloving are often not ideal, and a craniofacial resection is contraindicated as it seems to remove the bony barrier to local intracranial spread. Consequently an endonasal endoscopic approach is increasingly used for localized disease, and particularly for recurrence (14). Whichever approach is used, the surgeon should be aware of the possibility of amelanotic disease and satellite lesions (Fig. 16.17). A coagulating laser such as the argon or KTP may be useful for recurrences that produce epistaxis.

Despite the relative lack of radiosensitivity, some of the longest survivors are those receiving local surgical clearance and radiotherapy though it is difficult to demonstrate this statistically (42). However, radiotherapy is now offered postoperatively in most cases unless precluded by dissemination of disease or general health of the patient.

The overall prognosis is poor with more than 50% dead within 3 years and 66% dead within 5 years. Five-year survival rates of 6 to 31% have been quoted in the literature, but again the natural history of the disease makes 5-year survival meaningless and the patient is constantly at risk of death from this condition. In a cohort of 58 patients, survival ranged from 1 to 228 months with rapid loss within the first 36 months, irrespective of treatment. Five-year actuarial survival was 28%, falling to 20% at 10 years (Fig. 16.18). Palatal lesions have an even worse prognosis

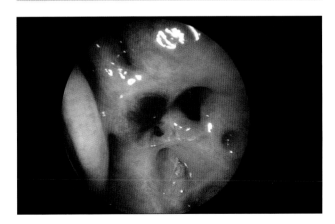

Figure 16.17 Endoscopic view showing recurrent malignant melanoma in posterior nasal cavity adjacent to middle turbinate.

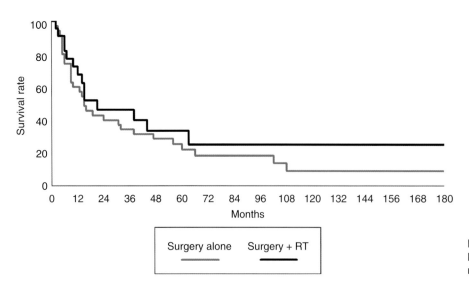

Figure 16.18 Actuarial survival Kaplan Meier curve in patients with malignant melanoma. *Source*: From Ref. 42.

with the majority of patients dead within 1 to 2 years from presentation. At present the use of palliative interleukins, interferon, and other chemotherapy are of unproven benefit in mucosal melanoma.

STAGING

Although the tumor node metastasis (TNM) classification has been applied to sinonasal malignancy (44), most tumors are T4 at presentation and a tumor infiltrating the skull base will inevitably have a different prognosis from one arising in the anterior floor of the maxillary sinus (45). The relatively low incidence of metastatic spread also limits the usefulness of the conventional TNM classification nor does it take into account information derived from modern imaging or the prognostic impact of improved oncologic resection, for example, by a craniofacial approach (Table 16.3).

INVESTIGATIONS
General Guidelines

Although sinonasal malignancy is rare, new and persistent nasal symptoms should always be investigated particularly if unilateral. Endoscopic examination of the nose may facilitate early detection of neoplasia. Care should be taken to adequately decongest the nose, and an attempt should always be made to examine beyond a septal deflection. All tissue removed during routine sinonasal procedures, for example, polypectomy should be submitted for histology.

Diagnostic Investigation

Adequate and representative tissue must be obtained for expert histological opinion. This is best performed under a general anesthetic and with the use of endoscopic techniques, it is rarely if ever necessary to transgress normal tissue planes by a sublabial or external incision. When lymphoma is suspected, fresh tissue may be required.

A diagnosis of "anaplastic" carcinoma should always be queried and tissue sent for immunohistochemistry.

Hematological investigations may be appropriate, for example, HIV test for Kaposi's sarcoma or lymphoma; blood films for chloroma (granulocytic sarcoma); anti-nuclear cytoplasmic antibody (ANCA), angiotensin converting enzyme (ACE), ESR etc. in the differential diagnosis of midline destructive lesions such as Wegener's granulomatosis or sarcoidosis.

Localizing Investigations

A combination of computed tomography (CT) and magnetic resonance imaging (MRI) provides an accuracy of 98% (46,47) in determining extent of disease. Direct coronal and axial CT with contrast enhancement demonstrates bone detail and best detects early cribriform plate erosion. MRI [three planar sections with gadolinium Diethylenetriamine pentaacetic acid (DTPA)] allows soft tissue differentiation between tumor, inflammation, mucus retention, and fibrosis (48).

For most malignant tumors, additional imaging of the body is not routinely required, but more extensive staging should be undertaken for poorly differentiated tumors such as sinonasal undifferentiated carcinoma, neuroendocrine carcinoma, and lymphomas require using CT, MRI, or positron emission tomography (PET)-CT (49). A chest X-ray and/or chest CT should be done in those with tumors such as adenoid cystic that have a tendency to spread to the lung. Similarly an ultrasound of the neck combined with a fine-needle aspiration is recommended for those tumors associated with higher rates of cervical metastases such as olfactory neuroblastoma and sinonasal undifferentiated carcinoma (50).

Follow-up is necessarily long-term, even lifelong and usually includes repeated MRI and endoscopic examination of the cavity, including biopsy under general anesthetic in response to clinical and radiological findings (Fig. 16.19). The use of a dedicated database may facilitate this process (51).

Table 16.3 TMN Classification (44)

Primary Tumor (T)

Maxillary sinus

TX	Primary tumor cannot be assessed
T0	No evidence of primary tumor
Tis	Carcinoma *in situ*
T1	Tumor limited to the maxillary sinus mucosa with no erosion or destruction of bone
T2	Tumor causing bone erosion or destruction including extension into the hard palate and/or middle nasal meatus, except extension to posterior wall of maxillary sinus and pterygoid plates
T3	Tumor invades any of the following: bone of the posterior wall of maxillary sinus, subcutaneous tissues, floor or medial wall of orbit, pterygoid fossa, ethmoid sinuses
T4a	Tumor invades anterior orbital contents, skin of cheek, pterygoid plates, infratemporal fossa, cribriform plate, sphenoid or frontal sinuses
T4b	Tumor invades any of the following: orbital apex, dura, brain, middle cranial fossa, cranial nerves other than maxillary division of trigeminal nerve V_2, nasopharynx, or clivus

Nasal cavity and ethmoid sinus

TX	Primary tumor cannot be assessed
T0	No evidence of primary tumor
Tis	Carcinoma in situ
T1	Tumor restricted to any one subsite, with or without bony invasion
T2	Tumor invading two subsites in a single region within the nasoethmoidal complex, with our without bony invasion
T4a	Tumor invades any of the following: anterior orbital contents, skin of the nose or cheek, minimal extension to anterior cranial fossa, pterygoid plates, sphenoid or frontal sinuses
T4b	Tumor invades any of the following: orbital apex, dura, brain, middle cranial fossa, cranial nerves other than V_2, nasopharynx, or clivus

Regional lymph nodes (N)

NX	Regional lymph nodes cannot be assessed
N0	No regional lymph node metastasis
N1	Metastasis in a single ipsilateral lymph node, 3 cm or less in greatest dimension
N2	Metastasis in a single ipsilateral lymph node, more than 3 cm but not more than 6 cm in greatest dimension, or in multiple ipsilateral lymph nodes, none more than 6 cm in greatest dimension, or in bilateral or contralateral lymph nodes, none more than 6 cm in greatest dimension
N2a	Metastasis in a single ipsilateral lymph node, more than 3 cm but not more than 6 cm in greatest dimension
N2b	Metastasis in multiple ipsilateral lymph nodes, none more than 6 cm in greatest dimension
N2c	Metastasis in bilateral or contralateral lymph nodes, none more than 6 cm in greatest dimension
N3	Metastasis in a lymph node, more than 6 cm in greatest dimension

Distant metastasis (M)

MX	Distant metastasis cannot be assessed
M0	No distant metastasis
M1	Distant metastasis

TREATMENT POLICY

General

There are three main objectives of the treatment of sinonasal malignancy:

1. curative resection of the tumor
2. reconstruction and rehabilitation
3. where cure cannot be achieved, a genuine attempt at palliation.

Specific

Surgery

In choosing the correct therapeutic modality it is important to understand the natural history of each individual histology.

The vast majority of patients therefore undergo some form of surgical excision be it lateral rhinotomy (and medial maxillectomy), midfacial degloving, some form of partial or total maxillectomy, total rhinectomy, or craniofacial resection with or without orbital clearance, and increasingly an entirely endoscopic resection in selected cases.

The lateral rhinotomy approach, attributed to Moure in 1902 (52) but described as early as 1848, gives excellent access to the nasal cavity, the entire frontoethmosphenoidal complex, and medial maxilla. Limiting the superior extent of the incision to the medial canthus and careful repair of the alar margin diminishes the cosmetic problems that originally limited its popularity. It is still often used for malignant melanoma but has been superseded in many other circumstances by endoscopic approaches or a midfacial degloving, which offer greater bilateral access and avoid external scars.

The midfacial degloving combines bilateral sublabial incisions with elevation of the soft tissues of the mid-third of the face via intercartilaginous incisions. Its main limitation is the time taken for careful closure to avoid vestibular stenosis and oroantral fistula and limited access to the frontal sinus. It is most often used in young patients, those with extensive benign neoplasia, and for malignancy of the nasal cavity and upper jaw where the skull base has not been compromised. It was popularized by Price et al. (53) and in a series of more than 170 patients we have experienced minimal long-term morbidity (54,55). It may of course be combined with a bicoronal incision for access to the anterior skull base (56). The Weber–Fergusson incision is now rarely employed except in those older patients with malignancy of the upper jaw requiring conventional radical maxillectomy with or without orbital clearance and for procedures such as the maxillary swing designed for access to the nasopharynx (57).

The craniofacial resection has been established as the "gold standard" for malignant tumors that involve the anterior skull base, facilitating a genuine oncologic resection of lesions that was hitherto impossible and was previously managed by total maxillectomy and orbital clearance (58). The craniofacial operation was originally described in 1954 (59) and was subsequently developed by Ketcham et al. (60) and Terz et al. (61) and more recently by Cheeseman and others (6,62). It is well recognized that the poor prognosis associated with malignant tumors of the nose and paranasal sinuses is largely a consequence of local recurrence or rather residual disease in the region of the skull base.

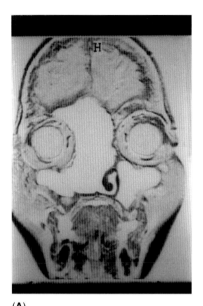

(A)

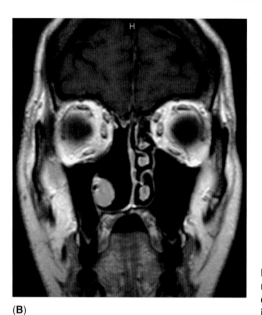

(B)

Figure 16.19 **(A)** Postoperative magnetic resonance imaging showing craniofacial cavity **(B)** postoperative magnetic resonance imaging showing endoscopic cavity.

A combined approach offers an oncologic resection with minimal morbidity and excellent cosmesis. Present experience indicates that a combination of radiotherapy and radical surgery offers the best prognosis for radiosensitive tumors with radical resection optimally performed 6 weeks following radiotherapy irrespective of response. The craniofacial resection also enables careful assessment of any extension of disease from the ethmoids into the orbit using frozen section evaluation of orbital periosteum. As a consequence of this, a proportion of eyes have been salvaged (6,63–65). If the orbital periosteum has been penetrated by disease, orbital clearance is performed, usually with preservation of the skin and orbicularis muscle that results in a skin-lined socket into which a prosthesis may be placed at a later date.

The craniofacial operation utilizes an extended lateral rhinotomy incision (or midfacial degloving with bicoronal incision) and provides access to the anterior cranial fossa via a shield-shaped window craniotomy, which can be replaced at the end of the procedure. Through the craniotomy, the frontal lobes and overlying dura are retracted as dissection of the dura is carried out on a wide front progressing posteriorly onto the smooth bone of the jugum sphenoidale, exposing cribriform plate, ethmoid, and orbital roofs. An en bloc removal of both ethmoid complexes and cribriform plate together with the perpendicular plate of the ethmoid can then be performed with additional resection of adjacent structures as appropriate. In cases where the medial bony wall of the orbit has been breached but the periosteum is intact, the compromised area of periosteum may be resected and grafted using a split-skin graft with preservation of the globe and its musculature. Similarly dura may be resected and repaired with fascia lata to which a thin fenestrated split-skin graft is applied. As for other radical sinus surgery, the surgical cavity is packed with ribbon gauze soaked in Whitehead's varnish (compound iodoform

paint: iodoform benzoin, prepared storax, tolu balsam, and solvent ether) which is removed under a short general anesthetic at 10 days (66). The standard closure can be modified using local flaps and bone grafts if required following excision of extensive anteriorly placed disease. The incision heals remarkably well, and the patients can be followed-up with regular examination under anesthesia combined with Gadolinium (Gd) MRI.

Rhinectomy is occasionally required for extensive nasal tumors, and the resulting defect is most conveniently repaired with a prosthesis that may be held in place by spectacles and tissue adhesive or osseointegrated implants.

The benefits of the rigid endoscope in the diagnosis, biopsy, and long-term follow-up of patients with sinonasal malignancy is self-evident. The ability to repair the skull base for CSF leaks and to undertake orbital decompression led to the application of endoscopic techniques, first to benign and more recently sinonasal malignancies either alone (14–16,67,68) or in combination with a craniotomy (69). The patients must be carefully selected and informed of the various options and the need for long-term follow-up. The aim must be to effect a complete wide-field resection including removal of skull base, lamina, dura, and orbital papyracea as appropriate, albeit piecemeal but providing clear margins ideally under frozen section control. If this is not possible, then an alternative approach must be employed as this definitively should not be regarded as a debulking to be followed by chemoradiation except in the presence of such extensive disease that only palliation is being considered.

Radiotherapy
External beam radiotherapy has been used generally in combination with surgery for SCC and other radiosensitive

tumors (70). Care is taken to protect the orbit, brain, and pituitary fossa while delivering an optimum therapeutic dose of approximately 60 Gy. This is important to avoid radiation-induced cataracts, keratosis, or retinal changes. Three-field external beam treatment is generally used. New techniques include hyperfractionation and IMRT.

Occasionally implants of radioactive gold or iodine have been used in the treatment of inoperable recurrent adenoid cystic carcinoma of the skull base, as has afterloading with irridium-192 for recurrence in the nasopharynx.

Chemotherapy

Of the three oncologic modalities—surgery, radiotherapy, and chemotherapy—chemotherapy has proved least useful in the treatment of sinonasal malignancies with the exception of mesenchymal tumors such as embryonal rhabdomyosarcoma and lymphoma. In the presence of extensive poorly differentiated SCC (Fig. 16.5) palliative chemotherapy has been given with some good effect with a reasonable tumor response for anything up to 18 months to 2 years. Indeed the optimal treatment of sinonasal undifferentiated carcinoma is chemoradiation. Marked tumor regression has also been produced with high dose intra-arterial cis-platinum combined with intravenous sodium thiosulphate as a neutralizing agent in some selected extensive SCC lesions (71), but there is no evidence that adjuvant chemotherapy has any significant effect. Remarkably good results have been published for the use of topical 5-fluorouracil in sinus cavities after surgical debulking for SCC of the maxilla (27,28) though they have not been reproduced from other centers.

Reconstruction and Rehabilitation

Although the clinician's primary goal is curative eradication of the malignancy, this should not be at the expense of the patient's appearance and function. Any disability consequent on major sinonasal surgery is immediately apparent and difficult to hide. In a study designed to assess perception of relative severity of 11 common facial disfigurements resulting from surgery, orbital exenteration and radical maxillectomy scored highest with rhinectomy only outweighed by mandibulectomy (72). In a study using a modified European Organisation for Research and Treatment of Cancer (EORTC) questionnaire a series of 49 patients who had undergone ablative surgery for a head and neck malignancy during the preceding 2 years were studied. This included 11 craniofacial patients who reported significant problems with vision, smell, taste, and headaches. High levels of fatigue were reported by this group (73), which has also been described in other studies (74) and could represent a somatic manifestation of psychological distress.

Patients undergoing radical maxillectomy require close liaison with an expert maxillofacial prosthodontist. The patient must be assessed preoperatively to obtain dental impressions and modify existing dentures so that a temporary obturator may be placed in the surgical cavity at the end of the procedure. This can be done using gutta percha molded to the self-retaining preprepared denture base (75). This will allow relatively normal speech and nutrition in the immediate postoperative period. A permanent hard acrylic or soft polymer obturator can be fashioned in due course.

A wide range of other repair options have been described (17) and algorithms developed for reconstruction (76). These range from a temporalis muscle flap to fill an orbital socket to microvascular free-tissue transfer combined with obturation which is the preferred option in many units following total maxillectomy +/− orbital exenteration (77,78). Combinations of muscle and bone have been described including rectus abdominis, latissimus dorsi, and scapula.

Osseointegration techniques have greatly facilitated the appearance and retention of intraoral and facial prostheses, after rhinectomy or orbital clearance. The Branemark system of osseointegrated implants uses titanium screws that become integrated into the skeleton and to which the prosthesis can be firmly attached by a press-stud or magnet arrangement (79). The screws can be implanted at the time of the resection or as a secondary procedure. They must be implanted in bone at least 3 to 4 mm in depth. Radiotherapy slows the process of integration, which may take up to 1 year in the orbital socket. This is much slower than in the intraoral cavity. A temporary prosthesis can be offered in the interim.

Palliation

Sinonasal malignancy, if left untreated, produces appalling disfigurement often accompanied by pain, bleeding, and blindness. It could also be argued that tumors such as malignant melanoma and adenoid cystic carcinoma carry an ultimately poor prognosis, and it is therefore more likely that treatment buys a symptom-free interval rather than cure. As the surgical procedures carry a minimal morbidity with good cosmesis and function, there are many instances where they may be undertaken without expectation of a curative excision. This is particularly true of craniofacial resection, and it is quite possible for patients to undergo several revision procedures during the course of their disease for example in chondrosarcoma of the skull base. This can provide the patient with long symptom-free periods and enable vision to be preserved by judicious orbital decompression.

Palliative radiotherapy (and chemotherapy) may also be appropriate for extensive radiosensitive tumors that have spread intradurally and/or affect the cavernous sinus and middle cranial fossa.

REFERENCES

1. Acheson ED, Cowdell RH, Hadfield E et al. Nasal cancer in woodworkers in the furniture industry. Br Med J 1968; ii: 587–96.
2. Wilhelmsson B, Drettner B. Nasal problems in wood furniture workers. A study of symptoms and physiological variables. Acta Otolaryngol 1984; 98: 548–55.
3. Drettner B, Wilhelmsson B, Lundh B. Experimental studies on carcinogenesis in the nasal mucosa. Acta Otolaryngol 1985; 99: 205–7.
4. Lund VJ. Malignancy of the nose and sinuses: epidemiological and aetiological considerations. Rhinology 1991; 29: 57–68.
5. Roush GC. Epidemiology of cancer of the nose and paranasal sinuses, current concepts. Head Neck Surg 1979; 2: 3–11.
6. Howard DJ, Lund VJ, Wei WI. Craniofacial resection for sinonasal neoplasia – a twenty-five year experience. Head Neck 2006; 28: 867–73.

7. Iannetti G, Valentini V, Rinna C et al. Ethmoido-orbital tumors: our experience. J Craniofac Surg 2005; 16: 1085–9.

8. Suárez C, Llorente JL, Fernández de León R et al. Prognostic factors in sinonasal tumors involving the anterior skull base. Head Neck 2004; 26: 136–44.

9. Carrillo JF, Guemes A, Ramirez-Ortega MC et al. Prognostic factors in maxillary sinus and nasal cavity carcinoma. Eur J Surg Oncol 2005; 31: 1206–12.

10. Dulguerov P, Jacobsen M, Allal A et al. Nasal and paranasal sinus carcinoma: are we making progress? A series of 220 patients and a systematic review. Cancer 2001; 92: 3012–29.

11. Bhattacharyya N. Cancer of the nasal cavity Survival and factors influencing prognosis. Arch Otolaryngol Head Neck Surg 2002; 128: 1079–83.

12. Lund VJ. Distant metastases from sinonasal cancer. In: Ferlito A, ed., Distant Metastases from Head and Neck Cancer: a multi-institutional view. ORL 2001; 63: 212–13.

13. Cantu G, Bimbi G, Miceli R et al. Lymph node metastases in malignant tumors of the paranasal sinuses: prognostic value and treatment. Arch Otolaryngol Head Neck Surg 2008; 134: 170–7.

14. Lund VJ, Howard DJ, Wei WI. Endoscopic resection of malignant tumors of the nose and sinuses. Am J Rhinol 2007; 21: 89–94.

15. Goffart Y, Jorissen M, Daele J et al. Minimally invasive endoscopic management of malignant sinonasal tumors. Acta Oto-Rhino-Laryngologica Belg 2000; 54: 221–32.

16. Stammberger H, Anderhuber W, Walch Ch. Possibilities and limitations of endoscopic management of nasal and paranasal sinus malignancies. Acta Otorhinolaryngol Belg 1999; 53: 199–205.

17. Suarez C, Ferlito A, Lund VJ et al. Management of the orbit in malignant sinonasal tumours. Head Neck 2008; 30: 242–50.

18. Weber AL, Stanton AC. Malignant tumours of the paranasal sinuses: radiologic, clinical and histopathologic evaluation of 200 cases. Head Neck Surg 1984; 6: 761–76.

19. Takasaka T, Kawamoto K, Nakamura K. A case-control study of nasal cancers. Acta Otolaryngol Suppl 1987; 435: 136–42.

20. Doll R, Morgan IG, Speizer FE. Cancer of the lung and sinuses in nickel workers. Br J Cancer 1970; 12: 32–41.

21. Harrison DFN. Snuff – its use and abuse. Br Med J 1964; ii: 1649–52.

22. Rankow RM, Conley J, Fodor P. Carcinoma of the maxillary sinus following thorotrast instillation. J Maxillofac Surg 1974; 2: 119–26.

23. Woodson GE, Robbins T, Michaels L. Inverted papilloma. Consideration in treatment. Arch Otolaryngol 1985; 111: 806–11.

24. Weymuller EA, Reardon EJ, Nash D. Comparison of treatment modalities in carcinoma of the maxillary sinus. Arch Otolaryngol 1980; 106: 625–9.

25. Har-El G, Hadar T, Krespi YP. An analysis of staging systems for carcinoma of the maxillary sinus. Ear Nose Throat J 1988; 67: 511–20.

26. Sisson GA, Toriumi DM, Atiyah RA. Paranasal sinus malignancy: a comprehensive update. Laryngoscope 1989; 99: 143–50.

27. Sakai S, Honki A, Fuchihata DD et al. Multidisciplinary treatment of maxillary sinus cancer. Cancer 1983; 52: 1360–4.

28. Knegt P, de Jong P, van Andel J et al. Carcinoma of the paranasal sinuses. Results of a prospective pilot study. Cancer 1989; 56: 57–62.

29. Harrison DFN, Lund VJ. Tumours of the Upper Jaw. London: Churchill-Livingstone, 1993.

30. Mills SE, Gaffey MJ, Frierson HF. Tumors of the Upper Respiratory Tract and Ear. Washington, DC: Armed Forces Institute of Pathology, 2000.

31. Howard DJ, Lund VJ. Reflections on the management of adenoid cystic carcinoma of the nose and paranasal sinuses. Otolaryngol Head Neck Surg 1985; 93: 338–40.

32. Lund VJ, Howard D, Wei W et al. Olfactory neuroblastoma Laryngoscope 2003; 113: 502–4.

33. Herrold K. Induction of olfactory neuroepithelial tumours in Syrian hamsters by diethynitrosamine. Cancer 1964; 17: 205–15.

34. Harrison DFN. Surgical pathology of olfactory neuroblastoma. Head Neck Surg 1984; 7: 60–4.

35. Rinaldo A, Ferlito A, Shaha AR et al. Esthesioneuroblastoma and cervical lymph node metastases: clinical and therapeutic implications. Acta Oto-Laryngologica 2002; 122: 125–221.

36. Kadish, S, Goodman M, Wang CC. Olfactory neuroblastoma: a clinical analysis of 17 cases. Cancer 1976; 37: 1571–6.

37. Lund VJ, Milroy CM. Olfactory neuroblastoma; clinical and pathologic aspects. Rhinology 1993; 31: 1–6.

38. Dulguerov P, Abdelkarim SA, Calcaterra TC. Esthesioneuroblastoma: a meta-analysis and review. Lancet Oncol 2001; 2: 683–8.

39. Diaz E, Johnigan R, Pero C. Olfactory neuroblastoma. The 22 year experience at one comprehensive cancer center. Head Neck 2005, 27: 138–249.

40. Kim D, Jo Y, Heo D et al. Neoadjuvant etoposide, ifosafamide and cisplatin for the treatment of olfactory neuroblastoma. Cancer 2004; 101: 2257–60.

41. Casiano RR, Numa WA, Falquez AM. Endoscopic resection of esthesioneuroblastoma. Am J Rhinol 2001; 15: 271–9.

42. Lund VJ, Howard DJ, Harding L et al. Management options and survival in malignant melanoma of the sinonasal mucosa. Laryngoscope 1999; 109: 208–11.

43. Holmström M, Lund VJ. Malignant melanoma of the nasal cavity following occupational exposure to formaldehyde. Br J Indust Med 1991; 48: 9–11.

44. American Joint Committee on Cancer: Cancer Staging Atlas Greene FL, Compton CC, Fritz AG, Shah JP, Winchester DP. Springer, 2006.

45. Cantu G, Solero CL, Miceli R et al. Which classification for ethmoid malignant tumors involving the anterior skull base? Head Neck 2005; 27: 224–31.

46. Lloyd GAS, Lund VJ, Howard DJ et al. Optimum imaging for sinonasal malignancy. J Laryngol Otol 2000; 114: 557–62.

47. Madani G, Morley SJ, Lund VJ et al. Imaging of malignant sinonasal tumours. Seminars in Ultrasound, CT MR 2009; 30: 25–38.

48. Lund VJ, Lloyd GAS, Howard DJ et al. Enhanced magnetic resonance imaging and subtraction techniques in the post-operative evaluation of craniofacial resection for sinonasal malignancy. Laryngoscope 1996; 106: 553–8.

49. Koshy M, Paulino A, Howell R et al. F-18 FDG PET-CT fusion in radiotherapy treatment planning for head and neck cancer. Head Neck 2005; 27: 494–502.

50. Collins B, Cramer H, Hearn S. Fine needle aspiration cytology of metastatic neuroblastoma. Acta Cytol 1997, 41: 802–10.

51. Trimarchi M, Lund VJ, Nicolai P et al. A database to collect and analyse clinical data and images of neoplasms of the sinonasal tract. Ann Otol Rhinol Laryngol 2004; 113: 335–7.

52. Moure EJ. Treatment of primitive malignant tumours of the ethmoid. Revue Hebdomadaire de Laryngologie 1902; 2: 401–12.

53. Price JC, Holliday MJ, Johns ME. The versatile midface degloving approach. Laryngoscope 1988; 98: 291–5.

54. Howard DJ, Lund VJ. The role of midfacial degloving in modern rhinological practice. J Laryngol Otol 1999; 113: 885–7.

55. Lund VJ Surgical management of mid-facial tumours – transfacial degloving, mid-facial degloving or endoscopic

approach. Curr Opin Otolaryngol Head Neck Surg 2001; 9: 95–9.

56. Shah J, Kraus DH, Arbit E et al. A craniofacial resection of the tumours involving the anterior skull base. Otolaryngol Head Neck Surg 1992; 106: 387–93.

57. Lam KH, Wei FL, Yue CP et al. Maxillary swing approach to the orbit. Head Neck Surg 1991; 13: 107–13.

58. Ganly I, Patel SG, Singh B et al. Craniofacial resection for malignant paranasal sinus tumors: Report of an International Collaborative Study. Head Neck 2005; 27: 575–84.

59. Smith RR, Klopp CT, Williams JM. Surgical treatment of cancer of the frontal sinus and adjacent areas. Cancer 1954; 7: 991–4.

60. Ketcham AS, Wilkins RH, Van Buren JM et al. A combined intracranial approach to the paranasal sinuses. Am J Surg 1963; 106: 698–703.

61. Terz JJ, Young HF, Lawrence W. Combined craniofacial resection for locally advanced carcinoma of the head and neck. Am J Surg 1980; 140: 613–24.

62. Cheesman AD, Lund VJ, Howard DJ. Craniofacial resection for tumours of the nasal cavity and paranasal sinuses. Head Neck Surg 1986; 8: 429–35.

63. McCary WS, Levine PA, Cantrell RW. Preservation of the eye in the treatment of sinonasal malignant neoplasms with orbital involvement. A confirmation of the original treatise. Arch Otolaryngol Head Neck Surg 1996; 122: 657–9.

64. Imola MJ, Schramm VL Jr. Orbital preservation in surgical management of sinonasal malignancy. Laryngoscope 2002; 112: 1357–65.

65. Nishino H, Ichimura K, Tanaka H et al. Results of orbital preservation for advanced malignant maxillary sinus tumors. Laryngoscope 2003; 113: 1064–9.

66. Lim M, Lew-Gor S, Sandhu G et al. Whitehead's varnish nasal pack. J Laryngol Otol 2007; 121: 592–4.

67. Castelnuova P, Battaglia P, Locatelli D et al. Endonasal micro-endoscopic treatment of malignant tumors of the paranasal sinuses and anterior skull base. Oper Tech Otolaryngol Head Neck Surg 2006; 17: 152–67.

68. Carrau R, Kassam A, Snyderman C et al. Endoscopic transnasal anterior skull base resection for the treatment of sinonasal malignancies. Oper Tech Otolaryngol Head Neck Surg 2006; 17: 102–10.

69. Thaler, ER, Kotapka M, Lanza D et al. Endoscopically assisted anterior cranial skull base resection of sinonasal tumors. Am J Rhinol 1999; 13: 303–10.

70. Raben A, Pfistr D, Harrison LB. Radiation therapy and chemotherapy in the management of cancers of the nasal cavity and paranasal sinuses. In: Kraus DH, Levine HL, eds. Nasal Neoplasia. New York: Thieme, 1997; 183–202.

71. Robbins KT, Storniolo AM, Hryniuk WM et al. "Decadose" effects of cisplatin squamous cell carcinoma of the upper aerodigestive tract. II. Clinical Studies. Laryngoscope 1996; 106: 37–42.

72. Dropkin MJ, Malgady RG, Scott DW et al. Scaling of disfigurement and dysfunction in postoperative head and neck patients. Head Neck Surg 1983; 6: 559–70.

73. Jones E, Lund VJ, Howard DJ. Quality of life in patients treated surgically for head and neck cancer. J Laryngol Otol 1992, 106: 238–42.

74. Lloyd S, Devesa-Martinez P, Howard, DJ et al. Quality of life of patients undergoing surgical treatment of head and neck malignancy. Clin Otolaryngol 2003; 28: 524–32.

75. Manderson RD. Prosthetics in head and neck surgery. In: McGregor IA, Howard DJ, eds. Head and Neck Surgery, Part 2, 4th ed. London: Butterworth-Heinemann, 1992; 576–92.

76. Cordeiro PG, Santamaria E. A classification system and algorithm for reconstruction of maxillectomy and midfacial defects. Plast Reconstr Surg 2000; 105: 2331–46.

77. Cordeiro PG, Santamaria E, Kraus DH et al. Reconstruction of total maxillectomy defects with preservation of the orbital contents. Plast Reconstr Surg 1998; 102: 1874–84.

78. Pryor SG, Moore EJ, Kasperbauer JL. Orbital exenteration reconstruction with rectus abdominis microvascular free flap. Laryngoscope 2005; 115: 1912–16.

79. Tjellstrom A. Osseointegrated systems and their application in the head and neck. Arch Otolaryngol Head Neck Surg 1989; 3: 39–70.

17

Juvenile Angiofibroma

Ian Witterick and Patrick J Gullane

DEFINITION AND HISTORICAL BACKGROUND

Juvenile angiofibroma is a rare benign but locally aggressive tumor originating in the region of the sphenopalatine foramen and presenting almost exclusively in adolescent males (1–7). Early descriptions of nasal masses by Hippocrates are believed to have included cases of angiofibromas (8). Chelius in 1847 described the presence of a fibrous nasal mass in the pubertal male (9). Chaveau writing in 1906 believed the site of origin of these lesions to be in the nasopharynx and coined the term "juvenile nasopharyngeal angioma." Friedberg's histological analysis of these tumors in the 1940s demonstrated them to be composed of connective tissue and vascular elements, and he amended the term to "juvenile nasopharyngeal angiofibroma" (10). The introduction of modern radiological techniques however further refined the understanding of the origin and growth patterns of these lesions, and it is currently believed that the site of origin is not within the nasopharynx but from the region of the sphenopalatine foramen (11,12). Hence "nasopharyngeal" has been dropped from the nomenclature, and these lesions are currently known as juvenile angiofibromas.

INCIDENCE

The true incidence of these lesions is unknown, but a figure of 0.05% of all head and neck tumors is often quoted (1,2). Some authors allude to a higher incidence in the Asian subcontinent, specifically India and Egypt (1). However Harrison believes that this can be explained on the grounds of local referral patterns to a few centers of expertise, rather than as a result of a definitive ethnic susceptibility (4).

The overwhelming majority of angiofibromas have been documented in adolescent males (2,13–15) with only a handful of histologically documented cases described in females (16–21). The mean age at presentation is 13 years with a range from 5 to 50 years (2,4,5,13).

ETIOLOGY

The etiological background of this tumor remains unresolved. Over the decades several authors have investigated the possibility of a tumor site in the nasopharynx whose growth patterns are under the influence of fluxes in circulating levels of sexual hormones. Brunner is credited with the identification of the site of origin of this tumor, based on the work he carried out in 1942 on full-term embryos (22).

He identified a region of endothelially lined vascular spaces in the fascia basilis of the sphenoid. These findings were later to be confirmed by Harrisons's work in 1987 (4). He demonstrated similar endothelial tissue in the region of the sphenopalatine foramen and the base of the pterygoid plates in male and female 24-week-old human fetuses. Investigators then hypothesized that growth of this vascular tissue was secondary to hormonal fluctuations taking place in the male during puberty. Martin in 1948 suggested that growth of the tumor tissue was due to a relative overproduction of estrogens or a lack of androgens (23). Schiff suggested tumor growth was due to an alteration in the pituitary androgen–estrogen axis (24). Walike and Mackay demonstrated that diethylstilboestrol decreased the growth potential of endothelial cells and stimulated the growth of fibrous tissue (25). They suggested therefore that this estrogen might cause regression of the angiofibroma. Maurice and Milad further subscribed to this theory in 1981 (26). They concluded that the angiofibroma arose from ectopic genital tissue, which grew under the influence of male sex hormones during puberty. Farag and co-workers studied tumor samples from seven males and presented their findings in 1987 (27). The results of their analysis led to the following observations, that the angiofibromatous tissue was not in fact ectopic sequestered genital tissue, but normal nasal mucosa that had an excess of androgen receptors and grew during puberty as a result of fluctuations in circulating levels of male sex hormones. To date however no definitive study is available that has quantified angiofibroma growth rates with changes in estrogen and androgen levels.

CLINICAL PRESENTATION

The clinical presentation is usually dependent on tumor site and local extension at the time of diagnosis (Table 17.1). Neel detailed the patterns of tumor spread, which takes place by submucosal extension and through local tissue planes of least resistance (11). The tumor can extend anteriorly into the nasal cavity, superiorly into the sphenoid sinus and the sella, laterally via the sphenopalatine foramen into the pterygomaxillary fossa, the infratemporal fossa, and the inferior orbital fissure. Tumor spread intracranially is via the sella or the foramen lacerum into the middle cranial fossa. The majority of patients present with unilateral nasal obstruction and spontaneous epistaxis (2–5,13,16,21,28). Patients with more extensive tumor spread may also present with hypernasal speech, proptosis, conductive hearing loss, cheek swelling, and cranial nerve deficits of III to VI (28).

Table 17.1 Presenting Complaints

Unilateral epistaxis
Nasal obstruction
Rhinorrhoea
Hypernasal speech
Serous otitis media
Maxillary swelling
Anosmia
Proptosis
Exophthalmos
Diplopia
Headaches
Neck mass
Cranial nerves III–VI deficits

Clinical examination should consist of endoscopic examination of the nasal cavity and the nasopharynx. The appearance of the tumor mass tends to reflect its vascularity and may appear as pale white if predominantly composed of fibrous tissue or dark red and fleshy if vascular. Nasendoscopy usually reveals a polypoid or submucosal mass filling the nasopharynx or obstructing the posterior nares. More extensive tumors may prolapse below the soft palate, cause diffuse swelling over the maxillary antrum, and extend into the upper neck and infratemporal fossa.

Once clinical evaluation is complete diagnosis is currently established using dual radiological imaging with contrast-enhanced high-resolution computed tomography (CT) scanning and gadolinium-enhanced magnetic resonance imaging (MRI) (29–32). The diagnosis is based on the location of the tumor and its pattern of spread, which can be accurately mapped out using contrast enhanced CT scanning (2,3,30,31). As the tumor originates in the region of the sphenopalatine foramen there is usually enlargement of this foramen on CT imaging (Fig. 17.1) (4). Tumor vascularity

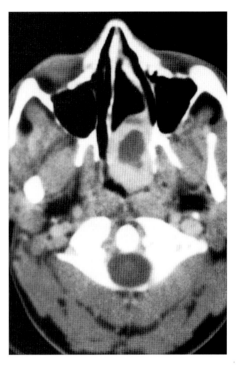

Figure 17.1 Computed tomography image of angiofibroma in the region of the pterygopalatine foramen.

is demonstrated by the presence of signal voids on MRI (Fig. 17.2) (32). Gadolinium-enhanced MRI clearly distinguishes tumor from surrounding tissue and is very sensitive in delineating intracranial extension; CT is also valuable in this context (Fig. 17.3). Biopsy of the mass continues to be contraindicated because of the risk of intractable hemorrhage and the fact that an accurate diagnosis can be safely

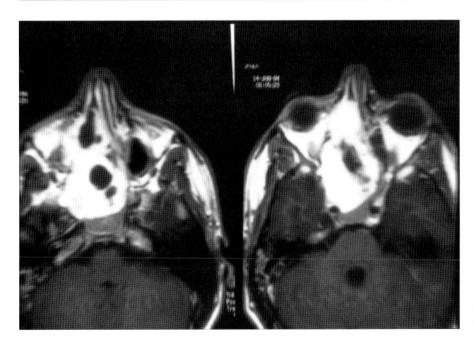

Figure 17.2 Magnetic resonance imaging with gadolinium enhancement demonstrating the highly vascular tumor with signal voids.

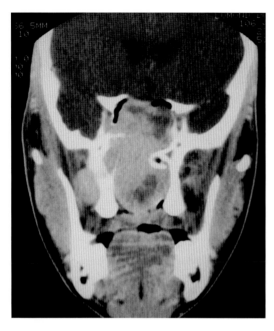

Figure 17.3 Computed tomography image demonstrating intracranial extension of angiofibroma.

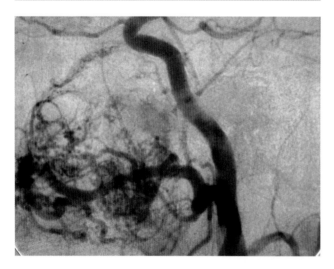

Figure 17.4 Angiogram demonstrating the blood supply of the angiofibroma.

established using current imaging modalities. The introduction of CT and MRI has eliminated the need to establish a diagnosis using angiography. Currently the role of angiography is in preoperative embolization to reduce tumor blood supply prior to surgery (Fig. 17.4).

Staging of the disease is based on the CT findings. The established staging systems are those of Sessions (1981) (3), Fisch (1983) (33), Chandler (1984) (2), Andrews (1989) (34), and Radkowski (1996) (35) (Table 17.2). Each system is based on the well-recognized patterns of tumor spread,

Table 17.2 Staging Systems for Juvenile Angiofibroma

Sessions et al. (3)	Ia Tumor limited to the nasopharynx and/or nares
	Ib Extension to one or more sinuses
	IIa Minimal extension into the pterygomaxillary fossa
	IIb Full occupation of the pterygomaxillary fossa
	III Intracranial extension
Fisch (33)	I Tumor limited to nasal cavity and nasopharynx with no bone erosion
	II Tumor invading the pterygomaxillary fossa and all sinuses, with bony destruction
	III Tumor invading the infratemporal fossa, orbit and parasellar region, remaining lateral to the cavernous sinus
	IV Tumors with extensive invasion of the cavernous sinus, optic chiasmal region or pituitary fossa
Chandler et al. (2)	I Tumor confined to the nasopharynx
	II Tumor extension to the nasopharynx and/or sphenoid sinus
	III Tumor extension into one or more of the following sites: maxillary antrum, ethmoid sinus, pterygomaxillary or infratemporal fossae, orbit, cheek
	IV Intracranial extension
Andrews (34)	I Tumor limited to the nasopharyngeal cavity; bone destruction negligible or limited to the sphenopalatine foramen
	II Tumor invading the pterygopalatine fossa or the maxillary, ethmoid, or sphenoid sinus with bone destruction
	III Tumor invading the infratemporal fossa or orbital region without intracranial involvement (a) or with intracranial extradural (parasellar) involvement (b)
	IV Intracranial intradural tumor without (a) or with (b) infiltration of the cavernous sinus, pituitary fossa, or optic chiasm
Radkowski (35)	Ia Limited to nose and/or nasopharynx
	Ib Extension into one or more sinuses
	IIa Minimal extension into the pterygopalatine fossa
	IIb Full occupation of the pterygopalatine fossa, displacing the posterior wall of the maxillary sinus forward. Lateral and/or anterior displacement of braches of the maxillary artery. Superior extension may occur, eroding orbital bones
	Involvement of the infratemporal fossa with or without extension to the cheek or posterior to the pterygoid plates
	IIIa Erosion of the skull base with minimal intracranial extension
	IIIb Erosion of the skull base with extensive intracranial extension with or without cavernous sinus invasion

and the higher the stage the more extensive the disease. Staging assists in planning management strategies and in the reporting of results, therefore the universal adoption of one staging system would allow for easier transfer of information and comparison of results between centers.

DIFFERENTIAL DIAGNOSIS

The diagnosis of juvenile angiofibroma is made on the basis of the clinical presentation, physical examination, and pattern of spread on CT imaging. However other lesions do present in the nasal cavity and nasopharynx, which give rise to nasal obstruction and epistaxis in this age group. Benign lesions such as simple nasal polyps can cause nasal obstruction, and an antrochoanal polyp can prolapse into the nasopharynx. Tumors that expand within the pterygo-palatine fossa and cause bowing of the posterior maxillary wall, such as rhabdomyosarcoma, hemangiopericytoma, and neurilemmomas must be differentiated from juvenile angiofibroma. Some of these lesions are also vascular with signal voids seen on MRI making the differential from juvenile angiofibroma difficult, and on occasion a tissue diagnosis may be necessary.

PATHOLOGICAL APPEARANCE

The macroscopic appearance of the angiofibroma is in part dependent on the varying amounts of fibrous to vascular elements within it. The mass can vary in appearance from pale white to red and fleshy with visible overlying vessels, which bleed on contact (Fig. 17.5). These tumors are non-encapsulated and spread by submucosal extension and local infiltration (11). The gross specimen is usually a lobulated mass with a base of varying width. The microscopic features of this tumor were defined by Sternberg in 1954 (36). He suggested that the tumor was a variant of an angioma because of the presence of vascular elements dispersed throughout a dense connective tissue network (Fig. 17.6). Electron microscopic studies carried out by McGavern and Taxy led them to conclude that the stromal cells may arise from fibroblasts or myofibroblasts, which are frequently seen in other fibroproliferative disorders (37,38). It has been suggested by certain authors that tumors with a predominantly fibrous composition on serial sectioning may represent the end stage of tumor involution.

NATURAL HISTORY OF THE DISEASE

Controversy still exists as to the natural progression of this disease (4). The literature supports the fact that angiofibroma is a disease predominantly of males (2,13–15) with only a handful of reported cases occurring in females (16–21). Patients tend to present when the tumor has grown to sufficient size to cause symptoms, which is usually during the adolescent years. The mean age at presentation is 13 years with a range from 5 to 50 years (2,4,5,13). There are no significant numbers of untreated control cases in the literature that have been serially followed with radiological imaging to support the theory that these tumors will eventually undergo involution and cease to grow. Despite this however there is a belief that tumor involution does in fact take place (39,40). Stansbie and Phelps (41) reported radiological documentation of intracranial tumor growth cessation in a patient who had undergone previous surgery. Weprin and Siemers (42) reported a single case of an 11-year-old boy with biopsy-proven angiofibroma who received no treatment but was followed with serial radiological imaging over an 11-year period. The patient was followed between 1978 and 1989, and during this period there was progressive involution of an originally extensive intracranial angiofibroma. A CT scan carried out in 1989 showed no evidence of tumor, thus confirming complete and spontaneous tumor resolution. These authors suggest that this case report adds weight to the theory that angiofibromas are hormone dependent, and postpubertal stabilization of sex hormone fluctuations can lead to involution of these tumors. However the overwhelming evidence suggests that these are locally aggressive tumors that will continue to grow and spread in the absence of adequate treatment, with a tendency to recur if incompletely excised (43,44).

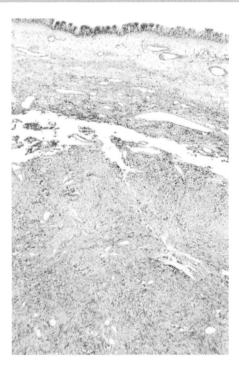

Figure 17.6 Microscopic pathological specimen.

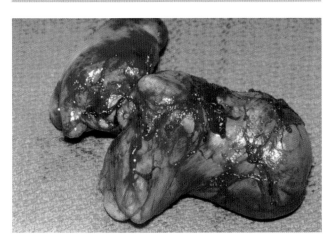

Figure 17.5 Macroscopic pathological specimen.

The potential for malignant transformation of the benign angiofibroma has also been alluded to in the literature. Makek et al. (45) reported a case of fibrosarcoma developing in a previously benign angiofibroma. However this patient had undergone four previous surgical resections and two courses of radiation treatment. They reviewed other case reports of malignant transformation and noted that all patients had received radiation treatment varying from 11 months to 21 years prior to malignant transformation. The majority of these lesions were reported as fibrosarcomas, which led Makek's group to conclude that the fibrous elements of the angiofibroma appeared to be the tissue most likely to undergo malignant transformation when exposed to radiation in the form of treatment. Of note is the fact that the Toronto group, which treated 55 patients with primary radiation, demonstrated no cases of malignant transformation within the tumor with a follow-up period ranging from 3 to 26 years (21).

MANAGEMENT

Surgery with preoperative embolization and postoperative radiotherapy for residual disease is currently practiced by most centers treating patients with angiofibromas. Historically numerous methods of treatment were employed in the management of this tumor, including cryosurgery (46), sclerotherapy, and electrocoagulation (24). Medical treatment using estrogen analogues had been in vogue in the 1970s and 1980s as a result of the various theories suggesting that tumor growth occurred in response to androgen stimulation (28,47–49). This form of therapy has now been largely abandoned.

Chemotherapeutic agents have been used by one center. Goepfert in 1985 treated five patients with two chemotherapeutic regimens. The first regimen was a combination of doxorubicin and dacarbazine. The second regimen was vincristine, dactinomycin, and cyclophosphamide. Tumor regression was recorded in all patients (50). Goepfert suggested that chemotherapeutic agents should be used in the management of residual disease where surgery or radiotherapy was not indicated. He also suggested that chemotherapeutic agents should be used in the setting of controlled trials.

Embolization

Angiofibromas are highly vascular lesions that derive their main blood supply from the external carotid system via the internal maxillary artery (Figs. 17.7 and 17.8). Additional supplies may be derived from the anterior branch of the ascending pharyngeal artery and the palatal branches of the external carotid system (51). As the tumor expands and spreads, it picks up blood supplies from the internal carotid system through the sphenoidal artery and the ophthalmic artery. Large tumors tend to receive a substantial blood supply from the arteries on the contralateral side.

Tumor removal without prior embolization has been reported to be associated with significant intraoperative blood loss, and there are reports of intraoperative mortalities secondary to hemorrhage (15). Robertson was the first to advocate preoperative embolization in the early 1970s (52). He proposed that occluding the vessels supplying the tumor would lead to less blood loss at the time of surgery. Since then many authors have published their results suggesting that preoperative embolization reduces blood loss and

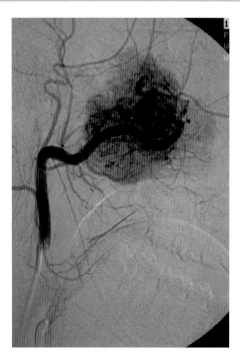

Figure 17.7 Preembolization angiogram.

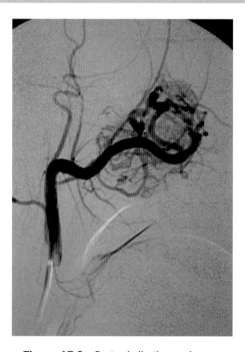

Figure 17.8 Postembolization angiogram.

assists in the ease of surgical resection as a result of a drier operative field (14,53–57).

Angiography with a view to embolization is recommended 48 to 72 hours prior to planned surgery (57). The material used to embolize the feeding vessels is either Gelfoam particles (51,53–54) of 1 mm in diameter or polyvinyl alcohol (58). Gelfoam is usually resorbed within a few weeks allowing the internal maxillary artery to recanalize partially or completely. Polyvinyl alcohol causes more permanent occlusion. Delay in performing surgery or the use of large particle size will adversely effect the success of embolization (57). Selective catheterization of the tumor feeding vessels requires the skill of an experienced interventional radiologist who is familiar with the blood supply to the face. Complications arising from embolization occur when there has been accidental embolization of cerebral vessels, ophthalmic vessels, and facial vessels, resulting in hemiparesis, blindness, and facial soft tissue and skin necrosis (51,59,60). However most reported series have few or no cases of permanent complications.

Radiation

The majority of centers treating angiofibromas will use adjunctive radiotherapy in the management of residual tumor following surgery or inoperable intracranial disease. The group from the Princess Margaret Hospital in Toronto has the largest experience of treating angiofibromas with primary radiotherapy (21). The outcome of 55 patients treated with primary radiotherapy, with a follow-up ranging from 3 to 26 years, was published in 1984 (21). Primary radiotherapy was as effective as primary surgery and posed no greater threat of serious morbidity. They state that with accurate CT imaging of the disease extent and using adequate radiation fields, control rates in excess of 80% could be achieved (Fig. 17.9). Their treatment protocol consists of external beam radiation of 3000 to 3500 cGy delivered over 3 weeks. Cummings emphasizes that tumor regression following radiation treatment takes place slowly, over a period of 12 to 20 months. Complete tumor regression, as demonstrated by clinical examination can be used as an index of control, as these patients rarely presented with recurrences.

Acute or late complications as a result of radiotherapy were infrequently encountered. Facial skeletal growth was not interfered with, and there were no cases of hypopituitorism. Two patients developed cataracts, as the orbit was involved with disease and therefore was in the field of radiation. Late tumor induction was recorded in two patients, with one case of radiation-induced thyroid cancer and one facial basal cell carcinoma. Intensity modulated radiation therapy has not been reported in large series of patients but may further reduce the chance of radiation induced complications (61).

Surgery

Primary surgical extirpation of angiofibromas is generally recognized as the mainstay of treatment. The surgical approach used will be determined by the stage of the disease as detailed from the clinical and radiological work-up. Surgery is tailored to the extent of the tumor, and the age and growth of the patient. From a realistic perspective, the choice of the surgical approach is based heavily on the surgeon's experience and training. However, several basic concepts are important including sufficient exposure of the tumor, the ability to effectively control bleeding, and trying to minimize postoperative facial scars, deformity, and growth of the facial skeleton (28).

The surgical approaches can be defined as endoscopic, transfacial, and transbasal/skull base approaches. The transfacial approaches can be further subdivided into transoral, transnasoethmoidal, and transmaxillary (62). The skull base approaches can be subdivided into the anterior and lateral approaches. Tumors involving the nasal cavity and extending anteriorly and inferiorly into the maxillary sinus can be approached through a midfacial degloving incision (Fig. 17.10) (63,64). This transoral approach described by Conley in 1979 sites an incision in the gingivobuccal sulcus spanning from one maxillary tuberosity to the other and extended into the pyriform aperture down to the periosteum (63). An osteotomy in the anterior maxillary wall is then performed to gain access to the tumor mass. Complete reconstruction of the facial skeleton is achieved at the end of the resection by fixation of the osteotomized bone segments.

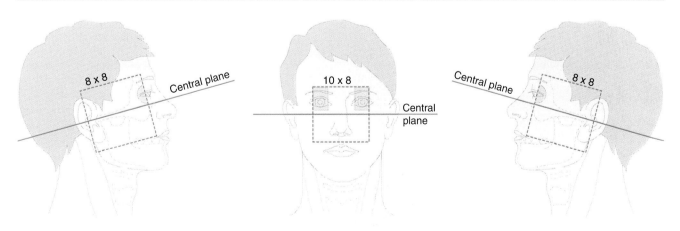

Figure 17.9 Radiation fields as graphically demonstrated by Cummings. *Source*: from Ref. 21.

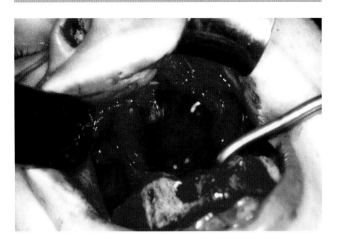

Figure 17.10   Facial degloving approach.

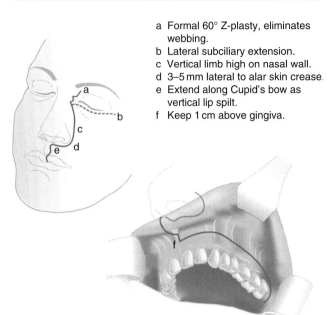

a   Formal 60° Z-plasty, eliminates webbing.
b   Lateral subciliary extension.
c   Vertical limb high on nasal wall.
d   3–5 mm lateral to alar skin crease.
e   Extend along Cupid's bow as vertical lip spilt.
f   Keep 1 cm above gingiva.

Figure 17.12   Approach via a Weber–Ferguson incision.

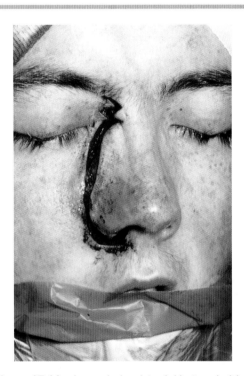

Figure 17.11   Approach via a lateral rhinotomy incision.

Minimal disruption of facial growth has been reported with this approach and the main complication is that of nasal aperture stenosis. This can be overcome by the judicious incorporation of Z-plasties into the rim incision.

Tumors that extend to involve the ethmoid sinus and the nasopharynx can be approached using a lateral rhinotomy incision with a mono or bilateral reflection of the nasal pyramid depending on the extent of the tumor (Fig. 17.11) (5,28,65,66). Again meticulous repositioning of the bony nasal pyramid is essential to achieve long-term satisfactory aesthetic results. Tumor that extends to involve the entire nasal cavity and the maxillary sinus with erosion of the

posterior wall of the sinus can be approached through a Weber–Ferguson incision (Fig. 17.12) (5,28). Wide exposure of the tumor is gained by complete removal of the frontal process of the maxilla, nasoantral wall below the inferior turbinate, lacrimal bone, lamina papyracea, and the anterior and posterior ethmoid cells up to the level of the cribriform plate. During this dissection care is taken to preserve the lacrimal sac and duct and the periosteum of the medial wall of the orbit.

Tumors where the main ethmoidal-sphenoidal extension involves the anterior skull base are approached through a bicoronal incision and an anterior craniofacial resection (67).

The incidence of tumor extension into the infratemporal fossa and the orbital apex and middle cranial fossa is quoted as being 10 to 20% (36,71). The treatment of intracranial extension is controversial (66). Fisch advocates a lateral skull base approach in the management of Fisch type III and type IV tumors, with a single lateral extradural approach to the middle cranial fossa (33). The frontal branch of the facial nerve, temporalis muscle, zygomatic arch, and masseter muscle are all displaced inferiorly to allow access to the infratemporal fossa. During tumor resection the internal carotid artery is visible at all times using this approach. Fisch states that with a lateral skull base approach it is possible to radically remove Fisch type III tumors, with subtotal removal of type IV tumors and postoperative radiotherapy used in the treatment of symptomatic intracranial residual disease (33). Some authors suggest that these type IV tumors are best managed with primary radiotherapy because of the greater morbidity and mortality associated with this type of surgical approach (28,66).

Transnasal endoscopic approaches for tumors that have extended to the nasal cavity, nasopharynx, paranasal

Table 17.3 Endoscopic Surgical Resection Results for Juvenile Angiofibromas

Author	Year	N	Age Range	Mean Age	Staging System	Stage	Prev OR	Endo	Endo Assist	F/U (mo) Mean (Range)	N Rec	Rx Rec
Carrau	2001	13	11–28	13	Not used	NS	4	7	8	34¶ (8–84)	2	Re OR
Scholtz	2001	7	10–37	16.9	Not used	NS		7	0	37.7 (12–60)	1	Re OR
Roger	2002	20	11–32	15*	Radkowski	I-4, II-7, IIIa-9	7			22¶ (NS)	2‡	Obs
Onerci	2003	12	12–20	16	Radkowski	Ib-1, IIa-2, IIb-4, IIc-1, IIIa-4		11	1	NS (6–36)	2‡	Obs
Wormald	2003	7	NS	14	Radkowski	I-1, IIa-2, IIb-3, IIc-1		7	0	45 (NS)	0	n/a
Nicolai	2003	15	13–30	15.8	Andrews	I-2, II-9, IIIa-3, IIIb-1	3	15	0	50 (24–93)	1	NS
Borghei	2006	23	10–26	16.2	Radkowski	Ia-5, Ib-9, IIa-4, IIb-5		23		33 (13–57)	1	Re-OR
Chen	2006	7	NS	19.7	Radkowski	Ia-1, IIa-2, IIc-1, IIIa-3		7	0	54 (28–84)	1	Re-OR
de Brito Macedo Ferreira	2006	9	9–20	15.2	Chandler	II-8 and III-1		8	1	NS (1–37)	0	n/a
Andrade	2007	12	9–22	NS	Andrews	I-8, II-4		12	0	24 (5–42)	0	n/a
Eloy	2007	6	11–23	17.2	Radkowski	Ia-1, Ib-1, IIb-4		6	0	67 (NS)	1	Re-OR

* = Median.
¶ = Median.
‡ = Residual or remnant tumor following resection.
Abbreviations: Endo = Endoscopic procedures; Endo assist = Endoscopically assisted procedures; F/U (mo) = Follow-up months; N = Number of patients; N Rec = Number of recurrences; NS = Not stated; n/a = Not applicable; Obs = Observation; Prev OR = Previous operation; Re-OR = Re-operation; Rx Rec = Treatment of recurrence.

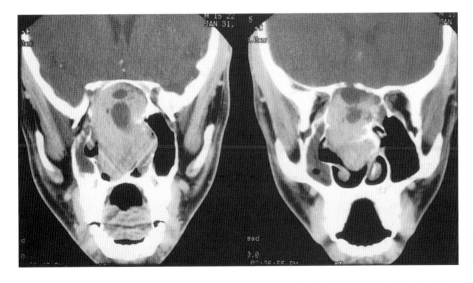

Figure 17.13 Computed tomography images demonstrating recurrence following treatment.

sinuses, and pterygopalatine fossa have been successful (Table 17.3). Involvement of the infratemporal fossa, anterior skull base, and orbit often require an open approach, but some authors report successful removal of these more extensive tumors by endoscopic surgery, even with minimal intracranial, extradural extension (68–72).

The recurrence rates following surgery in recent series range from 6 to 24% (Fig. 17.13) (73–76) in open approaches and 0 to 29% in endoscopic approaches (Table 17.3) (68–72,77–83). This is in comparison to rates of 61% recorded by Biller (84) in 1978 and 45% by Boles and Dedo (85) in

1976. The significant reduction in recurrence rates has been attributed to a better understanding of the disease process in combination with accurate preoperative staging with CT imaging.

FUTURE DEVELOPMENTS

Comprehensive genomic analysis has identified MDM2 and AURKA as novel amplified genes in juvenile angiofibromas (86). The fact that angiofibromas are highly vascular tumors has led several authors to investigate if their growth is regulated by angiogenic growth factors. Basic fibroblast growth factor, an angiogenic growth factor which stimulates endothelial cells, smooth muscle cells, and fibroblasts (87–89), has been identified in angiofibromas (90). Angiofibromas also have significant expression of matrix metalloproteinases that may have a role in tumor growth and angiogenesis (91).

Nagai et al. (92) localized transforming growth factor-b_1 (TGF-b_1) in the endothelial and fibroblast cells of angiofibromatous tissue. TGF-b_1 (93) induces various extracellular matrix proteins and vascular endothelial growth factor (VEGF). VEGF has been demonstrated to be involved in the regulation of normal and pathological angiogenesis (94–96). Nagai et al. concluded that TGF-b_1 may be involved in the development of fibrosis in angiofibromas and stimulate the production of VEGF leading to new blood vessel formation within the tumor. Platelet-derived growth factor B (97), a direct-acting angiogenic growth factor, has been identified by immunohistochemical analysis in angiofibromatous tumor tissue (92). This again suggests that v may contribute to the development of new blood vessel formation and fibrosis within the angiofibroma.

Inhibition of the expression of angiogenic growth factors by angiofibromas may lead to a reduction in tumor growth, or indeed tumor involution. The delivery of an antiangiogenic agent to the tumor bed, for example by selective angiography has potential for future use in the clinical setting.

REFERENCES

1. Batsakis JG. Tumours of the Head and Neck, 2nd ed. Baltimore: Williams and Wilkins, 1979; 296–300.
2. Chandler JR, Goulding R, Moskowitz L et al. Nasopharyngeal angiofibromas: staging and management. Ann Otol Rhinol Laryngol 1984; 93: 322–9.
3. Sessions RB, Bryan RN, Naclerio RM et al. Radiographic staging of juvenile angiofibroma. Head Neck Surg 1981; 3: 279–83.
4. Harrison DFN. The natural history, pathogenesis and treatment of juvenile angiofibroma. Arch Otolaryngol Head Neck Surg 1987; 113: 936–42.
5. Iannetti G, Belli E, De Ponte F et al. The surgical approaches to nasopharyngeal angiofibroma. J Cranio-Maxillofac Surg 1994; 22: 311–16.
6. Jacobsson MB, Petruson B, Svendsen P et al. Juvenile nasopharyngeal angiofibroma: a report of eighteen cases. Acta Otolaryngol 1988; 105: 132–9.
7. Mishra SC, Shukla GK, Bhatia N et al. A rational classification of angiofibroma of the post nasal space. J Laryngol Otol 1989; 103: 912–16.
8. Hippocrates. Complete works, Vol. 10 (Translated by E. Littre). Paris: JB Baillière, 1839–61.
9. Chelius JM. System of Surgery, Vol. 2. London: Henry Renshaw, 1847.
10. Friedberg SA. Vascular fibromas of the nasopharynx. Arch Otolaryngol 1940; 13: 313–26.
11. Neel HB, Whicker JH, Devine KD et al. Juvenile angiofibroma: review of 120 cases. Am J Surg 1973; 126: 547–56.
12. Lund VJ, Lloyd GAS, Howard DJ. Juvenile angiofibroma: imaging techniques in diagnosis. Rhinology 1989; 28: 97–102.
13. Antonelli AR, Cappiello J, Di Lorenzo D et al. Diagnosis, staging and treatment of juvenile nasopharyngeal angiofibroma (JNA). Laryngoscope 1987; 97: 1319–25.
14. Economou TS, Abermayor E, Ward PH. Juvenile nasopharyngeal angiofibroma: an update of the UCLA experience, 1960–1985. Laryngoscope 1988; 98: 170–5.
15. Ward PH. The evolving management of juvenile nasopharyngeal angiofibroma. J Laryngol Otol 1983; 8 (Suppl): 103–4.
16. Witt TR, Shah JR, Sternberg SS. Juvenile nasopharyngeal angiofibroma. A 30 year clinical review. Am J Surg 1983; 146: 521–5.
17. Finnerman WB. Juvenile nasopharyngeal angiofibroma in the female. Arch Otolaryngol 1951; 54: 620–3.
18. Parchet V. Nasopharyngeal angiofibromas in women. Ann Otolaryngol 1951; 68: 60–9.
19. Handousa A, Farig H, Elwi AM. Nasopharyngeal fibroma: clinico-pathological study of 70 cases. J Laryngol Otol 1954; 68: 647–66.
20. Osborn DA, Sokolovski A. Juvenile nasopharyngeal angiofibroma in an elderly female. Arch Otolaryngol 1981; 89: 602–3.
21. Cummings BJ, Blend R, Keane T et al. Primary radiation therapy for juvenile nasopharyngeal angiofibroma. Laryngoscope 1984; 94: 1599–605.
22. Brunner H. Nasopharyngeal fibroma. Ann Otol Rhinol Laryngol 1942; 51: 29–63.
23. Martin H, Ehrlich HE, Abels JC. Juvenile nasopharyngeal angiofibroma. Ann Surg 1948; 129: 513–36.
24. Schiff M. Juvenile nasopharyngeal angiofibroma: a theory of pathogenesis. Laryngoscope 1959; 69: 981–1016.
25. Walike JW, Mackay B. Nasopharyngeal angiofibroma: light and electron microscopic changes after stilbesterol therapy. Laryngoscope 1970; 79: 1108–13.
26. Maurice M, Milad M. Pathogenesis of juvenile nasopharyngeal fibroma. J Laryngol Otol 1981; 95: 1121–6.
27. Farag NM, Ghanimah SE, Ragie A et al. Hormone receptors in nasopharyngeal angiofibroma. Laryngoscope 1987; 97: 208–11.
28. Gullane PJ, Davidson J, O'Dwyer T et al. Juvenile angiofibroma: a review of the literature and a case series report. Laryngoscope 1992; 102: 928–33.
29. Davis KR. Embolization of epistaxis and juvenile nasopharyngeal angiofibromas. Am J Roentgenol 1987; 148: 209–18.
30. Weinstein MA, Levine H, Duchesneau PM et al. Diagnosis of juvenile angiofibroma by computed tomography. Radiology 1978; 126: 703–5.
31. Levine HL, Weinstein MA, Tucker HM et al. Diagnosis of juvenile nasopharyngeal angiofibroma by computed tomography. Otolaryngol Head Neck Surg 1979; 87: 304–10.
32. Lloyd GAS, Phelps PD. Juvenile angiofibroma: imaging by magnetic resonance, CT and conventional techniques. Clin Otolaryngol 1986; 59: 675–8.
33. Fisch U. The infratemporal fossa approach for nasopharyngeal tumours. Laryngoscope 1983; 93: 36–44.
34. Andrews C, Fisch U, Valavanis A et al. The surgical management of extensive nasopharyngeal angiofibromas with the infratemporal fossa approach. Laryngoscope 1989; 99: 429–37.
35. Radkowski D, McGill T, Healy GB et al. Angiofibroma. Changes in staging and treatment. Arch Otolaryngol Head Neck Surg 1996; 122: 122–9.
36. Sternberg SS. Pathology of juvenile nasopharyngeal angiofibroma. A lesion of adolescent males. Cancer 1954; 7: 15–28.
37. McGavern MH, Sessions DG, Dorfman RF et al. Nasopharyngeal angiofibroma. Arch Otolaryngol 1969; 90: 94–104.
38. Taxy JB. Juvenile nasopharyngeal angiofibroma: an ultrastructural study. Cancer 1977; 39: 1044–54.
39. Bahtia ML. Intracranial extensions of juvenile angiofibroma of the nasopharynx. J Laryngol Otol 1967; 81: 1395–403.
40. Jacobsson M, Petruson B, Ruth M et al. Involution of juvenile angiofibroma with intracranial extension. Arch Otolaryngol Head Neck Surg 1989; 115: 238–9.
41. Stansbie JM, Phelps PD. Involution of residual juvenile nasopharyngeal angiofibroma. J Laryngol Otol 1986; 100: 599–603.

42. Weprin LS, Siemers PT. Spontaneous regression of juvenile nasopharyngeal angiofibroma. Arch Otolaryngol Head Neck Surg 1991; 117: 796–9.

43. Bryan RN, Sessions RB, Horowitz BL. Radiographic management of juvenile angiofibromas. Am J Neuroradiology 1984; 93: 322–9.

44. McCombe A, Lund VJ, Howard DJ. Recurrence in juvenile angiofibroma. Rhinology 1990; 28: 97–102.

45. Makek MS, Andrews JC, Fisch U. Malignant transformation of a nasopharyngeal angiofibroma. Laryngoscope 1989; 99: 1088–92.

46. Maniglia AJ, Mazzarella LA, Minkowitz S et al. Maxillary sinus angiofibroma treated with cryosurgery. Arch Otolaryngol 1969; 89: 111–16.

47. Lee DA, Rao BR, Meyer JS et al. Hormonal receptor determination in juvenile nasopharyngeal angiofibromas. Cancer 1980; 46: 547–51.

48. Johns ME, MacLeod RM, Cantrell RW. Estrogen receptors in nasopharyngeal angiofibromas. Laryngosope 1980; 90: 628–34.

49. Johnson S, Kloster JH, Schiff M. The action of hormones on juvenile nasopharyngeal angiofibroma. Acta Otolaryngol 1966; 61: 143–59.

50. Goepfert H, Cangir A, Lee YY. Chemotherapy for aggressive juvenile nasopharyngeal angiofibroma. Arch Otolaryngol Head Neck Surg 1985; 111: 285–9.

51. Lasjaunias P, Picard L, Manelfe C et al. Angiofibroma of the nasopharynx. J Neuroradiology 1980; 7: 73–95.

52. Roberson GH, Biller H, Sessions DG et al. Presurgical embolization of the internal maxillary artery in juvenile angiofibroma. Laryngoscope 1972; 82: 1524–32.

53. Roberson GH, Price AC, Davis JM et al. Therapeutic embolization of juvenile angiofibroma. Am J Roentgenol 1979; 133: 657–63.

54. Pletcher JD, Newton TH, Deho HN et al. Preoperative embolization of juvenile nasopharyngeal angiofibromas of the nasopharynx. Ann Otol Rhinol Laryngol 1975; 84: 740–6.

55. Waldman SR, Levine HL, Astor F et al. Surgical experience with nasopharyngeal angiofibroma. Arch Otolaryngol 1983; 107: 677–82.

56. Steinberger SJ, Wetmore RF. Current management of juvenile nasopharyngeal angiofibroma. Trans Pa Acad Ophthalmol Otolaryngol 1984; 37: 65–70.

57. Siniluoto TMJ, Luotonen JP, Tikkakoski TA et al. Value of preoperative embolization in surgery for nasopharyngeal angiofibroma. J Laryngol Otol 1993; 107: 514–21.

58. Jacobsson M, Petruson B, Svendsen P et al. Juvenile nasopharyngeal angiofibroma. A report of eighteen cases. Acta Otolaryngol 1988; 105: 132–9.

59. Gay I, Elidan J, Gordon R. Oronasal fistula: a possible complication of preoperative embolization in the management of juvenile nasopharyngeal angiofibroma. J Laryngol Otol 1983; 97: 651–6.

60. Soong HK, Newman SA, Kumar AAJ. Branch artery occlusion. An unusual complication of external carotid embolization. Arch Ophthalmol 1982; 100: 1909–11.

61. Kuppersmith RB, Teh BS, Donovan DT et al. The use of intensity modulated radiotherapy for the treatment of extensive and recurrent juvenile angiofibroma. Int J Pediatr Otorhinolaryngol 2000; 52: 261–8.

62. Belmont J. The Le Fort osteotomy approach for nasopharyngeal and nasal fossa tumours. Arch Otolaryngol Head Neck Surg 1988; 114: 751–4.

63. Conley J, Price J. Sublabial approach to the nasal and nasopharyngeal cavities. Am J Surg 1979; 138: 615–18.

64. Casson PR, Bonnano PC et al. The midfacial degloving procedure. Plast Reconstr Surg 1974; 53: 102–13.

65. Pope T. Surgical approach to tumours of the nasal cavity. Laryngoscope 1989; 88: 912–16.

66. Bremer JW, Neel HB, De Santo LW et al. Angiofibroma treatment trends in 150 patients in 40 years. Laryngoscope 1986; 96: 1321–9.

67. Standefer J, Holt GR, Brown WE et al. Combined intracranial and extracranial excision of nasopharyngeal angiofibroma. Laryngoscope 1983; 93: 772–8.

68. Roger G, Tran Ba Huy P, Froelich P et al. Exclusively endoscopic removal of juvenile nasopharyngeal angiofibroma: trends and limits. Arch Otolaryngol Head Neck Surg 2002; 128: 928–35. Erratum in: Arch Otolaryngol Head Neck Surg 2003; 129: 88.

69. Onerci TM, Yucel OT, Ogretmenoglu O. Endoscopic surgery in treatment of juvenile nasopharyngeal angiofibroma. Int J Pediatr Otorhinolaryngol 2003; 67: 1219–25.

70. Nicolai P, Berlucchi M, Tomenzoli D et al. Endoscopic surgery for juvenile angiofibroma: When and how. Laryngoscope 2003; 113: 77–82.

71. Chen MK, Tsai YL, Lee KW et al. Strictly endoscopic and harmonic scalpel-assisted surgery of nasopharyngeal angiofibromas: eligible for advanced stage tumors. Acta Oto-Laryngologica 2006; 126: 1321–5.

72. Hofmannn T, Bernal-Sprekelsen M, Koele W et al. Endoscopic resection of juvenile angiofibromas – long term results. Rhinology 2005; 43: 282–9.

73. Jafek BW, Krekorian EA, Kirsch WM et al. Juvenile nasopharyngeal angiofibroma: management of intracranial extension. Head Neck Surg 1979; 2: 119–28.

74. Krekorian EA, Kato RH. Surgical management of nasopharyngeal angiofibroma with intracranial extension. Laryngoscope 1977; 87: 154–64.

75. Tandon DA, Bahadur S, Kacker SK et al. Nasopharyngeal angiofibroma: a nine year experience. J Laryngol Otol 1988; 102: 805–9.

76. Maharaj D, Fernandes CMC. Surgical experience with juvenile nasopharyngeal angiofibroma. Acta Otolaryngol (Stockh) 1988; 105: 132–9.

77. Carrau RL, Snyderman CH, Kassam AB et al. Endoscopic and endoscopic-assisted surgery for juvenile angiofibroma. Laryngoscope 2001; 111: 483–7.

78. Scholtz AW, Appenroth E, Kammen-Jolly K et al. Juvenile nasopharyngeal angiofibroma: management and therapy. Laryngoscope 2001; 111: 681–7.

79. Wormald PJ, Van Hasselt A. Endoscopic removal of juvenile angiofibromas. Otolaryngol Head Neck Surg 2003; 129: 684–91.

80. Borghei P, Baradaranfar MH, Borghei SH et al. Transnasal endoscopic resection of juvenile nasopharyngeal angiofibroma without preoperative embolization (Clinical report). Ear Nose Throat J 2006; 85: 740–3.

81. de Brito Macedo Ferreira LM, Gomes EF, Azevedo JF et al. Endoscopic surgery of nasopharyngeal angiofibroma. Revista Brasileira de Otorrinolaringologia 2006; 72: 475–80.

82. Andrade NA, Pinto JA, Nobrega MO et al. Exlusively endoscopic surgery for juvenile nasopharyngeal angiofibromas. Otolaryngol Head Neck Surg 2007; 137: 492–6.

83. Eloy P, Watelet JB, Hatert AS et al. Endonasal endoscopic resection of juvenile nasopharyngeal angiofibroma. Rhinology 2007; 45: 24–30.

84. Biller H.F. Juvenile nasopharyngeal angiofibroma. Ann Otol Rhinol Laryngol 1978; 87: 630–2.

85. Boles R, Dedo H. Nasopharyngeal angiofibroma. Laryngoscope 1976; 86: 364–70.

86. Schick B, Wemmert S, Bechtel U et al. Comprehensive genomic analysis identifies MDM2 and AURKA as novel amplified genes in juvenile angiofibromas. Head & Neck 2007; 29: 479–87.

87. Folkman J, Klagsbrun M. Angiogenic factors (Review). Science 1987; 235: 442.

88. Moscatelli D, Presta M, Rifkin DB. Purification of a factor from human placenta that stimulates capillary endothelial cell

protease production, DNA synthesis and migration. Proc Natl Acad Sci USA 1986; 83: 2091.

89. Gospodarowicz D, Neufeld G, Schweigerer L. Fibroblast growth factor (Review). Mol Cell Endocrinol 1986; 46: 187.

90. Schiff M, Gonzalez AM, Ong M et al. Juvenile nasopharyngeal angiofibromas contain an angiogenic growth factor: basic FGF. Laryngoscope 102: 1992; 940–5.

91. Duerr S, Wendler O, Aigner T et al. Metalloproteinases in juvenile angiofibroma--a collagen rich tumor. Hum Path 2008; 39: 259–68.

92. Nagai MA, Butugan O, Logullo A et al. Expression of growth factors, proto-oncogenes, and p53 in nasopharyngeal angiofibromas. Laryngoscope 1996; 106: 190–5.

93. Folkman J, Ling Y. Angiogenesis. J Biol Chem 1992; 267: 10931–4.

94. Ferrara N, Houck K, Jakeman L et al. Molecular and biological properties of the vascular endothelial growth factor family of proteins. Endocrinol Rev 1992; 13: 18–32.

95. Pertovaara L, Kaipainen A, Mustone T et al. Vascular endothelial growth factor is induced in response to transforming growth factor-b in fibroblastic and epithelial cells. J Biol Chem 1994; 269: 6271–4.

96. Rissau W. Angiogenesis is coming of age. Circ Res 1998; 82: 926–8.

97. Ross R, Raines EW, Bowen-Pope DF. The biology of platelet-derived growth factor (Review). Cell 1986; 46: 155.

18

Tumors of the Nasopharynx

Christopher M Nutting, Christopher P Cottrill and William I Wei

INTRODUCTION

Nasopharyngeal tumors are biologically distinct from the more common head and neck tumors and are characterized by their propensity for early lymphatic and distant metastatic spread. Anatomical constraints, together with widespread lymphatic permeation effectively exclude curative surgery. Radical radiotherapy is the mainstay of treatment for early disease and is combined with chemotherapy for advanced disease.

ANATOMY

The nasopharynx lies beneath the skull base, posterior to and continuous with the nasal cavities (Fig. 18.1A, B). It is lined in part by pseudostratified columnar respiratory-type epithelium and also in part by non-keratinizing stratified squamous epithelium.

Anatomical Relations

Roof and Posterior Wall

The sloping roof of the nasopharynx is continuous with the posterior wall. It is formed by the floor of the sphenoid sinus medially and the fibrocartilage of the foramina lacerum laterally (Fig. 18.1A, B). The cavernous sinus with the internal carotid artery and cranial nerves III, IV, V and VI lies immediately above the foramen lacerum on each side (Fig. 18.1C). The posterior wall overlies the basilar part of the occipital bone and the anterior arch of the atlas inferiorly. It is ridged, posteriorly, by the longus capitis muscles and beneath its fascial lining lie the medial retropharyngeal lymph nodes (Fig. 18.1D).

Lateral Walls

The eustachian (auditory) tubes gain access to the nasopharynx through its lateral walls, which are themselves formed by the pharyngobasilar fascia reinforced inferiorly by the superior constrictor muscles. Viewed from the nasal cavities the upper and posterior aspects of the eustachian tube orifices are marked by the cartilaginous tubal elevation behind which, on each side, lies the slit-like fossa of Rosenmüller. Immediately deep to the lateral wall lies the parapharyngeal space containing the internal carotid artery, cranial nerves IX, X, XI, XII, the internal jugular vein and lateral retropharyngeal lymph nodes (of Rouvière) (Fig. 18.1D).

The pharyngeal fascia and fibrous foramen lacerum offer little resistance to direct invasion by malignant tumors of the nasopharynx. This, along with the frequent involvement of lateral retropharyngeal nodes, explains the relatively common occurrence of cranial nerve palsies.

Floor

The floor of the nasopharynx is formed by the superior surface of the soft palate, which, in conjunction with the palatopharyngeal sphincter, serves to close the pharyngeal isthmus during swallowing, isolating the nasopharynx from the oropharynx below.

Lymphatic Drainage and Nerve Supply

The mucosa is raised into several folds by the underlying musculature and contains variable aggregations of lymphoid tissue. The most prominent of these, especially in children, is the pharyngeal tonsil (or "adenoids") lying in the midline and projecting forward from the junction of the roof and posterior wall. The rich submucosal lymphatic plexus drains primarily to the retropharyngeal, upper deep posterior cervical (junctional) and jugulodigastric node groups.

The nerve supply to the nasopharyngeal mucosa is derived from the maxillary division of the trigeminal nerve via a small branch, the pharyngeal nerve, which arises in the pterygopalatine fossa, close to the pterygopalatine ganglion.

PATHOLOGY

The pathological classification of nasopharyngeal tumors is described in Table 18.1. There have been many classifications proposed for nasopharyngeal carcinoma and the World Health Organization (WHO) originally described three types according to histology (1). In practical terms, however, epidemiological and clinical features broadly define two groups, the squamous cell carcinomas (SCC) of varying degrees of differentiation and the undifferentiated carcinomas of nasopharyngeal type (UCNT) (Fig. 18.2) (2–4). The WHO type 2 tumors are the most poorly defined with no clear morphological distinction between these and the undifferentiated carcinomas (3).

The term lymphoepithelioma describes a carcinoma with a reactive lymphocytic infiltrate where the epithelial component may form well-defined aggregates (Regaud pattern) or be diffusely interspersed with inflammatory cells (Schmincke pattern). As the lymphocytic infiltrate has no clear prognostic significance these tumors are best categorized according to the features of the epithelial component, which is invariably undifferentiated.

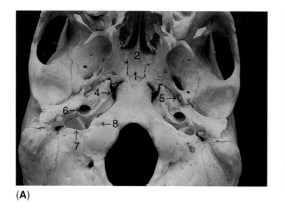

(A)

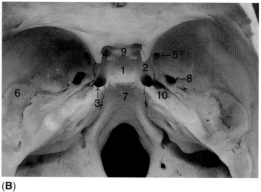

(B)

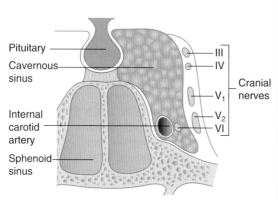

Pituitary
Cavernous sinus
Internal carotid artery
Sphenoid sinus

III
IV
V₁
V₂
VI

Cranial nerves

V₁ = Opthalmic division of V cranial nerve
V₂ = Maxillary division of cranial nerve
(C)

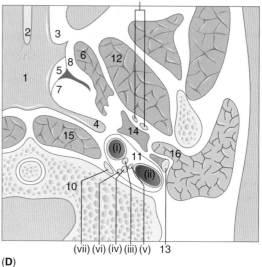

(vii) (vi) (iv) (iii) (v) 13
(D)

Figure 18.1

(A) Base of skull.
  1: roof of nasopharynx;
  2: posterior end of vomer;
  3: posterior end of inferior turbinates;
  4: foramen lacerum;
  5: eustachian tube orifice (bony portion);
  6: carotid canal;
  7: internal jugular canal;
  8: hypoglossal canal;

(B) Middle cranial fossa.
  1: sella turcica;
  2: carotid groove;
  3: foramen lacerum;
  4: optic canal;
  5: foramen rotundum;
  6: floor of middle cranial fossa;
  7: clivus;
  8: foramen ovale;
  9: optic chiasm;
  10: trigeminal ganglion impression.

(C) Cavernous sinus in coronal section

(D) Transverse section through the nasopharynx at the level of the atlas (C1).
  1: roof of nasopharynx;
  2: posterior end of vomer;
  3: posterior end of inferior turbinates;
  4: fossa of Rosenmüller;
  5: eustachian tube orifice;
  6: eustachian tube musculature;
  7: posterior eustachian tube cushion;
  8: anterior eustachian tube cushion;
  9: posterior wall of nasopharynx;
  10: C1;
  11: carotid sheath and its contents;
    i) internal carotid artery (ICA);
    ii) internal jugular vein (IJV);
    iii) cranial nerve IX;
    iv) cranial nerve X;
    v) cranial nerve XI;
    vi) cranial nerve XII;
    vii) sympathetic trunk;
  12: lateral pterygoid muscle;
  13: styloid process and musculature;
  14: parapharyngeal space;
  15: longus capitus;
  16: deep lobe of parotid;
  17: cranial nerve V (branches of mandibular division).

Table 18.1 Pathological Classification of Nasopharyngeal Tumors

Benign tumors
    Juvenile angiofibroma
Malignant tumors
    Nasopharyngeal carcinoma (NPC)   85%*
        WHO type 1–keratinizing squamous cell carcinoma
        WHO type 2–nonkeratinizing (differentiated) carcinoma
        WHO type 3–undifferentiated carcinoma
    Non-Hodgkin's lymphoma (Hodgkin's lymphoma rare)   10%*
    Adenoid cystic carcinoma
    Adenocarcinoma and minor salivary gland tumors
    Plasmacytoma
    Melanoma
    Sarcoma (especially rhabdomyosarcoma)
    Chordoma

*Approximate proportion of all malignant tumors.

NASOPHARYNGEAL CARCINOMA

Epidemiology and Pathogenesis

In the Western hemisphere (the Americas and Europe) nasopharyngeal carcinoma (NPC) is rare with an annual incidence of around 0.5/100,000, accounting for 1–2% of all head and neck cancers. In contrast, in southern China and Hong Kong the disease is endemic with annual incidence rates of up to 20–30/100,000 (5,6). This disparity is related to histopathological subtypes. In North American series keratinizing SCCs account for up to 68% of cases (7) while in the Far East over 95% are WHO type 2–3 (8). The incidence of UCNT is also high in Eskimo and Native Alaskan populations (9) and moderately increased in Malaysia, north Africa and southern Europe.

NPC probably results from a complex interaction of genetic and environmental factors. Familial clusters of NPC are reported in endemic areas and emigrants from these areas carry with them an increased risk (10), though this diminishes somewhat in successive generations (11). In ethnic Chinese, NPC is associated with the concurrence of human leukocyte antigen (HLA) types A2 and Bw46 (formerly Bsin2) (12). The phenotype B17 carries a similar relative risk and, like Bw46, is associated with benign conditions characterized by immune dysfunction such as autoimmune thyrotoxicosis and systemic lupus erythematosus. B17 is said to be associated with younger-onset disease and possibly carries a poorer prognosis (13). An HLA linkage study in affected sibling pairs suggests the presence of an NPC susceptibility gene closely linked to the HLA locus that may carry a relative risk of over 20 (14).

There is a strong association between UCNT and positive serology for Epstein–Barr virus (EBV) antigens (15). Antibody titres (particularly IgA) to the viral capsid antigen (VCA) and early antigen complex (EA) have been correlated with the stage of the disease (16) and a fall reflects tumor response to therapy. Persistently elevated or rising antibody titres predict for progression or recurrence (17,18). Clonal EBV DNA has been demonstrated in NPC as have the nuclear proteins necessary to ensure persistence of the viral genome with cell replication (19). These observations imply that the virus is present from the start of the neoplastic process and could contribute to it. The EBV latent membrane protein LMP1, for example, has oncogenic and growth-stimulating properties (19). It is conceivable that the genetic factors eluded to above influence the way in which an initial EBV infection is handled, allowing its persistence in a potentially oncogenic form. Recently, vaccines against EBV LMP1 (20) have entered clinical trials as an adjuvant to chemoradiotherapy.

Until recently it has been thought that SCC of the nasopharynx is biologically distinct from UCNT, with no EBV association. However, in situ hybridization techniques have now demonstrated the presence of EBV-encoded ribonucleic acid in all three histological types, though it is less abundant in well-differentiated tumors (21). Whether SCC is associated with the same risk factors as for other head and neck sites is unclear, though there is certainly evidence to suggest that heavy smoking further increases the risk of UCNT in endemic areas (22).

Environmental factors beyond EBV are likely to be important in UCNT. Ho (23) hypothesized that early childhood consumption of salted fish contributed to the high-risk of NPC in southern China and Hong Kong. This has been supported by a case-control study (24) and may also explain the high incidence of UCNT among Eskimos (9). Fish preservation by salting leads to the accumulation of potentially carcinogenic nitrosamines (23).

In general NPC affects a younger population than cancer at other head and neck sites. In endemic areas the

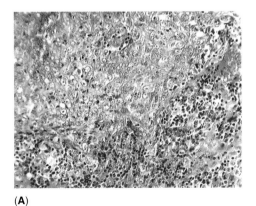

(A)

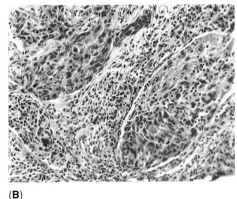

(B)

Figure 18.2 Photomicrographs of (A) undifferentiated carcinoma (UCNT) and (B) squamous cell carcinoma of the nasopharynx (hematoxylin and eosin). Both specimens show a background lymphocytic infiltrate illustrating that this is not a specific phenomenon.

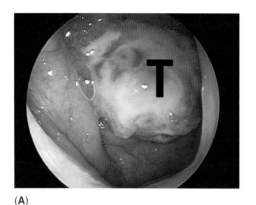

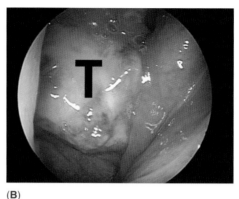

Figure 18.3 **(A)** Endoscopic view of an exophytic nasopharyngeal carcinoma (T), 0° endoscope inserted through the right nasal cavity. **(B)** Endoscopic view of the same tumor (T), 0o endoscope inserted through the left nasal cavity.

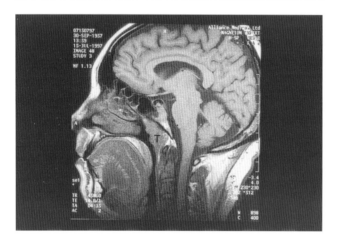

Figure 18.4 T1-weighted sagittal MR image showing a UCNT (T) occupying the roof and posterior wall of the nasopharynx.

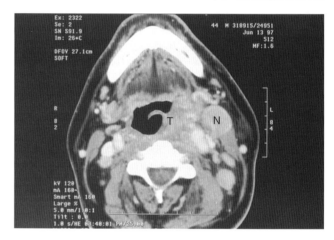

Figure 18.5 Contrast-enhanced CT scan showing invasion of the left lateral wall of the oropharynx by UCNT (T). Note the enlarged lymph nodes (N).

incidence rises from age 20 to peak in the fourth and fifth decades (22). In areas of lower risk the median age falls between the fifth and sixth decades but there is still a significant incidence in individuals under 30, giving rise to a bimodal distribution, with an initial peak between 15 and 25 years. All NPC types show a male predominance of around 3:1.

Natural History

The majority of tumors arise in the region of the fossa of Rosenmüller or roof of the nasopharynx (Fig. 18.3). By direct anterior extension the tumor may invade the posterior nasal cavity or extend inferiorly along the pharyngeal wall (Fig. 18.4), on to the soft palate or down to the tonsil (Fig. 18.5).

Involvement of the skull base at presentation has been reported in 35% of cases evaluated by CT scanning (25). The tumor may invade the sphenoid sinus or gain access to the cavernous sinus through the fibrous tissue floor of

the foramen lacerum (Fig. 18.6). Here cranial nerves III–VI are vulnerable, with V and VI being most frequently involved clinically (Fig. 18.7).

Parapharyngeal space involvement has been described in 35% to over 80% of cases (8,25–27). It may arise by direct tumor displacement, particularly adjacent to the eustachian tube where the lateral wall is relatively deficient (Fig. 18.8). Alternatively it can occur by expansion of involved retropharyngeal nodes (Fig. 18.9). Either case may progress to involvement of lower cranial nerves (CN IX–XII) where they lie adjacent to the major vessels in the posterior part of the parapharyngeal space. From the parapharyngeal space the tumor can gain access to the middle cranial fossa (Fig. 18.6) and cavernous sinus via the foramen ovale. Involvement of the pterygoid plates may lead to forward extension into the pterygopalatine fossa and beyond into the inferior orbital fissure. Alternatively tumor may invade the orbit via the ethmoid sinuses (Fig. 18.10).

In a report of 628 patients, 7% had involvement of one or more of cranial nerves II–VIII, while 3.5% had

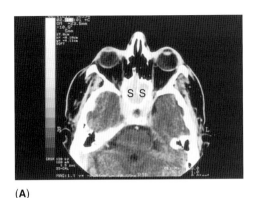

(A)

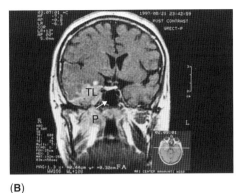

(B)

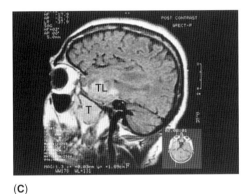

(C)

Figure 18.6 **(A)** Contrast-enhanced CT scan of the skull base showing tumor filling the sphenoid sinuses (S). **(B)** Gadolinium-enhanced coronal T1–weighted MR image showing UCNT in the right parapharyngeal space (P), extending through the foraminae of the skull base to involve the temporal lobe (TL) of the brain and cavernous sinus (arrow). **(C)** Sagittal image from the same series as **(B)**. Primary UCNT (T) with extension into temporal lobe (TL).

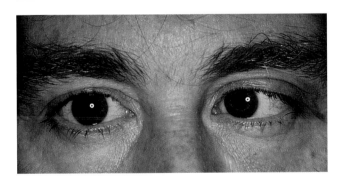

Figure 18.7 Right lateral rectus palsy.

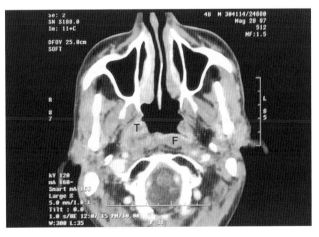

Figure 18.8 CT scan with intravenous contrast showing a right-sided nasopharyngeal carcinoma (T) displacing the parapharyngeal space. Note how the tumor has obliterated the right fossa of Rosenmüller as compared to the normal fossa (F) on the left.

involvement of the lower cranial nerves (IX–XII). Five patients had involvement of both groups (25). In a series of 378 patients reported from the M.D. Anderson Cancer Center, 8% had one or more cranial nerve palsies, with CN VI being the most commonly involved (28). In contrast, Lederman (29) described cranial nerve involvement in 26% of 218 patients at presentation and a similar figure (23.8%) was reported by Perez et al (30). Further lateral extension through the skull base can lead to sympathetic chain involvement and Horner's syndrome.

NPC is characterized by early and often bulky cervical lymph node involvement (Fig. 18.11). Large series report between 63% and 79% lymph node involvement (25,27,28, 30,31) with around 30% of patients having bilateral lymphadenopathy at diagnosis (28,30). There has been no obvious increase in the reported incidence with the now routine use of CT scanning (25,27), suggesting that nodal involvement is rarely subtle. The jugulodigastric (upper deep cervical) and posterior cervical (upper and middle) node groups are most frequently involved, followed by the middle deep cervical (28,30,32). Submental, occipital, or parotid nodal involvement is unusual. Intra-parotid lymph node metastases are rare.

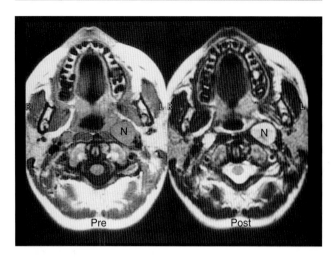

Figure 18.9   Paired T1-weighted MR images (pre- and postintravenous gadolinium) showing distortion of the left parapharyngeal space due to expansion of a retropharyngeal lymph node (N) by UCNT.

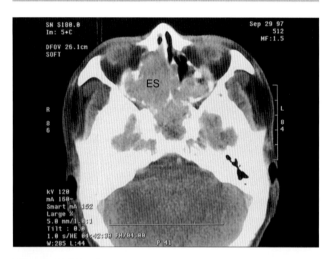

Figure 18.10   Contrast-enhanced CT scan showing expansion and destruction of the walls of the right ethmoid sinuses (ES) with extension of tumor into the right orbit.

A lack of correlation between the stage of the primary tumor and the extent of nodal involvement has been consistently reported (28,30,31) In keeping with this the nasopharynx is well recognized as a site of occult primary tumors in patients presenting with apparently isolated cervical lymphadenopathy. Cervical node relapse is reported to occur in 30% of untreated clinically node-negative necks (33).

Distant metastases are found in 3–6% of patients at presentation (31,34) but ultimately develop in around 40% (31,35). Bone is most commonly affected, followed by lung and liver. Bone marrow involvement is not uncommon in patients with metastatic disease and carries a poor prognosis (36). Lymph node metastases beyond the neck, and not necessarily in contiguity, may occur at presentation or on relapse (26).

Clinical Features

The most common presenting complaint is of a lump in the neck, reflecting the frequency of nodal involvement. The primary itself may cause nasal blockage, discharge, or bleeding, and obstruction of the auditory tube can lead to otitis media with effusion (Fig. 18.12) and otalgia. Bony destruction and expansion of the parapharyngeal space may result in a persistent deep-seated headache and direct invasion of CN V can give rise to trigeminal neuralgia.

Forward extension into the orbit can produce proptosis and diplopia as well as retro-orbital pain. With invasion of the cavernous sinus, palsies of CNs III, IV, and VI can also lead to diplopia or even complete ophthalmoplegia.

Involvement of the soft palate and pharyngeal wall may be evidenced by a sore throat or odynophagia. Difficulty in swallowing can also occur through compromise of the lower cranial nerves in the parapharyngeal space when it may be associated with mucosal hypoesthesia, disturbed taste, palatal incompetence, hemiglossal paralysis, and weakness of the muscles innervated by the spinal accessory nerve.

Metastatic disease may present as extra-regional lymphadenopathy, bone pain, respiratory symptoms, or hepatomegaly. Several paraneoplastic syndromes have been described with NPC including hypertrophic osteoarthropathy, pyrexia of unknown origin, and inappropriate antidiuretic hormone secretion. Metastatic disease may also be accompanied by a leukemoid peripheral blood picture (36).

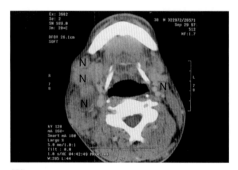

(A)

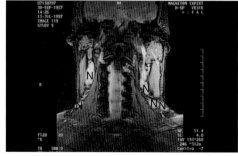

(B)

Figure 18.11   (A) Contrast-enhanced CT scan of the upper neck showing multiple involved nodes (N) in a patient with UCNT. (B) STIR sequence coronal MR image in a patient with bilateral lymphadenopathy (N) from UCNT.

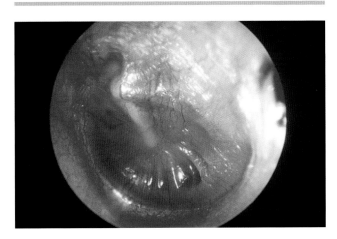

Figure 18.12 Chronic otitis media with effusion.

Table 18.2 Recommended Investigations in Nasopharyngeal Carcinoma

In all patients
    Direct nasopharyngoscopy and biopsy of primary tumor
    Full blood count
    Biochemistry profile including liver function tests and lactate
        dehydrogenase (LDH)
    Epstein–Barr virus serology (IgA anti-VCA, IgA anti-EA)
    Chest X-ray
    High resolution CT (with intravenous contrast) or MRI scan of the
        middle cranial fossa, skull base, nasopharynx, paranasal sinuses,
        neck and thoracic inlet
    Orthopantomogram
In patients with advanced nodal disease (UICC N3) or when metastatic
    disease is suspected
    Bone scan and plain radiographs of abnormal or symptomatic areas
    Liver ultrasound scan
Supplementary tests
    Baseline audiometry (if clinically indicated or prior to platinum
        chemotherapy)
    Creatinine or EDTA clearance (prior to platinum chemotherapy)

Clinical Assessment and Investigation

A full history, particularly with respect to neurological symptoms and complaints implicating metastatic disease is essential. As radiotherapy is the primary treatment modality it is important to assess dental health, and identify any potentially complicating factors, such as previous irradiation, smoking, alcohol abuse, and poor nutrition.

Physical examination should be directed toward nasal cavity and nasopharynx with the aid of a rigid endoscopic optical rod or flexible nasoendoscope noting the extent of the primary tumor, which may be grossly exophytic, or simply loss of definition of the fossa of Rosenmüller. Extension to the soft palate, pharyngeal wall and oropharynx should be sought by both inspection and palpation. Evidence of lower cranial nerve deficits may be apparent from palatal or glossal paralysis and atrophy. A full evaluation of the remaining cranial nerves should include visual assessment and examination of the tympanic membranes. The EBV is closely associated with NPC and the DNA of EBV are released into blood on necrosis of the cancer cells. Copies of EBV DNA have been found in plasma of patients with NPC (37). The quantity of DNA can be measured by real time quantitative polymerase chain reaction and this has been shown to escalate with more advanced stage (38). Its value in the early detection of recurrent NPC is however limited. In cases when the local or regional recurrence was still amenable to salvage treatment, only 67% had elevated copies (39).

The extent of nodal disease in the neck should be documented and further examination must include all other lymph node areas as these are potential sites of metastatic disease. Chest and abdominal examination should be directed towards the search for metastatic disease. Histological verification of a bulky tumor can be achieved through biopsy under local anesthetic and endoscopic guidance in the clinic. Smaller and less accessible tumors should be biopsied at examination under general anesthetic.

Appropriate imaging of the primary tumor is important not only for staging but for accurate radiotherapy planning. The choice between high resolution CT scanning and MRI is largely one of availability (40). Both techniques have their advantages and disadvantages in this setting and can be considered complementary. The superior spatial and contrast resolution of MRI make it the more sensitive investigation for the detection of subclinical tumors as well as for delineating soft tissue invasion in patients with extensive skull base disease. Consequently some authors consider it the modality of choice (41). However, bone involvement is more readily detected by CT and in a comparative study, more patients were up-staged by CT than MRI (42). If possible, patients should be imaged with both modalities. It is generally agreed that MRI is superior to CT for the detection of local recurrence and the imaging of treatment complications (40–42).

As indicated earlier, serology for EBV, particularly IgA directed towards VCA and EA can be useful diagnostically and may have a role in screening for asymptomatic NPC in high-risk populations (43). It can also be helpful in monitoring the response to therapy and in the diagnosis of relapse. The assay for IgG anti-ZEBRA antibodies is not in routine clinical use, though high titers appear to predict for the development of distant metastases (20). Less specific, high serum lactate dehydrogenase levels are also associated with metastatic disease (44).

A summary of the recommended investigations is given in Table 18.2. Screening for metastatic disease is indicated in patients with advanced nodal disease; any suspicious symptoms should be investigated. Finally, prior to embarking on radiotherapy a full dental assessment with completion of any restorative work is imperative.

Staging

A number of staging classifications have been proposed for NPC (23,45–48) but the two most commonly used have been those of Ho and the International Union Against Cancer (UICC) (1989). As outlined in Table 18.3 these classifications are based on different criteria, particularly with respect to the N stage. An analysis of CT-staged patients treated at the Prince of Wales Hospital, Hong Kong, suggests

Table 18.3 Staging Classifications for Nasopharyngeal Carcinoma

Ho (1978)		Prince of Wales Hospital (1991)		UICC (1989)		UICC (2002) (124)	
T1	Tumour limited to nasopharynx	T1	Tumour limited to nasopharynx	T1	Tumour limited to one wall of nasopharynx	T1	Tumour confined to nasopharynx
T2	Tumour beyond nasopharynx and into:	T2	Tumour beyond nasopharynx and into:	T2	Involvement of two or more walls of nasopharynx	T2	Tumour extends to soft tissues
n	Nasal fossa	n	Nasal fossa	T3	Invasion of nasal cavity and/or oropharynx	T2a	Tumour extends to oropharynx and/or nasal cavity without parapharyngeal extension*
o	Oropharynx	o	Oropharynx	T4	Invasion of skull base and/or cranial nerve(s)	T2b	Tumour with parapharyngeal extension*
P	Parapharyngeal region	T3a	Involvement of skull base and/or parapharyngeal region			T3	Tumour invades bony structures and/or paranasal sinuses
T3a	Bone involvement below skull base including floor of sphenoid sinus	T3b	Cranial nerve palsy			T4	Tumour with intracranial extension and/or involvement of the cranial nerves, fossa, infratemporal hypopharynx, orbit, or masticator space
T3b	Involvement of base of skull	T4	Intracranial extension				
T3c	Cranial nerve palsy						
T3d	Invasion of orbit, hypopharynx or infratemporal fossa						
N0	No palpable cervical nodes	N0	No palpable cervical nodes	N0	No palpable cervical nodes	N0	No regional lymph node metastasis
N1	Node(s) above skin crease extending laterally and backward from or just below thyroid notch	N1	Nodes above the supraclavicular fossa (N2f fixed nodes)	N1	Single unilateral node ≤3 cm	N1	Unilateral metastasis in lymph node(s), ≤6 cm, above the supraclavicular fossa
				N2a	Single ipsilateral node >3 cm ≤6 cm		
N2	Node(s) below skin crease but above supraclavicular fossa	N2	Supraclavicular fossa nodes (N3f fixed nodes)	N2b	Multiple ipsilateral nodes ≤6 cm	N2	Bilateral metastasis in lymph nodes, ≤6 cm, above the supraclavicular fossa
				N2c	Bilateral or contralateral nodes ≤6 cm	N3	Metastasis in lymph node(s)
N3	Supraclavicular nodes			N3	Node(s) >6 cm	N3a	>6 cm
						N3b	In the supraclavicular fossa
M0	No distant metastases	M0	No distant metastases	M0	No distant metastases	M0	No distant metastases
M1	Distant metastases	M1	Distant metastases	M1	Distant metastases	M1	Distant metastases
Stage grouping		**Stage grouping**		**Stage grouping**		**Stage groupings**	
I	T1 N0	Ia	T1 N0	I	T1 N0	0	Tis N0 M0
II	T2 and/or N1	Ib	T2 N0	II	T2 N0	I	T1 N0 M0
III	T3 and/or N2	IIa	T1–2 N1–N1f	III	T3 N0, T1–3 N1	IIA	T2a N0 M0
IV	N3 (any T)	IIb	T3 N0	IV	T4 N0–1	IIB	T1 N1 M0,
V	M1	IIIa	T3 N1–N1f		N2–3 (any T)		T2a N1 M0,
		IIIb	T1–2 N2–N2f		M1 (any T, any N)		T2b N0,N1 M0
		IVa	T3 N2–N2f, T4 any N M0			III	T1 N2 M0,
		IVb	M1 (any T any N)				T2a, T2b N2 M0,
							T3 N0, N1, N2 M0
						IVA	T4 N0, N1, N2 M0
						IVB	Any T N3 M0
						IVC	Any T Any N M1

Note: *Parapharyngeal extension denotes postero-lateral infiltration of tumor beyond the pharyngo-basilar fascia.

that the Ho classification is superior for the prediction of local failure, freedom from metastasis, and overall survival (49). A further refinement of the Ho classification, taking into account the prognostic significance of parapharyngeal involvement and intracranial extension, has been proposed by Teo (Table 18.3) (50). The major weakness of the 1989 UICC classification is the combination of a very heterogeneous group of patients in stage IV, while stages I and II are very similar in outcome and together account for only a small proportion of patients. These criticisms have been addressed in the 1997 and 2003 systems (Table 18.3) (47,51), which has also recognized the prognostic significance of supraclavicular node involvement as described by Ho (23).

Prognostic Factors

Age and Sex

There is considerable disagreement in the literature as to whether these represent significant prognostic factors. Several studies report that the survival of patients under 40 is better (52–54). Perez et al. (30) report poorer local control and survival in patients over 50, while others find no age effect (8,28). In a series of patients under 21, the prognosis was more favorable in those no more than 15 years old (55). Ho (56) did not find any influence of gender on prognosis, but several later studies have suggested that males fare worse both in terms of local control and survival (8,52–54).

Histological Subtype

It is difficult to generalize on the influence of histological subtypes from the published evidence. Part of the problem lies in the widely variable classifications used but more importantly, the large series from endemic areas include few differentiated SCCs. Perhaps as a result, these series show no significant effect of histology on survival (52–54). On the contrary, in a series from the Institut Gustave Roussy, in which half the patients had SCCs, the five-year disease-free survival was significantly better in those patients with UCNT (8). In support, two North American series suggest that histological subtype is a strong determinant of local control (28,57). One of these (28) found that histological subtype also predicated for regional control and indeed, that within the SCCs, the poorly differentiated (grade III) cases showed better local and regional control when compared to lower grade SCCs. Santos et al. (58) also report poorer local and regional control in SCC, reflected in worse five-year survival figures.

In the Mallinckrodt Institute series (30) histological subtype had no influence on disease-free and overall survival but local control of T2–T3 SCCs was considerably poorer (33%) than with other histological types (83%). In the same series undifferentiated carcinomas and lymphoepitheliomas were more frequently associated with distant metastases (41%) than either non-keratinizing (21%) or keratinizing (6%) SCCs.

Taking all of these observations together, a reasonable overview would be that stage for stage, local–regional control is more likely to be a problem with differentiated SCC while UCNT has a greater chance of failing distantly. Either scenario carries an ominous prognosis.

Recently three biomarkers—stathmin, 14-3-3sigma, and annexin 1—have been identified as of prognostic significance in NPC (59).

Disease Stage

The Ho classification is used in the large series reported from Hong Kong while Western centers employ the UICC system. Centers in mainland China and Taiwan have used different systems again [for example the Shanghai (52) and Huang (46)]. While the details of these various Chinese systems can be criticized (50) their stage groupings do predict for survival (31,46,52,53,56). There are no published series validating the 1989 UICC system, but in a comparative study from Hong Kong its predictive value proved inferior to the Ho system (49). In the absence of a unified system it is more instructive to consider the components of stage individually. Overall, the presence or absence of distant metastasis (M stage) is the dominant prognostic factor. In order to incorporate the various prognostic factors into the staging system, a revised American Joint Committee on Cancer (AJCC)/UICC staging system was published in 1997 (60). The T stage was revised and then graded according to the type of surrounding structures involved by the primary tumor in the nasopharynx. The N stage took into account the location as well as the size of the lymph nodes. This new staging system has been shown to stage patients precisely and to correlate with survival rates (61,62).

T Stage

Despite the number and variation of staging systems used, there is general agreement that the extent of the primary tumor is a strong predictor for local control (28,30,49,63). However, the value of subdividing disease confined to the nasopharynx (i.e., UICC 1989 T1 and T2) has been questioned (49,56) and systematic biopsy of all sub-sites has failed to demonstrate a correlation between the extent of involvement and local control (64). Nevertheless, discrepant local failure rates for UICC (1989) stages T1 and T2 have been reported (28,30). The 1997 revision of the UICC system no longer subdivides disease confined to the nasopharynx (Table 18.3).

The independent prognostic value of T stage for survival is unclear. Most series report outcomes for stage groupings from which it is impossible to determine the influence of primary stage, given the overriding effect of nodal involvement (see below). In multivariate analysis current T stage classifications offer a weak prognostic indicator (27,30,53,63). Notwithstanding this uncertainty there are clearly factors related to the extent of primary tumor that influence both local control and survival.

Cranial nerve involvement clearly predicts for increased risk of local and distant failure and poorer survival (54). Furthermore, it remains an independent predictor of poorer survival in multivariate analysis even when T stage does not (25,30). Similarly, it predicts for local failure independently of T stage (28). Involvement of the upper cranial nerves (II–VIII) is more ominous than the lower (IX–XII) (54). Invasion of the skull base in the absence of cranial nerve involvement is also associated with local and distant failure and a poorer outcome (28,54). Intracranial extension of the primary tumor predicts a very poor prognosis and is frequently associated with distant failure (25).

With the routine use of CT scanning it is clear that parapharyngeal extension (PPE) is common (27,65). Chua et al. (27) have defined three grades of involvement, with extensive PPE (grade 2–3) being associated with both local failure and distant metastases. The authors suggest that extensive PPE may lead to direct invasion of the vertebral (Batson's) venous plexus. Reporting the same association between PPE and metastatic disease, Teo et al. assert that extensive parapharyngeal tumor is difficult to distinguish from retropharyngeal nodal metastasis and that the latter may explain the link with distant metastasis (25).

N Stage

In the absence of clinically apparent distant metastases, cervical lymph node involvement is the strongest prognostic factor in NPC. The huge Hong Kong series clearly demonstrate the ability of Ho's levels of nodal involvement (23) to predict for distant failure and consequently survival (30,53,54). The 1989 UICC nodal classification also predicts for distant metastases (30) and both of these systems predict increasing regional failure with advanced nodal stage (28,54). In contrast, there appears to be no correlation between failure at the primary site and nodal stage (28,54).

In the 1970s Ho criticized the contemporary UICC system on its surgical basis. Though appropriate for the majority of head and neck cancers, it had little relevance to NPC and he was unable to demonstrate any prognostic significance for nodal laterality or fixity (56). Although none of the current systems include fixity, recent Hong Kong series suggest that this is indeed a prognostic factor (54,66,67), though of secondary importance to Ho's levels. The significance of maximum nodal size and laterality, on which the current UICC system (51) is based, remains controversial (54,66–69).

TREATMENT
Radiotherapy: Technique

Radiotherapy remains the primary treatment modality for NPC. The use of neoadjuvant and concomitant chemotherapy are increasingly applied, based on the results of a series of randomized clinical studies published in recent years (see below).

The challenge in planning successful and safe radiotherapy to the nasopharynx and the surrounding pathways of local invasion becomes obvious from a simple consideration of the anatomy. A radiation dose exceeding the tolerance of most normal tissues must be delivered to a site intimately related to the brainstem, temporal lobes, pituitary gland, and optic chiasm. Late radiation effects on other related structures such as the parotid glands, temporomandibular joints, and oropharyngeal musculature can contribute significantly to late morbidity.

In view of the necessarily narrow field margins and the proximity of critical structures, head and neck immobilization during treatment planning and delivery is essential. A standard is to use a plastic immobilization shell covering the full face, neck, and upper thorax in the supine position. The shell is drilled out or cut away over the treatment fields as far as practicable to retain the skin-sparing properties of the megavoltage treatment beams. A plastic

mouth bite may be used to depress the tongue away from the palate and out of the treatment volume.

Target Volume

Before treatment planning, an accurate assessment of the extent of the gross tumor volume (GTV) by a combination of clinical examination and CT and MRI scanning is essential. While gross tumor will need to be treated to a minimum dose of 70 Gy in 35 fractions or equivalent, clinically uninvolved sites at risk of microscopic disease need not be treated beyond 50–55 Gy, allowing sparing of adjacent sensitive structures. In modern radiotherapy practice three-dimensional radiotherapy planning techniques should be used. Diagnostic MRI can usefully be fused with radiotherapy planning CT scans to optimize imaging of the primary tumor site.

When the GTV is limited to the nasopharynx, the clinical target volume should include (bilaterally) the posterior quarter of the retro-orbit (i.e., behind the globe), the posterior half to one-third of the nasal cavity and adjacent maxillary sinus, the posterior ethmoid sinuses and the whole of the sphenoid sinus, the cavernous sinus with adjacent middle cranial fossa, the medial portion of the petrous temporal bone with the clivus and intervening fissure, the nasopharynx, the parapharyngeal tissues (including the medial pterygoid muscle, most of the adjacent lateral pterygoid muscle, the styloid process and jugular foramen), and the retropharyngeal space with the longus capitis muscle. Inferiorly the volume should include the whole of the soft palate and uvula with adjacent oropharynx. This volume will necessarily include the retro- and parapharyngeal nodes.

When there is extensive involvement of the nasal cavity the initial volume should include the whole of the nasal cavity, maxillary antrum, and all ethmoid sinuses bilaterally. Similarly, tumor extension down the lateral or posterior pharyngeal wall will require the primary volume to be extended inferiorly (see field arrangements below).

The areas of potential microscopic involvement have to be treated to a dose of at least 50 Gy. Delivering doses greater than this requires consideration of critical structures such as the optic nerves, spinal cord, and brainstem.

Given the propensity of nodal involvement in NPC, the majority of patients will require therapy to all cervical node groups, with the exception of the rarely involved submental nodes (32). In practice this means irradiation of both sides of the neck from the occiput to the sternal notch. Ho (56) questioned the need for elective nodal irradiation in clinically node-negative patients, quoting the results of a randomized study in which all cases of neck-only relapses in the unirradiated were successfully salvaged. The analysis, limited to T1N0 cases, showed no survival advantage for elective nodal irradiation. A further report from the same institute describing their subsequent experience with an observation policy in T1N0 (Ho) confirms successful salvage in the 30% of patients who relapsed in the neck (33). However, the survival of this group was lower than those not relapsing, with an increased rate of distant metastases. Since it is impossible to determine whether the neck relapses contributed to the distant failure and given the psychological morbidity of any disease recurrence, the authors now recommend elective nodal irradiation.

Conventional Technique: Field Arrangements and Radiation Dose

The fields are simulated and treated with the patient immobilized in the supine position with the neck fully extended (chin elevated). At the Royal Marsden Hospital the field arrangement is essentially that described by Ho (70) with minor modifications. The primary site is treated in two or three phases and the neck in one or two depending on the bulk of disease. These phases run in succession with no planned gaps in treatment. Our accepted maximum doses to critical normal tissues over a six to seven week course of treatment are: spinal cord and brainstem 45 Gy, optic nerve and retina 50 Gy and lens 10 Gy.

In patients with bulky cervical lymphadenopathy, particularly in the upper deep cervical or junctional region, or in those with extensive oropharyngeal involvement, the primary volume (as defined above) and both sides of the neck are treated in continuity with parallel opposed lateral fields extending inferiorly to the supraclavicular fossa (Fig. 18.13). In those patients where the position of the shoulders prevents irradiation of the lowest neck nodes with lateral fields a single anterior field with midline shielding is matched to the inferior border of the lateral fields. This volume is treated iso centrally to a maximum intersection dose of 30 Gy in 15 fractions of 2 Gy treating all fields daily over three weeks. It is our practice to use 5 or 6 MV photons for this phase. If there is a rapid response of the nodal disease this phase may be curtailed at 20 Gy in favor of an earlier switch to the second phase.

In the second phase of treatment the same patient position is adopted, though a new shell may be required if there has been a significant change in the contour of the neck. The primary volume (as defined above) is treated with small parallel opposed fields with lead shielding to the anterior orbit, mouth, brainstem, spinal cord, and posterior inferior corner of the field where it overlaps the neck fields (Fig. 18.14). This volume is treated to a further 20–30 Gy (depending on the phase 1 dose) in 2-Gy daily fractions to bring the total dose to 50 Gy at the intersection point. Whenever possible, high-energy photons should be used in order to improve sparing of the temporomandibular joints. During this phase both sides of the neck are treated with parallel opposed anterior and posterior fields with midline shielding to the spinal cord and larynx plus infraclavicular shielding bilaterally. With the neck extended the upper border of these fields runs across the angle of the mandible and the occiput (Fig. 18.14). Depending on the phase 1 dose the neck is treated to a further 30–40 Gy in daily 2-Gy fractions, specified at a point 3 cm lateral to the field center, 2.5 cm deep to the anterior skin surface (neck reference point). This brings the total neck dose to 60 Gy. The sites of originally involved nodes are thereafter boosted with electron fields of appropriate energy for the treatment depth to a total dose of 70 Gy or equivalent.

In the final phase of treatment to the primary site the volume is further reduced and localized to the site of the gross tumor at diagnosis with a 1–1.5 cm margin. This volume is treated with a three-field plan with an anterior field and two wedged opposed lateral fields (Fig. 18.15). This is treated to a further 20 Gy in daily fractions of 2 Gy (to a total dose of 70 Gy).

In patients without bulky nodal involvement we omit the initial large lateral fields, treating throughout with smaller lateral fields to the primary site (moving on to a three-field plan) with opposed anterior and posterior neck fields throughout. In the case of node-negative (on CT scan)

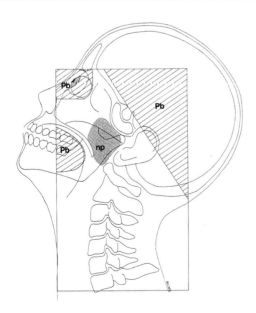

Figure 18.13 Diagram illustrating the borders and lead shielding (Pb) of the parallel-opposed lateral fields employed in the first phase of irradiation in NPC with bulky cervical lymphadenopathy. *Abbreviations*: np, nasopharynx.

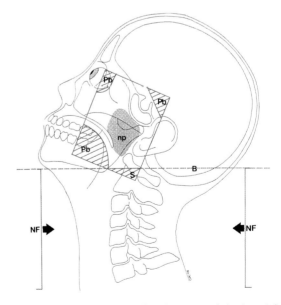

Figure 18.14 Diagram illustrating the extent of the lateral fields used to treat the nasopharynx and adjacent sites at risk of microscopic involvement. The upper border of the anterior and posterior parallel opposed neck fields (NF) is indicated (B) and the overlap is shielded (S). *Abbreviations*: Pb, lead shielding; np, nasopharynx.

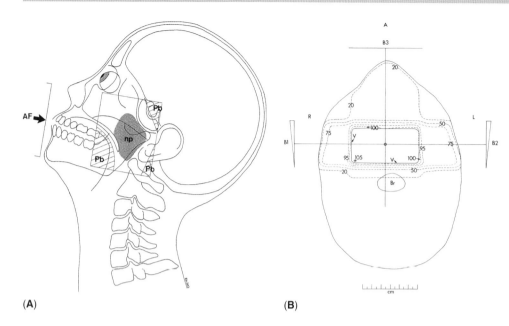

(A)   **(B)**

Figure 18.15 **(A)** Diagram indicating the field arrangement for the final phase of radiotherapy to the nasopharynx. AF: anterior field, Pb: lead shielding. **(B)** Dosimetry plan for the same field arrangement in a patient with bilateral parapharyngeal extension. The figures indicate percentage isodoses. *Abbreviations:* V, target volume; Br, brainstem.

well differentiated SCC the lower border of the neck fields lies at the inferior border of the thyroid cartilage.

Although this protocol is generally applicable the precise volume treated to each dose level should be individually tailored according to the clinical and imaging information available. For example, disease extending into the nasal cavity may need to be treated with a three-field plan throughout and disease extending into the paranasal sinuses certainly will. The final phase of treatment must take into account any disease extension into the parapharyngeal region, which, when involved, should be included with an adequate margin.

It is our practice to use megavoltage photon beams throughout, except for boosting the sites of nodal involvement. We have no experience in the use of mixed photon and (anterior) electron fields for the treatment of disease extending into the nasal cavity as detailed by Ho (70). Another technique outside of our experience but well described by the Hong Kong radiotherapists (54) is the use of a unilateral direct posterior oblique photon field to boost the parapharyngeal region. This is used at the end of a standard course of treatment and requires a new head cast with the patient's head turned to the contralateral side. The field lies behind the ipsilateral temporomandibular joint, anterior to the spinal cord, and below both temporal lobes and the opposite eye. A further dose of up to 20 Gy in 2-Gy fractions is given by this field (54). Examples of North American treatment techniques are described in detail by Fletcher and Million (71) and Perez (7).

Three Dimensional Conformal and Intensity-modulated Radiotherapy

Three-dimensional conformal radiotherapy has now become the standard for NPC to reduce the radiation dose to normal tissue structures with the aim of reducing radiation toxicity (72). The therapeutic advantage of conformal radiotherapy can also be used to increase radiation dose to the target with the aim of increasing tumor control rates within currently acceptable toxicity levels.

Intensity-modulated radiotherapy (IMRT) is a new method of radiation delivery which is becoming increasingly used to treat NPC. IMRT allows the delivery of radiation dose distributions with complex shapes, particularly where the required dose distribution is concave. This allows the delivery of high dose radiotherapy to tumors even when they are wrapped around a radiosensitive normal tissue structure such as the spinal cord or parotid gland (Fig. 18.16). The question of which head and neck tumors have the most to gain from an IMRT approach remains unanswered at present, but theoretical advantages have been demonstrated for, among others, tumors of the nasopharynx (73,74,75). Two small randomized clinical trials have recently been published to suggest that IMRT can reduce the rate of long term xerostomia in patients with nasopharyngeal carcinoma (76,77).

Radiation Dose, Technique, and Local Control

A considerable volume of literature discusses the question of a dose–response relationship in nasopharyngeal carcinoma (see Perez (7) for a detailed review). The evidence, such as it is, comes from retrospective reviews spanning the last five decades during which time there have been major changes in radiation oncology with the introduction of megavoltage treatment machines, the establishment of treatment simulation as standard practice, and the use of computerized dosimetry. Furthermore, major advances in radiation biology have led to considerable changes in fractionation in line with our current understanding of the basis of late tissue morbidity. Not surprisingly many studies spanning several decades have shown improvements in local control in later cohorts, often accompanied by increasing radiation doses. The difficulty in establishing a dose–response relationship from such data is illustrated by the study of Marks and co-workers (78) who felt that

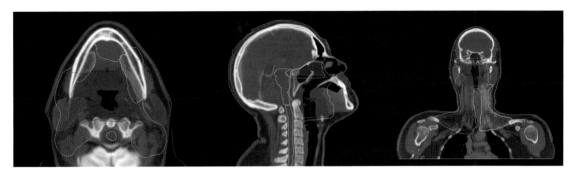

Figure 18.16 Shows the axial, sagittal, and coronal views of a typical IMRT plan for the nasopharynx. The figure shows the 95% isodose line (magenta) covering the PTV1 (dark blue), the 79.9% (yellow) isodose line covering the PTV2 (light blue). The figure also shows the sparing of the left parotid gland (magenta) and the right parotid gland (dark green).

improvement in local control owed more to technological advances than the increasing doses delivered. A later study from the same institute has suggested an improvement in local control for T1–T3 tumors treated to over 66 Gy, though very few patients received over 70 Gy (30). There was no corresponding improvement for T4 tumors. A recent retrospective study from the M.D. Anderson Cancer Center found no evidence of a dose effect in multivariate analysis (28).

The work of Yan and colleagues (79) has been cited as evidence of a dose–response effect. In a retrospective analysis they compared the outcome of patients with clinical evidence of residual disease at the primary site after standard treatment to 70 Gy who received no further therapy to those who were treated to a further 20–50 Gy with reduced fields. There was certainly improvement in the local control and five-year survival in the "boost" group but at the cost of increased severe radiation encephalomyelitis (17% vs. 5.5% in the "observed group").

One should be cautious in ascribing the reduced rates of distant metastases and better survival to the improved local control as the two groups were not well matched for advanced T and N stage. Unfortunately, those patients with T3–T4 tumors at diagnosis seemed to benefit less from the boost treatment.

One should balance these arguments for dose escalation against the high rates of local control (73% at five years) achieved by Lee and associates in over 4000 patients, the vast majority of whom were treated to 64–66 Gy. Local control was significantly worse in those patients treated to 55–59 Gy compared to 64 Gy or above. Perhaps more importantly, for patients who were staged and planned with CT, the five-year local control rates were 88% for T1 (Ho), 83% for T2 (Ho) and 67% for T3 (Ho).

There have been no prospective studies on dose escalation reported and these would certainly be difficult to run outside endemic areas. The advent of three-dimensional conformal planning is likely to bring with it improved dose distributions with more uniform delivery of currently prescribed doses to the target volume, with perhaps lower risks of normal tissue complications (80). In addition there is the potential for improved target definition with MRI. Improved dosimetry may therefore allow safe dose escalation

but as yet it is difficult to identify those patients who will benefit.

Brown and colleagues have suggested that proton therapy can improve tumor dose distribution at depth while reducing the dose received by adjacent normal tissues (81). Unfortunately, such therapy is expensive and not yet widely available. On the other hand the nasopharynx is one of the sites most likely to benefit from intensity-modulated radiation therapy (IMRT) for which the majority of modern linear accelerators can be adapted (82).

The results of the recent CHART study (continuous hyperfractionated accelerated radiation therapy) in head and neck cancers indicate that tumor cell repopulation during the course of treatment is a very real phenomenon (83). Accelerated radiotherapy thus offers an alternative approach to improving local control in NPC while hyperfractionation may improve the therapeutic ratio. Wang (84) has demonstrated that accelerated hyperfractionated treatment is feasible in NPC, with improved local control compared to historical controls treated once daily. There was no apparent increase in toxicity with the twice daily regimen. A prospective randomized study is needed to confirm these results.

In summary there may well be a modest dose–response effect between 55 and 70 Gy. However, in the absence of prospective data there is no clear indication to take the majority of patients beyond 70 Gy. Sadly, those patients who are at most risk of local relapse seem on present evidence to benefit least from dose escalation (30,79). Technological advances and novel fractionation regimens may, however, permit more effective delivery of current doses and allow the safe escalation of dose in those patients most at risk of local failure with current standard therapy.

Intracavitary Brachytherapy

Brachytherapy offers the potential for local delivery of high radiotherapy doses with rapid dose fall-off to spare neighboring normal tissues. In addition the use of low-dose rate sources confers the added advantage of the sparing effect of low-dose rate on late morbidity. Some authors advocate the routine addition of a brachytherapy boost to the nasopharynx after completion of external beam therapy to 60–70 Gy and describe appropriate after-loading techniques (59,85–87). Doses of 6–20 Gy in from one to three applications have been given using medium or high-dose rate systems. Wang (86) reported an improvement in local control with the addition of brachytherapy when compared to a non-randomized contemporary population, but the local failure rate in the latter was rather higher than one might expect from recent megavoltage external beam series (69).

From the published results it is not clear that the routine use of brachytherapy boosts confers any advantage over modern conformal external beam therapy. Tsao (88) advocates the selective use of brachytherapy in those patients with residual disease at the end of a standard course of external beam treatment and electively in all patients with well-differentiated SCC where the risk of local failure is increased. At the Royal Marsden Hospital we do not use brachytherapy in the initial management of NPC, reserving its use for recurrent disease.

Radiotherapy: Results of Treatment

The multiplicity of staging systems and heterogeneity of patient populations make it impossible to compare results across series. In addition, many retrospective reports include patients staged before the advent of CT and treated without simulation on orthovoltage machines. Table 18.4 shows the results of Lee and colleagues (69) who treated over 4000 patients with megavoltage irradiation between 1976 and 1985. Only 12 patients in this series had WHO type 1 tumors. The improved result in more recently treated patients is typical of many retrospective NPC series and reflects a combination of factors such as stage migration

Table 18.4 Actuarial local control rates for NPC treated with megavoltage irradiation

Stage (112)	All patients (N= 4128) control at 10 years	Patients treated 1976–1980 (N= 2010) control at 5 years	Patients treated 1981–1985 (N= 2118) control at 5 years
T1	74	77	83
T2	72	69	79
T3 (all)	61	64	67
T3a	72		
T3b	66		
T3c	50		
T3d	35		

Data from Ho (56).

after the introduction of CT scanning, improved target localization, and a degree of dose escalation. Table 18.5 illustrates the results from three Western series, with all patients retrospectively staged using the UICC 1989 system.

Patterns of Failure After Radical Radiotherapy

The time to failure is very consistent across the many series reported. Around 75% of recurrences, both locoregional and distant, occur within two years of treatment, 85–90% occurring within three years.

Thereafter there are a small number of relapses occurring out to five and even ten years.

Of 5037 patients treated at the Queen Elizabeth Hospital Hong Kong, half died of NPC (31). Forty-six percent of patients were known to be disease-free at the time of last follow-up or death. Thirty percent of patients had either persistent local disease or subsequently relapsed at the primary site and less than 15% of these were successfully salvaged by retreatment. Thirty-five percent of patients either had or developed distant metastases, the actuarial ten-year metastasis-free rate being 59%. As indicated in Table 18.6, there was a strong correlation between the cumulative incidence of metastasis and nodal stage at diagnosis. Of those developing distant metastases, just over 40% had associated local or regional failure.

In a more recent series of 628 patients from Hong Kong treated in the CT era, 185 (29.5%) had failed after two years of follow-up (89). Most of these (90) had developed distant metastases, three-quarters of whom had no evidence of local or regional recurrence. The two-year actuarial local failure rate was just 12.7% from a series in which 76% had primary disease beyond the nasopharynx. Patients with bulky (>4 cm) nodal disease were treated with neoadjuvant chemotherapy and all patients received bilateral neck radiotherapy. Of the 7% of patients who relapsed in the neck, the majority had associated local or distant failure.

In the Mallinckrodt Institute series of 143 patients, just over half died of NPC (30). Two-thirds of patients had evidence of local recurrence at the time of death and one-third had relapsed in the neck. Nineteen percent of patients developed distant metastases, two-thirds of whom had no evidence of locoregional recurrence at death. Of 256 patients treated at eight Veterans Administration Medical Centers from 1956 to 1978 only 10% were alive without evidence of recurrence at the time of reporting. Sixty-three percent had failed at the primary site and only 4% died from distant metastases with locoregional control (91). Once again distant failure correlated with nodal stage at diagnosis (Table 18.6). In a series from Memorial Sloan-Kettering

Table 18.5 Actuarial Local and Regional Control in Western NPC Series

Center	SCC*	LC at (years)	T1	T2	T3	T4	N0	N1	N2a	N2b	N2c	N3
Mallinckrodt (26) 1956–1986 (N = 143)	54	10	85	75	67	40	82	86	72†			72
Gustave Roussy (7) 1960–1991 (N = 308)	46	5	63	62	68	54	66	57	58	56	54	57
MD Anderson (24) 1954–1992 (N= 378)	51	5	93	79	68	53	95	94	91	80	77	71
		10	87	75	63	45	95	94	91	77	74	71

Abbreviation: LC: local control.
*Percentage squamous cell carcinoma in series.
†Figures for all N2 combined.

Table 18.6 Nasopharyngeal Carcinoma: Incidence of Distant Failure with Node Stage at Diagnosis

	N0	N1	N2	N3
Lee et al. (27) N = 5037 (Ho 1978 stage)	16	28	37	57
Petrovich et al. (91) N = 107 (AJC 1977 stage)	17	18	33	46

Cancer Center, just over half of 107 NPC patients relapsed and of these the primary site was the first site of failure in 60% (92). Hoppe and colleagues describe a 56% actuarial disease-free survival in 82 NPC patients. Of the 32 failures, 17 relapsed locally and 12 developed distant metastases with locoregional control (93).

It is very difficult to generalize over such widely different series. However, it is clear that both locoregional and distant failure are major causes of death in NPC. In endemic areas despite the high rates of local control in recent series, significant numbers of patients still succumb from distant metastases. In the West, where SCCs are more prevalent it would appear that local relapse is a more significant cause of failure.

Complications of Radiotherapy

The side effects of radiotherapy are conventionally termed "acute" or "early" if they occur during or within three months of completion of a course of radiotherapy. Some of these are reversible, depending on the total dose delivered. "Late" complications, developing at least three months and often years after a course of treatment are not reversible. The incidence increases with the total dose delivered and, unlike acute reactions, with increasing size of the individual daily fractions. It is likely that late reactions reflect the delayed expression of vascular damage with secondary ischemia and fibrosis. The incidence, diagnosis, and treatment of radiation complications in NPC have been reviewed in detail by Lee (94). In general the severity of acute reactions and the incidence of late complications increase with the size of the volume irradiated to high dose. Consequently, both are more likely to increase with advanced stages of disease.

Acute complications. The majority of patients develop acute mucositis and in many this is likely to be confluent within the high-dose region (28). Undernutrition and weight loss can easily occur as a result and close attention must be paid to the patient's diet. Salivary tissue responds rapidly to radiation and a transient early parotitis may occur that does not require specific therapy beyond reassurance (94). Early loss of salivary function is not uncommon and the majority of patients will develop some degree of long-term xerostomia (53,93). This, added to the common occurrence of reversible taste disturbance and anorexia will increase the potential for malnutrition. Nausea or vomiting, though rarely severe, can occasionally occur.

Even with the skin-sparing effects of megavoltage irradiation, most patients will develop some degree of skin reaction that may extend to moist desquamation (28).

Where possible the immobilization cast should be drilled out or cut away to minimize build-up effects. Finally, most patients describe some degree of malaise.

Late complications. With the close relationship of the nasopharynx to the CNS the potential for serious neurological complications is considerable. Such sequelae can take over two years to be expressed (95) and since a large number of patients will have relapsed by that time it is difficult to get a realistic impression of the true complication rates. Sanguineti and associates (28) have estimated the actuarial incidence of RTOG grade 3–5 late complications to be 16, 19 and 29% at 5, 10 and 20 years respectively. In their study 12 of 378 (3%) patients died as a result of late complications, though 11 of these were treated between 1954 and 1971, before the routine use of treatment simulation and megavoltage irradiation. Indeed, as a result of improved technique the ten-year actuarial incidence of severe (grade 4 and 5) late complications has dropped to 5% in their most recent cohort of patients.

Neurological damage occurred in 451 of the 5037 patients reported by Lee and co-workers (31) and accounted for all but three of the 62 radiation-induced fatalities. In a series from Beijing of NPC patients treated to doses of up to 90 Gy or more, the incidence of neurological complications was 18.4% (52). At conventional doses temporal lobe necrosis occurs in about 1% of patients (28,30) with a latent interval of four years (96). It may present with temporal lobe epilepsy, the features of raised intracranial pressure or more subtle symptoms such as personality changes (96). Few patients have specific neurological signs and MRI scanning is the investigation of choice (97). Early cases may respond to systemic steroids but these offer little benefit once extensive cystic change has occurred (96).

Late radiation damage to the brainstem or spinal cord can be equally devastating. It has been variably reported in 0–3% of cases (28,30,53) and generally presents with progressive spastic paraparesis. Most patients will have long-tract motor signs and again MRI is the investigation of choice (94). Sadly, there is little treatment to offer beyond rehabilitation and supportive care. With modern CT imaging and planning, accurate patient immobilization, and dosimetry this complication should be avoidable.

Other potential neurological complications include optic neuropathy and chiasmal damage, cranial nerve palsy, and retinopathy. Again these should be avoidable with careful planning and attention to normal tissue dose limits. The lower cranial nerves appear to be most vulnerable (53,93,95), presumably through late radiation changes in the parapharyngeal space.

Symptomatic hypopituitarism has been reported in 6% of cases (28), though much higher rates have been reported in patients investigated prospectively (98). Radiation damage to the hypothalamus is thought to be the underlying cause with the growth hormone axis the most commonly affected followed by the gonadotrophins, corticotrophin and thyroid-stimulating hormone (TSH) (98). Primary hypothyroidism may result from high-dose irradiation of the lower neck. Treating physicians should be aware of the possibility of long-term endocrine dysfunction in NPC survivors; periodic endocrine assessment is appropriate.

Serous otitis media has been reported in 7–18% of patients (52,93,95). Myringotomy is required where this is persistent. Of more concern is the recent report from Queen Mary Hospital Hong Kong in which prospective audiological assessment of treated NPC patients detected persistent sensorineural hearing loss (SNHL) in 24% of ears tested (99). High frequency was more affected than low frequencies. A similar number again developed transient SNHL. Fourteen percent of ears developed serous otitis media, the majority within two years. A particularly high incidence of persistent SNHL (46.9%) was found in those ears with serous otitis media, compared to those without (19%, $P = 0.0013$). There was no evidence of enhanced radiation-induced SNHL in those patients given neoadjuvant cisplatin. The authors suggest that the presence of a middle ear effusion is a marker for increased risk of damage to the inner ear. Clearly it is important to limit the radiation dose to the audiological apparatus as much as possible. Avoidance of specific structures such as the cochlea is possible using IMRT.

Of the soft tissue and bone complications, trismus is reported in 3–12% (28,52,78), moderate to severe neck fibrosis in 2–4% (28,30,95), and osteoradionecrosis (mandible, maxilla, skull base) in 2–3% (28,30). As in all head and neck sites where significant volumes of salivary tissue are irradiated to high dose, long-term xerostomia predisposes to dental caries and close attention to oral hygiene is essential. Finally, radiation-induced second malignancies, particularly osteosarcoma have been described in long-term survivors but with an incidence of less than 1%.

Radiotherapy for Local Recurrence

Although chemotherapy may offer some palliative benefit in locally recurrent disease it does not offer the prospect of long-term control (see below). Some cases may be amenable to local surgery, perhaps combined with brachytherapy as discussed later. For the majority of local recurrences re-irradiation offers the best hope for salvage. Obviously, given the risks of primary irradiation, retreatment to high dose carries a significant complication rate.

In the largest series of re-irradiated patients Lee and colleagues (100) report an actuarial five-year local salvage rate of 23% in 654 patients with local recurrence treated to a further 7.5–70 Gy (median 45.6 Gy) with external beam (82%), brachytherapy (6%), or a combination (12%). Despite close follow-up the majority of relapses were too bulky for brachytherapy alone. Fifty-one percent of patients responded completely, but over a third of these subsequently relapsed again after a median of one and a half years. Not surprisingly, salvage rates were better for more localized recurrences and were higher in those with less extensive primary tumors at first diagnosis. The estimated five-year complication-free rate was 52%. One or more serious late complications were recorded in 168 patients (26%) including 20 cases of temporal lobe necrosis. Thirteen of these individuals died as a result. Most of the other complications were in the soft tissues, such as trismus (16%) but two patients died after massive hemorrhage from telangiectatic mucosa. Late complications were fewer in those patients treated with more protracted fractionation (both courses) and in those treated by a combination of external beam and brachytherapy. There did not appear to be any association between the complication rate and the interval between courses of radiotherapy.

A report from the M.D. Anderson Cancer Center (101) describes a 35% actuarial five-year local control rate after re-irradiation to a median total dose of 112 Gy. Eight of the 53 patients developed severe complications that proved fatal in five. The overall five-year actuarial incidence of severe complications was 17%, reaching 39% in those patients receiving cumulative external beam doses of over 100 Gy. There was a suggestion of improved local control with fewer complications in those patients treated with a combination of external beam and intracavitary therapy. The authors found no dose–response relationship in this series, but in 51 patients retreated with external beam radiotherapy with or without brachytherapy, Wang (102) reported improved survival in those treated to 60 Gy or more. However, those treated to lower doses tended to have more advanced recurrences.

There is clearly a role for repeat irradiation in those patients with recurrent NPC. From the published experience it seems that few patients have sufficiently localized disease to be treated by brachytherapy alone, though a combination of external beam and brachytherapy is to be preferred where practicable. Radical treatment is necessary to achieve salvage rates of around 35%, perhaps higher in more selected cases. It is clearly important to exclude metastatic disease before embarking on such retreatments. For localized disease, a combination of surgery and perioperative brachytherapy is an option (141) that will be discussed later. Isolated nodal relapses in the neck can be managed as described below.

Chemotherapy

There is a large body of evidence (reviewed by Altun (8)) demonstrating that NPC is highly sensitive to chemotherapy. The most active regimens contain cisplatin and two widely employed schedules are outlined in Table 18.7 (103,104).

Neoadjuvant Chemotherapy

The rationale for combining primary (neoadjuvant or induction) chemotherapy with subsequent radiotherapy is twofold. First, cytotoxic reduction of bulky primary and nodal disease may enhance locoregional control and second, the eradication of systemic micrometastases at an early stage may reduce later distant relapses. Indeed, a number of studies have suggested that the addition of neoadjuvant chemotherapy can enhance local control and survival when compared to historical or non-randomized controls (105–107). In contrast, Tannock and colleagues were unable to demonstrate a long-term benefit from neoadjuvant chemotherapy despite a 75% response rate (108). Where side effects have been reported, chemotherapy seems to be tolerated by most patients and has not resulted in reductions of radiotherapy dose subsequently delivered.

Two randomized studies of neoadjuvant chemotherapy have been reported. In the first, Chan and colleagues (109) randomized 82 UCNT patients with Ho N3 or any N stage with nodal diameter of 4 cm or more, between their standard radiotherapy protocol and the same preceded and followed by chemotherapy. A modification of the Cisplatin

Table 18.7 Chemotherapy Regimens Used in Nasopharyngeal Carcinoma

BEC (93)	3-weekly cycle		
Bleomycin	15 IU	iv bolus	Day 1
Bleomycin	12 IU/m^2 per day	Continuous iv infusion	Days 1–5
Epirubicin	70 mg/m^2	iv bolus	Day 1
Cisplatin	100 mg/m^2	iv infusion	Day 1
PF (94)	3-weekly cycle		
Cisplatin	100 mg/m^2	iv infusion	Day 1
5–Fluorouracil	1000 mg/m^2	Continuous iv infusion	Days 1–5

See references for detailed schedules.

and 5 Fluoruracil (PF) schedule outlined in Table 18.7, in which the 5-fluorouracil was given for three rather than five days, was given for two cycles before the radiotherapy and for four cycles afterward. Sixty-five percent of patients responded to chemotherapy at the primary site and 81% in nodal disease. At the end of radiotherapy all of the combined arm patients were disease-free compared to 95% of the radiotherapy-only arm. The chemotherapy toxicity was much as one would anticipate for the regimen and there was no enhancement of the subsequent radiation toxicity. However, 46% of patients failed to complete the postradiation chemotherapy. After a median follow-up of 28.5 months there were no differences in two-year survival, locoregional relapse rate, distant metastatic rate, or relapse-free survival. While longer follow-up might reveal survival differences and the chemotherapy regimen could be criticized as suboptimal, the results suggest that a large survival benefit from induction chemotherapy is unlikely.

A second, larger, multicenter study has been reported by the International Nasopharynx Cancer Study Group (103). Using the Bleomycin, epirubicin and cisplatin (BEC) protocol (Table 18.7) developed at the Institut Gustave Roussy, 339 patients were randomized between three cycles of induction chemotherapy followed by radiotherapy or radiotherapy alone. The same radiotherapy technique and dose was employed in both arms. Over 90% of patients had UCNT and the majority were T3–T4, N2c–N3. There were 14 treatment-related deaths (8%) in the chemotherapy arm compared to two (1%) in the radiotherapy-only arm, though there was no enhancement of radiotherapy toxicity. Ninety-one percent of patients responded to the chemotherapy, with a complete response in 47%. After a median follow-up of 49 months, tumor progression, recurrence, or metastasis had occurred in 33% of the combined therapy patients compared to 55% of those receiving radiotherapy alone. The pattern of recurrence was the same in both groups suggesting that chemotherapy improved both locoregional control and distant failure rates. However, at the time of reporting there was no difference in overall survival. More time is needed to determine whether a true survival advantage has been masked by a short-term response of radiotherapy-only arm failures to salvage chemotherapy. The high chemotherapy-related death rate and relatively reduced compliance with radiotherapy in the combined arm may further hide a survival benefit from induction chemotherapy but the impression is that any advantage will be relatively small.

Concomitant Chemotherapy

Chemotherapy given during the course of radical radiotherapy offers the potential for radiation sensitization in the tumor as well as the possibility of eradicating micrometastases. It also offers the risk of enhanced toxicity, with radiotherapy delays or even dose reductions as a result. Huang and colleagues reported that the introduction of a number of different low-dose concomitant regimens involving cyclophosphamide, methotrexate, cisplatin, or bleomycin coincided with an improvement in local control and overall survival compared to historical series. However, many series report improved results over successive decades, for reasons discussed earlier, and without the use of chemotherapy. Turner and Tiver (110) report their experience with concomitant mitomycin C and 5-fluorouracil in 43 patients with advanced NPC. Over half of the radiotherapy courses were interrupted, for a median of two weeks, and there were two treatment-related deaths. With no obvious improvement over published results the authors could not support the continued use of this combined regimen. Souhami and Rabinowits (111) came to a similar conclusion after a trial of the same drugs with the addition of methotrexate. Again severe mucositis resulted in treatment interruptions and there was no clear improvement in survival.

The Radiation Therapy Oncology Group (RTOG) conducted a trial (RTOG 81-17) of cisplatin (100 mg/m^2 3-weekly × 3) given concomitantly with a standard course of irradiation for advanced SCC of the head and neck (112). This study includes a group of 27 patients with advanced NPC that has been reported separately in comparison with historical controls treated by radiation alone (113). All combined therapy patients reached a dose of at least 64.5 Gy while 19 of 27 completed three cycles of chemotherapy. A complete response at the end of therapy was seen in 24 (89%) and in all of those with poorly differentiated tumors. There was some degree of leukopenia in most patients, severe or life-threatening in four (15%). Moderate to severe mucositis occurred in 85% but there was no indication as to the frequency of treatment interruptions. However, in the main study the treatment time was over 70 days in 20% of those patients achieving over 64.5 Gy. There was a suggestion of improved local control and reduced distant failure in the stage IV NPC patients treated with combined therapy as compared to historical controls but the groups could not be considered directly comparable. The combined regimen formed the basis of the subsequent intergroup study (0099) discussed later.

Adjuvant Chemotherapy

The aim of adjuvant chemotherapy, given after radical radiotherapy, is to reduce the high distant metastatic failure rate. It is unlikely to contribute significantly to locoregional control. Once again there is a suggestion from retrospective series that the introduction of adjuvant chemotherapy into NPC treatment protocols has improved disease-free and overall survival compared with historical controls treated with radiation alone (114,115). In contrast, Teo and colleagues (116) found no reduction in distant metastases and indeed more rapid distant failure in a group of patients treated with both neoadjuvant and adjuvant platinum-based combination chemotherapy.

A large multicenter randomized trial coordinated by the Instituto Nazionale Tumori, Milan, failed to show any relapse-free or overall survival benefit for the addition of combination chemotherapy in patients in complete remission after radical radiotherapy for NPC (117). In the chemotherapy arm, patients received up to 12 cycles of vincristine, cyclophosphamide, and doxorubicin. Although there were some problems with compliance in the chemotherapy arm and the schedule did not include cisplatin, the results do argue against the routine use of adjuvant chemotherapy in NPC.

Combined Concomitant and Adjuvant Chemotherapy

The preliminary results of the Southwest Oncology Group coordinated Intergroup study 0099 with the Radiation therapy oncology group (RTOG) and Eastern Cooperative Oncology Group have been reported (118). Patients with UICC (1989) stages III and IV NPC were randomized between standard radical radiotherapy (70 Gy in 35 fractions over seven weeks) and the same with concomitant cisplatin (100 mg/m^2 day 1, 22, 43) followed by three cycles of adjuvant cisplatin plus 5-fluorouracil chemotherapy. The trial was closed prematurely on the advice of the Data Monitoring Committee when an interim analysis of 138 patients demonstrated a median progression-free survival of 13 months for the radiotherapy patients compared to 52 months for the combined arm. At a median follow-up of 40 months the median survival of the combined arm patients had not been reached, while that of the radiotherapy group was 30 months. There was an excess of deaths (39%) in the radiotherapy group compared to the combined arm (16%) with two-year actuarial survivals 55% and 80% respectively. There was apparently no increase in radiotherapy toxicity with concomitant cisplatin. This trial has been criticized on the basis that patients in the control arm of the trial had a lower survival rate than would have been expected from other Phase II experiences. The reasons for this are unclear.

Several further studies have confirmed the superiority of concomitant chemoradiotherapy in nasopharynx cancer, and this should now be regarded as the standard of care for stage III and IV patients (119–121).

Palliative Chemotherapy

It was the encouraging responses of recurrent and metastatic NPC to systemic chemotherapy that led to its investigation in primary therapy as previously discussed. Choo and Tannock (122) have summarized the Princess Margaret Hospital experience of palliative chemotherapy in recurrent and metastatic NPC. With the application of lymphoma-type and cisplatin-based regimens response rates of 70% could be achieved with at least two of 30 patients surviving in complete remission for over three years. In this retrospective review they were unable to demonstrate a survival benefit for more aggressive chemotherapy and could not comment on its palliative benefits beyond objective tumor responses. Al-Kourainy and colleagues (123) report a 76% response rate to platinum-containing regimens in 12 patients treated with recurrent disease. Half of those treated with the PF regimen (as Table 18.7 but 4-weekly) responded completely, with one of three complete remissions maintained for over five years.

Altun et al. (8) have described the evolution of palliative chemotherapy protocols at the Institut Gustave Roussy. Overall response rates of 50–75% have been achieved with platinum-based regimens including BEC (Table 18.7). Of 131 patients with metastatic disease treated between 1985 and 1991, 13 remained disease-free for more than two years and 11 of these were alive and in remission at up to 79 months. Long-term responses are described in both bony and visceral sites and it would seem that around 10% of patients will achieve durable remissions, perhaps cure with aggressive chemotherapy in metastatic disease. Obviously none of these regimens are without toxicity.

Surgery for Recurrent Nasopharyngeal Carcinoma
Recurrent or Persistent Disease in Cervical Lymph Node

With the frequent use of concurrent chemoradiation and the improved techniques of radiation the control of disease in the neck has markedly improved in recent years. The reported incidence of isolated failure in the neck lymph nodes was less than 5% (124). Those cervical lymph nodes that responded to the initial treatment might take up to three months to become clinically negative. Neck recurrence might present as persistent node following the chemoradiation or reappearance of the cervical lymph node after complete resolution following the initial treatment.

It is frequently difficult to confirm that the neck nodes harbor malignant cells after radiotherapy. Fine needle aspiration cytology examination has not been helpful, even when performed under ultrasonographic guidance; the yield is at best only 50%. Fluorodeoxyglucose (FDG) positron emission tomography (PET) has been shown to be superior in the detection of residual neck disease after radiation treatment of other head and neck cancers (125). If the presence of metastatic cancer in the cervical lymph node can be confirmed through functional imaging, or fine needle aspiration, or there is other evidence that the lymph node harbors malignant cells, such as clinical progression of the lymph node, then salvage therapy is indicated. There are a few salvage therapeutic options.

When these persistent or recurrent lymph nodes were managed with another course of external radiotherapy, an overall five-year survival rate of 19.7% has been reported (126). Retreatment of the neck with external beam radiotherapy also carries a high risk of tissue fibrosis and/or necrosis. Surgical salvage with radical neck dissection has achieved a five-year tumor local control rate of 66% in the neck with a five-year actuarial survival of 38% (127). The rationale for performing radical neck dissection for patients who might have only a single clinically evident persistent or recurrent lymph node is three-fold. Step serial section studies of radical neck dissection specimens have shown that there were three times more nodes with malignant cells in the specimen than clinically evident. Over 70% of these malignant nodes exhibit extracapsular spread and around 30% of these nodes were lying close to the spinal accessory nerve. Radical neck dissection was the recommended procedure for salvage of recurrent or persistent neck disease after radiotherapy (128). Three-quarters of the patients presented with a single enlarged node, with 86% presenting in cervical node levels II and upper V. In over half of the cases, the node

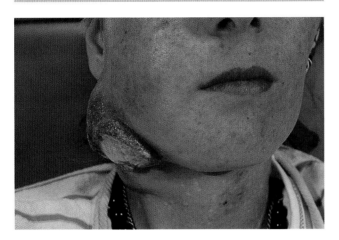

Figure 18.17 Fungating cervical lymphadenopathy.

was fixed to underlying structures or skin (Fig. 18.17 and Table 18.9).

Lymph node mobility was a significant prognostic factor affecting local control of disease and survival. This clinical feature suggested extracapsular spread and the malignant cells extending beyond the capsule to involve overlying neck skin, floor of the posterior triangle, and sometimes the carotid sheath. For these patients, even after the radical neck dissection, the resection margins were probably close. Further after-loading brachytherapy delivered to the tumor bed following radical neck dissection has been shown to be useful. Nylon tubes for the brachytherapy source were placed on the tumor bed accurately at the time of the neck dissection. The overlying skin which was included in the initial radiation field has to be replaced. The skin flap often used was the deltopectoral flap or the

Table 18.8 Surgical Approaches to the Nasopharynx

Type	Description	Reference
Anterior	Transnasal/transantral	Wilson
	Le Fort 1 maxillotomy	Belmont
Inferior	Palatal split	Fee et al.
	Transpalatal flap	Harrison et al.
	Transcervico-mandibulo-palatal	Morton et al. (130)
Lateral	Infratemporal	Fisch (132)
Anterolateral	Maxillary swing	Wei et al. (109)

Table 18.9 Surgical Findings on Neck Dissection for Cervical Node Relapse in NPC

Structures involved by tumour infiltration	Cases (%)
Sternomastoid muscle	26
Internal jugular vein	16
Floor of posterior triangle, carotid artery, vagus nerve	4
Disease adherent to but not infiltrating	
local structures (for example floor of posterior triangle, carotid artery)	28

Data from Wilson (108).

pectoralis major myocutaneous flap. With this adjuvant therapy, a similar tumor control rate was achieved compared to when radical neck dissection alone was performed for less extensive neck disease (129).

Disease in the Nasopharynx: Nasopharyngectomy

Primary surgery has been advocated where recurrent disease remains localized (130, 140). A number of approaches have been described (Table 18.8) and the results have been summarized by Morton and colleagues (130).

The nasopharynx is located in the center of the head, its adequate exposure to allow oncological extirpation of tumor in the region has been a challenge. Various surgeons have employed different approaches to remove the disease in the nasopharynx. The overall mortalities associated with all these salvage surgical procedures have been low. Hsu et al. (131) reported a 46% local cure rate after the selective use of surgery for recurrence. The results were described as excellent for recurrent stage T1(rT1), good for rT2, fair for rT3, and palliative for rT4. These results reflected the extent of recurrence; from the least extensive, that is the roof of the nasopharynx, towards the ethmoid and oropharynx and from there to the most severe manifestations of deep parapharyngeal and skull base involvement. Similarly, Fisch (132) was able to achieve local control in T1/2 recurrences but could only palliate T4 lesions where infiltration of the dura and cranial nerves prevented complete excision.

The various anterior and inferior approaches may give adequate visualization of the tumor but do not allow the resection of the tumor from the lateral aspects in an oncological fashion. Most recurrent nasopharyngeal carcinoma is situated in the lateral wall of the nasopharynx, occluding the fossa of Rosenmuller and closely associated with the crura of the eustachian tube. A curative oncological resection should include these structures. Step serial sectioning of nasopharyngectomy specimen has shown that the persistent or recurrent nasopharyngeal carcinoma exhibited extensive submucosal extension and a wide resection of the nasopharynx was essential to reach a favorable outcome (133). This could be achieved best with the anterolateral approach or the maxillary swing approach; after osteotomies, the maxilla attached to the anterior cheek flap could be swung laterally to expose the tumor in the nasopharynx (Fig. 18.18A). The procedure was first reported in 1991 (134). The original facial incision described started with the Ferguson Longmire incision and this continued between the two central incisor teeth onto the hard palate in the midline and then turned laterally along the posterior edge of the hard palate (Fig. 18.18B). In recent years, the palatal incision was modified to a curve incision along the inner border of the upper teeth (Fig. 18.18C). In this way, the osteotomy site on the hard palate and the wound over the palatal mucoperiosteum were in different planes, thus avoiding the formation of palatal fistula. After the appropriate osteotomies, the maxilla could be swung laterally but remained attached to the anterior cheek flap (Fig. 18.18D). This exposed the persistent or recurrent tumor in the nasopharynx (Fig. 18.18E); en bloc resection of the tumor was possible (Fig. 18.18F). After removing the tumor, the margins at the tumor bed could be checked (Fig. 18.18G); then the osteocutaneous complex was returned and fixed

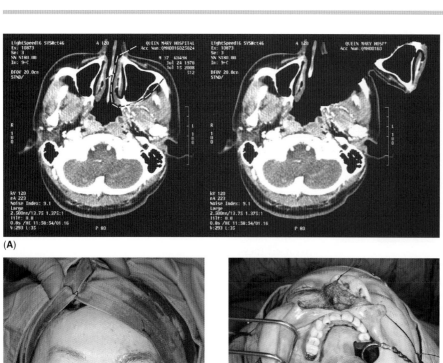

(A)

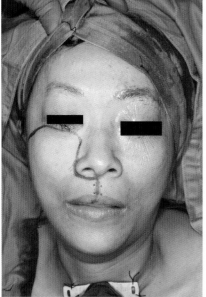

(B)

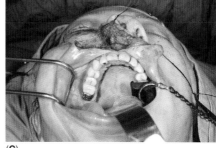

(C)

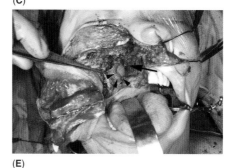

(E)

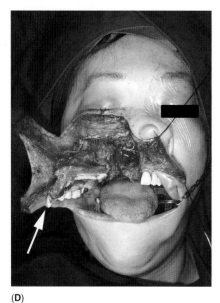

(D)

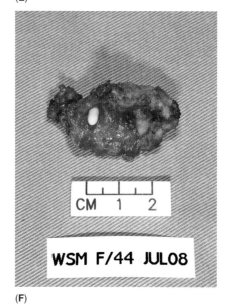

(F)

Figure 18.18   Schematic CT. (**A**) *Left*: The dotted line marks the osteotomy and the posterior part of the septum is divided. *Right*: The maxilla is swung laterally while remaining attached to the anterior cheek flap. Posterior part of the septum is removed. (**B**) The facial incision for maxillary swing approach to the nasopharynx as marked. (**C**) Incision on the palate is a curved incision along the inner border of the upper alveolus. Thus incision over the palatal mucoperiosteum and the osteotomy of the hard palate are in different planes. This reduces the incidence of palatal fistula. (**D**) The maxilla is swung laterally while remaining attached to the cheek flap (arrow). (**E**) The anterolateral approach exposed the tumor (arrow) situated in the fossa of Rosenmüller. The forceps is on the lateral crura of the eustachian tube, showing the opening of the tube (arrow heads). (**F**) En bloc resection of the tumor with the eustachian tube. A plastic tube is placed in the orifice of the auditory tympanic tube.

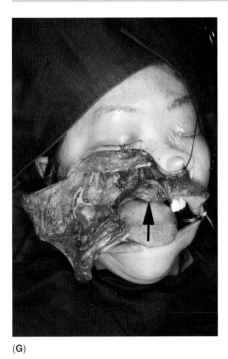

(G)

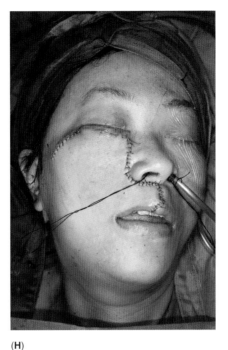

(H)

Figure 18.18 (*Continued*) (**G**) After removing the tumor, the tumor bed could be adequately examined. The palatal flap (arrow) can be seen to be viable. (**H**) At the completion of the resection, the osteocutaneous complex is returned, fixed to the rest of the facial skeleton and facial wound closed. A nasal pack and a nasogastric tube are inserted.

to the rest of the facial skeleton with miniplates and the facial wound closed (Fig. 18.18H).

When the recurrent or persistent tumor was localized in the nasopharynx without infiltration of skull base and could be removed with negative margins, the five-year actuarial control of tumor in the nasopharynx has been reported to be 65% and the five-year disease-free survival rate was around 54% (135,136). The long-term results including the functional aspect have been satisfactory (137). The main associated morbidity was a varying degree of trismus, which responded to passive stretching. In recent years with the modification of the incision on the palate, the complication of palatal fistula following this procedure has been eliminated (138).

SUMMARY

Nasopharyngeal cancer represents a pathologically and epidemiologically distinct entity. Surgery rarely has a role in its treatment, which is primarily chemoradiotherapy. Survival rates for locally advanced undifferentiated NPC is higher than for equivalent stage head and neck cancers at other sites. Recent advances in imaging and radiotherapy delivery are likely to improve outcomes in this important patient group (139).

REFERENCES

1. Shanmugaratnam K, Sobin LH. Histological typing of upper respiratory tract tumors. In: Shanmugaratnam K, Sobin LH, eds. International Histological Classification of Tumours: No 19. Geneva: World Health Organization, 1978; 32–3.
2. Micheau C, de The G, Orofiamma B et al. Practical value of classifying NPC into two major microscopical types. In: Grundman E, Krueger GRF, Ablashi DV, eds. Cancer Campaign, Volume 5: Nasopharyngeal Carcinoma. Stuttgart: Gustav Fisher, 1981; 51–7.
3. McGuire L, Suen M. Histopathology. In: van Hasselt A, Gibb A, eds. Nasopharyngeal Carcinoma. Hong Kong: The Chinese University Press, 1991; 91–9.
4. Nicholls JM. Nasopharyngeal carcinoma: Classification and histological appearances. Adv Anat Path 1997; 4: 71–84.
5. Yu M. Nasopharyngeal carcinoma: epidemiology and dietary factors. IARC Scientific Publications, 1991; 104.
6. Parkin DM, Whelan SL, Ferlay J et al., eds. Cancer Incidence in Five Continents, Vol. VII International Agency for Research on Cancer, Publication No. 143, 1997; 814–15.
7. Perez CA. Nasopharynx. In: Perez CA, Brady LW, eds. Principles and Practice of Radiation Oncology, 2nd edn. Philadelphia: JB Lippincott, 1992; 617–43.
8. Altun M, Fandi A, Dupuis O et al. Undifferentiated nasopharyngeal cancer (UCNT): Current diagnostic and therapeutic aspects. Int J Radiat Oncol Biol Phys 1995; 32: 857–87.
9. Lanier A, Bender T, Talbot M et al. Nasopharyngeal carcinoma in Alaskan Eskimos, Indians and Aleuts: a review of cases and study of Epstein–Barr virus, HLA, and environmental risk factors. Cancer 1980; 46: 2100–6.
10. Buell P. Nasopharynx cancer in Chinese of California. Br J Cancer 1965; 19: 459–70.
11. King H, Haenzel W. Cancer mortality among foreign and native-born Chinese in the United States. J Chron Dis 1972; 26: 623–46.
12. Chan S, Day N, Kunaratnam N et al. HLA and nasopharyngeal carcinoma in Chinese—a further study. Int J Cancer 1983; 32: 171–6.
13. Chan S, Day N, Khor T et al. HLA markers in the development and prognosis of NPC in Chinese. In: Grundman E, Krueger GRF, Ablashi DV, eds. Cancer Campaign, Volume 5: Nasopharyngeal Carcinoma. Stuttgart: Gustav Fischer, 1981: 205–11.
14. Lu S-J, Day N, Dagos L et al. Linkage of a nasopharyngeal carcinoma susceptibility locus to the HLA region. Nature 1990; 346: 470–1.

15. Henle W, Henle G, Ho JHC et al. Antibodies to Epstein–Barr virus in nasopharyngeal carcinoma, other head and neck neoplasms and control groups. J Nat Cancer Inst 1970; 44: 225–31.

16. Henle W, Ho JHC, Henle G et al. Antibodies to Epstein–Barr virus related antigens in nasopharyngeal carcinoma: comparison of active cases and long term survivors. J Nat Cancer Inst 1973; 51: 361–9.

17. Henle W, Ho JHC, Henle G et al. Nasopharyngeal carcinoma: significance of changes in Epstein–Barr virus-related antibody patterns following therapy. Int J Cancer 1977; 20: 663–72.

18. Fan H, Nicholls J, Chua D et al. Laboratory markers of tumour burden in nasopharyngeal carcinoma : a comparison of viral load and serological tests for Epstein-Barr virus. Int J Cancer 2004; 112: 1036–41.

19. Liebowitz D. Nasopharyngeal carcinoma: the Epstein–Barr virus association. Semin Oncol 1994; 21: 376–81.

20. Duraiswamy J, Sherritt M, Thomson S et al. Therapeutic LMP1 polyepitope vaccine for EBV-associated Hodgkin disease and nasopharyngeal carcinoma. Blood 2003; 101: 3150–6.

21. Pathmanathan R, Prasad U, Chandrika G et al. Undifferentiated, nonkeratinizing and squamous cell carcinoma of the nasopharynx. Variants of Epstein–Barr virus-infected neoplasia. Am J Pathol 1995; 146: 1355–67.

22. Lin T, Chang H, Chen C et al. Risk factors for nasopharyngeal carcinoma. Anticancer Res 1986; 6: 791–6.

23. Ho JHC. Stage classification of nasopharyngeal carcinoma: a review. In: de The G, Ito Y, eds. Nasopharyngeal carcinoma: Etiology and Control. Lyon: International Agency for Research on Cancer, 1978; 20: 94–114.

24. Yu M, Ho J, Lai S et al. Cantonese-style salted fish as a cause of nasopharyngeal carcinoma: report of a case-control study in Hong Kong. Cancer Res 1986; 46: 956–61.

25. Teo P, Shiu W, Leung S et al. Prognostic factors in nasopharyngeal carcinoma investigated by computed tomography. Radiother Oncol 1992; 23: 79–93.

26. Cvitkovic E, Bachouchi M, Armand J. Nasopharyngeal carcinoma: biology, natural history, and therapeutic implications. Haematol Oncol Clin North Am 1991; 5: 821–38.

27. Chua D, Sham J, Kwong D et al. Prognostic value of paranasopharyngeal extension of nasopharyngeal carcinoma. A significant factor in local control and distant metastasis. Cancer 1996; 78: 202–10.

28. Sanguineti G, Geara F, Garden A et al. Carcinoma of the nasopharynx treated by radiotherapy alone: determinants of local and regional control. Int J Radiat Oncol Biol Phys 1997; 37: 985–96.

29. Lederman M. Cancer of the Nasopharynx: Its Natural History and Treatment. Springfield, IL: Charles C. Thomas, 1961.

30. Perez C, Devinini V, Marcial-Vega V et al. Carcinoma of the nasopharynx: factors affecting prognosis. Int J Radiat Oncol Biol Phys 1992; 23: 271–80.

31. Lee A, Poon Y, Foo W et al. Retrospective analysis of 5037 patients with nasopharyngeal carcinoma treated during 1976–1985: overall survival and patterns of failure. Int J Radiat Oncol Biol Phys 1992; 23: 261–70.

32. Fletcher G, Million R. Malignant tumors of the nasopharynx. Am J Roentgenol Radium Ther Nucl Med 1965; 93: 44–55.

33. Lee A, Sham J, Poon Y et al. Treatment of stage I nasopharyngeal carcinoma: Analysis of the patterns of relapse and results of withholding elective neck irradiation. Int J Radiat Oncol Biol Phys 1989; 17: 1183–90.

34. Neel HI. Nasopharyngeal carcinoma: clinical presentation, diagnosis, treatment and prognosis. Otolaryngol Clin North Am 1985; 18: 479–90.

35. Ahmad A, Stefani S. Distant metastases of nasopharyngeal carcinoma: a study of 256 male patients. J Surg Oncol 1986; 33: 194–7.

36. Cvitkovic E, Bachouchi M, Boussen H et al. Leukemoid reaction, bone marrow invasion, fever of unknown origin, and metastatic pattern in the natural history of advanced undifferentiated carcinoma of nasopharyngeal type. J Clin Oncol 1993; 11: 2434–42.

37. Mutiranura A, Pornthanakasem W, Theamboonlers A et al. Epstein-Barr viral DNA in serum of patients with nasopharyngeal carcinoma. Clin Cancer Res 1998; 4: 665–9.

38. Lin JC, Wang WY, Chen KY et al. Quantification of plasma Esptein-barr virus DNA in patients with advanced stage nasopharyngeal carcinoma. N Eng J Med 2004; 350: 2461–70.

39. Wei WI, Yuen AP, Ng RW et al. Quantitative analysis of plasma cell-free Epstein-Barr virus DNA in nasopharyngeal carcinoma after salvage nasopharyngectomy: a prospective study. Head Neck 2004; 26: 878–83.

40. Kreel L, Ma H, Metreweli C. Imaging. In: van Hasselt C, Gibb A, eds. Nasopharyngeal Carcinoma. Hong Kong: The Chinese University Press, 1991.

41. Mancuso A. Imaging in patients with head and neck cancer. In: Million R, Cassisi N, eds. Management of Head and Neck Cancer: A Multidisciplinary Approach. Philadelphia: JB Lippincott, 1994.

42. King AD, Vlantis AC, Tsang RK et al. Magnetic resonance imaging for the detection of nasopharyngeal carcinoma. AJNR Am J Neuroradiol 2006; 27: 1288–91.

43. Yong-Sheng Z, Sham J, Ng M et al. Immunoglobulin A against viral capsid antigen of Epstein–Barr virus and indirect mirror examination of the nasopharynx in the detection of asymptomatic nasopharyngeal carcinoma. Cancer 1992; 69: 3–7.

44. Liaw C-C, Wang C-H, Huang J-S et al. Serum lactate dehydrogenase level in patients with nasopharyngeal carcinoma. Acta Oncol 1997; 36: 159–64.

45. Chang C, Liu T, Chang Y et al. Radiation therapy of nasopharyngeal carcinoma. Acta Radiolog Oncol 1980; 19: 433–438.

46. Huang S, Lui L, Lynn T-C. Nasopharyngeal cancer: study III. A review of 1206 patients treated with combined modalities. Int J Radiat Oncol Biol Phys 1985; 11: 1789–93.

47. UICC. TNM Atlas, 4th edn. Berlin: Springer-Verlag, 1997.

48. UICC. TNM Atlas, 3rd edn, 2nd rev. Berlin: Springer-Verlag, 1992.

49. Teo P, Leung S, Yu P et al. Comparison of the Ho's, UICC and AJC stage classification for nasopharyngeal carcinoma (NPC). Cancer 1991; 67: 434–9.

50. Teo P. Staging. In: van Hasselt C, Gibb A, eds. Nasopharyngeal Carcinoma. Hong Kong: The Chinese University Press, 1991.

51. Sobin LH, Wittekind Ch, eds. TNM Classification of malignant tumours, 6th edn. UICC/AJC. New York: John Wiley, 2002.

52. Qin D, Hu Y, Yan J et al. Analysis of 1379 patients with nasopharyngeal carcinoma treated by radiation. Cancer 1988; 61: 1117–24.

53. Sham J, Choy D. Prognostic factors of nasopharyngeal carcinoma: a review of 759 patients. Br J Radiol 1990; 63: 51–8.

54. Teo P, Yu P, Lee W et al. Significant prognosticators after primary radiotherapy in 903 nondisseminated nasopharyngeal carcinoma evaluated by computed tomography. Int J Radiat Oncol Biol Phys 1996; 36: 291–304.

55. Ingersoll L, Shiao Y, Donaldson S et al. Nasopharyngeal carcinoma in the young: A combined MD Anderson and Stanford experience. Int J Radiat Oncol Biol Phys 1990; 19: 881–7.

56. Ho JHC. An epidemiologic and clinical study of nasopharyngeal carcinoma. Int J Radiat Oncol Biol Phys 1978; 4: 183–98.

57. Hoppe R, Williams J, Warnke R et al. Carcinoma of the nasopharynx: the significance of histology. Int J Radiat Oncol Biol Phys 1978; 4: 199–205.

58. Santos J, Gonzalez C, Cuesta P et al. Impact of changes in the treatment of nasopharyngeal carcinoma: an experience of 30 years. Radiother Oncol 1995; 36: 121–7.

59. Cheng AL, Huang WG, Chen ZC et al. Identification of novel nasopharyngeal carcinoma biomarkers by laser capture microdissection and proteomic analysis. Clin Cancer Res 2008; 14: 435–45.

60. Fleming ID, Cooper JS, Henson DE et al., eds. AJCC Cancer Staging Manual, 5th edn. Philadelphia: Lippincott-Raven, 1997, 33–5.

61. Cooper JS, Cohen R, Stevens RE. A comparision of staging systems for nasopharyngeal carcinoma. Cancer 1998; 83: 213–19.

62. Özyar E, Yildiz F, Akyol FH et al. Comparison of AJCC 1988 and 1997 classifications for nasopharyngeal carcinoma. Int J Radiat Oncol Biol Phys 1999; 44: 1079–87.

63. Cellai E, Olmi P, Chiavacci A et al. Computed tomography in nasopharyngeal carcinoma: part II: impact on survival. Int J Radiat Oncol Biol Phys 1990; 19: 1177–82.

64. Sham J, Wei W, Nicholls J et al. Extent of nasopharyngeal carcinoma involvement inside the nasopharynx. Lack of prognostic value on local control. Cancer 1992; 69: 854–9.

65. Yu Z, Xu G, Huang Y et al. Value of computed tomography in staging the primary lesion (T-staging) of nasopharyngeal carcinoma (NPC): an analysis of 54 patients with special reference to the parapharyngeal space. Int J Radiat Oncol Biol Phys 1985; 11: 2143–7.

66. Sham J, Choy D, Choi P. Nasopharyngeal carcinoma: the significance of neck node involvement in relation to the pattern of distant failure. Br J Radiol 1990; 63: 108–13.

67. Lee A, Foo W, Chan D. Nasopharyngeal carcinoma: evaluation of N-staging by Ho and AJCC/UICC system. Int J Radiat Oncol Biol Phys 1994; 30(Suppl 1): 202.

68. Neel H, Taylor W, Pearson G. Prognostic determinants and a new view of staging for patients with nasopharyngeal carcinoma. Ann Otolaryngol Rhinol Laryngol 1985; 94: 529–37.

69. Lee A, Law S, Foo W et al. Nasopharyngeal carcinoma: local control by megavoltage irradiation. Br J Radiol 1993; 66: 528–36.

70. Ho JHC. Nasopharynx. In: Halnan K, ed. Treatment of Cancer. London: Chapman and Hall, 1982: 249–67.

71. Fletcher G, Million R. Nasopharynx. In: Fletcher G, ed. Textbook of Radiotherapy. Philadelphia: Lea and Febiger, 1980: 364–83.

72. Leibel SA, Kutcher GJ, Harrison LB et al. Improved dose distributions for 3D conformal boost treatments in carcinoma of the nasopharynx. Int J Radiat Oncol Biol Phys 1991; 20: 823–33.

73. Hunt MA, Zelefsky MJ, Wolden S et al. Treatment planning and delivery of intensity-modulated radiation therapy for primary nasopharynx cancer. Int J Radiat Oncol Biol Phys 2001; 49: 623–32.

74. Xia P, Fu KK, Wong GW et al. Comparison of treatment plans involving intensity-modulated radiotherapy for nasopharyngeal carcinoma. Int J Radiat Oncol Biol Phys 2000; 48: 329–37.

75. Sultanem K, Shu HK, Xia P et al. Three-dimensional intensity-modulated radiotherapy in the treatment of nasopharyngeal carcinoma: the University of California-San Francisco experience. Int J Radiat Oncol Biol Phys 2000; 48: 711–22.

76. Pow EH, Kwong DL, McMillan AS et al. Xerostomia and quality of life after intensity modulated radiotherapy vs conventional radiotherapy for early stage nasopharyngeal carcinoma: initial report on a randomized controlled clinical trial. Int J Radiat Oncol Biol Phys 2006; 66: 981–91.

77. Kam MK, Leung SF, Zee B et al. Prospective randomized study of intensity modulated radiotherapy on salivary gland function in early stage nasopharyngeal carcinoma patients. J Clin Oncol 2007; 25: 2873–9.

78. Marks J, Bedwinek J, Lee F et al. Dose-response analysis for nasopharyngeal carcinoma. An historical perspective. Cancer 1982; 50: 1042–50.

79. Yan J, Qin D, Hu Y et al. Management of local residual primary lesion of nasopharyngeal carcinoma (NPC): are higher doses beneficial? Int J Radiat Oncol Biol Phys 1989; 16: 1465–9.

80. Leibel S, Kutcher G, Harrison L et al. Improved dose distributions for 3D conformal boost treatments in carcinoma of the nasopharynx. Int J Radiat Oncol Biol Phys 1991; 20: 823–33.

81. Brown A, Urie M, Chisin R et al. Proton therapy for carcinoma of the nasopharynx: a study in comparative treatment planning. Int J Radiat Oncol Biol Phys 1989; 16: 1607–14.

82. Webb S. The Physics of Conformal Radiotherapy. Advances in Technology. Bristol: Institute of Physics Publishing, 1997.

83. Saunders M, Dische S, Barrett A et al. Randomised multi-centre trials of CHART vs. conventional radiotherapy in head and neck and non-small-cell lung cancer: an interim report. Br J Cancer 1996; 73: 1455–62.

84. Wang C. Accelerated hyperfractionation radiation therapy for carcinoma of the nasopharynx. Cancer 1989; 63: 2461–7.

85. Zhang Y, Liu T, Fi C. Intracavitary radiation treatment of nasopharyngeal carcinoma by the high dose rate afterloading technique. Int J Radiat Oncol Biol Phys 1989; 16: 315–318.

86. Wang C. Improved local control of nasopharyngeal carcinoma after intracavitary brachytherapy boost. Am J Clin Oncol 1991; 14: 5–8.

87. Kouvaris J, Plataniotis G, Sandilos C et al. Combined tele-therapy and intracavitary brachytherapy boost for the treatment of nasopharyngeal carcinoma. Radiother Oncol 1996; 38: 263–7.

88. Tsao S. Radiotherapy. In: van Hasselt C, Gibb A, eds. Nasopharyngeal Carcinoma. Hong Kong: The Chinese University Press, 1991.

89. Yu K, Teo P, Lee W et al. Patterns of early treatment failure in non-metastatic nasopharyngeal carcinoma: a study based on CT scanning. Clin Oncol 1994; 6: 167–71.

90. Choy D, Sham J, Wei W et al. Transpalatal insertion of radioactive gold grain for the treatment of persistent and recurrent nasopharyngeal carcinoma. Int J Radiat Oncol Biol Phys 1993; 25: 505–12.

91. Petrovich Z, Cox J, Middleton R et al. Advanced carcinoma of the nasopharynx. 2. Pattern of failure in 256 patients. Radiother Oncol 1985; 4: 15–20.

92. Vikram B, Mishra U, Strong E et al. Patterns of failure in carcinoma of the nasopharynx: I. Failure at the primary site. Int J Radiat Oncol Biol Phys 1985; 11: 1455–9.

93. Hoppe R, Goffinet D, Bagshaw M. Carcinoma of the nasopharynx. Eighteen years' experience with megavoltage radiation therapy. Cancer 1976; 37: 2605–12.

94. Lee A. Complications of radiation therapy. In: van Hasselt C, Gibb A, eds. Nasopharyngeal Carcinoma. Hong Kong: The Chinese University Press, 1991.

95. Mesic J, Fletcher G, Goepfert H. Megavoltage irradiation of epithelial tumors of the nasopharynx. Int J Radiat Oncol Biol Phys 1981; 7: 447–53.

96. Lee A, Ng S, Ho JHC et al. Clinical diagnosis of late temporal lobe necrosis following radiation therapy for nasopharyngeal carcinoma. Cancer 1988; 61: 1535–42.

97. Lee A, Cheng L, Ng S et al. Magnetic resonance imaging in the clinical diagnosis of late temporal lobe necrosis following radiotherapy for nasopharyngeal carcinoma. Clin Radiol 1990; 41: 24–41.

98. Lam K, Tse V, Wang C et al. Effects of cranial irradiation on hypothalamic-pituitary function: a 5–year longitudinal study in patients with nasopharyngeal carcinoma. Q J Med 1991; 78: 165–76.

99. Kwong D, Wei W, Sham J et al. Sensorineural hearing loss in patients treated for nasopharyngeal carcinoma: a prospective study of the effect of radiation and cisplatin treatment. Int J Radiat Oncol Biol Phys 1996; 36: 281–9.

100. Lee A, Foo W, Law S et al. Reirradiation for recurrent nasopharyngeal carcinoma: factors affecting the therapeutic ratio and ways for improvement. Int J Radiat Oncol Biol Phys 1997; 38: 43–52.

101. Pryzant R, Wendt C, Declos L et al. Re-treatment of nasopharyngeal carcinoma in 53 patients. Int J Radiat Oncol Biol Phys 1992; 22: 941–7.

102. Wang C. Re-irradiation of recurrent nasopharyngeal carcinoma: treatment techniques and results. Int J Radiat Oncol Biol Phys 1987; 13: 953–6.

103. International Nasopharynx Cancer Study Group. Preliminary results of a randomized trial comparing neoadjuvant chemotherapy (cisplatin, epirubicin, bleomycin) plus radiotherapy vs. radiotherapy alone in stage IV (≥N2, M0) undifferentiated nasopharyngeal carcinoma: a positive effect on progression-free survival. Int J Radiat Oncol Biol Phys 1996; 35: 463–9.

104. Dimery I, Peters L, Goepfert H et al. Effectiveness of combined induction chemotherapy and radiotherapy in advanced nasopharyngeal carcinoma. J Clin Oncol 1993; 11: 1919–28.

105. Khoury G, Paterson I. Nasopharyngeal carcinoma: a review of cases treated by radiotherapy and chemotherapy. Clin Radiol 1987; 38: 17–20.

106. Atichartakarn V, Kraiphibul P, Clongsusuek P et al. Nasopharyngeal carcinoma: result of treatment with cis-diamminedichloroplatinum II, 5 fluorouracil and radiation therapy. Int J Radiat Oncol Biol Phys 1988; 14: 461–9.

107. Garden A, Lippman S, Morrison W et al. Does induction chemotherapy have a role in the management of nasopharyngeal carcinoma? Results of treatment in the era of computerised tomography. Int J Radiat Oncol Biol Phys 1996; 36: 1005–12.

108. Tannock I, Payne D, Cummings B et al. Sequential chemotherapy and radiation for nasopharyngeal cancer: absence of long-term benefit despite a high rate of tumour response to chemotherapy. J Clin Oncol 1987; 5: 629–34.

109. Chan A, Teo P, Leung T et al. A prospective randomized study of chemotherapy adjunctive to definitive radiotherapy in advanced nasopharyngeal carcinoma. Int J Radiat Oncol Biol Phys 1995; 33: 569–77.

110. Turner S, Tiver K. Synchronous radiotherapy and chemotherapy in the treatment of nasopharyngeal carcinoma. Int J Radiat Oncol Biol Phys 1993; 27: 371–7.

111. Souhami L, Rabinowits M. Combined treatment in carcinoma of the nasopharynx. Laryngoscope 1988; 98: 881–3.

112. Marcial V, Pajak T, Mohuiddin M et al. Concomitant cisplatin chemotherapy and radiotherapy in advanced mucosal squamous cell carcinoma of the head and neck. Cancer 1990; 66: 1861–8.

113. Al-Sarraf M, Pajak T, Cooper J et al. Chemo-radiotherapy in patients with locally advanced nasopharyngeal carcinoma: a Radiation Therapy Oncology Group study. J Clin Oncol 1990; 8: 1342–51.

114. Rahima M, Rakowsky E, Barzilay J et al. Carcinoma of the nasopharynx. An analysis of 91 cases and a comparison of differing treatment approaches. Cancer 1986; 58: 843–9.

115. Tsujii H, Kamada T, Tsuji H et al. Improved results in the treatment of nasopharyngeal carcinoma using combined radiotherapy and chemotherapy. Cancer 1989; 63: 1668–72.

116. Teo P, Ho J, Choy D et al. Adjunctive chemotherapy to radical radiation therapy in the treatment of advanced nasopharyngeal carcinoma. Int J Radiat Oncol Biol Phys 1987; 13: 679–85.

117. Rossi A, Molinari P, Boracchi P et al. Adjuvant chemotherapy with vincristine, cyclophosphamide and doxorubicin after radiotherapy in local-regional nasopharyngeal cancer: results of a 4-year multicenter randomized study. J Clin Oncol 1988; 6: 1401–10.

118. Al-Sarraf M, LeBlanc M, Giri P et al. Superiority of chemoradiotherapy (CT-RT) vs. radiotherapy (RT) in patients (pts) with locally advanced nasopharyngeal cancer (NPC). Preliminary results of Intergroup 0099 (SWOG 8892, RTOG 8817, ECOG 2388) randomized study (meeting abstract). Proc Ann Meeting of the American Society of Clinical Oncology 1996; 15: A882.

119. Wee J, Tan EH, Tai BC et al. Randomised trial of radiotherapy vs concurrent chemoradiotherapy followed by adjuvant chemotherapy in patients with AJCC.IUCC stage III and IV nasopharyngeal cancer of the endemic variety. J Clin Oncol 2005; 23: 6730–8.

120. Lee AW, Lau WH, Tung SY et al. Preliminary results of a randomized study on therapeutic gain by concurrent chemotherapy for regionally advanced nasopharyngeal carcinoma: NPC-9901 trial by the Hong Kong Nasopharyngeal Cancer Study Group. J Clin Oncol 2005; 23: 6966–75.

121. Lee AW, Tung SY, Chan AT et al. Preliminary results of a randomized study (NPC-9902 trial) on therapeutic gain by concurrent chemotherapy and/or accelerated fractionation for locally advanced nasopharyngeal carcinoma. Int J Radiat Oncol Biol Phys 2006; 66: 142–51.

122. Choo R, Tannock I. Chemotherapy for recurrent or metastatic carcinoma of the nasopharynx. A review of the Princess Margaret Hospital experience. Cancer 1991; 68: 2120–4.

123. Al-Kourainy K, Crissman J, Ensley J et al. Excellent response to cis-platinum-based chemotherapy in patients with recurrent or previously untreated advanced nasopharyngeal carcinoma. Am J Clin Oncol 1988; 11: 427–30.

124. Huang SC, Lui LT, Lynn TC. Nasopharyngeal cancer: study III. A review of 1206 patients treated with combined modalities. Int J Radiat Oncol Biol Phys 1985; 11: 1789–93.

125. Yao M, Luo P, Hoffman HT et al. Pathology and FDG PET correlation of residual lymph nodes in head and neck cancer after radiation treatment. Am J Clin Oncol 2007; 30: 264–70.

126. Sham JS, Choy D. Nasopharyngeal carcinoma: treatment of neck node recurrence by radiotherapy. Australas Radiol 1991; 35: 370–3.

127. Wei WI, Lam KH, Ho CM et al. Efficacy of radical neck dissection for the control of cervical metastasis after radiotherapy for nasopharyngeal carcinoma. Am J Surg 1990; 160: 439–42.

128. Wei WI, Ho CM, Wong MP et al. Pathological basis of surgery in the management of postradiotherapy cervical metastasis in nasopharyngeal carcinoma. Arch Otolaryngol Head Neck Surg 1992; 118: 923–9.

129. Wei WI, Ho WK, Cheng AC et al. Management of extensive cervical nodal metastasis in nasopharyngeal carcinoma after radiotherapy: a clinicopathological study. Arch Otolaryngol Head Neck Surg 2001; 127: 1457–62.

130. Morton R, Liavaag P, McLean M et al. Transcervico-mandibulo-palatal approach for surgical salvage of recurrent nasopharyngeal cancer. Head and Neck 1996; 18: 352–8.

131. Hsu M, Ko J, Sheen T et al. Salvage surgery for recurrent nasopharyngeal carcinoma. Arch Otolaryngol Head Neck Surg 1997; 123: 305–9.

132. Fisch U. The infratemporal fossa approach for nasopharyngeal tumours. Laryngoscope 1983; 93: 36–43.

133. Wei WI. Carcinoma of the nasopharynx. Adv Otolaryngol Head Neck Surg 1998; 12: 119–32.

134. Wei WI, Lam KH, Sham JS. New approach to the nasopharynx: the maxillary swing approach. Head Neck 1991; 13: 200–7.

135. Wei WI. Nasopharyngeal cancer: current status of management. Arch Otolaryngol Head Neck Surg 2001; 127.

136. Wei WI. Cancer of the nasopharynx: functional surgical salvage. World J Surg 2003; 27: 844–848, 766–9.

137. Ng RW, Wei WI. Quality of life of patients with recurrent nasopharyngeal carcinoma treated with nasopharyngectomy using the maxillary swing approach. Arch Otolaryngol Head Neck Surg 2006; 132: 309–16.

138. Ng RW, Wei WI. Elimination of palatal fistula after the maxillary swing procedure. Head Neck 2005; 27: 608–12.

139. Wei WI, Sham JS. Nasopharyngeal carcinoma. Lancet 2005; 365: 2041–54.

140. Wei W, Ho C, Yuen P et al. Maxillary swing approach for resection of tumours in and around the nasopharynx. Arch Otolaryngol Head Neck Surg 1995; 121: 638–42.

141. Hall CE, Harris R, A'Hern R et al. Le Fort I osteotomy and low-dose rate Ir192 brachytherapy for treatment of recurrent nasopharyngeal tumours. Radiother Oncol. 2003; 66: 41–8.

19

Tumors of the Parapharyngeal Space

Rajan S Patel, Patrick J Gullane and Christine B Novak

INTRODUCTION

The parapharyngeal space is a highly complex potential space located bilaterally in the upper neck and contains numerous vital neurovascular structures. Tumors involving this space are extremely rare, comprising less than 1% of all head and neck neoplasms. A thorough knowledge of the anatomy of the parapharyngeal space is fundamental to understanding the routes of passage of lesions to and from the space, awareness of the clinical presentation of parapharyngeal tumors, selecting and interpreting radiological investigations, and to understanding and planning the most appropriate surgical approach to this region.

ANATOMY

As the name implies, the parapharyngeal space lies lateral to the pharynx and is most easily visualized as an inverted pyramid with its floor at the skull base and its apex at the attachment of the posterior belly of digastric to the greater cornu of the hyoid bone. It is defined superiorly by the inferior petrous temporal bone including the carotid canal, the jugular foramen, and the hypoglossal foramen, posteriorly by the carotid sheath, the prevertebral fascia covering the prevertebral musculature and the vertebrae, and laterally by the fascia overlying the pterygoid muscle, the deep lobe of the parotid, the posterior belly of the digastric muscle, and the ascending ramus of the mandible. These three osseous borders are rigid, thereby offering some resistance to spread of tumor. Anteriorly the parapharyngeal space is bounded by pterygomandibular raphe, and medially it abuts the buccopharyngeal fascia overlying the pharyngeal constrictors and the tensor and levator veli palatini (Fig. 19.1). The parapharyngeal space communicates with the retropharyngeal and submandibular spaces, which permit spread of tumor along fascial planes with minimal resistance. Lymphatics from the parapharyngeal space drain to the upper deep cervical lymph nodes.

The fascia extending between the styloid process and the tensor veli palatini divides the parapharyngeal space into pre-styloid and post-styloid spaces. The contents of these spaces are shown in Table 19.1.

Pre-styloid tumors are almost always of salivary origin and post-styloid lesions usually paraganglioma or neural in origin with occasional primary or secondary lymph node neoplasms found (Table 19.2).

PATHOLOGY

Parapharyngeal tumors consist of a heterogeneous group of tumors, which are mostly (80%) benign (1,3–5).

Salivary Gland Neoplasms

Salivary gland tumors are the most common primary lesions to develop in the parapharyngeal space and may arise from the deep lobe of the parotid, from minor salivary glands in the lateral pharyngeal wall, or ectopic salivary tissue in the parapharyngeal space (1,3-5).

Deep-Lobe Parotid Tumors

Approximately 10% of parotid tumors originate in the deep lobe of the gland and they are almost always benign pleomorphic adenomas (1,3–5). The most commonly reported malignancies are mucoepidermoid carcinomas, adenoid cystic carcinomas, and acinar cell carcinomas (1,3–5). Deep-lobe tumors may extend into the parapharyngeal space either directly through the stylomandibular tunnel, which is formed by the stylomandibular ligament posteroinferiorly and by the ascending ramus of the mandible anteriorly. Tumors passing through here have the classic "dumbbell" and are palpable as a retromandibular mass externally while displacing the tonsil and soft palate medially. Tumors arising from the retromandibular portion of the gland tend to pass behind the stylomandibular ligament, have a more rounded appearance, and become very large before causing symptoms.

Minor Salivary Gland Tumors

A smaller number of tumors arise from minor salivary glands in the mucosa of the lateral pharyngeal wall or in ectopic salivary tissue in the parapharyngeal space. These can be distinguished from deep-lobe tumors radiologically and pathologically as there is a layer of fat separating the tumor from the deep lobe of the parotid.

Paraganglioma

Paraganglioma are neuroendocrine neoplasms arising from paraganglia, which are aggregates of cells located within neuronal and vascular adventitia throughout the body. The largest collection of paraganglia is located in the adrenal

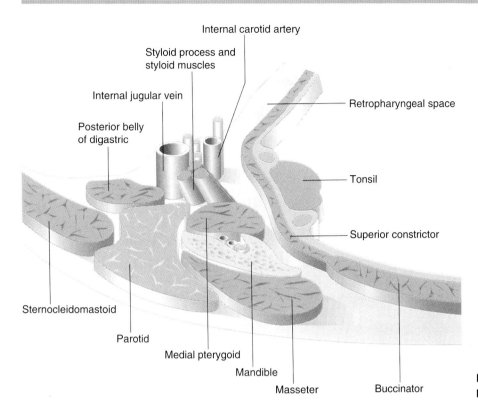

Figure 19.1 Normal anatomy of the parapharyngeal space.

Table 19.1   Normal Structures within the Parapharyngeal Space

Structure	Pre-styloid space	Post-styloid space
Vascular	Internal maxillary artery	Internal carotid artery Internal jugular vein
Nervous	Lingual nerve Inferior alveolar nerve Auriculotemporal nerve	Cranial nerve IX, X, XI, XII Cervical sympathetic trunk
Other	Loose areolar and adipose tissue	Lymph nodes

Table 19.2   Differential Diagnoses of Parapharyngeal Space Neoplasms (1,2)

	Group	Pathology
Pre-styloid (45%)	Salivary (45%)	Benign: pleomorphic adenoma Malignant: adenoid cystic carcinoma, carcinoma ex-pleomorphic adenoma, acinic cell carcinoma, mucoepidermoid carcinoma
Post-styloid (45%)	Paraganglioma (20%)	Carotid body tumor Glomus vagale
	Neurogenic (15%)	Neurilemmoma Neurofibroma
	Lymph nodes (10%)	Lymphoma Metastases
Others (10%)	Vascular	Hemangiopericytoma, angiosarcoma, hemangioma
	Connective Tissue	Rhabdomyosarcoma, lipoma, liposarcoma, fibrosarcoma, osteosarcoma

medulla, which secretes catecholamines in association with the sympathetic nervous system. Paraganglia within the head and neck are associated with the parasympathetic nervous system and are most predominant in the carotid body at the carotid bifurcation (6). Paraganglia also arise in the temporal bone along Arnold's nerve (the auricular branch of the vagus nerve), and Jacobson's nerve (the tympanic branch of the glossopharyngeal nerve), and at the jugular bulb. Carotid body and jugulotympanic paraganglioma comprise 80% of all head and neck paraganglioma, and vagal paraganglioma account for 5% (7). Paragangliomas have been reported in other head and neck sites including larynx (8), trachea (9), sympathetic trunk (10), and paranasal sinus (11).

Paragangliomas of extracranial origin give rise to two distinct lesions in different locations. Carotid body paraganglioma (carotid body tumors) tend to splay the carotid bifurcation, displacing the internal carotid artery posterolaterally and the external carotid artery anteromedially. As they enlarge, they tend to encase the carotid system; they may involve adjacent nerves such as the hypoglossal and vagus nerves, and eventually involve the parapharyngeal space. Vagal paraganglioma (glomus vagale) arise from one of the vagal ganglia; most commonly they originate from the inferior nodose ganglion displacing the carotid system anteromedially, without splaying the bifurcation, and extend into the post-styloid parapharyngeal space. Skull base involvement is less likely in these paraganglioma compared to those arising in the middle or superior vagal ganglia, which are generally associated with early skull base involvement and intracranial extension.

More women than men develop sporadic paraganglioma (ratio 3:1), and rarely (5%) these patients have multiple lesions (12). Patients living at high altitude have an increased risk of developing carotid paraganglioma secondary to chronic hypoxemia. This patient population has a female preponderance, low rate of bilaterality (5%), and positive family history (1%) (13). Emerging evidence implicates heredity in up to 50% of cases of head and neck paraganglioma (14). Patients with familial paraganglioma have an equal gender distribution, lower age of onset, higher rate of multicentricity (at least 25%), and are more likely to have paraganglioma of the carotid or vagus than at other sites (14–16).

Familial paraganglioma may occur as part of a familial tumor syndrome, such as Multiple Endocrine Neoplasia IIA or IIB, von Hippel Landau, and Carney triad (paraganglioma, pulmonary chondroma, and gastrointestinal stroma tumor) (14). Non-syndromic familial paraganglioma are thought to be related to mutations in the succinate dehydrogenase gene, which is inherited in an autosomal dominant pattern with incomplete penetrance, as the maternally derived gene is inactivated during female oogenesis. Three of four genes encoding subunits of the mitochondrial II complex—succinate dehydrogenase complex, subunit B, iron sulfur (Ip) (SDHB), succinate dehydrogenase complex, subunit C, integral membrane protein (SDHC), and succinate dehydrogenase complex, subunit D, integral membrane protein (SDHD)—have been implicated in the pathogenesis of hereditary head and neck paragangliomas (17–19). SDHD mutations are associated with multifocal paraganglioma, and SDHB with malignant paraganglioma (20). Affected men have a 50% chance of having an affected child, whereas affected women will not have an affected child, but may transmit an inactivated gene (21). Genetic counseling and radiological screening performed in family members of patients with paraganglioma can identify: 1) those at risk of disease, allowing for early identification and treatment, and 2) carriers, allowing their offspring to receive screening (14). Those found to have the paternal gene should undergo regular radiological screening.

Paragangliomas are solid neoplasms with a red-brown appearance and may be completely encapsulated. Histologically, clusters of chief cells and sustentacular cells are seen separated by a highly vascular fibrous stroma. Head and neck paraganglioma rarely (5%) secrete catecholamines unlike the histologically similar pheochromocytoma found in the adrenal medulla (22). Malignant paraganglioma occur rarely (5%) and are identified by the presence of regional or distant metastases or invasion of surrounding non-neuroendocrine structures (23). However, the multicentric nature of these tumors can make this diagnosis difficult.

Neurogenic Tumors

The parent cell of neurogenic tumors in the head and neck is probably the Schwann cell. They account for 20–30% of all parapharyngeal space lesions (24) and give rise to two distinct tumor types; neurilemmoma (schwannoma) and neurofibroma. The vagus and the cervical sympathetic trunk are the most commonly involved nerves. Most patients are asymptomatic and present with a mass in the neck.

Neurilemmoma

Neurilemmoma are the most common neurogenic tumor arising in the parapharyngeal space. They are solitary, slow-growing, well-encapsulated tumors, which occasionally may be associated with von Reklinghausen's neurofibromatosis (NF1). The associated nerve fibers are draped over the lesion and usually can be dissected from the tumor at surgery. Pain and neurological dysfunction are unusual but patients may experience paraesthesia following surgery. These tumors are rarely malignant.

Neurofibroma

Neurofibroma are unencapsulated and nerve fibers run through the tumor making it difficult to dissect them from the nerve of origin without sacrificing fibers. These lesions are associated with NF1 and are usually multiple and subcutaneous, but may also arise in the parapharyngeal space. Sarcomatous transformation occurs in fewer than 10% of lesions in patients with NF1, and is usually heralded by sudden growth or recurrence of the tumor after resection. Malignant neurofibrosarcoma invade adjacent tissues and may metastasize.

SYMPTOMS AND SIGNS

The parapharyngeal space is not easily accessible to routine clinical examination and generally remains silent until a pathological process progresses. Despite the wide variety of tumors involving the parapharyngeal space, they all tend to present in a similar manner (Table 19.3).

However, the onset of symptoms is often insidious and may be quite subtle. Most parapharyngeal space tumors present as a painless mass, although in some patients there may be local or radiating tenderness (Fig. 19.2). The boundaries of the parapharyngeal space permit tumor to spread most easily in a medial and inferior direction. Medial extension will produce displacement of the lateral pharyngeal wall and soft palate, while inferior extension produces a mass in the neck near the angle of the mandible. Tumors must be at least 3 cm in size before they are clinically detectable. Medial displacement of the tonsil and soft palate may cause partial upper airway obstruction with snoring, obstructive sleep apnea, dysphagia, or dysarthria as the presenting symptoms (Fig. 19.3). Paragangliomas and other vascular lesions may be pulsatile with audible bruits or present with pulsatile tinnitus due to the noise of turbulent vascular flow. Lesions of neural origin or glomus vagale may present with single or multiple cranial nerve palsies (IX to XII), particularly hoarseness and vocal cord palsy or Horner's syndrome. Large tumors may cause eustachian tube dysfunction and otitis media with effusion. Malignancy should be suspected with symptoms of pain, trismus, and cranial nerve neuropathies, particularly in the presence of a small mass (25).

A complete examination of the head, neck, and upper aerodigestive tract is required with particular attention to mobility of tumor, function of the facial nerve and other lower cranial nerves (IX to XII), and presence of bruits. Bimanual palpation of the oropharynx should be carried out when possible to determine the mobility and consistency of the tumor mass as well as to determine whether

Table 19.3 Presenting Symptoms and Signs of Parapharyngeal Space Tumors (1)

Symptoms	Frequency (%)
Intraoral/neck mass	85
Ear pressure or pain	36
Dysphagia	13
Hearing loss	11
Hoarseness	10
Facial or jaw pain	6
Facial nerve weakness, throat pain, pulsatile tinnitus, tongue paraesthesia, aspiration, headache, hypertension, syncope	<5

Signs	
Intraoral displacement of tonsil/soft palate	65
Neck mass (11% pulsatile)	58
Vocal cord paralysis/paresis	8
Hearing loss/OME	9
Palatal paralysis	5
Atrophic or fasiculating tongue	5
Horner's syndrome	2
Trismus	2

Abbreviation: OME, Otitis media with effusion.

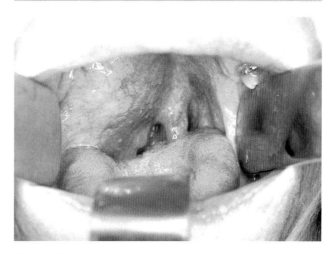

Figure 19.3 Intraoral view of a parapharyngeal tumor pushing the lateral wall of the pharynx medially (deep-lobe parotid tumor).

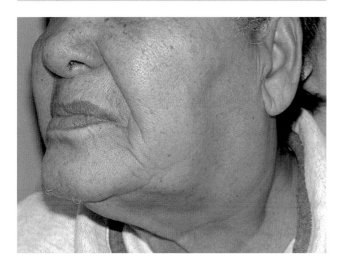

Figure 19.2 Patient with a left-sided neck mass, carotid body tumor.

there is significant tenderness or a pulsatile nature to the neoplasm.

INVESTIGATION

All patients with a mass in the parapharyngeal space should undergo assessment with either a CT scan or MRI of the neck to determine the size of the tumor and its relationship to surrounding structures (26). Tumors found in the pre-styloid space rarely need further investigation as almost all arise from the deep lobe of the parotid or minor salivary glands. Those arising in the post-styloid space often require angiography to help differentiate paraganglia from neural lesions and determine the vascularity of the tumor. Fine-needle aspiration (FNA) may be a valuable adjunct to

these investigations while incisional biopsy is to be discouraged due to seeding of some tumors and possible massive uncontrolled bleeding.

Radiology

It is generally acknowledged that MRI is superior to CT in the evaluation of parapharyngeal space lesions (25). MRI provides excellent soft tissue, vascular resolution, and tumor margin resolution as well as characterizing the tumor pathology, which provides a pre-operative diagnosis in 95% of parapharyngeal tumors (5,25,26). The only significant disadvantage of MRI is the lack of information about bone erosion at the skull base, which is provided by CT.

The pathology of the tumor may be evident from its inherent appearance on MRI and the way it displaces the carotid sheath and parapharyngeal fat. T1-weighted images are best for examining normal anatomy and tumor–fat interfaces, while T2-weighted images are best for assessing tumor margins and the tumor–muscle interface. Pre-styloid lesions tend to push the carotid artery posteriorly and the parapharyngeal fat medially and posteriorly (Figs. 19.4 and 19.5). Deep-lobe parotid tumors in this area have a homogeneous appearance with a moderate to high signal on T2-weighted images. Minor salivary gland tumors and ectopic salivary tissue can be differentiated from deep-lobe tumors as the fat plane is preserved between the deep-lobe of the parotid and the tumor. Post-styloid lesions push the carotid artery anteriorly and the parapharyngeal fat pad anteriorly and laterally (Figs. 19.6 and 19.7). Paragangliomas arising from the carotid body tend to splay apart the internal and external carotid arteries and have a "salt and pepper" appearance due to vascular flow voids. Schwannoma and neurofibroma tend to have a more homogeneous appearance with moderate to high signal on T2-weighted images. Lymph nodes have a characteristic radiological appearance. Malignancy should be suspected when there is loss of the normal tissue planes, invasion of the muscle, or replacement of the normal increased fat signal of the bone marrow and skull base on T1 images by lower density tumor signal (25).

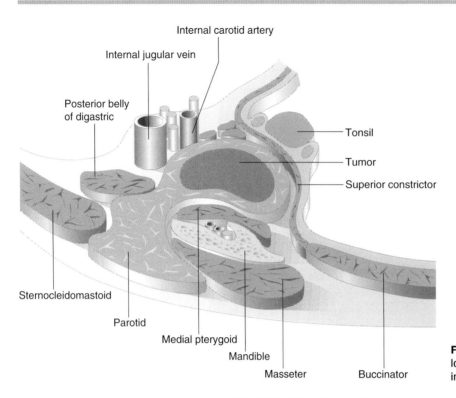

Figure 19.4 Location of a pre-styloid, deep-lobe parotid tumor in relation to other structures in the neck.

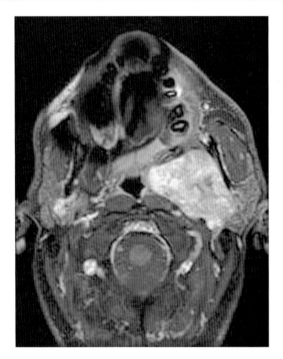

Figure 19.5 MRI of a deep-lobe parotid tumor.

Angiography

Angiography of all lesions suspected to be a paraganglioma in the post-styloid space is necessary to confirm the diagnosis, determine the vascularity of the tumor, and examine its relationship to the great vessels of the neck.

Carotid body paraganglioma splay apart the internal and external carotid arteries producing the so called "lyre" sign on angiography (Fig. 19.8), while glomus vagale are found more superiorly and tend to displace the carotid artery anteriorly. Angiography in patients with paraganglioma will identify major feeding vessels for possible embolization or ligation and pick up other clinically silent vascular lesions in the neck. It will also pick up an evidence of vessel invasion in patients with malignant parapharyngeal tumors. MRI angiography has been promoted as a non-invasive modality that provides excellent characterization of the vascular relations of the tumor. However, unlike angiography it does not provide information on the angioarchitecture of the lesion nor the dominant feeding vessels of the lesion. Angiography also offers a therapeutic option of embolizing the tumor feeding vessel, and provides information on multicentric lesions not visualized on MRI.

Cytology

Transcervical or transoral FNA cytology aids the diagnosis of many parapharyngeal lesions including salivary gland tumors and paraganglioma. However, schwannoma, spindle cell neoplasms, granulomatous inflammation, and other benign lesions may prove difficult to diagnose cytologically. It has been suggested that FNA cytology adds little to the management of parapharyngeal neoplasms as radiological investigations usually give an indication of the likely pathology (27).

Special Investigations

Head and neck paraganglioma rarely secrete catecholamines, but it is generally recommended that when the diagnosis

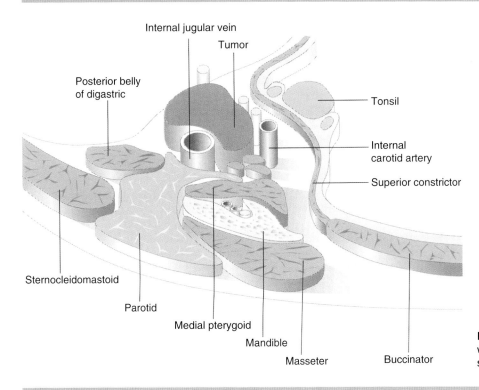

Figure 19.6 Location of a post-styloid, vagal neurilemmoma, in relation to other structures in the neck.

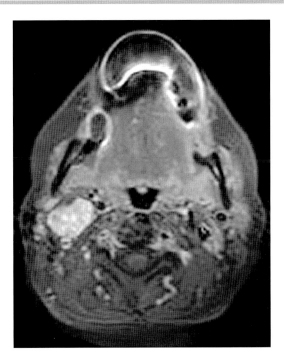

Figure 19.7 MRI of a vagal neurilemmoma.

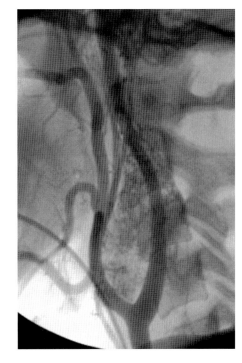

Figure 19.8 Angiogram of a carotid body tumor demonstrating the "lyre" sign due to splaying of the internal and external carotid artery.

is suspected 24-hour urinary catecholamine levels should be taken. This is particularly important in patients with multicentric lesions; a positive family history of paraganglioma; or with symptoms suggestive of excess catecholamines, such as hypertension, palpitations, flushing, tachycardia, nervousness, excessive sweating, nausea, diarrhea, or fatigue. Indium pentetreotide scanning has been recommended for detection of familial paraganglioma, since it utilizes a somatostatin radiolabel found in abundance in paraganglioma (28). This modality can be used to diagnose a parapharyngeal mass, as well as detect multicentric lesions elsewhere in the body.

MANAGEMENT

There is general consensus in the literature that salivary gland tumors, neurilemmoma, and neurofibroma should be treated surgically with postoperative radiation reserved for cases with malignant pathology. The management of paraganglioma, however, is more controversial. Decisions regarding treatment modality should consider the biological behavior, size, and site of the tumor; the age and medical status of the patient, and treatment related morbidity (29). The cranial neuropathy resulting from untreated neurogenic tumors is of gradual onset, which is less functionally disabling than the sudden loss that may result from surgery. Thus, since untreated non-functional paraganglioma rarely result in death, radiation or observation with interval surveillance radiographic scanning is a safe approach in elderly patients and those with significant medical comorbidity. Furthermore, advances in radiotherapy delivery have resulted in improved long-term control with acceptable morbidity, making it a primary treatment option (30,31).

Surgery is the mainstay of therapy for carotid body paraganglioma provided the patient is medically fit and familiar with the risks of resection (Table 19.4).

Morbidity related to surgical resection of these tumors relates to cranial nerve trauma, which increases with increasing tumor size, and tumor type (37,38). Other than cranial nerve injury, stroke is the most common major postoperative complication. Occasionally carotid reconstruction may be necessary to reduce the risk of stroke (Figs. 19.9 and 19.10).

Management of bilateral carotid paraganglioma presents a management dilemma because of the risk of bilateral vagus nerve injury and baroreflex failure syndrome, which may manifest as refractory hypertensive episodes (39). The treatment decision depends on the tumor stage, morbidity associated with therapy, and the pre-operative status of the vagus nerve. Whichever treatment modality is used the objective should be to preserve at least one vagal nerve. Generally we advocate resecting the larger tumor first and observing the contralateral tumor. If intervention is required for the contralateral carotid paraganglioma at a later date, we offer surgery provided the patient is medically fit and has a functioning vagal nerve on the previously operated side. Otherwise the patient is offered radiotherapy. However, the exception to this treatment paradigm involves a young patient with bilateral carotid paraganglioma. In these

Table 19.4 Results of Carotid Body Tumor Surgery

Reference	Year	Number of patients	Cranial nerve palsies (%)	CVA (%)	Local control (%)	Follow-up (years)
Nora (32)	1988	52	21	10	94	2-21
Rodriguez-Cuevas (13)	1998	80	18	4	NR	NR
Wang (33)	2000	28	41	0	100	2.9 (mean)
Plukker (34)	2001	35	26	NR	100	10 (median)
Luna-Ortiz (35)	2005	46	50	2	100	3 (median)
Sajid (36)	2007	95	19	1	96	1 (mean)

Abbreviation: NR, not reported.

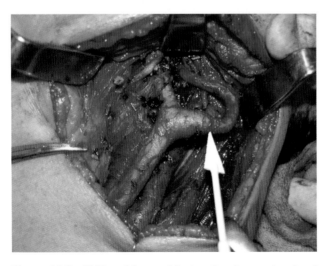

Figure 19.9 Kinking of the carotid artery, Doppler reveals reduced flow.

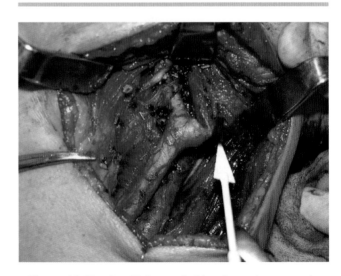

Figure 19.10 Carotid shortened with end to end anastomosis.

Table 19.5 Results of Vagal Paraganglioma Surgery

Reference	Year	Number of patients	Cranial nerve X palsy (%)	Multiple cranial nerve palsies	Local control (%)	Follow-up (years)
Netterville (41)	1998	40	100%	50%	100%	5.7 (mean)
Miller (40)	2000	16	88%	57%	81%	NR
Bradshaw (42)	2005	10	100%	60%	NR	NR

Abbreviation: NR, not reported.

patients, we prefer to avoid radiation-induced carotid arteriosclerosis and radiation-induced malignancies. Therefore, we would consider excising one side and proceed to a delayed excision of the contralateral carotid paraganglioma if vagal nerve function on the operated side is normal.

Cranial nerve morbidity occurs more frequently with vagal paraganglioma resection than with carotid body resection. Vagal paraganglioma surgery often results in sacrifice of the vagus nerve, and spared nerves frequently do not recover (40–42). Vagal paralysis is frequently associated with hypoglossal and glossopharyngeal nerve paralysis (Table 19.5) (40–42). Therefore, iatrogenic cranial neuropathy should be the main consideration when planning treatment, and other treatment options such as radiation or observation should be considered.

Radiation targets the vascular stroma of paraganglioma rather than the paraganglia cells themselves, which are radioresistant. Since resolution of tumors is rare, local control refers to stability (or regression) of tumor size and is generally associated with no improvement of neurological symptoms. Nevertheless, emerging evidence supports primary radiation therapy for carotid body paraganglioma and is based on a comprehensive review of the literature comprising over 1000 carotid body tumors (30,31). Using a regimen of 45–50 Gy in 25 fractions over four weeks, responses range from prevention of further growth to complete resolution of the tumor with minimal morbidity. Fewer than 10% of tumors fail to respond and tumor growth can be controlled in at least 75% of patients over a 20-year period. The main concern, particularly in younger patients, is the induction of second primary tumors.

Current literature generally advocates surgery for small to moderate size paraganglioma, particularly in younger patients, or those causing compressive symptoms. Radiation is generally reserved for older patients or those with high-risk lesions where the risk of complications from surgery is unacceptably high. Radiation is also recommended for residual or recurrent tumor after surgery and for patients with multiple paraganglioma where there is a risk of causing multiple cranial nerve palsies (43). A period of observation can also be considered in the elderly and high-risk patients, particularly those with multiple tumors. However many of these lesions eventually grow and cause significant symptoms, although they do not affect long-term survival (44).

Surgical Approaches
Transoral
The transoral approach, although direct and advocated by some in the past for small salivary gland tumors of the parapharyngeal space, does not permit control of major vessels and results in an unacceptably high level of seeding and recurrence (45,46). For this reason it can no longer be recommended.

Transcervical
The transcervical approach gains access to the parapharyngeal space through the lateral neck. This approach is ideal for small- to moderate-sized post-styloid lesions, such as paraganglioma and nerve sheath tumors, that do not abut the skull base because there is limited exposure superiorly and vascular control at the skull base is difficult to establish. After raising sub-platysmal flaps the marginal mandibular division of the facial nerve is identified and preserved, and major vessel control is established proximally and distally. To improve access, the submandibular gland can be resected, the digastric tendon and stylomandibular ligament may be divided, and the mandible dislocated anteromedially. Sub-adventitial dissection of paraganglioma is recommended to avoid excessive bleeding while taking care to avoid rupturing the carotid artery. Neurilemmoma may be shelled out from their capsule.

Transparotid-Cervical
The transparotid-cervical approach is similar to the transcervical approach, except the superficial lobe of the parotid is resected with facial nerve exposure prior to tumor resection (Fig. 19.11). This approach is best suited to deep lobe parotid lesions that extend into the neck and the parapharyngeal space. The facial nerve is dissected off the deep lobe of the parotid and mobilized to allow access to the parapharyngeal space. The same maneuver described above can be performed to improve access.

Transparotid/Cervical with Mandibulotomy
Greatly improved exposure for both of the above approaches may be gained by performing a parasymphyseal mandibulotomy and retracting the mandible laterally (Fig. 19.12). This is recommended for large tumors (>10 cm), recurrent tumors, malignancies of the oropharynx with parapharyngeal extension, and those which are vascular, or where carotid artery exposure at the skull base is required. For this approach, a tracheostomy is required to prevent postoperative airway obstruction from pharyngeal edema. A parasymphyseal mandibulotomy is performed and the intraoral mucosa is divided along the gingivolingual sulcus, taking care to identify and preserve the hypoglossal and lingual nerves. The parapharyngeal space is widely exposed and the lateral skull base can be accessed. Deep and superiorly based parapharyngeal masses can be removed.

is removed and the ear canal closed into a blind pouch. The jugular bulb and the internal carotid artery in the temporal bone can be drilled out providing distal access to the great vessels. With this exposure a tumor in the superior parapharyngeal space and the lateral skull base is readily accessed and removed. The eustachian tube is packed off with fat, fascia and bone dust and the facial nerve repositioned at the end of the procedure. For those tumors with intracranial extension a suboccipital cranio-tomy will provide access to the intracranial portion of the tumor.

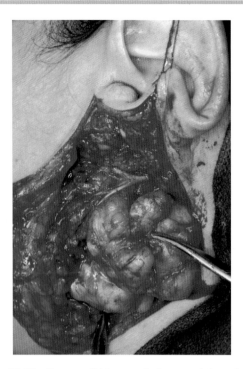

Figure 19.11 Transparotid transcervical approach to a deep-lobe parotid tumor.

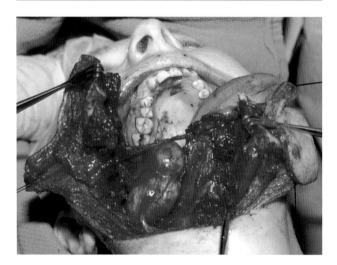

Figure 19.12 Transcervical approach with midline mandibulotomy for a large vagal neurilemmoma.

Infratemporal Fossa Approaches

For lesions extending into the jugular foramen and lateral skull base, such as vagal paraganglioma, an infratemporal fossa approach is required (Fisch type A). This involves extending the transparotid-cervical dissection to include a radical mastoidectomy and transposition of the facial nerve anteriorly after carefully dissecting it from its bony canal. The skin of the bony ear canal with the tympanic membrane

Preoperative Embolization

The efficacy of preoperative embolization of paraganglioma is controversial. Proponents of embolization cite lower blood loss and transfusion requirements (47). However, others argue that there is no significant difference in blood loss, transfusion requirement, operative time or perioperative morbidity. There is a small risk of cerebrovascular event or blindness during embolization, which should be performed within 48 hours of surgery to avoid the development of collateral tumor blood supply in the post-inflammatory phase.

Resection and Replacement of the Carotid Artery

In a few patients with large vascular tumors or those invading the major vessels of the neck, resection and replacement of the common or internal carotid artery may be required. Preoperative balloon occlusion testing and stable xenon-enhanced CT cerebral blood flow measurements will give an indication of the risk this poses to the patient and can significantly alter management (48).

Complications of Surgery

Neurovascular morbidity is the most common complication of surgery in the parapharyngeal space. Cranial nerve palsies occur postoperatively in up to 50% of patients, some due to traction or devascularization of the nerve, others due to deliberate sacrifice of an involved nerve. Cranial nerves VII, IX to XII and the sympathetic chain are at risk depending upon preoperative neural involvement by tumor, the location of the lesion, and the surgical approach. Unilateral vagal palsies are the most common problem and occur in almost all patients with vagal paraganglioma (49,50). They can present with any combination of dysphonia, dysphagia, or aspiration. Rehabilitation of the voice should wait until compensation from the other cord has occurred unless aspiration is a major problem. Gastrostomy feeding may be indicated prior to compensation. Resection of neurilemmoma involving the cervical sympathetic trunk may result in Horner's syndrome. Most patients can tolerate single cranial nerve palsy but multiple palsies are often disabling. Intimal damage to the common or internal carotid artery may result in a cerebrovascular accident and vascular damage at the time of surgery may require ligation of the internal or common carotid artery. Patients having surgery of the parapharyngeal space must be counseled about the risk of neurovascular damage, which is expected in a proportion of patients.

REFERENCES

1. Hughes KV III, Olsen KD, McCaffrey TV. Parapharyngeal space neoplasms. Head Neck 1995; 17: 124–30.
2. Pensak ML, Gluckman JL, Shumrick KA. Parapharyngeal space tumors: an algorithm for evaluation and management. Laryngoscope 1994; 104: 1170–3.
3. Carrau RL, Myers EN, Johnson JT. Management of tumors arising in the parapharyngeal space. Laryngoscope 1990; 100: 583–9.
4. Shahab R, Heliwell T, Jones AS. How we do it: a series of 114 primary pharyngeal space neoplasms. Clin Otolaryngol 2005; 30: 364–7.
5. Som PM, Curtin HD. Lesions of the parapharyngeal space. Role of MR imaging. Otolaryngol Clin North Am 1995; 28: 515–42.
6. Knight TT Jr, Gonzalez JA, Rary JM et al. Current concepts for the surgical management of carotid body tumor. Am J Surg 2006; 191: 104–10.
7. Sniezek JC, Netterville JL, Sabri AN. Vagal paragangliomas. Otolaryngol Clin North Am 2001; 34: 925–39, vi.
8. Del Gaudio JM, Muller S. Diagnosis and treatment of supraglottic laryngeal paraganglioma: report of a case. Head Neck 2004; 26: 94–8.
9. Michaelson PG, Fowler CB, Brennan J. Tracheal paraganglioma presenting with acute airway obstruction. Otolaryngol Head Neck Surg 2005; 132: 661–2.
10. Moyer JS, Wolf GT, Bradford CR. Current thoughts on the role of chemotherapy and radiation in advanced head and neck cancer. Curr Opin Otolaryngol Head Neck Surg 2004; 12: 82–7.
11. Mouadeb DA, Chandra RK, Kennedy DW et al. Sinonasal paraganglioma: endoscopic resection with a 4-year follow-up. Head Neck 2003; 25: 1077–81.
12. Myssiorek D. Head and neck paragangliomas: an overview. Otolaryngol Clin North Am 2001; 34: 829–36, v.
13. Rodriguez-Cuevas S, Lopez-Garza J, Labastida-Almendaro S. Carotid body tumors in inhabitants of altitudes higher than 2000 meters above sea level. Head Neck 1998; 20: 374–8.
14. Dundee P, Clancy B, Wagstaff S et al. Paraganglioma: the role of genetic counselling and radiological screening. J Clin Neurosci 2005; 12: 464–6.
15. Grufferman S, Gillman MW, Pasternak LR et al. Familial carotid body tumors: case report and epidemiologic review. Cancer 1980; 46: 2116–22.
16. van der Mey AG, Maaswinkel-Mooy PD, Cornelisse CJ et al. Genomic imprinting in hereditary glomus tumours: evidence for new genetic theory. Lancet 1989; 2: 1291–4.
17. Badenhop RF, Jansen JC, Fagan PA et al. The prevalence of SDHB, SDHC, and SDHD mutations in patients with head and neck paraganglioma and association of mutations with clinical features. J Med Genet 2004; 41: e99.
18. Mhatre AN, Li Y, Feng L et al. SDHB, SDHC, and SDHD mutation screen in sporadic and familial head and neck paragangliomas. Clin Genet 2004; 66: 461–6.
19. Pawlu C, Bausch B, Neumann HP. Mutations of the SDHB and SDHD genes. Fam Cancer 2005; 4: 49–54.
20. Neumann HP, Pawlu C, Peczkowska M et al. Distinct clinical features of paraganglioma syndromes associated with SDHB and SDHD gene mutations. JAMA 2004; 292: 943–51.
21. McCaffrey TV, Meyer FB, Michels VV et al. Familial paragangliomas of the head and neck. Arch Otolaryngol Head Neck Surg 1994; 120: 1211–16.
22. Schwaber MK, Glasscock ME, Nissen AJ et al. Diagnosis and management of catecholamine secreting glomus tumors. Laryngoscope 1984; 94: 1008–15.
23. Lee JH, Barich F, Karnell LH et al. National Cancer Data Base report on malignant paragangliomas of the head and neck. Cancer 2002; 94: 730–7.
24. Hamza A, Fagan JJ, Weissman JL et al. Neurilemmomas of the parapharyngeal space. Arch Otolaryngol Head Neck Surg 1997; 123: 622–6.
25. Miller FR, Wanamaker JR, Lavertu P et al. Magnetic resonance imaging and the management of parapharyngeal space tumors. Head Neck 1996; 18: 67–77.
26. Mafee MF, Raofi B, Kumar A et al. Glomus faciale, glomus jugulare, glomus tympanicum, glomus vagale, carotid body tumors, and simulating lesions. Role of MR imaging. Radiol Clin North Am 2000; 38: 1059–76.
27. Stoeckli SJ, Schuknecht B, Alkadhi H et al. Evaluation of paragangliomas presenting as a cervical mass on color-coded Doppler sonography. Laryngoscope 2002; 112: 143–6.
28. Myssiorek D, Palestro CJ. 111Indium pentetreotide scan detection of familial paragangliomas. Laryngoscope 1998; 108: 228–31.
29. Pellitteri PK, Rinaldo A, Myssiorek D et al. Paragangliomas of the head and neck. Oral Oncol 2004; 40: 563–75.
30. Hu K, Persky MS. The multidisciplinary management of paragangliomas of the head and neck, Part 2. Oncology (Williston Park) 2003; 17: 1143–53.
31. Hu K, Persky MS. Multidisciplinary management of paragangliomas of the head and neck, Part 1. Oncology (Williston Park) 2003; 17: 983–93.
32. Nora JD, Hallett JW Jr, O'Brien PC et al. Surgical resection of carotid body tumors: long-term survival, recurrence, and metastasis. Mayo Clin Proc 1988; 63: 348–52.
33. Wang SJ, Wang MB, Barauskas TM et al. Surgical management of carotid body tumors. Otolaryngol Head Neck Surg 2000; 123: 202–6.
34. Plukker JT, Brongers EP, Vermey A et al. Outcome of surgical treatment for carotid body paraganglioma. Br J Surg 2001; 88: 1382–6.
35. Luna-Ortiz K, Rascon-Ortiz M, Villavicencio-Valencia V et al. Carotid body tumors: review of a 20-year experience. Oral Oncol 2005; 41: 56–61.
36. Sajid MS, Hamilton G, Baker DM. A multicenter review of carotid body tumor management. Eur J Vasc Endovasc Surg 2007; 34: 127–30.
37. Hallett JW Jr, Nora JD, Hollier LH et al, Pairolero PC. Trends in neurovascular complications of surgical management for carotid body and cervical paragangliomas: a fifty-year experience with 153 tumors. J Vasc Surg 1988; 7: 284–91.
38. Weed DT, Netterville JL, O'Malley BB. Paragangliomas of the head and neck. In: Harrison LB, Sessions RB, Hong WK, eds. Head and neck cancer: a multidisciplinary approach. Philadelphia: Lippincott-Raven, 1999; 777–98.
39. Netterville JL, Reilly KM, Robertson D et al. Carotid body tumors: a review of 30 patients with 46 tumors. Laryngoscope 1995; 105: 115–26.
40. Miller RB, Boon MS, Atkins JP et al. Vagal paraganglioma: the Jefferson experience. Otolaryngol Head Neck Surg 2000; 122: 482–7.
41. Netterville JL, Jackson CG, Miller FR et al. Vagal paraganglioma: a review of 46 patients treated during a 20-year period. Arch Otolaryngol Head Neck Surg 1998; 124: 1133–40.
42. Bradshaw JW, Jansen JC. Management of vagal paraganglioma: is operative resection really the best option? Surgery 2005; 137: 225–8.
43. Carrau RL, Myers EN, Johnson JT. Management of tumors arising in the parapharyngeal space. Laryngoscope 1990; 100: 583–9.
44. van der Mey AG, Frijns JH, Cornelisse CJ et al. Does intervention improve the natural course of glomus tumors? A series of 108 patients seen in a 32-year period. Ann Otol Rhinol Laryngol 1992; 101: 635–42.

45. Work WP. Parapharyngeal space and salivary gland neoplasms. Otolaryngol Clin North Am 1977; 10: 421–6.

46. Work WP, Hybels RL. A study of tumors of the parapharyngeal space. Laryngoscope 1974; 84: 1748–55.

47. Persky MS, Setton A, Niimi Y et al. Combined endovascular and surgical treatment of head and neck paragangliomas—a team approach. Head Neck 2002; 24: 423–31.

48. de Vries EJ, Sekhar LN, Horton JA et al, Yonas H. A new method to predict safe resection of the internal carotid artery. Laryngoscope 1990; 100: 85–8.

49. Biller HF, Lawson W, Som P et al. Glomus vagale tumors. Ann Otol Rhinol Laryngol 1989; 98: 21–6.

50. Urquhart AC, Johnson JT, Myers EN et al. Glomus vagale: paraganglioma of the vagus nerve. Laryngoscope 1994; 104: 440–5.

20

Salivary Gland Neoplasms

Robert L Ferris, Jeffrey D Spiro and Ronald H Spiro

INTRODUCTION

The major and minor salivary glands of the head and neck can give rise to a diverse group of both benign and malignant neoplasms. Because of the low incidence, large number of different histologic subtypes (1), variety of potential sites, and the need for extended follow-up, an individual clinician is unlikely to accumulate significant personal experience with most types of salivary neoplasms. In this chapter, the etiology, incidence, pathology, and presentation of salivary tumors will first be reviewed. Treatment options and results will then be discussed, in an effort to provide insight into these varied and challenging neoplasms.

ANATOMIC CONSIDERATIONS

Parotid Gland

The paired parotid glands are located in close proximity to the cartilage of the external auditory canal, which lies posterior to the parenchyma of the gland. Anteriorly the gland abuts both the lateral and posterior border of the ramus of the mandible and the overlying masseter muscle, while inferiorly it rests medially on the posterior belly of the digastric muscle, as well as the sternomastoid muscle laterally. Medially the parotid is adjacent to the parapharyngeal space, while superiorly it reaches the arch of the zygoma (Fig. 20.1). Accessory parotid tissue is usually present anterior to the body of the gland along the course of Stenson's duct.

The facial nerve courses through the parotid gland, where it divides initially into an upper and lower division. The nerve then further divides into its five principal branches, but the exact pattern of arborization varies considerably, and surgeons need to be familiar with these common variations (2). Although there is no true anatomic separation, the parotid gland is arbitrarily divided into "superficial" and "deep" lobes by the plane of the facial nerve.

There are numerous lymph nodes located within, and adjacent to, the capsule of the parotid gland that serve as the first echelon of nodal drainage for the temporal scalp, portions of the cheek, the pinna, and the external auditory canal. For this reason, the parotid gland may harbor metastatic cutaneous malignancy from these sites. Efferent lymphatics from the gland communicate with lymph nodes of the upper and middle deep jugular chain.

Submandibular Gland

The paired submandibular glands are located in the anterior triangle of the neck, and are bounded superiorly and laterally by the body of the mandible. The mylohyoid muscle is located anterior to the gland, while the hyoglossus muscle lies medial to the gland. The platysma muscle overlies the lateral surface of the gland, and the hyoid bone is located inferiorly and medially. The submandibular (Wharton's) duct exits the gland medial to the mylohyoid muscle, then courses anteriorly and superiorly to empty into the anterior floor of the mouth.

Several important nerves lie in close proximity to the submandibular gland. The marginal branch of the facial nerve runs just deep to the platysma along the superolateral aspect of the gland. The lingual and hypoglossal nerves are located adjacent to the deep (medial) surface of the gland, while the nerve to the mylohyoid is adjacent to the superior aspect of the gland (Fig. 20.2). In addition to being at risk during surgery on the gland, these nerves provide potential pathways for perineural extension of malignant submandibular neoplasms.

Unlike the parotid gland, there are no lymph nodes within the parenchyma of the submandibular gland. There are, however, a number of lymph nodes in close proximity to the gland near the inferior border of the mandible and adjacent to the facial vessels. These nodes are the first echelon of drainage for portions of the lip and oral cavity, as well as facial skin, and drain in turn to the deep jugular chain of nodes. Pathologic enlargement of these nodes may be confused with a tumor of the submandibular gland, and metastatic cancer in these nodes may also involve the adjacent gland by direct extension.

Sublingual Glands

Located beneath the mucosa of the floor of the mouth, the small paired sublingual glands drain directly into the oral cavity through numerous small ducts. Tumors arising in the sublingual glands are usually difficult to distinguish from those arising in minor salivary glands located submucosally in the floor of the mouth.

Minor Salivary Glands

Small submucosal glands are located throughout the upper aerodigestive tract, and may give rise to salivary type neoplasms in locations such as the larynx, pharynx, and paranasal sinuses. These glands are found in highest concentration in the palate. Small rests of heterotopic salivary tissue can also be found within cervical lymph nodes, the mandible, the thyroid gland, and the middle ear, where they can give rise to salivary neoplasms in these unusual locations (3).

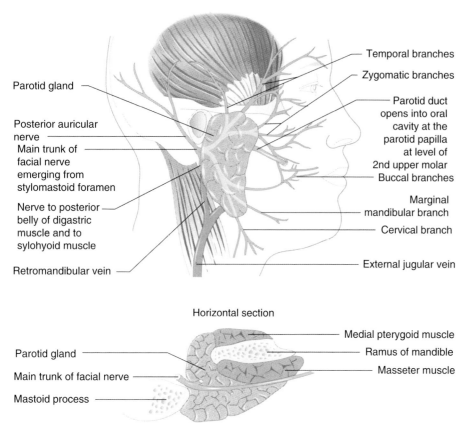

Figure 20.1 Anatomic relations of the parotid gland.

INCIDENCE AND ETIOLOGY

Malignant salivary neoplasms account for about 7% of epithelial cancers of the head and neck in the United States, with an annual incidence of about 1 per 100,000 population (4). A similar incidence is reported from both the United Kingdom and Denmark (5,6). Benign salivary neoplasms occur more frequently, but the precise incidence is difficult to quantify as they are obviously not included in cancer registry data.

The site distribution of salivary gland tumors in several large series is summarized in Figure 20.3 (7–9). The majority of salivary neoplasms originate in the parotid gland, while minor salivary gland and submandibular gland neoplasms are much less common. True primary tumors of the sublingual gland are quite unusual (10). The relative incidence of benign and malignant tumors in these various sites is depicted in Figure 20.4 (7–9,11–16). While most parotid neoplasms are benign, about half of submandibular tumors are malignant, and an even higher proportion of minor salivary neoplasms will be malignant. In examining the statistics concerning minor salivary tumors, one must consider the site within the upper aerodigestive tract, and the source of the data. Minor salivary tumors encountered outside the oral cavity are far more likely to be malignant, and reports from tertiary referral centers are also more likely to contain a higher proportion of patients with malignant tumors (14–16). Because the parotid gland is by far the most common site of origin, and a significant

majority of parotid tumors are benign, the most common salivary neoplasm typically encountered will be a benign parotid tumor.

In most cases, the etiology of salivary gland neoplasms remains obscure. There are, however, a number of predisposing factors that have been identified. Exposure to ionizing radiation has been implicated both in survivors of the atomic bomb explosion at Hiroshima and in individuals who received low-dose irradiation to the head and neck in childhood (17–20). Exposure to wood dust has been associated with an increased incidence of a clear cell variant of adenocarcinoma of the nasal cavity and paranasal sinuses, but it is not clear whether these tumors arise in submucosal glands or respiratory epithelium (21,22). Genetic factors are suggested by the increased incidence of salivary carcinoma in Eskimo families (23). One recent report correlates Warthin's tumor with cigarette smoking (24), while another study associates the use of aromatic amines contained in hair dye with salivary cancer (25).

HISTOLOGIC CLASSIFICATION

One of the more challenging aspects of salivary neoplasms is their varied histologic appearance (1). Most centers utilize a classification scheme based on the one originally described by Foote and Frazell (26). The system currently used at Memorial Sloan-Kettering Cancer Center is summarized in Table 20.1.

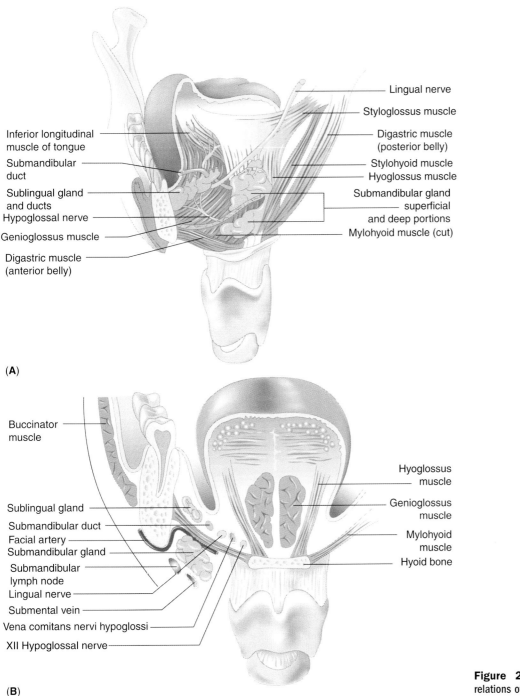

Inferior longitudinal muscle of tongue
Submandibular duct
Sublingual gland and ducts
Hypoglossal nerve
Genioglossus muscle
Digastric muscle (anterior belly)

Lingual nerve
Styloglossus muscle
Digastric muscle (posterior belly)
Stylohyoid muscle
Hyoglossus muscle
Submandibular gland superficial and deep portions
Mylohyoid muscle (cut)

(A)

Buccinator muscle

Sublingual gland
Submandibular duct
Facial artery
Submandibular gland
Submandibular lymph node
Lingual nerve
Submental vein
Vena comitans nervi hypoglossi
XII Hypoglossal nerve

Hyoglossus muscle
Genioglossus muscle
Mylohyoid muscle
Hyoid bone

(B)

Figure 20.2 **(A)** and **(B)** Anatomic relations of the submandibular gland.

Pleomorphic adenoma, or benign mixed tumor, is the most common salivary neoplasm overall, and the most frequently encountered benign salivary tumor in all sites. Warthin's tumor, or papillary cystadenoma lymphomatosum, is next in frequency among benign neoplasms. Other benign tumors are uncommon as a group. These include oncocytoma, monomorphic adenoma, and the benign lymphoepithelial lesion of Godwin (7–9,27,28).

Among malignant tumors, mucoepidermoid carcinoma, adenoid cystic carcinoma, adenocarcinoma, and malignant mixed tumor are most common. Acinic cell carcinoma, primary squamous carcinoma, and anaplastic carcinoma are encountered less frequently (7–9,11–16,27). Different histologic types of salivary cancer are more prevalent in certain salivary sites than in others. The relative incidence of various malignant tumors by salivary site according to pooled data from a number of large reported series is presented in Figure 20.5 for the parotid (5–9,29–35), submandibular (6–9,36–41), and minor salivary glands (7,9,15,42). Mucoepidermoid carcinoma is the most common malignant parotid neoplasm, while adenoid cystic carcinoma is the most frequently encountered submandibular malignancy. In minor salivary sites, these two types of salivary cancer have a similar incidence, followed closely by adenocarcinoma.

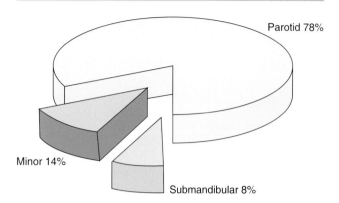

Figure 20.3 Distribution of salivary neoplasms by site (total of 8863 cases).

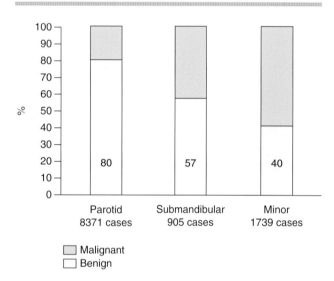

Figure 20.4 Relative proportion of benign versus malignant salivary neoplasms at various primary sites. Numbers under each site are total cases represented per site.

Table 20.1 Histologic Classification of Salivary Neoplasms

Benign
Pleomorphic adenoma
Warthin's tumor
Lymphoepithelial lesion
Oncocytoma
Monomorphic adenoma

Malignant
Mucoepidermoid carcinoma
Adenoid cystic carcinoma
Adenocarcinoma
Malignant mixed tumor
Acinic cell carcinoma
Epidermoid carcinoma
Anaplastic carcinoma

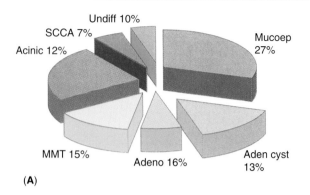

(A)

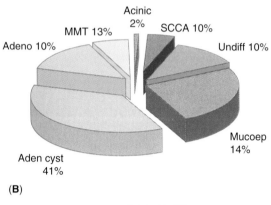

(B)

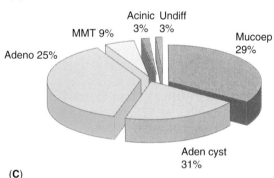

(C)

Figure 20.5 (A) Overview of malignant histology for parotid gland (total of 2331 cases). (B) Overview of malignant histology for submandibular gland (total of 499 cases). (C) Overview of malignant histology for minor salivary sites (total of 1107 cases). *Abbreviations*: Adeno, adenocarcinoma; Aden cyst, adenoid cystic carcinoma; Mucoep, mucoepidermoid carcinoma; MMT, malignant mixed tumor; Acinic, acinic cell carcinoma; SCCA, squamous carcinoma; Undiff: undifferentiated carcinoma.

The parotid gland may also be the site of metastases from cutaneous carcinoma arising in areas of the scalp or facial skin which drain to intraparotid lymph nodes. Squamous carcinoma or melanoma arising in these sites accounts for 70–80% of metastases to the parotid gland. While metastases from infraclavicular primary sites to the parotid may also occur, they are much less common (43–47).

BENIGN TUMORS
Pleomorphic Adenoma
This neoplasm was formerly known as a benign mixed tumor because it contains both epithelial and mesenchymal

elements. As noted above, it is the most common salivary neoplasm encountered overall, mainly because of its high incidence in the parotid gland. Pleomorphic adenomas are surrounded by a pseudocapsule, beyond which there are numerous microscopic extensions. This is one reason surgeons in the United States have avoided simple enucleation of these tumors, fearing an increase in local recurrence. Such recurrences are typically evident within five years of excision, but a significant proportion may occur ten years or more following excision (7,48).

Warthin's Tumor (Papillary Cystadenoma Lymphomatosum, Adenolymphoma)

This tumor is also known as cystadenolymphoma, and is rarely encountered outside the parotid gland, where it is the second most common benign neoplasm. The tendency for this neoplasm to occur in the parotid gland is a direct result of its histologic origin within lymph nodes inside the capsule of the parotid gland. Warthin's tumor tends to occur in the tail of the parotid gland in older male patients, and is also noted to be bilateral or multiple in a small but significant number of cases (49–51).

Oncocytoma

This is a rare benign tumor usually found in the parotid. It occurs in older women and is slow growing, attaining an average size of 3–4 cm. It is almost always solitary.

Monomorphic Adenomas

These tumors are similar in clinical presentation to pleomorphic adenomas and usually arise in the parotid gland. There are various types depending on the histological pattern and the cell of origin. The most common of these is the basal cell adenoma. Monomorphic adenomas usually arise in the lower part of the parotid gland and occur almost exclusively in males with a peak age incidence of 50–70 years.

MALIGNANT TUMORS

Salivary cancers can be divided into those believed to arise from the intercalated ducts, such as adenoid cystic carcinoma and adenocarcinoma, and those believed to originate from the secretory ducts, which include mucoepidermoid carcinoma and salivary duct carcinoma. A higher tumor grade appears to correlate with more aggressive behavior in mucoepidermoid carcinomas and adenocarcinoma not otherwise specified (37,52,53), but the relevance of grade to other subtypes, such as adenoid cystic carcinoma, is unclear (54,55,56).

Mucoepidermoid Carcinoma

As noted above, mucoepidermoid carcinoma is the most common malignant neoplasm encountered in the parotid gland, and the most prevalent salivary cancer overall. In the past, low-grade lesions with well defined glandular elements were not considered malignant because they metastasize so infrequently. In contrast, high-grade mucoepidermoid carcinoma may be nearly devoid of glandular features under the microscope, rendering it hard to distinguish from primary squamous carcinoma without the use of special stains to identify mucin-producing cells (57–64). High-grade lesions are aggressive and have a proclivity for regional metastases, with an incidence as high as 70% in one report (61). A recently described chromosomal translocation that results in a fusion gene product has been described in a subset of mucoepidermoid carcinomas, which appears to confer a better prognosis (65,66). Intermediate-grade lesions will display histologic and clinical features between the extremes noted above. The natural history of intermediate- and high-grade mucoepidermoid carcinoma is less protracted than that of many other types of salivary cancer, and five-year follow-up should be indicative of long-term cure in most cases.

Adenoid Cystic Carcinoma

This interesting neoplasm is notable for its protracted natural history, and its tendency toward both local recurrence and pulmonary metastases. As previously noted, it is the most common malignant neoplasm of the submandibular gland, and shares this distinction with mucoepidermoid carcinoma in minor salivary sites. If patients with adenoid cystic carcinoma are followed for extended periods, disease-related deaths are noted to occur even 20 or more years after treatment (67–69). Prolonged survival has also been observed in many patients with documented pulmonary metastases (70).

Adenoid cystic carcinoma can present a variety of histologic appearances, with solid, tubular and cribriform patterns described. In some centers, a grading system has attempted to correlate these subtypes with outcome, demonstrating a poor prognosis for the solid pattern, and a more favorable outcome for the tubular pattern (54,71–73). Other reports, including those from Memorial Hospital, demonstrate that differences in survival based on histologic grading disappear when follow-up exceeds 10 years (68,74,75). This suggests that histologic grading may correlate with the length of the disease-free interval, but not the ultimate disease outcome in adenoid cystic carcinoma (76).

Adenocarcinoma

Adenocarcinoma arising in salivary glands may assume a variety of appearances on microscopic examination, including papillary, ductal (resembling breast cancer), and mucinous histologic subtypes (77,78). In those studies where grading of salivary adenocarcinoma is performed, high-grade lesions are associated with a much worse prognosis than low-grade lesions (77–79). Survival data demonstrate a significant decline from five to ten years after treatment, which indicates the need for adequate long-term follow-up when assessing the results of treatment for this type of salivary cancer (77–79).

Salivary Duct Carcinoma

Salivary duct carcinoma is an aggressive tumor of the head and neck with a poor prognosis, first described in 1968 by Kleinsasser et al. (2) Salivary duct carcinoma affects a preponderance of men (4:1), usually in the fourth to sixth decades, occurring in more than 80% of cases in the parotid gland (4–5). Whereas this tumor usually begins de novo, studies suggest that it can arise as a component of carcinoma ex pleomorphic adenoma (see below). Salivary duct carcinoma shares significant morphologic and immunophenotypic overlap with ductal carcinoma of the breast, including HER-2/neu expression. Previous studies have detected HER-2/neu at the protein level in salivary duct carcinoma, suggesting a potential role for the HER2 blocking monoclonal antibody, trastuzumab, based therapy.

Malignant Mixed Tumor

This type of malignant salivary neoplasm is distinguished histologically by some features of pleomorphic adenoma in association with a malignant epithelial component, usually adenocarcinoma. There is some controversy as to the origin of these tumors, which are believed to arise either from a pre-existing benign mixed tumor (i.e., carcinoma-ex-pleomorphic adenoma) or to develop de novo (80–82). As with adenocarcinoma, disease-related deaths may occur 10 or more years after treatment, and adequate long-term follow-up is needed to correctly assess treatment results (80–82).

Acinic Cell Carcinoma

This uncommon salivary neoplasm is seldom encountered outside the parotid gland, and is generally associated with fairly indolent behavior. It is considered a low-grade malignancy, but higher grade variants occur (papillocystic). It has the capability to metastasize or recur locally, particularly if extensive at diagnosis or inadequately treated initially (53,55,83,84).

CLINICAL PRESENTATION AND EVALUATION
History

The most common presenting symptom of benign or malignant neoplasms arising in major salivary glands is an asymptomatic swelling. For minor salivary sites, the symptoms will vary according to the location, as summarized in Figure 20.6. Episodic swelling of major salivary glands accompanied by pain and related to salivary stimuli is suggestive of duct obstruction. One study estimates that 80–90% of submandibular gland enlargement is a result of inflammatory disease (85).

Pain is reported in 2.5–4% of patients with benign parotid tumors, and 10–29% of patients with parotid cancer, perhaps indicative of perineural invasion by tumor cells (5,6,33,86,87). The same symptom is reported in a few patients with benign submandibular neoplasms, and up to 50% of patients with malignant submandibular tumors (12,36–38). Pain is clearly more common with malignant salivary neoplasms, but it is not by itself diagnostic of malignancy. In general, the duration of symptoms tends to be shorter in those patients with malignant tumors. However, it is possible for patients with salivary cancer to present with an asymptomatic swelling that has been present for several years, or even a decade or more (7). Therefore, the fact that a salivary gland mass has been present for an extended period of time is no guarantee that it is benign.

Physical Findings

As previously noted, the location of a salivary mass is an important consideration, as the likelihood of malignancy is

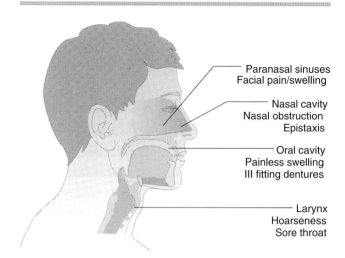

Figure 20.6   Typical symptoms of minor salivary tumors by site.

directly related to the site of origin. Most benign minor salivary gland tumors arise in the oral cavity, while neoplasms arising in other minor salivary sites are usually malignant (16). The size of a salivary tumor is important to document. Malignant neoplasms tended to be larger at presentation, but about half of the major salivary cancers treated at Memorial Hospital were 3 cm or less in size at diagnosis (7).

Although about 10% of parotid gland tumors arise medial to the plane of the facial nerve in the so-called deep "lobe" of the gland, more than three-fourths of these tumors will present as a typical external parotid mass, similar to typical neoplasms arising lateral to the nerve. The remainder will present with palatal or pharyngeal swelling, with or without a palpable external mass, as depicted in Figure 20.7 (88). Tumors arising in accessory parotid tissue will present as a mass in the cheek, near the anterior border of the masseter muscle and separate from the main body of the parotid gland, similar to Figure 20.8 (89).

Minor salivary tumors typically will present as a submucosal mass, but ulceration of the overlying mucosa is sometimes noted, particularly after trauma from dentures or previous biopsy (Fig. 20.9). If locally advanced, patients with lesions arising in the nasal cavity or paranasal sinuses may have facial swelling or displacement of the orbital contents. The true extent of minor salivary neoplasms arising in less accessible sites such as the paranasal sinuses is usually not appreciated on physical examination alone.

There are certain physical findings that help to distinguish benign from malignant major salivary neoplasms, as summarized in Figure 20.10. Fixation of the tumor to either skin or deep structures suggests extension of malignant disease outside the gland with invasion of surrounding tissues. With untreated parotid cancer, fixation to skin was noted in 9% of patients at Memorial Hospital, while fixation to deep tissues was noted in 13% of patients at the M.D. Anderson Hospital and 17% of patients at Memorial Hospital (86,90).

Weakness or paralysis of the facial nerve in a previously untreated patient almost always indicates that a tumor is malignant. While there are anecdotal reports of

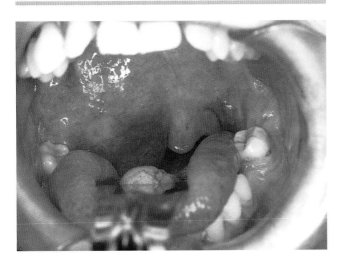

Figure 20.7 Medial displacement of the palate and tonsil seen with deep-lobe parotid tumors extending into the parapharyngeal space.

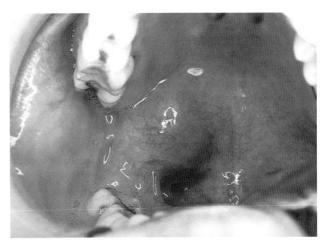

Figure 20.9 Minor salivary tumors usually present as asymptomatic swellings beneath intact mucous membranes. It is not possible clinically to distinguish this low-grade mucoepidermoid carcinoma in the right soft palate just posterior to the junction with the hard palate from a benign tumor arising in the same site.

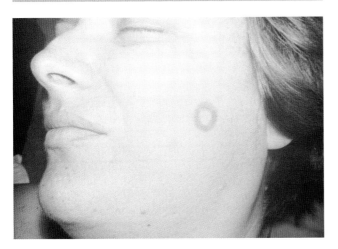

Figure 20.8 Typical location of a tumor arising in accessory parotid tissue anterior to the gland, in this instance an adenoid cystic carcinoma.

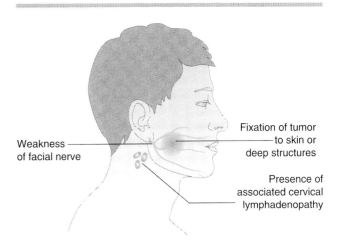

Figure 20.10 Physical findings indicative of malignancy in a major salivary neoplasm.

facial palsy in association with benign parotid neoplasms, some degree of facial nerve dysfunction has been noted in 9–25% of patients with previously untreated parotid cancer (5,6,11,86,87,90–92). This finding is usually associated with a poor prognosis, and is most commonly encountered in patients with adenoid cystic carcinoma, undifferentiated carcinoma, and squamous carcinoma (96,91,92).

The presence of nodal enlargement in association with a salivary tumor is another strong indicator of malignancy. Cervical node metastases are noted at presentation in 13–25% of patients with parotid cancer (5,32,86,90), and 14–33% of patients with submandibular gland cancer (36,41,93). In patients with malignant submandibular neoplasms one must be careful to distinguish direct extension to adjacent lymph nodes from actual lymphatic metastases. The histologic

subtypes of salivary cancer most likely to metastasize to regional lymph nodes are squamous carcinoma, high-grade mucoepidermoid carcinoma, high-grade adenocarcinoma, and malignant mixed tumor (33,36,86). In the Memorial Hospital experience with minor salivary cancer, regional node metastases were present initially in 14% of cases (16).

Diagnostic Imaging

Careful history and physical examination are often sufficient to establish the diagnosis and the extent of a tumor in the major salivary glands. If palpation of a major salivary lesion suggests fixation to adjacent structures, diagnostic imaging is indicated to better delineate the extent of disease. Deep-lobe parotid tumors involving the parapharyngeal space, and minor salivary tumors arising in the nasal cavity or paranasal sinuses, usually require radiographic evaluation to define the full extent of disease (Fig. 20.11). As a general guideline, these studies should only be obtained if they will directly impact the management of the patient.

Several imaging modalities may be useful to the clinician when evaluating a salivary gland tumor (94). In cases of suspected inflammatory disease in the submandibular gland, plain radiographs may demonstrate a calculus in the gland or in Warthin's duct. CT scans are best for the evaluation of cortical bone involvement by neoplasms, while MRI better visualizes soft tissue details, as well as medullary bone involvement. In the paranasal sinuses, MRI may also help to distinguish tumor from opacification of an obstructed sinus by fluid.

Fine-needle Aspiration Biopsy

Fine-needle aspiration biopsy (FNAB) provides an opportunity to obtain information about the histology of a salivary tumor prior to the initiation of treatment (95,96). In centers with an experienced cytopathologist, the distinction between benign and malignant neoplasms can be made with a high degree of reliability (97–100). The ability of aspiration cytology to provide an exact diagnosis varies widely between centers, particularly when dealing with a malignant salivary neoplasm (97–100).

FNAB is not essential for every patient. Those who have small, clinically obvious intraparotid tumors will be effectively treated by conventional subtotal parotidectomy regardless of the histologic diagnosis. Needle biopsy may have its greatest utility in the diagnosis of a submandibular mass, where it can help to distinguish neoplastic from more common inflammatory changes, which may spare the patient unnecessary surgery. Aspiration cytology may also differentiate a reactive lymph node adjacent to a salivary gland from a tumor within the gland itself. Caution must always be exercised in applying the results if the aspiration cytology is inconsistent with the clinical presentation.

Staging

Clinical staging of salivary cancer is essential when comparing treatment results and estimating prognosis. Some years ago, a staging system was devised for major salivary cancer that incorporated the size of the lesion and the presence

or absence of facial nerve palsy or fixation to adjacent structures (86). The current American Joint Committee on Cancer (AJCC) and International Union Against Cancer (UICC) staging systems, while more complex, still utilize these basic elements, as documented in Tables 20.2 (56,101). While there is no separate staging system for minor salivary cancer, a study from Memorial Hospital demonstrated that the staging system used for squamous carcinoma at various primary sites has similar prognostic value for minor salivary cancer arising in the same sites (102). This approach to minor salivary lesions has been incorporated in the current staging systems for salivary cancer (56,101).

Molecular Alterations in Salivary Malignancy

As the molecular understanding of salivary cancers grows, the number of potential targets and therapies increases. The epidermal growth factor receptor (EGFR), a transmembrane receptor involved in signal transduction, is commonly overexpressed and/or constitutively activated in a number of malignancies, and has been associated with aggressive malignant behavior. Expression of EGFR is common (>50% frequency) in both mucoepidermoid carcinoma (103,104) and salivary duct carcinoma (105,106), but less common in adenoid cystic carcinoma (103,104,106,107). HER-2, another member of the EGFR family of receptors, may undergo heterodimerization with EGFR, and in this way is involved in signal transduction. Trastuzumab, a monoclonal antibody targeting the HER-2 receptor, is effective in breast cancer that overexpresses HER-2 (108). Overexpression of HER-2 is more likely in cancers of excretory duct origin. It is commonly observed in salivary duct carcinoma (109–111) and occasionally seen in mucoepidermoid carcinoma (103,110,112), with a negative prognostic potential. In adenoid cystic carcinoma, both microvessel density, a measure of tumor angiogenesis, and tumor levels of vascular endothelial growth factor, along with the transcription nuclear factor κB (NF-κB), potent pro-angiogenic factors, have been shown to be prognostic of survival. Angiogenesis inhibitors thus may have a role in treatment of these tumors.

TREATMENT: SURGERY

Surgical resection is the principal form of treatment for both benign and malignant salivary tumors.

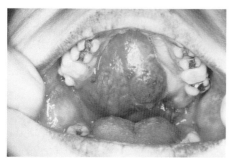

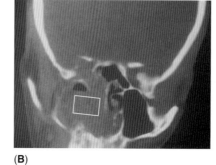

(A)   **(B)**

Figure 20.11   (A) Extensive adenoid cystic carcinoma presenting as a mass that replaces the entire palate in a 37-year-old woman. Radiographic imaging is essential in order to appreciate the true extent and origin of this tumor. (B) Coronal CT view shows clinically unsuspected destruction of the skull base and invasion of the anterior cranial fossa by a massive tumor that seems to have originated in the right maxillary antrum.

Table 20.2 AJCC and UICC Staging Systems for Salivary Cancer

AJCC staging system		UICC staging system	
Primary tumor (T)		*Primary tumor (T)*	
TX	Primary tumor cannot be assessed	TX	Primary tumor cannot be assessed
T0	No evidence of primary tumor	T0	No evidence of primary tumor
T1	Tumor 2 cm or less in greatest dimension	T1	Primary tumor 2 cm or less in greatest dimension; no extraparenchymal extension
T2	Tumor >2 cm but not >4 cm in greatest dimension	T2	Primary tumor >2 cm but not >4 cm; no extraparenchymal extension
T3	Tumor >4 cm but not >6 cm in greatest dimension	T3	Primary tumor >4 cm but not >6 cm and/or extraparenchymal extension without VII nerve involvement
T4	Tumor >6 cm in greatest dimension	T4	Primary tumor >6 cm and/or invades base of skull/VII nerve
All T categories are subdivided into:			
(a)	No local extension		
(b)	Evidence of local extension: invasion of skin, soft tissues, bone or nerve		
Regional lymph nodes (N)		*Regional lymph nodes (N)*	
NX	Regional nodes cannot be assessed	NX	Regional lymph nodes cannot be assessed
N0	No regional lymph node metastasis	N0	No regional lymph node metastasis
N1	Metastasis in single node 3 cm or less	N1	Metastasis to single ipsilateral node 3 cm or less
N2a	Metastasis in single ipsilateral node >3 cm but not >6 cm	N2a	Metastasis to single ipsilateral node >3 cm but not >6 cm
N2b	Metastasis in multiple ipsilateral nodes, none >6 cm	N2b	Metatasis to multiple ipsilateral nodes none >6 cm
N2c	Metatasis in bilateral or contralateral nodes, none >6 cm	N2c	Metastasis to bilateral/contralateral nodes none >6 cm
N3	Metastasis in lymph node >6 cm	N3	Metastasis to node >6 cm
Distant metastasis (M)		*Distant metastasis (M)*	
MX	Distant metastasis cannot be assessed	MX	Distant metastasis cannot be assessed
M0	No distant metastasis	M0	No distant metastasis
M1	Distant metastasis	M1	Distant metastasis
Stage grouping		*Stage grouping*	
Stage I	T1a or T2a/N0/M0	Stage I	T1 or T2/N0/M0
Stage II	T1b or T2b or T3a/N0/M0	Stage II	T3/N0/M0
Stage III	T3b or T4a/N0/M0	Stage III	T1 or T2/N1/M0
	Any T (except T4b)/N1/M0	Stage IV	T4/N0/M0
Stage IV	T4b/any N/M0		T3/N1/ M1
	Any T/N2 or N3/M0		T4/N1/M0
	Any T/Any N/M1		Any T/N2 or N3/M0
			Any T/Any N/M1

Benign Lesions

In general, surgical treatment of benign salivary tumors at any site consists of adequate local excision. Resection of minor salivary tumors must be tailored to the specific primary site in question, which is usually the oral cavity in patients with benign tumors (Fig. 20.12). Benign neoplasms arising in the submandibular gland can be resected through a simple excision of the gland itself, except in the case of the rare recurrent neoplasm in this location, which may require a more extended procedure.

The most common site for a benign salivary neoplasm is the parotid gland. In such cases, most surgeons in the United States, guided by the extent of the neoplasm, perform a partial or total resection of the superficial "lobe" of the parotid gland with exposure and preservation of the facial nerve (Fig. 20.13). Surgeons who have considerable experience with more limited extracapsular dissection of such lesions report very good results and few complications with these more conservative procedures (113,114). This approach should not be confused with enucleation, which has no role in surgical management of salivary neoplasms.

When a benign tumor arises in the "deep" lobe of the parotid gland, initial removal of the "superficial" lobe with identification and preservation of the facial nerve is usually required. Careful radiographic examination of whether the tumor arises from the superficial lobe and extends through

the stylomandibular tunnel is essential to determine whether this is necessary. Even sizable lesions in this location can then usually be excised through a transcervical approach, which may be facilitated by excision of the submandibular gland. Other approaches to the parapharyngeal space are described in Chapter 19. Tumors arising in accessory parotid tissue in the buccal space are best excised through a standard parotidectomy flap that is extended anteriorly, as described by Rodgers (Rodgers and Myers 1988) rather than an incision directly through the overlying cheek skin. Such an approach permits excision of the main parotid gland if the duct must be resected, and also facilitates identification of the buccal branch of the facial nerve (89,115).

In cases of recurrent pleomorphic adenoma of the parotid gland, the choice of secondary surgical procedure will depend on the extent of the initial surgery. In patients who have not yet had a formal superficial parotidectomy with nerve dissection, this procedure remains a good option. If the nerve has been previously dissected, subsequent dissection will be technically challenging because of scar tissue, and a higher incidence of nerve dysfunction should be expected. Sacrifice of all, or a portion, of the facial nerve may be necessary if recurrent benign disease is infiltrating nerve branches. Some authors have also advocated radiotherapy in diffuse recurrences and to attempt facial nerve preservation (116).

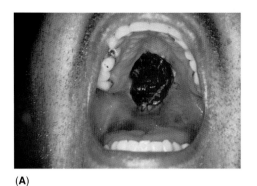

(A)

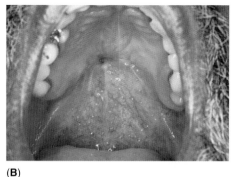

(B)

Figure 20.12 **(A)** Palatal defect remaining after removal of a benign pleomorphic adenoma down to the underlying bone. Wound was packed with xeroform gauze and allowed to heal by secondary intention. **(B)** Healed palate about 4 months later.

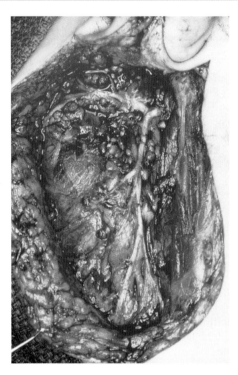

Figure 20.13 Operative field after a conventional subtotal parotidectomy that exposes the facial nerve and removes all of the gland lateral to it.

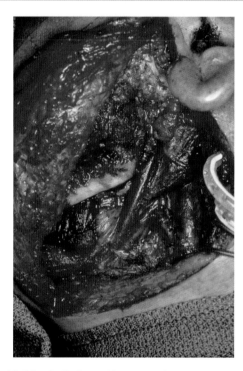

Figure 20.14 Radical parotidectomy performed in conjunction with a supraomohyoid neck dissection for a sizable, high-grade mucoepidermoid carcinoma. The resection has been extended to include the underlying masseter muscle, and the lower division of the facial nerve was included with the specimen. Nerve grafting is always performed if proximal and distal stumps can be identified.

Malignant Lesions: Parotid Gland

Surgery remains the mainstay of treatment for primary or metastatic cancer of the parotid gland. Excision of the lateral portion of the gland with dissection of the facial nerve is the minimum procedure utilized for early-stage lesions. In the case of a more extensive parotid cancer, the resection may need to be extended to include adjacent structures such as the mandible, zygoma, or temporal bone, as well as some or all of the facial nerve (Fig. 20.14). In general, these more extensive "radical" parotidectomies are associated with a poor outcome.

There has been a trend toward conservative management of the facial nerve in the surgical treatment of malignant parotid tumors, supported by the increasing use of

adjuvant irradiation. The incidence of sacrifice of either the entire nerve or a portion thereof varies from 29% to 40% in reported series (29,31,86,90). Most head and neck surgeons would currently advocate preservation of facial nerve branches unless they are adherent to or directly invaded by the tumor. This approach relies on the use of postoperative radiotherapy to control any microscopic residual disease. If major branches, or the main trunk, of the facial nerve must be sacrificed, cable grafting of the facial nerve should be accomplished immediately, utilizing branches of the cervical plexus or the sural nerve.

Malignant Lesions: Submandibular Gland

Simple excision of the submandibular gland may be sufficient in cases where the tumor is confined within the capsule of the gland. Given the high incidence of adenoid cystic carcinoma at this site, a more extensive regional resection is often required, which may include the adjacent muscles, the lingual or hypoglossal nerves, a portion of the mandible, or the floor of the mouth (Fig. 20.15). One study advocates a block dissection of the submandibular triangle as the minimal procedure in cases of submandibular cancer (37), but it is more reasonable to tailor the resection to the extent of the tumor. Depending on the histologic diagnosis, a supraomohyoid neck dissection may be appropriate as part of the initial treatment. In some reports, radical neck dissection has been employed in this setting, but the inclusion of the lowest jugular nodes, the posterior triangle lymphatics, and non-lymphatic structures remote from the gland adds little to the margins of resection adjacent to the gland itself. Moreover, any operation is not truly "radical" in patients with larger tumors unless the bed of the gland is included with the surgical specimen.

Malignant Lesions: Minor Salivary Glands

Malignant minor salivary neoplasms may arise at various sites in the upper aerodigestive tract, and surgical treatment will obviously vary depending on the site of origin. In general, these lesions are resected in a manner similar to that utilized for squamous carcinoma arising at the same primary site. This may require procedures as diverse as laryngectomy for a lesion arising in the larynx and maxillectomy for a lesion arising in the maxillary antrum.

Malignant Lesions: Neck Dissection

In those infrequent instances when a patient with salivary cancer presents with palpable nodal metastases, a comprehensive lymphadenectomy is clearly indicated. This may or may not preserve the accessory nerve. The approach to the clinically negative neck is more controversial. Because the incidence of regional metastases is relatively low for most types of salivary cancer, elective lymphadenectomy at Memorial Hospital is reserved for those patients with high-grade mucoepidermoid carcinoma or primary squamous carcinoma, which are known to have a high incidence of nodal involvement. Other approaches have been advocated, including routine sampling either of the primary tumor or of first echelon nodes at risk by frozen section (117–119).

Malignant Lesions: Intraoperative Frozen Section Analysis

As noted above, some surgeons advocate the use of intraoperative frozen section analysis of salivary neoplasms to guide decisions regarding the extent of resection, such as the need for elective regional lymphadenectomy. As with FNAB frozen section analysis is reliable in distinguishing benign from malignant neoplasm, but the ability to establish a precise histologic diagnosis depends upon the quality of the sample and the skill and experience of the pathologist (120–123). For this reason, caution is required when using information obtained by frozen section, particularly when the pathology report appears to conflict with the clinical findings.

TREATMENT: RADIATION THERAPY

Salivary neoplasms were once thought to be relatively resistant to radiotherapy, but experience acquired during the past two decades demonstrates that this treatment modality does have an important role (124). Radiotherapy has been most frequently employed as adjunctive treatment following surgery, usually in the setting of high-grade and/or advanced-stage lesions, where there is concern about adequacy of excision. The indications for postoperative radiotherapy in the treatment of salivary cancer are summarized in Table 20.3.

In addition to the use of more conventional beam energies, there is a growing experience with fast neutron radiation therapy. This form of teletherapy appears to offer biologic advantages specific to the treatment of malignant salivary neoplasms, particularly adenoid cystic carcinoma. It has been utilized primarily in the setting of recurrent or residual disease following surgery in inaccessible locations, such as the skull base, but may be more effective as a primary treatment for tumors in these difficult locations (125,126). Morbidity is a significant concern with neutron therapy, and more time and experience are necessary to better assess its role.

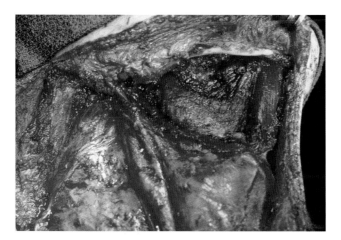

Figure 20.15 This 34-year-old man had a radical neck dissection for an adenoid cystic carcinoma of the right submandibular gland. Because the tumor involved adjacent tissues, the entire bed of the gland was removed en bloc with the neck specimen, including the mylohyoid, digastric, stylohyoid and hyoglossus muscles, lingual and hypoglossal nerves, and a portion of the overlying floor of the mouth.

Table 20.3 Indications for Postoperative Radiotherapy

High grade malignancy/unfavorable histology
Advanced clinical stage
Positive margins of resection
Recurrent disease
Positive neck nodes following neck dissection

TREATMENT: CHEMOTHERAPY

The proclivity for distant recurrence displayed by certain types of salivary cancer, particularly adenoid cystic carcinoma (ACC) and high-grade adenocarcinoma, highlights the need for effective systemic chemotherapy. Standard cytotoxic chemotherapies, including platinum or taxane-based regimens, have been studied as single or combined agents in patients with ACC and other histological subtypes. The European Organization for the Research and Treatment of Cancer (EORTC) has performed phase II trials in advanced or recurrent adenoid cystic carcinoma (98). The activity of cisplatin in ACC has been reported in three manuscripts, including a prospective phase II trial (51) and two retrospective case series (18,75). Two objective responses were observed in 13 patients in the prospective trial. In the United States, the Eastern Cooperative Oncology Group (ECOG) conducted a phase II trial in which paclitaxel was administered to patients with advanced, chemotherapy-naïve salivary gland cancers (34). No objective responses were observed in the 14 patients with ACC who were enrolled, while seven patients had stable disease as their best response. Taken together, these data suggest that some antitumor activity and symptom palliation are seen with single agents, including mitoxantrone, vinorelbine, and epirubicin in previously untreated patients. There are no data that patients previously treated with chemotherapy derive any benefit from further chemotherapy.

Despite expression of the target on a substantial fraction of tumors (127), no objective responses have been observed with agents targeting EGFR or HER-2 (2,36,39,59), including gefitinib (36), trastuzumab (39), imatinib (44,83), lapatinib (2), cetuximab (59), and bortezomib (9). (Table 20.3 below). Many patients enrolled in these trials had been previously treated with cytotoxic chemotherapy. Two clinical studies evaluated imatinib, an agent that targets the proto-oncogene tyrosine kinase (C-Kit) which is frequently expressed in ACC (44,83). Nevertheless, no objective responses were observed in a total of 27 patients who received imatinib alone (44,83). There are, however, case

reports of patients with ACC responding to doses of this agent similar to those used in the above-mentioned studies (7,28). Possible explanations for these disparate findings include the degree of overexpression of KIT and the proliferative rate of the tumors of the enrolled patients (28); additional study of this agent in selected patients appears warranted, but its routine use outside of a clinical trial is not supported by the data at this time.

Although recent phase II trials (Table 20.3) with a number of novel agents including gefitinib (36), trastuzumab (39), imatinib (44,83), lapatinib (2), cetuximab (59), and bortezomib (9) in salivary gland malignancies, predominantly adenoid cystic carcinoma, reported no objective response rates, the rate of stable disease generally exceeded 50%. A randomized study of a novel agent versus no therapy has yet to be performed in salivary gland malignancies. Nevertheless, the evaluation of novel agents should continue and, indeed, a number of clinical trials are ongoing or planned. For example, the ECOG has proposed a phase II trial of sorafenib, an inhibitor of multiple kinases, including vascular endothelial growth factor receptor, in incurable adenoid cystic carcinoma.

RESULTS

Benign Lesions

The results of primary surgery for benign salivary neoplasms are generally excellent. The reported recurrence rates for pleomorphic adenoma of the parotid gland are generally less than 5% (113,114,128,129). While surgeons in the United States favor superficial parotidectomy with facial nerve dissection as a minimum procedure, recent studies suggest no significant difference between this procedure and more limited excisions, in regard to both disease control and incidence of facial nerve injury (113,114).

When pleomorphic adenoma recurs following initial surgery, subsequent treatment is less successful and is, as expected, associated with higher morbidity. Control rates for surgery in this setting vary widely, perhaps as a result of variable follow-up (130–134); in one study one-third of

---

Table 20.3   Trials with Targeted Agents in Salivary Malignancies

Reference	Drug	Molecular target	# evaluable patients			Efficacy		Comments
			Total	ACC	Others	PR	SD	
Haddad 2003	Trastuzumab	HER-2	14	2	12	1 (MEC)	2 (SDC)	
Glisson 2005	Gefitinib	EGFR	28	19	9	0	10 / 19 ACC	In ACC: 5 / 19 had stable disease for >6 months
Hotte 2005	Imatinib	c-kit	15	15	0	0	9 / 15	6-month PFS 12.5 %; Median PFS 2.3 months
Agulnik 2006	Lapatinib	EGFR and HER-2	39	20	19	0	15 / 20 ACC 9 / 19 other	7 / 20 (35%) of ACC patients had SD ≥ 6 months; in ACC, median PFS 3.5 months*
Argiris 2006	Bortezomib	proteasome	25	25	0	0	17 / 25	6-month PFS 67%; median PFS 8.4 months
Licitra 2006	Cetuximab	EGFR	30	23	7	0	20 / 23 ACC	9 / 20 (45%) of patients ACC had SD ≥ 6 months; 6-month PFS 43 %

Abbreviations: ACC, adenoid cystic carcinoma; MEC, mucoepidermoid carcinoma; SDC, salivary duct carcinoma; PR, partial response; SD, stable disease; EGFR, epidermal growth factor receptor; pts, patients; PFS, progression-free survival.

second, or subsequent, recurrences occurred ten or more years after treatment (134). In prior reports, permanent dysfunction of all or part of the facial nerve occurred in 12–25% of cases following treatment for recurrent pleomorphic adenoma of the parotid gland (130–134). The use of radiotherapy has been suggested to help avoid sacrifice of facial nerve branches in this setting (135).

Malignant Lesions: General Considerations

Several important issues must be considered when analyzing the results of treatment for salivary cancer. The natural history of different types of malignant salivary tumors varies considerably. Five-year follow-up is adequate for most patients with intermediate or high-grade mucoepidermoid carcinoma and primary squamous carcinoma. Ten-year follow-up is needed in order to appreciate the indolent behavior of some malignant salivary tumors. Disease-related deaths from adenoid cystic carcinoma, for example, may occur 20 or more years following treatment. Survival must also be distinguished from cure; prolonged survival has been observed in patients with adenoid cystic carcinoma even in the presence of documented pulmonary metastases. Finally, the relatively small number of patients with salivary cancer of any specific type, stage, and site of origin means

that conclusions regarding treatment must be accepted with caution.

Malignant Lesions: Analysis by Histology or Grade

Histologic grade of salivary cancer is usually reflected in the clinical stage of the disease. When tumor grading is possible—as with mucoepidermoid, acinic cell, and adenocarcinomas—it is of definite prognostic significance. Survival by histologic grade for patients treated at Memorial Hospital is depicted in Figure 20.16. In two recent studies concerning prognostic variables in cancer of the parotid gland, histologic grade was identified as an important predictor of outcome (5,90). It should be noted that, in general, histologic grade tends to be reflected in the clinical stage of patients with salivary cancer; those patients with microscopically high-grade lesions usually present with advanced-stage lesions.

Survival curves for various types of salivary cancer treated at Memorial Hospital show significant variation (Fig. 20.17). Acinic cell carcinoma is associated with a favorable five-year survival of 76% to 100% in various reports (53,55,83,84). In one study, local recurrence was common in those patients with parotid lesions treated by local excision rather than formal superficial parotidectomy (53).

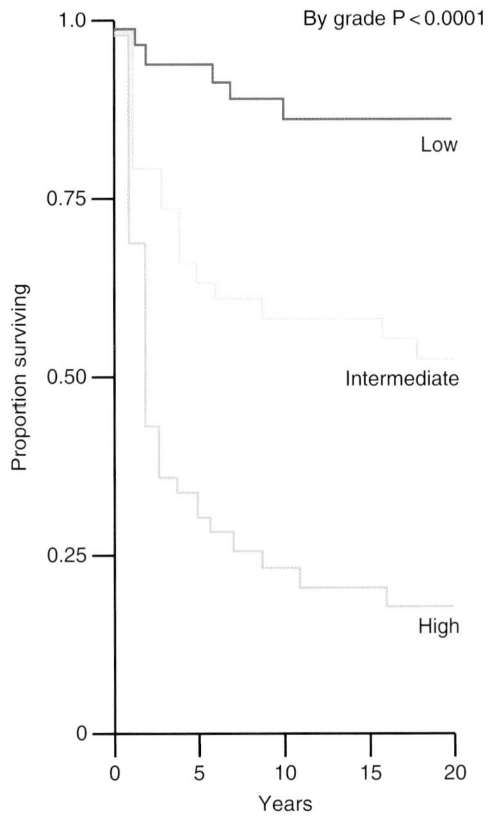

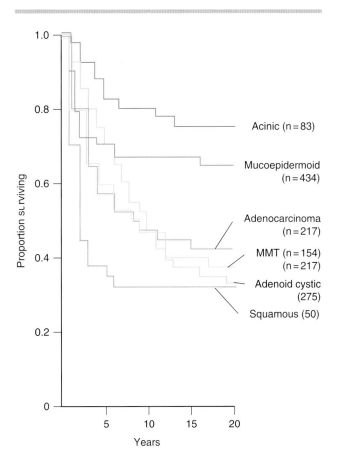

Figure 20.16 Differences in survival were significant when Memorial Hospital patients with salivary gland carcinoma were stratified according to the histologic grade of the primary tumor. Grading was possible for mucoepidermoid carcinomas, adenocarcinomas, acinic cell carcinomas, and squamous cell carcinomas.

Figure 20.17 Survival in Memorial Hospital patients treated for salivary gland carcinoma according to histologic diagnosis.

In patients with mucoepidermoid carcinoma, treatment results are usually reported by tumor grade, which is a highly significant prognostic indicator. Five-year survival varies from 76% to 100% in patients with low-grade lesions, but drops to 22–49% for high-grade lesions (58–64).

Five-year survival figures for adenoid cystic carcinoma vary from 50% to over 80%, but are particularly misleading (52,54,67–75). When follow-up is extended to 10 years, survival decreases to 29–67%, and then falls to about 25% after 15 years (68,69). Local recurrence is common, and distant metastases (usually pulmonary) occur in about half of all patients (70). As previously discussed, some studies suggest that grading of adenoid cystic carcinoma is of prognostic value, while other reports demonstrate that grade may correlate with disease-free interval, but not ultimate survival (52,54,71–75).

Overall five-year survival for patients with salivary adenocarcinoma is 76–85%, but falls to 34–71% after 10 years (77–79). As with mucoepidermoid carcinoma, histologic grading of adenocarcinoma correlates well with outcome, with high-grade lesions carrying a poor prognosis. Patients with malignant mixed tumor have a five-year survival of 31–65%, which diminishes to 23–36% when follow-up is extended to 10 years (80–82).

Malignant Lesions: Analysis by Clinical Stage

The extent of disease at presentation, as documented by clinical stage, is the strongest predictor of treatment outcome in salivary cancer. Clinical staging has been demonstrated to be predictive of outcome for both major and minor salivary gland cancers. Survival by stage for patients treated at Memorial Hospital is depicted in Figure 20.18 (7). Similar results have been reported from other centers in the United States. Recent multivariate analysis of data from the United Kingdom confirmed clinical stage as the most important independent predictive factor, with 10-year survival rates of 96%, 70%, 47%, and 19% reported for AJCC stages I through IV, respectively (6). Analysis of data on parotid cancer from Denmark revealed remarkably similar corrected survival rates of 85%, 69%, 43%, and 14% for UICC stages I through IV, respectively (5).

Malignant Lesions: Analysis by Treatment

While conventional beam radiotherapy alone is relatively ineffective as a primary treatment for salivary cancer, centers that utilize fast neutron radiotherapy to treat salivary gland cancer report more encouraging short-term results. This modality is often employed in cases of inoperable disease, as well as gross residual or recurrent disease following prior surgical resection. In one report, patients treated primarily with fast neutron radiotherapy had a 92% actuarial five-year locoregional control rate, leading the authors to suggest that surgical resection prior to neutron therapy be limited to those patients where disease-free margins can be achieved (126).

In patients with salivary cancer treated with surgery alone, treatment failure at the primary site is a significant problem. In a report from Memorial Hospital concerning patients treated some years ago when adjuvant radiotherapy was seldom used, the locoregional recurrence rates were 39%, 60%, and 65% for parotid, submandibular, and

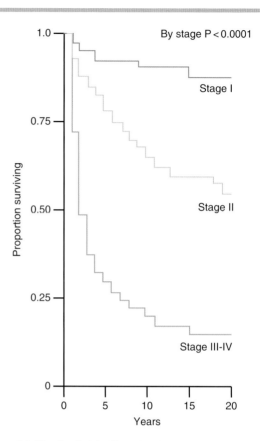

Figure 20.18 Survival in Memorial Hospital patients treated for salivary gland carcinoma according to clinical stage.

minor salivary primary sites, respectively. Isolated treatment failure in cervical lymph nodes was seldom a problem (7). In an effort to improve locoregional control rates for salivary cancer, the use of adjuvant radiotherapy has been increasing during the past two decades, particularly in those patients with advanced stage disease or other adverse prognostic findings.

Retrospective data from a number of centers suggests that the addition of postoperative radiotherapy improves the locoregional control of malignant salivary neoplasms, but prolonged survival has not been consistently demonstrated (31,32,42,79,87,136). This probably reflects, in part, treatment failure at distant sites, as well as a tendency to select those patients with less favorable presentation for adjuvant treatment. In recent reports from the M.D. Anderson Hospital, improvements in local control were most evident in patients with either parotid or submandibular cancer when the disease extended beyond the confines of the gland (90,93,137). In an attempt to overcome the selection bias inherent in retrospective studies, a matched-pair analysis of patients treated at Memorial Hospital with or without postoperative radiotherapy was performed (138). There was a significant improvement in both local control of disease and survival in those patients with stage III and IV disease who received combination therapy, but a similar benefit was not evident for patients with early stage disease.

REFERENCES

1. Westra WH. Diagnostic difficulties in the classification and grading of salivary gland tumors. Int J Radiat Oncol Biol Phys 2007; 69(2 Suppl): S49–51.
2. Katz AD, Catalano P. The clinical significance of the various anastamotic branches of the facial nerve: report of 100 patients. Arch Otolaryngol 1987; 113: 959–62.
3. Batsakis JG. Heterotopic and accessory salivary tissue. Ann Otol Rhinol Laryngol 1986; 95: 434–6.
4. National Cancer Institute, Biometry Branch. The Third National Cancer Survey: Advanced Three Year Report 1969–1971 Incidence. Bethesda, MD: National Cancer Institute, 1974.
5. Pedersen D, Overgaard J, Sogaard H et al. Malignant parotid tumors in 110 consecutive patients: treatment results and prognosis. Laryngoscope 1992; 102: 1064–9.
6. Renehan A, Gleave EN, Hancock BD et al. Long-term follow-up of over 1000 patients with salivary gland tumors treated in a single center. Br J Surg 1986; 83: 1750–4.
7. Spiro RH. Salivary neoplasms: overview of a 35 year experience with 2807 patients. Head Neck Surg 1986; 8: 77–84.
8. Eneroth CM. Salivary gland tumors in the parotid gland, submandibular gland, and the palate region. Cancer 1971; 27: 1415–18.
9. Eveson JW, Cawson RA. Salivary gland tumors: a review of 2410 cases with particular reference to histological types, site, age and sex distribution. J Pathol 1985; 146: 51–8.
10. Spiro RH. Treating tumors of the sublingual glands, including a useful technique for repair of the floor of the mouth after resection. Am J Surg 1995; 170: 457–60.
11. Woods JE, Cheng GC, Beahrs OH. Experience with 1360 primary parotid tumors. Am J Surg 1975; 130: 460–2.
12. Simons JN, Beahrs OH, Woolner LB. Tumors of the submaxillary gland. Am J Surg 1964; 108: 485–94.
13. Conley J, Myers EN, Cole R. Analysis of 115 patients with tumors of the submandibular gland. Ann Otol Rhinol Laryngol 1972; 81: 323–30.
14. Chaudry AP, Labay GR, Yamane GM et al. Clinicopathologic and histogenetic study of 189 intraoral minor salivary tumors. J Oral Med 1984; 39: 58–78.
15. Waldron CA, El-Mofty SK, Gnepp DR. Tumors of the intraoral minor salivary glands: a demographic and histologic study of 426 cases. Oral Surg Oral Med Oral Pathol 1988; 66: 323–33.
16. Spiro RH, Koss LG, Hajdu SI et al. Tumors of minor salivary origin: a clinicopathologic study of 492 cases. Cancer 1973; 31: 117–29.
17. Takeichi N, Hirose T, Yamamoto H. Salivary gland tumors in atomic bomb survivors, Hiroshima, Japan: I. Epidemiologic observation. Cancer 1976; 38: 2462–8.
18. Saku T, Hatashi Y, Takahara O et al. Salivary gland tumors among atomic bomb survivors, 1950–1987. Cancer 1997; 79: 1465–75.
19. Maxon HR, Saenger EL, Buncher CR et al. Radiation-associated carcinoma of the salivary glands: a controlled study. Ann Otol Rhinol Laryngol 1981; 90: 107–8.
20. Katz AD, Preston-Martin S. Salivary gland tumors and previous radiotherapy to the head and neck: report of a clinical series. Am J Surg 1984; 147: 345–8.
21. Klintenberg C, Olofsson J, Hellquist H et al. Adenocarcinoma of the ethmoid sinuses: a review of 28 cases with special reference to wood dust exposure. Cancer 1984; 54: 482–8.
22. Hadfield EH, Macneth NG. Adenocarcinoma of the ethmoids in furniture workers. Ann Otol Rhinol Laryngol 1971; 80: 699–703.
23. Merrick Y, Albeck H, Nielson NH et al. Familial clustering of salivary gland carcinoma in Greenland. Cancer 1986; 57: 2097–102.
24. Pinkston JA, Cole P. Cigarette smoking and Warthin's tumor. Am J Epidemiol 1996; 144: 183–7.
25. Spitz MR, Fueger JJ, Goepfert H et al. Salivary gland cancer: a case-control investigation of risk factors. Arch Otolaryngol Head Neck Surg 1990; 116: 1163–6.
26. Foote FW Jr, Frazell EL. Tumors of the major salivary glands. Cancer 1953; 6: 1065–133.
27. Marin VTW, Salmaso R, Onnis GL. Tumors of salivary glands: review of 479 cases with particular reference to histological types, site, age and sex distribution. Appl Pathol 1989; 7: 154–60.
28. Rodriguez-Bigas MA, Sako K, Razack MS et al. Benign parotid tumors: a 24 year experience. J Surg Oncol 1991; 46: 159–61.
29. Hodgkinson DJ. The influence of facial nerve sacrifice in surgery of malignant parotid tumors. J Surg Oncol 1976; 8: 425–32.
30. Friedman M, Levin B, Grybauskas V et al. Malignant tumors of the major salivary glands. Otolaryngol Clin North Am 1986; 19: 625–36.
31. Guillamondegui OM, Byers RM, Luna MA et al. Aggressive surgery in treatment for parotid cancer: the role of adjunctive postoperative radiotherapy. Am J Roentgenol 1975; 1213: 49–54.
32. Tu G, Hu Y, Jiang P et al. The superiority of combined therapy in parotid cancer. Arch Otolaryngol 1982; 108: 710–13.
33. Rafla S. Malignant parotid tumors: natural history and treatment. Cancer 1977; 40: 136–44.
34. Hollander L, Cunningham MP. Management of cancer of the parotid gland. Surg Clin North Am 1973; 53: 113–19.
35. Hugo NE, McKinney P, Griffith BH. Management of tumors of the parotid gland. Surg Clin North Am 1973; 53: 105–11.
36. Spiro RH, Hajdu SI, Strong EW. Tumors of the submaxillary gland. Am J Surg 1976; 132: 463–8.
37. Byers RM, Jesse RH, Guillamondegui OM et al. Malignant tumors of the submaxillary gland. Am J Surg 1973; 126: 458–63.
38. Lowe JT Jr, Farmer JC Jr. Submaxillary gland tumors. Laryngoscope 1974; 84: 542–52.
39. Trial ML, Lubritz J. Tumors of the submandibular gland. Laryngoscope 1974; 84: 1225–32.
40. Pyper PL, Beverland DE, Bell DM. Tumors of the submandibular gland. J R Coll Surg Edinb 1987; 32: 233–5.
41. Rafla S. Submaxillary gland tumors. Cancer 1970; 26: 821–6.
42. Chou C, Zhu G, Luo M et al. Carcinoma of the minor salivary glands: results of surgery and combined treatment. J Oral Maxillofac Surg 1996; 54: 448–53.
43. Conley J, Arena S. Parotid gland as a focus of metastasis. Arch Surg 1963; 897: 757–64.
44. Nicholas RD, Pinnock LA, Szymanowski RT. Metastases to parotid nodes. Laryngoscope 1980; 90: 1324–8.
45. Khurana VG, Mentis DH, O'Brien CJ et al. Parotid and neck metastases from cutaneous squamous cell carcinoma of the head and neck. Am J Surg 1995; 170: 446–50.
46. Jecker P, Hartwein J. Metastasis to the parotid gland: is a radical surgical approach justified? Am J Otolaryngol 1996; 17: 102–5.
47. Batsakis JG. Pathology consultation: metastases to major salivary glands. Ann Otol Rhinol Laryngol 1990; 99: 501–3.
48. Batsakis JG, Regezi JA. The pathology of head and neck tumors: salivary glands, part 3. Head Neck Surg 1979; 1: 260–71.
49. Chapnick JS. The controversy of Warthin's tumor. Laryngoscope 1983; 93: 695–716.
50. Eveson JW, Cawson RA. Warthin's tumor (cystadenolymphoma) of salivary glands: a clinicopathologic investigation of 278 cases. Oral Surg Oral Med Oral Pathol 1986; 61: 256–62.
51. Yoo GH, Eisele DW, Askin FB et al. Warthin's tumor: a 40 year experience at the Johns Hopkins Hospital. Laryngoscope 1994; 104: 799–803.

52. Szanto PA, Luna MA, Tortoledo E et al. Histologic grading of adenoid cystic carcinoma of the salivary glands. Cancer 1984; 54: 1062.

53. Oliveira P, Fonseca I, Soares J. Acinic cell carcinoma of the salivary glands: a long term follow-up study of 15 cases. Eur J Surg Oncol 1992; 18: 7–15.

54. Grahne B, Lauren C, Holsti LR. Clinical and histologic malignancy of adenoid cystic carcinoma. J Laryngol Otol 1977; 91: 743–9.

55. Spafford PD, Mintz DR, Hay J. Acinic cell carcinoma of the parotid gland: review and management. J Otolaryngol 1991; 20: 262–6.

56. American Joint Committee on Cancer. Manual for Staging of Cancer, 4th edn. Philadelphia: JB Lippincott, 1992.

57. Batsakis JG, Regezi JA. The pathology of head and neck tumors: salivary glands, part 2. Head Neck Surg 1979; 1: 167–80.

58. Eneroth CM, Hjertman L, Moberger G et al. Mucoepidermoid carcinomas of the salivary glands with special reference to the possible existence of a benign variety. Acta Otolaryngol 1972; 73: 68–74.

59. Spiro RH, Huvos AG, Berk R et al. Mucoepidermoid carcinoma of salivary gland origin: a clinicopathologic study of 367 cases. Am J Surg 1978; 136: 461–8.

60. Healey WV, Perzin KH, Smith L. Mucoepidermoid carcinoma of salivary gland origin: classification, clinicopathologic correlation and results of treatment. Cancer 1970; 26: 368–88.

61. Evans HL. Mucoepidermoid carcinoma of salivary glands: a study of 69 cases with special attention to histologic grading. Am J Clin Pathol 1984; 81: 696–701.

62. Nascimento AG, Amaral ALP, Prado LAF et al. Mucoepidermoid carcinoma of salivary glands: a clinicopathologic study of 46 cases. Head Neck Surg 1986; 8: 409–17.

63. Hicks MJ, el-Naggar AK, Flaitz CM et al. Histocytologic grading of mucoepidermoid carcinoma of major salivary glands in prognosis and survival. Head Neck 1995; 17: 89–95.

64. Plambeck K, Friedrich RE, Hellner D et al. Mucoepidermoid carcinoma of the salivary glands: clinical data and follow-up of 52 cases. J Cancer Res Clin Oncol 1996; 122: 177–80.

65. Tonon G, Modi S, Wu L et al. t(11;19)(q21;p13) translocation in mucoepidermoid carcinoma creates a novel fusion product that disrupts a Notch signaling pathway. Nat Genet 2003; 33: 208–13.

66. Okabe M, Miyabe S, Nagatsuka H et al. MECT1-MAML2 fusion transcript defines a favorable subset of mucoepidermoid carcinoma. Clin Cancer Res, 2006; 12: 3902–7.

67. Batsakis JG, Regezi JA. The pathology of head and neck tumors: salivary glands, part 4. Head Neck Surg 1979; 1: 340–9.

68. Spiro RH, Huvos AG, Strong EW. Adenoid cystic carcinoma of salivary origin. Am J Surg 1974; 128: 512–20.

69. Blank C, Backsoom A, Eneroth CM et al. Adenoid cystic carcinoma of the parotid gland. Acta Radiol 1967; 6: 177–96.

70. Spiro RH. Distant metastasis in adenoid cystic carcinoma of salivary origin. Am J Surg 1997; 174: 495–8.

71. Eby LS, Johnson DS, Baker HW. Adenoid cystic carcinoma of the head and neck. Cancer 1972; 29: 1160–8.

72. Matsuba HM, Simpson JR, Mauney M, Thawley SE. Adenoid cystic carcinoma: a clinicopathologic correlation. Head Neck Surg 1986; 8: 200–4.

73. Perzin KH, Gullane P, Clairmont AC. Adenoid cystic carcinomas arising in salivary glands: a correlation of histologic features and clinical course. Cancer 1978; 42: 265–82.

74. Spiro RH, Huvos AG. Stage means more than grade in adenoid cystic carcinoma. Am J Surg 1992; 165: 623–8.

75. Nasimento AG, Amaral ALP, Prado LAF et al. Adenoid cystic carcinoma of salivary glands: a study of 61 cases with clinicopathologic correlation. Cancer 1986; 57: 312–19.

76. Seethala RR, Hunt JL, Baloch ZW et al. Adenoid cystic carcinoma with high-grade transformation: a report of 11 cases and a review of the literature. Am J Surg Pathol 2007; 31: 1683–94.

77. Spiro RH, Huvos AG, Strong EW. Adenocarcinoma of salivary origin: a clinicopathologic study of 204 patients. Am J Surg 1982; 144: 423–31.

78. Kemp BL, Batsakis JG, el-Naggar AK et al. Terminal duct adenocarcinomas of the parotid gland. J Laryngol Otol 1995; 109: 466–8.

79. Simpson JR, Matsuba HM, Thawley SE et al. Improved treatment of salivary gland adenocarcinomas: planned combined surgery and irradiation. Laryngoscope 1986; 96: 904–7.

80. Spiro RH, Huvos AG, Strong EW. Malignant mixed tumors of salivary origin: a clinicopathologic study of 146 cases. Cancer 1977; 39: 388–96.

81. LiVolsi VA, Perzin KH. Malignant mixed tumors arising in salivary glands: I. Carcinomas arising in benign mixed tumors: a clinicopathologic study. Cancer 1977; 39: 2209–30.

82. Gerughty RM, Scofield HH, Brown FM et al. Malignant mixed tumors of salivary origin. Cancer 1969; 24: 471–86.

83. Spiro RH, Huvos AG, Strong EW. Acinic cell carcinoma of salivary origin: a clinicopathologic study of 67 cases. Cancer 1978; 41: 924–35.

84. Batsakis JG, Chinn EK, Weimert TA et al. Acinic cell carcinoma: a clinicopathologic study of 35 cases. J Laryngol Otol 1979; 93: 325–40.

85. Galia LJ, Johnson JT. The incidence of neoplastic versus inflammatory disease in major salivary gland masses diagnosed by surgery. Laryngoscope 1981; 91: 512–16.

86. Spiro RH, Huvos AW, Strong EW. Cancer of the parotid gland: a clinicopathologic study of 288 primary cases. Am J Surg 1975; 130: 452–9.

87. Borthune A, Kjellevold, Kaalhus O et al. Salivary gland malignant neoplasms: treatment and prognosis. Int J Radiat Oncol Biol Phys 1986; 12: 747–54.

88. Nigro MF, Spiro RH. Deep lobe parotid tumors. Am J Surg 1977; 134: 523–7.

89. Johnson FE, Spiro RH. Tumors arising in accessory parotid tissue. Am J Surg 1979; 138: 576–8.

90. Frankenthaler RA, Luna MA, Lee SS et al. Prognostic variables in parotid cancer. Arch Otolaryngol Head Neck Surg 1991; 117: 1251–6.

91. Eneroth CM. Facial nerve paralysis: a criterion of malignancy in parotid tumors. Arch Otolaryngol 1972; 95: 300–4.

92. Conley JJ, Hamaker RC. Prognosis of malignant tumors of the parotid gland with facial paralysis. Arch Otolaryngol 1975; 101: 39–41.

93. Weber RS, Byers RM, Petit B et al. Submandibular gland tumors: adverse histologic factors and therapeutic implications. Arch Otolaryngol Head Neck Surg 1990; 116: 1055.

94. Weissman JL. Imaging of the salivary glands. Semin Ultrasound CT MR 1995; 16: 546–68.

95. Seethala RR, LiVolsi VA, Baloch ZW. Relative accuracy of fine-needle aspiration and frozen section in the diagnosis of lesions of the parotid gland. Head Neck 2005; 27: 217–23.

96. Alphs HH, Eisele DW, Westra WH. The role of fine needle aspiration in the evaluation of parotid masses. Curr Opin Otolaryngol Head Neck Surg 2006; 14: 62–66.

97. Lindberg RD, Ackerman M. Aspiration cytology of salivary gland tumors: diagnostic experience from six years of routine laboratory work. Laryngoscope 1976; 86: 584–9.

98. O'Dwyer P, Farrar WB, James AG et al. Needle aspiration biopsy of major salivary gland tumors: its value. Cancer 1986; 57: 554–7.

99. Layfield LJ, Tan P, Glasgow BJ. Fine needle aspiration of salivary gland lesions: comparison with frozen sections and histologic findings. Arch Pathol Lab Med 1987; 111: 346–53.

100. Atula T, Greenman R, Laippala P et al. Fine-needle aspiration biopsy in the diagnosis of parotid gland lesions: evaluation of 438 biopsies. Diagn Cytopathol 1996; 15: 185–90.

101. International Union Against Cancer. TNM Classification of Malignant Tumors, 5th edn. New York: Wiley-Liss, 1997.

102. Spiro RH, Thaler HT, Hicks WS et al. The importance of clinical staging of minor salivary tumors. Am J Surg 1991; 162: 330–6.

103. Gibbons MD, Manne U, Carroll WR et al. Molecular differences in mucoepidermoid carcinoma and adenoid cystic carcinoma of the major salivary glands. Laryngoscope 2001; 111: 1373–8.

104. Katopodi E, Patsouris E, Papanikolaou VKA et al. Immunohistochemical detection of epidermal growth factor and its receptor in salivary gland carcinomas. Oral Surg Oral Med Oral Pathol Oral Radiol Endod 2003; 95: 266–8.

105. Fan CY, Melhem MF, Hosal AS et al. Expression of androgen receptor, epidermal growth factor receptor, and transforming growth factor alpha in salivary duct carcinoma. Arch Otolaryngol Head Neck Surg 2001; 127: 1075–9.

106. Locati LD, Perrone F, Losa M. Treatment relevant immunophenotyping of 139 salivary gland carcinomas. Ann Oncol, in press.

107. Shintani S, Funayama T, Yoshihama Y et al. Expression of *c-erbB* family gene products in adenoid cystic carcinoma of salivary glands: an immunohistochemical study. Anticancer Res 1995; 15: 2623–6.

108. Slamon DJ, Leyland-Jones B, Shak S et al. Use of chemotherapy plus a monoclonal antibody against HER2 for metastatic breast cancer that overexpresses *HER2*. N Engl J Med 2001; 344: 783–92.

109. Etges A, Pinto DS, Kowalski LP et al. Salivary duct carcinoma: immunohistochemical profile of an aggressive salivary gland tumor. J Clin Pathol 2003; 56: 914–18.

110. Glisson B, Colevas AD, Haddad R et al. *HER2* expression in salivary gland carcinomas: dependence on histological subtype. Clin Cancer Res 2004; 10: 944–6.

111. Hellquist HB, Karlsson MG, Nilsson C. Salivary duct carcinoma—a highly aggressive salivary gland tumor with overexpression of *c-erbB-2*. J Pathol 1994; 172: 35–44.

112. Press MF, Pike MC, Hung G et al. Amplification and overexpression of *HER-2/neu* in carcinomas of the salivary gland: correlation with poor prognosis. Cancer Research 1994; 54: 5675–82.

113. McGurk M, Renehan A, Gleave EN et al. Clinical significance of the tumor capsule in the treatment of parotid pleomorphic adenomas. Br J Surg 1996; 83: 1747–9.

114. Prichard AJ, Barton RP, Narula AA. Complications of superficial parotidectomy versus extracapsular lumpectomy in the treatment of benign parotid lesions. J R Coll Surg Edinb 1992; 37: 155–8.

115. Afify SE, Maynard JD. Tumors of the accessory lobe of the parotid gland. Postgrad Med J 1992; 68: 461–2.

116. Chen AM, Garcia J, Bucci K et al. Recurrent pleomorphic adenoma of the parotid gland: long-term outcome of patients treated with radiation therapy. Int J Radiat Oncol Biol Phys 2006; 66: 1031–5.

117. Ball ABS, Fish S, Thomas JM. Malignant epithelial parotid tumors: a rational treatment policy. Br J Surg 1995; 82: 621–3.

118. Johns ME. Parotid cancer: a rational basis for treatment. Head Neck Surg 1980; 3: 132–44.

119. Krause CJ. The management of parotid neoplasms. Head Neck Surg 1981; 3: 340–3.

120. Hillel AD, Fee WE. Evaluation of frozen section in parotid gland surgery. Arch Otolaryngol 1983; 109: 230–2.

121. Wheelis RF, Yarrington CT Jr. Tumors of the salivary glands: comparison of frozen section diagnosis with final pathologic diagnosis. Arch Otolaryngol 1984; 110: 76–7.

122. Granick MS, Erickson ER, Hanna DC. Accuracy of frozen section diagnosis in salivary gland lesions. Head Neck Surg 1985; 7: 465–7.

123. Rigval NR, Miller P, Lore JM et al. Accuracy of frozen section diagnosis in salivary gland lesions. Head Neck Surg 1985; 7: 465–7.

124. Terhaard CH. Postoperative and primary radiotherapy for salivary gland carcinomas: indications, techniques, and results. Int J Radiat Oncol Biol Phys 2007; 69(2 Suppl): S52–5.

125. Krull A, Schwarz R, Engenhart R et al. European results in neutron therapy of malignant salivary gland tumors. Bull Cancer Radiother 1996; 83(Suppl): 125–9.

126. Buchholz TA, Laramore GE, Griffen BR et al. The role of fast neutron therapy in the management of advanced salivary gland malignant neoplasms. Cancer 1992; 69: 2779–88.

127. Cornolti G, Ungari M, Morassi ML et al. Amplification and overexpression of *HER2/neu* gene and *HER2/neu* protein in salivary duct carcinoma of the parotid gland. Arch Otolaryngol Head Neck Surg 2007; 133: 1031–6.

128. Leverstein H, van der Wal JE, Tiwari RM et al. Surgical management of 246 previously untreated pleomorphic adenomas of the parotid gland. Br J Surg 1997; 84: 399–403.

129. Laccourreye H, Laccourreye O, Cauchois R et al. Total conservative parotidectomy for primary benign pleomorphic adenoma of the parotid gland: a 25 year experience with 229 patients. Laryngoscope 1994; 104: 1487–94.

130. O'Dwyer PJ, Farrar WB, Finkelmeier WR et al. Facial nerve sacrifice and tumor recurrences in primary and recurrent benign parotid tumors. Am J Surg 1986; 152: 442–5.

131. Conley JJ, Clairmont AA. Facial nerve in recurrent benign pleomorphic adenoma. Arch Otolaryngol 1979; 105: 247–51.

132. Fee WE, Goffinet DR, Calcaterra JC. Recurrent mixed tumors of the parotid gland: results of surgical therapy. Laryngoscope 1978; 88: 265–73.

133. Phillips PP, Olsen KD. Recurrent pleomorphic adenoma of the parotid gland: report of 126 cases and a review of the literature. Ann Otol Rhinol Laryngol 1995; 104: 100–4.

134. Niparko JK, Beauchamp ML, Krause CJ et al. Surgical treatment of recurrent pleomorphic adenoma of the parotid gland. Arch Otolaryngol 1986; 112: 1180–4.

135. Samson MJ, Metson R, Wang CC et al. Preservation of the facial nerve in the management of recurrent pleomorphic adenoma. Laryngoscope 1991; 101: 1060–2.

136. Fu KK, Leibel SA, Levine ML et al. Cancer of the major and minor salivary glands. Cancer 1977; 40: 2882–90.

137. Garden AS, El-Naggar AK, Morrison WH et al. Postoperative radiotherapy for malignant tumors of the parotid gland. Int J Radiat Oncol Biol Phys 1997; 37: 79–85.

138. Armstrong JG, Harrison LB, Spiro RH et al. Malignant tumors of major salivary origin: a matched pair analysis of the role of combined surgery and postoperative radiotherapy. Arch Otolaryngol Head Neck Surg 1990; 116: 290–3.

21

Management of Tumors of the Temporal Bone

David A Moffat

INTRODUCTION

Tumors involving the temporal bone are rare but present with symptoms similar to inflammatory ear disease. A high index of suspicion is required for the early diagnosis of malignant tumors. Pain, bleeding from the ear canal, and facial palsy may herald the onset of malignancy. Local extension of tumor to structures surrounding the temporal bone occurs early and often silently, and as a result, most tumors present at a relatively advanced stage. The prognosis of treated squamous cell carcinoma (SCC) of the temporal bone is determined primarily by the extent of local disease at diagnosis. Combined treatment of tumors limited to the external auditory canal (EAC) can result in a moderate five-year survival, but advanced cancer has a very poor prognosis.

The surgical management of patients with temporal bone cancer is a major undertaking involving resection of major structures and high treatment morbidity. Treatment is best carried out by a multidisciplinary team skilled in dealing with the complex regions of the temporal bone and skull base.

SURGICAL ANATOMY

The anatomy of the temporal bone and adjacent regions is complex and contains the organs of hearing and balance; the cranial nerves responsible for facial movement, speech, and swallowing; and the major vessels providing arterial supply and venous drainage to the cranium and brain. The temporal bone is in turn surrounded by important structures of the face and infratemporal fossa, the dura of the middle and posterior cranial fossae and underlying brain and upper neck and cervical spine. A conceptual organization of the various compartments of the temporal bone is important in understanding the spread of temporal bone cancer and forms the anatomical basis of the previously described en bloc resections of the temporal bone.

The tympanic membrane and promontory of the middle ear form the medial resection margins for tumors arising in the EAC. Small tumors limited to the lateral portion of the external canal can be excised en bloc with a sleeve resection of the external canal and adjacent conchal bowl (Fig. 21.1). The tympanic membrane forms the medial limit of the resected margin.

More medially arising EAC tumors can be removed by lateral temporal bone resection (LTBR) (1) where the medial limit is formed by the promontory of the first turn of the cochlea and the resection includes the tympanic membrane (Fig. 21.1). Tumors extending into or involving

the middle ear can be removed by subtotal temporal bone resection by including the otic capsule in the resection (STBR) (2–4). Total temporal bone resection (TTBR) (5,6) for tumors involving the petrous apex includes removing the complete temporal bone (Fig. 21.1). Extended temporal bone resection (ETBR) with supraomohyoid neck dissection for advanced and recurrent cancer has been recently advocated (6). Infratemporal fossa skull base approaches have been designed for resection of tumors involving the jugular foramen (7). The normal anatomical structures contained within each compartment determine the functional deficits associated with resections of tumors arising within these regions. Excision of the external ear by sleeve resection and LTBR results in cosmetic deformity and moderate conductive hearing loss. When resection of middle ear tumors by STBR includes the otic capsule, total hearing loss, transient vertigo, facial nerve palsy, and risk of cerebrospinal fluid (CSF) leak result. Extension of the resection inferiorly to include the neurovascular compartments of the jugular foramen results in sacrifice of the lower cranial nerves and the additional deficits of dysphonia and dysphagia with risk of aspiration. Resection of the surrounding structures such as mandible and infratemporal fossa, dura and overlying brain, facial and lower cranial nerves, internal carotid artery (ICA) (6,8,9) and dural venous sinuses is possible, but the morbidity of the resection is considerably increased. Careful preoperative planning is required prior to deciding which resection is applicable and difficult intraoperative decisions may be required before extending the resection limits to surrounding anatomical regions.

GENERAL CONSIDERATIONS

Age

Temporal bone cancer tends to affect the 50- to 60-year-old age group predominantly, although younger ages have been reported, particularly with tumors of the middle ear (10). A typical mean age is 72.6 within a range of 56–98 (11). Sarcomas are limited to children.

Incidence

Little information is available on the incidence of temporal bone malignancy as few centers deal with enough cases to gain a large experience with the patterns of disease. In Britain the age adjusted incidence is 1/1,000,000 per year for women, and 0.8/1,000,000 per year for men (12). Expressed as a fraction of all otological complaints the incidence is in the region of 0.025–0.005% (10,13,14). The prevalence has been reported as 0.006% (15).

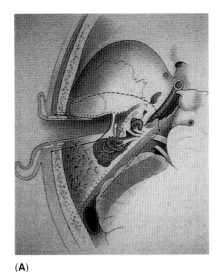

(A)

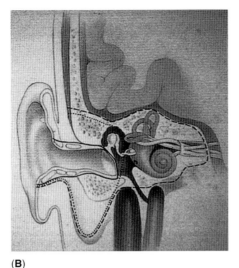

(B)

Figure 21.1 (A, B) The concept of en bloc resection of the temporal bone is illustrated in the axial and coronal planes. Sleeve resection of the external auditory canal (solid line) is rarely indicated for small lesions of the EAC. Lateral temporal bone resection (dotted line) is indicated for most cancers limited to the EAC. Total temporal bone resection (dashed line) is indicated for advanced temporal bone cancer and is performed by a combination of en bloc and piecemeal resection techniques, rather than neatly as shown in this diagram. (Reproduced from the *Atlas of Neuro-otology and Skull Base Surgery*; Robert K. Jackler MD; Mosby 1996, with kind permission of the editor).

Gender

The gender proportion is near to equal (16), although many studies have shown a slight female preponderance, ratio of 1:1.2 (17).

Etiology

Etiological factors implicated in the development of temporal bone cancer have been studied. Temporal bone cancer can be divided into two major groups: (1) laterally arising in the skin of the external ear involving the pinna and lateral third of the EAC. Exposure to ultraviolet radiation is thought to be the major etiological factor in this group (18) and while this is well documented with regards to the pinna, there is no evidence base for this in relation to the external auditory canal (2). In more medially arising external auditory canal tumors and middle ear cancer, chronic inflammation is likely to be the major etiology, as about half of these cancers are associated with a long history of chronic discharge (17,19). Radiation associated tumors are well described in the literature. In the temporal bone these arise following initial radiotherapy for lesions in close anatomical proximity, for example, nasopharyngeal carcinoma. Lustig (20) reports a latency time with a mean of 12.9 years post treatment and Goh (21) a latency of 15 years. Occupational factors such as radiation exposure in watch dial makers (22,23), frost bite (18), and a possible link with aflatoxin generated by fungi in the EAC (17), as well as prolonged topical exposure to chlorinated disinfectants (24) have been proposed as etiological factors.

CLASSIFICATION
Sites of Temporal Bone Cancer

To some extent this classification is artificial as advanced tumor involves multiple sites and it is difficult to identify the site of origin (Table 21.1).

Table 21.1 Sites of Temporal Bone Cancer

	Lewis (13)	Nelms and Paparella (25)	Conley and Schuller (26)
Auricle (%)	60	85	60–70
External canal (%)	30	12	20–30
Middle ear (%)	10	1.5	10

Histology

The most common type of malignancy arising in the temporal bone is squamous carcinoma. Adenocarcinoma is much less common and other histopathological types are very rare. (Table 21.2).

Most malignant tumors of the temporal bone arise from the epithelial elements of the EAC and middle ear. Metastasis to the temporal bone occurs by hematogenous spread, usually to marrow-containing regions, commonly the petrous apex (28), or by direct extension from the nasopharynx and parotid gland. Hematological malignancies such as lymphoma, leukemia and eosinophilic granuloma can also involve the temporal bone and should be considered in multiple or bilateral lesions.

Non-neoplastic destructive temporal bone lesions and benign neoplasm need to be differentiated from malignant tumors of the temporal bone. They include fibrous dysplasia (29–31), osteoradionecrosis, necrotizing otitis externa (32–34), sarcoid, Paget's disease and giant cell tumor of bone. Careful evaluations with multiple deep-tissue biopsies are required to avoid sampling error and confirm the tissue diagnosis prior to planning definitive treatment.

NATURAL HISTORY AND MECHANISMS OF SPREAD OF MALIGNANT TUMORS

Spread tends to occur via extension through the numerous vascular, neural, and natural foramina between the temporal bone and surrounding structures (Figs. 21.2 and 21.3).

Table 21.2   Histology of Primary Temporal Bone Cancers. Adapted from Krespi et al. (27)

	Conley (1965)*	Lewis (1982)*	Tucker (1965)*	Kuhel (1995)†	
Squamous cell carcinoma	24	86	68	82.2	
Adenocarcinoma	4	2	1	8.8 (including adenoid cystic carcinoma)	
Basal cell carcinoma	1	8	–	5.6	
Metastasis	–	–	8	–	–
Sarcoma	5	2	6	–	
Melanoma	–	–	–	–	0.4
Miscellaneous	2	2	6	0.4	
Total no. of cases	36	100	89	>500	

*Absolute numbers.
†percentages.

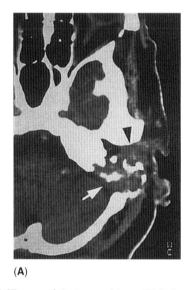
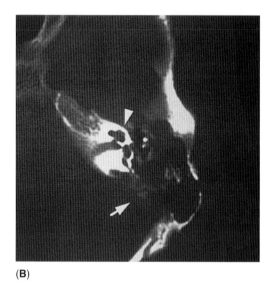

(A)   **(B)**

Figure 21.2   Axial CT scans of the temporal bone. **(A)** In the contrast-enhanced scan the apparent limits of the tumour can be seen. Involvement of the lateral temporal bone with margins extending to the pinna and periauricular skin, the temporomandibular joint (black arrow head) and the posterior fossa dura and sigmoid sinus (white arrow) is shown. **(B)** The posterior fossa bony plate has been destroyed (white arrow). In the bone window CT settings the otic capsule structures including the cochlea (arrow head) are well preserved. The otic capsule is highly resistant to cancerous invasion and involvement of the cochlea and semicircular canals usually occurs late in the untreated history of temporal bone malignancy. In this case the patient presented with a 60dB hearing loss and intact cochlear and vestibular function. Cancer of the temporal bone spreads primarily by direct extension and is usually found to be more extensive at operation than shown by preoperative imaging.

Extension is multidirectional such that deep local spread to surrounding areas may be present but unsuspected at the time of surgery. This may account for the high incidence of local recurrence following surgery (11). Invasion of blood vessels in the skin of the EAC causes recurrent bloody otorrhoea, the most common presenting symptom of EAC cancer. Lateral extension along the subcutaneous plane gives the appearance of thickened edematous external canal skin (Figs. 21.3A,D). Circumferential spread with extension to the conchal bowl may occur and give rise to an appearance similar to chronic otitis externa.

Anterior extension to the temporomandibular joint (Fig. 21.2A), parotid gland, and infratemporal fossa occurs via the fissures of Santorini, the petrosquamous fissure, and preformed defects of the external canal (foramen of Hüschke), presenting with preauricular swelling and trismus. Involvement of the root of the zygoma with extension

to the masseter muscle and subsequent downward extension to the mandible and infratemporal fossa occurs in advanced cancer. Inferior extension to the jugular foramen, foramen magnum, cervical vertebrae, and upper neck, results in fullness and lower cranial nerve palsies. Medial growth through the tympanic membrane with extension of tumor into the middle ear cleft (Fig. 21.3A–F) allows spread via the pneumatized spaces of the temporal bone. Extension to the petrous apex, internal carotid artery (ICA) (35) and nasopharynx via the eustachian tube can easily occur. The internal carotid artery and otic capsule bone are highly resistant to tumor invasion and involvement of the labyrinth occurs late, resulting in sensorineural hearing loss (SNHL) and vertigo (Fig. 21.2). Extension to the internal auditory canal (IAC) may occur through the vestibule.

Superior extension to the epitympanic space and thin bone of the tegmen tympani will involve the middle

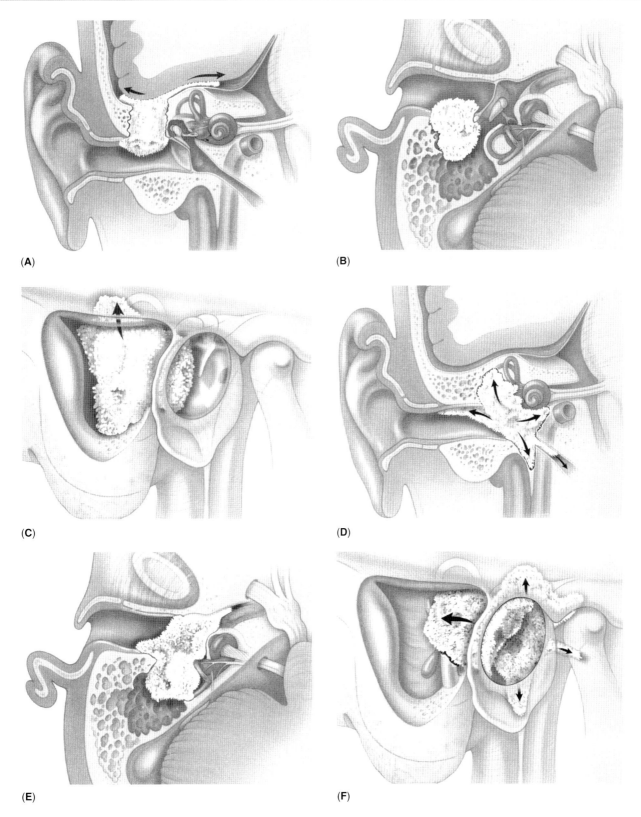

(A)

(B)

(C)

(D)

(E)

(F)

Figure 21.3 (**A**) Coronal section of an advanced temporal bone SCC demonstrating superior spread through the tegmen with involvement of dura and temporal lobe of the brain. (**B**) Axial section of the lesion showing its posterior extent in the mastoid. (**C**) Parasagittal section illustrating superior spread into the middle cranial fossa. (**D**) Coronal section of a very advanced temporal bone SCC illustrating the lines of spread within the temporal bone: superiorly, medially and laterally. (**E**) Axial view of the lesion demonstrating spread anteriorly, posteriorly, medially and laterally. (**F**) Parasagittal view showing anterior, posterior, superior and inferior spread. (Fig. 18.3 'Squamous cell carcinoma', Chapter 5, page 71 in *Tumors of the Ear and Temporal Bone* – Eds: Jackler and Driscoll, 2000, Lippincott Williams and Wilkins. Reproduced with kind permission of the editors.)

fossa dura and temporal lobe and is the most common route of intracranial spread (Fig. 21.3). This is suggested by persistent deep temporal headache. Posterior extension to the retroauricular sulcus and mastoid occurs through preformed defects of the EAC or direct bony erosion (Fig. 21.3). Involvement of the posterior fossa dura can occur from the mastoid.

Lymphatic Spread

The skin of the external ear canal has a sparse lymphatic network. Drainage is to the preauricular, mastoid, subparotid and subdigastric nodes initially, and then to deep upper cervical nodes (36,37). Clinically evident metastatic spread to regional lymph nodes is not common at the time of presentation (10–15%) (6,38–40) and is seen only in advanced cancer and has a very poor prognosis (41). Extension via peritubal lymphatics to the nasopharynx may occur with involvement of the retropharyngeal nodes. Lymphatic micrometastasis may be a cause for early regional treatment failure (11). Adenoid cystic carcinoma (ACC), basal cell carcinoma (BCC), and squamous cell carcinoma (SCC) have a particular propensity for perineural spread. The predominant nerve at risk is the facial nerve. Spread distally extends to the stylomastoid foramen and to the extratemporal facial nerve. Extension to the parotid segment of the facial nerve can selectively involve branches of the facial nerve and produce weakness in a particular region of facial musculature. Medial spread leads to the geniculate ganglion, intracranial portions of the facial nerve, and brain stem. Spread along the greater superficial petrosal nerve (GSPN) can occur and lead to involvement of the floor of the middle cranial fossa.

Hematogenous spread of temporal bone cancer to distant sites is rare at the time of presentation, and indicates incurable disease. Metastases in the lung and bone are the most common sites and may occur with squamous cancer, adenoid cystic carcinoma, adenocarcinoma, and sarcoma.

Metastasis to the temporal bone by hematological spread from tumors at distant sites occurs but is uncommon.

The petrous apex is the most common location for metastasis due to the presence of vascular bone marrow (28). Metastasis to the middle ear, mastoid and external canal also occurs. Presenting symptoms are pain, hearing loss, mass in the external auditory canal, and facial numbness (10,41,44). The most likely primary sites are breast, lung, kidney, prostate, salivary, pharynx or nasopharynx, gastrointestinal tract, and the occult primary (45).

Hematological malignancies such as lymphoma, leukemia and eosinophilic granuloma can also involve the temporal bone and should be considered in multiple or bilateral lesions. Intracranial spread by direct extension of tumor from the middle ear occurs and is typical of advanced sarcoma. Meningeal spread produces multiple cranial nerve palsies (46,47).

CLINICAL PRESENTATION

Pain, bleeding, discharge, facial palsy, and hearing loss are the most common presenting symptoms of temporal bone cancer. A high index of suspicion is required for early diagnosis of malignancy as these symptoms are typical of inflammatory ear disease and both conditions can co-exist (32,34), although the pain tends to be more severe in malignant disease and bleeding is relatively uncommon in chronic inflammatory disease. The range of symptoms and signs associated with the presentation of temporal bone cancer are shown in Table 21.3. Otoscopy reveals an exophytic lesion that is friable and bleeds on contact. Tumors can bear a similar appearance to chronic suppurative otitis media with granulation tissues, but malignant tumors tend to be predominantly exophytic (Fig. 21.4).

CLINICAL ASSESSMENT

The aim of preoperative assessment is to confirm the diagnosis of malignancy, define the extent of disease, and formulate a treatment plan. This is achieved with history taking,

Table 21.3 Clinical Presentation of Temporal Bone Cancer

	Leonetti et al. (48)* (N (%))	Kuhel et al. (37)† (%)	Pensak et al. (37) (%)
Symptoms			
Pain	19 (74)	51	60
Hearing loss	18 (69)	29	20
Headache	12 (46)		
Facial numbness	8 (31)		
Hoarseness	3 (12)		
Dysphagia	1 (4)		
Vertigo/tinnitus		15	
Signs			
Ear canal mass	26 (100)	37	
Bloody otorrhea	18 (69)	61	60
Facial paralysis	13 (50)	16	35
Cranial nerve defects	8 (31)		10
Parotid, neck mass	7 (27)		
Temporal mass	4 (15)	19	

*26 cases.
†442 cases.

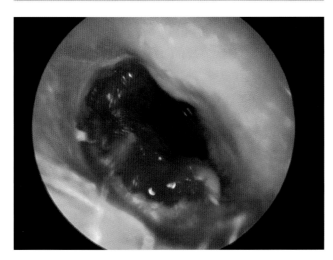

Figure 21.4 The otoscopic appearance of an SCC of the external auditory canal. This exophytic bleeding ulcerated mass in the posterior and inferior aspect of the EAC is characteristic of this pathology. The surrounding canal skin is edematous due to carcinomatous involvement. A high degree of suspicion is required to diagnose cancer of the EAC early as the presenting symptoms and appearances can easily be mistaken for otitis externa and indeed the two conditions often co-exist. *Source*: From *Squamous cell carcinoma of the temporal bone: current evidence for radiotherapy alone and surgery with postoperative radiotherapy*. In: *Recent Advances in Otolaryngology 8*; DA Moffat, J Keir and H Sudhoff, Royal Society of Medicine Publishers, 2008.

thorough physical examination, imaging, and biopsy. The length of the history and the rate at which symptoms develop give some idea of the extent of local spread and the degree of malignancy of the tumor. A long history of aural discharge suggests cancer associated with inflammatory ear disease (Marjolin's ulcer). Pulsatile tinnitus suggests a tumor of vascular origin, such as a glomus tumor, or a middle ear vascular anomaly, or a dural arteriovenous abnormality. Deep headache raises the suspicion of dural involvement. Facial weakness indicates invasion of the facial nerve. The onset of vertigo and SNHL indicates invasion of the labyrinth, and the development of speech and swallowing problems heralds involvement of the lower cranial nerves in the jugular foramen. The onset of trismus due to involvement of the temporomandibular joint, pterygoid muscles, or mandible suggests advanced disease that has spread anteriorly. The appearance of periauricular and parotid swelling is a grave sign.

Clinical examination includes careful microscopic examination of the location of tumor and its visible extent. Particular note is made of facial weakness, trismus, periauricular swellings and regional lymph node enlargement. Cranial nerve deficits are carefully recorded. Thorough assessment of hearing and balance function is recorded clinically and documented with audiometry.

General physical examination is carried out to detect distant spread. Assessment of the patient's nutritional and mental state gives some idea of the patient's general response to major surgery. Detailed assessment is made of co-existing illnesses and the patient's overall fitness for general anaesthesia.

INVESTIGATIONS

Biopsy

External canal lesions offer an opportunity for direct biopsy, but if a vascular tumor or vascular anomaly is suspected biopsy is best deferred until clinical and radiological assessments including carotid arteriography have been completed.

Multiple deep biopsies should be taken to avoid a sampling error. Results that return a report of chronic inflammation when there is suspicion of malignancy should be repeated as neoplastic and inflammatory disease commonly co-exist (32,34).

Imaging

Imaging is mandatory as part of the preoperative assessment and provides information on the nature of destructive temporal bone lesions and the extent of local and regional spread. CT scanning and MRI are complementary in the assessment of temporal bone tumors. The positive signal given by bone allows high-resolution CT (1 mm cuts or less) in the axial and coronal planes to provide accurate delineation of the extent of the destruction of the bone. MRI, on the other hand, where bone gives a negative signal impressively demonstrates soft tissue involvement such as dura, temporal lobe, brain, or pterygoid muscle especially when enhanced with gadolinium diethylenetriaminepentaacetic acid (Gd-DTPA). The presence of distant metastasis can be assessed with chest X-ray and skeletal survey. Accurate postoperative imaging aids in the planning of radiotherapy fields and identifies patients with recurrent disease for palliative treatment.

Computerized Tomography

High-resolution CT scanning in the axial and coronal planes is excellent for identifying bony erosion of the temporal bone and adjacent skull base (39,49) because bone gives a positive signal (Fig. 21.5). The bony architecture of the lesion may indicate the nature of the tumor. A diffuse ground glass appearance is suggestive of fibro-osseous dysplasia, an onion skin appearance is associated with giant cell tumors of the temporal bone, and Paget's disease has the specific radiological appearance of demineralized bone. Erosion of the external canal, mastoid cortex, tegmen, or petrous apex may indicate previously unsuspected deeper disease. Involvement of regional lymph nodes with tumor can be seen with ring enhancement of enlarged nodes (50).

Magnetic Resonance Imaging

The high sensitivity and specificity of postcontrast MRI scanning is useful in defining the extent of intracranial and soft tissue involvement. In MRI bone has a negative signal. Involvement of the dura and brain is an important prognostic indicator and high resolution MRI scanning in the axial and coronal planes with Gd-DTPA enhancement is mandatory (Fig. 21.6). Extension to the infratemporal fossa, and spread to regional lymph node groups can be identified (39,49). Tissue confirmation of the nature of disease is required prior to embarking on definitive treatment.

Angiography

Advanced disease involving the petrous apex may involve the intrapetrous carotid artery (ICA) (35) although this is

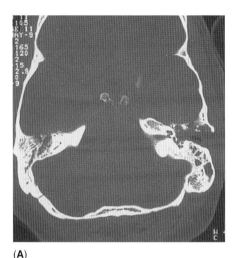 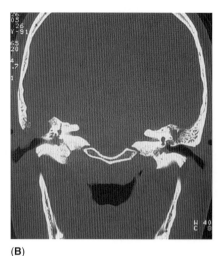

(A)   **(B)**

Figure 21.5 (A, B) Axial CT scan of extensive SCC of left temporal bone demonstrating marked bony erosion anteriorly and laterally (Fig. 21.5A). The coronal CT in the same patient shows marked erosion of the superior surface of the temporal bone and soft tissue filling the external auditory canal (Fig. 21.5B).

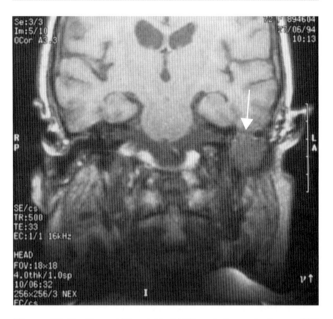

Figure 21.6 Coronal T1-weighted MRI scan demonstrating an SCC of the left temporal bone eroding the superior surface of the bone with dural involvement (white arrow). At surgery the tumour was noted to have invaded the temporal lobe of the brain.

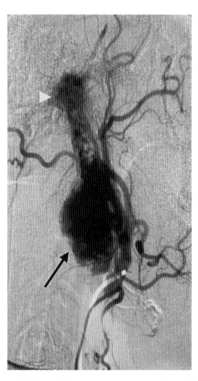

Figure 21.7 Right carotid arteriogram showing the multicentric nature of some glomus tumour types. This patient has a glomus tympanicum (white arrow head) and a carotid body tumour (black arrow) on the same side.

a rare finding at surgery and the ICA is relatively resistant to invasion by temporal bone tumors. Angiography is used preoperatively to assess the internal carotid artery and delineate the vascular pattern of the cerebral arterial anatomy (Fig. 21.7). Use of balloon occlusion techniques or cross-flow studies to demonstrate adequate contralateral cross-flow, suggests that safe en bloc resection of the internal carotid artery can take place (8,9). Confirmation of contralateral venous drainage allows safe resection of the sigmoid/jugular venous complex without risk of cerebral edema. Vascular anomalies and glomus jugular tumors can be diagnosed preoperatively, without need for biopsy and provide an

opportunity for preoperative embolization with coils and feathers.

Ultrasound

The role of ultrasound is limited to the assessment of the relationship of neck masses to the great vessels and assisting in guided percutaneous biopsy of neck nodes.

Other Imaging Techniques

Distant spread to lung, bone, and liver can be assessed preoperatively with chest X-ray and bone scan or skeletal survey. Technetium scanning is useful in excluding inflammatory conditions of the skull base as a cause of symptoms (32,34). Indium-labeled white-cell scanning can help in the diagnosis of inflammatory disease of the temporal bone.

STAGING

Several staging systems for malignancy involving the external ear have been proposed but currently no universally accepted system exists. Ideally a preoperative staging system should allow the extent of tumor to be easily categorized, aid in planning treatment, and be useful as a basis for evaluating the outcomes of treatment. A widely accepted staging system would facilitate the comparison of results between centers.

In 1985 Stell and McCormick (51) proposed a staging system for cancer involving the EAC and middle ear based on the anatomical origin of the tumor (external auditory canal or middle ear) and the extent of local spread, evaluated using clinical assessment, facial nerve status, and imaging. This staging system was later revised by Clark et al. (Table 21.4) (52).

More recently, Arriaga et al. (53) devised a staging system that conformed to the American Joint Cancer Committee's TNM classification providing a prediction of outcome based on the stage of the disease. Preoperative clinical and CT findings emphasized the extent of local disease as the major prognostic indicator, the adverse effect of regional lymph node spread, and the need for preoperative imaging to assess the extent of local disease (Table 21.5).

Hirsch (54) modified the staging system to upgrade the importance of facial nerve involvement. He believes that facial nerve involvement is a defining feature of a T3 carcinoma. For the facial nerve to be clinically involved the tumor must have invaded the medial wall of the middle ear cavity or extended beyond the boundaries of the mastoid into the infra-temporal space to invade the nerve at the stylomastoid foramen.

Moffat (41,42) in his series did not find facial nerve involvement to be a significant prognostic indicator.

N Status

Involvement of lymph nodes is a poor prognostic finding (41,42) and automatically places the patient in a higher category, that is, stage III (T1, N1) or stage IV (T2, 3 and 4, N1) disease.

M Status

Distant metastasis indicates a very poor prognosis and immediately places a patient in the stage IV category.

TREATMENT POLICY

Treatment of temporal bone malignancy is a major undertaking. Accurate preoperative assessment; organization of necessary specialist resources for surgical resection and reconstruction by a multidisciplinary team; postoperative recovery; and rehabilitation are all necessary. Provision must be made for delivery of radiotherapy and long-term follow-up.

Principles of Surgical Resection

Two contrasting approaches to temporal bone resection have been developed. The application of either is dependent on the extent of local disease and the particular preferences of different individual units.

Early Lesions

The principle of en bloc resection when applied to localized, small tumors confined to the EAC allows the utilization of a lateral temporal bone resection (LTBR), which may realistically remove small EAC lesions leaving a clear margin of normal surrounding tissue. Careful preoperative assessment of the extent of tumor is required, but few cancers are discovered early enough for en bloc surgical resection to be applied as the sole treatment modality—especially since these tumors are so aggressive.

Advanced Lesions

The feasibility of planned en bloc resections for advanced lesions has been challenged. The multidirectional spread of locally advanced cancer (44) does not allow the accurate preoperative assessment of the local extent of the tumor. Preoperative imaging commonly underestimates the extent of tumor and this has a critical prognostic significance. Total temporal bone resection en bloc may lead to vascular compromise of the brain stem as a result of sacrifice of the intrapetrous internal carotid artery as well as VII, IX, X, XI and XII cranial nerve palsies. Many surgeons in the field think that this may be unacceptable because there is no definitive evidence that it improves the ultimate prognosis.

One technique of surgical excision that has been proposed for these lesions by many skull-base surgeons is

Table 21.4 Staging System: Clark's Modification of Stell et al.'s Proposal (52)

T1	Tumor limited to site of origin
T2	Tumor extending beyond site of origin indicated by facial paralysis or radiological evidence of bone destruction
T3	Involvement of parotid gland/temporomandibular joint/skin (i.e., extracranial)
T4	Involvement of dura/base of skull (i.e., cranial)

Table 21.5 Staging System (53)

T1	Tumor limited to the EAC without bony erosion or evidence of soft tissue extension
T2	Tumor with limited EAC erosion (not full thickness) or radiological findings consistent with limited (<0.5 cm) soft tissue involvement
T3	Tumor eroding the osseous EAC (full thickness) with limited (<0.5 cm) soft tissue involvement of middle ear and/or mastoid, or causing facial paralysis at presentation.
T4	Tumor eroding the cochlea, petrous apex, medial wall of middle ear, carotid canal, jugular foramen, or dura, or with extensive (>0.5 cm) soft tissue involvement

step-wise removal of visible disease (3,6,15,39,53,54). Initial bloc resection is followed by piecemeal removal of residual tumor and the petrous apex is removed with a high speed drill. The theoretical risk of dissemination of tumor cells has not been substantiated, but most clinicians would consider it wise to recommend postoperative radiotherapy. The technique acknowledges that en bloc resection of deeper tissues is not possible in view of the anatomy and the vital structures within and adjacent to the temporal bone. Considerable intraoperative decision-making about the limits of resection is required. No comparison of the two techniques has been made as yet.

Management of the Neck

Since involvement of the local lymph nodes draining the temporal bone is an important prognostic indicator, management of the neck is an integral part of disease treatment. Resection of regional lymph nodes as part of the en bloc principle, can be accomplished by adding a supraomohyoid neck dissection and a total parotidectomy (16).

Supraomohyoid Neck Dissection

Clinically negative neck disease warrants treatment with a supraomohyoid neck dissection (16). This allows staging of the disease for postoperative radiotherapy and it also allows control of the great vessels of the neck and access to the skull base to be obtained. Exposed vessels are then preserved for anastomosis with the free flap repair.

Parotidectomy

The parotid gland contains the first echelon of nodes draining the external auditory canal. In T1 and T2 lesions a superficial parotidectomy is recommended and in T3 and T4 lesions a total parotidectomy (16) with an extended temporal bone resection is the treatment of choice.

Extended temporal bone resections

Extension of the resection to include dura, brain, parotid, ascending ramus and head of the mandible, and infratemporal fossa plus or minus the ICA (8,9,41,42), is possible but greatly increases the morbidity of the surgical procedure (5,6,8,56). An extended resection, however, with total temporal bone removal, and inclusion of the surrounding structures, including parotid gland, head and ascending ramus of mandible, local venous sinuses, lower cranial nerves, and supraomohyoid neck dissection followed by radiation has shown improved survival rates for recurrent and advanced de novo squamous cancer of the temporal bone (6,41,42) (Fig. 21.8).

RECONSTRUCTION

Extended temporal bone surgical resection leaves a large triangular composite defect with many different tissue types to be reconstructed (41,42). Lateral temporal bone resection will still leave a large defect in view of the necessary sacrifice of the pinna, which needs to be excised with a margin of healthy tissue in an 8 × 3 × 6-cm oval (41,42). The depth or medial extent of the defect will obviously be less than that of a total or extended temporal bone resection but nonetheless the defect to be reconstructed is considerable. Each reconstructive situation is unique and careful pre- and intraoperative consideration of the reconstructive options is needed (57).

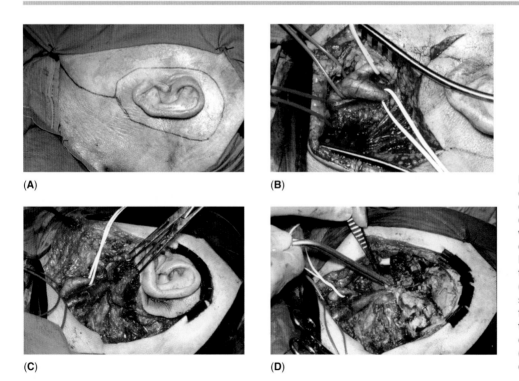

(A) (B) (C) (D)

Figure 21.8 (A) Incision marked out for extended temporal bone excision. (B) First step is to place colored slings around the great vessels in order to ensure vascular control and identify cranial nerves IX, X, XI, and XII prior to completing the supra-omohyoid neck dissection. (C) Wide access and good visualisation of the jugular and carotid foramina and skull base is essential before completing the en bloc extended temporal bone excision. (D) View of the large defect on completion of the resection.

Major issues of cosmesis, the durability of the repair particularly post-irradiation, and the detection of recurrent tumor need to be taken into account. Watertight closure of the CSF pathways is essential to avoid meningitis. Vascularized (57–61) or revascularized free flaps (62–64) are commonly used and satisfy most of the demands for reconstruction. Commonly used flaps include local and regional rotation flaps, and free tissue flaps. The utilitarian scalp rotation (Fig. 21.9) and nape flaps have a good blood supply and may be indicated in the elderly where the duration of

the procedure is important in reducing risk. Vascularized pedicled flaps including latissimus dorsi and trapezius flaps (57,60) (Fig. 21.10A, B) have been used. The Chinese free forearm flap based on the distal radial artery has been used, but the modified Chinese flap just distal to the antecubital fossa and based on the recently described anterior cubital artery (62) (Fig. 21.11) is a more useful flap; it is larger and has been employed very successfully. In recent years free lateral upper arm and thigh flaps have been used when possible. Free lateral upper arm flaps are used in

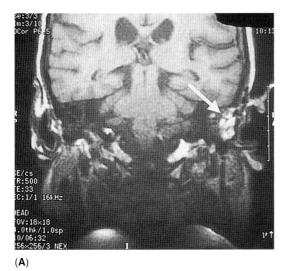

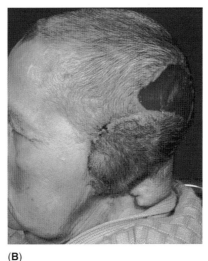

(A)   (B)

Figure 21.9 (A) Coronal T1-weighted MRI scan showing extensive SCC of left temporal bone (white arrow); (B) shows the patient postoperatively following a total temporal bone resection and scalp rotation flap.

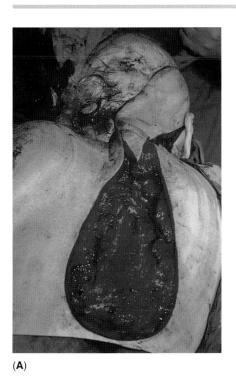

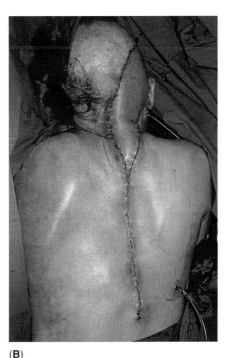

(A)   (B)

Figure 21.10 (A) Trapezius vascular pedicled flap, raised and inserted to cover defect; (B) immediately postoperatively.

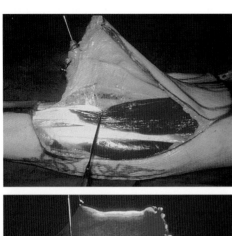

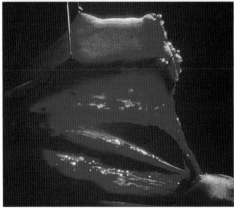

(A)

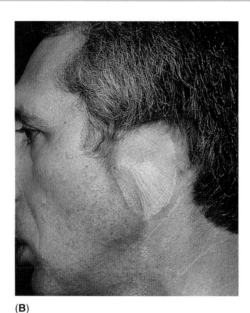

(B)

Figure 21.11 Modified Chinese free flap based on the anterior cubital artery. **(A)** This flap is larger and more useful than the flap based on the distal radial artery. **(B)** The good cosmetic result can be seen 2 years later.

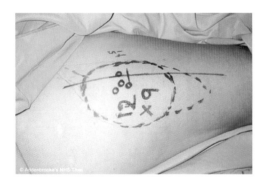

Figure 21.12 Free antero-lateral thigh flap marked out pre-operatively. *Source:* From *Squamous cell carcinoma of the temporal bone: current evidence for radiotherapy alone and surgery with postoperative radiotherapy.* In *Recent Advances in Otolaryngology 8*; David A. Moffat, James Keir and Holger Sudhoff, Royal Society of Medicine Publishers, 2008.

females since there is enough subcutaneous fat to be able to close the defect primarily obviating the need for split skin grafting of the donor site. In the male there is little subcutaneous fat and, therefore, the upper lateral thigh flap is used (57,64) (Fig. 21.12).

REHABILITATION

Following surgery patients may be left with several problems that require rehabilitation. The cosmetic appearance and residual neurological deficits need to be carefully assessed. Adequate consideration needs to be given to the psychological and nutritional state of the patient recovering from major surgery. Much of the management of neurological deficits is supportive as most defects become functionally compensated with time.

Vertigo resulting from labyrinthectomy is transient, with compensation occurring within a few weeks. Loss of hearing is rarely a major problem as the hearing thresholds in the contralateral ear are usually within normal limits. A BICROS hearing aid can be used with a prosthetic pinna.

Early postoperative management of facial weakness resulting from facial nerve resection aims to provide corneal protection. Initial treatment with lubricant ointment such as Lacrilube and the provision of a clear eye shield at night and artificial tears during the day provides adequate corneal protection. Medium term but temporary corneal protection results from the partial ptosis produced with botulinum toxin injection to the orbicularis oculus. Tarsorrhaphy or insertion of a gold weight to the upper tarsal plate provides longer term corneal protection. For permanent facial weakness a variety of facial nerve procedures, including grafting, and static or dynamic muscle, nerve, and tendon transfers can be used (65,66).

Laryngeal function may be severely compromised by acute loss of the lower cranial nerves IX, X, XI and XII, and further exacerbated by facial nerve palsy. This may result in oral incompetence, hypoglossal palsy—causing poor tongue control—and mandibular resection interfering directly with mastication. Marked dysphagia due to a palsy of the glossopharyngeal nerve will produce pooling of saliva in the ipsilateral pyriform fossa with spillover into the larynx and the concomitant risk of aspiration pneumonia. In the early postoperative phase nutrition is provided with alimentary feeds via a nasogastric tube or percutaneous endoscopic gastrostomy. As control of swallowing improves an oral diet of varying consistency can be introduced. A few patients do not gain full laryngeal compensation and aspiration continues to be a major problem. Speech improves greatly with compensation of the contralateral vocal cord, which may swing over the midline, particularly in young patients. Dysphonia tends to increase during the day but vocal quality may be acceptable. In many patients, however, the dysphonia warrants injection of the vocal fold with fat (temporary) or Teflon (permanent), or medialization of the vocal cord with thyroplasty surgery.

Consideration needs to be given to cosmesis in these patients. Provision of a hair piece may be useful in disguising the operated area particularly after scalp rotation flaps where there is a defect of the scalp that will require split skin grafting. A customized plastic pinna carefully constructed and attached to the flap with tissue adhesive has found favor with many patients in order to improve cosmesis (Fig. 21.13). Rarely is there enough surrounding bone remaining to attach osseointegrated titanium posts but if there is, consideration should be given to attaching a titanium bar (Fig. 21.14) to which the plastic pinna prosthesis can be fixed. This is a clearly more robust alternative to tissue adhesive.

THE ROLE OF RADIOTHERAPY IN TEMPORAL BONE CANCER

Radiotherapy can be given with one of three aims: as single-modality curative treatment, as a part of combined modality treatment, or with palliative intent.

Curative Radiotherapy

Although radiotherapy alone is adequate treatment for early lesions of the pinna, it is generally accepted that radiotherapy as a definitive single modality treatment is inadequate treatment for squamous carcinoma of the external auditory canal and middle ear, and for advanced lesions (10,67).

Combined Treatment

In most centers radiotherapy is given as part of a planned combined treatment with surgery regardless of the extent of the tumor or the status of tumor-free margins (67,68). Commonly used regimes are planned with fields to include the local area of resection and regional nodal groups. Dosage regimens depend on the tolerance of the surrounding tissues to radiation. Total dosages vary from 5000 cGy in 20 fractions over four weeks, to 6000–7000 cGy in 30–35 fractions over six to seven weeks. Complications of irradiation include otitis externa, cartilage necrosis, hearing loss, facial weakness, brain softening and osteoradionecrosis. Postoperative irradiation following an extended temporal bone resection has produced encouraging survival results in advanced and

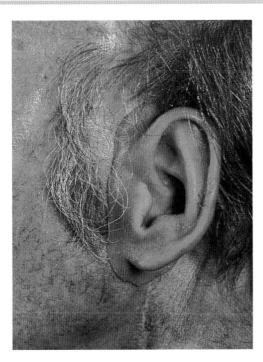

Figure 21.13 Customized prosthetic pinna attached with tissue adhesive provides good cosmesis.

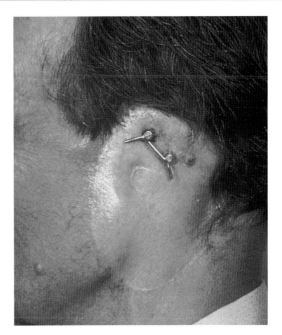

Figure 21.14 Osseointegrated titanium posts allow the fixation of a titanium bar to which a prosthetic pinna can be attached more securely. Unfortunately owing to the extensive nature of the surgery necessitated in SCC of the temporal bone this is rarely possible.

recurrent cancer (6,41,42). This can be administered even in those patients who have received pre-operative radiotherapy as sole or part primary treatment; the extended temporal bone resection removes the previously irradiated field (41,42).

PALLIATION
Surgical Palliation
In view of the difficulty in assessing the extent of an SCC of the temporal bone preoperatively—namely the likely underestimate of the size and degree of infiltration on imaging—it may not be possible to completely excise the lesion even with extended temporal bone resection. Some surgeons, therefore, are of the opinion that surgery is not indicated for advanced lesions. The results that have been achieved with ETBR and postoperative radiotherapy would be justification for radical surgical treatment and indeed there is an argument for ETBR as a palliative procedure to obviate bone pain and lessen the likelihood of tumor fungation.

Palliative Radiotherapy
Palliation aims to control the distressing symptoms of pain, discharge, and bleeding. Debulking the tumor will increase the likelihood of successful palliation with radiotherapy. The efficacy of radiotherapy in controlling these symptoms is not known and may not be superior to simple treatments of adequate analgesics and aural toilet.

Radiotherapy given as treatment for glomus tumors decreases the vascularity of the tumors and commonly halts their growth. It is effective treatment for decreasing the pulsatile tinnitus.

Role of Chemotherapy
Chemotherapy has not been used successfully in SCC of the temporal bone, but topical 5-fluorouracil may have a place in the palliation of fungating tumors. Cryotherapy with a liquid nitrogen spray has also been used for palliation of fungating tumors.

PROGNOSIS AND OUTCOME

It is difficult to meaningfully compare the treatment outcome of temporal bone malignancy for several reasons. Temporal bone malignancy is so rare that no one center has extensive experience with treatment. Lack of universally accepted staging systems and the wide variety of treatment protocols applied make comparison of results difficult. No prospective study comparing different treatment protocols has been carried out as yet. Despite these limitations, an analysis of the previously reported outcomes of 144 cases of temporal bone cancer by Prasad and Janecka (69) allows broad generalizations concerning the nature of temporal bone cancer and its treatment to be reached.

The local extent of tumor at diagnosis is an important prognostic indicator. In most studies the cure rate is high when the disease remains lateral to the tympanic membrane. When disease is detected early and limited to the external canal a lateral temporal bone resection can be performed. More extensive disease extending into the middle ear and surrounding structures including dura, brain, pterygoid muscles, otic capsule, and carotid carries a worse prognosis and hence surgery must be tailored to the disease stage. Review of the literature by Prasad and Janecka (69) demonstrated when disease had extended into the middle ear a lateral temporal bone resection offered a 28.7% survival whereas a more extensive subtotal temporal bone resection had a 41.7% five-year survival. More recently the cure rates for T3 and T4 tumors are reported between 35–47% (41,42). This highlights the importance of aggressive en bloc resection.

Moffat (6) in an early review in 1997 reported his data on 15 patients who underwent either a lateral temporal bone resection or for more advanced disease extended temporal bone resection. He achieved an overall outcome of 47.5% five-year survival. A more recent review in 2005 (41) of 39 patients revealed that survival for stage I and II disease was 100% and for stage III and IV disease was 43% (41). This again demonstrated the increased survival of early stage disease and the importance of early diagnosis and aggressive surgical management.

Moffat (41,42) and Moody (70) both recommend an en bloc resection and Moody proposes that a prospective protocol be developed in which each skull base unit follows a progression of treatment that is specific for each stage of the disease based on a consistent staging system. For early lesions a modified temporal bone resection or a lateral temporal bone resection (LTBR) is performed, with more advanced lesions a subtotal temporal bone resection (STBR) or a total temporal bone resection (TTBR) should be the treatment of choice. Moffat takes a more aggressive approach than this and states that the minimal procedure for disease lateral to the tympanic membrane should be a LTBR and superficial parotidectomy. For T3 and T4 disease an extended temporal bone resection and total parotidectomy with facial nerve sacrifice offers the greatest chance of cure (41,42).

Local recurrence is the most common sequel of treatment failure (83%), followed by locoregional failure (9%), regional failure alone (5.5%) and distant metastasis associated with regional failure (2%) (73). Half the recurrences are in the first 12 months following treatment, and 85% of recurrences occur within three years of treatment (74). Recent evidence suggests that treatment for advanced and recurrent cancer in the form of extended temporal bone resection and postoperative radiotherapy results in improved five-year survival rates of 47% (6). In this study all recurrences occurred within the first 12 months after treatment implying that for salvage surgery if the patient survives a year then there is a high chance of cure.

Specific Outcome Issues
Nodal Disease
Twenty-three percent of the 39 patients in Moffat's series (41,42) had nodal disease at presentation, confirmed by histology following a Crile's radical neck dissection. This was the most significant prognostic indicator in his series as survival in this group at two years was 0%. Death was always due to local recurrence and hence these authors believe that nodal disease is a good indicator of aggressive disease.

Histology
Undifferentiated tumors had a poorer prognostic outcome than moderately and well-differentiated tumors in all the

series reviewed (41,42). This is consistent with previous reports in the literature. Positive histological margins at the time of resection, not surprisingly, are a poor prognostic indicator in this locally aggressive disease. Death in these patients usually occurs within 12 months.

Dural and Cerebral Involvement

Dural involvement has always indicated a poor prognosis and Gillespie again supported this. In Moffat's series (41) dural involvement alone was not a significant prognostic indicator. Brain involvement is usually associated with a poor outcome. One patient, however, remains alive 11 years after an extended temporal bone resection and a partial temporal lobe resection.

Carotid Invasion

Invasion of the carotid artery signifies extensive disease progression. Both Gillespie (71) and Moffat no longer consider carotid resection. In the series described by Moffat of the seven patients with perivascular involvement of the carotid only one is alive at a follow up of six months. Gillespie (71) reports two patients with carotid involvement both of whom have died of their disease within months of treatment. Moody (70) successfully resected the carotid in one patient who is still alive, but no comment was made with regards to neurological status in this case.

De Novo Versus Salvage

Moffat analysed his patients according to their previous management. If they had undergone any treatment at another institution then further treatment was considered salvage. Those patients with no previous treatment were defined as de novo cases. Although the numbers were too small to make any statistical analysis the trend showed poorer outcomes for the salvage patients with a comparable stage of disease. This would support the concept that the first treatment protocol offers the greatest chance of cure and should be aggressive.

Radiation-associated Tumor (RAT)

Lim (72) reviewed 18 patients with radiation-associated tumors. Of these 83% had SCC. This was not statistically significant, but the trend was for the RAT to have a poorer prognosis. There was a statistical significance in their disease-free survival period.

Quality of Life

There has been limited work on patient perceived outcomes of what is often referred to as debilitating and disfiguring surgery. Kwok (75) has reported on a series of patients of whom a large number had undergone temporal bone resection for carcinoma. His patients retrospectively underwent a quality of life assessment. The cure rates were comparable with those in the world literature. Kwok (75) reports that "quality of life may be affected when the patients' condition is severe enough to cause ongoing physical symptoms, communication difficulties and social disturbances: yet for many patients poorer form and function are not invariably associated with poorer quality of life."

SUMMARY OF NON-SQUAMOUS CELL CARCINOMA LESIONS

Epithelial Carcinoma

Basal cell carcinoma (BCC) is the most common cutaneous malignancy. It has a propensity for deep local invasion and perineural spread with metastases being rare. Primary melanoma of the temporal bone is extremely rare with a very poor prognosis. Glandular tumors are one of three types: adenoid cystic, adenocarcinoma, or mucoepidermoid. Adenoid cystic carcinomas are the most common glandular tumors (76,77). Adenocarcinomas are usually well-differentiated low-grade papillary cancers (78) that arise from the middle ear mucosa or possibly endolymphatic sac (79). The long-term prognosis for high-grade adenocarcinoma and mucoepidermoid carcinoma is poor. In contrast, survival after adenoid cystic carcinoma can be lengthy even in the presence of metastases (76,81–83).

Chondrosarcoma

Chondrosarcoma of the temporal bone is extremely rare. These tumors may be indolent and present late. They tend to invade locally and metastasize late. They may extend outside the temporal bone and into the cerebellopontine angle. Radical surgery and postoperative radiotherapy is the treatment of choice.

Rhabdomyosarcoma

These are rare aggressive tumors almost exclusively limited to childhood age groups. Only 100 cases of rhabdomyosarcoma (RMS) of the ear were reported to 1975 (84,85). The mean age at presentation is five years (86). Until recently the prognosis has been extremely poor, but following the multimodality treatment (surgical resection, followed by radiotherapy and chemotherapy) protocol recommended by The Intergroup Rhabdomyosarcoma Study Committee treatment outcomes have greatly improved (87). Mean survival from diagnosis is 2.8 years and 11 of 24 patients were alive at five years (88). Recurrent sarcoma tends to spread early to the lungs and bone, and intracranially to involve multiple cranial nerves.

Benign/Malignant Glomus Tumors

The incidence of large benign glomus tumors (Fisch types B,C,D) is 1 per 1.3 million of the population (89). Ten percent are of multicentric origin (90). Rarely do they metastasize to local lymph nodes and to distant sites, or are frankly malignant. Malignant glomus tumors are extremely rare and occur 40 times less frequently than benign lesions (1 per 52 million population) (89). Glomus jugulare tumors are twice as common in females as in males. Although they are usually non-chromaffin paragangliomata with no endocrine function there has been an increasing number of reports of vasoactive tumors and it is important to carry out a urinary assay of the metabolites dopamine and 3-methoxy-4-hydroxy mandelic acid (vanillylmandelic acid [VMA]: normal up to 7 mg per 24 hours).

Surgery is the primary treatment since other modalities will not eradicate the tumor and are not curative. Standard otological approaches for glomus tumors arising in the middle ear cleft are adequate. Small glomus tympanicum tumors can be excised permeatally after raising a Rosen's flap and a KTP laser assists control of the vascular pedicle. Larger tympanicum tumors should be approached via an extended facial recess approach so that adequate control of the jugular bulb can be achieved. For larger tumors arising from the jugular bulb region, a combination of otological and skull-base techniques is necessary to gain control of the carotid artery and sigmoid-jugular complex. The trans- and infratemporal fossa approach is very satisfactory (89). The major postoperative problems arise from possible loss of cranial nerve function (VII, IX, X, XI, and XII may be affected in varying degrees), and facial paralysis, laryngeal dysfunction, aspiration, and CSF leak. These complications can lead to considerable morbidity. Large glomus jugulare tumors in young people are more aggressive and have a propensity to recur. In this group postoperative radiotherapy is indicated. It may also be necessary if there is doubt about the totality of the surgical excision. Careful regular and prolonged follow-up is mandatory.

External beam radiation as a primary treatment modality is effective in reducing the growth rate and vascularity of glomus tumors, and can be used as palliative therapy in those unfit for surgery. It may slow down or stop the tumor from growing. Most commonly relieved symptoms are tinnitus, vertigo, bleeding and pain (75). Hearing loss and cranial nerve function rarely change. Moderate dosages are effective, 3500 cGy over 3 weeks, with response rates being between 75% and 100% (91–93). Osteoradionecrosis of the temporal bone may ensue in varying degrees in the longer term as a result of the endarteritis obliterans produced by the radiation. In its mildest and most common form this is just an otitis externa, but rarely extensive necrosis of the temporal bone can occur with sequestrum formation.

Carotid arteriography and embolization with coils and feathers is a useful adjunct to surgery and should be performed two or three days preoperatively. Substantial reduction in intraoperative blood loss can be achieved with a reduced operative risk of diffuse intravascular coagulopathy. Embolization as a stand alone procedure may be considered to control growth rate and ameliorate troublesome symptoms such as pulsatile tinnitus. The outcome of combined embolization and radiotherapy is uncertain at the present time.

Benign Destructive Lesions (Giant Cell Tumors, Fibro-osseous Dysplasia and Paget's Disease)

A wide range of benign neoplasms and non-neoplastic destructive lesions can present with symptoms mimicking temporal bone cancer. These conditions rarely involve the otic capsule and a wide margin of normal bone or soft tissue is not required. Surgical principles in these situations must be individualized but aim to preserve the otic capsule and facial nerve. Conventional surgical approaches developed for inflammatory ear disease are applicable.

Metastases

These may be asymptomatic and discovered incidentally as a solitary or multiple solid temporal bone lesions. Metastases to the EAC (10,43,44) and middle ear have been reported. They present as conductive hearing loss due to eustachian tube dysfunction or involvement of the ossicular chain or

tympanic membrane. Treatment must be individualized and is generally palliative. Localized radiotherapy or chemotherapy appropriate to tumor type may be beneficial.

REFERENCES

1. Conley JJ, Novack AJ. The surgical treatment of tumour of the ear and temporal bone. Arch Otolaryngol 1960; 71: 635–52.
2. Campbell E, Volk BM, Burkland CW. Total resection of the temporal bone for malignancy of the middle ear. Ann Surg 1951; 134: 397–404.
3. Ward GE, Loch WE, Lawrence W. Radical operation for carcinoma of the external auditory canal and middle ear. Am J Surg 1951; 82: 169–78.
4. Parsons H, Lewis JS. Subtotal resection of the temporal bone for malignancy of the middle ear. Cancer 1954; 7: 995–1001.
5. Hilding DA, Selker R. Total resection of the temporal bone for carcinoma. Arch Otolaryngol 1969; 89: 636–45.
6. Moffat DA, Grey P, Ballagh RH et al. Extended temporal bone resection for squamous cell carcinoma. Otolaryngol Head Neck Surg 1997; 116: 617–23.
7. Fisch U, Fagan P, Valavanis A. The infratemporal fossa approach for the lateral skull base. Otolaryngol Clin North Am 1984; 17: 513–52.
8. Graham MD, Sataloff RT, Kemink JL et al. Total en bloc resection of the temporal bone and carotid artery for malignant tumors of the ear and temporal bone. Laryngoscope 1984; 94: 528–33.
9. Sataloff RT, Myers DL, Lowry LD et al. Total temporal bone resection for squamous cell carcinoma. Otolaryngol Head Neck Surg 1987; 96: 4–14.
10. Crabtree JA, Britton BH, Pierce MK. Carcinoma of the external auditory canal. Laryngoscope 1976; 86: 405–15.
11. Spector JG. Management of temporal bone carcinomas: a therapeutic analysis of two groups of patients and long-term follow-up. Otolaryngol Head Neck Surg 1991; 104: 58–66.
12. Morton RP, Stell PM, Derrick PP. Epidemiology of cancer of the middle ear cleft. Cancer 1984; 53: 1612–17.
13. Lewis JS. Cancer of the ear: a report of 150 cases. Laryngoscope 1960; 70: 551–79.
14. Conley JJ. Cancer of the middle ear and temporal bone. N Y State J Med 1974; 74: 1575–9.
15. Kinney SE, Wood BG. Malignancies of the external ear canal and temporal bone: surgical techniques and results. Laryngoscope 1987; 97: 158–64.
16. Kuhel WI, Hume CR, Selesnick SH. Cancer of the external auditory canal and temporal bone. Otolaryngol Clin North Am 1996; 29: 827–52.
17. Johns ME, Headington JT. Squamous cell carcinoma of the external auditory canal. A clinico-pathologic study of 20 cases. Arch Otolaryngol 1974; 100: 45–9.
18. Nager G. Adenocarcinoma of the middle ear. In: Pathology of the Ear and Temporal Bone. Baltimore: Williams and Wilkins, 1993.
19. Austin JR, Stewart KL, Fawzi N. Squamous cell carcinoma of the external auditory canal. Therapeutic prognosis based on a proposed staging system. Arch Otolaryngol Head Neck Surg 1994; 120: 1228–32.
20. Lustig LR, Jackler RK, Lanser MJ. Radiation-induced tumours of the temporal bone. Am J Otol 1997; 18: 230–5.
21. Goh YH, Chong VF, Low WK. Temporal bone tumours in patients irradiated for nasopharyngeal neoplasm. J Laryngol and Otol 1999; 113: 222–8.
22. Beal DD, Lindsay JR, Ward PH. Radiation induced carcinoma of the mastoid. Arch Otolaryngol 1965; 81.
23. Rubin RJ, Thaler SU, Holzer N. Radiation induced carcinoma of the temporal bone. Laryngoscope 1977; 87: 1613–21.

24. Monem SA, Moffat DA, Frampton MC. Carcinoma of the ear: a case report of a possible association with chlorinated disinfectants. J Laryngol Otol 1999 Nov; 113: 1004–7.

25. Nelms CR Jr, Paparella MM. Early external auditory canal tumors. Laryngoscope 1968; 78: 986–1001.

26. Conley J, Schuller DE. Malignancies of the ear. Laryngoscope 1976; 86: 1147–63.

27. Krespi YP, Levine TM. Management of tumours of the temporal bone. In: Alberti PW, Rubin RJ, eds. Otologic Surgery and Medicine. New York: Churchill Livingstone, 1988; 1409–22.

28. Procter B, Lindsay JR. Tumours involving the petrous pyramid of the temporal bone. Arch Otolaryngol 1947; 46: 180–94.

29. Fries JW. The roentgen features of fibrous dysplasia of the skull and facial bones. A critical analysis. Ther Nucl Medi 1957; 77: 71–88.

30. Nager GT, Kennedy DW, Kopstein E. Fibrous dysplasia: a review of the disease and its manifestations in the temporal bone. Ann Otol Rhinol Laryngol Suppl 1982; 92: 1–52.

31. Lambert PR, Brackmann DE. Fibrous dysplasia of the temporal bone: the use of computerised tomography. Otolaryngol Head Neck Surg 1984; 92: 461–67.

32. Mattucci KF, Setzen M, Galantich P. Necrotizing otitis externa occurring concurrently with epidermoid carcinoma. Laryngoscope 1986; 96: 264–6.

33. Al Shihabi BA. Carcinoma of temporal bone presenting as malignant otitis externa. J Laryngol Otol 1992; 106: 908–10.

34. Grandis JR, Hirsch BE, Yu VL. Simultaneous presentation of malignant external otitis and temporal bone cancer. Arch Otolaryngol Head Neck Surg 1993; 119: 687–9.

35. Michaels L, Wells M. Squamous cell carcinoma of the middle ear. Clin Otolaryngol 1980; 5: 235–48.

36. Jesse RH, Goepfert H, Lindberg RD et al. Combined intra-arterial infusion and radiotherapy for the treatment of advanced cancer of the head and neck. Am J Roentgenol Radium Ther Nucl Med 1969; 105: 20–5.

37. Pensak ML, Willging JP. Tumours of the temporal bone. In: Jackler RK, Brackmann DE, eds. Neurotology. St Louis: Mosby, 1994; 1049–57.

38. Arena S, Keen M. Carcinoma of the middle ear and temporal bone. Am J Otol 1988; 9: 351–6.

39. Arriaga M, Curtin HD, Takahashi H et al. The role of preoperative CT scans in staging external auditory meatus carcinoma: radiologic-pathologic correlation study. Otolaryngol Head Neck Surg 1991; 105: 6–11.

40. Hahn SS, Kim JA, Goodchild N et al. Carcinoma of the middle ear and external auditory canal. Int J Radiat Oncol Biol Phys 1983; 9: 1003–7.

41. Moffat DA, Wagstaff SA, Hardy DG. The outcome of radical surgery and postoperative radiotherapy for squamous carcinoma of the temporal bone Laryngoscope 2005 Feb; 115: 341–7.

42. Moffat DA, Wagstaff SA. Squamous cell carcinoma of the temporal bone. Curr Opin Otolaryngol Head and Neck Surg 2003; 11: 107–11.

43. Sadek SA, Dixon NW, Hardcastle PF. Metastatic carcinoma of the external auditory meatus secondary to carcinoma of the rectum. A case report. J Laryngol Otol 1983; 97: 459–64.

44. Goldman NC, Hutchison RE, Goldman MS. Metastatic renal cell carcinoma of the external auditory canal. Otolaryngol Head Neck Surg 1992; 106: 410–11.

45. Imamura S, Murakami Y. Secondary malignant tumors of the temporal bone. A histopathologic study and review of the world literature. Nippon Jibiinkoka Gakkai Kaiho 1991; 94: 924–37.

46. Dehner LP, Chen KT. Primary tumors of the external and middle ear. III. A clinico-pathologic study of embryonal rhabdomyosarcoma. Arch Otolaryngol 1978; 104: 399–403.

47. Tefft M, Fernandez C, Donaldson M et al. Incidence of meningeal involvement by rhabdomyosarcoma of the head and neck in children: a report of the Intergroup Rhabdomyosarcoma Study (IRS). Cancer 1978; 42: 253–8.

48. Leonetti JP, Smith PG, Kletzker GR et al. Invasion patterns of advanced temporal bone malignancies. Am J Otol 1996; 17: 438–42.

49. Grossman CB, ed. The temporal region. In: Magnetic Resonance Imaging and Computed Tomography of the Head and Spine. Baltimore: Williams and Wilkins, 1990; 281–307.

50. Yousem DM, Som PM, Hackney DB et al. Central nodal necrosis and extracapsular neoplastic spread in cervical lymph nodes: MR imaging versus CT. Radiology 1992; 182: 753–9.

51. Stell PM, McCormick MS. Carcinoma of the external auditory meatus and middle ear. Prognostic factors and a suggested staging system. J Laryngol Otol 1985; 99: 847–50.

52. Clark LJ, Narula AA, Morgan DA et al. Squamous carcinoma of the temporal bone: a revised staging. J Laryngol Otol 1991; 105: 346–8.

53. Arriaga M, Curtin H, Takahashi H. Staging proposal for external auditory meatus carcinoma based on preoperative clinical examination and computed tomography findings. Ann Otol Rhinol Laryngol 1990; 99: 714–21.

54. Hirsch, BE. Staging system revision. Arch Otolaryngol Head Neck Surg 2002; 128: 93–4.

55. Shih L, Crabtree JA. Carcinoma of the external auditory canal: an update. Laryngoscope 1990; 100: 1215–18.

56. Gacek RR, Goodman M. Management of malignancy of the temporal bone. Laryngoscope 1977; 87: 1622–34.

57. Moncrieff MD, Hamilton SA, Lamberty GH et al. Reconstructive options after temporal bone resection for squamous cell carcinoma. J Plast Reconstr Aesthet Surg 2007; 60: 607–14. Epub 2007 Jan 31.

58. McGregor IA, Jackson IT. The extended role of the deltopectoral flap. Br J Plast Surg 1970; 23: 173–85.

59. Bakamjian VY, Long M, Rigg B. Experience with the medially based deltopectoral flap in reconstructive surgery of the head and neck. Br J Plast Surg 1971; 24: 174–83.

60. McCraw JB, Magee WP Jr, Kalwaic H. Uses of the trapezius and sternomastoid myocutaneous flaps in head and neck reconstruction. Plast Reconstr Surg 1979; 63: 49–57.

61. Ariyan S, Cuono CB. Myocutaneous flaps for head and neck reconstruction. Head Neck Surg 1980; 2: 321–45.

62. Lamberty BGH, Cormack GC. The ante-cubital fasciocutaneous flap. Br J Plast Surg 1983; 36: 428–33.

63. Jones NF, Schramm VL, Sekhar LN. Reconstruction of the cranial base following tumour resection. Br J Plast Surg 1987; 40: 155–62.

64. Malata CM, Tehrani H, Kumiponjera D et al. Use of anterolateral thigh and lateral arm fasciocutaneous free flaps in lateral skull base reconstruction. Ann Plast Surg 2006; 57: 169–75.

65. May M. Facial reanimation after skull base trauma. Am J Otol 1985; Suppl: 62–7.

66. May M, Croxson GR, Klein SR. Bell's palsy: management of sequelae using EMG rehabilitation, botulinum toxin, and surgery. Am J Otol 1989; 10: 220–9.

67. Lederman M. Malignant tumours of the ear. J Laryngol Otol 1965; 79: 85–119.

68. Wang CC. Radiation therapy in the management of carcinoma of the external auditory canal, middle ear, or mastoid. Radiology 1975; 116: 713–15.

69. Prasad S, Janecka IP. Efficacy of surgical treatments for squamous cell carcinoma of the temporal bone: a literature review. Otolaryngol Head Neck Surg 1994; 110: 270–80.

70. Moody SA, Hirsch BE, Myers EN. Squamous cell carcinoma of the external auditory canal: an evaluation of a staging system. Am J Otol 2000; 21: 582–8.

71. Gillepsie MB, Francis HW, Chee N et al. Squamous cell carcinoma of the temporal bone: a radiographic-pathologic correlation. Arch Otolaryngol Head Neck Surg 2001 Jul; 127: 803–7.

72. Lim LH, Goh YH, Chan M et al. Malignancy of the temporal bone and external auditory canal. Otolaryngol Head Neck Surg 2000; 122: 882.

73. Prasad S, Janecka IP. Malignancies of the temporal bone-radical temporal bone resection. In: Brackmann DE, ed. Otologic Surgery. Philadelphia: WB Saunders, 1994; 49–62.

74. Harwood AR, Keane TJ. Malignant tumours of the temporal bone and external ear: medical and radiation therapy. In: Alberti PW, Rubin RJ, eds. Otologic Surgery and Medicine. New York: Churchill Livingston, 1988; 1389–408.

75. Kwok HC, Morton RP, Chaplin JM et al. Quality of life after parotid and temporal bone surgery for cancer. Laryngoscope 2002 May; 112: 820–3.

76. Pulec JL. Glandular tumors of the external auditory canal. Laryngoscope 1977; 87: 1601–12.

77. Perzin KH, Gullane P, Conley J. Adenoid cystic carcinoma involving the external auditory canal. A clinico-pathologic study of 16 cases. Cancer 1982; 50: 2873–83.

78. Glasscock ME III, McKennan KX, Levine SC et al. Primary adenocarcinoma of the middle ear and temporal bone. Arch Otolaryngol Head Neck Surg 1987; 113: 822–4.

79. Heffner DK. Low-grade adenocarcinoma of probable endolymphatic sac origin. A clinicopathologic study of 20 cases. Cancer 1989; 64: 2292–302.

80. Wetli CV, Pardo V, Millard M et al. Tumors of ceruminous glands. Cancer 1972; 29: 1169–78.

81. Dehner LP, Chen KT. Primary tumors of the external and middle ear. Benign and malignant glandular neoplasms. Arch Otolaryngol 1980; 106: 13–19.

82. Cannon CR, McLean WC. Adenoid cystic carcinoma of the middle ear and temporal bone. Otolaryngol Head Neck Surg 1983; 91: 96–9.

83. Hicks GW. Tumors arising from the glandular structures of the external auditory canal. Laryngoscope 1983; 93: 326–40.

84. Feldman BA. Rhabdomyosarcoma of the head and neck. Laryngoscope 1982; 92: 424–40.

85. Naufal PM. Primary sarcomas of the temporal bone. Arch Otolaryngol 1973; 98: 44–50.

86. Wiatrak BJ, Pensak ML. Rhabdomyosarcoma of the ear and temporal bone. Laryngoscope 1989; 99: 1188–92.

87. Raney RB Jr, Lawrence W Jr, Maurer HM et al. Rhabdomyosarcoma of the ear in childhood. A report from the Intergroup Rhabdomyosarcoma Study-I. Cancer 1983; 51: 2356–61.

88. Mandell LR. Ongoing progress in the treatment of childhood rhabdomyosarcoma [published erratum appears in Oncology (Huntingt) 1993 Mar; 7: 104]. Oncology (Huntingt) 1993; 7: 71–83.

89. Moffat DA, Hardy DG. Surgical management of large glomus jugulare tumours: infra- and trans-temporal approach. J Laryngol Otol 1989; 103: 1167–80.

90. Bickerstaff ER, Howell JS. The neurological importance of tumours of the glomus jugulare. Brain 1953; 76: 576–93.

91. Tidwell TJ, Montague ED. Chemodectomas involving the temporal bone. Radiology 1975; 116: 147–9.

92. Kim JA, Elkon D, Lim ML et al. Optimum dose of radiotherapy for chemodectomas of the middle ear. Int J Radiat Oncol Biol Phys 1980; 6: 815–19.

93. Wang CC. Paraganglioma of the head and neck. In: Radiation Therapy of Head and Neck Neoplasms. Boston: John Wright, 1983; 279.

22

Management of Thyroid Cancer

Ian Ganly, Nishant Agrawal, Robert M Tuttle, Snehal G Patel and Jatin P Shah

INTRODUCTION

Thyroid malignancy is the most common endocrine malignancy. The worldwide incidence of thyroid cancer is approximately 140,000 (1). Recently, in some regions of the world the incidence of thyroid cancer has been increasing. Evidence, however, supports that the increase in incidence appears to be due to improved detection rather than an increase in the true occurrence, and may reflect differences in access to healthcare (2).

Thyroid cancers encompass varied histologies ranging from the indolent, well-differentiated papillary thyroid cancer to the highly aggressive anaplastic carcinoma. The distinct tumor types are associated with characteristic epidemiological, clinical, and prognostic features. Unlike most head and neck tumors, thyroid cancer is more common in women and often follows a protracted natural history. The majority are differentiated carcinomas with a spectrum of papillary and follicular types that are unique in their potential for targeted therapy with radioactive ^{131}I. Cure can be achieved with surgery and adjuvant therapy but there is controversy regarding optimal treatment necessary to eradicate the disease and yet minimize potential morbidity.

Rarer tumors include medullary carcinoma arising from the parafollicular cells which is treated surgically, and thyroid lymphoma and aggressive anaplastic carcinoma, for which external beam radiotherapy and chemotherapy are of value. The thyroid may also be the site of metastases or may be invaded directly by squamous cell carcinoma of the hypopharynx or larynx.

SURGICAL ANATOMY

The thyroid gland develops from the pharyngeal pouch. It starts in the region of the foramen cecum at the base of the tongue and descends to the lower neck during embryogenesis. As the thyroid gland descends into the neck, it is associated with a tract called the thyroglossal duct. The thyroid gland lies within the pretracheal fascia in the anterior neck, and consists of two symmetrical pear-shaped lobes united in the midline by an isthmus that overlies the second to fourth tracheal rings (Fig. 22.1). There is often a pyramidal lobe, which may extend (usually to the left) up to the superior border of the thyroid cartilage. The thyroid gland is attached to the trachea and cricoid cartilage by Berry's ligament. This ligament is thickened pretracheal fascia with several coursing veins.

Anatomical variations (3,4) include absence of one of the lobes (0.03%) or the isthmus (0.02%), and ectopic thyroid tissue in the posterior tongue (lingual thyroid 0.02%), anywhere along the course of the thyroglossal tract (0.01%), or in other sites (0.01%). These less common sites include the larynx, trachea (5), and mediastinum. Very rarely ectopic thyroid may represent the only existing thyroid tissue. Malignant change most commonly occurs in the gland itself but may develop in ectopic sites. Thyroid tissue found in cervical lymph nodes (lateral aberrant thyroid) is almost invariably metastatic from an occult, well-differentiated thyroid carcinoma.

Vascular Supply

The arterial supply to the thyroid gland (4) is from the superior thyroid artery (the first branch of the external carotid artery) and the inferior thyroid artery (from the thyrocervical trunk of the subclavian artery). The venous drainage is through three veins, the superior, middle, and inferior thyroid veins. The superior and middle thyroid veins drain into the internal jugular vein and the inferior thyroid vein into the brachiocephalic vein. An intimate knowledge of the anatomical course, relations, and variations of the superior and inferior thyroid pedicles is essential for safe thyroid surgery (Fig. 22.2).

Recurrent Laryngeal Nerve

The recurrent laryngeal nerves innervate the intrinsic laryngeal musculature, except the cricothyroid muscle. In addition, the nerves also provide sensory innervation to the glottic larynx. The recurrent laryngeal nerves branch from the vagus low in the neck and descend into the superior mediastinum. On the left side the nerve loops around the ligamentum arteriosum at the level of the aortic arch and ascends in a more medial position toward the cricothyroid membrane. On the right side the nerve loops around the subclavian artery and ascends in a lateral to medial direction toward the tracheo-esophageal groove. At the lower pole of the thyroid gland the right recurrent laryngeal nerve is therefore slightly more lateral than on the left. On both sides, the nerve lies close to the branches of the inferior thyroid artery. In most cases the nerve lies posterior to the artery but several anatomical variations occur, including passing anterior to the artery or between the branches of the artery (Fig. 22.3). The nerve may also be non-recurrent in 0.3-08% of cases, more commonly on the right side traversing medially in a loop directly from

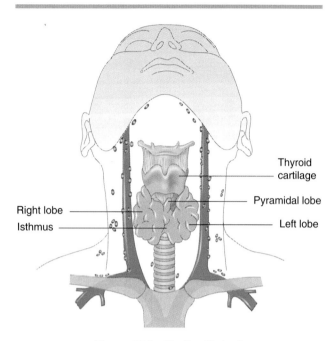

Figure 22.1   The thyroid gland.

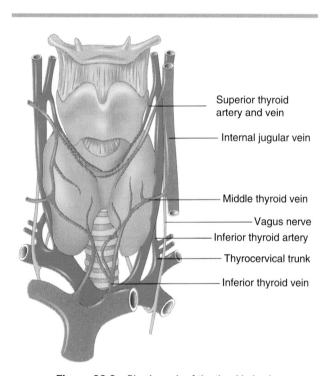

Figure 22.2   Blood supply of the thyroid gland.

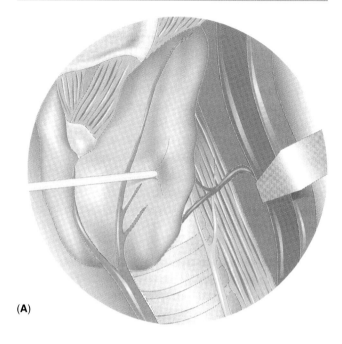

(A)

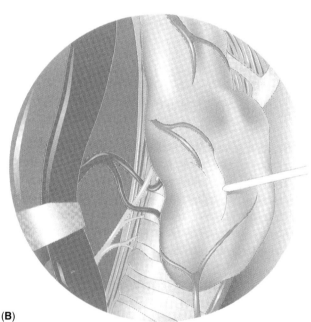

(B)

Figure 22.3   Relationship of the recurrent laryngeal nerve to the inferior thyroid artery. (A) Left side; (B) right side.

the vagus nerve (Fig. 22.4). This anomaly is associated with a retro-esophageal right subclavian artery.

The close anatomical relationship of the recurrent laryngeal nerve to the thyroid gland is clinically important because

1. Potential involvement of the nerve by thyroid tumors is a useful clinical and prognostic sign; laryngoscopy

should always be carried out either with a mirror or fiberoptic endoscope prior to any thyroid surgery to document vocal fold motion.

2. Paralysis of the nerve may or may not cause significant voice problems.

3. The risk to the nerve during thyroid surgery depends not only on the site and pathology of the tumor but also on the experience of the surgeon. The more common sites of injury are the area of Berry's ligament or the area where the nerve crosses the inferior thyroid artery (6).

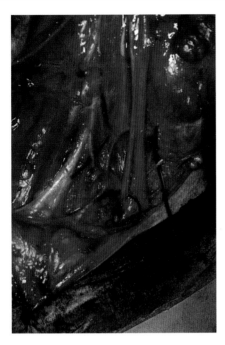

Figure 22.4 Non-recurrent recurrent laryngeal nerve (on the right side). Blue markers also identify the vagus and phrenic nerves.

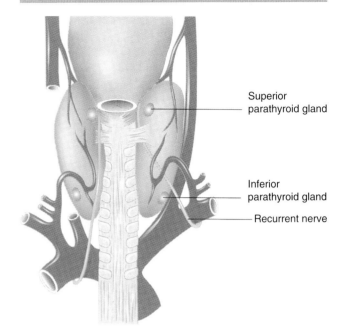

Figure 22.5 Common positions of the parathyroid glands.

Superior Laryngeal Nerve

The superior laryngeal nerve divides into an external and internal branch before entering the larynx. The external branch of the superior laryngeal nerve innervates the crico-thyroid muscle and lies posterior and medial to the superior laryngeal pedicle. This branch should be carefully identified and preserved when tying off the superior laryngeal artery and vein. It is particularly vulnerable with mass ligation of the superior pole. Damage to the nerve will cause alteration of the voice typically with loss of high pitch and deepening of tone due to loss of vocal cord tension control. The internal branch pierces the thyrohyoid membrane and provides sensory innervation to the supraglottic larynx.

Parathyroid Glands

There are four parathyroid glands, two superior and two inferior. The inferior parathyroid glands arise from the third branchial pouch and the superior parathyroid glands arise from the fourth branchial pouch. The relationship of the parathyroid glands to the thyroid is clinically important (Fig. 22.5). The superior glands are more consistent in location while the inferior glands are more variable. The blood supply to the parathyroid glands is predominantly from branches of the inferior thyroid artery. Every attempt should be made during surgery to identify and preserve some functioning parathyroid tissue and its respective blood supply. The anatomical relations are discussed in more detail elsewhere in this book.

Lymphatic Drainage

The thyroid gland has a rich lymphatic network (4), which connects freely between both lobes and drains into the

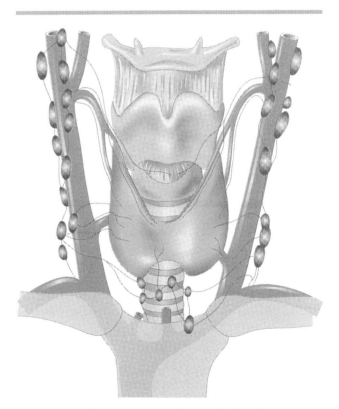

Figure 22.6 Lymphatic drainage of the thyroid gland.

following lymph node groups: pericapsular, pretracheal (delphian), tracheo-esophageal (paratracheal, level VI), deep cervical chain (levels II, III and IV), posterior triangle (level V, occipital and supraclavicular), retropharyngeal, and retro-esophageal (Fig. 22.6).

ENDOCRINOLOGY

Hormone Production

The production of the hormones thyroxine (T4) and triiodothyronine (T3) by the thyroid gland is regulated by the secretion of thyroid-stimulating hormone (TSH, thyrotropin) from the pituitary gland, which in turn is influenced by thyrotropin-releasing hormone (TRH) from the hypothalamus. TSH binds to receptors on the plasma membrane of thyroid epithelial cells. Through a signal transduction cascade, mediated by adenyl cyclase, cyclic AMP, and protein kinases, thyroid cell division, and hormone production are stimulated. T3 and T4 are then incorporated and stored as thyroglobulin (Tg) in the colloid. When released into the circulation, T3 and T4 are released from thyroglobulin and then exist in either a free form or bound form to thyroid hormone binding globulin. The level of T3 and T4 in the circulation then acts in a negative feedback loop to downregulate the level of TSH and TRH from the pituitary gland and hypothalamus, respectively. The levels of T3 and T4 can be measured in the blood by radioimmunoassay. As well as T3 and T4, the thyroid gland secretes another hormone called calcitonin. This is a hormone synthesized by the parafollicular cells of the thyroid gland.

Tumor Markers

Thyroglobulin is secreted by well-differentiated carcinoma cells and following total thyroidectomy, subsequent radioiodine ablation, and T4 suppression therapy, the Tg level should be undetectable. Tg assay during follow-up is therefore a helpful tumor marker. Increased levels are associated with tumor recurrence or metastases. In medullary thyroid carcinoma (MTC), which arises from the parafollicular cells, calcitonin also acts as a tumor marker following total thyroidectomy.

Growth Factors

Under normal conditions thyroid follicular cell activity is regulated by a number of extracellular growth factors that either stimulate or inhibit growth. They mediate their effects through receptors on the cell surface and also via a number of intracellular signal transduction pathways. Each step in the pathway is controlled genetically by a number of growth-promoting proto-oncogenes and growth-inhibiting tumor suppressor genes (7). The principle factors influencing thyroid growth are listed in Table 22.1.

EPIDEMIOLOGY

Incidence

The true incidence of thyroid cancer is difficult to quantify due to varying data provided by the different screening methodologies that include palpation, ultrasound, and pathological examination. The prevalence of occult thyroid carcinoma in some adult populations may be as high as 5–10% (8) but the incidence of clinically evident thyroid carcinoma is only 0.05%. In a European population the incidence varies between 1.75 per 100,000 population (0.00175%) for males and 6.38 (0.00638%) for females (9). This implies that only 1–2% of occult carcinomas evolve into overt tumor during life, similar to the situation in prostatic carcinoma. The world-wide incidence (4) is in the

Table 22.1   Thyroid Growth Factors

Stimulators	Inhibitors
Thyroid stimulating hormone (TSH)	Iodine
Growth hormone (GH)	Lithium
Iodine deficiency	Vitamin A
Vitamin C	Transforming growth factor beta (TGF-beta)
Epidermal growth factor (EGF)	
Fibroblastic growth factors (FGF 1 and 2)	
Interleukin 1	
Prostaglandin E2	

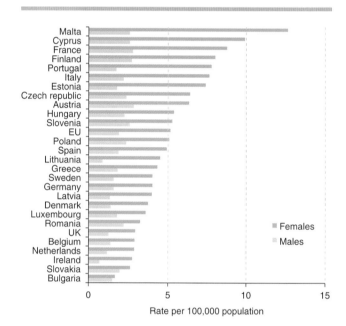

Figure 22.7   Age-standardised incidence rates, thyroid cancer, by sex, EU, 2002 estimates.

range of three to four per 100,000 population per annum, although this does vary widely, with the highest being in Iceland and Hawaii (15 per 100,000 per annum). In 2002 there were 19,034 new cases of thyroid cancer diagnosed in the European Union (EU). The highest incidence rate was in Malta, where the female rate was more than seven times higher than the rate of the lowest ranking country, Bulgaria (12.6 versus 1.7 per 100,000 females). More cases occur in females aged 15–44 than in any other age group. Age-standardized rates for the UK are lower than the EU average (Fig. 22.7).

Mortality Rate

The overall figure for thyroid carcinoma is four per million per annum, giving an average mortality rate of 10% (4), but this does vary widely depending on many factors.

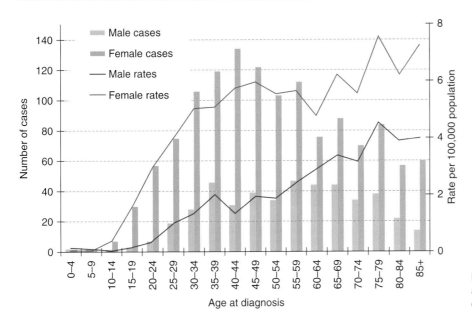

Figure 22.8 Numbers of new cases and age specific incidence rates, by sex, thyroid cancer, UK, 2005.

Age and Sex Ratio

Thyroid cancer incidence rates rise steadily with age. The rates are highest in those over age 75 but almost half of all cases occur in people aged less than 50 years (Fig. 22.8). Sex ratio varies with histological type (4), but in general, unlike squamous cell carcinoma of the head and neck, tumors are more common in females. For differentiated and anaplastic thyroid carcinomas the female to male ratio is 3:1 and for medullary carcinoma the ratio is 4:3.

Trends

In the UK the age-standardized incidence rates have increased slightly from 1.9 to 2.6 per 100,000 population between 1996 and 2005. Male incidence rates have remained around 1.4 per 100,000 male population over this period. There has been a larger increase in female incidence rates, from 2.5 to 3.8 per 100,000 population (Fig. 22.9). Despite this increase there has been a steady decline in the mortality rate since 1975 and this has remained steady at four per million per annum (Fig. 22.10).

AETIOLOGY
Previous Radiation

The most important risk factor in differentiated thyroid carcinoma is previous irradiation (10,11) especially before the age of 16. Therapeutic irradiation may have been given previously for thymic enlargement or other benign conditions in childhood, for example, hemangioma, keloid, tinea infection, or acne. The increase in thyroid carcinoma in Belarussian children after the Chernobyl disaster in 1986 is well documented (12,13,14). This has been characterized by a high incidence in boys giving an almost equal sex ratio, increased aggressiveness with intra-glandular tumor dissemination (92%), capsular and soft tissue invasion

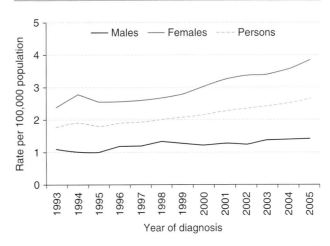

Figure 22.9 Age-standardized (European) incidence rates, thyroid cancer, by sex, UK, 1993–2005.

(89%), and cervical node metastases (88%) (12). Papillary carcinoma was diagnosed in 99% of cases. The short latent period of –four to six years (mean 5.8) is similar to that seen in the United States five years after large releases of ^{131}I from nuclear plants and atomic weapons tests (15). Diagnostic and therapeutic use of ^{131}I, on the other hand, has not been shown to be carcinogenic (16).

Genetic Predisposition

A family history (4,17) of thyroid cancer is found in 5% of patients with papillary carcinoma and 30% of patients with medullary tumors. Genetic factors are also associated with

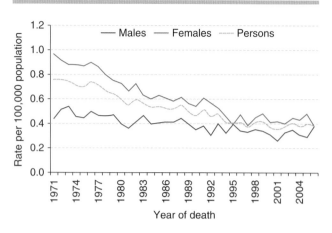

Figure 22.10 Age-standardized (European) mortality rates, thyroid cancer, by sex, UK, 1971–2006.

Table 22.2 Classification of Malignant Thyroid Tumors

Tumor type	Incidence (%)
Differentiated follicular cell-derived carcinomas	
Papillary carcinoma	70–80
Follicular carcinoma	10–20
Hurthle cell carcinoma	2–10
Parafollicular cell-derived carcinomas	
Medullary carcinoma	
Sporadic	4–6
Familial	2–3
Anaplastic (undifferentiated) carcinoma	
Giant cell, small cell and spindle cell variants	5–10
Other primary thyroid tumours	
Lymphoma	1
Others (squamous cell carcinoma, sarcoma)	
Secondary cancer to the thyroid from kidney, breast, colon, melanoma	1

Gardner's syndrome (familial colonic polyposis) and Cowden's disease.

Other Factors

Other factors which show an increased incidence of thyroid carcinoma are geographical distribution (2), history of Hashimoto's disease (4,18,19) and iodine content of the diet. In several surveys a positive correlation has also been found between increasing parity and incidence of differentiated thyroid carcinoma (12).

PATHOLOGICAL CLASSIFICATION OF THYROID TUMORS

The vast majority of thyroid swellings are due to cystic degenerative changes but there are a number of benign tumors, the most common being follicular cell adenoma, then Hurthle cell adenoma, and the rare teratoma. Malignant tumors may arise from the follicular cells (papillary, follicular, anaplastic), the parafollicular cells (medullary), or the stroma (lymphoma, sarcoma). Papillary carcinoma is by far the most common type of malignant thyroid tumor (70–80%), followed by follicular (10–20%), medullary carcinoma (5–10%), and anaplastic carcinoma (2–10%). Other tumors include poorly differentiated carcinoma (0.4–10%), Hurthle cell carcinoma (2–5%), lymphoma, and metastases (Table 22.2). These cancers can be classified according to their behavior into low, intermediate, and high degree of malignancy (Table 22.3).

Malignant Tumors from Follicular Cells
Well-differentiated Thyroid Carcinoma

Well-differentiated thyroid cancer can be divided into papillary thyroid cancer (PTC) and follicular thyroid cancer (FTC). PTC is the most frequent thyroid cancer. It is often multifocal, nonencapsulated, and spreads through the lymph nodes. FTC is usually unifocal, encapsulated, and spreads via the bloodstream to distant organs and rarely to the lymph nodes.

Table 22.3 Correlation Between Degree of Malignancy and Histology

Degree of malignancy		
Low	Intermediate	High
Papillary carcinoma	Poorly differentiated carcinoma	Anaplastic carcinoma
Follicular carcinoma (minimally invasive)	Follicular carcinoma (widely invasive)	
Hurthle cell carcinoma (minimally invasive)	Hurthle cell carcinoma (widely invasive)	

Papillary carcinoma. The nuclear features of papillary carcinoma are nuclear clearing, grooves, and pseudoinclusions. PTC can be divided into classical PTC, follicular variant (FVPTC), tall cell variant (TCV), and rare variants such as sclerosing variant and columner cell variant.

Classical PTC. Papillary carcinoma (Fig. 22.11A) typically affects the young female, with a mean age at diagnosis of 35–45 years. The overall sex ratio is three females to one male but is 9:1 in Japan (4). There is a high incidence of multifocality and bilateralism (4), reported as 30–87.5% (20). Spread of disease is usually to paratracheal and cervical lymph nodes initially, and much later to the mediastinal lymph nodes. Distant metastasis usually occurs late and is limited to the lungs and rarely the bones (4). Although the disease often follows an indolent course with an overall 20-year survival of 90–95% (21), it tends to be more aggressive in later life and may progress rapidly after remaining localized for years (18,22). The main features are summarized in Table 22.4.

Follicular variant. This is the most common subset and is found in 9–22% of patients with PTC (23,24). The variant comprises follicles whose cells have features of papillary carcinoma. Recent work has subclassified this variant into nonencapsulated/infiltrative form and encapsulated

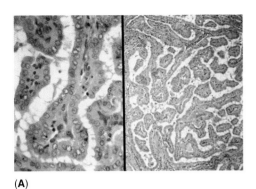

(A)

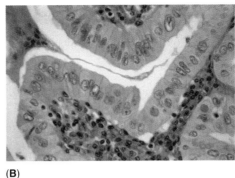

(B)

Figure 22.11 Histological features of papillary carcinoma. **(A)** Papillary; **(B)** tall cell variant.

Table 22.4 Features of Papillary Carcinoma

Commonest type – 80%
Typically females 35–45 years
Sex ratio F:M 3:1 (Japan 9:1)
Multifocality and bilateralism 30–87%
Pure papillary 3%: mixed pap/foll 97%
Lymph node metastases in 50%
Late distant metastases to lungs (+bones)
20 year survival 90–95%

noninvasive form (25). The encapsulated noninvasive form is three to four times more common than the infiltrative form. The nonencapsulated infiltrative form has a much higher incidence of lymph node spread (65% versus 5%) making it resemble classical PTC in its behavior. In contrast, encapsulated noninvasive form has a behavior much closer to that of follicular tumors (i.e., follicular adenoma and carcinoma). The behavior of this form is determined by the extent of capsule and vascular invasion. In general this form has a very low rate of capsule and vascular invasion and as such can be managed safely with lobectomy alone (25,26).

Tall cell variant Tall cell variant (Fig. 22.11B) is characterized by tumor composed of >50% tall cells (tall cell height at least twice its width), eosinophilic cytoplasm, and nuclear features characteristic of PTC. It is the most common of the aggressive variants of PTC and accounts for 10% of all cases of PTC (27). It has a higher recurrence rate and poorer survival than classical PTC. Previous work suggested this was because of older age at presentation, larger tumor size, and the presence of extrathyroidal extension (ETE). However, a recent paper (27) reported that TCV without ETE is biologically a more aggressive tumor than classical PTC without ETE, independent of age, gender, and tumor size. This study showed a higher rate of regional lymph node metastases at presentation in the TCV group compared to the classical PTC group (67% versus 40%, p = 0.004). TCV without ETE also more commonly invaded the capsule than classical PTC without ETE (52% versus 23%, p = 0.0004). The aggressive behavior of TCV may be due to high expression of Muc 1,

a protein which promotes cellular dissociation and oncogenic progression (28) or due to a higher prevalence of B-RAF mutations (29).

Diffuse sclerosing variant (DSPTC) First described in 1985 (30), DSPTC accounts for 2–6% of all PTC (31,32). The disease is more common in females with a mean age at diagnosis of 27 years. There is a high incidence of cervical metastases at presentation (70%). Clinically there is diffuse thyroid enlargement which can be mistaken for subacute or chronic thyroiditis (31). Histologically DSPTC has numerous psammoma bodies, extensive interstitial fibrosis, and a heavy lymphocytic infiltrate. It is the infiltrative growth pattern of DSPTC that is the characteristic feature (31). DSPTC appears to have the same favorable prognosis as classical PTC, though longer follow-up data is still necessary to clarify this. Given the propensity for this tumor to infiltrate intrathyroidal lymphatics and the high rate of nodal metastases total thyroidectomy and neck dissection to remove central or lateral neck nodes is recommended.

Columner cell variant (CCV) First described by Evans in 1986, CCV is defined as a tumor where the cell height is at least twice the width with the presence of prominent nuclear stratification (33,34). It is rare accounting for only 0.015–0.2% of all PTCs (34). It is further classified into encapsulated and nonencapsulated forms. The encapsulated form has an excellent prognosis (34). In contrast the nonencapsulated form is associated with extrathyroidal extension in 67% of cases, distant metastases in 87% of cases and mortality of 67% (35).

Follicular carcinoma. Follicular carcinoma is defined as a malignant thyroid tumor with features of follicular cell differentiation (4). The disease is usually unifocal, with less than 2% of cases bilateral. There is often a preexisting history of multinodular goiter and geographically occurrence is more frequent in iodine deficient areas. However, it is almost always a solitary tumor and rarely may be clinically occult. Follicular carcinoma affects a slightly older age group (mean 40–50 years) with a sex ratio similar to that of papillary carcinoma of three females to one male.

Often it is very well differentiated, with minimal or even nonexistent cellular pleomorphism. Histological recognition is dependent on the identification of capsular or

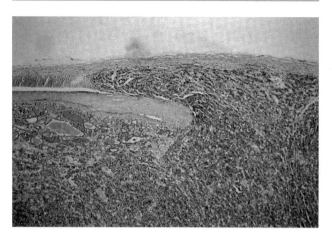

Figure 22.12 Histological features of follicular carcinoma showing capsular invasion.

Table 22.5   Features of Follicular Carcinoma

10% thyroid tumors
Older age group 40–50 years
Sex ratio F:M 3:1
Solitary and unifocal – bilateral cases in 2%
Pre-existing MNG or iodine deficient area
Vascular invasion (lungs, bones, brain)
Survival 80–85% at 10 years, 70–75% at 20 years

vascular invasion (Fig. 22.12.) (4,21,22,36). This makes differentiation from follicular adenoma, which often has some degree of cellular pleomorphism, unreliable by needle biopsy and even by frozen section (21,22).

Prognosis is still good with adequate treatment but not as good as papillary carcinoma, with a mean 10-year survival of 80–85%, and 20-year survival of 70–75% (4,37). Spread is blood borne to the lungs, bones, and rarely the brain or liver with lymphatic spread being unusual (Table 22.5). They can be classified into minimally invasive and widely invasive depending on the extent of capsule and vascular invasion. Minimally invasive tumors are encapsulated tumors with microscopic foci of capsule and vascular invasion. These tumors have an excellent prognosis with a 10-year survival over 95%. In contrast the widely invasive variant has gross invasion of the capsule and extensive vascular invasion. These tumors have a much poorer prognosis with a 25–50% mortality rate at 10 years.

Hurthle cell carcinoma (Oxyphilic variant of follicular carcinoma) Hurthle cell carcinoma is the malignant counterpart of Hurthle cell adenoma, also known as oncocytoma (38). It is characterized by plump cells with intensely eosinophilic cytoplasm and large vesicular nuclei. The WHO recommends that it be included as the oxyphilic variant of follicular carcinoma (39,40). It can also be classified into minimally invasive and widely invasive variants depending on the extent of capsule and vascular invasion (41).

Poorly Differentiated Thyroid Carcinoma (PDTC)

Poorly differentiated carcinomas are a group of tumors with an intermediate position with regard to histology and prognosis. The histological definition is controversial however. Some authors define these tumors on the basis of a solid, trabecular or sclerotic growth pattern. This includes the poorly differentiated "insula" thyroid carcinoma first described by Langhans (42). Others rely on histologic grading in terms of the presence of mitosis and necrosis irrespective of the growth pattern and cell type (43,44). At Memorial Sloan Kettering Cancer Center, PDTC are defined on the basis of the presence of necrosis and/or a high mitotic rate. A recent study by Hiltzik et al. (44) on 58 patients defined as PDTC, 74% patients developed disease recurrence and the overall five-year survival was 60%. Multivariate analysis showed that extrathyroid extension was an independent predictor for recurrence and survival in these patients. Rivera et al. reported that 46% of radioactive iodine refractory PET positive thyroid carcinomas are poorly differentiated carcinomas (45).

Anaplastic Carcinoma

Anaplastic carcinoma is a highly malignant tumor that appears partially or totally undifferentiated on light microscopy but has epithelial differentiation on ultrastructural or immunohistochemical grounds (2). It is a highly lethal form of thyroid cancer, which is rapidly progressive and presents late, typically with respiratory obstruction. There are three histological variants: small cell, spindle cell, and giant cell, with increasingly poor prognosis. However, many previously labeled small cell carcinomas have been subsequently proven on histochemical staining to be malignant lymphomas (4), that corresponds with the better prognosis.

Anaplastic carcinoma can arise from a preexisting papillary or follicular carcinoma (4,46) or multinodular thyroid. There is early spread to the cervical and mediastinal lymph nodes, lungs, liver, and bones. Typically elderly females are affected, with a mean age at presentation of 60–75. The sex ratio is three females to one male (4). Prognosis is dismal, with a mean overall survival of three to six months from time of diagnosis.

Malignant Tumors from Parafollicular Cells
Medullary Carcinoma

MCT arises from parafollicular or calcitonin secreting C cells. It comprises 5–10% of thyroid malignancies and the cells usually contain calcitonin granules (4). There is no benign counterpart but C cell hyperplasia may have the potential of malignant transformation.

MCT was first described as a sporadic form in 1959 and its association with familial multiple endocrine neoplasia (MEN) syndromes was recognized by Sipple in 1961. In MEN 2A syndrome, MCT is associated with hyperparathyroidism and/or pheochromocytoma, being transmitted by an autosomal dominant gene (Table 22.6). The medullary carcinoma is present in all affected family members, although a palpable thyroid swelling may not become evident before the age of 40 years (47).

MEN 2B syndrome is less common but the carcinoma is more aggressive, being associated with pheochromocytoma and a marfanoid appearance. There are also multiple

Table 22.6 MEN Syndromes

	2a	2b	FMTC
MTC	+	+	+
Phaeo	+	+	–
Parathyroid	+	–	–

mucosal neuromas affecting the lips, tongue (Fig. 22.13), oropharynx, and large bowel. Approximately 20% of MCT are familial (FMCT) inherited as an autosomal dominant condition with no associated endocrinopathy (48).

Fifty to seventy percent of MEN-associated tumors are multifocal but the sporadic form is more often unifocal. Familial forms of the disease are usually more indolent than the sporadic type, with the exception of MEN (4,39,49,50). Molecular studies have revealed the presence of the RET proto-oncogene mutation in MCT. Screening of family members is performed for RET positive patients. If the family members are positive, prophylactic total thyroidectomy is considered.

The mean age at presentation is 40–60 years for sporadic disease but 15–20 years for MEN-associated medullary carcinoma (4). Lymph node metastases (often bilateral) are frequently present at diagnosis. Distant metastases may also be present in the lungs, bones, or liver (4).

Prognosis is worse than that of follicular carcinoma. It is dependent on tumor subtype (non-MEN familial > MEN-associated > sporadic > MEN) and stage at presentation, being worse if lymph node metastases are present.

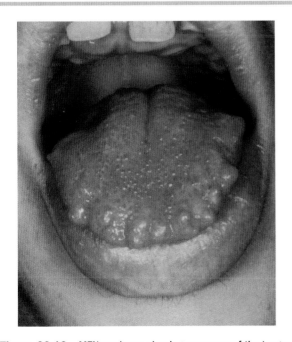

Figure 22.13 MEN syndrome showing neuromas of the tongue.

With adequate treatment the overall mean 10-year survival is 75–80% and 20-year survival is 60–65% (4,49,50).

Malignant Tumors from Stromal Cells
Thyroid Lymphoma

Primary thyroid lymphoma constitutes less than 1% of all thyroid malignancies. Almost all are non-Hodgkin's lymphomas, usually of B cell phenotype and of large cell morphology (4,51). Secondary lymphoma to the thyroid is five times more common. Systemic "B" symptoms are rare.

Thyroid lymphoma spreads within the gland initially, replacing most or all of it. It is usually of diffuse pattern but may be nodular. Regional lymphatic spread is common to the cervical and mediastinal nodes. Eighty percent arise in preexisting Hashimoto's disease. However, only a very small percentage of patients with Hashimoto's thyroiditis develop malignant lymphoma (4).

Similarly to anaplastic carcinoma thyroid lymphoma typically affects the elderly female, with the mean age at presentation of 65–75 years and a sex ratio of three females to one male (4). It is of great importance to distinguish thyroid lymphoma from anaplastic carcinoma due to their somewhat similar presentation yet different treatment and prognosis. Stage I involves the thyroid gland only; any regional lymph node involvement above the diaphragm becomes stage II (52).

MOLECULAR BIOLOGY OF THYROID CARCINOGENESIS

A summary of the important genetic events in thyroid carcinogenesis is shown in Table 22.7.

Table 22.7 Genetic Events in Thyroid Carcinogenesis

Gene	Tumor histology	Prevalence
RET (point mutations)	MTC (hereditary)	Germline: >95%
RET (point mutations)	MTC (sporadic)	Somatic: 50%–80%
RET rearrangements	PTC	Sporadic: ~20%
		Radiation-associated: 50-80%
BRAF mutation	PTC	30–70%
	PDTC	0–15%
	ATC	10–35%
RAS mutation	PTC	~10%
	FTC	~45%
	PDTC	20–35%
	ATC	50–60%
PIK3CA point mutation or amplification	FTC	10–30%
	ATC	25–45%
PTEN loss or point mutation	FTC	8–10%
	ATC	~6%
TP53 loss or point mutation	PTC	0–5%
	FTC	0–9%
	PDTC	20–25%
	ATC	60–70%
CTNNB1 point mutation	PDTC	0–25%
	ATC	Up to 65%
PPARG rearrangement	FTC	~25–60%

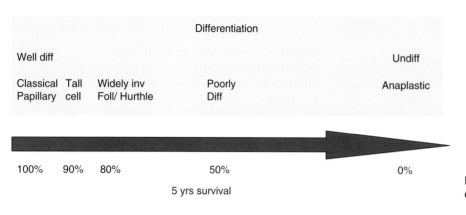

Differentiation

Well diff   Undiff

Classical Tall   Widely inv   Poorly   Anaplastic
Papillary cell   Foll/ Hurthle   Diff

100%   90%   80%   50%   0%

5 yrs survival

Figure 22.14 Correlation between dedifferentiation and survival.

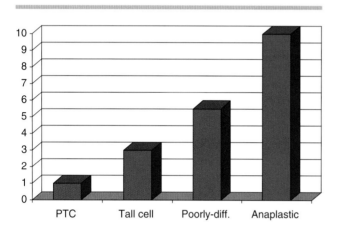

Figure 22.15 Relationship between number of chromosomal abnormalities and histology. *Source*: From Wreesmann, Ghosslin, Singh Am J Pathol 2002, Cancer Res 2004.

Thyroid Cancers Derived from Follicular Thyroid Cells

As in other tumor types, there is now evidence to suggest that thyroid cancer progresses through the accumulation of chromosomal aberrations from well-differentiated PTC to poorly differentiated cancer to anaplastic cancer. (Figs. 22.14 and 22.15). These chromosomal aberrations result in the accumulation of somatic mutations in tumor suppressor genes and oncogenes. Oncogenic activation of RET and NTRK1, tyrosine kinases, and B-RAF, serine threonine kinases, lead to the activation of mitogen activated protein kinase (MAPK), leading to stimulation of cell division in PTC (53, 54). Follicular neoplasms are frequently associated with activation of Ras. Mutations of the tumor suppressor *TP53* occur in most anaplastic thyroid carcinomas (53,55). There are two main pathways which are important in thyroid carcinogenesis. These are the RET/RAS/RAF/MAPK pathway and the PI3K/Akt/PTEN pathway (Fig. 22.16).

RET/RAS/RAF/MAPK Pathway and Thyroid Carcinogenesis

BRAF mutations, RAS mutations and RET/PTC rearrangements are mutually exclusive in thyroid carcinomas

indicating that just one activating event in this pathway is required for tumorigenesis (56).

BRAF mutations and thyroid cancer. RAF proteins are serine-threonine protein kinases. There are three isoforms: ARaf, BRaf, and CRaf. BRaf is the predominant isoform in thyroid cells. Raf proteins are recruited to the plasma membrane by GTP-bound Ras leading to phosphorylation and activation of Raf. Raf then phosphorylates and activates MEK which then phosphoryates and activates MAPK. This signals cellular proliferation and gene expression. Mutations of the BRaf gene occur in 15–30% of all cancers (57) and are most frequent in thyroid carcinoma (36–53%) (56,58,59). Over 85% of BRaf mutations cause a single amino acid substitution of valine by glutamate at position 600. This BRaf[V600E] mutation results in BRaf being rendered active resulting in a gain of function effect. BRaf[V600E] is found only in PTC, poorly differentiated carcinoma and anaplastic carcinoma derived from PTC. It is absent in follicular adenomas and goiters and therefore can be used to differentiate nodules of indeterminate nature on fine needle aspirate (60). These mutations also result in suppression of thyroid peroxidase, sodium iodide symporter, and thyroglobulin mRNA which means that BRaf[V600E] PTC tumors are more likely to be radioiodine refractory and FDG-avid (61).

RAS mutations and thyroid cancer. Three RAS genes are important in cancer pathogenesis: HRas, KRas and NRas. These proteins are plasma membrane GTPases that transduce activation signals from cell surface tyrosine kinase receptors to Raf. The rate limiting step in Ras activation is the exchange of bound GDP to GTP. This is a very slow step but is facilitated by guanine nucleotide exchange factors such as Sos proteins. When growth factors bind to tyrosine kinase receptors, the receptors dimerize and become autophosphorylated. This allows proteins with SH2 domains (such as Grb2) to bind which in turn bind to Sos proteins. This then activates RAS by exchanging GDP for GTP. Activated Ras therefore exists in a GTP-RAS bound state. This in turn can activate Raf again by phosphorylation. Point mutations in RAS that increase affinity for GTP or inactivate its GTPase function result in the protein being switched on permanently. This mutation occurs in 30% of human cancers making RAS the most

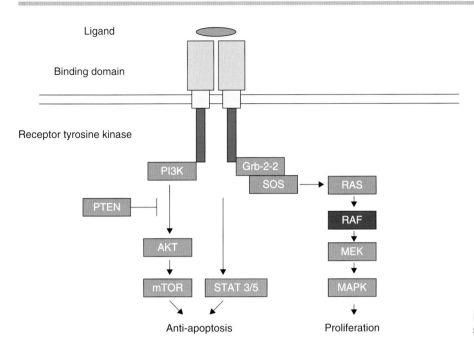

Figure 22.16 Receptor tyrosine kinase signal transduction in thyroid carcinogenesis.

widely mutated human proto-oncogene. Mutations of all three RAS oncogenes have been reported in thyroid cancer. These mutations are most common in follicular carcinoma (45%) and uncommon in PTC (10%). They are also common in anaplastic carcinoma (50–60%) and poorly differentiated carcinoma (25–35%) (62,63).

RET/PTC rearrangements and thyroid cancer. RET is not expressed in normal follicular thyroid cells. However, many papillary carcinomas express chimeric RET molecules resulting from chromosomal rearrangements that fuse the RET TK domain to a partner gene found in PTC. The resulting RET/PTC oncogene produces a kinase protein that can then act on the RAS/RAF/MAPK pathway driving tumorigenesis. RET/PTC1 and RET/PTC3 are the most common rearrangements. These genes are found in 20–30% of adult sporadic papillary carcinomas. They are found more frequently in sporadic papillary carcinoma from children and young adults (40–79%) (64). Radiation exposure has been implicated in the development of the RET/PTC rearrangements because 80% of tumors removed from children with papillary carcinoma affected by the Chernobyl nuclear accident have these rearrangements (64).

PI3K/Akt/PTEN Pathway and Thyroid Carcinogenesis

Phosphatidylinositol 3 kinase (PI3K) is a major mediator of cell proliferation and growth. It is a kinase composed of a p85 regulatory and p110 catalitic subunits. Ligand bound receptor tyrosine kinases recruit PI3K to the cell membrane which results in the recruitment and activation of the serine-threonine protein kinase Akt via phosphylation. Akt plays a cardinal role in regulating cell proliferation (by suppression of p21 and activation of cyclin D), angiogenesis (by activation of VEGF and HIF-1α), apoptosis

(antiapoptosis by phosphorylating Forkhead, Bad and procaspase 9), protein translation (by phosphorylation of mTOR) (65). The phosphatase PTEN (phosphatase and tensin homolog deleted on chromosome ten) blocks activation of Akt by PI3K and acts to switch off this pathway (66).

In thyroid cancer, this pathway can be activated by activation of PI3K, Akt or by loss of PTEN. Loss of PTEN is mutually exclusive with activation of PI3K indicating that only one genetic event is required to activate this pathway. PI3K is activated by activating mutations of PIK3CA (which encodes the p110 catalytic subunit of PI3K). These mutations are found in 23% of anaplastic thyroid cancer, 8% well-differentiated follicular and 2% well-differentiated PTC (67). In human thyroid cancer, there are increased levels of total and phosphorylated Akt with higher levels in regions of capsular invasion suggesting Akt is important in invasion and progression (68). Inactivating mutations of PTEN occur in Cowden's syndrome (69), where germline mutations in PTEN confer predisposition to FTCs. Sporadic mutation in PTEN are rare in thyroid cancer but this gene can be inactivated by promotor hypermethylation. This mechanism of inactivating PTEN occurs in up to 25% of anaplastic thyroid cancers but less frequently in well-differentiated thyroid cancer (70,71).

p53

In well-differentiated thyroid carcinoma, p53 mutations are rare (0–9%) but are very common in poorly differentiated (17–38%) and anaplastic carcinoma (67–88%). p53 mutations are therefore a late event in thyroid carcinogenesis and is associated with progression and more aggressive phenotype (72).

β Catenin and E-cadherin

β catenin (encoded by the CTNNB1 gene) and E-cadherin are cell adhesion molecules that bind together to form adheren junctions. E—cadherin expression is high in normal thyroid tissue but decreased in undifferentiated thyroid carcinomas probably due to gene promoter methylation (73). β catenin mutations are present in poorly differentiated (25%) and anaplastic (65%) carcinomas but not well-differentiated carcinomas (74). Thus both loss of E-cadherin expression and acquisition of β catenin mutations is associated with thyroid carcinoma dedifferentiation and disease progression (75).

PPARγ

Peroxisome proliferator activated receptor γ (encoded by the PPARγ gene on chromosome 3p25) is a nuclear receptor involved in cell cycle control and apoptosis. The thyroid transcription factor PAX8 can be activated by a chromosomal rearrangement with this gene resulting in increased cell proliferation of thyroid tissue resulting in carcinoma. The PAX8/ PPARγ chimeric gene has been identified in 50% of human follicular carcinomas, follicular thyroid adenomas, and follicular variant of PTC (76,77).

Thyroid Cancer Derived from Parafollicular Cells (MTC)

There is a strong association between mutations of the RET gene and the development of MTC. The RET gene is localized on chromosome 10q and encodes a transmembrane receptor tyrosine kinase that is mainly expressed in precursor cells of the neural crest and urogenital tract. It is essential for the early development of the autonomic nervous system. In the normal thyroid, RET is expressed by parafollicular cells but not follicular cells. In these cells it activates numerous intracellular pathways involved in cell proliferation and survival including the RAS/RAF/MAPK pathway, PI3K/Akt pathway, and Src/JAK/STAT pathway. MTC results from activating point mutations in the RET gene that results is permanent activation of these pathways resulting in uncontrolled cell proliferation. Different mutations are associated with the familial and sporadic forms and are associated with different risks.

MTC can occur in sporadic form (75% cases) or as a familial syndrome (25%) as mentioned before. Sporadic MTCs harbor somatic RET protooncogene mutations in up to 40–80% of cases. In familial MTC, 95% of cases have germline RET mutations. Almost all relevant RET mutations are located in exons 10, 11, 13, 14, 15, and 16. MEN2A mutations cause aminoacid substitutions of the extracellular cysteines at codons 609, 611, 618, 620, 630, and 634. Mutation of codon 634 accounts for 85% of all mutations identified in MEN2A (78). MEN2B is associated with mutations that affect the intracellular tyrosine kinase domain, usually at codons 918, 883, and 922. Mutation of codon 918 accounts for 95% of all mutations identified in MEN2B (78). FMTC is associated with mutations that affect the extracellular cysteines at codons 609, 611, 618, and 620. Mutation of codon 634 has never been reported in FMTC. Somatic RET mutations are found in sporadic MTC. The most common mutation is at codon 918 (80%).

These mutations have different transforming activity. The mutation with the highest transforming activity is at codon 918. This accounts for the fact that sporadic MTC has a worse prognosis than its MEN2A counterparts.

MTC has nearly 100% penetrance in MEN2 syndromes and FMTC, but the aggressiveness and clinical course differ between the different types of MEN2. The only available treatment that can prevent metastatic MTC in MEN2 carriers is prophylactic thyroidectomy. Delaying thyroidectomy until puberty or later carries a high risk of allowing MTC to develop and metastasize. Recently the American Thyroid Association (ATA) classified mutations into groups A–D according to risk (D being most aggressive). Patients with level D mutations (codon 883, 918) should undergo prophylactic total thyroidectomy within the first year of life. Patients with level C (codon 634) should have a thyroidectomy before age five. Patients with level B mutations (codons 609, 611, 618, 620, 630) and level A mutations (codons 768, 790, 791, 804, 891) may have their surgery after the age of five provided that they have a normal calcitonin level, normal ultrasound, and family history indicates less aggressive behavior (79).

CLINICAL PRESENTATION

The suspicious symptoms and associated features are summarized in Tables 22.8 and 22.9. In addition, careful examination of the patient may reveal signs that further increase the suspicion of malignancy (Table 22.10).

Table 22.8 Symptoms of Thyroid Cancer

Thyroid nodule (10–50% of solitary nodules)
Cervical lymphadenopathy
Hoarseness
Haemoptysis
Stridor
Dysphagia/'globus'
Hyperthyroidism
Diarrhoea (MTC)

Table 22.9 Associated Factors in Thyroid Cancer

Clinical presentation	
Age: nodules	<14 yrs – 50% malignant
	>50 yrs – 45% malignant
Sex: nodules (FNA)	M – 29% malignant
	F – 4% malignant
Previous irradiation	
Genetic factors –	Gardner's syndrome (FCP)
	Cowden's disease
Papillary Ca and breast, ovarian and CNS malignancies	

Table 22.10 Clinical Signs of Malignancy

Hard, fixed or irregular thyroid swelling
Cervical lymphadenopathy
Recurrent laryngeal nerve palsy

Solitary Thyroid Nodule

Differentiated thyroid carcinoma most commonly presents in a euthyroid patient as a "solitary thyroid nodule" identified either on clinical examination or as an incidental finding on ultrasound scan, computerized tomography (CT) scan, or PET scan. Ten to fifty percent of solitary thyroid nodules may be malignant. Age at presentation is important in someone with a thyroid nodule. In patients under 14 years of age or over 50 years of age, approximately 50% of solitary nodules are malignant (Table 22.9). Small nodules are usually asymptomatic but larger swellings usually cause discomfort in the anterior lower neck with "globus-type" symptoms and, less commonly, tracheal and/or esophageal compression.

Cervical Lymphadenopathy

The other frequent presentation is of cervical lymphadenopathy in a patient with an asymptomatic or occult primary. These nodes may be cystic in up to 30% of patients. Nodes may also appear in someone with a long-standing goiter.

Hoarseness and Dysphagia

Less commonly, tumors may present with a vocal cord palsy, dysphagia, or in rare instances with hemoptysis (5). Anaplastic carcinoma and lymphoma usually present with more rapid onset of swelling and stridor.

Other Symptoms

In patients with medullary carcinoma, symptoms such as diarrhea may be present (Table 22.8).

INVESTIGATIONS
Fine-needle Aspiration Cytology

Fine-needle aspiration cytology (FNAC) has become the key investigation in the workup of thyroid nodules (21,22,80,81,82) and is indicated in the evaluation of all thyroid nodules. It is a safe, easy, inexpensive, and reliable test that will effectively distinguish between neoplastic (potentially malignant) lesions and degenerative (probably benign) disease with an accuracy of up to 95%. Since its introduction the incidence of malignancy in patients undergoing surgery for nodular disease has increased from 10% to 50% because of increased accuracy of preoperative diagnosis. The number of patients subjected to thyroid surgery has also fallen from 67% to 43% (81). Even in experienced hands 10–15% of aspirations are inadequate or non-diagnostic, but this may be reduced by half by repeated aspirations or by ultrasound-guided FNAC. Typical results of FNAC are shown in Table 22.11. It is important to note that while the diagnosis of malignancy is reliable

Table 22.11 Results of Thyroid FNAC

Degenerative conditions (75%)
  Thyroid cyst
    Fluid should be sent for cytological assessment
  Degenerative or colloid nodule
    <1% risk of malignancy

Neoplastic conditions (4% positive; 11% suspicious)
  Papillary neoplasm
    99% accuracy in positive reports
    60% accuracy in suspicious reports
  Follicular neoplasm
    Unreliable for distinguishing between follicular adenoma and well-differentiated follicular carcinoma: excision required
  Medullary carcinoma
    Reliable diagnosis when combined with calcitonin staining
  Anaplastic carcinoma
    Usually diagnostic but may not distinguish from lymphoma or metastatic carcinoma
  Lymphoma
    Open biopsy required for immunocytochemistry
  Other specific tumors

Inconclusive (10%)
  FNAC should be repeated (under ultrasound guidance)

Table 22.12 Cytology Classification (THY) of Thyroid Masses

Cytology classification (THY) of thyroid masses		
Classification	Cytology diagnosis	Action
Thy1	Non-diagnostic	FNAC should be repeated
Thy2	Non-neoplastic	FNAC should be repeated 3–6 months apart
Thy3	Follicular lesion/suspected follicular neoplasm	Surgical intervention– lobectomy
Thy4	Suspicious of malignancy	Surgical intervention– lobectomy or total
Thy5	Diagnostic of malignancy	Surgical intervention– lobectomy or total

on FNAC, a negative result cannot rule out malignancy because of sampling error. Classification of FNAC results with recommended actions are shown in Table 22.12. FNAC is also invaluable in assessing any associated cervical lymphadenopathy.

Ultrasonography

High-frequency real-time high-resolution ultrasonography (up to 3 mm resolution with 7 MHz or 10 MHz probe) is currently the most sensitive method for evaluating thyroid nodules (83), and is ideally used in combination with FNAC in preliminary assessment. An ultrasound maybe performed as the initial evaluation of a thyroid mass to distinguish between a solid and cystic mass. Less than 5% of cystic thyroid nodules are malignant, but this is higher for recurrent and large cysts. It also effectively distinguishes a solitary thyroid nodule from the dominant nodule in a multinodular goiter. Ultrasound is effective in assessing the size and position of cervical lymphadenopathy (83,84). It is also useful in identifying and sampling clinically non-palpable incidentalomas and an apparently occult primary tumor in patients presenting with metastatic nodes. Ultrasound is helpful in following masses/nodules that are managed nonsurgically and to evaluate for recurrence in the thyroid bed during follow-up.

Radionuclide Scanning
Thyroid Scintigraphy
Thyroid scintigraphy was previously the most commonly used investigation for thyroid nodules. Technetium 99m is taken up by the thyroid and is readily available but uptake is low and scans are neither sensitive nor specific, although the information provided in terms of "hot" or "cold" nodules may be helpful. Iodine-123 is ideal but its cost and availability restrict its use. These scans are no longer used as first-line investigation of thyroid nodules but remain invaluable for whole-body imaging following total thyroidectomy for well-differentiated carcinoma.

18-FDG-PET
Not all patients with thyroid cancer will have radioiodine avid tumors, although thyroglobulin levels are elevated. This is particularly the case with tumors with dedifferentiation such as poorly differentiated thyroid carcinoma, tall cellvariant, and Hurthle cell carcinoma (85,86). In these patients, 18- FDG-PET is useful during follow-up to detect locoregional recurrence and distant metastases.

Other Radionucleotides
In medullary carcinoma a variety of scanning agents including pentavalent dimercaptosuccinic acid and

metaiodobenzylguanidine may locate in recurrent or metastatic disease (Fig. 22.17). However, they are not taken up by tumor cells as readily as ^{131}I in differentiated carcinoma and positive scans occur in only 30% of tumors.

Computerized Tomography and Magnetic Resonance Imaging (MRI)
CT and MRI scanning do not have a role in the routine diagnosis of thyroid malignancy (21,22), but once the diagnosis is made can provide invaluable information to assess extrathyroid involvement of the larynx, trachea, pharynx, esophagus, and carotid sheath (Figs. 22.18 and 22.19). They may also help to identify possible neck disease,

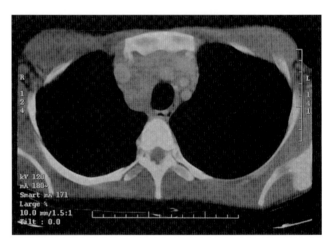

Figure 22.18 Large papillary carcinoma mediastinal nodes resected by thoracocervical approach.

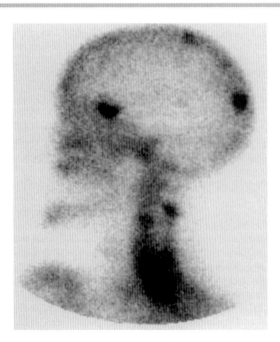

Figure 22.17 Metastases from MTC shown on mIBG scan.

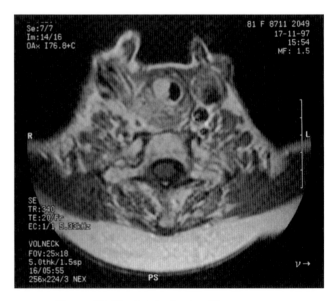

Figure 22.19 Intratracheal papillary carcinoma.

Table 22.13 Indications for CT/MR Scanning

Neck	Possible bilateral lobe involvement
	Extrathyroid invasion of trachea, larynx, esophagus, carotid
	Lymph node involvement
Thorax	Retrosternal spread
	Superior mediastinal nodes
	Pulmonary metastases in MTC/anaplastic carcinoma
Abdomen	Exclusion of phaeochromocytoma in MTC
	Liver metastases in MTC/anaplastic carcinoma
	Lymphoma staging

and to assess the superior mediastinum for retrosternal spread or nodal metastases. They are essential for evaluation of recurrent thyroid tumors. In MCT and lymphoma they are indicated for exclusion of pheochromocytoma and staging, respectively (Table 22.13).

The main disadvantage of CT scanning is the necessary administration of iodine contrast, which can block subsequent use of diagnostic or therapeutic radioiodine for six months. MRI involves neither radiation nor iodine and with increasing diagnostic ability is the investigation of choice in differentiated carcinoma.

CT or MRI scanning of the mediastinum is indicated when mediastinal lymphadenopathy is suspected. A plain chest radiograph is adequate as preoperative screening for pulmonary metastases, which may need confirmation by whole thoracic CT.

CT scanning of the abdomen is part of the metastatic screen for medullary and anaplastic carcinoma as well as lymphoma (49,50) but not indicated for papillary or follicular carcinoma.

Blood Tests

Thyroid function tests (i.e., serum free T4 and TSH) should be requested for all patients with thyroid disease. Thyroid autoantibodies (anti-microsomal and anti-thyroglobulin) are indicated if Hashimoto's disease or thyroid lymphoma is suspected.

Tumor markers, thyroglobulin (87) for papillary/follicular carcinoma, and calcitonin and carcinoembryonic antigen (CEA) for medullary carcinoma have a proven role in monitoring and follow-up (88). Calcitonin is also helpful in initial diagnosis.

Other Screening Investigations

Indirect or fiberoptic laryngoscopy to assess vocal cord mobility and/or intra-tracheal disease is indicated for all patients with suspected thyroid malignancy. It is mandatory for both preoperative and postoperative assessment.

Serum calcium and 24-hour urinary catecholamines are indicated in all patients with medullary carcinoma to screen for MEN 2 (49,50,89). Indium-111 octreotide scanning is reliable in excluding an associated pheochromocytoma. Serum calcium should also be measured prior to any thyroid surgery and postoperatively to monitor possible parathyroid deficiency.

Previously, if MEN 2 was diagnosed, all first degree relatives were screened by clinical examination, thyroid ultrasound, serum calcitonin with pentagastrin stimulation, serum calcium, and 24-hour urinary catecholamines (49,50,90). Since the identification of the RET mutation, it is now preferable to refer the index case to a clinical geneticist.

EVALUATION OF THE SOLITARY THYROID NODULE

A solitary thyroid nodule is defined as "any discrete macroscopic intra-thyroidal lesion that is clearly distinguishable from the adjacent normal thyroid parenchyma" (21). This is usually diagnosed on ultrasound or scan; its clinical significance and management is based on the principle of confirmation or exclusion of cancer (21,36). Solitary thyroid nodules comprise two histological groups.

1. Degenerative lesions: cysts, degenerative colloid nodules;
2. Neoplastic lesions: (a) benign: follicular adenoma, Hurthle cell adenoma, teratoma; (b) malignant: papillary, follicular, medullary or anaplastic carcinoma.

The frequency of thyroid nodules compared with the relative scarcity of thyroid cancer makes it a priority to reduce the number of thyroid explorations for benign disease (21,22,36). However, the overall incidence of malignancy in patients presenting with thyroid nodules is 10%. This is increased when stratified for age and sex (4,22,91). (Females under 50 years, 10%; over 50 years, 30%; males under 50 years, 15%; over 50 years, 45%.) It is also important clinically to distinguish a true solitary thyroid nodule from the dominant nodule in a multinodular goiter (4,92) since the latter carries a much lower risk of malignancy of <1%.

The main issue surrounding the evaluation of a solitary thyroid nodule is to determine whether the nodule is malignant. As customary, a careful history and physical examination may reveal details that are suggestive of malignancy. Factors that suggest a malignant process include age, history of head and neck irradiation/radiation exposure, rapid growth, compressive symptoms, family history of thyroid cancer, nodule >4 cm, fixation, lateral neck mass, and vocal cord paralysis. Although most patients with a thyroid nodule are euthyroid, the functional status of the thyroid gland is assessed by checking thyroid function tests. Fine needle aspiration (FNA) with or without ultrasound guidance has become the standard diagnostic methodology to evaluate a thyroid nodule (92). FNA allows classification as benign in 60–75% of cases, indeterminate in 10–30% of cases, insufficient in 10–30% of cases, and malignant in 3–5% of cases (93). Ultrasound has become the imaging modality of choice to evaluate thyroid nodules. Ultrasound can detect nodules as small as 3 mm in diameter. Patterns that predict malignancy include hypoechogenicity (solid), heterogeneity, irregularity, intranodular vascularity, and microcalcifications. Indeterminate usually encompasses a follicular neoplasm that cannot be definitively categorized as benign or malignant. A strategy for the evaluation of a solitary thyroid nodule is shown in Figure 22.20 (22,36).

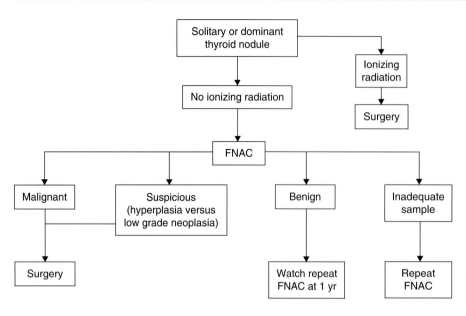

Figure 22.20 Evaluation of a solitary or dominant thyroid nodule.

Table 22.14 TNM Staging for Thyroid Carcinoma

Primary tumor

Tx	Primary tumor cannot be assessed
T0	No evidence of primary tumor
T1	Tumor 1 cm or less in greatest dimension, limited to the thyroid
T1a	Unifocal
T1b	Multifocal
T2	Tumor 1–4 cm in greatest dimension, limited to the thyroid
T2a	Unifocal
T2b	Multifocal
T3	Tumor >4 cm in greatest dimension, limited to the thyroid
T3a	Unifocal
T3b	Multifocal
T4	Tumor of any size, extending beyond the thyroid capsule
T4a	Unifocal
T4b	Multifocal

Regional lymph nodes

Nx	Regional lymph nodes cannot be assessed
N0	No regional lymph node metastasis
N1a	Metastasis in ipsilateral cervical lymph node(s)
N1b	Metastasis in midline, contralateral or bilateral cervical lymph node(s) or metastasis in mediastinal lymph node(s)

Metastases

M0	No metastases
M1	Metastases present

Table 22.15 Stage Grouping for Thyroid Carcinoma

(a) Papillary or follicular carcinoma in patients aged 45 years or older

Stage I	T1	N0	M0
Stage II	T2–3	N0	M0
Stage III	T4	N0	M0
	T1–3	N1	M0
Stage IV	T1–4	any N	M1

(b) Papillary or follicular carcinoma in patients under 45 years of age

Stage I	T1–4	N0	M0
Stage II	T1–4	any N	M1

(No stage III or IV)

(c) Medullary carcinoma, any age

Stage I	T1	N0	M0
Stage II	T2–4	N0	M0
Stage III	T1–4	N1	M0
Stage IV	T1–4	any N	M1

(d) Anaplastic carcinoma, any age

Stage IV	T1–4	any N	M0–1

(No stage I, II or III; all cases are stage IV)

TNM STAGING SYSTEMS

In thyroid cancer, the TNM staging system is primarily based on pathologic findings from retrospective studies, as there is no level 1 evidence from prospective randomized trials. The most recent update of TNM was in 2002 (Table 22.14) (39). Lang et al. concluded that the TNM staging system is the most reliable and consistent system compared to the other scoring systems described above (94).

Taking into account the histology and age factors, thyroid carcinomas can be arranged into various stage groupings as shown in Table 22.15. Tumor staging is one of the most important prognostic factors for patients with well-differentiated thyroid cancer. Gulcelik et al. (95) reported 10-year overall survival of 98% for stage I, 91% for stage II, 80% for stage III, and 41% for stage IV. Disease-free survival was 91%, 71%, 66%, and 14% for stage I–IV, respectively.

The histological grading (Grades I, II, III) of thyroid carcinoma is also an influential factor. One of the limitations of the TNM staging system is the lack of grade as a prognostic factor. In particular, identification of tall cell, insular, and poorly differentiated thyroid cancer portends a poor prognosis. Lymphomas have a complex grading system and classification (96); in the thyroid they are predominantly of non-Hodgkin's B cell type.

PROGNOSTIC FACTORS

The prognosis of patients with thyroid cancer is related to the histology (Fig. 22.14). The 10-year survival is 98% for papillary carcinoma, 92% for follicular carcinoma, 80% for medullary carcinoma, and 13% for anaplastic carcinoma (97). For each histologic type, other prognostic factors have been identified. The significance of various prognostic factors such as age in differentiated thyroid cancer was recognized by Sloan in 1954 (98) and later by the EORTC group in 1979 (99). Although a consensus has not emerged, a number of staging systems have been proposed in an attempt to predict outcome and to help tailor treatment and extent of surgery (Table 22.16). These schemes are based on multivariate analysis of retrospective data (37,99,100,101) that have resulted in identification of important prognostic factors that include gender, histology, size, grade, presence of nodal and distant metastases, extent of tumor, and completeness of resection. Five of the most widely used are summarized below.

AGES (Mayo Clinic, 1987)

Age >40; histological Grade >1; Extrathyroid extension; Size >3 cm

Hay et al. (101) proposed this prognostic system in which patients were divided into four groups that correlate with progressively shorter survival, according to their prognostic score (PS) which was calculated from a formula based on these four risk factors. Eighty-five percent of the total cohort was in group I whose 20-year cause-specific mortality was only 1%. The mortality for stages II, III, and IV were 20%, 67%, and 87%, respectively. Histologic grade is used infrequently and thus MACIS was introduced.

AMES (Lahey Clinic, 1988)

Age >40 for males or >50 for females; Metastasis; Extrathyroid extension; Size >5 cm

Cady introduced this simpler scheme (101) dividing patients into high risk (AMES factors present) and low risk (AMES factors absent) groups. Those who are over the age limit and who have any of the other adverse risk factors are classified as high risk, while all others including all patients below the age limit are classified as low risk. Only 5% of patients in the low-risk group but 55% in the high-risk group developed recurrent disease, with a cause specific mortality of 1.8% and 46%, respectively. It was calculated that the 40-year survival was 95% for the low-risk group and 45% for the high-risk group of patients.

GAMES (Memorial Sloan Kettering Cancer Center, 1992)

Histological Grade >2; Age >45 years; distant Metastasis; Extension beyond the thyroid capsule; Size >4 cm

The controversy over extent of thyroid surgery was addressed by Shah et al (101,102,103). In low-risk groups total thyroidectomy offered no survival advantage over lobectomy. Staging of patients into high- and low-risk patient and tumor-risk groups provides criteria for justifying partial rather than total thyroidectomy (Tables 22.17 and 22.18).

MACIS (Mayo Clinic, 1993)

Metastasis; Age >40; Completeness of resection; extrathyroid Invasion; Size.

Hay et al. (104) revised their earlier staging system because grading of tumors was not universally used. Patients were similarly divided into four risk groups and the prognostic score calculated (Table 22.19). Using the MACIS scoring system the 20-year mortality was 1% in group I, 11% in group II, 44% in group III, and 76% in group IV (Table 22.20).

Table 22.16 Staging Systems for Thyroid Cancer

Age (Sloan, 1954)
Age, sex, histology, size, mets (EORTC, 79)
Age, grade, extent, size (AGES, Hay, 1987)
Age, mets, extent, size (AMES, Cady, 1988)
Grade, age, mets, extent, size (GAMES, Shah, 1996)
Mets, age, completeness of resection, invasion, size
  (MACIS, Hay, 1993)
TNM system (UICC, 1992)

Table 22.17 High- and Low-risk Prognostic Factors

High risk	Low risk
Females >45 yrs	Females <45 yrs
Males	Small size T1
Size: Papillary >1.5 cm	Complete excision
Size: Follicular >1 cm	No nodes/mets
Incomplete resection	Low grade histology
Extrathyroid spread	Papillary
Local and distant mets	
High-grade follicular	

Table 22.18 Conservation Surgery

Low-risk pt + low-risk tumour – lobectomy
High-risk pt + low-risk tumour – ?lobectomy
Low-risk pt + high-risk tumour } Total
High-risk pt + high-risk tumour } Thyroidectomy
Total thyroidectomy for all tumours >1.5 cm

Table 22.19 MACIS Scoring System

PS = 0 (if no metastases) or + 3 (if metastases present)
　　+3.1(if age is <40) or 0.08 × age (if age 40+)
　　+1 (if incomplete resection)
　　+1 (if extrathyroid invasion)
　　+0.3 × tumor size (in cm)

Table 22.20 Mortality for MACIS Groups

Group	PS	Mortality (%)
I	<6	1
II	6–6.99	11
III	7–7.99	44
IV	8+	76

DAMES (Karolinska Institute, 1992)

DNA ploidy; Age >40 for females and >50 for males; Metastasis; Extension beyond the thyroid capsule; Size >5 cm.

This was based on a study (105) which showed that the assessment of tumor nuclear DNA content added prognostic value to the existing AMES risk group system.

TREATMENT

The general management of a patient presenting with a thyroid mass is outlined in Figure 22.21. If malignancy is proven the subsequent management is governed by appropriate specific protocols depending on the histology (Figs. 22.22–22.25). Surgery remains the optimal initial treatment for papillary, follicular, and medullary carcinoma, providing the best chance of cure. Radiotherapy is the main option for anaplastic carcinoma and thyroid lymphoma.

There remain two important challenges in the surgical management of thyroid lesions.

1. *Reducing the benign to malignant ratio for thyroid operations.* Palpable thyroid nodules are found in 3–8% of adults, the incidence increasing with age and 50% have nodules on ultrasonic or CT imaging. In contrast, thyroid carcinoma is designated as a rare cancer (less than 1% of all cancers), with a low mortality rate. There is, therefore, a need to identify the minority of patients with nodules who carry a significant risk of malignancy.
2. *Fine tuning the extent of surgery according to prognostic indices.* With the different tumor types and the wide variation in natural history and biological behavior, treatment must be tailored so that while ensuring the best chance of cure, it is not so aggressive as to cause unnecessary morbidity in those patients with better prognosis.

There are also other controversial aspects of management that continue to be debated.

1. *Lobectomy or total thyroidectomy?* The extent of surgical resection remains controversial. Lobectomy with isthmusectomy is advocated for early papillary and follicular carcinoma with good prognostic indices (26) but others

favor a minimum of total or near-total thyroidectomy (21,22,106). The authors practice a policy of risk stratification in deciding the extent of surgery.

2. *Node plucking or proper node dissection?* The extent of neck dissection is also still debated. "Node plucking" or "berry picking'" operations are almost certainly inadequate, such that the minimum operation should be some form of modified radical or selective neck dissection (21,22) depending on node status.
3. *TSH suppression?* Postoperative TSH suppression therapy is indicated in all patients with well-differentiated thyroid malignancy (21,22). For patients with other tumors, physiological thyroid hormone replacement is required to achieve a normal TSH level.
4. *Radioactive iodine?* Radioiodine has played an important role in the management of differentiated thyroid carcinoma for over 50 years (107). In addition to its use as a diagnostic aid to assess possible sites of residual thyroid tissue or tumor, it can be used in a therapeutic role for the treatment of known inoperable residual or metastatic cancer, or in an ablative setting to destroy normal residual thyroid tissue after thyroid surgery. The rationale for radioiodine ablation (108,109) includes subsequent iodine treatment of any residual cancer as well as improvement in the sensitivity of subsequent radionuclide scanning and thyroglobulin monitoring.
5. *External beam radiotherapy?* It is also the main therapeutic modality for anaplastic carcinoma and thyroid lymphoma. It is used, when indicated, in addition to radioiodine therapy.
6. *Chemotherapy?* Cytotoxic chemotherapy has shown little potential in thyroid cancer apart from thyroid lymphoma. Medullary carcinoma is the only other thyroid tumor to demonstrate significant response to chemotherapy (110) where it has a palliative role.

MANAGEMENT OF PAPILLARY CARCINOMA

Surgery

Management of the Primary

Partial thyroidectomy versus total thyroidectomy? There is continued controversy concerning the extent of thyroid resection, some advocating a more conservative approach for low-risk groups (103) while others would recommend total thyroidectomy for all patients who are diagnosed preoperatively for the reasons given in Table 22.21. In a disease where at least 80% of patients are cured regardless of the extent of surgery, the higher potential morbidity rates associated with total thyroidectomy must be weighed against the small increase in cure rate and reduction in recurrence. Retrospective studies have shown some value in separating patients into high- and low-risk groups (37,101,103,104) while others have recommended total (or near-total) thyroidectomy for tumors over 1.5 cm in size (Table 22.18) (21,22,107). Our group traditionally divides patients into low-, intermediate-, and high-risk groups based on the GAMES scoring system. The intermediate group has two sub-groups: low-risk patients with high-risk tumors and high-risk patients with low-risk tumors. The long term survival is 99% in the low-risk group, 85% in the intermediate-risk group, and 57% in the high-risk

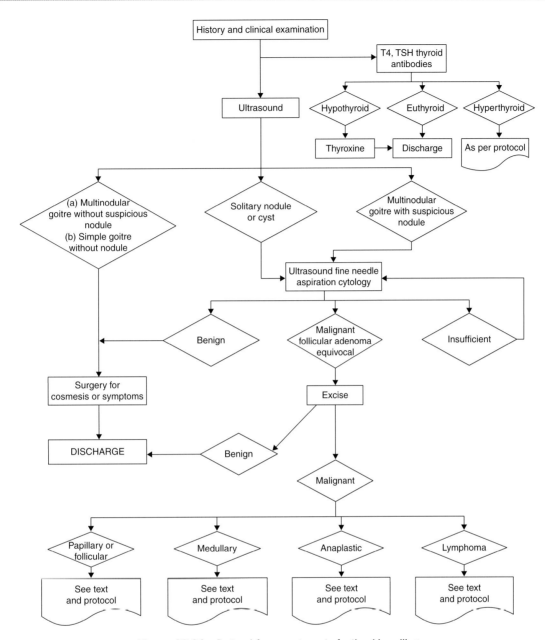

Figure 22.21 Protocol for management of a thyroid swelling.

group (102). The decision of a total thyroidectomy versus lobectomy should be based on risk group analysis and intra-operative findings. In most cases, an ipsilateral lobectomy and isthmusectomy is sufficient for the low-risk group. In high-risk patients, total thyroidectomy to facilitate adjuvant radioiodine ablation and eradication of all gross disease is imperative.

Postoperative diagnosis of papillary carcinoma. When the diagnosis of papillary carcinoma is made postoperatively after lobectomy in a patient with good prognostic indices/low-risk tumor, it is acceptable to adopt a "wait and see" policy with close clinical follow-up.

Management of the Neck

The first echelon lymph nodes for thyroid cancer are the central lymph node compartment (level VI) lymph nodes. These are bound by the hyoid bone superiorly, sternal notch inferiorly, and the carotid arteries laterally. Subdivisions are the pretracheal, paratracheal, precricoid (delphian), and supramediastinal nodes. From the central compartment, metastatic spread is to the lateral compartment nodes, most commonly levels II–IV and less commonly to level V, level I, and retropharyngeal lymph nodes. However, skip metastases to the lateral nodes can occur in 2–19% of cases bypassing the central nodes. This may suggest a direct route of spread from the thyroid

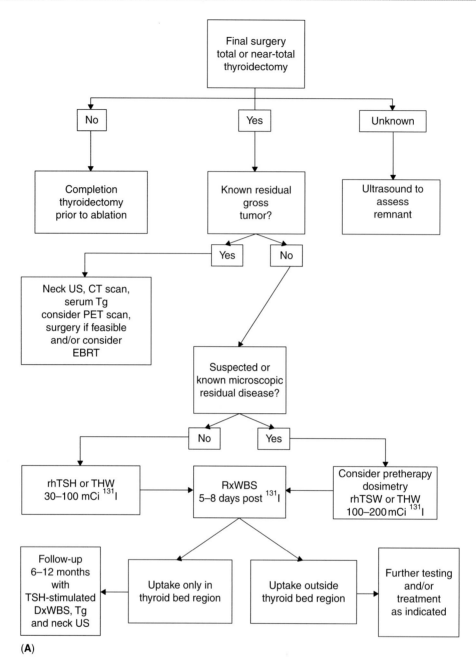

(A)

Figure 22.22   **(A)** Protocol for remnant ablation for differentiated thyroid carcinoma after total or near-total thyroidectomy. *Abbreviations*: EBRT, external beam radiotherapy; DXWBS, diagnostic whole body scan; RXWBS, treatment whole body scan; rhTSH, recombinant human TSH; THW, thyroid hormone withdrawal.

to the lateral compartment or alternatively failure to identify micrometastases in the central compartment lymph nodes.

In patients with a clinically negative neck, the incidence of occult micrometastases neck ranges from 30–70% (111,112,113). The incidence depends on the size of the primary (26% in tumors <1 cm and 66% in tumors >1 cm). Machens et al. (114) reported the central nodes and lateral nodes were involved in 29% each, whereas Wada et al. (114) reported 61% for the central compartment and 40% for the

lateral compartment. Mirallie (115) reported that the paratracheal nodes were the most common site involved (50%). Shaha (116) reported on 1038 patients at MSKCC and reported 56% of patients had a clinically positive neck at the initial evaluation. Given the fact that lymph node metastases are so common it may seem somewhat surprising that thyroid cancer has a 93–98% 10 year survival rate (117). There remains controversy about the impact of nodal metastasis on survival. Several studies suggest there is no decrease in survival in the presence of nodal disease,

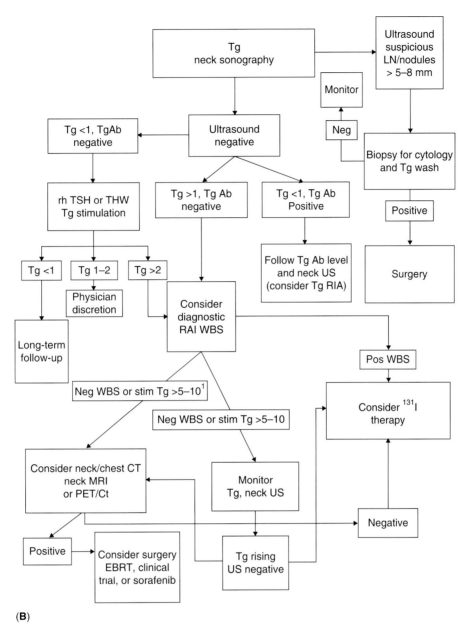

Figure 22.22 *(Continued)* **(B)** Longer term follow-up of patients with differentiated thyroid carcinoma, 6–12 months after remnant ablation. *Abbreviations*: Tg, thyroglobulin; LN, lymph node; TgAb, Tg antibodies; TgRIA, Tg radioimmuno assay; RAIWBS, radioactive iodine whole body scan.

especially in the population of patients less than 45 years of age (118,119). Other studies report a reduced survival (120,121,122). Nodal size greater than 3 cm and extracapsular spread are poor prognostic signs (123). The management of the neck therefore is a controversial subject.

Ultrasound is excellent for the evaluation of thyroid nodules (124) and for evaluation of the neck for paratracheal and lateral neck nodes in thyroid cancer (125). Indeed, this is the investigation of choice for neck node evaluation in thyroid cancer.

Elective treatment of the neck.

Central compartment of neck Due to the high incidence of occult metastases, many have recommended elective treatment of the central compartment lymph nodes. In a case control study of 195 patients having central compartment neck dissection, the 10-year survival was greater in the group having neck dissection compared to those who did not (98.4% versus 89–92%) (126). Lee et al. (127) suggested that only the ipsilateral central compartment need be dissected for tumors less than 2 cm; posttreatment

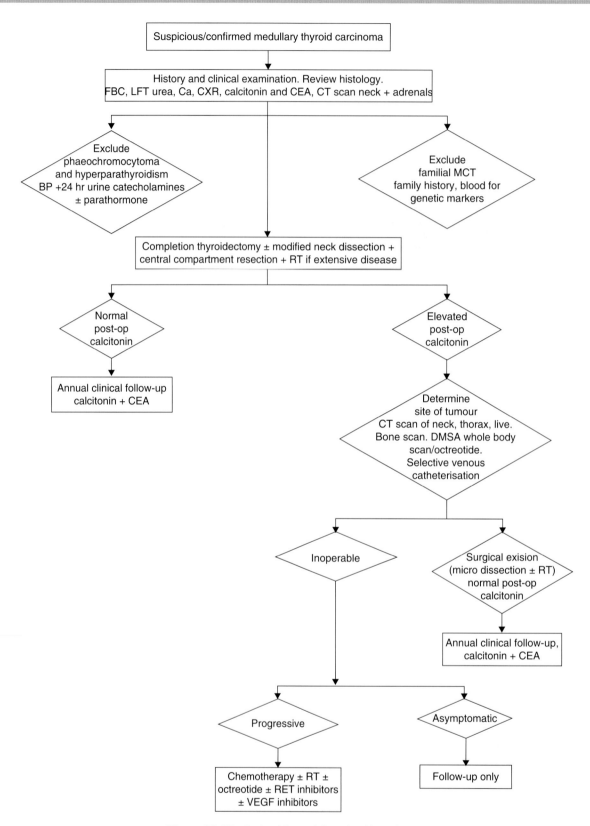

Figure 22.23 Protocol for medullary thyroid carcinoma.

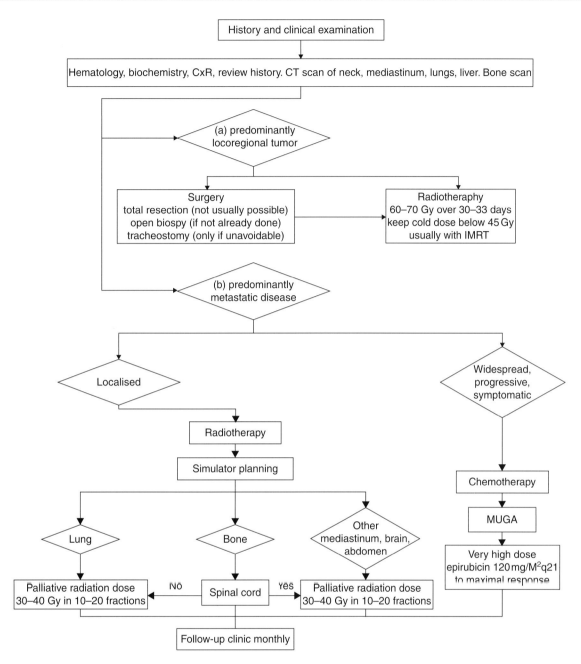

Figure 22.24 Protocol for anaplastic thyroid carcinoma.

thyroglobulin levels for patients having ipsilateral versus complete central compartment were equivalent. Other authors suggest that adjuvant radioactive iodine therapy may be an alternative treatment (128) because central compartment dissection is associated with a high incidence of temporary and permanent hypoparathyroidism as well as increasing the risk of damage to the recurrent laryngeal nerves. As such, dissection of the central compartment should only be done if any nodes appear enlarged or suspicious. Our policy is to carry out a therapeutic tracheo-esophageal groove clearance only when paratracheal nodal disease is demonstrated clinically or radiologically, or palpable disease is found at operation.

Lateral compartment of neck Treatment of the clinically negative lateral neck remains a controversial topic. Even though occult metastases are seen in up to 40% of patients (115), studies have shown that in patients having a lateral neck dissection and those that do not, the regional recurrence rates were equivalent, suggesting that routine radioactive iodine therapy is sufficient to treat occult metastatic disease (115,129). Elective treatment of the lateral neck is therefore not standard practice.

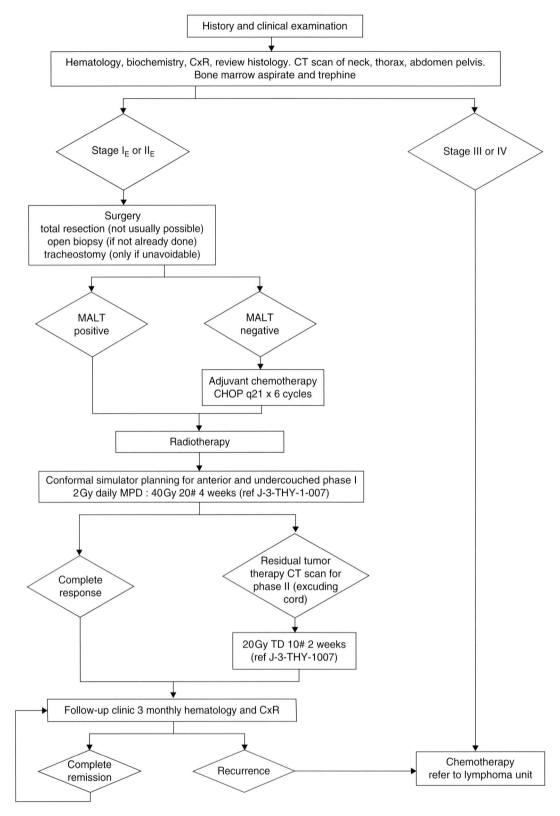

Figure 22.25 Protocol for primary lymphoma of the thyroid.

Table 22.21 Advantages of Total Thyroidectomy

Multifocal disease exists histologically in up to 87.5% of cases (20)

Locoregional recurrence is higher after unilateral lobectomy (25%) compared with bilateral lobectomy (6%)

Any residual tumour has the potential to transform to anaplastic carcinoma (4,46)

Although differentiated thyroid carcinoma tends to follow an indolent course irrespective of the extent of treatment, this slow progression of disease is deceptive and survival after 15 years has been shown to be significantly lower in patients treated non-radically, with cause-specific mortality occuring up to 40 years after initial treatment

Follow-up with thyroglobulin and radioiodine scans are easier to interpret after total thyroidectomy (21)

Complications of hypoparathyroidism and recurrent laryngeal nerve injury are minimal in experienced hands

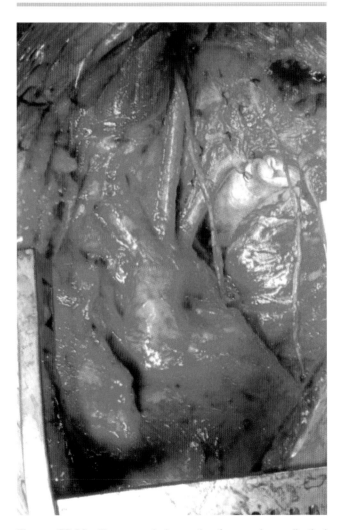

Figure 22.26 Thoraco-cervical resection for superior mediastinal disease.

Treatment of the clinically positive neck.

Central compartment of neck Clinically apparent nodal metastases in the central compartment from differentiated thyroid cancer are treated with central compartment neck dissection. Therapeutic dissection is carried out as far down the mediastinum as required so that all palpable disease is removed. If superior mediastinal disease is detected (Fig. 22.18) preoperatively or at the primary operation it is preferable to resect this down to the arch of the aorta either through a transcervical or combined thoracocervical approach (130) (Fig. 22.26).

Lateral compartment of neck If nodes are present in the lateral compartment, then a lateral neck dissection should also be carried out. Patients who have positive lateral nodes but no nodes in the central compartment clinically, that is, skip metastases, are treated with a combined lateral and central neck dissection. A recent study by Khafif et al. (131) reported that in patients with positive nodes in the lateral neck compartment 84% of these patients will also have positive nodes in the central compartment. The main debate is over what type of lateral neck dissection should be carried out. Several studies have shown that multiple neck levels are involved when the lateral neck is clinically positive (132,133,134). This is an argument against "berry picking" or superselective neck dissection as this may lead to a higher rate of missed disease and recurrent operations. It is recommended that a modified radical neck dissection type III be carried out for the positive neck. In a study of 44 neck dissections in 39 patients, all patients had levels II–V dissected; the incidence of metastases was 52% in level II, 57% in level III, 41% in level IV, and 21% in level V (135). Roh et al. (136) reported 76% level IV and 70% level IIA and III nodes were involved, 17% of level IIb, 4% in level I, 16% in the infraaccessory compartment of level V, but 0% in the supraaccessory nerve compartment of level V. These authors therefore recommended dissection of levels II–V including level IIb but sparing the supraaccessory compartment of level V. In contrast, however, a study by Turanli (135) comparing mRND type III to selective neck dissection (levels II–IV) showed no differences in disease-free survival, overall survival, or local recurrence at 80 months follow-up.

It is our policy to carry out a selective neck dissection (levels II–V) with preservation of the internal jugular vein, the sternocleidomastoid, cervical sensory plexus (C2, 3, 4), and accessory nerve if not clinically involved at operation. Level I can be spared if there are no pathologic nodes in the region. If previous nodectomy has been performed with positive histology, a completion modified radical neck dissection is carried out to clear all potentially involved nodes. After an open biopsy, sacrifice of the sternocleidomastoid muscle and internal jugular vein is sometimes necessary.

Locally Advanced Papillary Cancer

For more extensive tumor involving the larynx, trachea, esophagus, or common carotid artery, there is controversy concerning potential functional morbidity associated with wide radical excision against likelihood of cure. For unresectable disease initial therapy consists of total thyroidectomy with maximal debulking of the tumor followed by radioiodine therapy +/– external beam radiotherapy

(52,136). Occasionally iodine-negative progressive or recurrent disease may demand more radical surgery comprising partial or total laryngectomy, esophagectomy, tracheal, or carotid artery resection with appropriate reconstruction. Long-term disease control and prolonged survival may be achieved (137,138,139).

Adjuvant Radioactive Iodine
Indications
Radioactive iodine (RAI) remnant ablation (Fig. 22.22A). has an ablative function (destruction of residual thyroid tissue that will allow very sensitive disease detection with TG and an improved ability to verify a patient has no evidence of disease) and an adjuvant therapy function (destruction of microscopic residual thyroid cancer in an effort to decrease recurrence and improve survival). In the low-risk patient, surgical removal of all tumor results in high cure rates and very low recurrence rates that are unlikely to be improved with routine use of RAI ablation. However, in the high-risk group a combined approach using surgery followed by radioactive iodine is indicated (140,141). Data regarding the use of routine RAI ablation in the intermediate-risk patients is conflicting with some authors suggesting a benefit in terms of decreased recurrence rates and perhaps even a decrease in disease specific mortality. It is now clear that not all patients with thyroid cancer need RAI. Our approach is to risk stratify the patients based on the usual clinico-pathological features and consider RAI ablation only for intermediate- and high-risk patients.

Subsequent Radioiodine Therapy
Residual inoperable disease can be treated by repeated therapeutic doses of radioiodine every six months until all tumor has been eradicated (52). This regime has been shown to be safe with no significant increased incidence of pulmonary fibrosis, subfertility, or abnormal birth history (52,142,143), provided that the following precautions are taken.

1. All patients undergoing radioiodine therapy should have undergone total or near-total thyroidectomy so as to reduce the dose of radioactivity to the minimum.
2. Existing pregnancy must be excluded at the time of iodine administration. Conception should be delayed for both male and female patients for six months thereafter.
3. Liberal fluid intake and frequent micturition during isotope therapy achieve rapid renal excretion of surplus radioactivity. A laxative should routinely be prescribed to reduce dose to the bowel.
4. Iodine-rich foods as well as iodine-based contrast radiography should be avoided for three weeks prior to radioiodine therapy to make it more effective.
5. Lemon drops or bitter sweets will stimulate secretion of saliva and reduce dose to the salivary glands, minimizing subsequent xerostomia.
6. Repeat doses should be prescribed only when therapeutic benefit can be demonstrated.

However, a small risk of second malignancies has been reported during long term follow-up of patients receiving more than 300–400 mCi cumulated activities of RAI. The risk is very small and should not deter the clinician from using RAI when clinically indicated but does indicate that RAI should be used cautiously in low-risk patients who are least likely to benefit from treatment beyond surgery and thyroid hormone suppression (144,145,146).

External Beam Radiotherapy
External beam radiotherapy using megavoltage photons to a dose of 60 Gy over six weeks can be given in addition if there is incomplete surgical resection of tumor or high-risk patient and tumor (147). This has been shown to significantly decrease the locoregional recurrence rate in such patients from 23% to 11% at five years.

Follow-up
Detection of Recurrence
The serum thyroglobulin level should be measured and the patient put on TSH suppression for life. Follow-up includes annual clinical examination and thyroglobulin assay for life. Elevated thyroglobulin levels in patients on suppressive therapy may be an indicator of persistent/recurrent disease. In many cases, the trend of thyroglobulin is most helpful. Thyroglobulin levels are reliable in the absence of thyroglobulin antibodies. Skeletal and pulmonary metastases, versus lymphatic metastases, are associated with the highest levels of thyroglobulin. Radioiodine scintigraphy can be used to localize the site of recurrence. Anatomical localization can be carried out by ultrasound, noncontrast CT, or by MRI (Fig. 22.22B).

Treatment of Recurrent Papillary Carcinoma
Recurrence of differentiated thyroid carcinoma occurs in up to 25% of patients and in many instances is due to incomplete or inadequate primary treatment. Historically many patients have been treated with less than total thyroidectomy and "node picking," with reliance on postoperative radioactive iodine to eradicate microscopic or even macroscopic cervical, paratracheal, or mediastinal nodal disease which is present in up to 80% of patients. Appropriate head and neck training in selective and modified radical neck dissection techniques is essential. Referral to an appropriate specialist should be considered before a patient's disease is deemed inoperable.

At initial presentation potential nodal disease and upper aerodigestive tract involvement should be properly assessed by a thorough head and neck examination with CT or MR of the neck and mediastinum so that optimal complete eradication of disease can be achieved at the first operation. Recurrent papillary carcinoma should be reassessed by clinical examination, indirect laryngoscopy, and imaging. All locoregional disease should be excised where possible followed by repeat radioiodine treatment +/− external beam radiotherapy. In the older patient with intra-laryngotracheal disease (Fig. 22.19), satisfactory prolonged palliation may be achieved with endoscopic resection rather than recourse to total laryngectomy (5). Radical locoregional surgery may occasionally be necessary (21,22, 139,140,141).

MANAGEMENT OF FOLLICULAR CARCINOMA AND HURTHLE CELL CARCINOMA

The management of follicular carcinoma is similar to that of papillary carcinoma, including radioiodine ablation, with minor differences.

1. All follicular neoplasms diagnosed on FNAC should be regarded as potential follicular carcinomas and subjected to lobectomy and isthmusectomy with frozen section, proceeding to total thyroidectomy if malignancy is confirmed. It is, however, very difficult to diagnose carcinoma on frozen section because this can be determined only on demonstration of capsular or vascular invasion (Fig. 22.12). In most cases the procedure is terminated and paraffin section awaited. If cancer is subsequently confirmed we would usually advocate completion thyroidectomy followed by radioactive iodine ablation.
2. Minimally invasive follicular or Hurthle cell carcinoma less then 2 cm in size in low-risk patients can be treated by thyroid lobectomy and isthmusectomy. Tumors greater than 4 cm are usually treated by total thyroidectomy. For tumors between 2 and 4 cm in size in low-risk patients treatment is at the discretion of the physician and patient.
3. Widely invasive follicular or Hurthle cell carcinoma of any size should be treated by total thyroidectomy.
4. Palpable or suspicious central compartment or lateral neck nodes should be treated in a similar manner to PTC.

MANAGEMENT OF MEDULLARY CARCINOMA
Surgery
The minimum initial treatment for medullary carcinoma is total thyroidectomy, bilateral central compartment (level VI) lymph node dissection, and ipsilateral selective neck dissection (levels II–V) (Fig. 22.23) (21,22,49,146). Limited superior mediastinal disease can be resected through the neck incision but occasionally a thoracocervical approach with upper median sternotomy (131) is required. The aim is surgical clearance of all macroscopic and microscopic disease (22,49,146).

External Beam Radiotherapy
This modality is reasonably effective for treating surgically unresectable residual or recurrent disease, in which case a high dose of at least 60 Gy over six weeks is required (49,50,148,149,150). Adjuvant irradiation is recommended for extrathyroidal disease, extensive nodal involvement, or extracapsular spread.

Chemotherapy
Apart from lymphoma, medullary carcinoma is the only thyroid cancer to show any significant response to cytotoxic chemotherapy, with a partial response rate of up to 60% (111). However, response is short-lived and toxicity from drugs such as doxorubicin is severe. With no demonstrable survival benefit, its role is palliative, used in the context of unresectable, progressive, and symptomatic disease. Other active drugs include cisplatin, carboplatin, and etoposide but combination chemotherapy has not been shown to be of benefit (111). A less toxic agent can be selected initially, escalating to a more toxic drug when a previously responsive tumor develops resistance. There are many ongoing clinical trials with small molecule inhibitors.

Follow-up and Detection of Recurrence
Routine follow-up consists of 6-monthly clinical examination together with measurement of calcitonin and CEA levels (49,111,148) for the first five years, and annually thereafter (49,151). If the postoperative calcitonin and CEA levels are normal or undetectable at six months, this usually indicates a good chance of cure. False positives do occur, and a frequent scenario is that of a calcitonin level that, although lower than it was preoperatively, remains elevated (149) without any obvious macroscopic disease. An elevated serum calcitonin six months after surgery signals residual/recurrent disease.

Patients with serum calcitonin levels above 100 pg/ml should undergo a workup to evaluate for residual/recurrent disease. An ultrasound of the neck, CT of the thorax and abdomen, plus bone scanning will be necessary for surveillance of metastatic disease. Frequently no site of tumor can be documented and such patients should be simply followed-up annually and considered for surgery if a resectable metastasis subsequently becomes apparent.

MANAGEMENT OF ANAPLASTIC CARCINOMA
Surgery
The vast majority of cases present at an advanced inoperable state. It is important to differentiate this from thyroid lymphoma, which can present similarly but which has a different prognosis and management. Occasionally isthmusectomy may relieve respiratory obstruction but open biopsy and tracheostomy are preferably avoided in order to minimize the risk of fungation (Fig. 22.24) (46). Nevertheless, airway control, preferably cricothyroidotomy (152), and nutritional access may be indicated.

External Beam Radiotherapy
This is the only worthwhile modality of treatment (147). Survival is not prolonged but airway and swallowing obstruction can be relieved or avoided. Radiotherapy is given using wide fields extending from both mastoids down to the carina, including both sides of the neck and supraclavicular fossa. A dose of 50–60 Gy over –five to six weeks is necessary to achieve worthwhile regression (46,147). Accelerated treatment comprising two fractions each day over a shorter period of time may be more effective.

Chemotherapy
Although radiotherapy response usually follows high-dose treatment most patients die from widespread metastases within six months. Although no effective systemic therapy exists, paclitaxel is the most effective chemotherapeutic agent for anaplastic thyroid cancer. Combination with radiosensitizing agents such as doxorubicin, may increase local response rate. Enrollment in ongoing clinical trials offers another potential therapeutic option.

Combination Therapy

A recent study reported good results with combined modality treatment involving aggressive surgical debulking, postoperative accelerated radiotherapy, and combination chemotherapy (153), but this regimen requires further evaluation.

MANAGEMENT OF THYROID LYMPHOMA

Surgery

The only surgical management for primary lymphoma of the thyroid (Fig. 22.25) is a generous open biopsy to determine accurate diagnosis by immunocytochemistry. Lymphoma is managed primarily by external beam radiation and chemotherapy. Mucosa-associated lymphoid tissue (MALT) status should be assessed by the histological pattern (51,147).

External Beam Radiation and Chemotherapy

Stage I and II Disease

The principles of treatment are similar to that of other non-Hodgkin lymphomas (52,154). For stage I and MALT-positive disease this consists of a dose of 40 Gy external beam radiotherapy, given over four weeks to both sides of the neck and mediastinum. For stage I MALT negative and all stage II patients this should be preceded by combination cytotoxic chemotherapy such as the CHOP regime (cyclophosphamide, doxorubicin, vincristine, and prednisolone) (51,111).

Stage III and IV Disease

Patients with stage III and IV disease are treated with more intensive primary chemotherapy followed by radiotherapy to sites of initial bulk disease (51).

REFERENCES

1. Pisani P, Bray F, Parkin DM. Estimates of the world-wide prevalence of cancer for 25 sites in the adult population. Int J Cancer 2002; 97: 72–81.
2. Davies L, Welch HG. Increasing incidence of thyroid cancer in the United States, 1973–2002. JAMA. 2006; 295: 2164–7.
3. Williams ED, Toyn CE, Harach HR. The ultimobranchial gland and congenital thyroid abnormalities in man. J Pathol 1989; 159: 135–41.
4. Rosai J, Carcanjiu ML, DeLellis RA. Tumours of the thyroid gland. In: Atlas of tumor pathology. Washington, DC: Armed Forces Institute of Pathology, 1992.
5. See ACH, Patel SG, Montgomery PQ et al. Intralaryngotracheal thyroid: ectopic thyroid disease or invasive carcinoma? J Laryngol Otol 1998; 112: 673–6.
6. Loré JM Jr. Practical anatomical considerations in thyroid tumor surgery. Arch Otolaryngol 1983; 109: 568–74.
7. Wynford-Thomas D. Thyroid cancer. In: Nemoine N, Neoptolemus J, Cooke T, eds. Cancer: a molecular approach. Oxford: Blackwell Scientific, 1994; 192–222.
8. Pelzzo MR, Piotto A, Rubello D et al. High prevalence of occult papillary thyroid carcinoma in a surgical series for benign thryoid disease. Tumori 1990; 76: 255–7.
9. Delisle MJ, Schvartz C, Theobald S et al. Cancers of the thyroid. Value of a regional registry on 627 patients diagnosed, treated and followed by a multidisciplinary team. Ann Endocrinol Paris 1996; 57: 41–9.
10. Calandra DB, Shah KH, Lawrence AM et al. Total thyroidectomy on irradiated patients. A 20 year experience in 206 patients. Ann Surg 1985; 202: 356–60.
11. Schneider AB, Pinsky S, Bekerman C et al. Characteristics of 108 thyroid cancers detected by screening in a population with a history of head and neck irradiation. Cancer 1980; 46: 1291–7.
12. Abelin T, Averkin JI, Egger M et al. Thyroid cancer in Belarus post-Chernobyl: improved detection or increased incidence? Soz-Praventivmed 1994; 39: 189–97.
13. Nikiforov Y, Gnepp DR. Pediatric thyroid cancer after the Chernobyl disaster. Pathomorphologic study of 84 cases (1991–1992) from the Republic of Belarus. Cancer 1994; 74: 748–66.
14. Buglova EE, Kenigsberg JE, Sergeeva NV. Cancer risk estimation in Belarussian children due to thyroid irradiation as a consequence of the Chernobyl nuclear accident. Health-Physics 1996; 71: 45–9.
15. Mangano JJ. A post-Chernobyl rise in thyroid cancer in Connecticut, USA. Eur J Cancer Prev 1996; 5: 75–81.
16. Salabe GB. Aetiology of thyroid cancer: an epidemiological overview. Thyroidology 1994; 6: 11–19.
17. Lote K, Anderson K, Nordal E et al. Familial occurrence of papillary thyroid carcinoma. Cancer 1980; 46: 1291–7.
18. Chesky VE, Hellwig CA, Welch JW. Cancer of the thyroid associated with Hashimoto's disease: an analysis of 48 cases. Am J Surg 1962; 28: 678–85.
19. Ott RA, Calandra DB, McCall A et al. The incidence of thyroid carcinoma in patients with Hashimoto's thyroiditis and solitary cold nodules. Surgery 1985; 98: 1202–6.
20. Russel WO, Ibanez ML, Clark LR et al. Thyroid carcinoma: classification, intraglandular dissemination and clinicopathological study based on whole organ sections of 80 glands. Cancer 1968; 16: 1425–60.
21. Hay ID, Klee GG. Thyroid cancer diagnosis and management. Clin Lab Med 1993; 725–34.
22. Tezelman S, Clark OH. Current management of thyroid cancer. Adv Surg 1995; 28: 191–21.
23. Passler C, Prager G, Scheuba C et al. Follicular variant of papillary thyroid carcinoma: a long term follow-up. Arch Surg 2003; 138: 1362–6.
24. Tielans ET, Sherman SI, Hruban RH et al. Follicular variant of papillary thyroid carcinoma. A clinicopathologic study. Cancer 1994; 73: 424–31.
25. Liu J, Singh B, Tallini G et al. Follicular variant of papillary thyroid carcinoma: a clinicopathologic study of a problematic entity. Cancer 2006; 107: 1255–64.
26. Rosai J, Carcangiu ML, Delellis RA. Follicular carcinomas. Papillary carcinomas. In: Rosai J, Sobin LH, eds. Tumors of the thyroid gland/Atlas of Tumor Pathology. Washington, DC: Armed Forces Institute of Pathology, 1992: 49–121.
27. Ghossein RA, Leboeuf R, Patel KN et al. Tall cell variant of papillary thyroid carcinoma without extrathyroid extension: Biologic behaviour and clinical implications. Thyroid 2007, 17: 655–61.
28. Wreesman VB, Sieczka EM, Socci ND et al. Genome wide profiling of papillary thyroid cancer identifies MUC1 as an independent prognostic marker. Cancer Res 2004; 64: 3780–9.
29. Adeniran AJ, Zhu Z, Gandhi M et al. Correlation between genetic alterations and microscopic features, clinical manifestations, and prognostic characteristics of thyroid papillary carcinomas. Am J Surg Pathol 2006; 30: 216–22.
30. Vickery AL, Carcangiu ML, Johannessen JV et al. Papillary carcinoma. Semin Diagn Pathol 1985; 2: 90–100.
31. Fujimoto Y, Obara T, Ito Y et al. Diffuse sclerosing variant of papillary carcinoma of the thyroid. Clinical importance,

surgical treatment, and follow-up study. Cancer 1990; 66: 2306–12.

32. Soares J, Limbert E, Sobrinho-Simoes M. Diffuse sclerosing variant of papillary thyroid carcinoma. A clinicopathologic study of 10 cases. Pathol Res Pract 1989; 2: 200–6.

33. Evans H. Columnar-cell carcinoma of the thyroid. A report of two cases of an aggressive variant of thyroid carcinoma. Am J Clin Pathol 1986; 1: 77–80.

34. Wenig B, Thompson L, Adair C et al. Thyroid papillary carcinoma of columnar cell type: a clinicopathologic study of 16 cases. Cancer 1998; 4: 740–53.

35. Sywak M, Pasieka J, Ogilvie T. A review of thyroid cancer with intermediate differentiation. J Surg Oncol 2004; 86: 44–54.

36. Mazzaferri EL. Management of a solitary thyroid nodule. New Engl J Med 1993; 328: 553–9.

37. Cady B, Rossi R. An expanded view of risk group definition in differentiated thyroid carcinoma. Surgery 1988; 104: 947–53.

38. Tallini G, Carcangio ML, Rosai J. Oncocytic neoplasm of the thyroid gland. Acta Pathol 1992; 42: 305–11.

39. Hernenak P, Sobin LH. Thyroid carcinoma. In: TNM classification of malignant tumours: International Union against Cancer, 4th edn. New York: Springer-Verlag, 1987.

40. Hedinger C, Williams ED, Sobin LH. Histological typing of thyroid tumors. In: International classification of tumours, 2nd edn. World Health Organization, New York: Springer-Verlag, 1988; 11.

41. Stojadinovic A, Ghossein RA, Hoos A et al. Hürthle cell carcinoma: a critical histopathologic appraisal. J Clin Oncol 2001; 19: 2616–25.

42. Carcangiu ML, Zampi G, Rosai J. Poorly differentiated "insular" thyroid carcinoma. A reinterpretation of Langhans' "wucherinde Struma." Am J Surg Pathol 1984; 8: 655–68.

43. Volante M, Landolfi S, Chiusa L et al. Poorly differentiated carcinomas of the thyroid with trabecular, insular and solid patterns: a clinicopathologic study of 183 patients. Cancer 2004; 100: 950–7.

44. Hiltzik D, Carlson DL, Tuttle RM et al. Poorly differentiated thyroid carcinomas defined on the basis of mitosis and necrosis. A clinicopathologic study of 58 patents. Cancer 2006; 106: 1286–95.

45. Rivera M, Ghossein RA, Schoder H et al. Histopathologic characterization of RAI refractory PET positive thyroid carcinomas. Cancer 2008; 113: 48–56.

46. Tan RK, Finley RK, Driscoll D et al. Anaplastic carcinoma of the thyroid: a 24 year experience. Head Neck 1995; 17: 41–7.

47. Dunn JM, Farndon JR. Medullary thyroid carcinoma. Br J Surg 1993; 80: 6–9.

48. Watkinson J. The management of thyroid tumors. Personal communication.

49. Moley JF. Medullary thyroid cancer. Surg Clin North Am 1995; 75: 405–20.

50. Gautvik KM. Medullary carcinoma of the thyroid: an update of diagnostic and prognostic factors. Scand J Clin Lab Invest 1991; 51: 85–9.

51. Tupchong L, Hughes F, Harmer CL. Primary lymphoma of the thyroid: clinical features, prognostic factors and results of treatment. Int J Radiat Oncol Biol Phys 1986; 12: 1813–21.

52. Harmer CL. Thyroid cancer. In: Horwich A, ed. Oncology: a multidisciplinary textbook. London: Chapman and Hall, 1995: 565–83.

53. Fagin JA. Challenging dogma in thyroid cancer molecular genetics—role of RET/PTC and BRAF in tumor initiation. J Clin Endocrinol Metab 2004; 89: 4264–6.

54. Xing M. BRAF mutation in thyroid cancer. Endocr Relat Cancer 2005; 12: 245–62.

55. Fagin JA, Matsuo K, Karmakar A et al. High prevalence of mutations of the p53 gene in poorly differentiated human thyroid carcinomas. J Clin Invest 1993; 91: 179–84.

56. Kimura ET, Nikiforova MN, Zhu Z et al. High prevalence of BRAF mutations in thyroid cancer: genetic evidence for constitutive activation of the RET/PTC-RAS-BRAF signaling pathway in papillary thyroid carcinoma. Cancer Res 2003; 63: 1454–7.

57. Davies H, Bignell GR, Cox C et al. Mutations of the BRAF gene in human cancer. Nature 2002; 417: 949–54.

58. Soares P, Trovisco V, Rocha AS et al. BRAF mutations and RET/PTC rearrangements are alternative events in the etiopathogenesis of PTC. Oncogene 2003; 22: 4578–80.

59. Xu X, Quiros RM, Gattuso P et al. High prevalence of BRAF gene mutation in papillary thyroid carcinomas and thyroid tumor cell lines. Cancer Res 2003; 63: 4561–7.

60. Cohen Y, Rosenbaum E, Clark DP et al. Mutational analysis of BRAF in fine needle aspiration biopsies of the thyroid: A potential application for the preoperative assessment of thyroid nodules. Clin Cancer Res 2004; 10: 2761–5.

61. Mian C, Barollo S, Pennelli G et al. Molecular characteristics in papillary thyroid cancers (PTCs) with no 131I uptake. Clin Endocrinol 2008; 68: 108–16.

62. Vasko V, Ferrand M, Di Cristofaro J et al. Specific pattern of RAS oncogene mutations in follicular thyroid tumors. J Clin Endocrinol Metab 2003; 88: 2745–52.

63. DeLellis RA. Pathology and genetics of thyroid carcinoma. J Surg Oncol 2006; 94: 662–9.

64. Ciampi R, Nikiforov YE. RET/PTC rearrangements and BRAF mutations in thyroid tumorigenesis. Endocrinology 2007; 148: 936–41.

65. Mitsiades CS, Mitsiades N, Koutsilieris M. The Akt pathway: molecular targets for anti-cancer drug development. Curr Cancer Drug Targets 2004; 4: 235–56.

66. Wu X, Senechal K, Neshat MS et al. The PTEN/MMAC1 tumor suppressor phosphatase functions as a negative regulator of the phosphoinositide 3-kinase/Akt pathway. Proc Natl Acad Sci U S A 1998; 95: 15587–91.

67. Garcia-Rostan G, Costa AM, Pereira-Castro I et al. Mutation of the PIK3CA gene in anaplastic thyroid cancer. Cancer Res 2005; 65: 10199–207.

68. Shinohara M, Chung YJ, Saji M et al. AKT in thyroid tumorigenesis and progression. Endocrinology 2007; 148: 942–7.

69. Liaw D, Marsh DJ, Li J et al. Germline mutations of the PTEN gene in Cowden disease, an inherited breast and thyroid cancer syndrome. Nat Genet 1997; 16: 64–7.

70. Alvarez-Nunez F, Bussaglia E, Mauricio D et al. PTEN promoter methylation in sporadic thyroid carcinomas. Thyroid 2006; 16: 17–23.

71. Frisk T, Foukakis T, Dwight T et al. Silencing of the PTEN tumor-suppressor gene in anaplastic thyroid cancer. Genes Chromosomes Cancer 2002; 35: 74–80.

72. Dobashi Y, Sugimura H, Sakamoto A et al. Stepwise participation of p53 gene mutation during dedifferentiation of human thyroid carcinomas. Diagn Mol Pathol 1994; 3: 9–14.

73. Smith JA, Fan CY, Zou C et al. Methylation status of genes in papillary thyroid carcinoma. Arch Otolaryngol Head Neck Surg 2007; 133: 1006–11.

74. Garcia-Rostan G, Camp RL, Herrero A et al. Beta-catenin dysregulation in thyroid neoplasms: down-regulation, aberrant nuclear expression, and CTNNB1 exon 3 mutations are markers for aggressive tumor phenotypes and poor prognosis. Am J Pathol 2001; 158: 987–96.

75. Nikiforov YE. Genetic alterations involved in the transition from well-differentiated to poorly differentiated and anaplastic thyroid carcinomas. Endocr Pathol 2004; 15: 319–27.

76. Kroll TG, Sarraf P, Pecciarini L et al. PAX8-PPARgamma1 fusion oncogene in human thyroid carcinoma [corrected]. Science 2000; 289: 1357–60.

77. Dwight T, Thoppe SR, Foukakis T et al. Involvement of the PAX8/peroxisome proliferator-activated receptor gamma rearrangement in follicular thyroid tumors. J Clin Endocrinol Metab 2003; 88: 4440–5.

78. Jimenez C, Gagel RF. Genetic testing in endocrinology: lessons learned from experience with multiple endocrine neoplasia type 2 (MEN2). Growth Horm IGF Res 2004; 14(Suppl A): S150–7.

79. Kloos R, Eng C, Evans D et al. Medullary thyroid cancer: management guidelines of the American Thyroid Association. Thyroid, 2009; in press.

80. Hamburger JI, Hussain M, Nishiyama R et al. Increasing the accuracy of fine needle biopsy for thyroid nodules. Arch Pathol Lab Med 1989; 113: 1035–9.

81. Gharib H, Goellner JR, Johnson DA. Fine needle aspiration biopsy of the thyroid: a 12 year experience with 11,000 biopsies. Clin Lab Med 1993; 13: 3.

82. Goellner JR, Gharib H, Melton LJ III et al. Fine needle aspiration cytology of the thyroid. Acta Cytol 1987; 31: 587–90.

83. Solbiati L, Cioffi V, Ballerati E. Ultrasonography of the neck. Radiol Clin North Am 1992; 30: 941–54.

84. Katz JF, Kane RA, Reyes J et al. Thyroid nodules: sonographic pathologic correlation. Radiology 1984; 151: 741–5.

85. Chandrakanth A, Hsu JF, Ghossein RA et al. Histological aggressiveness of fluorodeoxyglucose positron-emission tomogram (FDG–PET) detected incidental thyroid carcinomas. Ann Surg Oncol 2007; 14: 3210–15.

86. Al-Nahhas A, Khan S, Gogbashian A et al. 18F-FDG PET in the diagnosis and follow-up of thyroid malignancy. In Vivo 2008; 22: 109–14.

87. Lindegard MW, Paus E. Thyroglobulin in patients with differentiated thyroid carcinoma. Scand J Clin Lab Invest 1991; 51: 79–84.

88. Palmer BV, Harmer CL, Shaw HJ. Calcitonin and carcino-embryonic antigen in the follow up of patients with medullary carcinoma of the thyroid. Br J Surg 1984; 71: 101–4.

89. Gagel RF, Tashjian AH, Cummings T et al. The clinical outcome of prospective screening for multiple endocrine neoplasia. N Engl J Med 1988; 318: 478–84.

90. Ponder BAJ, Finer N, Coffrey R et al. Family screening in medullary thyroid carcinoma without a family history. Quart J Med 1988; 252: 299–308.

91. Belfiore A, Sava L, Runello F et al. Solitary automatously functioning thyroid nodules and iodine deficiency. J Clin Endocrinol Metab 1983; 56: 283–7.

92. Cibas ES, Alexander EK, Benson CB et al. Indications for thyroid FNA and pre-FNA requirements: a synopsis of the National Cancer Institute Thyroid Fine-Needle Aspiration State of the Science Conference. Diagn Cytopathol 2008; 36: 390–9.

93. Belfiore A, La Rosa GL. Fine-needle aspiration biopsy of the thyroid. Endocrinol Metab Clin North Am 2001; 30: 361–400.

94. Lang BH, Chow SM, Lo CY et al. Staging systems for papillary thyroid carcinoma: a study of 2 tertiary referral centers. Ann Surg 2007; 246: 114–21.

95. Gulcelik MA, Gulcelik NE, Kuru B et al. Prognostic factors determining survival in differentiated thyroid cancer. J Surg Oncol 2007; 96: 598–604.

96. Rhys Evans PH. Tumours of the oropharynx and lymphomas of the head and neck. In: Kerr A, ed. Scott Brown's disease of the ear, nose and throat. London: Butterworth, 1996; 14.

97. Gilliland FD, Hunt WC, Morris DM et al. Prognostic factors for thyroid carcinoma. A population-based study of 15,698 cases from the Surveillance, Epidemiology and End Results (SEER) program 1973–1991. Cancer 1997; 79: 564–73.

98. Sloan W. Of the origin, characteristics and behavior of thyroid carcinoma. J Clin Endocrinol Metab 1954; 14: 1309–35.

99. Byar DP, Green SB, Dor P et al. A prognostic index for thyroid carcinoma: A study of the EORTC thyroid cancer co-operative group. Eur J Cancer 1979; 15: 1033–41.

100. Hay ID, Grant CS, Taylor WF et al. Ipsilateral lobectomy versus bilateral lobar resection in papillary thyroid carcinoma: a retrospective analysis of surgical outcome using a novel prognostic scoring system. Surgery 1987; 102: 1088–95.

101. Shah JP, Loree TR, Dharker D et al. Prognostic factors in differentiated carcinoma of the thyroid gland. Am J Surg 1992; 164: 658–61.

102. Shah JP, Loree TR, Dharker D et al. Lobectomy versus total thyroidectomy for differentiated carcinoma of the thyroid gland: a matched-pair analysis. Am J Surg 1993; 166: 331–4.

103. Shah JP. Thyroid and parathyroids. In: Shah JP, ed. Head and neck surgery, 2nd edn. New York: Mosby Wolfe, 1996; 393–429.

104. Hay ID, Bergstralh EJ, Goellner JR et al. Predicting outcome in papillary thyroid carcinoma: development of a reliable prognostic scoring system in a cohort of 1779 patients treated surgically at one institution during 1940 through 1989. Surgery 1993; 114: 1088–97.

105. Pasieka JL, Zedenius J, Auer G et al. Addition of nuclear DNA content to the AMES risk group classification for papillary thyroid carcinoma. Surgery 1992; 112: 1154–9.

106. Vickery JL. Thyroid papillary carcinoma: pathological and philosophical controversies. Am J Surg Pathol 1983; 7: 797–807.

107. Seidlin SM, Marinelli LD, Oshry E. Radioactive iodine therapy: effect on functioning metastases of adenocarcinoma of the thyroid. JAMA 1946; 132: 838–45.

108. Wong JB, Kaplan MM, Meyer KB et al. Ablative radioiodine therapy for apparently localised thyroid carcinoma: a decision analytic perspective. Endocrinol Metab Clin North Am 1990; 19: 635–44.

109. Harmer CL, McCready VR. Thyroid cancer: differentiated carcinoma. Cancer Treat Rev 1996; 22: 161–77.

110. Hoskin PJ, Harmer CL. Chemotherapy for thyroid cancer. Radiother Oncol 1987; 187–94.

111. Qubain SW, Nakano S, Baba M et al. Distribution of lymph node micrometastases in pN0 well differentiated thyroid carcinoma. Surgery 2002; 13: 249–56.

112. Attie JN, Khafif RA, Steckler RM. Elective neck dissection in papillary carcinoma of the thyroid. Am J Surg 1971; 122: 464–71.

113. Machens A, Hinze R, Thomusch O et al. Pattern of nodal metastases for primary and reoperative thyroid cancer. World J Surg 2002; 26: 22–8.

114. Wada N, Duh QY, Sugino K et al. Lymph node metastasis from 259 papillary thyroid microcarcinomas: frequency, pattern of occurrence and recurrence, and optimal strategy for neck dissection. Ann Surg 2003; 237: 399–407.

115. Mirallie E, Vissset J, Sagan C et al. Localisation of cervical node metastases of papillary thyroid carcinoma. World J Surg 1999; 23: 970–3.

116. Shaha AR, Shah JP, Loree TR. Risk group stratification and prognostic factors in papillary carcinoma of thyroid. Ann Surg Oncol 1996; 3: 534–8.

117. Hundahl SA, Fleming ID, Fremgen AM et al. A National Cancer Data Base report on 53,856 cases of thyroid carcinoma treated in the US, 1985–1995. Cancer 1998; 83: 2638–48.

118. Hughes CJ, Shaha AR, Shah JP et al. Impact of lymph node metastasis in differentiated thyroid carcinoma of the thyroid: a matched pair analysis. Head Neck 1996; 18: 127–32.

119. Sato N, Oyamatsu M, Koyama Y et al. Do the level of nodal disease according to the TNM classification and the number of involved cervical nodes reflect prognosis in patients with differentiated carcinoma of the thyroid gland? J Surg Oncol 1998; 69: 151–5.

120. Scheumann GF, Gimm O, Wegener G et al. Prognostic significance and surgical management of locoregional lymph node metastases in papillary thyroid cancer. World J Surg 1994; 18: 559–67.

121. Lundgren CI, Hall P, Dickman PW et al. Clinically significant prognostic factors for differentiated thyroid carcinoma: a population based, nested case control study. Cancer 2006; 106: 524–31.

122. Sugitani I, Yanagisawa A, Shimizu A et al. Clinicopathologic and immunohistochemical studies of papillary thyroid microcarcinoma presenting with cervical lymphadenopathy. World J Surg 1998; 22: 731–7.

123. Kitajiri S, Hiraumi H, Hirose T et al. The presence of large lymph node metastasis as a prognostic factor of papillary thyroid carcinoma. Auris Nasus Larynx 2003; 30: 169–74.

124. Fish SA, Langer JE, Mandel SJ. Sonographic imaging of thyroid nodules and cervical lymph nodes. Endocrinol Metab Clin North Am 2008; 37: 401–17, ix.

125. Langer JE, Mandel SJ. Sonographic imaging of cervical lymph nodes in patients with thyroid cancer. Neuroimaging Clin N Am 2008; 18: 479–89, vii–viii.

126. Tisell LE, Nilsson B, Molne J et al. Improved survival of patients with papillary thyroid carcinoma after surgical microdissection. World J Surg 1996; 20: 854–7.

127. Lee YS, Kim SW, Kim SW et al. Extent of routine central lymph node dissection with small papillary thyroid carcinoma. World J Surg 2007; 31: 1954–9.

128. Cooper DS, Doherty GM, Haugen BR et al. Management guidelines for patients with thyroid nodules and differentiated thyroid cancer. Thyroid 2006; 16: 109–42.

129. Ito Y, Jikuzono T, Higashiyama T et al. Clinical significance of lymph node metastasis of papillary thyroid carcinoma located in one lobe. World J Surgery 2006; 30: 1821–8.

130. Ladas G, Rhys Evans PH, Goldstraw P. Anterior cervical transsternal approach for the resection of benign tumors of the thoracic inlet. Ann Thorac Surg 1999; 67: 785–9.

131. Khafif A, Ben-Yosef R, Abergel A et al. Elective paratracheal neck dissection for lateral metastases from papillary carcinoma of the thyroid: is it indicated? Head Neck 2008; 30: 306–10.

132. Pingpank JF Jr, Sasson AR, Hanlon AL et al. Tumor above the spinal accessory nerve in papillary thyroid cancer that involves lateral neck nodes: a common occurrence. Arch Otolaryngol Head Neck Surg 2002; 128: 1275–8.

133. Kupferman ME, Patterson M, Mandel SJ et al. Patterns of lateral neck metastasis in papillary thyroid carcinoma. Arch Otolaryngol Head Neck Surg 2004; 130: 857–60.

134. Roh JL, Kim JM, Park CI. Lateral cervical lymph node metastases from papillary thyroid carcinoma: pattern of nodal metastases and optimal strategy for neck dissection. Annals of Surg Oncol 2007; 15: 1177–82.

135. Turanli S. Is the type of dissection in lateral neck metastasis for differentiated thyroid carcinoma important? Otolaryngol Head Neck Surg 2007; 136: 957–60.

136. Tubiana M, Haddad E, Schlumberger M et al. External radiotherapy in thyroid cancers. Cancer 1985; 55: 2062–71.

137. Breaux E, Guillamondegui OM. Treatment of locally invasive carcinoma of the thyroid: how radical? Am J Surg 1980; 140: 514–18.

138. Ballantyne AJ. Resections of the upper aerodigestive tract for locally invasive thyroid cancer. Am J Surg 1994; 168: 636–9.

139. Friedman M, Shelton VK, Skolnick GM et al. Laryngotracheal invasion by thyroid carcinoma. Ann Otol Rhinol Laryngol 1982; 91: 363–7.

140. Mazzaferri EL, Jhiang SM. Long term impact of initial surgical and medical therapy on papillary and follicular thyroid cancer. Am J Med 1994; 97: 418–28.

141. Young RL, Mazzaferri EL, Rahe AJ et al. Pure follicular thyroid carcinoma: impact of therapy in 214 patients. J Nucl Med 1977; 21: 733–7.

142. Sarker SD, Beierwaltes WH, Gill SP et al. Subsequent fertility and birth histories of children and adolescents treated with iodine 131 for thyroid cancer. J Nucl Med 1976; 17: 460–4.

143. Edmonds CJ, Smith T. The long term hazards of the treatment of thyroid cancer with radioiodine. Br J Radiol 1985; 59: 45–51.

144. Brown AP, Chen J, Hitchcock YJ et al. The risk of second primary malignancies up to three decades after the treatment of differentiated thyroid cancer. J Clin Endocrinol Metab 2008; 93: 504–15.

145. Rubino C, de Vathaire F, Dottorini ME et al. Second primary malignancies in thyroid cancer patients. Br J Cancer 2003; 89: 1638–44.

146. Subramanian S, Goldstein DP, Parlea L et al. Second primary malignancy risk in thyroid cancer survivors: a systematic review and meta-analysis. Thyroid 2007; 17: 1277–88.

147. Harmer CL, Bidmead M, Shepherd S et al. Radiotherapy planning techniques for thyroid cancer. Br J Radiol 1998; 71: 1069–75.

148. Harmer CL. External beam therapy for thyroid cancer. Ann Radiol 1977; 20: 791–800.

149. Steinfield AD. The role of radiation therapy in medullary cancer of the thyroid. Radiology 1977; 123: 745–9.

150. Tissel LE, Hansson G, Jansson S et al. Reoperation in the surgical treatment of asymptomatic metastasizing medullary thyroid carcinoma. Surgery 1986; 99: 60–6.

151. Van Heerden JA, Grant CS, Gharig H et al. Long term course of patients with persistent hypercalcitoninemia after apparent curative primary surgery for medullary thyroid carcinoma. Ann Surg 1990; 212: 395–9.

152. Shaha AR. Airway management in anaplastic thyroid carcinoma. Laryngoscope 2008; 118: 1195–8.

153. Tennvall J, Lundell G, Hallgust P et al. Combined doxorubicin, hyperfractionated radiotherapy and surgery in thyroid carcinoma: Report on 2 protocols, the Swedish Anaplastic Thyroid Carcinoma Group. Cancer 1994; 74: 1348–54.

154. Harmer CL. Radiotherapy in the management of thyroid cancers. Ann Acad Med Singapore 1996; 25: 413–19.

23

Tumors of the Parathyroid Glands

Bill Fleming, John Lynn, Peter H Rhys Evans and Andrew C H See

INTRODUCTION

Parathyroid tumors are a common endocrine problem, but only account for a small percentage of head and neck neoplasms. The overwhelming majority are benign adenomas that present as primary hyperparathyroidism. Parathyroid carcinomas are extremely rare and usually are associated with a florid history of severe hypercalcemia. Patients with a malignant tumor are also more likely to have a palpable mass in the neck.

The incidence of hyperparathyroidism is increasing due to the routine inclusion of serum calcium measurement in biochemical assays, the ready availability of plasma intact parathyroid hormone (PTH) levels, and higher resolution ultrasound scanning. Diagnosis is often made in apparently asymptomatic cases, but treatment is important even in this group because of the increased risk of premature death from hypertension and cardiovascular disease in patients with few symptoms and only marginally raised serum calcium. Surgical treatment is also more frequent, even in the elderly, with the adoption of minimally invasive techniques for excision, the advent of better anesthetic agents, such as remifentanil, and the use of intraoperative PTH estimation, making successful surgery more likely.

SURGICAL ANATOMY
Embryology and Position

The four parathyroid glands arise embryologically from the third and fourth branchial pouches and in the adult human occupy a rather variable position in the anterior neck and mediastinum.

The superior parathyroids arise together with the lateral thyroid gland from the fourth branchial pouch and in the adult occupy a relatively constant position, usually adjacent to the upper pole of the thyroid gland. Eighty percent are adjacent to the cricoid behind the thyroid gland, 15% lie behind the thyroid, 3% in the retro-esophageal and retropharyngeal positions and 1% above the thyroid upper pole (1,2). Fifty percent of superior parathyroids lie beneath the capsule of the thyroid glands, but true intrathyroid parathyroids are very rare.

The inferior parathyroids paradoxically arise from the third branchial pouch together with the thymus gland and descend to a much more variable position. Fifty percent lie adjacent to the lower thyroid pole near the point of entry of the inferior thyroid artery (i.e., "normal" position) and a further 20% are beside the thyroid in variable position or alongside the trachea. A further 25% are within the thymus

and 2% are ectopic, lying anywhere up to and including the hyoid superiorly, the pulmonary hilum in the posterior mediastinum inferiorly, and the carotid sheaths bilaterally. Although 25% of inferior parathyroid glands are intrathymic, the vast majority of these (95%) lie in the superior thymic tongue, which is almost always accessible from the neck (1,2).

The most important thing to remember in parathyroid anatomy is the relationship of the parathyroids to the plane of the recurrent laryngeal nerve (Fig. 23.1). Superior glands lie behind the plane of the nerve, so when ectopic tend to travel down posteriorly into the retropharyngeal or retroesophageal area. Inferior glands lie in front of the plane of the nerve and so tend to be found in the anterior mediastinum if ectopic. The position of the inferior thyroid artery is inconstant and of little use in locating a missing gland. In addition there is positional symmetry of the upper glands in 80% of cases and in 70% of inferior glands.

Number

Reports of missing parathyroid glands are probably more likely to be due to occult than truly missing glands, but supernumerary parathyroid glands have been reported in 2–6.5% of adults (2). Anatomical studies of parathyroid glands have typically shown an incidence of 0.2–0.6% with two glands, 5–13% with three glands, 80–91% with four glands, 4–5% with five glands, and 0.5% with six glands (3,4). Cases with seven and even eight glands have been reported.

Macroscopic Appearance

Sir Richard Owen, conservator of the Hunterian Museum of the Royal College of Surgeons of England was the first to describe the parathyroid gland in an Indian rhinoceros as a "small compact yellow glandular body attached to the thyroid at the point where the veins emerge" (5). In humans the reddish brown glands are sometimes difficult to distinguish from adjacent fat lobules; they typically measure $6 \times 3 \times 2$ mm in size and weigh 30–40 mg (3).

CLINICOPATHOLOGICAL FEATURES
General Considerations
Presentation

The vast majority of parathyroid tumors are functional adenomas and therefore present with primary hyperparathyroidism (HPT). In the author's experience however, up to 70% of patients now present without symptoms or with only vague maladies such as muscle pain, joint pain, or fatigue,

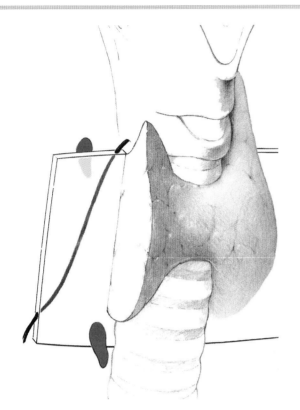

Figure 23.1 Diagram illustrating the coronal plane of the recurrent laryngeal nerve and the relationship of the upper parathyroid behind this plane, and the lower parathyroid in front of the plane of the nerve. *Source*: Modified from Randolph GW (2003) *Surgery of the Thyroid and Parathyroid Glands*. Elsevier Science, USA, p. 277.

after having been picked up on biochemical screening. The classically described presentation of "stones, bones, moans, and groans" is rarely encountered. Very few parathyroid tumors grow sufficiently large to actually present as a lump in the neck, and when palpable are more likely carcinoma.

In the first author's series at the Hammersmith Hospital of 152 patients the median calcium level at presentation was 2.79 (range 2.13–4.12), but 17% presented with severe hypercalcemia with a serum calcium over 3.00 mmol/l. Parathyroid hormone levels ranged from 3.3 to 668 (normal range 1.5–6.6).

Parathyroid carcinoma is rare, occurring in less than 1%, and 50–75% have a palpable neck mass (6,7). The presence of a recurrent laryngeal nerve palsy is also suspicious of carcinoma. Nevertheless it is usually difficult to distinguish the different tumor types clinically, and because the preoperative management is similar, parathyroid tumors tend to be considered and managed together as a group at this stage.

Secondary hyperparathyroidism is a compensatory condition in response to the hypocalcemic state seen in a multitude of conditions like vitamin D deficiency, severe chronic intestinal malabsorption, and chronic renal failure. It can sometimes progress to tertiary hyperparathyroidism in which the parathyroid glands become autonomously functioning, hyperplastic, or adenomatous. This is most commonly seen in patients with end-stage renal failure, and

results in marked hyperparathyroidism, requiring surgical treatment for the parathyroid glands.

Epidemiology

The annual incidence of primary HPT is not known precisely as multichannel auto-analyzers pick up more patients with hypercalcemia. The incidence in men is about 0.3%, and in women 1–3%, affecting 1 in 500 women over 40 years of age and 2.6% of postmenopausal females (8). In the authors' series the average age at presentation was 58 years, ranging from 20 to 88 years. Adenomas were twice as common in females, but the incidence of carcinoma was equal in both sexes.

Genetic Predisposition

No discernible etiological factor has been identified in most cases of parathyroid neoplasia, but adenomas are usually monoclonal, suggesting a mutation in a progenitor cell is an important step (9). The genetic defects are not entirely clear as yet, but probably several are required to produce a parathyroid tumor. Multiple endocrine neoplasia (MEN) types 1 and 2 are associated with an inherited genetic predisposition for parathyroid hyperplasia. A loss of alleles on chromosome 11 results in parathyroid tumors in some patients with MEN1, and also in some cases of solitary adenomata (9–12).

The normal gene appears to inhibit tumor formation and parathyroid glands from patients with gene depletion are unusually large. Primary hyperparathyroidism affects up to 90% of the MEN1 gene carriers and it appears to be a multiglandular disorder with a high propensity for recurrence after parathyroid surgery (13). Seventy percent of excised glands show nodular hyperplasia, which appears to be more commonly associated with recurrence and 30% have diffuse hyperplasia.

There is also a hereditary syndrome of hyperparathyroidism (frequently from parathyroid cancers) and the development of fibro-osseous tumors of the maxilla or mandible. The jaw tumor syndrome is associated with loss of heterozygosity of chromosome 1q, which contains the *HRPT2* gene. Affected patients will usually have developed parathyroid adenomas by the age of 40, and 5% will develop parathyroid carcinoma. Half of the cases develop fibro-osseous tumors in the jaw (14).

Prognostic Factors

Successful excision of the parathyroid adenoma(s) is the definitive curative treatment in primary HPT with resolution well over 95% in experienced hands. In parathyroid carcinoma, a multivariate analysis of 95 patients showed that prognosis was improved if the tumor was resected en bloc, occurred at a younger age, or had better histopathology and DNA ploidy (15). Other prognostic factors include time to recurrence and the presence of metastatic disease (16,17).

Parathyroid Adenoma

Parathyroid adenoma is the most common cause of primary HPT. The vast majority of adenomas are solitary, but multiple adenomas do exist and it is important to be able to discern this with imaging prior to surgery if a focused

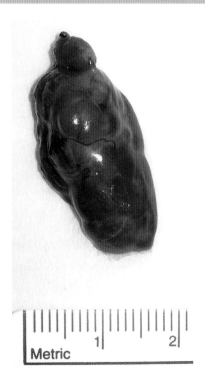

Figure 23.2 Large parathyroid adenoma.

approach is contemplated. In the authors' series of 152 patients there was a single adenoma in 75% of cases, but this can increase to 80–85% in other series. The size of a parathyroid adenoma is extremely variable, from 50 mg to more than 11 g in the authors' series, and does not correlate with activity or calcium levels (Fig. 23.2).

The typical gross appearance is that of a soft reddish-brown or tan-colored gland, often embedded in fat. The surgeon should be able to visually distinguish it not only from lobules of fat, which are yellow and float in saline (Wang's test), but also from thyroid nodules, which are firmer and redder in color, and lymph nodes, which are a grayish pink and intermediate in consistency. Adenomas are more commonly found in the inferior glands.

Microscopically most consist of large chief cells arranged in sheets or in a pseudoglandular pattern, with absent or minimal intracellular or intercellular fat. Often the nuclei may be pyknotic or pleomorphic, which should not be mistaken for mitoses that are the hallmark of carcinoma.

Asymmetric Hyperplasia

Double adenoma is a rare event and can be confused with a variant of asymmetric hyperplasia that affects only two glands. True double adenoma occurs when there are two abnormal and two normal glands, without evidence of MEN or familial HPT, and the patient is cured by removal of the two affected glands. The classification of patients with more than one but less than four enlarged parathyroid glands has been debated for some time, particularly whether double adenoma actually exists or is a form of asymmetric hyperplasia. The latter implies that the patient is at risk of recurrent or persistent HPT from the two remaining glands,

and should be carefully followed up to rule out multiglandular disease. Asymmetric hyperplasia occurred in 7% of the Hammersmith series of patients.

Microadenoma

Another extremely rare entity is parathyroid microadenoma, characterized by a small but active parathyroid tumor that does not exceed the normal parathyroid weight. It may be overlooked during initial neck exploration, and is usually only located at the second or third exploration when no enlarged glands have been found.

Parathyroid Hyperplasia

Diffuse hyperplasia affecting all glands, as a cause for primary hyperparathyroidism, is diagnosed extremely rarely since the advent of minimally invasive scan-directed surgery. The incidence is now less than 5%, having been around 15% in the era of routine full exploration of the neck. This is difficult to explain but may be because of over diagnosis at full exploration, with enlargement of some glands possibly related to vitamin D deficiency and in fact non-functional. It may also be possible that focused surgery is missing some cases of multiple adenoma and these cases will recur in time.

Chief cell or nodular hyperplasia accounts for 80–85% of parathyroid hyperplasia that involves all four (or more) glands. The glands are smaller than those in parathyroid adenomas and are typically 0.5–1 g in size, but can range up to 10 g. There is often marked variation in size of the individual glands and not infrequently patients can present confusingly with one markedly enlarged gland and three slightly enlarged or almost normal-sized glands.

Microscopically they consist of cords, sheets, or follicular arrangements of chief cells, not unlike adenomas. Nodular chief-cell hyperplasia is the usual pathology of the parathyroids in MEN1 syndrome. There is also minimal intracellular fat as seen in adenomas, but there is a variable amount of intercellular stromal fat cells. Clear cell hyperplasia is a relatively uncommon form of parathyroid hyperplasia: macroscopically they tend to be very large, usually 5–10 g, but range up to 50–60 g in size. Microscopically they consist of sheets of large pale vacuolated clear or "water" cells. They are not known to be associated with MEN.

Parathyroid Carcinoma

These are rare tumors occurring in 0.5–4% of HPT patients (6), and usually present with marked hyperparathyroidism. Non-functioning tumors account for only a small proportion and tend to be far more aggressive and are usually incurable. This is probably because they are not associated with hypercalcemia and therefore escape early clinical detection. Although routine calcium screening has led to an increased incidence of HPT there has not been a corresponding rise in the incidence of parathyroid cancer (18).

The preoperative clinical differentiation between parathyroid carcinoma and adenoma is often difficult but clinical features suggesting carcinoma include: (a) severely elevated serum calcium levels (usually >3.5 mmol/l), (b) grossly elevated serum PTH levels (usually greater than four times normal), (c) palpable tumor (>2 cm in 50% of cases), and (d) voice change suggestive of vocal cord palsy (16,17).

However these features are not totally reliable and the possibility of malignancy may only arise intraoperatively.

Carcinomas are hard, gray-white, and large with an average weight of about 10 g. They often adhere to adjacent structures and sometimes are encased within a fibrous or inflammatory-like reaction. More advanced tumors may invade surrounding structures, such as the thyroid, larynx, pharynx, trachea, esophagus, or carotid sheath. It can be extremely difficult to differentiate carcinoma from atypical parathyroid adenoma (APA). Vascular invasion, true capsular or tissue invasion, and the presence of recurrence are needed for an unequivocal diagnosis of malignancy. In contrast, the presence of broad fibrous bands, mitotic figures, trabecular growth pattern, and atypical nuclear features may be found in both malignancy and APA (19). Needle biopsy is usually unreliable and even frozen section confirmation is often difficult. Final diagnosis usually rests on the finding of vascular or tissue invasion at the postoperative paraffin section.

Parathyroid carcinoma spreads both via the lymphatics and hematogenously. Cervical lymph node metastases are rare at the time of presentation, and lymphadenectomy may not be justified unless pathological nodes are seen at surgery (19). Distant blood-borne metastases do occur, usually in the lungs, and sometimes in the liver or bones, but are rarely the first presentation of parathyroid cancer (2,6,20). They are, however, a frequent cause of persistent hypercalcemia after surgery.

Local recurrence occurs in 28–50% of cases and if it occurs within two years of initial surgical treatment the long-term prognosis is very poor (15,17). Overall five-year survival is reported as up to 85%, but is better in patients in whom en bloc resection of the tumor is achieved (21–23). Most patients who die from disease succumb to the complications of hypercalcemia rather than to local disease progression.

INVESTIGATIONS AND PREPARATION
General Guidelines
Parathyroid tumors most commonly present with primary HPT, manifested by hypercalcemia together with an elevated PTH level. This may be associated with diseases of the respective target organs, such as renal (urinary calculi) and less often skeletal (osteitis cystica) or pancreatic (acute or chronic pancreatitis) disorders. The other common presentation is that of tertiary hyperparathyroidism, usually in patients with end-stage renal disease.

Patient evaluation should begin with a careful and thorough history and physical examination including the assessment of the evidence of target organ involvement, previous history of thyroid or parathyroid surgery, voice change, and the presence of a neck mass or cervical lymphadenopathy or both.

The subsequent investigation and preparation of a patient with a parathyroid tumor is best divided into four categories

1. confirmation of diagnosis and assessment of target organ involvement,
2. make the patient safe for surgery by managing hypercalcemia,
3. tumor localization to allow focused surgery, and
4. staging investigations if carcinoma suspected.

1. Diagnostic Investigations
Laboratory Tests
The basic investigations for the diagnosis of primary hyperparathyroidism are serum levels of calcium, corrected for albumin concentration, phosphate, and PTH. Primary HPT would show hypercalcemia associated with a low serum phosphate and an elevated PTH level, a combination that would in most cases be practically diagnostic. Hypercalciuria occurs in up to 75% of patients and can help to exclude familial hypercalcemic hypocalciuria where the calcium receptor has been reset and there is no parathyroid tumor.

Serum intact PTH elevation is diagnostic of a parathyroid tumor, but may also be elevated in the presence of vitamin D deficiency, so this also needs to be measured. Ectopic sources of PTH are extremely rare, the most common source being lung and renal carcinoma, which in some cases may be occult. There is at present no good tumor marker for parathyroid carcinoma. PTH is a good marker for detecting parathyroid tumors, and for postsurgical monitoring and follow-up, but it does not distinguish well between carcinoma and other parathyroid tumors. Although it has been said that serum PTH levels are usually greater than four times the normal range in carcinoma patients and rarely so in other tumors, this is not invariably the case (17).

Screening Tests
Screening for target organ involvement may be required, depending on how the patient had presented, and would include: chest X-ray; kidney, ureter, and bladder (KUB) X-ray; and serum amylase and alkaline phosphatase.

2. Treatment of Hypercalcemia
If the patient presents with severe hypercalcemia, with a corrected serum calcium above 3mmol/l, then intervention is required to lower the level and make the patient safe for anesthesia. In the authors' experience 17% of patients presented with a serum calcium above 3mmol/l. There are a number of strategies to lower serum calcium.

1. Increase fluid intake either orally if hypercalcemia is mild, or intravenously if more severe.
2. Loop diuretics such as furosemide in combination with adequate hydration can be an effective short-term measure.
3. Bisphosphonates such as pamidronate are extremely effective, but have a long-lasting effect that can make postoperative hypocalcemia a problem for some weeks or even months.
4. Dialysis can be used to quickly lower the calcium but the effect is short-lived.
5. Surgery to remove the tumor is obviously the best way of permanently lowering the calcium to safe levels.
6. Intractable severe hypercalcemia is often the terminal event in uncontrolled metastatic parathyroid carcinoma, with death resulting from cardiac arrhythmias, renal failure, or coma due to central nervous system depression. Tumor debulking in this situation is the most effective treatment if feasible.

7. The use of a calcimimetic drug, such as cinacalcet, can also be very effective, but is only available for use in the treatment of renal hyperparathyroidism and for the treatment of hypercalcemia in parathyroid carcinoma.

3. Localizing Investigations
a. Preoperative

General considerations. There has been a huge shift in the view of surgeons regarding preoperative investigation to localize a parathyroid tumor. Until recently localization investigations were indicated for recurrent or persistent primary HPT (24–28), but were not generally performed before initial neck exploration (29–31). As patients have called for less invasive surgery and as the quality of high resolution ultrasound and Sestamibi scanning has improved, scan-directed minimally invasive surgery has become the preferred operation in most cases. In the past we agreed with the view of the endocrine radiologist Dr J. Doppman, suggesting that "the only localization study needed by a patient undergoing initial parathyroid surgery is to locate an experienced parathyroid surgeon" (32). Our firm view now, however, is that patients undergoing initial parathyroid surgery should only locate an experienced parathyroid surgeon who is using localization studies.

All patients with a confirmed diagnosis of primary hyperparathyroidism should undergo preoperative high resolution ultrasound and ^{99m}Tc-Sestamibi scanning as a minimum. This can localize abnormal parathyroids in about 80% of cases and allow the use of minimally invasive surgical techniques, even under local anesthetic and sedation. Bilateral neck exploration is confined to patients who have no localization or non-concordant scans. It may in fact be better to go on to more invasive tests such as angiography and venous sampling in those patients who fail to have their abnormal gland localized with ultrasound or Sestamibi, but this is controversial. Preoperative localization studies do have limitations, as they may fail to identify asymmetric hyperplasia or ectopic glands and are less accurate in patients with hyperplasia.

The most frequent causes of failure to successfully treat primary HPT are an inadequate initial exploration and the presence of ectopic glands. A significant correlation between the chances of success and the experience of the surgeon has been documented and it is suggested by the authors that a minimum of 20 procedures per year is necessary to achieve acceptable results.

Ultrasonography. High-resolution real-time ultrasound (US) using high-frequency probes (7 MHz or 10 MHz) provides an excellent non-invasive and cost-effective method for detecting parathyroid tumors. Parathyroid adenomata are sonolucent and demonstrate vascularity at color Doppler measurement. More recently studies have been undertaken in the additional use of ultrasound contrast agents such as microbubbles to improve accuracy (33). Preoperative US has a sensitivity of around 80% in the unexplored neck, but is less accurate (40%) in patients who have previously undergone attempted parathyroidectomy. Reported sensitivity varies from 43% to 92%, largely depending on the presence of more than one adenoma, ectopic glands out of the range of view, and the experience of the radiologist (34,35) (Fig. 23.3).

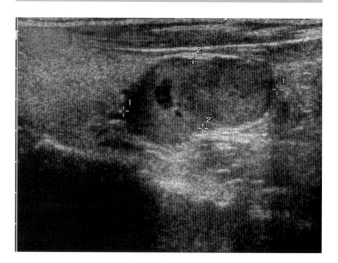

Figure 23.3   Ultrasound localization of a parathyroid adenoma.

Radionuclide scanning. The classic technique of thallium technitium subtraction scanning (^{201}Tl/^{99m}Tc) has proven to be a useful and relatively non-invasive method for localizing parathyroid tumors in both the neck and the mediastinum, but has been largely superseded by ^{99m}Tc-Sestamibi scanning, which has greater sensitivity of over 80% (36,37). Scanning can detect up to 87% of single adenomas, 55% of abnormal glands in multiglandular disease, and up to 75% of persistent and recurrent lesions in the previously explored neck (37). Sestamibi was originally developed as a blood pool scanning agent but is now used to localize parathyroids that concentrate the Sestamibi in their metabolically active mitochondria (Fig. 23.4). It has the advantage over ultrasound of being able to localize ectopic glands, particularly in the mediastinum. The addition of single photon emission computed tomography (SPECT) can also enhance accuracy.

CT scanning. This has not been shown to be as sensitive as ultrasound in detecting neck lesions and is more costly. It is more successful in detecting adenomas in ectopic sites such as the superior mediastinum and tracheo-esophageal groove and in patients who have undergone previous surgical exploration. CT may also help to identify pulmonary and hepatic metastases in patients with malignant disease. Sensitivity ranges from 41% to 86% with an average of 63% (32).

MRI. This is best confined to localizing ectopic glands in the chest as it is poor at distinguishing adenomata in the neck, which have a similar signal intensity to thyroid tissue. As with CT scanning, MRI offers good resolution for tumors in the superior mediastinum and paratracheal area and in patients with persistent hypercalcemia after surgical parathyroid exploration. A review of six recent studies showed an average sensitivity of 74%, which is better than other modalities (32).

Positron emission tomography (PET) scanning. PET scanning with ^{11C}methionine may be useful in a highly select group of patients with recurrent or persistent HPT. PET offers a sensitivity of 83% and an accuracy of 88% in

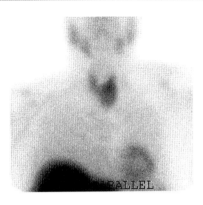

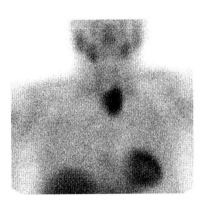

Figure 23.4 Sestamibi scan of a parathyroid adenoma in the left lower position.

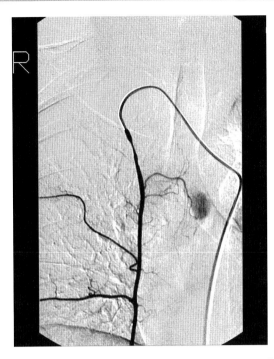

Figure 23.5 Angiography illustrating a parathyroid adenoma in the mediastinum.

successfully locating a parathyroid adenoma (38,39). It is expensive, however, and has limited availability, confining its use to a very small group of cases.

Parathyroid angiography and venous sampling. Before re exploration is undertaken after failure to extract a parathyroid adenoma at initial surgery, the diagnosis needs to be reconfirmed and the ultrasound and Sestamibi scan repeated. Further investigations depend on the circumstances, but more invasive techniques are usually indicated. Parathyroid angiography and selective venous sampling have a high sensitivity in localizing "lost" glands, approaching 95% in our series (Fig. 23.5).

Almost all enlarged glands are hypervascular, which produces a characteristic angiographic blush, making this technique highly sensitive, when combined with venous sampling, for PTH. With a reported sensitivity of 90–95%, it can be used in parathyroid adenoma patients after failed initial surgery, but also prior to re-exploration for renal hyperparathyroidism (40,41).

b. Intraoperative Techniques

Methylene blue. Intraoperative localization of parathyroids is becoming less of an issue with accurate scan-directed techniques and the increasing experience of parathyroid surgeons working in dedicated endocrine surgical centers. The use of intraoperative intravenous dyes such as methylene blue to selectively stain the parathyroid glands is still popular in the United Kingdom with some surgeons but the authors have not found it useful.

Frozen section. Immediate frozen section of any tissue removed from the neck is useful to confirm that parathyroidectomy has been achieved and a thyroid nodule or lymph node has not been removed instead. This is particularly so in the confined spaces of a scan-directed minimally invasive approach.

Intraoperative PTH estimation. Another useful adjunct to successful surgery is the quick intraoperative assay of the biologically active N-terminal fragment of PTH, which has a half-life of only 3–6 minutes. A fall in PTH to normal levels intraoperatively will confirm the removal of the offending parathyroid lesion, particularly in single adenoma or where the preoperative scans are not concordant (42,43). There is some debate about whether the intraoperative quick PTH does add value to surgical decision making, as the equipment is not widely available and is expensive (43,44). Care also needs to be taken in patients with asymmetric hyperplasia or four-gland disease as the PTH may drop but not return to normal.

4. Staging and Screening Investigations of Suspected Parathyroid Carcinoma

Patients who are suspected preoperatively to have parathyroid carcinoma should be screened for metastatic disease with a chest X-ray, liver ultrasound, and a bone scan. Those who have confirmed carcinoma whose PTH levels fall to within normal levels postoperatively require no further investigation. If this is not the case, appropriate staging investigations would include CT or MRI scans of the neck, thorax, and abdomen and, if not already done, a bone scan (45–47). All patients with parathyroid hyperplasia should undergo additional screening for MEN syndrome.

TREATMENT OF PARATHYROID TUMORS
Indications for Primary Parathyroid Surgery
Surgery is the mainstay of treatment for all parathyroid tumors, with three main objectives: a normal calcium and PTH with no supplements, a perfect voice, and a good scar. The possibility of using local anesthesia and undergoing the operation as an outpatient are bonuses to the principal objectives.

Patients presenting with classic hyperparathyroid symptoms of "painful bones, renal stones, psychic moans, abdominal groans, and fatigue overtones" are likely to be already developing complications of hypercalcemia and surgery is plainly indicated.

These patients, however, are less frequently encountered and an increasing number of asymptomatic patients are being picked up with minimally elevated levels of calcium. There is some debate as to whether these patients should be carefully followed-up or should undergo surgery. The National Institute of Health (NIH) Consensus Development Conference in 1990 and revisions in 2002 provided some guidelines (48,49), but the authors feel that all patients with hypercalcemia and primary hyperparathyroidism should undergo parathyroidectomy for the following reasons.

1. Symptoms may be subtle, especially psychiatric symptoms, which may only become evident postoperatively.
2. Approximately 25% of asymptomatic patients treated without surgery have progression of disease (50).
3. Approximately 50% of conservatively treated patients become symptomatic, with 6% developing renal stones, 5% bone disease, and 5% psychological problems (51).
4. Psychiatric symptoms affect almost two-thirds of patients with HPT and many of these are reversed following surgery (50).
5. Limited evidence suggests increased mortality from cardiovascular disease (53,54).
6. Glucose control is improved in diabetics with hyperparathyroidism (55).
7. Minimally invasive surgery is safe and has a high rate of cure in experienced hands.
8. The cost of long-term follow-up far exceeds the cost of surgical cure.

Parathyroid Surgery
There are a number of different methods of surgical parathyroidectomy and each has advantages and disadvantages. Surgical identification of all four glands is not necessary if the parathyroid tumor has been carefully localized by preoperative imaging before surgery. Scan-directed minimally invasive parathyroidectomy is possible in approximately 80% of cases, leaving traditional open exploration of all four glands for those patients who have not been localized or who have other indications for full exploration, such as MEN syndrome, renal hyperparathyroidism, or use of lithium.

If a second normal gland is seen during focused scan-directed parathyroidectomy, no further exploration is undertaken, although a caveat to this approach is to remember

that only 30% of double adenomas are ipsilateral. If a second gland is found to be abnormal however, further exploration is indicated and all four glands must be visualized.

The standard management of parathyroid hyperplasia is subtotal parathyroidectomy, which consists of the removal of the three most abnormally large glands and the partial removal of the remaining more normal looking gland, preserving its blood supply intact. Alternatively this remnant can be removed from the neck and auto-transplanted into a forearm muscle, so that further neck exploration is not needed in the future should hyperparathyroidism recur. In cases of renal hyperparathyroidism where the patient is unlikely to ever have a renal transplant, total parathyroidectomy with calcium and vitamin D replacement is preferred as there is a 75% chance of recurrence of HPT if these patients have auto-transplantation. In all cases thymectomy should be performed as a significant number of patients have rests of parathyroid tissue within the substance of the thymus.

1. Traditional Open Parathyroidectomy
Bilateral exploration of the neck allows an assessment of all four glands when localization has been unsuccessful preoperatively or there is suspected hyperplasia. It enables the surgeon to identify the parathyroids, remove the affected gland(s), and mark the remaining glands with Ligaclips™ to aid identification if further surgery is needed in the future. Bilateral exploration also has the advantage of being able to diagnose hyperplasia, but the disadvantage of a larger wound and the potential for greater morbidity as both recurrent laryngeal nerves and all parathyroids can be damaged.

It is worth remembering that parathyroids tend to be symmetrically placed on each side of the neck, and most are situated in the normal anatomical positions. The position of the parathyroids is related to the plane of the recurrent laryngeal nerves: superior glands lie posterior to the plane and inferior glands anterior to this plane. Any excised gland should be subject to frozen section to confirm successful resection of a parathyroid.

When a gland cannot be found, it is usually a missing inferior gland, as these are more variable in position. In this case a thymectomy should be performed as the gland is often to be found embedded within the thymus (Fig. 23.6). If the thymus is not present it raises the possibility of an

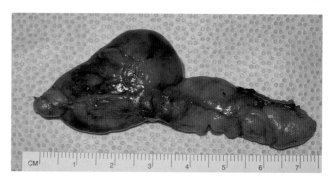

Figure 23.6 Large parathyroid adenoma embedded within the thymus gland.

undescended parathyroid and a search should be made more superiorly. Failing that, the carotid sheath must be opened and explored, and thought given to a possible intrathyroid adenoma, necessitating a hemithyroidectomy. The search for a missing superior gland is aided by taking down the superior thyroid pedicle and also searching along the trachea-esophageal groove, as ectopic superior glands are likely to have descended posteriorly.

2. Scan-directed Minimally Invasive Parathyroidectomy (MIP)

This approach has rapidly become the favored approach in recent years and is indicated in the majority of patients (approximately 80%) who undergo successful localization with preoperative imaging (Fig. 23.7). It allows a small focused incision over the affected gland (which can be facilitated by skin marking at prior ultrasound), either a lateral collar incision or one placed along the line of the anterior border of the sternocleidomastoid muscle. The latter is particularly useful in the elderly patient undergoing exploration under local anesthesia.

Confirmation with frozen section, and ideally intraoperative PTH if available aids the success rate of this technique, which should be greater than 95%. The authors strongly advocate the use of intraoperative nerve monitoring and a headlight to protect the recurrent laryngeal nerve. The advantages of this technique are the excellent cosmetic result and minimal morbidity, against the small possibility of missing asymmetric hyperplasia.

3. Minimally Invasive Video-Assisted Parathyroidectomy (MIVAP)

This technique was developed by Miccoli and colleagues and requires no gas insufflation (56,57). It uses a central neck incision and an endoscope as an aid to visualization, and has the advantage of allowing access to both sides of the neck. It is difficult to master, however, with longer operating times and greater expense. It also carries a higher rate of recurrent laryngeal nerve injury, and is not suitable for repeat

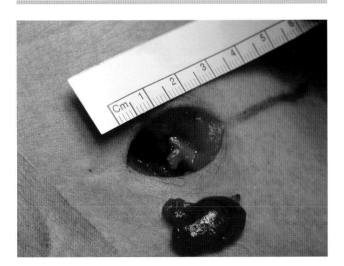

Figure 23.7 Scan directed focused parathyroidectomy.

parathyroidectomy where scarring has obliterated the surgical planes.

Ikeda in Japan has taken the operation even further in order to remove any scarring from the neck (58). This technique uses a sub-mammary or axillary approach, but has not become popular because of the higher complication rates and a steep learning curve.

4. Radio-Guided Parathyroidectomy

This technique has been popularized by Norman and relies on the capability of parathyroid tumors to take up Sestamibi (59). This is administered to the patient two hours prior to surgery and a handheld gamma probe is used to detect the tumor and confirm its removal. This technique has not become popular in many centers, but in our experience it may be useful in those patients who are initially Sestamibi negative. The higher dose of Sestamibi may make the tumor easier to locate with the handheld probe than after the lower dose used for the scan. It can be useful in locating deep, ectopic, or recurrent tumors, but it is a costly technique and logistically difficult.

5. Endoscopic Parathyroidectomy

This technique requires three or four incisions in the neck and gas insufflations, but does give a good view of the structures. Access to the opposite side requires another three incisions, which has meant the technique is not favored, particularly when the difficult learning curve, higher cost, slower operating time, and higher complication rates are taken into account.

Management of Parathyroid Carcinoma
Surgical Management

The only effective and potentially curative treatment for parathyroid carcinoma is surgery. The surgeon should be alerted to the possibility prior to operation by the severe symptoms and the presence of a palpable neck mass. Preoperative imaging should give further clues, particularly if there is evidence of invasion or nodal metastases. Minimally invasive techniques should be avoided in this situation and a traditional exploration adopted allowing good exposure. Any lesion suspicious of a carcinoma should probably be treated as one, recognizing that it can be very difficult to distinguish from an atypical parathyroid adenoma (19). This means an en bloc resection, including the ipsilateral thyroid lobe and isthmus and any adherent structure (16,17). Clearance of the ipsilateral tracheo-esophageal groove lymph nodes (level VI) is also necessary. Frozen section can be utilized, but this is not definitive in the majority of cases because of the difficult histological criteria for diagnosis (19,20).

When locally invasive parathyroid cancer is encountered the lesion should be resected as thoroughly as possible, even at the expense of the integrity of the recurrent laryngeal nerve, larynx, trachea, esophagus, or carotid artery (16,17,45,46,60). This is because an incompletely resected carcinoma will inevitably result in early recurrence, and complete resection will not be possible in recurrent cases (47). Radical surgery should only be carried out, however, after histological confirmation. If frozen section is not definitive, then resection should be delayed until a confirmatory paraffin section report is obtained.

The role of elective cervical lymph node clearance is controversial and some authors advocate a routine radical neck dissection at the time of parathyroid surgery for carcinoma. We would advocate a selective neck dissection (level VI) for N0 disease and a modified radical neck dissection only in the presence of gross cervical node involvement (23,60).

Non-Surgical Treatment

Adjuvant external beam radiotherapy may have a place in the management of parathyroid carcinoma as the rate of local recurrence is lower independent of the disease stage or type of surgery (21,61). There has been no established routine role for chemotherapy in the management of parathyroid carcinoma and rarely has it been of benefit (17,62). Newer therapies such as immunotherapy have shown promise in achieving hormonal, biochemical, and clinical improvements in a patient with metastatic parathyroid cancer by immunizing the patient against PTH (63).

Calcimimetics such as cinacalcet, which act by blocking the calcium sensing receptor, have proven very successful in controlling the severe hypercalcemia seen in metastatic and recurrent parathyroid carcinoma (64,65).

Metastatic Parathyroid Carcinoma

The principle of aggressive debulking should apply equally to metastatic parathyroid carcinoma for two important reasons.

1. Parathyroid carcinoma even at an advanced stage behaves in an indolent, slowly progressive fashion, and meaningful palliation for prolonged duration, often many years, can be achieved by aggressive tumor debulking.
2. Patients who die of advanced parathyroid carcinoma almost invariably do so as a result of the uncontrolled hypercalcemia rather than from an invasive carcinoma.

All surgically resectable disease should be removed or debulked as thoroughly as possible, to the extent of a thoracotomy for lung metastasis or hepatic resection for liver metastasis (45–47,66,67).

Recurrent Parathyroid Carcinoma

Recurrence of parathyroid carcinoma is usually heralded by the reappearance of hypercalcemia and an elevated PTH. The patient should have their serum calcium aggressively treated by medical management to get the level down to as close to 3 mmol/l as possible, which lowers the potential anesthetic risk. A complete diagnostic reassessment is required, including a Sestamibi scan to look for locoregional recurrence in the neck, as well as CT or MRI scans of the neck, thorax, and abdomen, and a bone scan. Although recurrent disease is essentially incurable, aggressive debulking can achieve palliation for a long time (45–47,66,67). It is vital, however, that the extent of disease is well-localized before surgical intervention, and that "blind" neck explorations are not attempted.

Complications After Parathyroidectomy
Hungry Bone Syndrome and Postoperative Hypocalcemia

This temporary but troublesome postoperative condition is due to the reversal of parathyroid osteodystrophy, and must be anticipated in every case of parathyroid resection, particularly in patients who are vitamin D deficient. It can be particularly prolonged if the patient has been treated with bisphosphonates before surgery, or if bone disease is extensive and the hyperparathyroidism has been severe.

Patients may need intravenous calcium given on the first postoperative night, but this should never be given by a peripheral IV line as extravasation of the calcium infusion can have devastating effects on the skin and subcutaneous tissues of the arm. It is usually possible to treat hypocalcemia without IV calcium, however, but patients may need to take calcium and vitamin D oral supplementation for weeks or months after surgery. This is not usually a problem in asymptomatic patients picked up on biochemical screening or in those with minimal symptoms and no end-organ damage.

Strategies After Failed Parathyroid Exploration

Occasionally, exploration of the neck fails to reveal the tumor. In the case of a focused approach, immediate conversion to standard neck exploration should be done, allowing all four parathyroids to be visualized. If after exploring within the normal boundaries of a cervical parathyroid exploration (the hyoid superiorly, the carotid sheaths bilaterally, and the thymus gland inferiorly) the affected gland remains elusive, then it is probably best to close the neck and investigate further. If three glands are identified, as is most often the case, they should be marked with a Ligaclip™, and an ipsilateral thymectomy and thyroid lobectomy—on the side of the missing parathyroid—carried out in the hope that the occult gland is within one of these glands.

The lost inferior gland is most often to be found in the thymus, which is easily accessible from a standard cervical incision. Another common location is within the thyroid gland, more usually the site of a missing upper rather than lower gland. Missing superior glands have often passed down behind the esophagus in the trachea-esophageal groove, but can also be found higher up in the neck. Taking down the superior pole of the thyroid and dividing the superior part of the sternothyroid muscle can aid exposure. In the event that all these strategies fail then the parathyroid must be considered to be ectopic and may be in the chest. Before contemplating re-exploration it is mandatory to localize the missing gland and the best method of doing so is with parathyroid angiography and venous sampling.

Mediastinal Exploration

If the lost gland is located in the anterior upper mediastinum, which occurs in approximately 1% of cases, then exploration can be carried out usually by manubrial split. Full sternotomy is rarely necessary, except if the gland is lower down in the aorto-pulmonary window, which may require a more radical dissection. Mediastinal exploration is not indicated at first operation because the pathologist may locate the missing gland in the thymus or thyroid at paraffin section, and the adenoma's blood supply may inadvertently be disrupted during dissection of the neck, turning an apparently negative exploration into a successful result.

If the patient is unsuitable for further mediastinal exploratory surgery, then the tumor may be suitable for embolization at angiography. This usually works best when there is a single feeding vessel that can be selectively catheterized (68,69).

CONCLUSION

Parathyroid surgery using minimally invasive scan-directed techniques is highly successful in treating hyperparathyroidism, with success rates approaching 98% in the Hammersmith series. Even in experienced hands up to 5% of patients have persistent or recurrent hypercalcemia following primary parathyroid surgery due to occult or ectopic disease. This figure is significantly higher, however, if exploration is undertaken by an inexperienced or occasional parathyroid surgeon, emphasizing the need to concentrate expertise in fewer specialized centers.

REFERENCES

1. Wang CA. The anatomical basis of parathyroid surgery. Ann Surg 1976; 183: 271–5.
2. Castleman B, Roth SI. Tumours of the parathyroid gland. In: Atlas of Tumour Pathology. Washington, DC: Armed Forces Institute of Pathology, 1978.
3. Gilmour IR. The gross anatomy of the parathyroid glands. J Pathol 1938; 46: 133–48.
4. Graney DE. Thyroid and parathyroid anatomy. In: Cumming CW, Fredrickson JM, Harker LA et al. eds. Otolaryngology—Head and Neck Surgery. St Louis: CV Mosby, 1986; 2469–73.
5. Owen R. On the anatomy of the Indian rhinoceros (Rh. Unicornis, L). Trans Zoo Soc Lond 1862; iv: 31–58.
6. Koea JB, Shaw JH. Parathyroid cancer: biology and management. Surg Oncol 1999; 8: 155–65.
7. Stojadinovic A, Hoos A, Nissan A et al. Parathyroid neoplasms: clinical, histopathological, and tissue microarray-based molecular analysis. Hum Pathol 2003; 34: 54–64.
8. Lundgren E, Rastad J, Thurfjell E et al. Population-based screening for primary hyperparathyroidism with serum calcium and parathyroid hormone values in menopausal women. Surgery 1997; 121: 287–94.
9. Arnold A, Staunton CE, Kim HG et al. Monoclonality and abnormal PTH genes in parathyroid adenomas. N Engl J Med 1988; 318: 658–62.
10. Thakker RV, Bouloux P, Wooding C et al. Association of parathyroid tumours in multiple endocrine neoplasia type 1 with loss of alleles on chromosome 11. N Engl J Med 1989; 321: 218–24.
11. Friedman E, Sakaguchi K, Bale AE et al. Clonality of parathyroid tumours in familial multiple endocrine neoplasia type 1. N Engl J Med 1989; 321: 213–18.
12. Mowschenson PM, Silen W. Developments in hyperparathyroidism. Curr Opin Oncol 1990; 2: 95–100.
13. Hellman P, Skogseid B, Juhlin C et al. Findings and long-term results of parathyroid surgery in multiple endocrine neoplasia. World J Surg 1992; 16: 718–23.
14. Szabo J, Heath B, Hill VM et al. Hereditary hyperparathyroidism-jaw tumor syndrome: the endocrine tumor gene HRPT2 maps to chromosome 1q21-q31. Am J Hum Genet 1995; 56: 944–50.
15. Sandelin K, Auer G, Bondeson L et al. Prognostic factors in parathyroid cancer: a review of 95 cases. World J Surg 1992; 16: 724–31.
16. Van Heerden JA, Weiland LH, ReMine K et al. Cancer of the parathyroid glands. Arch Surg 1979; 114: 475–80.
17. Anderson BJ, Samaan NA, Vassilopoulou-Sellin R et al. Parathyroid carcinoma: features and difficulties in diagnosis and management. Surgery 1983; 94: 906–15.
18. Shane E, Bilezikian JP. Parathyroid carcinoma: a review of 62 patients. Endocr Rev 1982; 3: 218–26.
19. Ippolito G, Palazzo FF, Sebag F et al. Intraoperative diagnosis and treatment of parathyroid cancer and atypical parathyroid adenoma. Br J Surg 2007; 94: 566–70.
20. Schantz A, Castleman B. Parathyroid carcinoma. A study of 70 cases. Cancer 1973; 31: 600–5.
21. Clayman GL, Gonzalez HE, El-Naggar A et al. Parathyroid carcinoma: evaluation and interdisciplinary management. Cancer 2004; 100: 900–5.
22. Van-Heerden JA, Grant CS. Surgical treatment of primary hyperparathyroidism: an institutional perspective. World J Surg 1991; 15: 688–92.
23. Grandberg PO, Cedermark B, Farnebo LO et al. Parathyroid tumours. Curr Probl Cancer 1985; 9: 1.
24. Levin KE, Clark OH. The reasons for failure in parathyroid operations. Arch Surg 1989; 124: 911–15.
25. Clark OH, Okerlund MD, Moss AA et al. Localization studies in patients with persistent or recurrent hyperparathyroidism. Surgery 1985; 98: 1083–94.
26. Shen W, Duren M, Morita E et al. Reoperation for persistent or recurrent primary hyperparathyroidism. Arch Surg 1996; 131: 861–7.
27. Cheung PS, Borgstrom A, Thompson NW. Strategy in re-operative surgery for hyperparathyroidism. Arch Surg 1989; 124: 676–80.
28. Rodriquez JM, Tezelman S, Siperstein AE et al. Localization procedures in patients with persistent or recurrent hyperparathyroidism. Arch Surg 1994; 129: 870–5.
29. Whelan PJ, Rotsein LE, Rosen IB et al. Do we really need another localizing technique for parathyroid glands? Am J Surg 1989; 158: 382–4.
30. Tibblin S, Bondesson A-G, Uden P. Current trends in the surgical treatment of solitary parathyroid adenoma: a questionnaire study from 53 surgical departments in 14 countries. Eur J Surg 1991; 157: 103–7.
31. Doppman JL, Miller DL. Localization of parathyroid tumours in patients with asymptomatic hyperparathyroidism and no previous surgery. J Bone Miner Res 1991; 6: 153–9.
32. Doppman JL. Preoperative localization of parathyroid tissue in primary hyperparathyroidism. In: Belizikan JP, Malcus R, Levine MA (eds.) The Parathyroids 2nd ed. Academic Press, New York: 2001; 475–86.
33. Cosgrove D. Future prospects for Sonovue and CPS. Eur Radiol 2004; 14 Suppl 8: P116–24.
34. Lucas RJ, Welsh RJ, Glover JL. Unilateral neck exploration for primary hyperparathyroidism. Arch Surg 1990; 125: 982–4.
35. Lloyd MN, Lees WR, Milroy EJ. Pre-operative localization in primary hyperparathyroidism. Clin Radiol 1990; 41: 239–43.
36. Weber CJ, Vansant J, Alazraki N. Value of technitium 99m sestamibi iodine 123 imaging in reoperative parathyroid surgery. Surgery 1993; 114: 1011–18.
37. Pattou F, Huglo D, Proye C. Radionuclide scanning in parathyroid diseases. Br J Surg 1998; 85: 1605–16.
38. Otto D, Boerner AR, Hofmann M et al. Pre-operative localization of hyperfunctional parathyroid tissue with 11C-methionine PET. Eur J Nuc Med Mol Imaging 2004; 31: 1405–12.
39. Beggs AD, Hain SF. Localization of parathyroid adenomas using 11C-methionine positron emission tomography. Nuc Med Commun 2005; 26: 133–6.

40. Seehofer D, Steinmuller T, Rayes N et al. Parathyroid hormone venous sampling before reoperative surgery in renal hyperparathyroidism: comparison with noninvasive localization procedures and review of the literature. Arch Surg 2004; 139: 1331–8.

41. Reidel MA, Schilling T, Graf S et al. Localization of hyperfunctioning parathyroid glands by selective venous sampling in reoperation for primary or secondary hyperparathyroidism. Surgery 2006; 140: 907–13.

42. Barczynski M, Konturek A, Cichon S et al. Intraoperative parathyroid hormone assay improves outcomes of minimally invasive parathyroidectomy mainly in patients with a presumed solitary parathyroid adenoma and missing concordance of preoperative imaging. Clin Endocrinol (Oxf) 2007; 66: 878–85.

43. Stalberg P, Sidhu S, Sywak M et al. Intraoperative parathyroid hormone measurement during minimally invasive parathyroidectomy: does it "value-add" to decision-making? J Am Coll Surg 2006; 203: 1–6.

44. Gawande AA, Monchik JM, Abbruzzese TA et al. Reassessment of parathyroid hormone monitoring during parathyroidectomy for primary hyperparathyroidism after 2 preoperative localization studies. Arch Surg 2006; 141: 381–4.

45. Flye MW, Brennan MF. Surgical resection of metastatic parathyroid carcinoma. Ann Surg 1981; 193: 425–32.

46. Fujimoto Y, Obara T, Ito Y et al. Localization and resection of metastatic parathyroid carcinoma. World J Surg 1986; 10: 539–47.

47. Sandelin K, Tullgren O, Farnebo LO. Clinical course of metastatic parathyroid cancer. World J Surg 1994; 18: 594–8.

48. Potts JT. Proceedings of the NIH consensus development conference on diagnosis and management of asymptomatic primary hyperparathyroidism. J Bone Miner Res 1990; 6: 9–13.

49. Bilezikian JP, Potts JT Jr, Fuleihan Gel-H et al. Summary statement from a workshop on asymptomatic primary hyperparathyroidism: a perspective for the 21st century. J Clin Endocrinol Metab 2002; 87: 5353–61.

50. Silverberg SJ, Shane E, Jacobs TP et al. A 10-year prospective study of primary hyperparathyroidism with or without parathyroid surgery. N Eng J Med 1999; 341: 1301–2.

51. Scholz DA, Purnell DC. Asymptomatic primary hyperparathyroidism: 10 year prospective study. Mayo Clin Proc 1981; 56: 473–8.

52. Carty SE, Norton JA. Management of patients with persistent or recurrent primary hyperparathyroidism. World J Surg 1991; 15: 716–23.

53. Palmer M, Adami HO, Bergstrom R et al. Mortality after operation for primary hyperparathyroidism. A follow-up of 441 patients operated on from 1956–1979. Surgery 1987; 102: 1–7.

54. Stefenelli T, Mayr H, Bergler-Klein J et al. Primary hyperparathyroidism: incidence of cardiac abnormalities and partial reversibility after successful parathyroidectomy. Am J Med 1993; 95: 197–202.

55. Richards ML, Thompson NW. Diabetes mellitus with hyperparathyroidism: another indication for parathyroidectomy? Surgery 1999; 126: 1160–6.

56. Miccoli P, Bendinelli C, Vignali E et al. Endoscopic parathyroidectomy: report of initial experience. Surgery 1998; 124: 1077–80.

57. Miccoli P, Bendinelli C, Berti P et al. Video-assisted versus conventional parathyroidectomy in primary hyperparathyroidism: a prospective randomised study. Surgery 1999; 126: 1117–22.

58. Ikeda Y, Takami H, Sasaki Y et al. Endoscopic neck surgery by the axillary approach. J Am Coll Surg 2000; 191: 336–40.

59. Norman J, Chheda H. Minimally invasive parathyroidectomy facilitated by intraoperative nuclear mapping. Surgery 1997; 122: 998–1004.

60. Wang CA, Gaz RD. Natural history of parathyroid carcinoma. Am J Surg 1985; 193: 522.

61. Munson ND, Foote RL, Northcutt RC et al. Parathyroid carcinoma: is there a role for adjuvant radiation therapy? Cancer 2003; 98: 2378–84.

62. Chahinian AP, Holland JF, Marinescu A et al. Case report. Metastatic non-functioning parathyroid carcinoma: ultrastructural evidence of secretory granules and response to chemotherapy. Am J Med Sci 1981; 282: 80–4.

63. Betea D, Bradwell AR, Harvey TC et al. Hormonal and biochemical normalization and tumor shrinkage induced by anti-parathyroid hormone immunotherapy in a patient with metastatic parathyroid carcinoma. J Clin Endocrinol Metab 2004; 89: 3413–20.

64. Dong BJ. Cinacalcet: an oral calcimimetic agent for the management of hyperparathyroidism. Clin Ther 2005; 27: 1725–51.

65. Silverberg SJ, Rubin MR, Faiman C et al. Cinacalcet hydrochloride reduces the serum calcium concentration in inoperable parathyroid carcinoma. J Clin Endocrinol Metab 2007; 92: 3803–8.

66. Dubost C, Jehanno C, Lavergne A et al. Successful resection of intrathoracic metastases from two patients with parathyroid carcinoma. World J Surg 1984; 8: 547–56.

67. Iihara M, Okamoto T, Suzuki R et al. Functional parathyroid carcinoma: long-term treatment outcome and risk factor analysis. Surgery 2007; 142: 936–43.

68. Miller DL, Doppman JL, Chang R et al. Angiographic ablation of parathyroid adenomas: lessons from a 10-year experience. Radiology 1987; 165: 601–7.

69. McIntyre RC Jr, Kumpe DA, Liechty RD. Reexploration and angiographic ablation for hyperparathyroidism. Arch Surg 1994; 129: 499–503.

24

Sarcomas of the Head and Neck

Brian O'Sullivan and Patrick J Gullane

INTRODUCTION

Sarcomas of the head and neck (HN) are rare tumors of connective tissue origin that comprise less than 1% of head and neck malignancies. They arise in any soft tissue or osseous tissues of the region and may be found in patients of any age or gender. Unfortunately, HN sarcomas do not traditionally exhibit the high local control rates seen in similar histologies elsewhere and this may be the reason for their poorer survival. This has been attributed to the traditional inability to deliver intensive treatments because of their location among the critical anatomy of the head and neck.

In practice, treatment has inevitably drawn extensively from knowledge learned from the management of these tumors in other anatomic sites, most notably the extremities. The members of a sarcoma team ideally should have the expertise to provide the full range of approaches necessary for cases presenting to their center. Surgery with or without radiotherapy (RT) is almost exclusively the mainstay of local management of soft tissue sarcoma (STS). The respective roles of both have been evaluated in randomized trials for extremity lesions; these principles also apply to the management of certain bone tumors. The indication for adjuvant systemic treatments relies for the most part on published meta-analyses for STS that included head and neck STS patients and some overviews for HN osteosarcoma. The available reports that address head and neck sarcoma are also problematic for numerous reasons that include small study size, retrospective uncontrolled management assessments, frequent inclusion of pediatric with adult cases, various histological subtypes, admixture of patients with locally recurrent and primary presentation patients, and a wide range of study time periods. These methodological problems make interpretation of data for individual patient decision-making more difficult. In this chapter we shall present the essential elements involved in understanding the diagnostic and treatment requirements for this rare and varied group of head and neck malignancies using evidence drawn to a great degree from their more common counterparts in other anatomic regions.

NATURAL HISTORY OF SARCOMAS
Local Disease Extent

Unlike other sarcomas where local salvage options are often available when disease recurs, death from head and neck lesions is as often a consequence of uncontrolled local disease as it is from metastases. These tumors also present in multiple ways depending on the numerous potential anatomic sites and whether bone, vascular, or neural invasion is evident. Lesions may originate in the upper aero-digestive tract, paranasal sinus, and skull base with symptoms referable to these areas (e.g., nasal symptoms including obstruction or discharge and ocular proptosis from direct invasion in paranasal sinus tumors; cranial nerve abnormalities in lesions arising in the skull base or masticator space; alteration of voice or airway compromise for laryngeal and hypopharyngeal lesions). Tumors originating in the subcutaneous tissues of the face, neck, or scalp can initially present with a superficial mass or with bleeding.

Most STS spread in a longitudinal direction within the muscle groups where they originate. They generally respect barriers to tumor spread, such as bone, interosseous membrane, major fascial planes, etc, and this feature should be exploited in planning tissue preserving approaches to management. As they extend, lesions invade muscle and contiguous structures ultimately enveloping major neurovascular structures or other vital anatomy. The extending border comprises an outer perimeter of edematous tissue intermixed with a reactive zone of neovascularity with interspersed tumor satellites and pseudopodia. This surrounding area is generally termed the "pseudocapsule", and may encourage erroneous interpretation of anatomic disease containment that encourages enucleation. Such operations, frequently termed "shell out" procedures, almost invariably mean that residual disease remains, together with the requirement for further resection that is frequently more complicated in nature due to contamination of the adjacent tissues.

Bone and cartilage tumors often present with pain in addition to symptoms of mass and compression. Pain generally relates to infiltration and expansion of bone. In low-grade lesions, pain may be characterized as a prolonged aching sensation over a period of several years. Lesions of the jaw often present as a slow growing mass or with looseness of dentition. Because of their potential also to arise in the skull base, airway cartilages, and paranasal sinuses, these osseous lesions may manifest with a wide variety of presenting symptoms.

Metastatic Involvement

Most sarcomas present with localized disease with metastasis being present in fewer than 10% of cases at the time of diagnosis and initial treatment. Generally the patient is asymptomatic and staging investigations are needed to demonstrate the metastatic process. The predominant risk is to the lungs. Regional lymph node involvement is unusual but is represented most frequently in certain STS histological sub-types, most notably rhabdomyosarcomas, epithelioid sarcomas, alveolar soft part, angiosarcomas, and clear cell and synovial sarcomas. Rarely, bone sarcomas may also present with regional lymph node disease, which carries a very adverse outcome (Fig. 24.1). Remote bone marrow metastases may be evident, but are seen almost exclusively in rhabdomyosarcoma with associated lymphadenopathy or in Ewing's sarcoma. The latter also preferentially spreads to bone, and osteosarcoma rarely demonstrates bone metastases in the absence of lung involvement.

Site Specificity of Histological Subtypes

Most mesenchymal lesions found in head and neck soft tissues are not exclusive to the head and neck generally. Despite this, sarcoma subtypes appear to exhibit certain preferences for different topographic regions in the head and neck (1). In adult STS, the four most common groups are lesions in the neck (including larynx/pharynx), where liposarcoma, malignant peripheral nerve sheath tumor (MPNST), and synovial sarcoma predominate; scalp and facial skin, where angiosarcoma and dermatofibrosarcoma protuberans are most frequent; sinonasal tract, where MPNST and hemangiosarcoma predominate, followed by myxofibrosarcoma, and frequently rhabdomyosarcoma; and the oral cavity, where leiomyosarcoma and rhabdomyosarcoma are most often encountered. In children and adolescents, the vast majority of soft tissue malignancies are rhabdomyosarcomas (1).

Head and neck osteosarcomas account for about 5% to 10% of all osteosarcoma and are the most common malignant bone tumors. Head and neck osteosarcoma occurs in the third and fourth decades of life, where long bone osteosarcoma predominates in the teenage years. The mandible (40%) and maxilla are the most frequent bones involved although other skull bones may be affected (2). Chondrosarcoma comprises approximately 10% of malignancies of bone and is the second most common sarcoma of bone. Most (60%) arise from miscellaneous "head and neck bones" or "sino-nasal" sites, with some predilection for the clivus and petrous temporal bones; approximately 8% originate in the mandible. Almost one-quarter arise from the laryngotracheal cartilages (3).

Ewing's sarcoma appears to arise from pluripotent mesenchymal tissue, although a neuro-ectodermal origin is suspected. It amounts to about 10% of bone tumors. Swelling and pain in the jaw are the most common presentations. Radiology reveals an osteolytic lesion with sun-ray spicules of periosteal bone. It may also appear as a permeative lesion with an aggressive onion-skin type of periosteal reaction. Pathologic features of this small, blue, round cell tumor include nuclei with smooth contour and small nuclei with electron-lucent zones in the cytoplasm, which are lakes of glycogen. It is exceptionally rare in the head and neck and experience in its management remains anecdotal. A cooperative study of 301 Ewing's sarcoma cases recruited only six lesions affecting skull bones (2%), and three (1%) in the clavicles (4).

THE MULTIDISCIPLINARY MANAGEMENT APPROACH

A consistent approach to these rare diseases allows comparison of treatment approaches from center to center and ensures quality of care. An essential component to accomplish this is the implementation of multidisciplinary teams consisting of surgeons, radiation oncologists, medical oncologists, pathologists, and radiologists, along with support disciplines that allow for the optimal care of these complex cases (5). With a multidisciplinary team, all members ideally would see the patient and participate in formulating a treatment plan prior to implementation of any component of therapy.

Part of the multidisciplinary approach must also include an appreciation of the principles for safe acquisition of diagnostic tissues, as well as review of pathology

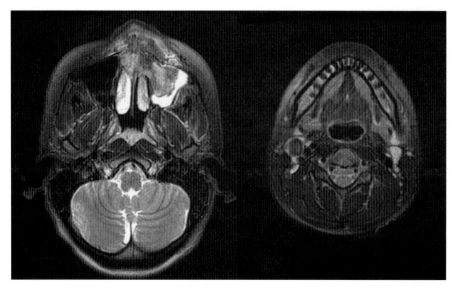

Figure 24.1 T2 Fat sat magnetic resonance axial images of an osteosarcoma with origin in the left maxilla of a teenage girl. Note the soft tissue mass in the pre-maxilla, palate, and the nasal fossa in addition to disease in the left maxillary sinus (*left image*). There is an unequivocal contralateral right sided level 2 lymph node that was proven to represent one of three involved nodes in that region at the time of subsequent surgery following induction chemotherapy. The patient also had a single metastasis that involved a vertebral body that was subsequently resected, as were the primary and disease in the neck. All sites of disease showed substantial pathological response to chemotherapy.

by an experienced pathologist as discussed later. (See "Diagnostic Pitfalls" below). Another practical but important factor is that the radiation oncologist ideally should be aware of—and preferably have an opportunity to see the patient prior to—any surgery being performed. Otherwise, imaging and pathology details may be lacking or inadequate, and precisely appreciating the original tumor characteristic for accurate postoperative adjuvant treatment may not be possible. The consequence of a fragmented radiotherapy service with significantly compromised outcome was evident in a study that addressed an extremity STS subsite in one particular center. There the local failure rate was 28% compared to two other centers where the local failure ranged from 5% to 10%. At the centers with lower failure rates treatment and consultation was restricted to sarcoma specialist radiation oncologists working in the same multidisciplinary setting as the surgeons (6).

A recent report evaluated outcome in 4205 operative cases of STS. It showed that high volume centers (those in the upper one-third of case volume in a geographic region) had better survival outcomes in numerous sites, including the head and neck, which comprised 12 % of the cases studied (7). Smaller centers may have more difficulty formulating a multidisciplinary team with all necessary components of care, including access to an effective multidisciplinary cancer conference that meets frequently and regularly. This is especially so for head and neck sarcoma management where the case volume is low. It may be preferable to have linkage with the main sarcoma team at the center so that treatment protocols and pathology expertise are maintained as consistently as possible. We have found the latter approach to be essential in our practice even though both the overall sarcoma referral and the head and neck program are of substantial size.

CLASSIFICATION OF HEAD AND NECK SARCOMAS
Histologic Classification

Soft tissues tumors comprise a heterogeneous group with varied histology, location, and behavior. Traditionally, the classification has been based on morphologic similarities between neoplastic cells and a putative normal tissue counterpart that is considered the tissue of origin (Table 24.1). More recent understanding of the biology and pathogenesis of these lesions indicates that they do not necessarily arise from the tissue type from which each derives its name (8). The techniques of electron microscopy, immunohistochemistry, and cytogenetics have been applied in the diagnosis and classification of these tumors; evolving techniques in molecular biology are beginning to become essential companions to the pathologic evaluation of sarcomas.

Tumors of bone are somewhat more specific regarding the tissue of origin, although rarely osteosarcoma and chondrosarcoma are also found in extraskeletal soft tissue sites (Table 24.1), thereby further emphasizing the elusive problem of reliably identifying a putative tissue of origin, whether it arises in bone or soft tissues. In practice, however, tumors of bone are divided into osteosarcomas, where the hallmark is the production of malignant osteoid by the tumor and the origin is almost exclusively from bone; chondrosarcoma arising from cartilage or bone; and the very rarely encountered Ewing's sarcoma, which like other "bone histologies" can also be found in soft tissue.

Traditionally electron microscopy has been useful in refining the diagnosis yielded by light microscopy; for example, it allows recognition of cellular details such as cross striations for rhabdomyosarcoma even in many poorly differentiated lesions. In general its use has declined with the improvements in immunohistochemistry though it has retained a role because few antibodies are completely specific or entirely sensitive (9). Thus immunohistochemistry allows the recognition of epithelial cells, muscle cells, Schwann cells, endothelial cells, and others but also has limitations. As neoplastic cells transform, they express epitopes that are not present on cells for which the tumor is named. For example, a rhabdomyosarcoma may at times express cytokeratin or S100, and a synovial sarcoma only rarely arises from synovial tissue. Despite its shortcomings, immunohistochemistry remains a pivotal component in confirming a diagnosis of head and neck sarcoma. As discussed below, molecular biological techniques are becoming the preferred means of understanding the pathogenesis and behavior of sarcomas, and the specific chromosomal aberrations found in certain types of sarcoma can be exploited for diagnosis (Table 24.2).

From the foregoing comments, it may seem that sarcomas generally, including those arising in the head and neck, could be most easily subdivided into those arising from "soft tissue" and those arising from "bone." Underlying this simple approach, however, is a complicated array of histological subtypes. In addition, all of subtypes manifesting in other anatomic sites are also to be found in the head and neck. The paragraphs that follow will discuss some pathological issues relevant to some histological STS subtypes that are also relevant to the management of head and neck sarcoma. This includes some discussion of the pathological principles related to classification of the most common traditional histological subtype—malignant fibrous histiocytoma (MFH). Now a diagnosis of exclusion, it lacks unique specificity or characteristics within the head and neck region. We also address pathological features of some less common tumors with clinical patterns that are relatively unique to the head and neck. These include rhabdomyosarcoma as the commonest pediatric STS found in the head and neck; angiosarcoma, which is enormously problematic in the scalp and facial skin of older patients; and hemangiopericytoma, a rare tumor with a relatively consistent presentation in the naso-ethmoid region. We also discuss two STS subtypes, synovial sarcoma and dermatofibrosarcoma protruberans (DFSP), which have characteristic molecular signatures of importance to diagnosis and potentially to treatment.

Malignant Fibrous Histiocytoma (MFH)

Since the late 1970s malignant fibrous histiocytoma (MFH) has borne the mantle of most common soft tissue sarcoma of middle and late adulthood and therefore warrants specific mention in this chapter. Originally described in the 1960s, the term MFH was used to describe a group of sarcomas deemed to be derived from a mixed histiocytic and fibroblastic lineage. The existence of "malignant fibrous histiocytoma" as a distinct entity is now considered controversial and at best is regarded as a heterogeneous group of tumors without a specific known line of differentiation. Most of these tumors were considered to be a variable

Table 24.1   Histologic Classification of Soft Tissue Sarcoma

FIBROUS TUMORS
Fibromatoses
    Superficial fibromatoses
        a. Palmar and plantar (DuPuytren's contracture fibromatoses
        b. Penile (Peyronie's fibromatosis)
        c. Knuckle pads
    Deep fibromatoses
        a. Abdominal fibromatosis (abdominal desmoid)
        b. Extraabdominal fibromatosis (extraabdominal desmoid)
        c. Intraabdominal fibromatosis (intraabdominal desmoid)
        d. Mesenteric fibromatosis (including Gardner's syndrome)
        e. Infantile (desmoid-type) fibromatosis

Fibrosarcoma
        a. Adult fibrosarcoma
        b. Inflammatory fibrosarcoma

FIBROHISTIOCYTIC TUMORS
Dermatofibrosarcoma protuberans (including pigmented form,
    Bednar tumor)

Malignant fibrous histiocytoma
        a. Storiform-pleomorphic
        b. Myxoid (myxofibrosarcoma)
        c. Giant cell (malignant giant cell tumor of soft parts)
        d. Inflammatory

LIPOMATOUS TUMORS
Atypical lipoma
Liposarcoma
        a. Well-differentiated liposarcoma
            (i.)   Lipoma-like liposarcoma
            (ii.)   Sclerosing liposarcoma
            (iii.) Inflammatory liposarcoma
        b. Dedifferentiated liposarcoma
        c. Myxoid / round cell liposarcoma
        d. Pleomorphic liposarcoma

SMOOTH MUSCLE SARCOMAS
    Leiomyosarcoma
    Epithelioid leiomyosarcoma

SKELETAL MUSCLE SARCOMAS
    Rhabdomyosarcoma
        a. Embryonal rhabdomyosarcoma
        b. Botryoid rhabdomyosarcoma
        c. Spindle cell rhabdomyosarcoma
        d. Alveolar rhabdomyosarcoma
        e. Pleomorphic rhabdomyosarcoma

Rhabdomyosarcoma with ganglionic differentiation
(ectomesenchymoma)

MALIGNANT TUMORS OF BLOOD AND LYMPH VESSELS
    Epithelioid hemangioendothelioma
    Angiosarcoma and lymphangiosarcoma
    Kaposi's sarcoma

MALIGNANT PERIVASCULAR TUMORS
    Malignant glomus (glomangiosarcoma) tumor
    Malignant hemangiopericytoma

MALIGNANT SYNOVIAL TUMORS
    Malignant giant cell tumor of tendon sheath

MALIGNANT NEURAL TUMORS
    Malignant peripheral nerve sheath tumor (MPNST)
    (neurofibrosarcoma)
        a. Malignant Triton tumor (MPNST with rhabdomyosarcoma)
        b. Glandular MPNST
        c. Epithelioid MPNST
    Malignant granular cell tumor
    Primitive neuroectodermal tumor
        a. Neuroblastoma
        b. Ganglioneuroblastoma
        c. Neuroepithelioma (peripheral neuroectodermal tumor)

PARAGANGIOLIONIC TUMORS
    Malignant paraganglioma

EXTRASKELETAL CARTILAGINOUS AND OSSEOUS TUMORS
    Extraskeletal chondrosarcoma
        a. Myxoid chondrosarcoma
        b. Mesenchymal chondrosarcoma
    Extraskeletal osteosarcoma

PLURIPOTENTIAL MALIGNANT MESENCHYMAL TUMORS
    Malignant mesenchymoma Alveolar soft part sarcoma
    Epithelioid sarcoma
    Malignant extrarenal rhabdoid tumor
    Desmoplastic small cell tumor
    Ewing Sarcoma – extraskeletal
    Clear cell sarcoma (melanoma of soft parts)
    Gastrointestinal stromal tumors
    Synovial sarcoma
        a. Biphasic synovial sarcoma
        b. Monophasic synovial sarcoma

Source: Fletcher CDM, Unni K, Mertens K, eds. World Health Organization Classification of Tumors: Pathology and Genetics of Tumors of Soft Tissue and Bone. IARC Press (International Agency for Research on Cancer) publishers, Lyon, France. Single 2002 (118). Benign lesions other than fibromatosis and atypical lipoma are not included in the present tabulation.

storiform and/or pleomorphic phenotype, or to be one of four rarer additional types: myxoid, the next most common subtype; giant cell; inflammatory; and angiomatoid, a rare variant and the only one to survive contemporary reclassification. Reclassification of many tumors in this group has afforded better prognostication and the old term "MFH" is generally considered obsolete today. This was reviewed in detail recently (10). Current nomenclature recognizes the entities undifferentiated high grade pleomorphic sarcoma (previously storiform-pleomorphic "MFH"); and myxofibrosarcoma (formerly myxoid "MFH"), which is now the most

common sarcoma of older adults, peaking in incidence in the 7th and 8th decades. It must be differentiated from other sarcoma containing myxoid areas, such as pleomorphic liposarcoma. In the end, the feature that sets these lesions apart is the absence of a defined line of differentiation; hence they have evolved to be a diagnosis of exclusion. For the purpose of this review they do not have particular relevance to the head and neck, although reports appear from time to time suggesting potential uniqueness in the head and neck, either based on anatomic origin or on etiology (e.g., as radiation induced lesions) (11). We would

Table 24.2.   Selected Cytogenetic Abnormalities in Sarcoma – Adapted from Antonescu et al. (13)

Histologic subtype	Usual translocations	Genes involved
Alveolar sarcoma of soft parts	t(X; 17)(p11; q25)	TFE3-ASPL
Angiomatoid fibrous histiocytoma	t(12; 16),(p13; p11)	FUS-ATF1
Chondrosarcomas extraskeletal myxoid	t(9; 22),(q22; q12.2)	EWS-CHN
Clear cell sarcoma	t(12; 22)(q13; q12)	EWS-ATF1
Congenital fibrosarcoma	t(12; 15)(p13; q25)	ETV6-NTRK3
Dermatofibrosarcoma protuberans	t(17; 22)(q22; q13)	COL1A1-PDGFB
Desmoplastic small round-cell tumor	t(11; 22)(p13; q12)	EWS-WT1
Endometrial stromal sarcoma	t(7; 17),(p15; q21)	JAZF1-JJAZ1
Ewing's/peripheral primitive neuroectodermal tumor	t(11; 22),(q24; q12)	EWS-FLI1
Extraskeletal myxoid chondrosarcoma	t(9; 22),(q22; q12)	EWS-NR4A3
Fibromyxoid sarcoma, low grade	t(7; 16),(q33; p11)	FUS-CREB3L2
Inflammatory myofibroblastic tumor	t(1; 2),(q22; p23)	TPM3-ALK
Myxoid liposarcoma	t(12; 16)(q13; p11)	FUS-DDIT3
Rhabdomyosarcoma (alveolar)	t(2; 13)(q35; q14) t(1; 13)(p36,q14)	PAX3(or7)-FOXO1A
Synovial sarcoma	t(X; 18)(p11.2; q11.2)	SYT/SSX1 or SSX2

Note: Gene nomenclature evolves at least as rapidly as pathological terminology.

submit that they do not have any remarkable associations and their management should adhere to the general strategies outlined later.

Rhabdomyosarcoma

The rhabdomyosarcoma (RMS) classification recognizes embryonal, botryoid, alveolar, and pleomorphic subtypes for both childhood and adult cases. Rhabdomyosarcoma can be recognized on light microscopy by the presence of cross striations within cytoplasmic fibrils of spindle shaped cells that typically demonstrate immunostaining for myogenic markers (12). Seventy percent of RMS can be classified as embryonal and 20% alveolar and the remainder are variants, including the uncommon pleomorphic subtype. The latter is almost never seen in the pediatric population and is not considered in those classifications; there is debate about whether it truly represents part of the disease process, and it may fall into the 'MFH' type categories described above.

Embryonal RMS has variable amounts of primitive spindle or round cells in a myxoid background. These rhabdomyoblasts appear in a variety of unusual shapes termed "tadpole" or "strap" cells. Cross striations on light microscopy can be seen in half of these cells. The botryoid RMS is felt to be a variant of embryonal RMS and only accounts for 5% of cases. It is defined as a tumor having polypoid morphology with the presence of subepithelial aggregates of malignant cells, which is referred to as the cambium layer. Botryoid tumors have a particularly favorable prognosis. A diagnosis of alveolar RMS is made if the tumor has alveolar-like spaces that are filled with round malignant, eosinophilic cells. Presence of any amount of alveolar morphology in the lesion qualifies it to be alveolar RMS. The presence of alveolar morphology has been identified as a poor prognosticator. There is also a solid variant of this tumor that lacks alveolar spaces but is still included in this subtype. The presence of sheets of anaplastic cells warrants a diagnosis of pleomorphic RMS. Generally the diagnosis of the less favorable alveolar subtype is based on the identification of the characteristic chromosomal

translocations t(2; 13)(q35; q14) and t(1; 13)(p36,q14) and their fusion products (Table 24.2) (13).

Angiosarcoma

Angiosarcoma is an especially devastating form of head and neck sarcoma. The majority of angiosarcomas are considered to originate from the endothelium of the blood vasculature (14). Koch and colleagues recently outlined the pathological features, which can range from well-differentiated to poorly differentiated lesions. They are typically composed of an accumulation of an irregular or sinusoidal pattern of vessel with vascular spaces lined by a single row of atypical endothelium that may also be several layers thick. Highly cellular lesions can manifest as sheets of cells with vascular space obliteration that contribute solid components as vascular channels are effaced by the crowding of cells. High-grade, poorly differentiated lesions can be comprised of undifferentiated cells and disordered architecture, making them difficult to discern from other histologies, though the hallmark clinical presentation and behavior generally leaves little doubt about the diagnosis. By immunohistochemistry, these tumors are usually positive for factor VIII-related antigen, vimentin, CD34, and CD31 (15).

It is suggested that angiogenesis and vascular permeability play a central role in the development of angiosarcomas. This is likely influenced by vascular endothelial growth factor A (VEGF-A), which plays a significant role in angiogenesis and vascular permeability. VEGF-A induces angiogenesis by acting through a tyrosine kinase receptor predominantly found on vascular endothelial cells including VEGF receptor-1. VEGF-A acts to enhance the growth of tumors by promoting a more extensive blood-vessel supply and increasing the probability of hematogenous metastases. Similarly, it has been proposed that angiogenesis and vascular permeability play a central role in development of angiosarcomas, suggesting a role for VEGF-A in the pathogenesis of angiosarcomas (14), thereby opening the potential for molecular targeted agents in the future. (See "Targeted Approaches").

Hemangiopericytoma

To clinicians, hemangiopericytoma is a confusing entity, in particular since pathologists have had difficulty informing them about whether these lesions will behave in a relatively indolent or aggressive manner. Fletcher has indicated that unlike most so-called hemangiopericytomas elsewhere, these head and neck lesions, typically originating in the nasal cavity or paranasal sinuses, are of true pericytic origin (1), and that perhaps this provides a distinction from apparently similar lesions in other anatomic sites. Potentially, this may explain the more favorable behavior of the head lesions compared to others; alternatively, the putative, less detrimental behavior may merely be a reflection of the fact that these tumors likely present earlier within the confines of the naso-ethmoid region due to earlier resulting symptoms, and are therefore smaller than their counterparts elsewhere. Histologically, tumor cells are arranged around relatively prominent, small, thin-walled blood vessels. The vessels form a "staghorn pattern" and contain perivascular hyalinization. Most cases show immunohistochemical positivity for actin. Factor XIIIa and CD34 positivity are also described. Mitoses are generally rare. The main composition is of relatively monomorphic spindled or ovoid cells with eosinophilic cytoplasm and bland nuclei, thus giving a rather myxoid appearance.

Synovial Sarcomas

Synovial sarcomas are tumors of pluripotential mesenchymal cells. There is little resemblance between synovial membranes and synovial sarcoma and the tumor rarely originates from synovial tissue. It has been suggested that the name of this sarcoma subtype should be modified (16). These tumors are composed of two morphologically distinct types of cells that form a characteristic biphasic pattern. The biphasic synovial sarcoma includes epithelial cells with a surrounding spindle or fibrous component. The spindle cells stain positive for keratin and epithelial membrane antigen. Vimentin is demonstrable in spindle cells but absent in epithelial cells. S-100 staining may give positive results. Monophasic synovial sarcomas of both fibrous and epithelial types are recognized, although the monophasic epithelial variant of synovial sarcoma is extremely rare. Synovial sarcomas contain a characteristic chromosomal translocation that is the gold standard in establishing the diagnosis, with the observation that 100% of biphasic and 96% of monophasic synovial sarcomas possess the specific t(X; 18)(p11; q11) translocation (Table 24.2).

Dermatofibrosarcoma Protuberans

Dermatofibrosarcoma protuberans (DFSP), as the name suggests, is an elevated nodular ("protruberant") lesion arising from the dermis with characteristic slow but persistent growth over many years. Infiltration can take place along connective tissue septae, between adnexae, and interdigitating with lobules of subcutaneous fat. A uniform population of slender fibroblasts is arranged in a monotonous storiform pattern with little nuclear pleomorphism and low mitotic activity. DFSP is composed of densely packed spindle cells arranged in a storiform or cartwheel pattern. CD34 staining is extensively positive in nearly all cases and has been used to confirm the diagnosis in less common situations where the storiform pattern is obscured by myxoid areas. DFSP subtypes include the Bednar tumor, which has melanin-containing cells along with the standard spindle cells of this neoplasm. Approximately 10% to 15% of all DFSPs contain areas of fibrosarcoma (DFSP-FS), and such cases tend to exhibit more aggressive behavior. More than 90% of DFSP are characterized by the t(17; 22) (q22; q13) reciprocal chromosomal translocation that is now becoming the hallmark feature of the diagnosis. This rearrangement leads to constitutive activation of the platelet-derived growth factor receptor (PDGFR) as a result of deregulated ligand expression, the potential utility of which is discussed later. (See "Targeted Approaches").

Grading of Sarcoma

In the diagnostic pathology of sarcoma, the actual histologic subtype of sarcoma is usually overshadowed in prognostic importance by the designation of pathologic grade (Fig. 24.2). Grade provides a means to identify cases at greatest risk for distant metastasis when combined with other factors. This is important because it provides a means to consider many patients for more intensive treatment approaches, or at least permits a rational approach to clinical trial design to evaluate the role of systemic adjuvant treatments to prevent distant metastases.

In STS many grading schemes have been proposed and validated as efficacious and have been reviewed in detail (17). The three-tier system proposed by the French Federation of Cancer Centers is precisely defined, easy to use, and is the most widely employed. The French system relies on a relatively balanced evaluation of parameters (differentiation score, mitoses, necrosis), but its greatest limitation lies in the assignment of a differentiation score. Roughly defined as the extent to which a lesion resembles normal tissue, differentiation score has little applicability for tumors that ostensibly have no normal tissue. It is also recognized that no system performs perfectly in all sarcomas. In their recent review Deyrup and Weiss highlighted problems, including the fact that some STS do not lend themselves well to grading. These include (1) those in which grade provides no additional information (e.g., well-differentiated liposarcoma/atypical lipomatous neoplasm, Ewing's sarcoma); (2) "ungradable" histological subtypes (e.g., epithelioid sarcoma, clear cell sarcoma, angiosarcoma); and (3) sarcomas that have traditionally been graded, but where this characteristic does not appear to differentiate these lesions prognostically (e.g., malignant peripheral nerve sheath tumor) (17).

Controversies surrounding grading seem to be less pronounced in bone tumors. Osteosarcomas are graded according to the cell type and relative anaplasia of the stromal component of the tumor. Increasingly, anaplastic tumors are given higher grades with the least well differentiated tumors appearing of highest grade. High-grade tumors (grade 3 or 4) generally comprise conventional (osteoblastic), telangiectatic, and dedifferentiated tumors. Chondroblastic and fibroblastic tumors are usually lower grade (grade 1 or 2). In general it is perceived that head and neck osteosarcoma have a lower potential for metastatic spread compared to other sites and this may relate to differences in the proportion of these osteosarcoma subtypes in the region.

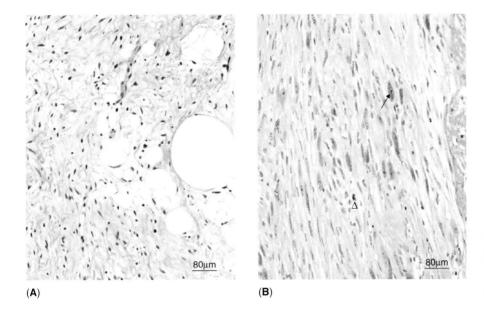

Figure 24.2 Photomicrographs of **(A)** low grade sarcoma showing low cellularity and very little nuclear atypia and **(B)** high grade sarcoma showing nuclear atypia (↑), mitotic activity (arrowhead), and necrosis (*).

(A)   **(B)**

Most chondrosarcomas have a clearly dominant grade. Typically grade is classified according to cellularity, nuclear features, and mitotic activity (18). Low-grade (well-differentiated) chondrosarcomas may be difficult to discriminate histologically from benign cartilaginous lesions because they have the consistency of hyaline cartilage. For chondrosarcoma, well-differentiated appearance (grade 1) is associated with longevity and favorable prognosis.

Myxomatous changes with cystic degeneration in the tumor correlates well with a low or medium histological grade. An absence of cartilaginous lobulation and the presence of spindle cell forms is characteristic of high-grade (grade 3) malignancy and heralds an unfavorable prognosis.

While sarcoma-specific risk stratification schemes that include multiple prognostic factors have been proposed and debated, the central importance of pathologic grading for sarcoma has remained indisputable. This principle has contributed to the acceptance of the critical role of grading in the ongoing assessment of these patients to a degree that it is included in the classification of disease extent discussed below. Importantly, Ewing's sarcoma has generally been classified as high grade in the staging classification.

Molecular Biology of Sarcomas

Contemporary appreciation of the molecular pathogenesis and behavior of sarcomas suggests that these lesions are divisible into two major genetic groups: (1) those possessing specific genetic alterations and usually simple karyotypes, such as reciprocal chromosomal translocations (e.g., SS18-SSX1 or SS18-SSX2 in synovial sarcoma); and (2) sarcomas with nonspecific genetic alterations and complex unbalanced karyotypes (13).

The first group, those characterized by specific recurrent chromosomal translocations, comprise approximately one-third of all sarcomas and the resulting product of the specific gene fusions usually encode aberrant chimeric transcription factors. These translocations are often the only cytogenetic abnormalities and appear to be pathogenetically important; however, while successful cloning of most genes involved in recurrent translocations has taken place, there remains a paucity of information about the downstream targets mediating oncogenic transformation. In general, the promiscuous pairing of a proximal gene that contributes a promoter and functional domain, with a distal gene possessing a DNA binding domain that confers target specificity, determines the phenotype of various soft tissue sarcomas. Most translocations result in the production of a tumor-specific RNA that encodes a novel transcription factor that plays a role in oncogenesis in mesenchymal cells.

One uncommon mechanism results in a chimeric autocrine growth factor and, as discussed earlier, is evident in DFSP where the t(17; 22)(q22; q13) translocation involving the COL1A-PDGFB genes provides a therapeutic target for response to the tyrosine kinase inhibitor, imatinib. Therefore these mechanisms represent opportunities for future management opportunities. (See "Targeted Treatments"). At this time however, they are typically used in a diagnostic manner to identify a particular subtype of tumor. This is the case for synovial sarcomas, nearly all of which exhibit the t(X; 18)(p11.2; q11.2) translocation, and can be distinguished from other tumors with similar morphology, such as a malignant peripheral nerve sheath tumor. Another example is the fusion product PAX3–FOXO1A arising from the t(2; 13)(q35; q14) translocation expressed in alveolar rhabdomyosarcoma (Table 24.2) (13).

The remaining two-thirds of soft tissue sarcomas lack a recurrent genetic signature and are characterized by numerous aberrations, including chromosomal losses and gains. Most adult spindle cell and pleomorphic sarcomas belong to this group. At the molecular level, this sarcoma subset features a high prevalence of p53 checkpoint alterations, including p53 inactivating mutations, homozygous deletion of CDKN2A, MDM2 amplifications, etc. Unfortunately, most cases with complex karyotypes and multiple aberrations do not have a consistent correlation with pathological or clinical parameters. There also appears to be no indication in most of these lesions that detectable genetic alterations might be useful either for diagnosis or prognosis (19).

Bone tumors are similarly heterogeneous with respect to molecular characteristics. Ewing's sarcoma belongs to the group associated with unique chromosomal translocations that give rise to specific fusion transcripts. For example, 85% of Ewing's sarcoma are associated with the t(11; 22)(q24; q12) translocation resulting in the fusion of the EWS and FLI1 genes (Table 24.2) and less commonly the (21; 22)(q22; q12) translocation that generates the EWS-ERG fusion gene. The most common malignant bone tumor, osteosarcoma, on the other hand, does not have any specific translocations or other molecular genetic abnormalities that can serve as diagnostic or tumor-specific markers of disease. RB1 and p53 genes, including related pathways such as MDM2, are frequently altered in sporadic osteosarcomas. Equally, analysis of chondrosarcoma shows substantial heterogeneity with respect to karyotypic complexity, and in truth the exact mechanisms underlying the development and progression of these heterogeneous tumors remain largely unknown (18).

DIAGNOSTIC EVALUATION AND STAGE CLASSIFICATION

Principles and Method of Biopsy

In general all soft tissue masses deep to the investing fascia should be considered to be sarcoma until proven otherwise. The same vigilance is needed for bone lesions, but here the opinion of an experienced diagnostic radiologist is also required. Both bone and soft tissue lesions should be staged with cross-sectional imaging before the biopsy to avoid compromising the planning of appropriate management. Open incisional biopsy of deep tumors is usually preferred over excisional biopsy to minimize the difficulty of the "unplanned" excision without the benefit of preoperative imaging and regard for margins. This undesirable approach was shown to increase the rate of local recurrence in sarcomas of the extremities and would also apply to head and neck sarcomas (20).

The biopsy should be carefully designed in order to facilitate subsequent surgical removal and adjuvant therapy. The biopsy track should be excised afterwards or alternatively may be included in the radiotherapy target volume of preoperative treatment. The open approach is normally recommended because it provides sufficient tissue for traditional histologic analysis as well as immunohistochemistry, electron microscopy, molecular assessment, and cytogenetics. Tumor cells are capable of spread and implantation along tissue planes facilitated by extravasated blood from the surgical site. Therefore the biopsy should be accomplished through the smallest incision possible with absolute hemostasis. Some disadvantages of this approach may include complications and potential delay in initiation

of neoadjuvant therapies if there are wound problems. The possibility also exists for poorly designed incisional biopsies to breach natural barriers to tumor growth, such as muscle fascia and periosteum that provide local containment of tumor (21). Fine needle aspiration biopsy (FNAB) can be a useful technique but these tumors are rare, complex, and difficult to diagnose even in experienced hands. Despite this, there is growing experience in diagnosis of sarcomas using core-needle biopsy or fine-needle aspiration biopsy. These techniques have been advocated by some groups for both soft tissue and bone lesions (21–23) and may be considered if the expertise is available. Anatomically based guidelines for core needle biopsy of bone lesions in other sites are available but there are no similar recommendations for head and neck lesions (24,25).

FNAB is useful for establishing the presence of recurrence (both local and metastatic) but its use as a primary diagnostic tool is controversial and should probably only be used where a cytopathologist with extensive experience in sarcoma is available. Core needle biopsy under local anesthesia provides a more consistent tissue specimen and cell preparation compared to FNAB. In our experience, open biopsy of soft tissue sarcoma is rarely indicated but yields a diagnosis when needle biopsy is unsuccessful (about 10 % of cases). Since diagnosis and grading are increasingly based on tissue obtained by core needle biopsy, new challenges have presented themselves for pathologists. The use of neoadjuvant therapy, especially, eliminates the possibility of accurate grading later when the lesion is resected. Grading on needle biopsies may need to be limited to a two-tier grading system, namely low- versus high-grade, especially since this is what is used in the stage classifications. A close dialogue with clinicians to resolve ambiguities may enhance accuracy (17).

The evaluation of rhabdomyosarcoma and Ewing's sarcoma frequently also includes additional needle-based tissue examination in the form of a bone marrow aspiration and biopsy. In the case of parameningeal rhabdomyosarcoma, cerebrospinal fluid is examined because of the unusual pattern of spread of these tumors and the implication this knowledge has on their management.

Imaging

Accurate, highly sophisticated imaging to delineate tumor extent for diagnostic, surgical, and radiotherapeutic planning is essential to the management of sarcoma. Plain radiography, bone scan, angiography, computed tomography (CT), magnetic resonance imaging (MRI), and positron emission tomography (PET) are generally not helpful in determining the diagnosis but all may contribute in different ways to delineation of the extent of local involvement. We have recently discussed the imaging characteristics of STS in detail (26).

Plain radiography remains useful to establish a differential diagnosis for primary bone tumors but is of little value in the evaluation of STS. Osteosarcoma is a highly aggressive lesion with permeative change, cortical breakthrough, and usually an associated soft-tissue mass (Fig. 24.1). The majority of conventional osteosarcomas also demonstrate an osteoid matrix. Particularly important is the ability of CT to accurately delineate bony anatomy surrounding the tumor. This is crucial in preoperative planning for ablation and reconstruction. CT is also important in assisting in differential diagnosis because MRI is insensitive to certain features such as calcification. Unfortunately, only axial images can be obtained directly by CT with sagittal and coronal reformatted images losing some detail.

The multiplanar imaging and soft tissue detail rendered by MRI makes this modality ideal for staging and treatment planning of both soft tissue and bone sarcomas of the head and neck. Although MRI is highly accurate in delineating the extent of a soft tissue or bony abnormality, it continues to be non-specific. The majority of soft tissue sarcomas will appear as low signal intensity on T1-weighted images and high on T2. These features are non-specific and require a biopsy for diagnosis.

Technetium scintigraphy is the traditional examination of choice for evaluating the entire skeleton to determine whether there are multiple lesions. It is particularly important for diseases with high propensity for bone metastasis such as Ewing's sarcoma. Occasionally, intrapulmonary osteoblastic metastases may be demonstrated.

Positron emission tomography (PET) has an emerging role in the evaluation of bone and soft tissue sarcomas (26–29). It uses radiotracers specific for biologic processes to produce images of regional tissue metabolism with fluorodeoxyglucose, the most commonly employed radiotracer for this purpose. New tracers are being evaluated that may refine the differing roles for PET imaging that include evaluation of: (1) the grade and extent of local disease including the potential for "skip" lesions in adjacent bone; (2) the presence of regional or distant metastases; and (3) the response to initial (i.e., neoadjuvant) treatment as a surrogate to prognosticate on future outcome. It does seem that high versus low-grade lesions may be distinguished and may even provide an imaging technique for biopsy guidance; in addition, response prediction to induction treatments seems to be possible (26–29). While the latter is of interest, it does not truly influence management. Little change in approach is possible, other than to withhold chemotherapy in patients who have not responded well to that point. Generally this would be considered unusual, especially in younger patients. The value following preoperative treatment in STS seems especially unrewarding. Additional radiotherapy is not normally administered following the initial course, and in the case of chemotherapy there remains substantial controversy as to whether it is contributing realistically to outcome. As discussed later for the treatment of osteosarcoma, enhancing the intensity of subsequent adjuvant chemotherapy in the absence of adequate pathological response to induction chemotherapy following resection has been suggested, but evidence for the value of this approach does not exist.

Despite the preceding discussion, the contribution of PET imaging to routine management is currently uncertain. It remains clear, however, that the most common metastatic spread pattern is to the lungs. Consequently, imaging of the chest is necessary. A chest radiograph is used for low-grade lesions, but CT of the chest is always necessary for high-grade tumors.

Diagnostic Pitfalls

In considering a diagnosis of sarcoma of the head and neck, beyond acquiring and interpreting adequate and timely imaging, the ability to achieve an accurate diagnosis may be confounded in several additional ways (1). In the adult especially, nonsarcomatous head and neck lesions may often show spindle cell morphology. These are frequently identified by the synonyms spindle cell or sarcomatoid squamous cell carcinoma, or alternatively may represent malignant melanoma of spindle cell or desmoplastic types. Because of this, the clinician must be vigilant, especially if there are cutaneous or mucosal lesions, or the clinician is confronted with a patient presenting with a mass in the parotid. The latter, especially if the patient is a middle-aged or older white male, may mimic sarcoma in a metastatic lymph node. Both squamous cell carcinoma and melanoma metastases from facial skin or scalp primaries are considerably more frequent than a sarcoma in this location.

If cytology alone is used, confidence in the pathological diagnosis may be a problem. This also applies, however, to small biopsies that may be more frequent in the head and neck because of anatomic constraints in obtaining tissue. In such cases, crush artifact may further influence interpretation. Lehnhardt et al. recently showed that expert pathology opinion was essential for optimal treatment of sarcoma and remains a source of concern even when expertise is present. Discordance in diagnosis (i.e., tumor entity and grading) was apparent in excess of 70% of cases among pathologists in private clinics, slightly fewer in general hospital pathology departments, and in 66% of cases in an academic environment. It only improved to 30% in a sarcoma reference center, even when punch or needle biopsies were not being considered. Inexperience of the pathologist was considered a strong factor leading to discrepant diagnosis, thereby warranting a recommendation for routine expert second opinion (30).

Stage Classification of Sarcomas

The International Union Against Cancer/American Joint Committee on Cancer (UICC/AJCC) TNM staging system is the most widely employed staging system for classifying extent of disease in sarcomas. The staging systems are outlined for soft tissue sarcoma in general (Table 24.3), rhabdomyosarcoma (Tables 24.4 and 24.5) and bone sarcomas (Table 24.6). In both STS and bone sarcoma, pathologic grading also provides an important prognostic measure and has been incorporated in the TNM staging system, which is an exception within the overall cancer stage classification (31,32). In STS lesions, histological grade and tumor size are the primary determinants of clinical stage (Table 24.3). Tumor size is further substaged as "a" (superficial tumor arising outside the investing fascia) or "b" (a deep tumor that arises beneath the fascia, such as in muscle, or invades the fascia). Notwithstanding these comments, the sarcoma TNM system is optimally designed to stage extremity tumors. While patients with head and neck sarcoma present with earlier T-category size and favorable pathology grade, the patient survival may be offset by the more complicated anatomical sites of origin.

One characteristic that appears misplaced in the sarcoma TNM system is the impact of isolated lymph node metastases. These are currently considered of sufficiently ominous significance to be regarded as equivalent to distant metastasis within the Stage IV group. Since the last edition of TNM, data from the Royal Marsden Hospital,

Table 24.3 International Union Against Cancer (UICC) and American Joint Committee on Cancer (AJCC) TNM classification (6ᵗʰ Edition) of soft tissue sarcomas (31,32)

Primary Tumor (T)

TX	Primary tumor cannot be assessed
T0	No evidence of primary tumor
T1	Tumor 5 cm or less in greatest dimension
	T1a superficial tumor
	T2b deep tumor
T2	Tumor more than 5 cm in greatest dimension
	T2a superficial tumor
	T2b deep tumor

Regional Lymph Nodes (N)

NX	Regional lymph nodes cannot be assessed
N0	No regional lymph node metastasis
N1	Regional lymph node metastasis

Distant Metastasis (M)

MX	Distant metastasis cannot be assessed
M0	No distant metastasis
MI	Distant metastasis

Stage Grouping

Stage I	G1-2	T1a, 1b, 2a, 2b	N0	M0
Stage II	G3-4	T1a, 1b, 2a	N0	M0
Stage III	G3-4	T2b	N0	M0
Stage IV	Any G	Any T	N1	M0
	Any G	Any T	N0	M1

Note: Superficial tumor is located exclusively above the superficial fascia without invasion of the fascia; deep tumor is located either exclusively beneath the superficial fascia, superficial to the fascia with invasion of or through the fascia, or both superficial yet beneath the fascia.
Abbreviation: G, Grade.

Table 24.4 IRSG Postsurgical Grouping Classification

Group 1: Localized disease, completely excised and no residual microscopic disease
  A. Confined to the site of origin, completely resected
  B. Infiltrating beyond site of origin, completely resected

Group 2: Total gross resection
  A. Gross resection with evidence of microscopic local residual disease
  B. Regional disease with involved lymph nodes, completely resected with no microscopic residual disease
  C. Microscopic local and/or nodal residual disease

Group 3: Incomplete resection or biopsy with gross residual disease

Group 4: Distant metastases

Table 24.5 International Society of Pediatric Oncology (SIOP) Presurgical Staging Classification (Clinical and Radiological Staging)

Stage	Tumor	Node	Metastases
I	T1a or T1b	N0, NX	M0
II	T2a or T2b	N0, NX	M0
III	Any T	N1	M0
IV	Any T	N1	M1

Abbreviations: T1, Confined to the anatomic site of origin; T2, Extension and/or fixation to surrounding tissue; (a), ≤5 centimeters in diameter; (b), >5 centimeters in diameter; NX, Unknown nodal status; N0, No nodes present clinically; N1, Regional nodes present; M0, No distal metastasis; M0, Metastasis present.
Source: From Ref. 58.

Table 24.6 International Union Against Cancer (UICC) and American Joint Committee on Cancer (AJCC) TNM classification (6ᵗʰ Edition) of bone sarcomas (31,32)

Primary Tumor (T)

TX	Primary tumor cannot be assessed
T0	No evidence of primary tumor
T1	Tumor (maximum dimension) ≤8 cm at time of diagnosis
T2	Tumor (maximum dimension) >8 cm at time of diagnosis
T3	Skip metastases-two discontinuous tumors in the same bone with no other distant metastasis

Regional Lymph Nodes (N)

NX	Regional lymph nodes cannot be assessed
N0	No regional lymph node metastasis
N1	Regional lymph node metastasis to be considered equivalent to distant metastatic disease (See M1b below)

Distant Metastasis (M)

MX	Distant metastasis cannot be assessed
M0	No distant metastasis
M1	Distant metastasis
	M1a = Lung only metastases
	M1b = All other distant metastases including lymph nodes

Stage Grouping

Stage	IA	G1,2	T1	N0	M0
Stage	IB	G1,2	T2	N0	M0
Stage	IIA	G3,4	T1	N0	M0
Stage	IIB	G3,4	T2	N0	M0
Stage	III	Any G	T3	N0	M0
Stage	IVA	Any G	AnyT	N0	M1a
Stage	IVB	Any G	AnyT	N0/N1	M1b

Note: Because of the rarity of lymph node involvement in sarcomas, the designation NX may not be appropriate and could be considered N0 if no clinical involvement is evident.
Abbreviation: G, Grade.

United Kingdom and the Princess Margaret Hospital, Canada have shown that the prognosis of this small subgroup of STS patients have a prognosis similar to Stage III disease (large, deep, and high-grade lesions) (33,34) and therefore will be included within the Stage III group in the next edition of the TNM. This is important for head and neck surgeons and radiation oncologists, who should consider these patients as potential candidates for curative treatment using locoregional treatment approaches in the same manner that they would for other head and neck cancers.

In addition the rarity of lymph node involvement in sarcoma makes the NX designation in applying the classification less appropriate compared to epithelial malignancy of the head and neck. The N0 designation is more appropriate for situations in which lymph node involvement is not clinically evident, even when the lymph nodes have not been examined pathologically, since only certain histological subtypes have a realistic risk of regional node involvement. This principle is acknowledged explicitly in the TNM classification of STS (31,32).

Rhabdomyosarcoma differs from other STS in that the designation of disease extent has traditionally been by a postoperative surgical classification developed by the North American Intergroup Rhabdomyosarcoma Study Group (IRSG) more than two decades ago (Table 24.4). This is not always relevant in the head and neck since such lesions will frequently be treated with aggressive protocols that use chemotherapy and radiotherapy without surgery. In general, the contemporary era has also witnessed protocols where chemotherapy is initiated well in advance of surgery. Subsequent reliance on a surgical staging system that describes the extent of disease at diagnosis is a major problem. The International Society of Pediatric Oncology (SIOP) has suggested a pre-surgical TNM staging system more in keeping with contemporary TNM staging for soft tissue sarcoma (Table 24.5). Both use a T-category break-point at 5 cm and one of these two pre-treatment approaches may be accepted more uniformly in the future.

The bone tumor TNM classification (Table 24.6) considers maximum lesion size (with a break point at 8 cm) and the presence of discontinuous tumors in the same bone without other distant metastasis (31,32). Of interest metastases to non-pulmonary sites are distinguished from M1 disease based on lung involvement alone.

TREATMENT OF SOFT TISSUE SARCOMAS
Surgery (With or Without Radiotherapy)

The invasive nature of STS requires a surgical margin approximating 2 cm in dimension, unless an intact barrier to tumor spread exists within a region with a closer surgical margin. Generally this will be provided by intact fascia in the radial distribution of the lesion, though bone or other skeletal anatomy may also provide the protection needed. In the HN, these margin recommendations are rarely achievable due to constraints posed by the desire to preserve functional anatomy and minimize cosmetic changes. There is an additional need to target any biopsy track or regions of previous incomplete resection within the planned surgical excision, unless they are otherwise encompassed in a preoperative radiotherapy volume. Lesions judged not to be resectable with secure margins on the basis of their presentation and proximity to critical anatomy, or due to the wish to preserve functional anatomy or cosmetic outcome, should be considered for adjuvant RT to achieve optimal local control (Fig. 24.3). Therefore the extent of the surgery needed may be modified when RT is applied strategically in situations where surgery alone would have been sufficient but would have needed a wider excision. In other circumstances, a conservative function sparing operation may again be accomplished using RT, though RT is frequently needed irrespective of the form of operation (conservative or ablative) if there has been prior contamination of tissues from prior ill-advised and unsuccessful excision attempts or by previous aberrant biopsy procedures.

In determining the risk of local failure, the presence of disease at the edge of the surgical margin has traditionally been considered an adverse prognostic factor that is not reliably reversed by the use of radiotherapy. While this is generally correct, there are some exceptions. Most notably we have shown that a "planned positive margin" at

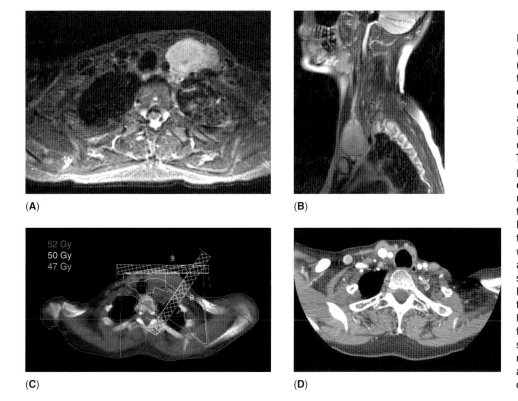

(A) (B) (C) (D)

Figure 24.3 Axial (**A**) and sagittal (**B**) view magnetic resonance images (MRI) of the neck in a 45-year-old female presentation of a dentritic cell sarcoma in the low neck with carotid artery juxtaposition and deviation of medial structures that include the trachea. Patient required combined surgery and radiotherapy. To minimize dose to brachial plexus, preoperative radiotherapy was delivered with three-dimensional conformal radiotherapy in 2001, prior to the availability of intensity modulated radiotherapy (IMRT) in our center. The radiotherapy treatment plan with superimposed isodose lines for a course of 50 Gy in 25 fractions is shown (**C**); the yellow cross cross-hatch shapes schematically depict the direction of the two conformal beams and their customized wedge filters (**C**). The MRI images show the stigma from the necessary surgical resection, but the patient remains asymptomatic and disease-free with eight-year follow-up (**D**).

a small area juxtaposed to a critical structure, such as a neurovascular bundle, is not associated with an adverse risk of recurrence provided the resection in that location of the margin is performed carefully to contain the contamination, and provided there has been properly administered adjuvant radiotherapy pre or postoperatively. These data were studied in extremity STS, but the principle is also applicable to the head and neck (35). The situation should be distinguished from a positive resection margin in soft tissue, such as in muscle where there can be wider dissemination of tumor cells.

Rare exceptions to the use of surgery in STS include many rhabdomyosarcomas where exquisite RT and chemotherapy sensitivity makes this unnecessary and the overwhelming risk is distant metastasis to bone marrow, meninges, and lung typically. Scalp and facial angiosarcomas often pose an overwhelming challenge to surgery due to the improbable ability to achieve useful margins in advanced lesions. Such tumors are frequently managed with RT or chemotherapy on a palliative basis.

Elective neck management with surgery or RT is rarely indicated in HN sarcomas due to the rarity of lymph node involvement, particularly for those histologies that require surgery. Some rare histological subtypes (i.e., rhabdomyosarcoma, clear cell, epithelioid and potentially synovial sarcoma and angiosarcoma) have a greater risk of regional lymph node involvement.

Radiotherapy Approaches
Evidence for Radiotherapy
Assuming that RT is required, the principles and evidence for its use are the same for HN STS as in other anatomic sites. Adjuvant RT was widely adopted for the management of soft tissue sarcoma following the observation that RT in combination with conservative excision could achieve equivalent results to more ablative surgery. The landmark observation was a trial that randomized high-grade sarcoma of the extremities to receive amputation versus a limb-sparing operation followed by adjuvant RT (36). Conservative surgical resection with or without adjuvant RT were compared in two further randomized clinical trials that showed approximately 20% absolute improvement in local control when RT is combined with surgery (37,38). Of interest, no improvement in local control was evident from the use of brachytherapy (BRT) in low-grade tumors in the trial reported by Pisters and colleagues (37). This unexpected result was not evident in the second trial reported by Yang and colleagues where external beam RT was used as the adjuvant treatment (38). These data are important for the general treatment of STS, though no randomized trials have been undertaken for HN sarcomas.

The advantage of a combined RT and surgery approach is also evident in one series where local control was 52% in those treated with surgery alone versus 90% in those treated with the combination (39). Another report showed that head and neck STS patients with either clear surgical margins or microscopic residuum had similar local control rates (26% and 30% failure, respectively) provided RT was administered (40). Finally, we also reported a prospective series of high risk cases treated on a consistent protocol by a limited number of radiation oncologists using preoperative RT (41). The local control result

approached 90%, which is comparable to extremity sarcoma of similar histology and is superior to historical series with less consistent approaches at our institution (40,41).

In the general use of radiotherapy, the same principles apply to the management of the neck as in the case of surgery. Thus elective neck treatment is only indicated for certain histological subtypes.

Pre- vs. Post-operative External Beam Radiotherapy
The scheduling of RT (pre- vs. post-operative) remains controversial due to the balance of different inherent trade-offs from the two approaches (42). For preoperative RT our policy has been to encompass gross tumor, including peritumoral edema where possible, to a dose of 50 Gy in 25 fractions over five weeks to be followed by surgery four to six weeks later. For postoperative RT planning, the high risk target area includes the surgical field containing all tissues handled during the surgical procedure, including scars and drain sites. A reducing field approach is ultimately used to deliver a dose of 60–66 Gy in the postoperative setting. The volume and doses are larger in postoperative compared to preoperative RT according to principles accepted for the radiobiology and clinical requirements for control of these lesions (42).

We conducted a randomized trial comparing preoperative and postoperative RT in extremity soft tissue sarcoma that showed that local control was equivalent in both groups (93%) (43). Our trial also uncovered concern about preoperative RT due to the increased risk of wound complications in some anatomic extremity sites, but not in others (43). Similarly, we found this was very uncommon in a separately undertaken prospective trial of head and neck STS (41). In the combined RT and surgery approach to head and neck STS, which also applies to other tumors such as chondrosarcoma, preoperative RT seems particularly suited, because of the smaller RT volumes and lower doses, to critical anatomy where wide margins cannot be obtained. This is especially notable in proximity to ocular structures (Fig. 24.4). At present, our guidelines for using preoperative RT are: (1) the need to maximally restrict RT volumes in some anatomic sites, (2) the desire to minimize RT dose in some situations (e.g., where critical neurological tissues are in close proximity), and (3) a desire to not irradiate new tissues, especially complex reconstructions that may be vulnerable to the effects of high dose postoperative RT.

Brachytherapy
Brachytherapy (BRT) is less widely used in the management of STS compared to external beam RT but is nonetheless effective. Very few reports in HN lesions exist to draw from, and in general, cases may not always be selected similarly for external beam and BRT protocols. BRT has several theoretical advantages over external beam radiotherapy, including reduced scatter to normal tissues, shorter delay between surgery and radiation therapy, and a much shorter time required to deliver a tumoricidal dose. For the delivery, afterloading catheters are placed in the tissue bed 1 cm apart, to cover the tumor bed and an additional 2 cm, approximately, around the margins (44).

Although theoretically BRT could possibly reduce the volume to be treated, in practice the volumes resemble

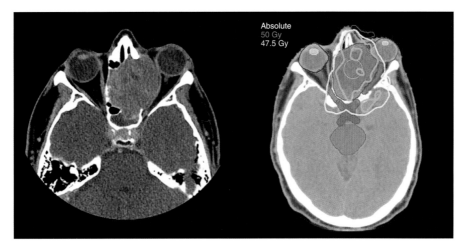

Figure 24.4 Axial computerized image of a base of skull chondrosarcoma in a 65-year-old male adjacent to ocular structures including the optic nerves and chiasm. The absence of calcification in the lesion suggested this was not an osteosarcoma, although chondroblastic osteosarcoma was included in the differential diagnosis following trans-nasal biopsy. Because of the lesion's location the patient was treated with preoperative intensity modulated radiotherapy (IMRT) to a dose of 50 Gy in 25 fractions to maximally spare the optic structures in terms of the dose and volume to these critical structures and the adjacent brain. The right-hand image shows an axial representation of the IMRT plan with the target region shown in red surrounded by the relevant isodose curves. This patient subsequently underwent cranio-facial resection with clear margins. The pathology, however, indicated that the diagnosis was a chondroblastic osteosarcoma and he was then treated with postoperative chemotherapy.

the coverage used in preoperative RT. Most experience has been with monotherapy low-dose rate treatments to 45 to 50 Gy at 0.45 Gy/hour with the skin dose restricted to doses of 20 to 25 Gy. BRT doses of 15 to 20 Gy are used if combined with external beam to a dose of 45 to 50 Gy. BRT requires specific technical expertise with surgical support and should ordinarily not be used as a sole RT method in the presence of the following: involved resection margins, low-grade histology, proximity of tumor to skin, and complex anatomic locations where the zone of risk is difficult to access (44). It also cannot be used if it requires high-dose placement juxtaposed against vulnerable anatomic structures, such as bone, peripheral nerves, or cranial nerves. These conditions of use probably at least partially explain why it is proportionately underused in the HN compared to extremity STS.

High Precision Radiotherapy Techniques

One of the challenges during treatment of head and neck tumors, especially sarcoma, is to selectively target areas of the volume to avoid delivering doses to vulnerable regions, while at the same time maintaining high dose gradients between target and normal tissues. Intensity modulated radiotherapy (IMRT) can be especially useful in those situations where adjuvant doses are relatively high to complex volumes, and normal tissue protection is desirable. Until recently particle beam approaches were the only method of treating complex tumors at the skull base with high-dose RT. Presently stereotactic fractionated RT or IMRT may provide similar outcomes. Despite the use of relatively close RT margins (1.5-cm margin), IMRT has provided a three-year actuarial local control of 95%, and regional node control rate of 90%, in 28 younger patients aged 1 to 29 years (median age 8 years) with rhabdomyosarcoma (45).

Combs et al. have also reported excellent outcomes using IMRT and fractionated stereotactic RT in children with head-and-neck-rhabdomyosarcoma with a low incidence of treatment-related side effects (46).

Radiotherapy Alone

RT alone may be the only option of management in selected adverse presentations in the HN where surgical management is not feasible. In a series addressing unresected STS, the five-year local control rate was 51% for small lesions (47). Doses of at least 63 Gy are recommended, and probably 70 Gy in 35 fractions should be administered if technically feasible. These data were obtained in predominantly non-head and neck sites, although one-quarter of the cases were in the head and neck in the report from Kepta and colleagues (47).

An exception to the almost universal need for combined surgery and RT in STS is in the treatment of rhabdomyosarcoma where, because of the unusually radio-responsive nature of these lesions, control can be expected using RT alone combined with chemotherapy. This treatment is discussed later.

Angiosarcoma, unfortunately, is well represented in the head and neck (accounting for approximately half of all angiosarcomas), especially in the scalp or facial skin. Local control is an overwhelming problem because of the difficulty determining the optimal extent of surgical and RT margins in these apparently multifocal tumors. Local recurrence beyond the treatment areas seems to be almost invariable. It remains uncertain if wide surgical excision is benefiting many of these typically elderly patients. Palliative RT alone may be the optimal approach for many patients. (See "Specific situations").

Systemic Approaches
Adjuvant Chemotherapy in Adult STS

Adjuvant chemotherapy is controversial in STS other than for specific histologies such as rhabdomyosarcoma, or potentially for larger synovial sarcoma where a good response is expected though the true value is uncertain. An individual patient data meta-analysis from the 1568 patients randomized in 14 trials addressed the role of doxorubicin-based adjuvant chemotherapy in STS (48). The results favored the use of adjuvant chemotherapy from the standpoint of recurrence-free survival and distant metastases, but not for overall survival (p = 0.12). HN STS were included to varying degrees in half of the studies (49–55). In the largest trial (n = 468), that of the EORTC, relapse-free survival was significantly better (56% vs. 43% for controls; p = 0.007) and local recurrence was significantly reduced by chemotherapy (17% versus 31%; p = 0.01) (54). This favorable finding appeared to be confined to HN and trunk tumors, and may provide an opportunity to improve local control in a situation where it has traditionally not been as satisfactory as in extremity STS.

Since the publication of the meta-analysis, a further study addressed very adverse tumors (confined to large high-grade lesions) and compared no systemic treatment to a very intensive cytotoxic regimen (five cycles of 4'-epidoxorubicin 60 mg/m² days 1 and 2 and ifosfamide 1.8 g/m² days 1 through 5, with hydration, mesna, and granulocyte colony-stimulating factor). The disease-free and overall survival rates were statistically improved at preliminary analysis. By the time of publication, however, the metastatic rate in both arms of the randomized trial was virtually identical (44% and 45%) (56). Unfortunately this raises the question whether the potential value of aggressive chemotherapy may largely be in delaying the manifestation of distant metastasis, but not in their prevention.

Chemotherapy for Pediatric Rhabdomyosarcoma

In childhood rhadomyosarcoma, chemotherapy has facilitated local management due to the excellent response in addition to local effect from RT, and is discussed in more detail later. (See "Specific Situations"). The demonstration of activity of vincristine, actinomycin D, and cyclophosphamide (VAC) against rhabdomyosarcoma led to pioneering studies of chemotherapy combined with surgery and radiation. The Intergroup Rhabdomyosarcoma Study Group (IRSG) has completed several studies to answer major therapeutic questions regarding this disease (57). Current research efforts are even exploring the potential of relying on chemotherapy as the sole therapy given the devastating local sequelae of RT that may arise in young children (58).

Targeted Approaches

Proven therapeutic molecular targets have remained elusive in sarcoma (59). Several possibilities are emerging, however, that may offer opportunities in this regard.

Bevacizumab, a humanized monoclonal antibody to vascular endothelial growth factor (VEGF), is an attractive agent to consider in angiosarcoma given its ability to inhibit tumor growth. Koontz et al. recently reported promising results in two patients using neoadjuvant bevacizumab combined with radiation therapy (60). Follicular dendritic cell sarcoma is a rare, malignant, non-lymphoid cell-derived tumor that originates from B-lymphoid follicles of nodal and extranodal sites. Surgery and RT are the mainstay of treatment for localized disease. Classic lymphoma and sarcoma regimens have shown dismal responses in the metastatic setting. An imatinib based combination recently has been reported to provide a potential therapeutic strategy (61).

The recent observations of response to imatinib (STI 571, Gleevec®) in DFSP predicted by the presence of the t(17; 22) translocation (Table 24.2) provides possibilities for molecular target therapies in the future (62). For this tumor, however, one should recall the excellent control rates seen with surgery alone or combined with radiotherapy. These targeted approaches are generally applicable to situations where surgery and radiotherapy are not feasible approaches.

Summary of Outcomes for STS of the Head and Neck

In a systematic literature review of HN STS, Mendenhall et al. showed that the local control rate after surgery alone or combined with RT is approximately 60% to 70% (63). The probability of local control is influenced by histologic grade, tumor size, and surgical margins, and appears to be improved by adjuvant RT. Distant metastasis rates approximate 20% to 30 % and survival rates are approximately 50% to 60 % (63–66).

TREATMENT OF BONE SARCOMAS
Surgery

Surgery accomplished with clear resection margins is the foundation of local treatment of osteosarcoma and chondrosarcoma. Neoadjuvant chemotherapy is indicated in the case of osteosarcoma but not in chondrosarcoma. RT as a local adjuvant to surgery has a role in high risk chondrosarcoma but data justifying this approach are far less prevalent for osteosarcoma. Management of the neck is rarely necessary though uncommonly patients may have lymph node metastases (Fig. 24.2).

The local resection should be planned with a very clear definition of tumor extent, particularly the intramedullary component; preoperative imaging is essential for this. As with STS any biopsy scars or other access routes for disease to "track" from the primary site should also be excised, especially if the contaminated area is not intended for inclusion in an RT target volume. It is important to emphasize that wide excision beyond the pseudocapsule is especially required for chondrosarcomas, which tend to have microscopic fingerlike extensions and a notorious propensity to seed the wound with later nodular recurrence if the tumor is violated. Intraoperatively, tumor clearance is confirmed by pathological examination of marrow biopsy at the resection site; similarly verification of completeness of resection is recommended in high risk areas, such as tissues adjacent to neuro-vascular structures in proximity to the tumor.

Chondrosarcoma is the most common sarcoma of the larynx and usually presents with a long history from a mass originating on the posterior cricoid lamina eventually resulting in airway compromise and voice dysfunction. These patients are generally older males (>50 years), and usually have low-grade lesions. Complete laryngectomy is virtually always curable, but more conservative and single modality surgery may be more appropriate when possible in such low grade tumors given the excellent survival rates (67,68). Recent advocates have suggested that total laryngectomy should be reserved for recurrent lesions and rare cases of voluminous high-grade chondrosarcoma of the larynx (69,70). In some cases we have also provided postoperative radiotherapy for patients with a high risk of late relapse and those who have chosen to avoid repeated surgery in the future.

Chondrosarcoma of the skull, especially those arising in the petrous temporal bone or clivus, are often also low-grade in type. Surgery is indicated but proximity to critical anatomy, including the internal carotid artery, brain stem, and the optic nerves make surgery problematic. RT is commonly performed on an adjuvant basis or alone as outlined in the "Radiotherapy" section (Fig. 24.4).

In Ewing's sarcoma, surgery is indicated in expendable bones to permit radiotherapy to be avoided entirely in low-volume disease. It is also important to minimize the use of RT in young patients when possible, especially in children. Any concern about resection margins, however, is an indication that radiotherapy is needed, which ideally can be administered with lower doses since the gross disease will have been resected. In addition, whenever a partial bone resection is undertaken, radiotherapy is indicated to the microscopic areas and a boost applied to any gross residual disease. We feel that very large volume disease is an indication for combined treatment (surgery and radiotherapy). Small volume disease is best managed with radiotherapy as the sole local modality, unless disease is limited and surgery can be accomplished with wide enough margins to obviate the need for radiotherapy. This would be most unusual in the head and neck, where the size of tumors is not extreme as it often is in other anatomic sites.

Radiotherapy
Osteosarcoma
Radiotherapy is not ordinarily used in osteosarcoma of the head and neck. After surgery with involved resection margins in HN osteosarcoma, revision surgery is advisable when feasible because the outlook for these patients is bleak, and adjuvant RT does not appear to confer the high rates of local control seen in STS and in most other tumors. The literature is scant in this area and concludes that outcome with RT is unrewarding due to a preponderance of unresectable lesions or the presence of residual disease after surgery. Reports have suggested that RT either confers no significant value (71), or is associated with worse outcome due to case selection (72,73).

Despite the generally pessimistic views expressed in the literature, DeLaney and colleagues described an overall local control rate at five years of 68% (+/−8.3%) in 41 osteosarcoma patients in whom surgical resection with widely negative margins was not possible (74). In 17 of these patients the tumor arose in the head and neck, and in eight it was of spinal origin. The authors concluded that RT can enhance local control of osteosarcoma and appears most effective in situations in which only microscopic or minimal residual disease is being treated (74).

At present the literature does not provide convincing evidence that RT as a sole modality is useful for the local

management of osteosarcoma, and it is typically reserved for palliation. Even in this setting it is often not helpful.

Chondrosarcoma
Radiotherapy for chondrosarcoma may be used with similar indications to those used for STS. In general the approaches are similar except that BRT is not a realistic option in bone lesions, largely due to concerns about toxicity to bone and the technical configuration of implants in the locations under discussion. Both adjuvant RT, or RT as a sole modality, should follow similar principles as for external beam RT for STS regarding planning, dose-fractionation parameters, and target volumes. The efficacy of the approach is similar to STS and is ordinarily reserved for situations with disease located close to critical anatomy such as the spinal cord (75). RT is most often used in lesions that are grade 2 or higher when surgical margins are compromised (76,77) although it is acknowledged that opinions vary as to its value. It was used as a component of management in more than 20% of cases in a large National Cancer Data Base (NCDB) report.[3]

RT as sole modality for chondrosarcomas in difficult locations, such as the clival regions, can be accomplished with proton beam RT or IMRT. Ten-year control rates of 70% to 80% have been reported from experienced centers using proton beam RT. Indications include the need to sacrifice critical vascular supply in clival lesions, or particular situations where the lesion is of small volume. The combination of surgical debulking and high-dose precision RT results in durable local control in a large proportion of skull base chondrosarcomas (in excess of 80%) with modest late toxicity (78). The outcome of lesions <25 ml in volume is especially good if adequate doses are administered with a combination of photons and protons (e.g., to approximately 70 Cobalt Gray Equivalent [CGE]) (79). Others have reported similar impressive results in smaller series with either protons or fractionated stereotactic RT (80,81).

Schulz-Ertner et al. recently reported the outcome of 54 patients with gross residual low- and intermediate-grade chondrosarcomas of the skull base treated with carbon ion RT. The actuarial local control rates were 96.2% and 89.8% at three and four years; overall survival was 98.2% at five years. Only one patient had grade 3 toxicity (82).

Ewing's Sarcoma
In Ewing's sarcoma radiotherapy alone is effective, but local control is a problem in bulky disease. Because children are commonly affected, influences on bone growth, and second malignancies following radiotherapy are a concern (83). Surgery should therefore also be considered in the management of individual situations. Radiotherapy target volumes traditionally included the entire bone involved, as well as any extraosseous soft tissue component of the tumor. Because induction chemotherapy is frequently used, treatment planning should be based on the original tumor volume before chemotherapy. Classically an initial 5 cm margin beyond disease and bone has been recommended for Ewing's sarcoma, although the need to spare tissues in children has stimulated an evolution to more conservative target definitions. As in STS and chondrosarcoma head and neck planning, treatments should be tailored to suit the anatomic region in question and any anticipated toxicities,

while bearing in mind the age of the patient. Care must be taken to protect critical organs in the head and neck and the "classic" approach will rarely be used. Additional boost to the original area of visualized gross disease is also highly recommended.

Doses of at least 50 Gy in 1.8–2 Gy per fraction are ordinarily employed for gross Ewing's disease and need to be tailored to the critical organs at risk, the bulk of disease at the start of chemotherapy, the response to chemotherapy, and the completeness of any surgical resection. Generally, conventional daily fractionated radiotherapy is used, but studies of smaller dose per fraction altered fractionation are underway to assess ability to minimize late responding tissue damage.

Chemotherapy
Osteosarcoma
Prior to the introduction of systemic adjuvant chemotherapy for the treatment of osteosarcoma, less than 20% of patients survived more than five years. In addition, within six months of salvage treatment that included pulmonary metastasectomy, further recurrence manifested in 50% of patients, almost exclusively in the lungs. With the introduction of chemotherapy to surgical management, long-term disease-free survival and overall survival rates exceeded 60%. Conclusive proof of this survival advantage became available from the results of two small randomized clinical trials that compared surgery alone to surgery followed by chemotherapy in patients presenting with localized high-grade osteosarcoma (84,85).

Frequently, a three-drug chemotherapy regimen comprising doxorubicin, cisplatin, and high-dose methotrexate is used. The strategy for localized disease today also involves neoadjuvant chemotherapy for approximately 10 weeks followed by definitive surgery, followed by additional adjuvant chemotherapy. A major reason for this approach is to permit a determination about whether more aggressive combinations of chemotherapy will improve outcome for poor histologic responders determined after resection. In truth, this strategy originated from the need to delay surgery for limb osteosarcoma in order to allow time to manufacture a limb prosthesis, thereby allowing the subsequent pathology specimen to be evaluated for pathological response to chemotherapy. This practice subsequently concluded that patients with pathologically responding tumors fared more favorably than those whose tumors did not respond as well. Surgeons also were more comfortable attempting limb preservation techniques following chemotherapy. Evidence that modifying chemotherapy to address poor response is advantageous awaits study. There is also no evidence that the induction approach is superior compared to postoperative chemotherapy. This strategy may be of benefit in head and neck tumors where the circumstances may differ compared to limb tumors, and where it may be advantageous to proceed with earlier surgery. The latter is potentially important if the diagnosis is in doubt, as may happen when attempting to distinguish a chondrosarcoma from a chondroblastic osteosarcoma.

In contrast to extremity osteosarcoma, prospective studies in the HN are lacking and the approaches are inconsistent. As a result, disagreement exists about the role of chemotherapy in treating seemingly more favorable osteosarcomas of the mandible and maxilla as compared to extremity lesions. Two independent overviews of the retrospective data regarding the role of adjuvant chemotherapy were reported simultaneously (71,72). As discussed earlier, both studies suggested RT was unhelpful. Kassir and colleagues, however, concluded that the role of chemotherapy in HN osteosarcoma remains unproven (72), while Smeeles and colleagues maintained that chemotherapy does improve survival (71). These two studies differed in that one accepted all non-metastatic patients, while Smeeles et al. restricted entry to those studies that reported on the status of surgical margins (86). In a National Cancer Data Base (NCDB) report, no substantial difference in the five-year survival rate was noted between treatment with surgery alone (74.7%) and surgery with adjuvant chemotherapy (71.3%).[2]

Chondrosarcoma
In contrast with osteosarcoma, chemotherapy is not ordinarily a component of chondrosarcoma management. The exception is in the mesenchymal subtype, a small round cell tumor, where chemotherapy was used in the majority of mesenchymal chondrosarcoma cases (57.5%) in the NCDB series[3] and has been our policy at Princess Margaret Hospital (87).

Ewing's Sarcoma
In Ewing's sarcoma, chemotherapy is critical to the improvements that have been witnessed in management outcomes in recent decades. The classic approach is a four-drug regimen consisting of vincristine, actinomycin-D, cyclophosphamide, and doxorubicin (VACA). More recent modifications have included the substitution of ifosfamide for cyclophosphamide (VAIA) especially in higher risk patients (4).

Treatment is generally administered for 12 cycles (over 36 months), and, as already implied, usually precedes local management. Care must be taken to avoid sensitizing agents such as actinomycin-D and doxorubicin with radiotherapy.

Summary of Outcomes in Bone Tumors
Osteosarcoma
Overall reported survival rates remain disappointing, generally being in the 30% to 40% range, with occasional small series projecting survival in the order of 70% (Table 24.7)

Table 24.7 Outcome in Osteosarcoma of the Head and Neck (selected series)

Author (year)	No. cases	Local control (5 yr)	Overall Survival (5 yr)
Mark (1991) (88)	18	10/18	50%
Ha (1999) (119)	27	NA	55%
Kassir (1997) (72) (meta-analysis)	173	NA	37%
Smeele (1997) (86) (meta-analysis)	201	NA	NA
Oda (1997) (73)	13	11/13	72%
Smith 2003 (2)	496	NA	59.7%

Table 24.8 Disease-specific Survival Rates by Grade, Anatomical Site, Age, Size, and Margin Status from the National Cancer Database Report on Osteosarcoma of the Head and Neck (Number of Cases = 496)

		1 Year	2 Year	3 Year	4 Year	5 Year
Grade	Low 1–2	93.8	90.4	78.6	74.3	74.3
	High 3–4	75.3	60.0	45.9	42.3	42.3
Anatomical site	Skull/facial bones	79.9	67.0	58.1	56.7	56.7
	Mandible	94.4	83.4	78.0	70.1	65.3
Age	<30 yrs	93.0	83.6	74.8	71.0	68.7
	30–60 yrs	86.6	79.8	71.0	67.2	64.8
	>60 yrs	63.4	44.5	38.2	34.4	34.4
Tumor size	<3 cm	83.6	83.6	74.0	69.1	69.1
	3–6 cm	95.4	88.0	77.4	74.4	66.5
	>6 cm	64.7	38.8	38.8	25.9	25.9
Histologic type	Osteoblastic	84.5	72.3	63.7	60.8	58.5
	Chondroblastic	96.6	88.5	83.4	78.1	78.1
Surgical margins	Clear	95.3	87.9	81.2	78.7	75.4
	Residual disease	60.8	50.6	31.7	31.7	31.7

Source: From Ref. 2.

Table 24.9 Disease-specific Survival Rates (%) by Grade and Anatomical Site from the National Cancer Database Report on Chondrosarcoma of the Head and Neck (Number of Cases = 400)

	1 Year	2 Year	3 Year	4 Year	5 Year
Grade					
1–2	97.6	97.6	96.2	93.2	93.2
3–4	90.9	90.9	79.6	67.3	67.3
Anatomical site					
Head and Neck bones	96.7	96.7	94.6	92.4	92.4
Laryngotracheal	95.8	95.8	93.3	88.0	88.0
Sinonasal	93.9	93.9	93.9	87.5	87.5
Head and Neck soft tissue	100	93.6	93.6	80.2	80.2

Source: From Ref. 3.

(72,73,86,88). The recent NCDB report showed a five-year disease specific survival rate of 59.7% (2). Factors associated with a poor prognosis were age older than 60 years; nonmandibular tumor location; tumor size >6 cm; histologic type of tumor; advanced disease stage; nonsurgical initial therapy; and positive margins of resection. The five-year survival figures for some of these factors are shown (Table 24.8).

Chondrosarcoma

In the NCDB, survival rates appeared similar regardless of the site of disease and are profoundly influenced by the grade of the lesion. The five-year disease-specific rates generally exceed 80%. The beneficial outcomes are clearly related to the fact that grade 1 (50%) and grade 2 (37%) were the predominant subtypes with grades 3 and 4 representing only 8% and 4% respectively. Superior outcome is evident for patients with lower-grade tumors (93.2%) compared with higher-grade tumors (67.3%) (*p* = .0265) (Table 24.9) (3). Individual series have not traditionally reported as favorable outcomes for the higher grade lesions. For example, the UCLA group reported a five-year disease free survival of 90% for low grade tumors and 14% for high grade tumors (89), while the M.D. Anderson Hospital reported a

90% five-year survival for grade 1 lesions versus 43% for grade 3 (90).

Ewing's Sarcoma

With the use of intensive induction chemotherapy approaches already mentioned, and use of radiotherapy in local management, along with surgery or both followed by additional chemotherapy, five-year survival ranges from 50 to 75%, depending on the risk category (4). The most common site of failure remains distant disease (4). We would emphasize that, with the current state of knowledge, chemotherapy alone should not be regarded as a standard to control gross tumor.

SPECIFIC SITUATIONS

The preceding discussion provides a general framework for the management of HN sarcomas. While in practice they are managed according to the principles noted, anatomic constraints imply that practitioners must use clinical judgment in choosing a local treatment strategy that suits the needs of the case. A general principle that seems most relevant to the head and neck is the compelling focus on tissue preservation due to the functional and cosmetic sensitivities involved and the influence this has on management outcome. In addition, numerous histological subtypes and clinical variants exist under the combined rubrics of soft tissue and bone malignancies and certain modifications are necessary to take account of different clinical and pathological characteristics. The sections that follow will summarize management specifics related to either individual sarcoma subtypes with unique characteristics in the head and neck, or present common sarcoma problems that are equally applicable to head and neck practice.

Rhadomyosarcoma

Rhabdomyosarcoma (RMS) is the most common soft tissue sarcoma in children younger than 15 years. Thirty-four percent of all pediatric rhabdomyosarcomas occur in the head and neck (91). These are divided by location into parameningeal (50%) for tumors originating in the nasopharynx, nasal cavity, paranasal sinuses, middle ear, mastoid, pterygoid fossa, or any parameningeal site with extension into a parameningeal location; orbital (25%); and non-orbital non-parameningeal (25%) (12).

RMS is rare in the adult patient where the median age at initial presentation is in the mid-twenties. The primary site of origin in adults can be variable but the majority occur in the ethmoid sinuses. The site of origin is important because it provides information concerning patterns of spread and relapse. Thus orbital lesions, while presenting

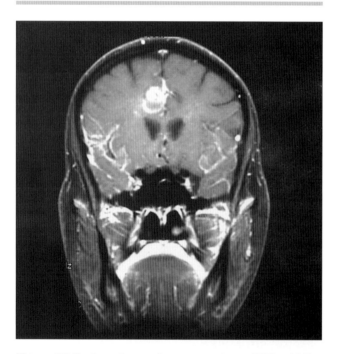

Figure 24.5 Coronal magnetic resonance image (MRI) exhibiting one of the hallmark intracranial changes of leptomeningeal relapse in an adult male patient treated for a rhabdomyosarcoma of the ethmoid sinus with extensive lymph node involvement. Diffuse non-nodular enhancement of the supratentorial cortex can be found in the brain, spine, or both and is often referred to as cake icing or zuckerguss (the German translation for sugar icing).

with dramatic early orbital content displacement, rarely manifest regional node metastasis or distant disease. In contrast, parameningeal sites provide significant risk of intracranial extension and cerebrospinal fluid (CSF) metastasis (Fig. 24.5) as well as distant disease. Adult patients appear to have especially aggressive lesions and early distant metastases to bone marrow, leptomeningeal sites, lung, and the breasts in female patients may occur. Attention to these regions is required in the staging work-up. It remains unresolved why tumors are so much more aggressive in adults than children and result in a higher overall mortality rate (92).

As summarized earlier, management is based on the principles of intensive chemotherapy, generally administered in a neoadjuvant basis, followed by concurrent chemoradiotherapy. The modern treatment of pediatric rhabdomyosarcoma has improved survival rates from 30% to 70% (57). The rates exceed 80% for embryonal, and are somewhat lower for alveolar and lower again for undifferentiated lesions. Good prognostic factors include head and neck location, stage 1 or 2 lesions, and low tumor grade. Poor prognostic factors include age younger than 1 year, alveolar histology, and high tumor grade. In patients with completely resected tumors (group I) it is evident that irradiation can be omitted from treatment protocols and that vincristine and actinomycin D (VA) chemotherapy is as effective as VAC. Non-alveolar residual microscopic disease (group II) can be controlled in 90% of patients with irradiation and cyclic-sequential VA chemotherapy. Patients with gross residual disease are treated with irradiation and chemotherapy with VAC, yielding a 52% survival. The unsatisfactory prognosis of patients with alveolar histology has been largely addressed with the use of aggressive chemotherapy. Specifically, VAC with doxorubicin and cisplatin results in 80% five-year survival (93).

The role of surgery is controversial given the great sensitivity of these lesions to chemotherapy and radiotherapy. It should only be performed at diagnosis in the absence of metastasis to lymph nodes or distant sites since prompt chemotherapy is the most critical intervention required to realize a favorable outcome. Subsequent surgery to achieve local control following initial chemotherapy should be conservative. In the young adult, where growth arrest and structural abnormalities from radiotherapy are not at issue, we only recommend surgery for the smallest lesions in favorable sites in the primary non-salvage situation. Frequently, radiotherapy would also be added to sterilize the field and treat potential lymph node regions since this risk is prodigious in our experience of treating young adults.

Radiotherapy alone (meaning with chemotherapy) or as an adjunct to surgery is a very effective strategy to effect local control, achieving rates on the order of 90%. Doses on the order of 50 Gy, and where possible, doses in the 45 Gy range are used. In the full grown patient our usual approach is to prescribe 60 to 70 Gy during six to seven weeks to sites of gross disease, while administering 50 Gy to potential areas of involvement, including the nodal regions at risk.

In the young child it is highly desirable to keep doses to a minimum. As a consequence, research is exploring the lower dose limits that can be used safely. The potential to use doses less then 40 Gy is being considered while there is also concern that this may be insufficient, especially for adverse situations such as the alveolar subtype or in the face of overt clinical disease.

Dermatofibrosarcoma Protuberans

DFSP is not infrequently seen in the skin of the scalp, face, and neck. The indolent and slowly growing nature of these lesions may result in them being hidden and undetected under the scalp hair for many years in young adults. Although borderline to low grade in histological appearance, DFSP has a propensity for local recurrence after simple excision. Fibrosarcomatous change may be seen with multiple recurrences over many years thereby reinforcing the need to achieve tumor control as well as to optimize cosmesis. For this reason, Mendenhall and colleagues recently suggested that the optimal treatment for DFSP is resection with wide margins, which carries a likelihood of local control exceeding 90%. Patients with positive or close surgical margins have an elevated risk of local recurrence after resection alone, but postoperative radiotherapy results in local control rates exceeding 85% in such patients. Radiotherapy alone for gross disease has also been shown to be an effective approach in patients for whom surgery was not considered to be an option (94). Another approach that has recently received significant support is Mohs micrographic surgery, which some authors propose carries an increased likelihood of local control compared to wide local excision. Paradisi et al. recently pooled results from the literature and reported six recurrences out of 463 cases for Mohs (1.3%, 95% CI 0.5–2.8%) and 288 recurrences out of 1394 cases for wide local excision (20.7%, 95% CI 18.6-22.9%) (95). Despite optimal surgical management, distant metastases may develop in up to 5% of patients. Activation of PDGFR provides the rationale for targeted inhibition as a treatment strategy for patients with unresectable locally advanced or metastatic DFSP that we discussed earlier (See "Targeted Treatments") (62).

Angiosarcoma

Angiosarcomas are tumors of vascular tissue that can arise in any area of the body but most frequently occur in the dermal tissues of the head and neck and manifest typically on the scalp (about 50%) or facial skin. These neoplasms commonly present as purple bruise like lesions in elderly men, and are rarely seen in patients of African origin (64). The macules usually become nodular, may coalesce, and may ulcerate. Frank bleeding is often an ongoing and major problem and often results in chronic oozing through dressings. A particularly difficult aspect of management is the apparent multifocal nature that makes judgement regarding the area of risk and accurate definition of margins for both surgical or radiotherapy ablation nearly impossible. The clinical examination must be meticulous because it is the only real means of identifying the deceptive areas of multifocal involvement that may exist (96). Frequently individual patches coalesce into flat masses measuring up to 6 cm in dimension, though this is variable and can be greater. Metastasis is common if patients survive sufficiently long, and is seen most typically in regional lymph nodes and in the lungs.

As implied above, angiosarcoma is a rare, difficult to treat, and usually lethal tumor (97,98). It is traditionally managed using wide local excision and postoperative radiotherapy, but despite aggressive treatment, this disease is marked by a tendency for local recurrence, multifocality, and poor survival. Lateral extension through the dermis makes assessment of surgical margins difficult; the rate of clear margins in a recent series was only 21.4% (97). Younger patients and those who have less extensive disease fare better. Postoperative radiation therapy should be employed routinely because it may lead to improved survival, though the median actuarial survival remains disappointing at 28.4 months (97). Buschmann and colleagues recently suggested a modified approach to surgical management based largely on the difficult diagnosis, often delayed therapy, and the rapid formation of metastases with the presumption that the tumor has already spread at the time of the initial presentation. The average survival period after resection of the external table immediate reconstruction by a split skin graft was 17.5 months (99). It may be equally valid to treat some of these patients with radiotherapy alone or with chemotherapy instead of with surgery (96,100,101). Our experience is that they are frequently radioresponsive, but lesions recur at the edge of the radiotherapy target volume rather than centrally. Some authors have suggested novel techniques, such as interstitial methods, combined with chemotherapy for certain anatomic problems (102). For more usual presentations, radiotherapy techniques remain challenging for these patients due to the large and convex surface of the scalp and the desire to avoid irradiating underlying brain beyond tolerance. Newer approaches that combine intensity modulated radiotherapy (IMRT) with other techniques are now available (103) and are generally our preferred approach (Fig. 24.6). Patients with advanced disease have a poor prognosis, but there can be dramatic responses to chemotherapy in a minority of patients; recent reports of the value of paclitaxel are the most promising (104,105).

Hemangiopericytoma

Classically this tumor occurs in the nasal cavity or sinuses (most often ethmoid sinus) of middle-aged adults of either sex and generally forms a relatively small (<5 cm) polypoid mass. While rare it remains specific to the sino-nasal region and has a somewhat unpredictable character (106). These tumors may have infiltrating margins, which may account for why approximately one-third of patients develop local recurrence, but this is usually indolent and nondestructive. Isolated cases pursue a malignant (metastasizing) course.

Presenting symptoms include a painless mass in the neck or soft tissues of the face. Sinonasal hemangiopericytoma presents with nasal obstruction and epistaxis and appears as a grey polypoid mass that bleeds briskly on manipulation. Wide local excision is the treatment of choice with some authorities advocating preoperative embolization. Although this is a low-grade malignancy, metastases have been reported in 3% of cases with a 3.3% incidence of death. Metastases are to lung, bone, and rarely to locoregional lymph nodes.

Kaposi's Sarcoma

Kaposi's sarcoma (KS) is the most frequent malignant lesion in patients infected with the human immunodeficiency

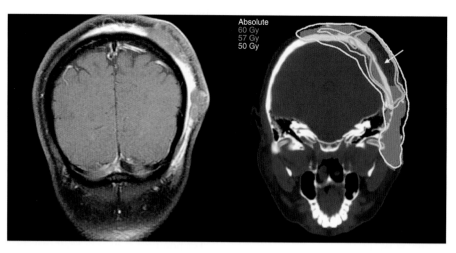

Figure 24.6   Magnetic resonance image (MRI) of the cranium showing a multifocal angiosarcoma of the scalp (*left image*). Note the prominent contiguous signal change remote from separate mass lesion decisions. This patient underwent a resection involving resection of the outer table of the skull and complex soft tissue reconstruction. Resection margins were clear of disease. The intervening tissues between the masses showed areas of atypical vascular proliferation progressing to low-grade angiosarcoma with vascular channels dissecting between the collagen fibers and corresponding to the altered signal areas in the MRI adjacent to the separate tumors masses. The right-hand image shows a post-operative radiotherapy plan using intensity modulated radiotherapy (IMRT) to spare the underlying intracranial contents. A dose of 50 Gy in 25 fractions was administered to the wider areas of abnormal signal and encompassing the original areas of gross disease using IMRT (see the yellow 50 Gy isodose line encompassing the turquoise region intended to receive 50 Gy). The original sites of overt disease prior to resection received an additional dose of 10 Gy in 5 fractions using electron beam to a total of 60 Gy in 30 fractions as shown (red region with arrow) for one of the lesions on this slice of the IMRT plan.

virus (HIV). Formerly as many as 95% of all patients with acquired immune deficiency syndrome (AIDS) had KS in the cutaneous or visceral forms. In the United States, KS is 10 times more common in homosexual men with HIV than in other subgroups with HIV and was originally the most common initial complication of HIV infection in homosexual men. Although KS is primarily a cutaneous disease, extracutaneous spread is common: the oral cavity and oropharynx are typical areas of involvement in the head and neck in addition to cosmetically disturbing lesions of the facial skin. Lesions of the hard palate are the most common intraoral manifestation. They may vary in appearance from red to violaceous nodules, macules, or plaques. Cutaneous lesions are divided into patch, plaque, or nodular stages. Other sites, especially the gastrointestinal (GI) tract, lungs, and lymph nodes, are often involved.

Treatment must be individualized for patients with KS. Local disease can often be treated with observation or cosmetic make-up. Treatment options depend greatly on the extent of tumor, the rate of growth, human immunodeficiency virus type I (HIV-I) viral load, and host factors (CD4+ T-lymphocyte count and overall medical condition). The clinical course of AIDS-related KS is highly variable, ranging from minimal stable disease to explosive growth. Limited cutaneous disease may be treated with topical alitretinoin gel, intralesional chemotherapy, radiation therapy, laser therapy, or cryotherapy. Often the lesion may be ablated but blood stained dermal and epidermal tissue changes may take much longer to resolve and the cosmetic problem persists for some time. The use of liposomal anthracyclines (daunorubicin and doxorubicin) and paclitaxel have facilitated management of patients in whom systemic therapy is warranted (107).

Fortunately, following the widespread use of highly active antiretroviral therapy (HAART) there has been a marked decline in new cases of Kaposi's sarcoma. Between 1984 and 2006, 596 cases of incident Kaposi sarcoma (KS) cases were identified among 12,959 people with HIV/AIDS in the Swiss HIV Cohort Study. Of the 596, 52 were among HAART users and in 33 (or 63.5%) of these HIV/AIDS patients, KS arose among those who had stopped treatment or used HAART for less than six months. In this study the hazard ratio for KS declined steeply in the first months after HAART initiation and continued to be low seven to ten years thereafter (HR, 0.06; 95% CI, 0.02–0.17) (108). Authors have also observed a reduction in the rate of AIDS related tumors in otolaryngology settings (109).

Liposarcoma

Liposarcoma merits comment since it is one of the most common soft tissue sarcomas, although it has traditionally been second to the now reclassified MFH subtype. The head and neck is a rare site for liposarcoma, comprising 4% of all liposarcomas; it does not have any particular predisposition to the region or unusual behavior pattern in this anatomic setting. In this setting, the neck is the single most common location, although 38% of cases involve the larynx/pharynx. The supraglottis is the most common subsite in the larynx. There are four types of liposarcoma described. The well differentiated liposarcoma is a neoplasm of borderline malignancy, which is usually readily resectable and has a very favorable biology even when excised marginally. Myxoid liposarcomas contain an abundant mucinous stroma with a network of capillaries. This subtype is generally low-grade and rarely metastasizes though can be unpredictable. It also possesses a unique molecular signature characterized by the existence of the t(12; 16)(q13; p12) translocation and the molecular phenotype of individual lesions may be used to track the lineage of unusual and late metastases found in this tumor type (110). Thus this histological subtype has a number of unusual characteristics, including a propensity to develop late onset and remote soft tissue metastases, and late bone metastases prior to lung lesions. This subtype also, however, exhibits unusually high sensitivity to radiotherapy (111). The latter is considered a reason for the excellent local control in this subtype of sarcoma (112) though this does not apply specifically to the head and neck.

In a recent report of head and neck liposarcomas from the M.D. Anderson Cancer Center both disease-specific and overall survival rates were higher in patients with well differentiated or myxoid tumors compared to patients with round cell or pleomorphic tumors. This report agrees with previous findings. In fact, crude disease-specific survival was 100% for well differentiated liposarcomas and myxoid liposarcomas versus 60% for round cell tumors and only 45% for pleomorphic liposarcomas. This finding highlights the importance of obtaining grading and histologic subtype information to accurately prognosticate and select appropriate treatment. Treatment with surgical excision offers the best control rate and radiotherapy is used according to the principles described earlier for soft tissue sarcoma.

Synovial Sarcoma

Synovial sarcomas tend to occur in young patients between the second and fifth decades of life, but can be found in any patient or site. In the head and neck they may arise in relation to the prevertebral areas from the skull base to the hypopharynx, and many involve the parapharyngeal space. Synovial sarcoma must be distinguished from other calcifying tumors (e.g., lower neck lesions need to be distinguished from thyroid neoplasms, which may also exhibit calcification) since approximately 10% of them may exhibit calcification, with or without ossification. Radiology reveals calcification in up to one-third of cases with very high signal intensity on T2 MRI. The largest institutional series of synovial sarcomas was recently reported from the M.D. Anderson Cancer Center. The most common presenting complaint in the series was neck pain and the subsequent detection of a mass (113). This seemed to relate to the origin of a mass within the paraspinal muscles, which had adverse outcome compared to lesions arising in the upper aerodigestive tract, traditionally considered to be the most common site of involvement. In this small series (n = 40), 25 (63%) experienced a recurrence (12 local, 7 distant, and 6 both local and distant). Local recurrence appeared related to the biphasic histologic subtype, skull base location, large size, and involved resection margins, though statistical power was insufficient to achieve significance.

Local treatment follows the general principles of soft tissue sarcoma treatment with adequate excision and adjuvant radiotherapy when appropriate, with or without adjuvant chemotherapy. This histologic subtype exhibits more favorable responses to chemotherapy than most other histologic subtypes, as is apparent when treating metastatic disease. The disease also has a reputation for higher risk of lymph node metastasis, although varying rates have been identified (e.g., 1.4% to 13.7%) (16).

Radiation-Induced Sarcoma

Radiation-induced sarcoma of the head and neck (RISHN) is a long-term complication of treatment. The rarity of this tumor is reflected in the very few reported series. Diagnosis and management is extremely challenging, but should follow the principles outlined for the management of local recurrence in cases who have previously received radiotherapy. Thus surgery is the mainstay of treatment with appropriate attention to cosmesis and function preservation where possible. This requires recognition of the challenges posed by the close proximity of tumor to important regional structures and the technical difficulties of operating in an irradiated area. Judicious use of radiotherapy—potentially with brachytherapy or highly conformed external beams—may add to the outcome of the individual case. Chemotherapy may also be considered as an adjuvant given the potential that it may enhance local control in STS when other treatments cannot be applied as aggressively as necessary. It certainly should be considered for rhabdomyosarcoma and osteosarcoma (114).

Salvage for Recurrent Disease

In a study of 307 patients treated at the National Cancer Institute, isolated pulmonary metastatic disease was the most common pattern of initial recurrence (52%), followed by isolated local recurrence (20%). In this series, 45% of patients remained disease-free after surgical treatment of the first recurrence (115). Detection and management of recurrent disease is an important element of the treatment of sarcomas since a realistic potential exists for both local and metastatic salvage. In the head and neck, further local treatment options for local recurrence are problematic due to the anatomic proximity to critical anatomy, including major neurovascular structures. It is also important to bear in mind that these lesions could also represent radiation-induced sarcomas and the clinical setting needs to be considered in judging this distinction. A schema for the management of locally recurrent sarcoma is provided (Table 24.10).

Table 24.10 Schema for the Management of Locally Recurrent Sarcoma, Modified from Catton et al. (120)

Context of local recurrence	Recommended approach
No prior chemotherapy and/or radiotherapy	Consider combined approach with external beam radiotherapy. In osteogenic sarcoma consider induction chemotherapy with pathologic response assessment
Prior radiotherapy	Combined approach with brachytherapy
Critical structure involvement	Consider preoperative radiotherapy Ablative approach may need to be considered
In the presence of metastases	Multiple metastases – palliative treatment possibly including aggressive local treatment Few resectable metastases – local management as for non metastatic context with metastasectomy

Sarcomas commonly metastasize to lung, making pulmonary metastasectomy an important consideration in head and neck sarcomas due to the fact that pulmonary metastases are not necessarily indicative of incurable disease. In 70% of patients metastases will be confined to the lungs and in 80% of these they will be in the peripheral lung thereby lending themselves for wedge excision. In a multicenter EORTC study of 255 patients undergoing resection of pulmonary metastases for soft tissue sarcoma, a 38% five-year survival was achieved post- metastasectomy (116). Favorable prognostic factors in this group included low-grade histology, negative margins, and age less than 40 years. CT has replaced other modalities for the detection of pulmonary metastases. Patients are selected for metastasectomy in the context of a controlled primary in the absence of uncontrolled extrathoracic metastases, provided the pulmonary lesion is deemed amenable to surgery in the face of adequate pulmonary reserve (117).

CONCLUSIONS

The treatment of patients with sarcomas of the head and neck remains challenging due to the diverse histology, variable sites of presentation, and the requirements of multimodality therapy. Improvements in the care of these patients require the collaborative effort of multidisciplinary teams working together. Centralization and organization of resources should permit the accrual of sufficient patients to create and maintain programs for the appropriate investigation and treatment of these complex problems. The head and neck offers the additional challenges of anatomic constraints unique to this area. The close proximity of vital structures makes the resection of sarcomas in the head and neck extremely difficult in many situations. The importance of adjuvant treatment for this disease cannot be overstated because of these anatomic constraints. The psychological and functional problems associated with major resections in the head and neck creates additional challenges. Reconstructive efforts with the use of free tissue transfer have significantly improved the cosmetic, functional, and psychological outcomes of these patients. Newer radiotherapy techniques have also facilitated management. Along with future prospects for molecular targeting, we are beginning to witness the introduction of novel systemic agents with specific activity against certain tumor types. All of these approaches in combination with one another can be expected to lead to improved outcomes for these patients.

REFERENCES

1. Fletcher CD. Distinctive soft tissue tumors of the head and neck. Mod Pathol 2002; 15: 324–30.
2. Smith RB, Apostolakis LW, Karnell LH et al. National Cancer Data Base report on osteosarcoma of the head and neck. Cancer 2003; 98: 1670–80.
3. Koch BB, Karnell LH, Hoffman HT et al. National cancer database report on chondrosarcoma of the head and neck. Head Neck 2000; 22: 408–25.
4. Paulussen M, Ahrens S, Dunst J et al. Localized Ewing tumor of bone: final results of the cooperative Ewing's Sarcoma Study CESS 86. J Clin Oncol 2001; 19: 1818–29.
5. Wiklund T, Huuhtanen R, Blomqvist C et al. The importance of a multidisciplinary group in the treatment of soft tissue sarcomas. Eur J Cancer 1996; 32A: 269–73.
6. Pradhan A, Cheung YC, Grimer RJ et al. Does the method of treatment affect the outcome in soft-tissue sarcomas of the adductor compartment? J Bone Joint Surg Br 2006; 88: 1480–6.
7. Gutierrez JC, Perez EA, Moffat FL et al. Should soft tissue sarcomas be treated at high-volume centers? An analysis of 4205 patients. Ann Surg 2007; 245: 952–8.
8. Fletcher CD. The evolving classification of soft tissue tumours: an update based on the new WHO classification. Histopathology 2006; 48: 3–12.
9. Fisher C. The comparative roles of electron microscopy and immunohistochemistry in the diagnosis of soft tissue tumours. Histopathology 2006; 48: 32–41.
10. Nascimento AF, Raut CP. Diagnosis and management of pleomorphic sarcomas (so-called "MFH") in adults. J Surg Oncol 2008; 97: 330–9.
11. Wang CP, Chang YL, Ting LL et al. Malignant fibrous histiocytoma of the sinonasal tract. Head Neck 2009; 31: 85–93.
12. O'Sullivan B, Bell RS, Bramwell VHC. Sarcomas of the soft tissues. In: Souhami RL, Tannock I, Hohenberger P et al., eds. Oxford Textbook of Oncology, 2nd edn. Oxford: Oxford University Press, 2002; 2495–523.
13. Antonescu CR. The role of genetic testing in soft tissue sarcoma. Histopathology 2006; 48: 13–21.
14. Itakura E, Yamamoto H, Oda Y et al. Detection and characterization of vascular endothelial growth factors and their receptors in a series of angiosarcomas. J Surg Oncol 2008; 97: 74–81.
15. Koch M, Nielsen GP, Yoon SS. Malignant tumors of blood vessels: angiosarcomas, hemangioendotheliomas, and hemangiopericytomas. J Surg Oncol 2008; 97: 321–9.
16. Brennan MF, Singer S, Maki RG et al. Soft tissue sarcoma. In: DeVita VT, Lawrence T, Rosenberg SA, eds. Principles and Practice of Oncology, 8th edn. Philadelphia: Lippincott Williams & Wilkins, 2008; 1741–93.
17. Deyrup AT, Weiss SW. Grading of soft tissue sarcomas: the challenge of providing precise information in an imprecise world. Histopathology 2006; 48: 42–50.
18. Bovee JV, Cleton-Jansen AM, Taminiau AH et al. Emerging pathways in the development of chondrosarcoma of bone and implications for targeted treatment. Lancet Oncol 2005; 6: 599–607.
19. Borden EC, Baker LH, Bell RS et al. Soft tissue sarcomas of adults: state of the translational science. Clin Cancer Research 2003; 9: 1941–56.
20. Noria S, Davis A, Kandel R et al. Residual disease following unplanned excision of soft-tissue sarcoma of an extremity. J Bone Joint Surg Am 1996; 78: 650–5.
21. Domanski HA. Fine-needle aspiration cytology of soft tissue lesions: diagnostic challenges. Diagn Cytopathol 2007; 35: 768–73.
22. Soderlund V, Skoog L, Unni KK et al. Diagnosis of high-grade osteosarcoma by radiology and cytology: a retrospective study of 52 cases. Sarcoma 2004; 8: 31–6.
23. Skoog L, Pereira ST, Tani E. Fine-needle aspiration cytology and immunocytochemistry of soft-tissue tumors and osteo/chondrosarcomas of the head and neck. Diagn Cytopathol 1999; 20: 131–6.
24. Liu PT, Valadez SD, Chivers FS et al. Anatomically based guidelines for core needle biopsy of bone tumors: implications for limb-sparing surgery. Radiographics 2007; 27: 189–205; discussion 206.
25. Espinosa LA, Jamadar DA, Jacobson JA et al. CT-guided biopsy of bone: a radiologist's perspective. AJR Am J Roentgenol 2008; 190: W283–9.

26. Robinson E, Bleakney RR, Ferguson PC et al. Oncodiagnosis panel, 2007: multidisciplinary management of soft-tissue sarcoma. Radiographics 2008; 28: 2069–86.

27. Ioannidis JP, Lau J. 18F-FDG PET for the diagnosis and grading of soft-tissue sarcoma: a meta-analysis. J Nucl Med 2003; 44: 717–24.

28. Brenner W, Bohuslavizki KH, Eary JF. PET imaging of osteosarcoma. J Nucl Med 2003; 44: 930–42.

29. Tewfik JN, Greene GS. Fluorine-18-deoxyglucose-positron emission tomography imaging with magnetic resonance and computed tomographic correlation in the evaluation of bone and soft-tissue sarcomas: a pictorial essay. Curr Probl Diagn Radiol 2008; 37: 178–88.

30. Lehnhardt M, Daigeler A, Hauser J et al. The value of expert second opinion in diagnosis of soft tissue sarcomas. J Surg Oncol 2008; 97: 40–3.

31. Greene FL, Page D, Norrow M et al. AJCC Cancer Staging Manual, 6th edn. New York: Springer; 2002.

32. Sobin L, Wittekind WH. TNM Classification of Malignant Tumours, 6th edn. New York: Wiley-Liss; 2002.

33. Behranwala KA, A'Hern R, Omar AM et al. Prognosis of lymph node metastasis in soft tissue sarcoma. Ann Surg Oncol 2004; 11: 714–19.

34. Riad S, Griffin AM, Liberman B et al. Lymph node metastasis in soft tissue sarcoma in an extremity. Clin Orthop Relat Res 2004; 426: 129–34.

35. Gerrand CH, Wunder JS, Kandel RA et al. Classification of positive margins after resection of soft-tissue sarcoma of the limb predicts the risk of local recurrence. J Bone Joint Surg [Br] 2001; 83-B: 1149–55.

36. Rosenberg SA, Tepper J, Glatstein E et al. The treatment of soft-tissue sarcomas of the extremities: prospective randomized evaluations of (1) limb-sparing surgery plus radiation therapy compared with amputation and (2) the role of adjuvant chemotherapy. Ann Surg 1982; 196: 305–15.

37. Pisters PW, Harrison LB, Leung DH et al. Long-term results of a prospective randomized trial of adjuvant brachytherapy in soft tissue sarcoma. J Clin Oncol 1996; 14: 859–68.

38. Yang JC, Chang AE, Baker AR et al. Randomized prospective study of the benefit of adjuvant radiation therapy in the treatment of soft tissue sarcomas of the extremity. J Clin Oncol 1998; 16: 197–203.

39. Tran LM, Mark R, Meier R et al. Sarcomas of the head and neck. Prognostic factors and treatment strategies. Cancer 1992; 70: 169–77.

40. Le Vay J, O'Sullivan B, Catton C et al. An assessment of prognostic factors in soft-tissue sarcoma of the head and neck. Arch Otolaryngol Head Neck Surg 1994; 120: 981–6.

41. O'Sullivan B, Gullane P, Irish J et al. Preoperative radiotherapy for adult head and neck soft tissue sarcoma: assessment of wound complication rates and cancer outcome in a prospective series. World J Surg 2003; 27: 875–83.

42. Pisters PW, O'Sullivan B, Maki RG. Evidence-based recommendations for local therapy for soft tissue sarcomas. J Clin Oncol 2007; 25: 1003–8.

43. O'Sullivan B, Davis A, Turcotte R et al. Pre-operative versus post-operative radiotherapy in soft issue sarcoma of the limbs: a randomized trial. The Lancet 2002; 359: 2235–41.

44. Nag S, Shasha D, Janjan N et al. The American Brachytherapy Society recommendations for brachytherapy of soft tissue sarcomas. Int J Radiat Oncol Biol Phys 2001; 49: 1033–43.

45. Wolden SL, Wexler LH, Kraus DH et al. Intensity-modulated radiotherapy for head-and-neck rhabdomyosarcoma. Int J Radiat Oncol Biol Phys 2005; 61: 1432–8.

46. Combs SE, Behnisch W, Kulozik AE et al. Intensity Modulated Radiotherapy (IMRT) and Fractionated Stereotactic Radiotherapy (FSRT) for children with head-and-neck-rhabdomyosarcoma. BMC Cancer 2007; 7: 177.

47. Kepka L, Delaney TF, Suit HD et al. Results of radiation therapy for unresected soft-tissue sarcomas. Int J Radiat Oncol Biol Phys 2005; 63: 852–9.

48. The sarcoma meta-analysis collaboration. Adjuvant chemotherapy for localised resectable soft-tissue sarcoma of adults: meta-analysis of individual data. Lancet 1997; 350: 1647–54.

49. Wilson RE, Wood WC, Lerner HL et al. Doxorubicin chemotherapy in the treatment of soft-tissue sarcoma. Combined results of two randomized trials. Arch Surg 1986; 121: 1354–9.

50. Alvegard TA, Sigurdsson H, Mouridsen H et al. Adjuvant chemotherapy with doxorubicin in high-grade soft tissue sarcoma: a randomized trial of the Scandinavian Sarcoma Group. J Clin Oncol 1989; 7: 1504–13.

51. Antman K, Ryan L, Borden E. Pooled results from three randomized adjuvant studies of doxorubicin versus observation in soft tissue sarcoma: 10 year results and review of literature. In: Salmon SE, ed. Adjuvant Therapy of Cancer. Vol VI. Philadelphia: WB Saunders, 1990; 529–43.

52. Baker LH. Adjuvant therapy for soft tissue sarcomas. In: Ryan JR BL, ed. Recent concepts in sarcoma treatment. Dordecht: Kluwer Academic Publishers, 1988; 131–6.

53. Glenn J, Kinsella T, Glatstein E et al. A randomized, prospective trial of adjuvant chemotherapy in adults with soft tissue sarcomas of the head and neck, breast, and trunk. Cancer 1985; 55: 1206–14.

54. Bramwell V, Rouesse J, Steward W et al. Adjuvant CYVADIC chemotherapy for adult soft tissue sarcoma—reduced local recurrence but no improvement in survival: a study of the European Organization for Research and Treatment of Cancer Soft Tissue and Bone Sarcoma Group. J Clin Oncol 1994; 12: 1137–49.

55. Ravaud A, Bui NB, Coindre JM. Adjuvant chemotherapy with Cyvadic in high risk soft tissue sarcoma: A randomized prospective trial. In: Salmon SE, ed. Adjuvant Therapy of Cancer. Vol VI. Philadelphia: WB Saunders, 1990; 556–66.

56. Frustaci S, Gherlinzoni F, De Paoli A et al. Adjuvant chemotherapy for adult soft tissue sarcomas of the extremities and girdles: results of the Italian randomized cooperative trial. J Clin Oncol 2001; 19: 1238–47.

57. Raney RB, Maurer HM, Anderson JR et al. The Intergroup Rhabdomyosarcoma Study Group (IRSG): Major fessons from the IRS-I through IRS-IV studies as background for the current IRS-V treatment protocols. Sarcoma 2001; 5: 9–15.

58. Stevens MCG. Malignant mesenchymal tumours of childhood. In: Souhami RL, Tannock I, Hohenberger P et al., eds. Oxford textbook of oncology, 2nd edn. Oxford: Oxford University Press, 2002; 2525–38.

59. Wunder JS, Nielsen TO, Maki RG et al. Opportunities for improving the therapeutic ratio for patients with sarcoma. Lancet Oncol 2007; 8: 513–24.

60. Koontz BF, Miles EF, Rubio MA et al. Preoperative radiotherapy and bevacizumab for angiosarcoma of the head and neck: two case studies. Head Neck 2008; 30: 262–6.

61. Azim HA, Elsedewy E, Azim HA Jr. Imatinib in the treatment of follicular dendritic sarcoma: a case report and review of literature. Onkologie 2007; 30: 381–4.

62. McArthur GA, Demetri GD, van Oosterom A. Molecular and clinical analysis of locally advanced dermatofibrosarcoma protuberans treated with imatinib: Imatinib Target Exploration Consortium Study B2225. J Clin Oncol 2005; 23: 866–73.

63. Mendenhall WM, Mendenhall CM, Werning JW et al. Adult head and neck soft tissue sarcomas. Head Neck 2005; 27: 916–22.

64. Sturgis EM, Potter BO. Sarcomas of the head and neck region. Curr Opin Oncol 2003; 15: 239–52.

65. Singh RP, Grimer RJ, Bhujel N et al. Adult head and neck soft tissue sarcomas: treatment and outcome. Sarcoma 2008; 2008: 1–5.

66. Penel N, Mallet Y, Robin YM et al. Prognostic factors for adult sarcomas of head and neck. Int J Oral Maxillofac Surg 2008; 37: 428–32.

67. Kozelsky TF, Bonner JA, Foote RL et al. Laryngeal chondrosarcomas: the Mayo Clinic experience. J Surg Oncol 1997; 65: 269–73.

68. Lewis JE, Olsen KD, Inwards CY. Cartilaginous tumors of the larynx: clinicopathologic review of 47 cases. Ann Otol Rhinol Laryngol 1997; 106: 94–100.

69. Sauter A, Bersch C, Lambert KL et al. Chondrosarcoma of the larynx and review of the literature. Anticancer Res 2007; 27: 2925–9.

70. Bathala S, Berry S, Evans RA et al. Chondrosarcoma of larynx: review of literature and clinical experience. J Laryngol Otol 2008; 122: 1127–9.

71. Smeele LE, Kostense PJ, van der Waal I et al. Effect of chemotherapy on survival of craniofacial osteosarcoma: a systematic review of 201 patients. Journal of Clinical Oncology 1997; 15: 363–7.

72. Kassir RR, Rassekh CH, Kinsella JB et al. Osteosarcoma of the head and neck: meta-analysis of nonrandomized studies. Laryngoscope 1997; 107: 56–61.

73. Oda D, Bavisotto LM, Schmidt RA et al. Head and neck osteosarcoma at the University of Washington. Head Neck 1997; 19: 513–23.

74. DeLaney TF, Park L, Goldberg SI et al. Radiotherapy for local control of osteosarcoma. Int J Radiat Oncol Biol Phys 2005; 61: 492–8.

75. Malawar MM, Hellman LJ, O'Sullivan B. Sarcomas of bone. In: DeVita VT, Lawrence T, Rosenberg SA, eds. Principles and practice of oncology, 8th edn. Philadelphia: Lippincott Williams & Wilkins, 2008; 1794–833.

76. Harwood AR, Krajbich JI, Fornasier VL. Radiotherapy of chondrosarcoma of bone. Cancer 1980; 45: 2769–77.

77. McNaney D, Lindberg RD, Ayala AG et al. Fifteen year radiotherapy experience with chondrosarcoma of bone. Int J Radiat Oncol Biol Phys 1982; 8: 187–90.

78. DeLaney TF, Trofimov AV, Engelsman M et al. Advanced-technology radiation therapy in the management of bone and soft tissue sarcomas. Cancer Control 2005; 12: 27–35.

79. Hug EB, Loredo LN, Slater JD et al. Proton radiation therapy for chordomas and chondrosarcomas of the skull base. J Neurosurg 1999; 91: 432–9.

80. Noel G, Habrand JL, Mammar H et al. Combination of photon and proton radiation therapy for chordomas and chondrosarcomas of the skull base: the Centre de Protontherapie D'Orsay experience. Int J Radiat Oncol Biol Phys 2001; 51: 392–8.

81. Debus J, Schulz-Ertner D, Schad L et al. Stereotactic fractionated radiotherapy for chordomas and chondrosarcomas of the skull base. Int J Radiat Oncol Biol Phys 2000; 47: 591–6.

82. Schulz-Ertner D, Nikoghosyan A, Hof H et al. Carbon ion radiotherapy of skull base chondrosarcomas. Int J Radiat Oncol Biol Phys 2007; 67: 171–7.

83. Paulussen M, Ahrens S, Lehnert M et al. Second malignancies after Ewing tumor treatment in 690 patients from a cooperative German/Austrian/Dutch study. Ann Oncol 2001; 12: 1619–30.

84. Eilber F, Giuliano A, Eckardt J et al. Adjuvant chemotherapy for osteosarcoma: a randomized prospective trial. J Clin Oncol 1987; 5: 21–6.

85. Link MP, Goorin AM, Miser AW et al. The effect of adjuvant chemotherapy on relapse-free survival in patients with osteosarcoma of the extremity. N Engl J Med 1986; 314: 1600–6.

86. Smeele LE, Snow GB, van der Waal I. Osteosarcoma of the head and neck: meta-analysis of the nonrandomized studies. Laryngoscope 1998; 108: 946.

87. Harwood AR, Krajbich JI, Fornasier VL. Mesenchymal chondrosarcoma: a report of 17 cases. Clin Orthop 1981: 144–8.

88. Mark RJ, Sercarz JA, Tran L et al. Osteogenic sarcoma of the head and neck. The UCLA experience. Arch Otolaryngol Head Neck Surg 1991; 117: 761–6.

89. Mark RJ, Tran LM, Sercarz J et al. Chondrosarcoma of the head and neck. The UCLA experience, 1955–1988. Am J Clin Oncol 1993; 16: 232–7.

90. Finn DG, Goepfert H, Batsakis JG. Chondrosarcoma of the head and neck. Laryngoscope 1984; 94: 1539–44.

91. Pappo AS, Shapiro DN, Crist WM et al. Biology and therapy of pediatric rhabdomyosarcoma. J Clin Oncol 1995; 13: 2123–39.

92. La Quaglia MP, Heller G, Ghavimi F et al. The effect of age at diagnosis on outcome in rhabdomyosarcoma. Cancer 1994; 73: 109–17.

93. Pappo AS, Shapiro DN, Crist WM. Rhabdomyosarcoma. Biology and treatment. Pediatr Clin North Am 1997; 44: 953–72.

94. Mendenhall WM, Zlotecki RA, Scarborough MT. Dermatofibrosarcoma protuberans. Cancer 2004; 101: 2503–8.

95. Paradisi A, Abeni D, Rusciani A et al. Dermatofibrosarcoma protuberans: wide local excision vs. Mohs micrographic surgery. Cancer Treat Rev 2008; 34: 728–36.

96. Asgari MM, Cockerell CJ, Weitzul S. The head-tilt maneuver: a clinical aid in recognizing head and neck angiosarcomas. Arch Dermatol 2007; 143: 75–7.

97. Pawlik TM, Paulino AF, McGinn CJ et al. Cutaneous angiosarcoma of the scalp: a multidisciplinary approach. Cancer 2003; 98: 1716–26.

98. Kohler HF, Neves RI, Brechtbuhl ER et al. Cutaneous angiosarcoma of the head and neck: report of 23 cases from a single institution. Otolaryngol Head Neck Surg 2008; 139: 519–24.

99. Buschmann A, Lehnhardt M, Toman N et al. Surgical treatment of angiosarcoma of the scalp: less is more. Ann Plast Surg 2008; 61: 399–403.

100. Holloway CL, Turner AR, Dundas GS. Cutaneous angiosarcoma of the scalp: a case report of sustained complete response following liposomal Doxorubicin and radiation therapy. Sarcoma 2005; 9: 29–31.

101. DeMartelaere SL, Roberts D, Burgess MA et al. Neoadjuvant chemotherapy-specific and overall treatment outcomes in patients with cutaneous angiosarcoma of the face with periorbital involvement. Head Neck 2008; 30: 639–46.

102. de Keizer RJ, de Wolff-Rouendaal D, Nooy MA. Angiosarcoma of the eyelid and periorbital region. Experience in Leiden with iridium192 brachytherapy and low-dose doxorubicin chemotherapy. Orbit 2008; 27: 5–12.

103. Bedford JL, Childs PJ, Hansen VN et al. Treatment of extensive scalp lesions with segmental intensity-modulated photon therapy. Int J Radiat Oncol Biol Phys 2005; 62: 1549–58.

104. Schlemmer M, Reichardt P, Verweij J et al. Paclitaxel in patients with advanced angiosarcomas of soft tissue: a retrospective study of the EORTC soft tissue and bone sarcoma group. Eur J Cancer 2008; 44: 2433–6.

105. Penel N, Bui BN, Bay JO et al. Phase II trial of weekly paclitaxel for unresectable angiosarcoma: the ANGIOTAX Study. J Clin Oncol 2008; 26: 5269–74.

106. Koscielny S, Brauer B, Forster G. Hemangiopericytoma: a rare head and neck tumor. Eur Arch Otorhinolaryngol 2003; 260: 450–3.

107. Dezube BJ. Acquired immunodeficiency syndrome-related Kaposi's sarcoma: clinical features, staging, and treatment. Semin Oncol 2000; 27: 424–30.

108. Franceschi S, Maso LD, Rickenbach M et al. Kaposi sarcoma incidence in the Swiss HIV Cohort Study before and after highly active antiretroviral therapy. Br J Cancer 2008; 99: 800–4.

109. Campanini A, Marani M, Mastroianni A et al. Human immunodeficiency virus infection: personal experience in changes in head and neck manifestations due to recent anti-retroviral therapies. Acta Otorhinolaryngol Ital 2005; 25: 30–5.

110. Antonescu CR, Elahi A, Healey JH et al. Monoclonality of multifocal myxoid liposarcoma: confirmation by analysis of TLS-CHOP or EWS-CHOP rearrangements. Clin Cancer Res 2000; 6: 2788–93.

111. Pitson G, Robinson P, Wilke D et al. Radiation response: an additional unique signature of myxoid liposarcoma. Int J Radiat Oncol Biol Phys 2004; 60: 522–6.

112. Guadagnolo BA, Zagars GK, Ballo MT et al. Excellent local control rates and distinctive patterns of failure in myxoid liposarcoma treated with conservation surgery and radiotherapy. Int J Radiat Oncol Biol Phys 2008; 70: 760–5.

113. Harb WJ, Luna MA, Patel SR et al. Survival in patients with synovial sarcoma of the head and neck: association with tumor location, size, and extension. Head Neck 2007; 29: 731–40.

114. Patel SG, See AC, Williamson PA et al. Radiation induced sarcoma of the head and neck. Head Neck 1999; 21: 346–54.

115. Potter DA, Glenn J, Kinsella T et al. Patterns of recurrence in patients with high-grade soft-tissue sarcomas. J Clin Oncol 1985; 3: 353–66.

116. van Geel AN, Pastorino U, Jauch KW et al. Surgical treatment of lung metastases: The European Organization for Research and Treatment of Cancer-Soft Tissue and Bone Sarcoma Group study of 255 patients. Cancer 1996; 77: 675–82.

117. Rusch VW. Surgical techniques for pulmonary metastasectomy. Semin Thorac Cardiovasc Surg 2002; 14: 4–9.

118. Fletcher CDM, Unni K, Mertens K, eds. World Health Organization Classification of Tumours: Pathology and genetics of tumours of soft tissue and bone. Lyon, France: IARC Press (International Agency for Research on Cancer); 2002.

119. Ha PK, Eisele DW, Frassica FJ et al. Osteosarcoma of the head and neck: a review of the Johns Hopkins experience. Laryngoscope 1999; 109: 964–9.

120. Catton C, Swallow CJ, O'Sullivan B. Approaches to local salvage of soft tissue sarcoma after primary site failure. Semin Radiat Oncol 1999; 9: 378–88.

25

Non-melanoma Skin Cancer

Rajan S Patel, Danny J Enepekides, Jamil Asaria and Patrick J Gullane

EPIDEMIOLOGY

Non-melanoma skin cancer (NMSC) is the most common malignancy worldwide. It is of particular relevance to the head and neck surgeon as sun-exposed regions of the head and neck are the most frequently involved sites for the development of NMSC (70–80% of cases). The vast majority of NMSC is basal cell carcinoma (BCC), which comprises 75% of cases, while cutaneous squamous cell carcinoma (cSCC) accounts for 20% of NMSC. A wide variety of additional non-melanoma skin tumors arise from other cell types present in skin, such as lymphocytes, vascular endothelial cells, Merkel cells, mesenchymal stromal cells, and cells forming the adnexal structures. These entities are quite rare relative to BCC and cSCC and will not be discussed in this chapter. Although the mortality from NMSC is relatively low, the morbidity and cost associated with treatment is substantial (1). Furthermore, the incidence of NMSC has increased markedly since the 1960s and continues to rise (2). This is generally believed to be a consequence of increased cumulative ultraviolet exposure and is related to an increasingly elderly population, change in outdoor activities, and depletion of the atmospheric ozone layer (3).

The worldwide incidence of NMSC is difficult to determine as the cancer is not typically followed in tumor registries; however, populations of fair-skinned individuals in proximity to the equator are at particular risk. The highest incidence rates by far are seen in Australia and Newzeland with between 1% and 2% of the population developing NMSC per year (4).

ETIOLOGY

While sun exposure is the primary etiologic agent in the formation of NMSC, additional risk factors include genetic predisposition, predisposing skin lesions, immunosuppression, and trauma. Genetic syndromes associated with the development of NMSC are characterized by conditions that decrease protection and cellular repair mechanisms against sun exposure, including xeroderma pigmentosum, nevoid basal cell syndrome, albinism, epidermodysplasia veruciformis, and porokeratosis (5). Certain predisposing skin lesions, such as nevus sebaceous, actinic keratosis, and cutaneous horns can undergo malignant transformation and thus warrant appropriate treatment (6,7).

Immunosuppression is a significant risk factor for NMSC. This patient population has dramatically increased in size as a consequence of anti-rejection regimens associated with organ transplantation and treatment with immunosuppressive pharmacologic agents for rheumatologic and autoimmune diseases, and HIV. These patients are at markedly increased risk of developing NMSC, including tumors of a more aggressive and invasive behavior. Additionally, while the ratio of BCC to cSCC in the general population is approximately 4:1, in the transplant population, cSCC is twice as common as BCC (8).

CLINICOPATHOLOGICAL FACTORS AND PROGNOSIS

BCC is comprised of five different histological types. Nodular BCC is the most common subtype and is characterized by a raised pearly rolled edge with surface telangiectasia often with a central ulcer. Superficial BCC is the least aggressive subtype and is characterized by scaly, dry, erythematous, circular plaques. Basosquamous BCC has some histological features of cSCC and occasionally metastasizes making it the most aggressive subtype. Morpheic (sclerosing) BCC is a locally aggressive tumor with an indistinct border rendering margin control challenging. Pigmented BCC contains melanin, tends to occur in dark skinned populations, and is often confused with melanoma (9).

cSCC is characterized by nests of epidermal cells consisting of varying proportions of normal and anaplastic squamous cells. Poorly differentiated cSCC, determined by increasing proportions of anaplastic cells, is associated with more aggressive disease. Adenosquamous cSCC is a histological variant characterized by solid and gland-like epithelial proliferations that extend into the dermis. These tumors most often affect the exposed head and neck of elderly patients and have a similar malignant potential to typical cSCC. Spindle cell and clear cell cSCC are other histological variants, which occur rarely.

Survival is ultimately influenced by the development of regional and distant metastases (10,11). Distant metastases are rare (12). While nodal metastasis from BCC occurs extremely rarely, the rate of nodal metastasis from cSCC of the head and neck is difficult to determine because of the lack of prospectively maintained tumor registries and the wide variability of retrospectively reported rates reflecting biases in referral practice, but it is likely to occur in fewer than 5% of cases (13–18). Several clinicopathological features known to increase the risk of locoregional failure will be discussed (Tables 25.1 and 25.2).

Table 25.1 Risk Factors for Local Recurrence of Basal Cell Carcinoma

	Low-risk	High-risk
Size	Low-risk location <20 mm High-risk location <6 mm	Low-risk location >20 mm High-risk location >6 mm
Location	Cheeks, forehead, scalp, and neck	"Mask areas" of face
Borders	Well-defined	Poorly defined
Primary vs. recurrent	Primary	Recurrent
Immunosuppression	Absent	Present
Pathology	Nodular and superficial variants	Basosquamous variant
Perineural involvement	Absent	Present

Table 25.2 Risk Factors for Locoregional Recurrence of Squamous Cell Carcinoma

Clinical	Low-risk	High-risk
Size	Low-risk location <20 mm High-risk location <6 mm	Low-risk location >20 mm High-risk location >6 mm
Location	Cheeks, forehead, scalp, and neck	"Mask areas" of face
Borders	Well-defined	Poorly defined
Primary vs. Recurrent	Primary	Recurrent
Immunosuppression	Absent	Present
Site of prior radiation or chronic inflammation	Absent	Present
Rapidly growing tumor	Absent	Present
Neurological symptoms	Absent	Present
Pathology		
Degree of differentiation	Well differentiated cSCC	Moderately or poorly differentiated cSCC, Adenosquamous, desmoplastic variants
Depth	Clark level I, II, III, or <4 mm	Clark level IV, V, or >4 mm
Perineural invasion	Absent	Present

Tumor Thickness and Depth of Invasion

Strong evidence exists that tumor thickness and depth of invasion is associated with development of nodal metastasis. In a large series of head and neck cSCC, patients with tumors thicker than 4 mm or Clark level IV–V, had a regional metastatic rate of 46% compared with 7% in patients with thinner tumors (12). Several other studies have reported similar findings utilizing the same tumor thickness/depth of invasion thresholds (19–21).

Tumor Grade

Poorly differentiated lesions have the greatest metastatic potential (19,22). In a series of 571 patients, the rate of metastasis in poorly differentiated tumors was significantly higher compared to other tumor grades (17% vs. 4%; p = .004) (22). Similarly, desmoplastic cSCCs have a greater risk of regional nodal metastasis (18,23).

Tumor Size

Several studies have cited head and neck cSCC diameter greater than a threshold size of 2 cm (>T1) as predictive of regional metastasis (12,19–22,24), with lesions greater than 2 cm having triple the metastatic potential of smaller lesions (12). Another series has reported a median size of 15 mm in a series of 135 patients with metastatic cSCC (25), leading some to suggest that tumor size alone is a weak predictor of metastasis (11,26).

Anatomical Site

The parotid gland is considered the basin for metastatic lymphatic nodal involvement from cSCCs located on or around the ear, cheek, and frontotemporal skin and scalp. These lesions and those on the lower lip display a high propensity to nodal metastasis (12,14,16,24,27–29).

Perineural and Lymphovascular Invasion

The incidence of perineural spread in cSCC is approximately 4% to 14% (12,30). Studies have shown a significantly higher rate of nodal metastasis in cSCC (35% vs. 15%; p < .0005) and lip squamous cell carcinoma (SCC) (41% vs. 5%; p < .0001) for patients with perineural invasion compared with those without (28,30). In another study, the presence of perineural invasion independently predicted for poorer three-year disease-specific survival (64% vs. 91%; p = .002) (10). Although, the presence of lymphovascular invasion has been shown to independently predict for nodal metastasis, its impact on outcome is more uncertain (24).

Recurrent Squamous Cell Carcinoma

Several studies report a high incidence of local recurrences (39% to 50%) in patients with regional metastases, which may indicate that recurrent cSCCs are biologically more aggressive than primary cSCCs (12,14,16). This finding is consistent with a recent study reporting that recurrent cSCCs were significantly larger (2.4 cm vs. 1.5 cm) and more likely to involve perineural invasion (24% vs. 10%), lymphovascular invasion (17% vs. 8%), and invade beyond the subcutaneous tissues (30% vs. 10%) (10).

Immunosuppression

Immunosuppression as a consequence of management of organ transplantation or systemic disease, such as chronic lymphocytic leukemia, is associated with development of NMSC, usually cSCC (31,32). Since the risk of disease is related to the duration of immunosuppression (66% risk at 24 years) (32), patients are typically affected at an earlier age and have a tendency to develop more new cSCC. Development of metastasis in immunosuppressed patients is estimated at 13%, more than twice the rate in immunocompetent patients (12), and occurs at a smaller lesion size and depth of invasion threshold than in immunocompetent patients (33).

Table 25.3 AJCC Staging System for Non-melanoma Skin Cancer (34)

Primary Tumor (T)

TX	Primary tumor cannot be assessed
T0	No evidence of primary tumor
Tis	Carcinoma in situ
T1	Tumor 2 cm or less in greatest dimension
T2	Tumor more than 2 cm but not more than 5 cm in greatest dimension
T3	Tumor not more than 5 cm in greatest dimension
T4	Tumor invades deep extradermal structures (i.e., cartilage, skeletal muscle, or bone)

Regional Lymph Nodes (N)

NX	Regional lymph nodes cannot be assessed
N0	No regional lymph node metastasis
N1	Regional lymph node metastasis

Distant Metastasis (M)

MX	Distant metastasis cannot be assessed
M0	No distant metastasis
M1	Distant metastasis

Combined staging

Stage 0	Tis	N0	M0
Stage I	T1	N0	M0
Stage II	T2 and T3	N0	M0
Stage III	T4	N0	M0
	Any T	N1	M0
Stage IV	Any T	Any N	M1

Abbreviation: AJCC, American Joint Committee on Cancer

STAGING

The present TNM staging for NMSC (34) (excluding eyelid, vulva, and penis) is outlined in Table 25.3. The current staging system has been challenged with regard to its tumor and nodal classification. The current tumor staging relates to two-dimensional size only, and does not include depth of invasion. Indeed, size alone has been found to be a poor predictor of outcome, and lesions with a thickness of greater than 4 mm have a greater propensity for lymph node metastasis (19). Furthermore, a small NMSC that involves nasal or auricular cartilage would be staged T4, whereas a tumor with much larger surface area in an alternate location would be staged as a T3.

The nodal staging, currently represented by N0 or N1, results in marked heterogeneity among patients with nodal disease. Alternate staging systems have been proposed based on data that demonstrate worse prognosis in patients with both parotid and neck metastasis than those with involvement of parotid nodes only (35,36). Additionally, patients with cervical nodes greater than 3 cm in diameter, or with multiple positive neck nodes, have been shown to have worse prognosis (36). Accordingly, revised nodal staging systems incorporating size and number of regional nodes, as well as division of nodes according to parotid and cervical distribution, have been proposed.

DIAGNOSIS

BCC most commonly afflicts patients between the ages of 40 and 60 years. However, the demographics have been shifting toward a younger age of incidence likely associated with societal trends related to sunbathing. Men are more commonly affected than females, and people of Fitzpatrick Skin Type I or II are at higher risk than those with darker skin color. The typical appearance of a BCC is that of a nodular, raised lesion with pearly, rolled borders. The lesions are often characterized by a surface translucence, an opalescent nature, and telangiectasia.

cSCC also presents more commonly in men than in women with a ratio of 3:1. Again, fair-skinned individuals who burn easily are at highest risk and the sun-exposed regions of the head and neck are most commonly affected. The lesions may present with a variety of clinical morphologies. Invasive cSCC is generally seen as a raised, firm, red-pink, keratotic papule, most commonly located in a sun-exposed region. Larger lesions may present with erosion or ulceration and may be deeply invasive at the time of presentation.

Approximately 2–3% of cSCC spread to regional lymph nodes in the head and neck, particularly to nodes in the parotid bed. Patients at increased risk of regional metastasis include those with tumors larger than 2 cm or depth greater than 4 mm to 5 mm, perineural invasion, immunocompromised state, and recurrent tumors (25).

To confirm the clinical diagnosis of NMSC, an adequate biopsy specimen is essential. The preferred method of biopsy is a punch or incisional biopsy that passes beneath the depth of the epidermis. An adequately deep biopsy specimen is imperative in order to provide a sample that will allow for the assessment of depth of invasion. It is reasonable to completely excise small lesions located in non-critical areas.

TREATMENT OF THE PRIMARY TUMOR

The appropriate management of NMSC of the head and neck requires complete eradication of the primary tumor with maximal preservation of function and cosmesis. This is achieved based on the extent of the primary tumor and the desires and comorbidities of the individual patient. Although the vast majority of NMSC are cured with relatively simple treatment, when advanced their management can present a formidable challenge to the head and neck surgeon and have a tremendous impact on the patient's quality of life. Whereas cure rates for early NMSC of the head and neck exceed 95% (37), advanced disease continues to be associated with mortality rates of up to 70% (38,39). Therefore, early diagnosis and appropriate management is paramount.

Therapeutic modalities for NMSC of the head and neck can be divided into two broad categories: non-excisional and excisional. Non-excisional modalities, aside from radiation therapy, include cryosurgery, curettage and electrodessication, laser therapy, topical chemotherapy, or immune modulators; non-excisional modalities are reserved for small, low-risk, or superficial lesions. Excisional techniques include conventional surgical excision and Moh's micrographic surgery. Unlike the previous group, excisional therapies are based on complete histologic clearance of the primary tumor and have the advantage of providing prognostic information about the primary, such as the presence of lymphovascular or perineural spread.

Non-excisional Therapy

Non-excisional treatments, aside from radiation therapy, should be reserved for the management of small low-risk NMSC. They are relatively simple, well-tolerated and inexpensive therapies that, when used appropriately, result in excellent cure rates. Although these therapies prevent microscopic assessment of tumor, biopsy of all suspected malignancies or recurrent skin lesions must always be performed prior to definitive management.

Cryosurgery

Cryosurgery, as the name implies, uses extreme cold to ablate lesions of the skin. This treatment modality should only be considered for the management of pre-malignant lesions (e.g., nevus sebaceous, actinic keratosis) and small, well-demarcated, low-risk histologically confirmed NMSC. Cryosurgery requires rapid cooling of the lesion to at least $-50°C$. Liquid nitrogen is the most commonly used cryogen. The treatment is relatively well-tolerated but frequently requires local anesthesia. In order to eradicate disease, the entire thickness of tumor must reach tumoricidal temperatures. Intradermal temperature probes and dermal ultrasound have been used in an attempt to increase treatment effectiveness (40).

Cryosurgery may be used to treat actinic keratosis, seborrheic keratosis, solar lentigo, and low-risk cutaneous basal cell and squamous cell carcinomas. When treating malignant disease, a margin of at least 5 mm should be included in the treatment field (40–42). This increases the likelihood that the freeze zone encompasses the entire lesion. This management approach requires the patient to undergo multiple treatments.

Cryosurgery frequently results in hypopigmentation and, therefore, is best suited for fair-skinned individuals. It also destroys hair follicles and should only be used on non-hair-bearing skin (i.e., not scalp, eyebrow, beard, etc). It is absolutely contraindicated for the treatment of sclerosing BCC, recurrent BCC, or recurrent cSCC, or in cases where histology is needed. It should also be avoided in areas with compromised circulation, underlying cartilage, uncertainity in postoperative healing, or important nearby structures, such as the eyelids, nasal tip, and alae. Alternative treatments should be considered in patients with connective tissue disease, cryoglobulinaemia, cold urticaria, or heavily pigmented skin. Following treatment patients often experience localized discomfort, erythema, blistering, and sloughing as the wound heals by secondary intention. Severe scarring is uncommon.

When used in appropriately selected patients, cryosurgery may offer excellent control of low-risk small and well-demarcated cutaneous BCC and cSCC. Five-year cure rates for highly selected lesions range from 90% to 98% and depend on the skill and experience of the treating physician (41,42). A recent study of 2000 patients, treated by a single physician for primary or recurrent basal cell and squamous cell carcinoma, showed that cryosurgery was associated with a 30-year cure rate of 98.6% (40). It should be stated that despite these excellent results, cryosurgery is most appropriate for the management of benign skin lesions.

Curettage and Electrodessication

Curettage and electrodessication is frequently employed to treat small superficial NMSC. This technique takes advantage of the textural interface that exists between tumor and normal dermis. As such it is not indicated for tumors that extend to fat. It is also contra-indicated for the treatment of lesions in hair-bearing skin because it may inadequately treat tumor extending down follicular structures. A sharp curette is used to remove tumor until its interface with the tougher dermis is reached. Following removal of friable tumor the base is electrodessicated with a cautery device or excision. High tumoricidal temperatures are applied to kill any remaining tumor cells. As is the case with all non-excisional techniques, margins are not assessed microscopically. Frequently, following electrodessication the base of the wound is re-curetted. This step can be repeated in order to decrease the likelihood of recurrence. Should subdermal fat be encountered during the procedure, the lesion should be surgically excised to microscopically negative margins. The results with this technique are highly operator dependent. Wounds are allowed to heal by secondary intention and frequently result in hypertrophic scars. Curettage and electrodessication should be avoided in the cosmetically sensitive areas of the face.

This technique should be limited to small (<2 cm) low-risk BCC and cSCC. Curettage and electrodessication should be avoided when tumors are recurrent, ill-defined, extend deeper than the superficial dermis, or are located in high-risk areas. It is contraindicated for the treatment of morphea-type (i.e., sclerosing) BCC (43,44).

Cure rates are excellent when curettage and electrodessication is used to treat appropriately selected BCC and cSCC. Five-year cure rates for BCC and cSCC are 92% and 96%, respectively (45,46). Recurrence rates as high as 17.6%, however, have been reported with tumors located in high-risk areas, such as the nose, central third of the face, auricle, and periorbital skin (47). This discrepancy highlights the importance of patient selection.

Light Therapies

Laser surgery. Lasers have been successfully used to treat both pre-malignant and malignant lesions of the skin. Full-face laser resurfacing using CO2 or Erbium: YAG lasers have shown promise in treating multifocal actinic keratosis and likely preventing the development of cSCC. Iyer et al. demonstrated that following full-face laser resurfacing, 87% of patients with multifocal actinic keratosis remained lesion-free for at least a year, falling to 58.3% at two years (48).

Photodynamic therapy. This is another form of light therapy that has shown promise for the treatment of superficial NMSC. Photodynamic therapy requires activation of photosensitizers that preferentially accumulate within cancer cells. Once activated by light at wavelengths matching their specific absorption, these photosensitizers produce singlet oxygen that is then capable of killing cells directly, sublethal mutagenesis, and induction of apoptosis. Photosensitizers may be administered systemically, or in the case of skin lesions, topically. Topical application is ideally suited for management of cutaneous lesions as it permits selective treatment of the area of concern and avoids systemic toxicity. For the purposes of NMSC treatment, the two most commonly used topical photosensitizers are methyl aminolevulinate (MAL) and 5-aminolevulinic acid (ALA). Both are converted to protoporphyrin IX once absorbed into skin, and accumulate in the membranes of mitochondria and other intracellular organelles. Protoporphyrin activated by laser light at wavelengths between 450–750 nm. Absorption into the deep dermis is limited and it is currently recommended that photodynamic therapy be reserved for the treatment of superficial lesions. Maximal absorption and intracellular accumulation of MAL and ALA requires time (at least three hours under an occlusive dressing). Patients typically experience mild pain, irritation, and erythema following treatment.

The results with photodynamic therapy have been encouraging. Complete clearance of superficial BCC and cSCC is common. Rhodes et al. demonstrated a 90% complete response rate for small nodular BCC treated with topical ALA-photodynamic therapy with 74% remaining disease-free at two years (49). Similarly, treatment of Bowen's disease resulted in 88% complete response rates (50). Recurrence rates for NMSC, however, remain high, up to 31% and 52% for superficial BCC and cSCC in situ, respectively (51,52). Effectiveness may increase when combined with other non-excisional therapies including curettage. Photodynamic therapy should not be considered for the treatment of thick tumors, lesions with aggressive histology, recurrent cancer, or lesions in high-risk areas (53). In properly selected patients, this treatment modality offers a good non-surgical alternative with excellent cosmetic results.

Local Chemotherapy

Topical 5-fluorouracil. The anti-metabolite 5-fluorouracil (5-FU) interferes with DNA synthesis through the inhibition of thymidylate synthetase. It has been used extensively for the successful management of actinic keratosis. Its use for invasive BCC and cSCC remains controversial. It may be considered for a highly select group of patients. Due to poor absorption, topical 5-FU should only be used for the treatment of very superficial BCC in patients unsuitable for other more conventional treatments. Gross et al. reported a 90% histologic cure rate in a series of 31 superficial BCC of the trunk and limbs using 5% 5-FU applied twice daily for up to 12 weeks (54). Similar results have been reported for topical 5-FU treatment of superficial cSCC and Bowen's disease (55).

Intralesional 5-FU has also been used for treatment of Bowen's disease, BCC and cSCC of the head and neck. Although considered experimental therapy, intralesional 5-FU has successfully treated deeper lesions. This requires repeated injections over 6 to 10 weeks. In a series of 122 patients with biopsy-proven BCC, injectable 5-FU was associated with a 90% histologically confirmed tumor clearance rate and very acceptable toxicity (56).

Most patients experience a brisk inflammatory response in the treatment field. An erythematous rash with crusting and small superficial ulcerations is common. Although uncomfortable, the rash quickly resolves following cessation of treatment. Typically, patients are left with a smooth complexion several weeks after therapy. Systemic complications are very rare.

Intra-lesional interferon alpha. Interferon alpha (IFNα is a cytokine that has been successfully used for the treatment of BCC. It promotes apoptosis in BCC by up-regulating the CD-95 ligand-receptor interaction and through stimulation of IL-2 and IL-10. Similar effects have been reported

in cSCC in vitro (57). Clinical experience with intra-lesional IFNα has demonstrated reasonable efficacy for treatment of BCC. Complete long-term response rates of 50–98% have been reported (58). Multiple injections are required and patients frequently report flu-like symptoms including fever, myalgia, and headache.

Bostanci et al. treated 20 histologically proven BCC with intra-lesional IFNα.

Injections were given three times per week for three weeks and biopsies were taken eight weeks later. Of the 20 lesions, 11 (55%) achieved a complete clinical and histological response, six showed partial response, two remained stable, and one lesion increased in size. Complete responders were followed for seven years and only one lesion recurred (59). Tucker et al. treated 50 patients with 98 biopsy-proven superficial and nodular BCC with peri-lesional and intra-lesional IFNα. Sixty-eight of 98 tumors were followed for at least 10 years. Kaplan-Meier estimated cure rates at 5 and 10 years were 98% (60).

Results with intra-lesional IFNα have been variable. This treatment is experimental and should be reserved for patients refusing or unable to tolerate more conventional therapies. Currently, experience is largely limited to treatment of BCC and should not be extrapolated to include cSCC.

Imiquimod. Imiquimod is an immune response modulator currently approved by the U.S. Food and Drug Administration for the treatment of actinic keratosis, superficial BCC, and external genital warts (44). Imiquimod is an imidazoquinolone that binds to the cell surface toll-like receptor 7 and induces production of pro-inflammatory cytokines including IFNα, tumor necrosis factor alpha, and IL-12. These cytokines in turn mediate its anti-tumoral effects and promote a TH-1 mediated immune response to the tumor (61). When applied topically imiquimod induces a localized inflammatory response. This usually results in erythema, edema, and superficial ulceration, scabbing, and crusting within the treatment field. This may be associated with pain or burning. Acute toxicity may necessitate short breaks in therapy but rarely necessitates discontinuation of imiquimod. Although uncomfortable and unsightly, the development of this inflammatory response seems to correlate with the effectiveness of treatment. Systemic toxicity is rare but includes the development of fever, myalgia, nausea, and rigors. Imiquimod should be avoided in individuals with pre-existing autoimmune disease. Hypersensitivity reactions have been reported.

Imiquimod is applied directly to the skin by the patient. Complete clinical response rates ranging from 52% to 100% have been reported and seem to depend on the frequency of application and the duration of treatment (44). Although associated with the highest response rates, twice daily treatment results in significant local toxicity. The current recommended dosing schedule for the treatment of superficial BCC is once daily application of 5% imiquimod cream to the affected skin five days per week for six weeks. This regimen is associated with 80–88% complete response rates for appropriately selected superficial BCC (62–64).

Although currently approved only for the treatment of superficial BCC, imiquimod has also been used to treat nodular BCC, Bowen's disease, and superficial cSCC with varying effectiveness. Clearance rates of 71–76% have been reported for nodular BCC treated for 6 to 12 weeks with

5% imiquimod cream (63). Increased effectiveness has been reported when imiquimod is combined with pre-treatment curettage alone or curettage and electrodessication. Tilman et al. reported results with a series of 45 lesions, 23 BCC and 22 cSCC. The majority were high-risk lesions located on the head and neck. Many had curettage prior to imiquimod therapy. Three months following completion of treatment, biopsies revealed persistent disease in three cases (2 BCC and 1 SCC). During a median follow-up of 26 months only one additional cSCC recurred (61).

Imiquimod is also an effective treatment for carcinoma in situ and dysplastic skin in high-risk individuals. Its use has been investigated for the prevention of cSCC in solid organ transplant patients. In a randomized, placebo-controlled trial, 5% imiquimod therapy resulted in a 62.1% complete clearance rate of actinic keratosis in heart, kidney, and liver transplant patients. Furthermore, none of the patients experienced graft rejection or a deterioration of graft function during treatment. In this high-risk patient population, topical imiquimod therapy should be considered once dysplastic skin changes become evident, especially in patients with a history of cSCC (65).

Imiquimod has become a valuable treatment modality for low-risk superficial BCC and premalignant skin changes. It has also shown promise for the treatment of superficial cSCC and nodular BCC. At present, its use, alone or in combination with curettage and electrodessication, should be reserved for the prevention of cutaneous malignancy in at-risk individuals and for the treatment of low-risk BCC and cSCC in patients considered poor candidates for surgical excision.

Radiotherapy

External beam radiation therapy is included among the non-excisional therapies, but unlike the others should not be considered a treatment exclusively for low-risk lesions. Radiation is a powerful tool and plays a very important role in the management of advanced disease. With regard to primary treatment, the appropriateness of its use for low-risk lesions has been controversial. Postoperative adjuvant radiotherapy remains essential in the management of advanced primary disease and in cases associated with regional metastases. There is no question that radiotherapy represents a very effective treatment modality for superficial BCC and cSCC of the head and neck. Orthovoltage X-ray or electron beam fractionated irradiation has been associated with cure rates of 90% for small BCC and cSCC of the head and neck (66,67). Treatment is protracted, usually requiring weeks of therapy and costing at least five times as much as conventional surgery; however, in elderly patients who are not operative candidates or for treatment of lesions in cosmetically sensitive areas it is an excellent form of primary therapy (Figs. 25.1 and 25.2).

Primary radiotherapy in appropriately selected low-risk NMSC is associated with overall recurrence rates of 8.7% and 10% for BCC and cSCC, respectively (12,47). These excellent results are limited to superficial lesions with favorable histology. When compared to nodular BCC, sclerosing BCC is not as well-controlled, with Kaplan-Meier five-year recurrence rate estimates of 8.2% versus 27.2%, respectively (68). Advanced disease is also associated with much lower local-control rates. In a series of 85 patients with 88 T4 head

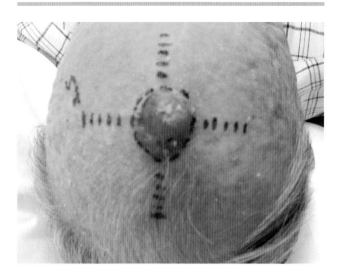

Figure 25.1 Patient with a large scalp squamous cell carcinoma who refused surgery.

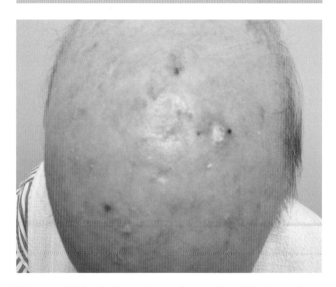

Figure 25.2 Patient shown 3 months following primary radiotherapy.

and neck BCC or cSCC treated with primary radiotherapy, Othman et al. reported five-year and 10-year local control rates of 53% and 49%, respectively. When surgical salvage was included five-year and 10-year local control rates increased to 90% and 85%, respectively (69). This study and others have highlighted the need for multimodality therapy in advanced cases of NMSC (70,71). It was recommended that postoperative adjuvant radiation therapy be considered for lesions amenable to complete surgical resection with acceptable cosmesis and function; however, in poor surgical candidates with significant medical comorbidities or primaries that are unlikely to be completely resected, primary radiotherapy is a very valuable and effective treatment option, especially when combined with salvage surgery.

One of the greatest disadvantages of primary fractionated radiotherapy is the length of treatment, which typically lasts four to five weeks. For many elderly patients with medical comorbidities this represents a significant treatment obstacle. In order to circumvent this problem, altered dosage and scheduling regimens have been investigated. The effectiveness of single fraction radiotherapy was assessed in a series of 1005 BCC and cSCC, 97% of which were located in the head and neck. All were treated at a single institution with 10-year follow-up. Overall five-year disease-free and radionecrosis-free survival was 90% and 84%, respectively. There was no significant difference in control rates when comparing doses of 20 Gy and 22.5 Gy. However, necrosis rates were significantly lower with the lower dose. Radionecrosis required surgical intervention in 16% of cases (72). Although certainly not conventional, single fraction radiotherapy may be considered for non-surgical patients unfit to receive multiple treatments whose tumors are less than 3 cm in diameter.

Compared to surgery, primary radiotherapy may provide better cosmetic results in certain aesthetically sensitive areas of the face including the nose, ears, and lips; however, the treatment is associated with long term sequelae including dermal atrophy, telangiectasia, hypo- and hyperpigmentation, and in-field second primary carcinomas. For this reason, current practice guidelines recommend considering primary radiation for patients over 50 years of age or those who are poor candidates for surgery. Radiation is contraindicated in patients with genetic disease predisposing to cutaneous malignancy (basal cell nevus syndrome and xerodverma pigmentosum) and connective tissue disease.

Adjuvant radiation therapy should be considered for deep lesions invading muscle, nerve, bone, or cartilage, and recurrent lesions located in high-risk areas.

Excisional Therapy

Surgical excision of NMSC of the head and neck, unlike the aforementioned techniques, permits the surgeon to assess the completeness of resection through microscopic evaluation of margins. Although these techniques may be applied to just about any primary, there are specific instances where each is indicated. In general, conventional surgical excision, with intraoperative or postoperative margin analysis, is indicated in either low-risk lesions or for advanced cancers. Mohs micrographic surgery is indicated for non-advanced recurrent tumors or non-advanced high-risk lesions.

Mohs Micrographic Surgery

Mohs micrographic surgery is considered the gold-standard treatment for non-advanced recurrent and non-advanced high-risk NMSC. This technique, developed in the 1940s by Dr. Frederick Mohs, is labor-intensive and highly specialized. The procedure permits complete resection of cancer with minimal destruction of normal tissue. Unlike conventional surgical margins, which are randomly assessed and therefore permit sampling error, close to 100% of peripheral and deep margins are examined during Mohs surgery. Conventional surgery resects visible tumor along with a cuff or margin of normal tissue to encompass the entire cancer.

The width of the margin is determined by the size and histologic subtype of the lesion. Unfortunately, BCC and cSCC may exhibit extensive microscopic radial growth patterns, with fingers of tumor following nerve, blood vessels, and periosteum far beyond a lesion's visible or palpable limits. Unlike simple surgical excision, which assumes the predetermined margin will encompass disease, Mohs micrographic surgery allows the surgeon to map, microscopically follow, and completely resect tumor. By mounting and sectioning peripheral and deep margins in the horizontal plane, essentially 100% of the periphery is assessed. This ability to completely resect cancer permits patients to safely undergo immediate reconstruction.

Studies have quite clearly demonstrated that Mohs surgery for non-advanced recurrent and non-advanced high-risk NMSC of the head and neck is superior to standard resection or radiotherapy. Traditional surgical resection is associated with five-year recurrence rates of 10.1%, 10.9%, and 18.7% for primary BCC of the head and neck and cSCC of the lip and ear, respectively (12,47,73). This is in sharp contrast to the five-year recurrence rates seen with Mohs micrographic surgery; 1%, 3.1%, and 5.3% for the same three groups, respectively (12,47,73). In the case of recurrent BCC the difference in five-year recurrence rates is even more striking; 5.6% and 17.4% for Mohs surgery and traditional resection, respectively. Similarly, Mohs excision of recurrent cSCC yields five-year recurrence rates of 6.7% as compared to 23.3% with traditional surgery (12,47,73). Other differences between the two techniques include the cost and length of the procedures. Although Mohs surgery frequently is described as more costly, Bialy et al. recently demonstrated that once the additional cost of re-resection to achieve negative margins with traditional surgery is included, Mohs surgery is cost-comparable to surgical resection (74). Mohs excision remains a more time consuming treatment, particularly with larger or more invasive lesions that may require multiple passes to completely excise.

Mohs surgery is currently indicated for the treatment of recurrent and high-risk BCC and cSCC of the head and neck. This would include sclerosing (morpheaform) BCC, cancers with ill-defined borders or perineural spread, or those located in high-risk areas, including the periorbital and canthal regions, the eyelids, the central third of the face, the nasal alae and columella, the auricular helix, and post-auricular sulcus. In general, Mohs surgery should be reserved for lesions greater than 2 cm in diameter (43). Although cancers involving cartilage or bone cannot be completely removed with Mohs surgery, this treatment modality can certainly be part of a multidisciplinary approach. For example, in lesions involving the nasal tip including cartilage or bone, Mohs surgery can be used to clear the soft tissue component of the cancer and conventional surgery with postoperative margin control can be used to deal with the remainder of the cancer. Such an approach provides the greatest chance of local control and may be augmented with the addition of postoperative radiation therapy, if indicated.

Conventional Surgery

Traditional surgical excision of NMSC of the head and neck remains the most common treatment for low-risk lesions. It is fast, safe, well-tolerated and, in most cases, provides excellent cosmetic results. Surgical excision with intra-operative or, more frequently, postoperative margin analysis is an excellent and very effective form of treatment for lesions less than 2 cm in size located in low-risk areas of the head and neck (43). The effectiveness of this treatment is entirely dependent on taking appropriate surgical margins. Excision margins for NMSC should be wide enough to encompass the entire tumor the majority of the time, but should not be excessive and result in unnecessary sacrifice of normal tissue. There are many recommendations in the literature ranging from 0.3 to 1 cm and 0.4 to 1.5 cm for BCC and cSCC measuring less than 2 cm, respectively. Clearly, tumor specific features, such as histologic subtype, grade, and location affect these numbers and the surgeon must appreciate all of these factors.

Wolf et al. demonstrated that a margin of 0.4 cm will completely remove low-risk BCCs with a 95% five-year cure rate (75). Low-risk lesions are defined as tumors less than 2 cm in size, with well-defined borders and favorable histology, located in low- to intermediate-risk areas. For larger lesions, Mohs surgery is recommended and, if simply resected, surgical margins must be much wider.

Adequate surgical margins for SCC have also been evaluated and depend on careful assessment of the primary. Size of the primary is an important consideration. Rowe et al. demonstrated in a large meta-analysis of 2939 cSCC (2234 cases were less than 2 cm and 705 were greater than 2 cm) that the diameter of the primary was very important. Lesions less than 2 cm in diameter had a recurrence rate of 7.4% as compared to 15.2% for larger cancers (12,47). Brodland et al. also demonstrated in series of cSCC undergoing Mohs surgery, that a margin of 0.4 cm completely excised 95% of cancers less than 2 cm in diameter. For larger lesions, a margin of 0.6 cm was required (76). Similarly, differentiation of the tumor impacts the width of excision margins. In the meta-analysis by Rowe et al., poorly differentiated cancers recurred more frequently than well to moderately differentiated tumors, 28.6% versus 13.6%, respectively. This confirms clinical experience that poorly differentiated lesions require wider margins (12). Exactly how much wider has never been prospectively assessed, but in such cases communication between surgeon and pathologist is crucial. Finally, location is a very important consideration. In Brodland's study, lesions less than 2 cm in size located in high-risk areas such as the ears, eyelids, scalp, nasal alae, and lips required 0.6 cm margins in order to achieve histologic clearance of the cancer in 95% of cases. Taken together, this data suggests that for low-risk cSCC a margin of at least 0.4 cm is required increasing to 0.6 cm when small tumors are located in high-risk areas (12). Furthermore, larger size and more aggressive histology require wider margins and extremely careful margin analysis.

Although Mohs surgery offers far more inclusive assessment of surgical margins, communication between surgeon and pathologist, along with accurate sampling and labelling of at-risk margins by the surgeon, can definitely increase the completeness of traditional surgical excision and help identify patients requiring additional treatment. In a prospective randomized trial comparing Mohs surgery and standard surgical resection of BCC, Smeets et al. suggested that recurrence rates were similar for both (77).

The study demonstrated that surgical excision was initially incomplete in 18% and 32% of primary and recurrent BCC, respectively; however, when identified and retreated, the results of surgical excision were equivalent to Mohs surgery. Long-term assessment of control rates for both groups are required, but the study highlights the frequency of incomplete resection and the effectiveness of careful margin analysis (77).

Special Considerations

Non-melanotic skin cancer of the head and neck can be an incredibly challenging disease to manage when advanced or recurrent, highlighting the need for appropriate initial therapy. There are several situations that deserve special attention and frequently require a multidisciplinary approach. These include involvement of the orbit, temporal bone, skull base, and midface, as well as extensive perineural invasion. Unlike the majority of NMSC, these tumors are associated with poor prognosis and significant morbidity. Distant metastases from NMSC of the head and neck are uncommon, even in the setting of advanced local disease. Therefore, the majority of patients dying from NMSC of the head and neck do so as a result of local-regional disease progression and consequently suffer the pain, disfigurement, and dysfunction that accompany it.

Orbit. Involvement of the orbit by NMSC occurs as a result of perineural spread, lymphovascular spread, or direct invasion. Regardless of cause, this is most frequently seen in the setting of recurrent periorbital cancer. Management of orbital invasion frequently requires orbital exenteration. This results in disfigurement and remains an emotionally charged issue. BCC and cSCC located on the eyelids, brow, and periorbital skin are high-risk and deserve aggressive initial therapy in order to avoid secondary involvement of the orbit. In a large series of basal cell and squamous cell eyelid carcinomas treated with primary surgical resection, initial surgical excision was incomplete in 12% to 25%. Morpheaform lesions and tumors located at the medial canthus were incompletely excised 15% to 35% of the time (78,79). These results highlight the need for aggressive initial therapy. In most cases these cancers should be treated with Mohs surgery.

Orbital involvement may be quite insidious and diagnosis requires a heightened index of suspicion. Evaluating periorbital skin cancer requires careful examination of the orbit, including cranial nerve examination. When present, perineural spread is most frequently clinically associated with either the trigeminal or facial nerves. Patients with restricted extraocular muscle movements or cranial nerve findings invariably have extensive disease and poor prognosis. CT and MRI examination of the orbit and skull base are indicated whenever orbital invasion is suspected (Figs. 25.3 and 25.4).

Operability of such tumors depends primarily on the posterior extent of disease. Tumors that involve the orbital apex or cavernous sinus are most often inoperable. In such cases, primary radiotherapy may be the most appropriate treatment, although local control rates are poor. Tumors that invade orbital fat, muscle, or the globe are managed with orbital exenteration, appropriate reconstruction, and adjuvant radiation therapy. Overall five-year survival is

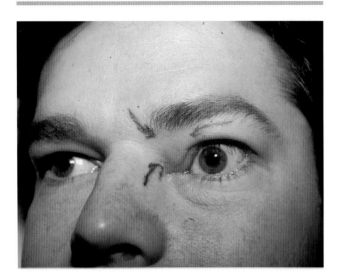

Figure 25.3 Patient with recurrent squamous cell carcinoma of the left medial canthus causing orbital displacement and diploplia.

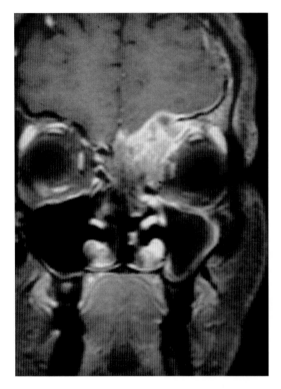

Figure 25.4 MRI of the same patient showing extensive orbital invasion.

55% but may be far worse if there is extensive perineural spread (30). Reconstruction of orbital exenteration defects is best accomplished with split thickness skin grafting and prosthetic rehabilitation. Advanced disease may also require resection of orbital bone, the skull base, or paranasal sinuses. Such extensive disease may be associated with regional

metastases and frequently necessitates free flap reconstruction. Other indications for free flap reconstruction include previous irradiation, extensive associated midface or frontal craniofacial defects, and patient preference.

Temporal bone. NMSC of the auricle and post-auricular sulcus may invade the temporal bone through medial extension down the external auditory canal or less frequently by direct invasion of the mastoid. These cancers, if undetected or improperly treated, can invade the middle ear space and eventually involve the infratemporal fossa, inner ear, petrous apex, or middle fossa. Advanced disease is extremely difficult to successfully treat and is associated with very poor prognosis. Management of NMSC involving the temporal bone is not significantly different than the treatment of primary temporal bone malignancy. The most appropriate initial treatment is surgical resection. The type of temporal bone resection is entirely dependent on the medial extent of tumor. Lesions confined to the bony external auditory canal are best managed with lateral temporal bone resection, which consists of removal of the entire bony and cartilaginous external auditory canal, tympanic membrane, malleus, and incus. Cancers that extend to the middle ear cleft require subtotal temporal bone resection, which includes resection of the inner ear; finally, those that invade the inner ear or petrous apex require total temporal bone resection. Such extensive tumors are associated with very poor local control rates and survival.

In a large meta-analysis of temporal bone cancer, Prasad and Janecka confirmed that tumors of the lateral canal were most appropriately managed by some form of lateral temporal bone resection (80). The analysis also questioned the aggressive surgical management of disease extending deeply into the inner ear or to the petrous apex (80). More recent experience with cutaneous malignancy involving the temporal bone has validated an aggressive approach with complete surgical resection and postoperative adjuvant radiotherapy producing overall survival rates ranging between 63% and 77% (81,82). Tumors with extensive perineural involvement, positive resection margins, extension to the inner ear or petrous apex, or invasion into the middle or infratemporal fossa do not fare so well.

Midface. Tumors of the central third of the face have the potential to spread insidiously along the embryonal fusion planes of the maxilla and premaxilla (83). These periosteal planes allow cancers of the columella, nasal tip, and nasal vestibule to spread and involve the floor of the nose, septum, and lateral nasal walls ultimately leading to paranasal sinus and anterior skull base invasion. Such aggressive disease often requires radical surgical resection including subtotal or total rhinectomy. In order to prevent the development of such advanced disease, NMSC of the central third of the face require curative initial treatment.

As previously mentioned, the majority of such cancers are most appropriately managed with Mohs surgery. The success of Mohs surgery, however, is often hampered by bone or cartilage invasion. Such tumors are most appropriately dealt with by conventional surgical excision; however, an alternate approach combines Mohs with conventional surgery. Soft tissue margins may be cleared by the Mohs surgeon and, following discussion with the head and neck surgeon, the remainder of the cancer can be resected using intraoperative frozen sections to guide the excision. Tumors that involve the second division of the trigeminal nerve require special attention as they may spread to the pterygomaxillary space, orbital apex, and cavernous sinus. The majority of such tumors require postoperative radiation therapy. Primary radiation should be reserved for poor surgical candidates and unresectable disease.

The psychosocial impact of rhinectomy should not be underestimated. Fortunately, prosthetic rehabilitation, reconstructive surgery, or a combination of the two offers these patients excellent cosmetic and functional restorations. Despite the success of reconstructive surgery, the temptation to perform immediate or early nasal or maxillary reconstruction in high-risk cancers should be avoided. Recurrence rates for such cancers are quite high with five-year disease free survival for advanced disease approaching 30% (84). Early reconstruction may delay the discovery of recurrent disease. Furthermore, recurrence deep to a soft tissue or composite flap means sacrifice of the patient's best reconstructive option. Currently, delayed reconstruction is recommended for patients with aggressive tumor histology, extensive perineural spread, significant bone invasion, or questionable margins, or those for whom postoperative radiation is indicated. Given that the majority of recurrences develop within 18 to 24 months, it is advised to wait at least a year before reconstruction. Many patients interested in surgical reconstruction may be prosthetically rehabilitated during this time. In fact, prosthetic restoration may be preferable in these high-risk patients as it allows easy visualization of the resection margins and permits early diagnosis of recurrence. Resections involving large or complex segments of the midface may require immediate reconstruction despite the risk of buried recurrence. These patients should have a baseline CT and MRI performed at the completion of therapy and be followed with serial imaging.

Perineural spread. Perineural spread is a very significant issue in the evaluation and treatment of NMSC of the head and neck. High-risk cancers of the face are in particularly close proximity to the relatively superficial branches of the facial and trigeminal nerves. Fortunately, perineural spread is associated with fewer than 5% of all BCC and cSCC (85,86). It is most frequently seen in the setting of recurrent tumors and more commonly associated with cSCC and morpheaform BCC. Not only does perineural spread increase the risk of local recurrence and regional metastases, it has a significant negative impact on prognosis.

Early diagnosis of perineural spread demands a heightened index of suspicion and careful evaluation of the patient and often patients will initially complain of formication. This may progress to paraesthesia or dysaesthesia. Unfortunately, once patients develop pain, numbness, or motor deficits extensive perineural involvement is likely. Only 30–40% of patients with histologic evidence of perineural spread will have documented preoperative signs or symptoms (87). The facial nerve and second division of the trigeminal nerve are most frequently involved. Careful history taking with particular attention paid to the progression of neuropathic symptoms often suggests the tumor's path of spread and helps with evaluation of preoperative imaging. Unfortunately, perineural spread may be quite insidious and present years after treatment of the primary tumor. It is essential to monitor patients carefully following treatment of high-risk lesions and evaluate new signs and symptoms appropriately.

CT and MRI complement each other and are used to evaluate patients with locally advanced skin cancers. However, with regards to perineural spread, MRI is the gold standard due to its unsurpassed soft tissue resolution and multiplanar capabilities. CT may demonstrate foraminal widening and helps assess for regional node metastases but will not detect early perineural spread (Fig. 25.5A). MRI findings suggestive of perineural spread include thickening or enlargement of nerve, obliteration of normal fat planes surrounding a nerve, and asymmetrical nerve enhancement (Figs. 25.5B, 25.5C, and 25.5D). Although centripetal spread toward the skull base and central nervous system is clinically most important, distal spread may also occur and should be considered in every case. Skip metastases along the nerve are also possible and may be difficult to detect and treat.

The extent of perineural spread, and whether it is incidental or not, is a very important prognostic factor. In a series of cSCC treated with Mohs excision, the incidental finding of perineural spread along small peripheral unnamed nerve branches did not negatively impact survival (88). Five-year overall survival was 89% and none of the patients received postoperative radiation therapy (88). In another series, projected 10-year survival rates for patients with invasion of named nerves or positive perineural margins was 62% compared to 93% when perineural margins were negative and the nerves involved were unnamed and incidentally found (89). Galloway et al. correlated pre-treatment radiographic findings to outcome in 45 patients with clinically evident perineural spread from head and neck NMSC. Ten patients had no radiographic evidence of perineural spread, 14 patients had minimal or moderate peripheral disease, and 21 patients had either central or macroscopic disease. Minimal to moderate disease was defined as abnormal enhancement of nerve without enlargement, or enlargement of peripheral nerve up to two or three times normal size. Macroscopic disease implied an increase in size greater than three times normal. Five-year local control in the imaging negative group was 76%, compared to 57% and 25% in the minimal to moderate peripheral involvement and macroscopic or central involvement groups, respectively. Similarly, overall five-year survival was 90%, 50%, and 58% in the three respective cohorts (90).

Current evidence suggests that significant perineural spread is best managed with an aggressive multidisciplinary approach. Complete surgical resection, if possible, followed by adjuvant radiation therapy is the treatment of choice. Alternatively, primary radiation should be offered to unresectable patients. This must include treatment of regional lymphatics because up to 16% of patients will have clinically evident metastases or will harbor occult disease (85,87–90). There is no evidence to support the addition of concurrent chemotherapy at this time. Unfortunately, resecting extensive perineural disease often requires radical surgery that may include orbital exenteration, maxillectomy, or skull base surgery. Perineural spread is often significantly more extensive than preoperative imaging suggests. The decision to operate and the choice of surgical approach must take this into account. Disease at the skull base often extends intracranially to involve the Gasserian ganglion or cavernous sinus. This frequently results in incomplete

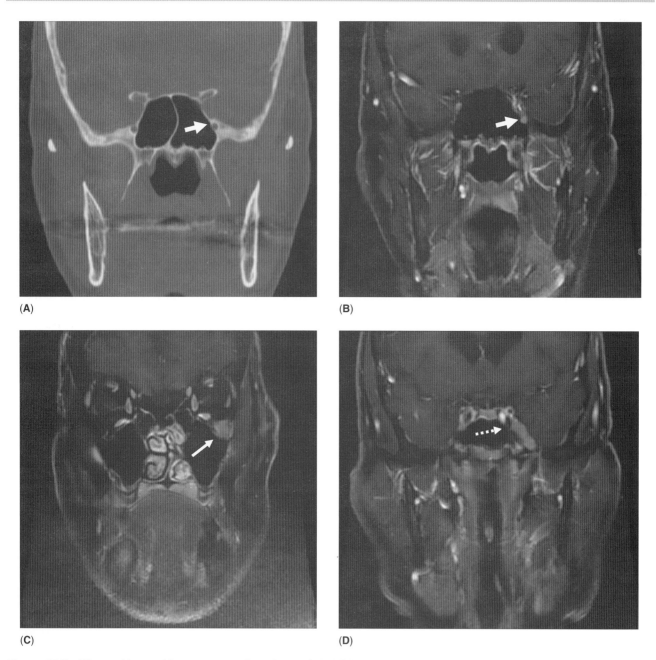

(A)

(B)

(C)

(D)

Figure 25.5   72 year old man with a squamous cell carcinoma of the left lower eyelid with perineural spread. Note the normal appearance of foramen rotundum on CT (arrow in **A**) despite the obvious perineural invasion seen on MRI (arrow in **B**). Note the expansion of the infraorbital nerve (arrow in **C**), and perineural extension via V2 through the pterygopalatine space to the cavernous sinus (arrow in **D**).

resection and positive perineural margins. The benefit of such aggressive surgery in the setting of extensive peripheral perineural disease is questionable and should only be considered for patients capable of receiving adjuvant radiation. Surgery is not indicated when there is preoperative evidence of cavernous sinus invasion.

The skull base. Skull base involvement by NMSC is typically a late phenomenon and seen in the setting of recurrent cancers that have been incompletely treated.

It represents a tremendous therapeutic challenge because most patients have had prior aggressive therapy including surgery and, frequently, radiation. The ability to provide meaningful intervention depends on the extent and location of disease, the comorbidities of the patient, and the ability to offer multimodality treatment. Skull base involvement may result from direct spread, perineural spread, or perivascular spread. Frequently, all three are present. The cause of skull base invasion is a very important consideration and impacts decision making significantly. Tumors that result in radiographically evident perineural disease typically extend well beyond the limits suggested by MRI. Once intracranial, they often involve the Gasserian ganglion or cavernous sinus and complete resection is usually impossible.

Skull base resection for NMSC of the head and neck is a formidable undertaking and requires a multidisciplinary team including head and neck oncology, microvascular reconstructive surgery, neurosurgery, radiation oncology, medical oncology, and skilled support staff. These procedures are associated with high perioperative morbidity rates and significant mortality. Resection is frequently associated with extensive disfigurement and functional insult. Once thought of as inappropriate, skull base resection for selected NMSC has gained acceptance facilitated by the advent of microsurgery.

The results of craniofacial resection for NMSC were assessed by Backous et al. in an effort to identify prognostic factors and determine long-term survival (91). A cohort consisting of 20 cSCC and 15 BCC cases was retrospectively reviewed. All living patients were followed for 10 years. Twenty-one patients underwent craniofacial resection alone and an additional 28.6% received adjuvant postoperative radiotherapy. There were two perioperative deaths and 37.1% of patients suffered early surgical complications. The overall disease specific survival rate was 20%. Two- and five-year survival was significantly better with BCC (92% and 76%) compared to SCC (54% and 24%). There were no long-term survivors of SCC with intracranial disease. Regardless of histology, intracranial extension, perineural spread, and prior radiotherapy significantly decreased five-year survival. It was concluded that craniofacial resection was warranted in highly select patients whose disease was deemed resectable (91).

In 2007 the International Skull Base Society spearheaded a multinational collaborative study to further assess the results of craniofacial resection for NMSC of the head and neck (92). The study group consisted of 17 institutions, all of which are considered centers of excellence in skull base surgery. This retrospective study assessed craniofacial resection in 106 patients with BCC and 14 with cSCC. The perioperative complication and mortality rates were 35% and 4%, respectively. Five-year disease specific survival was 75%. This is significantly better than previously reported and likely reflects the preponderance of BCC in the study population and may also reflect the experience and skill of the treating surgeons and institutions. Complete resection to negative microscopic margins was possible in 74% of cases. When final resection margins were negative or close, five-year disease specific survival was 82% as compared to 46.1% when margins were positive. Once again, five-year disease specific survival was superior in BCC compared to cSCC (79.3% vs. 28.6%). Tumors that invaded bone or dura were associated with five-year disease specific survival rates of 69.8% and 66.5%, respectively. Regardless of histology, however, brain invasion was universally fatal. The results clearly demonstrate that appropriately selected patients benefit from such an aggressive approach.

At present, craniofacial resection for NMSC should be considered for all cancers involving bone or dura, without evidence of significant intracranial perineural spread, without brain invasion, and without involvement of vital structures including the carotid artery and optic chiasm.

Tumors that do not meet these criteria should be dealt with non-operatively. Current evidence does not support resection of the carotid artery or cavernous sinus for NMSC. In these situations palliation is best accomplished with non-operative therapy.

MANAGEMENT OF THE NECK

Regional metastasis from BCC is extremely rare but does occur, particularly from tumors displaying squamous differentiation. Although most cSCC is curable by treatment of the primary lesion alone, a minority may metastasize and ultimately result in death from disease. Since the presence of regional nodal metastasis is a key prognosticator for survival, management of the neck is crucial in the treatment paradigm of patients with high-risk cSCC (10,13,16, 20,71). Metastases to the parotid and neck lymphatics occurs in up to 5% of patients, with certain clinicopathological factors known to increase the risk of regional metastases, namely tumor diameter >2 cm, invasion depth >4 mm, poorly differentiated tumors, recurrent tumors, immunosuppression, and site (ear, lip, scar, and non–sun-exposed skin) (12).

Sentinel Lymph Node Biopsy

Sentinel lymph node biopsy (SLNB) involves a limited dissection of first echelon node(s), or sentinel node(s), to which a particular tumor site drains. The sentinel nodes are mapped and located preoperatively utilizing lymphoscintigraphy, identified intraoperatively, surgically excised, and examined histologically. The potential advantage of SLNB is that it may provide an accurate method of predicting the metastatic disease status of the neck thereby eliminating the requirement and potential morbidity related to elective neck dissection (END). Nevertheless, its value in improving survival outcomes is currently unproven. Enthusiasm for this technique in melanoma, which has a higher metastatic rate to regional nodes (15% to 20%), is considerably greater than in cSCC, which has a lower metastatic rate (5%). Nevertheless, there may be a role in patients with high-risk cSCC. Studies reporting the value of SLNB in cSCC, however, lack control groups and comprise fewer than 40 patients with adequate follow-up data (93). Therefore, at present, use of SLNB in cSCC remains investigational, and the question of whether early detection of subclinical nodal metastasis with SLNB results in prolonged disease-free or overall survival remains unanswered.

Treatment of the Parotid Gland

Since patients with metastatic cutaneous SCC involving the parotid have a relatively high incidence of clinical (26%) as well as occult (35%) neck disease, neck dissection should be performed in conjunction with parotid surgery (Figs. 25.6 and 25.7). Several studies have demonstrated more favorable outcomes following parotidectomy, neck dissection, and adjuvant irradiation in this disease (36,94). Parotidectomy with facial nerve sacrifice confers no locoregional control advantage compared to facial-nerve-sparing parotidectomy followed by adjuvant irradiation (36).

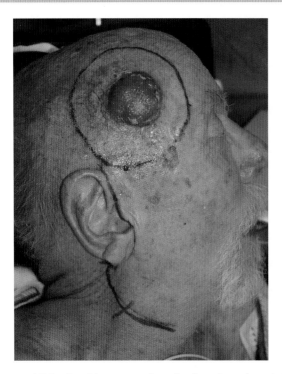

Figure 25.6 Parotidectomy and neck dissection planned for cutaneous squamous cell carcinoma of the parietal scalp.

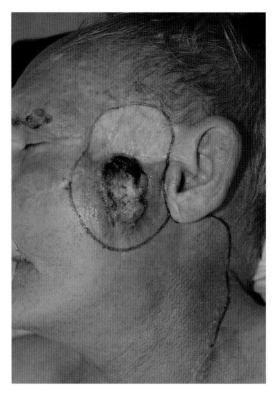

Figure 25.7 Parotidectomy and neck dissection planned for cutaneous squamous cell carcinoma of the pre-auricular skin.

Elective Neck Treatment

The value of elective neck dissection (END) of regional nodal lymphatics in patients with high-risk cSCC without nodal disease (N0) is controversial. Proponents of END argue that since the location of regional metastasis from head and neck cSCC is generally predictable, END serves as a diagnostic staging procedure allowing the microscopic detection of occult metastases (95). Accordingly, END provides valuable information that guides prognosis and the need for adjuvant regional treatment. Theoretically, END in patients with occult disease may have a therapeutic role improving survival by eliminating progression of occult disease to clinically apparent nodal disease and reducing the rate of distant metastases. Any potential survival advantage of END, however, has not been adequately investigated and this lack of evidence is the crux of the current controversy concerning the use of END in cSCC. Although elective irradiation is an option there is no high level evidence supporting this practice.

The importance of treating the neck in patients with parotid metastases is well-documented (96). Recent evidence suggests that neck level II is at greatest metastatic risk in the presence of parotid metastases, with up to 79% of pathologically involved nodes located at this level. In addition to dissection of level II, the authors propose a paradigm for identifying other levels at risk of occult disease based on the anatomical location of the primary cutaneous lesion. The recommendation is to perform a supraomohyoid neck dissection, including the external jugular nodes, for an anterolateral primary; and in the case of a posteriorly located primary, include level V (97).

Therapeutic Neck Treatment

There are no randomized controlled studies comparing disease outcome following different combinations of treatment in the setting of clinical neck disease. Those studies that do exist contain heterogeneous groups with respect to tumor and patient characteristics. Nevertheless, emerging evidence from several recent studies advocates the use of neck dissection and adjuvant radiotherapy with more favorable locoregional relapse rates (20% to 27%) compared with surgery alone (43% to 57%) (35,71). The largest series also reports disease-specific survival advantage at five years in those patients treated with a combined modality approach (73%) compared with surgery alone (54%) (71). Although some data supports the use of selective neck dissection with adjuvant irradiation in patients with limited neck disease (98), the current recommendation is a comprehensive neck dissection (97).

REFERENCES

1. Housman TS, Feldman SR, Williford PM et al. Skin cancer is among the most costly of all cancers to treat for the Medicare population. J Am Acad Dermatol 2003; 48: 425–9.
2. Glass AG, Hoover RN. The emerging epidemic of melanoma and squamous cell skin cancer. JAMA 1989; 262: 2097–100.

3. Ridky TW. Nonmelanoma skin cancer. J Am Acad Dermatol 2007; 57: 484–501.

4. Diepgen TL, Mahler V. The epidemiology of skin cancer. Br J Dermatol 2002; 146(Suppl 61): 1–6.

5. Shumrick KA, Coldiron B. Genetic syndromes associated with skin cancer. Otolaryngol Clin North Am 1993; 26: 117–37.

6. Ehrig T, Cockerell C, Piacquadio D et al. Actinic keratoses and the incidence of occult squamous cell carcinoma: a clinical-histopathologic correlation. Dermatol Surg 2006; 32: 1261–5.

7. Mencia-Gutierrez E, Gutierrez-Diaz E, Redondo-Marcos I et al. Cutaneous horns of the eyelid: a clinicopathological study of 48 cases. J Cutan Pathol 2004; 31: 539–43.

8. Berg D, Otley CC. Skin cancer in organ transplant recipients: epidemiology, pathogenesis, and management. J Am Acad Dermatol 2002; 47: 1–17.

9. Bigler C, Feldman J, Hall E et al. Pigmented basal cell carcinoma in Hispanics. J Am Acad Dermatol 1996; 34: 751–2.

10. Clayman GL, Lee JJ, Holsinger FC et al. Mortality risk from squamous cell skin cancer. J Clin Oncol 2005; 23: 759–65.

11. Nolan RC, Chan MT, Heenan PJ. A clinicopathologic review of lethal nonmelanoma skin cancers in Western Australia. J Am Acad Dermatol 2005; 52: 101–8.

12. Rowe DE, Carroll RJ, Day CL Jr. Prognostic factors for local recurrence, metastasis, and survival rates in squamous cell carcinoma of the skin, ear, and lip. Implications for treatment modality selection. J Am Acad Dermatol 1992; 26: 976–90.

13. Epstein E, Epstein NN, Bragg K et al. Metastases from squamous cell carcinomas of the skin. Arch Dermatol 1968; 97: 245–51.

14. Jol JA, van Velthuysen ML, Hilgers FJ et al. Treatment results of regional metastasis from cutaneous head and neck squamous cell carcinoma. Eur J Surg Oncol 2003; 29: 81–6.

15. Moller R, Reymann F, Hou-Jensen K. Metastases in dermatological patients with squamous cell carcinoma. Arch Dermatol 1979; 115: 703–5.

16. Tavin E, Persky M. Metastatic cutaneous squamous cell carcinoma of the head and neck region. Laryngoscope 1996; 106: 156–8.

17. Czarnecki D, Staples M, Mar A et al. Metastases from squamous cell carcinoma of the skin in southern Australia. Dermatology 1994; 189: 52–4.

18. Breuninger H, Schaumburg-Lever G, Holzschuh J et al. Desmoplastic squamous cell carcinoma of skin and vermilion surface: a highly malignant subtype of skin cancer. Cancer 1997; 79: 915–19.

19. Cherpelis BS, Marcusen C, Lang PG. Prognostic factors for metastasis in squamous cell carcinoma of the skin. Dermatol Surg 2002; 28: 268–73.

20. Kraus DH, Carew JF, Harrison LB. Regional lymph node metastasis from cutaneous squamous cell carcinoma. Arch Otolaryngol Head Neck Surg 1998; 124: 582–7.

21. Rodolico V, Barresi E, Di Lorenzo R et al. Lymph node metastasis in lower lip squamous cell carcinoma in relation to tumour size, histologic variables and p27Kip1 protein expression. Oral Oncol 2004; 40: 92–8.

22. Breuninger H, Black B, Rassner G. Microstaging of squamous cell carcinomas. Am J Clin Pathol 1990; 94: 624–7.

23. Petter G, Haustein UF. Histologic subtyping and malignancy assessment of cutaneous squamous cell carcinoma. Dermatol Surg 2000; 26: 521–30.

24. Moore BA, Weber RS, Prieto V et al. Lymph node metastases from cutaneous squamous cell carcinoma of the head and neck. Laryngoscope 2005; 115: 1561–7.

25. Veness MJ, Palme CE, Morgan GJ. High-risk cutaneous squamous cell carcinoma of the head and neck: results from 266 treated patients with metastatic lymph node disease. Cancer 2006; 106: 2389–96.

26. Veness MJ, Porceddu S, Palme CE et al. Cutaneous head and neck squamous cell carcinoma metastatic to parotid and cervical lymph nodes. Head Neck 2007; 29: 621–31.

27. Lai SY, Weinstein GS, Chalian AA et al. Parotidectomy in the treatment of aggressive cutaneous malignancies. Arch Otolaryngol Head Neck Surg 2002; 128: 521–6.

28. Frierson HF Jr, Cooper PH. Prognostic factors in squamous cell carcinoma of the lower lip. Hum Pathol 1986; 17: 346–54.

29. O'Brien CJ. The parotid gland as a metastatic basin for cutaneous cancer. Arch Otolaryngol Head Neck Surg 2005; 131: 551–5.

30. Goepfert H, Dichtel WJ, Medina JE et al. Perineural invasion in squamous cell skin carcinoma of the head and neck. Am J Surg 1984; 148: 542–7.

31. Mehrany K, Byrd DR, Roenigk RK et al. Lymphocytic infiltrates and subclinical epithelial tumor extension in patients with chronic leukemia and solid-organ transplantation. Dermatol Surg 2003; 29: 129–34.

32. Sheil AG, Disney AP, Mathew TH et al. De novo malignancy emerges as a major cause of morbidity and late failure in renal transplantation. Transplant Proc 1993; 25: 1383–4.

33. Martinez JC, Otley CC, Stasko T et al. Defining the clinical course of metastatic skin cancer in organ transplant recipients: a multicenter collaborative study. Arch Dermatol 2003; 139: 301–6.

34. AJCC. The AJCC cancer staging manual, 6th edn. 2002. New York: Springer. Ref Type: Pamphlet.

35. Audet N, Palme CE, Gullane PJ et al. Cutaneous metastatic squamous cell carcinoma to the parotid gland: analysis and outcome. Head Neck 2004; 26: 727–32.

36. O'Brien CJ, McNeil EB, McMahon JD et al. Significance of clinical stage, extent of surgery, and pathologic findings in metastatic cutaneous squamous carcinoma of the parotid gland. Head Neck 2002; 24: 417–22.

37. Miller DL, Weinstock MA. Nonmelanoma skin cancer in the United States: incidence. J Am Acad Dermatol 1994; 30: 774–8.

38. Kaldor J, Shugg D, Young B et al. Non-melanoma skin cancer: ten years of cancer-registry-based surveillance. Int J Cancer 1993; 53: 886–91.

39. Lai SY, Weber RS. High-risk non-melanoma skin cancer of the head and neck. Curr Oncol Rep 2005; 7: 154–8.

40. Kuflik EG. Cryosurgery for skin cancer: 30-year experience and cure rates. Dermatol Surg 2004; 30: 297–300.

41. Graham GF, Clark LC. Statistical analysis in cryosurgery of skin cancer. Clin Dermatol 1990; 8: 101–7.

42. Kuflik EG. Cryosurgery for cutaneous malignancy. An update. Dermatol Surg 1997; 23: 1081–7.

43. Miller SJ. The National Comprehensive Cancer Network (NCCN) guidelines of care for nonmelanoma skin cancers. Dermatol Surg 2000; 26: 289–92.

44. Neville JA, Welch E, Leffell DJ. Management of nonmelanoma skin cancer in 2007. Nat Clin Pract Oncol 2007; 4: 462–9.

45. Kopf AW, Bart RS, Schrager D et al. Curettage-electrodesiccation treatment of basal cell carcinomas. Arch Dermatol 1977; 113: 439–43.

46. Sheridan AT, Dawber RP. Curettage, electrosurgery and skin cancer. Australas J Dermatol 2000; 41: 19–30.

47. Rowe DE, Carroll RJ, Day CL Jr. Long-term recurrence rates in previously untreated (primary) basal cell carcinoma: implications for patient follow-up. J Dermatol Surg Oncol 1989; 15: 315–28.

48. Iyer S, Friedli A, Bowes L et al. Full face laser resurfacing: therapy and prophylaxis for actinic keratoses and non-melanoma skin cancer. Lasers Surg Med 2004; 34: 114–19.

49. Rhodes LE, de Rie M, Enstrom Y et al. Photodynamic therapy using topical methyl aminolevulinate vs surgery for nodular basal cell carcinoma: results of a multicenter randomized prospective trial. Arch Dermatol 2004; 140: 17–23.

50. Salim A, Leman JA, McColl JH et al. Randomized comparison of photodynamic therapy with topical 5-fluorouracil in Bowen's disease. Br J Dermatol 2003; 148: 539–43.

51. Fien SM, Oseroff AR. Photodynamic therapy for non-melanoma skin cancer. J Natl Compr Canc Netw 2007; 5: 531–40.

52. Marmur ES, Schmults CD, Goldberg DJ. A review of laser and photodynamic therapy for the treatment of nonmela-noma skin cancer. Dermatol Surg 2004; 30: 264–71.

53. Braathen LR, Szeimies RM, Basset-Seguin N et al. Guidelines on the use of photodynamic therapy for nonmelanoma skin cancer: an international consensus. International Society for Photodynamic Therapy in Dermatology, 2005. J Am Acad Dermatol 2007; 56: 125–43.

54. Gross K, Kircik L, Kricorian G. 5% 5-Fluorouracil cream for the treatment of small superficial Basal cell carcinoma: efficacy, tolerability, cosmetic outcome, and patient satisfaction. Dermatol Surg 2007; 33: 433–9.

55. Cox NH, Eedy DJ, Morton CA. Guidelines for management of Bowen's disease. British Association of Dermatologists. Br J Dermatol 1999; 141: 633–41.

56. Miller BH, Shavin JS, Cognetta A et al. Nonsurgical treatment of basal cell carcinomas with intralesional 5-fluorouracil/epi-nephrine injectable gel. J Am Acad Dermatol 1997; 36: 72–7.

57. Buechner SA, Wernli M, Harr T et al. Regression of basal cell carcinoma by intralesional interferon-alpha treatment is mediated by CD95 (Apo-1/Fas)-CD95 ligand-induced suicide. J Clin Invest 1997; 100: 2691–6.

58. Acarturk TO, Edington H. Nonmelanoma skin cancer. Clin Plast Surg 2005; 32: 237–48.

59. Bostanci S, Kocyigit P, Alp A et al. Treatment of basal cell carcinoma located in the head and neck region with intrale-sional interferon alpha-2a: evaluation of long-term follow-up results. Clin Drug Investig 2005; 25: 661–7.

60. Tucker SB, Polasek JW, Perri AJ et al. Long-term follow-up of basal cell carcinomas treated with perilesional inter-feron alfa 2b as monotherapy. J Am Acad Dermatol 2006; 54: 1033–8.

61. Tillman DK Jr, Carroll MT. Topical imiquimod therapy for basal and squamous cell carcinomas: a clinical experience. Cutis 2007; 79: 241–8.

62. Geisse J, Caro I, Lindholm J, Golitz L, Stampone P, Owens M. Imiquimod 5% cream for the treatment of superficial basal cell carcinoma: results from two phase III, randomized, vehicle-controlled studies. J Am Acad Dermatol 2004; 50: 722–33.

63. Huber A, Huber JD, Skinner RB Jr et al. Topical imiquimod treatment for nodular basal cell carcinomas: an open-label series. Dermatol Surg 2004; 30: 429–30.

64. Tyring S, Conant M, Marini M et al. Imiquimod; an international update on therapeutic uses in dermatology. Int J Dermatol 2002; 41: 810–16.

65. Ulrich C, Bichel J, Euvrard S et al. Topical immunomodula-tion under systemic immunosuppression: results of a multi-centre, randomized, placebo-controlled safety and efficacy study of imiquimod 5% cream for the treatment of actinic keratoses in kidney, heart, and liver transplant patients. Br J Dermatol 2007; 157(Suppl 2): 25–31.

66. Silverman MK, Kopf AW, Gladstein AH et al. Recurrence rates of treated basal cell carcinomas. Part 4: X-ray therapy. J Dermatol Surg Oncol 1992; 18: 549–54.

67. Voss N, Kim-Sing C. Radiotherapy in the treatment of dermatologic malignancies. Dermatol Clin 1998; 16: 313–20.

68. Zagrodnik B, Kempf W, Seifert B et al. Superficial radio-therapy for patients with basal cell carcinoma: recurrence rates, histologic subtypes, and expression of p53 and Bcl-2. Cancer 2003; 98: 2708–14.

69. Al Othman MO, Mendenhall WM, Amdur RJ. Radiotherapy alone for clinical T4 skin carcinoma of the head and neck with surgery reserved for salvage. Am J Otolaryngol 2001; 22: 387–90.

70. Veness MJ, Palme CE, Smith M et al. Cutaneous head and neck squamous cell carcinoma metastatic to cervical lymph nodes (nonparotid): a better outcome with surgery and adju-vant radiotherapy. Laryngoscope 2003; 113: 1827–33.

71. Veness MJ, Morgan GJ, Palme CE et al. Surgery and adjuvant radiotherapy in patients with cutaneous head and neck squamous cell carcinoma metastatic to lymph nodes: combined treatment should be considered best practice. Laryngoscope 2005; 115: 870–5.

72. Chan S, Dhadda AS, Swindell R. Single fraction radiotherapy for small superficial carcinoma of the skin. Clin Oncol (R Coll Radiol) 2007; 19: 256–9.

73. Rowe DE, Carroll RJ, Day CL Jr. Mohs surgery is the treatment of choice for recurrent (previously treated) basal cell carcinoma. J Dermatol Surg Oncol 1989; 15: 424–31.

74. Bialy TL, Whalen J, Veledar E et al. Mohs micrographic surgery vs traditional surgical excision: a cost comparison analysis. Arch Dermatol 2004; 140: 736–42.

75. Wolf DJ, Zitelli JA. Surgical margins for basal cell carcinoma. Arch Dermatol 1987; 123: 340–4.

76. Brodland DG, Zitelli JA. Surgical margins for excision of primary cutaneous squamous cell carcinoma. J Am Acad Dermatol 1992; 27: 241–8.

77. Smeets NW, Krekels GA, Ostertag JU et al. Surgical excision vs Mohs' micrographic surgery for basal-cell carcinoma of the face: randomised controlled trial. Lancet 2004; 364: 1766–72.

78. Nemet AY, Deckel Y, Martin PA et al. Management of peri-ocular basal and squamous cell carcinoma: a series of 485 cases. Am J Ophthalmol 2006; 142: 293–7.

79. Griffiths RW. Audit of histologically incompletely excised basal cell carcinomas: recommendations for management by re-excision. Br J Plast Surg 1999; 52: 24–8.

80. Prasad S, Janecka IP. Efficacy of surgical treatments for squamous cell carcinoma of the temporal bone: a literature review. Otolaryngol Head Neck Surg 1994; 110: 270–80.

81. Moore MG, Deschler DG, McKenna MJ et al. Management outcomes following lateral temporal bone resection for ear and temporal bone malignancies. Otolaryngol Head Neck Surg 2007; 137: 893–8.

82. Pfreundner L, Schwager K, Willner J et al. Carcinoma of the external auditory canal and middle ear. Int J Radiat Oncol Biol Phys 1999; 44: 777–88.

83. Panje WR, Bumsted RM, Ceilley RI. Secondary intention healing as an adjunct to the reconstruction of mid-facial defects. Laryngoscope 1980; 90: 1148–54.

84. Ampil FL, Nathan CO, Lian TF et al. Salvage treatment of recurrent skin cancer of the midface. Am J Clin Oncol 2002; 25: 580–2.

85. Ballantyne AJ, McCarten AB, Ibanez ML. The extension of cancer of the head and neck through peripheral nerves. Am J Surg 1963; 106: 651–67.

86. Cottel WI. Perineural invasion by squamous-cell carcinoma. J Dermatol Surg Oncol 1982; 8: 589–600.

87. McCord MW, Mendenhall WM, Parsons JT et al. Skin cancer of the head and neck with clinical perineural invasion. Int J Radiat Oncol Biol Phys 2000; 47: 89–93.

88. Lawrence N, Cottel WI. Squamous cell carcinoma of skin with perineural invasion. J Am Acad Dermatol 1994; 31: 30–3.

89. McCord MW, Mendenhall WM, Parsons JT et al. Skin cancer of the head and neck with incidental microscopic perineural invasion. Int J Radiat Oncol Biol Phys 1999; 43: 591–5.

90. Galloway TJ, Morris CG, Mancuso AA et al. Impact of radio-graphic findings on prognosis for skin carcinoma with clini-cal perineural invasion. Cancer 2005; 103: 1254–7.

91. Backous DD, DeMonte F, El Naggar A et al. Craniofacial resection for nonmelanoma skin cancer of the head and neck. Laryngoscope 2005; 115: 931–7.

92. Maghami EG, Talbot SG, Patel SG et al. Craniofacial surgery for nonmelanoma skin malignancy: report of an international collaborative study. Head Neck 2007; 29: 1136–43.

93. Ross AS, Schmults CD. Sentinel lymph node biopsy in cutaneous squamous cell carcinoma: a systematic review of the English literature. Dermatol Surg 2006; 32: 1309–21.

94. Bron LP, Traynor SJ, McNeil EB et al. Primary and metastatic cancer of the parotid: comparison of clinical behavior in 232 cases. Laryngoscope 2003; 113: 1070–5.

95. Martinez JC, Cook JL. High-risk cutaneous squamous cell carcinoma without palpable lymphadenopathy: is there a therapeutic role for elective neck dissection? Dermatol Surg 2007; 33: 410–20.

96. O'Brien CJ, McNeil EB, McMahon JD et al. Incidence of cervical node involvement in metastatic cutaneous malignancy involving the parotid gland. Head Neck 2001; 23: 744–8.

97. Vauterin TJ, Veness MJ, Morgan GJ et al. Patterns of lymph node spread of cutaneous squamous cell carcinoma of the head and neck. Head Neck 2006; 28: 785–91.

98. Gooris PJ, Vermey A, de Visscher JG et al. Supraomohyoid neck dissection in the management of cervical lymph node metastases of squamous cell carcinoma of the lower lip. Head Neck 2002; 24: 678–83.

26

Cutaneous Melanoma of the Head and Neck

Kerwin Shannon and Christopher J O'Brien

EPIDEMIOLOGY

In countries with substantially Caucasian populations, the incidence of cutaneous melanoma has risen sharply over recent decades (1–5), with the greatest increases seen in elderly men (2). Epidemiological investigations suggest that increasing melanoma rates are real and due primarily to increased exposure to ultraviolet radiation, rather than a consequence of more complete reporting. Mortality trends in white populations have also been increasing but less steeply than incidence rates (1). An improvement in overall survival has been observed, however (6), attributed to earlier detection (7).

Approximately 10–20% of cutaneous malignant melanomas arise on the skin of the head and neck (4,8). In a series of 998 patients with cutaneous melanoma of the head and neck treated at the Sydney Melanoma Unit (SMU), the male to female ratio was 3:2 and the age incidence fairly evenly distributed through the adult decades (9). Melanoma rarely occurs during childhood and adolescence. Table 26.1 shows the distribution of head and neck cutaneous melanoma by subsite. The most common individual primary site, at the SMU is the face. Other researchers have also found a similar preponderance of facial melanoma on subsite analysis (9–11).

ETIOLOGY AND RISK FACTORS

Melanoma is predominantly a disease of people whose origins are European (12) and the major cause of melanoma is sun exposure (13,14). The incidence of melanoma is highest in the white population of Australia and even within this population the incidence of melanoma increases with proximity to the equator (15). Interestingly, indoor workers are more frequently affected than outdoor workers, as are people of higher socioeconomic status (16). This is not consistent with a simple dose-response relationship between sun exposure and melanoma. Instead, intermittent intense exposure on a recreational basis is associated with the development of melanoma (17–19). Overall, the greatest risk appears to be associated with sunburn in childhood or adolescence (17). Clearly, eliminating excessive exposure to sunlight is important and current guidelines on melanoma prevention advise sunscreen use to supplement physical protection (20). Whether or not the use of even broad spectrum sunscreens reduces the risk of melanoma is unclear, but some concerns that sunscreen use may actually increase melanoma risk have proved unfounded (21).

The presence of large numbers of pigmented nevi is also known to be a risk factor for the development of melanoma. In a survey of over 4500 melanoma patients, 81% reported a change in the appearance of a pre-existing mole as the initial manifestation (22). Furthermore, numbers of both common and atypical nevi have been found to correlate with individual melanoma risk (23). Large congenital nevi, in particular those greater than 19 cm in diameter, are also predisposed to malignant change and transition to melanoma (24). The presence of atypical or dysplastic nevi is associated with increased risk of melanoma. These may be familial and individuals with multiple atypical nevi, also called dysplastic nevus syndrome, should be closely monitored (25). Individual atypical nevi, however, should not be regarded as being high-risk precursors since the likelihood of transformation for any given lesion is low (25).

A family history of melanoma is a significant risk factor, increasing an individual's risk at least threefold, and by 35 to 70 times if there are three or more affected first-degree relatives (26,27). Only occasionally, however, is the disease due to an identifiable, inheritable genetic mutation (28).

CLINICOPATHOLOGICAL FACTORS AND PROGNOSIS

Cutaneous melanoma of the head and neck may be classified into three main histological categories: nodular melanoma superficial spreading melanoma and lentigo maligna melanoma (Figs. 26.1–26.4). Nodular malignant melanoma has a predominantly vertical growth phase. Superficial spreading and lentigo maligna melanoma have a prolonged radial (or lateral) growth phase but may develop nodules over time. Lentigo maligna melanoma occurs particularly on the sun-exposed skin of elderly patients (29). The clinical utility of this classification is doubtful, however, since the histological types tend to have similar prognoses after correcting for tumor thickness (30). While the SMU series demonstrated that lentigo maligna melanoma has a significantly better prognosis when all other factors were adjusted for (9), this has not been confirmed by other research (8).

Desmoplastic melanoma and neurotropic melanoma are variant forms that comprise less than 1% of all melanoma and have a propensity to occur in the head and neck (31,32). The majority of these are not pigmented and have the appearance of a slowly enlarging, scar-like lesion. Histologically the usual appearance is one of proliferating spindle cells within a dense collagenous stroma. The neurotropic variant has a marked tendency for perineural and endoneural invasion (32,33).

Table 26.1 Distribution of Head and Neck Melanoma According to Subsite

Subsite	Primary melanomas (%)
Face	47
Neck	29
Scalp	15
Ear	10

Source: From Ref. 9.

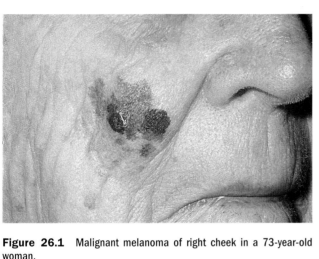

Figure 26.1 Malignant melanoma of right cheek in a 73-year-old woman.

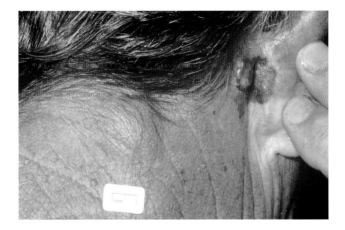

Figure 26.2 Nodular melanoma in the right postauricular area, metastatic involvement of the right occipital node.

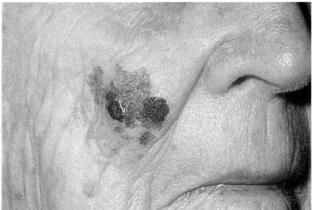

Figure 26.3 Superficial spreading melanoma of the left ear.

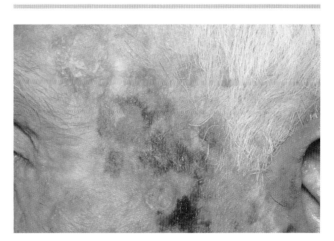

Figure 26.4 Lentigo maligna melanoma of the temple in an elderly male.

The likelihood of regional metastasis, distant metastasis, and therefore survival is influenced by a number of clinical and pathological characteristics of the primary melanoma. These are summarized in Table 26.2, where the chi-squared increment gives the relative importance of each prognostic factor, while simultaneously accounting for the contribution of the other listed factors.

Tumor Thickness and Level of Invasion

In the absence of distant and regional node metastases, tumor thickness is the most important pathological prognostic indicator in cutaneous melanoma (Table 26.2), and this applies equally in the head and neck as it does elsewhere (9–12). Breslow first identified the significance of this third tumor dimension in 1970. The upper reference

Table 26.2 Prognostic Factors in Localized (Stage i and ii)
Cutaneous Malignant Melanoma

Factor	X^2 increment
Tumor thickness	244.3
Ulceration	189.5
Age	45.6
Site	41.0
Level	32.7
Sex	15.1

Source: From Ref. 35.

Table 26.3 Tumor thickness and disease-specific survival in
998 patients with cutaneous melanoma of the head and neck

Thickness (mm)	5-year survival (%)	10-year survival(%)
<0.76	91	87
0.76–1.49	87	75
1.5–3.99	71	59
>4.0	57	48

Source: From Ref. 9.

point is the superficial aspect of the granular cell layer of
the epidermis and, in the case of ulceration, the base of
the ulcer. The lower reference point is the deepest point of
tumor invasion (34). A typically inverse relationship between
tumor thickness and survival was found in evaluating
998 patients with cutaneous melanoma of the head and
neck treated at the SMU (Table 26.3) (9). Thicker lesions
are more likely to be associated with lymph node and
distant metastases on presentation and subsequently thereafter
(34,35). Clark level of invasion has prognostic significance
only in that subset of patients with tumors less than
1mm in thickness (35).

Tumor Ulceration

Tumor ulceration has been shown to be independently associated
with a worse prognosis in a number of studies
(8–11,30). O'Brien et al. found the 10-year survival in patients
with head and neck melanoma with ulcerated lesions was
52%, compared with 72% for non-ulcerated melanomas (9).
Data compiled by the Melanoma Staging Committee of the
American Joint Committee on Cancer (AJCC) has shown the
presence of ulceration of the primary to be associated with
poorer outcome both in patients with localized disease and
in those with nodal metastases (35).

Mitotic Rate

Although not currently included in the AJCC staging system,
tumor mitotic rate has been shown to be an important
independent prognostic factor and possibly more powerful
than ulceration (36,37).

Anatomical Site

Some researchers have found that patients with scalp
melanoma have an especially poor prognosis (9,38–40). In
the SMU series, patients with scalp melanoma had a 10-year

Table 26.4 Survival According to Anatomical Subsite in 998 patients
with Cutaneous Melanoma of the Head and Neck

Site	5-year survival (%)	10-year survival (%)
Face	80	69
Scalp	59*	45*
Ear	81	61
Neck	80	72

*$P < 0.001$.
Source: From Ref. 9.

survival of 45%, significantly worse than patients with
lesions at other sites. This difference was confirmed on
multivariate analysis (Table 26.4). Fisher (8) and Andersson
et al (11), however, found no significant difference in outlook
for the head and neck subsites after adjusting for depth
and presence of ulceration.

Regional Lymph Node Involvement

Involvement of regional lymph nodes by melanoma leads
to a significant decrease in five- and 10-year survival (8,9).
This remains true even when only a small focus of tumor
is discovered in a node, and the status of sentinel nodes
has emerged as the most significant indicator of prognosis
(41). Factors most influencing outcome in patients with
nodal disease include the number of involved nodes, the
tumor burden in the nodes (macroscopic vs. microscopic)
and the presence or absence of ulceration in the primary
(35). In a series of patients treated at Duke University,
those with pathologically proven regional disease, following
elective lymph node dissection (clinically negative, pathologically
positive), had no better survival than those with
clinically apparent regional disease (clinically positive, pathologically
positive) (8). In a series of patients undergoing neck
dissection for cutaneous melanoma at the SMU, patients with
histologically positive nodes (clinically apparent or occult)
had five- and 10-year survival rates of 48% and 34%, respectively,
whereas those with histologically negative nodes had
survival rates of 75% and 67% (42). An updated series from
the same unit continues to show the worsening prognosis
as more involved nodes are found (43). A single involved
node carries a five-year survival of 50% whereas involvement
of more nodes worsens the prognosis significantly
(44), as demonstrated in Fig. 26.5.

Distant Metastases

There remains no effective treatment for distant metastatic
disease; survival in stage IV disease is measured in months
rather than years (35). No prognostic features in the AJCC
analysis separated survival by more than a few months. The
site of metastases has some influence, with metastases at
non-visceral sites (skin, subcutaneous tissues, and distant
lymph nodes) showing a better survival rate at one year
(59%) than those occurring in the viscera. Visceral sites of
metastases were most commonly lung, brain, liver, and
bone. Isolated lung metastases appeared to show improved
survival (57%) when compared to other viscera (41%) at
one year, but this difference disappeared during the second
year (35). An elevated serum lactate dehydrogenase (LDH)

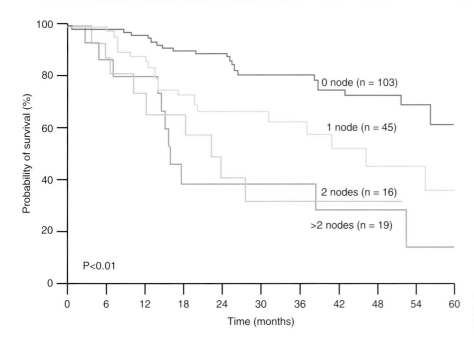

Figure 26.5 Influence of number of nodes involved with melanoma on survival. *Source:* From Ref. 77.

has been found to be a significant independent predictor of poorer survival, even after accounting for site and number of metastases (45–48).

Age

In general, younger patients who have melanoma have a better prognosis than their older counterparts (8,9,11,39,44). Advancing age also correlates with increased tumor thickness (35,44).

Gender

Virtually all studies have demonstrated a better prognosis in melanoma for women than their male counterparts (1,8,10,39). Part of the reason for better survival rates is that melanoma is more commonly observed on the extremities in women and these tumors have a better survival rate than lesions on the trunk or head and neck (44). Furthermore, in a study of cutaneous melanoma of the head and neck, women had less melanoma of the scalp than men (8).

STAGING

Staging of melanoma (Tables 26.5 and 26.6) should be according to the 2002 AJCC system (49). The "length by width" classification of the primary tumor, which correlates with prognosis in most tumor types, is replaced with thickness, which is more predictive of outcome. Clinical "T" classification is not therefore possible. Excisional biopsy and histopathological examination are necessary for proper staging.

The current staging system incorporates staging information obtained by elective lymphadenectomy and sentinel node biopsy through definitions of clinical and pathological

staging. The N classification is determined by the number of nodes involved, and whether they are micrometastases or macrometastases. Node size has not been convincingly shown to have independent prognostic value (50,51).

Satellite lesions and subcutaneous nodules within 2 cm of the primary tumor are no longer considered in the T category. Lesions around the primary, and in-transit metastases between the primary and the draining lymph nodes, are all thought to represent intra-lymphatic metastases, and have equally poor survival outcomes (50). They are classified as N2c in the absence of synchronous nodal metastases, and N3 when occurring in combination with involved nodes.

Three "M" categories are included. This is justified by the differing prognosis of patients who have skin, subcutaneous, or distant nodal involvement as the sole site of distant metastatic disease, when compared to those with lung metastases alone, or to those with other visceral metastases. This category also includes a serum marker, LDH level, found to be one of the most predictive independent markers of reduced survival regardless of the site and number of metastases (45,46,48).

Much work is ongoing to determine the prognostic significance of a number of host and tumor-related factors, most notably mitotic rate, which might be incorporated into subsequent revisions of the staging system (52). The AJCC Melanoma Committee has reconvened in preparation for a revision of the staging system due to be published in 2009.

DIAGNOSIS

Clinical Diagnosis

The aim in clinical diagnosis is to identify malignant melanoma in its earliest stage of development when it is readily curable. Generally, small malignant melanomas are

Table 26.5 Melanoma Staging

Primary Tumor (T)

TX	Primary tumor cannot be assessed (eg. Shave biopsy or regressed melanoma)
T0	No evidence of primary tumor
Tis	Melanoma *in situ*
T1	Melanoma ≤ 1.0 mm in thickness with or without ulceration
T1a	Melanoma ≤ 1.0 mm in thickness and level II or III, no ulceration
T1b	Melanoma ≤ 1.0 mm in thickness and level IV or V or with ulceration
T2	Melanoma 1.01–2.0 mm in thickness with or without ulceration
T2a	Melanoma 1.01–2.0 mm in thickness, without ulceration
T2b	Melanoma 1.01–2.0 mm in thickness, with ulceration
T3	Melanoma 2.01–4.0 mm in thickness with or without ulceration
T3a	Melanoma 2.01–4.0 mm in thickness, without ulceration
T3b	Melanoma 2.01–4.0 mm in thickness, with ulceration
T4	Melanoma > 4.0 mm in thickness with or without ulceration
T4a	Melanoma > 4.0 mm in thickness, no ulceration
T4b	Melanoma > 4.0 mm in thickness, with ulceration

Regional Lymph Nodes (N)

NX	Regional lymph nodes cannot be assessed
N0	No regional lymph nodes
N1	Metastasis in one lymph node
N1a	Clinically occult (microscopic) metastases
N1b	Clinically apparent (macroscopic) metastases
N2	Metastasis in two to three regional nodes or intra-lymphatic regional metastases *without* nodal metastases.
N2a	Clinically occult (microscopic) metastases
N2b	Clinically apparent (macroscopic) metastases
N2c	Satellite or in-transit metastasis *without* nodal metastasis
N3	Metastasis in four or more regional nodes, or matted metastatic nodes, or in-transit metastasis or satellite(s) *with* metastasis in regional node(s)

Distant Metastasis (M)

MX	Distant metastasis cannot be assessed
M0	No distant metastasis
M1	Distant metastasis
M1a	Metastasis to skin, subcutaneous tissues or distant lymph nodes
M1b	Metastasis to lung
M1c	Metastasis to all other visceral or distant metastasis at any site associated with an elevated serum lactate dehydrogenase (LDH)

Table 26.6 Clinical Stage Grouping

Stage 0	Tis	N0	M0
Stage IA	T1a	N0	M0
Stage IB	T1b	N0	M0
	T2a	N0	M0
Stage IIA	T2b	N0	M0
	T3a	N0	M0
Stage IIB	T3b	N0	M0
	T4a	N0	M0
Stage IIC	T4b	N0	M0
Stage III	Any T	N1	M0
	Any T	N2	M0
	Any T	N3	M0
Stage IV	Any T	Any N	M1

Diagnostic Biopsy

The technique of choice is a total excisional biopsy with narrow margins, incorporating subcutaneous fat. This allows assessment of the whole lesion and accurate microstaging. Following excisional biopsy, primary closure is preferable to local flaps or skin grafting. Incisional or punch biopsy should be reserved for larger lesions, or those located in a functionally and aesthetically sensitive area.

Diagnostic Work-up

Careful clinical assessment of the regional lymph nodes is essential for management planning. The parotid region nodes deserve particular attention. These nodes drain the face, anterior scalp, and ear. The occipital and postauricular nodes also require careful palpation along with the other levels of the neck. Where level IV and level V nodes are involved the axilla should also be examined (56).

Because of the low return from anatomical imaging techniques for the detection of disseminated disease in patients who have clinical stage I or II disease, extensive diagnostic testing has not been proven cost-effective (57,58). All patients should have liver function tests, including serum LDH, and a chest X-ray, but CT scanning should be reserved for symptomatic or high-risk patients. Studies have focused on positron emission tomography (PET) in the evaluation of high-risk patients (59–61). PET has greater sensitivity than whole body CT in the detection of metastatic disease, but false-positive scans do occur with PET in association with acute inflammatory processes, including that associated with surgical wound healing. Its use is not recommended in initial staging, and PET is less sensitive than sentinel node biopsy in the detection of occult nodal metastases (62–64). PET is used prior to contemplating major salvage surgery in the setting of disease recurrence where it has been shown to influence clinical management in nearly half of patients (59,65,66).

TREATMENT OF MELANOMA

The objectives of treatment for patients with melanoma include the control of local disease and prevention, where possible, of distant spread. Unfortunately, the absence of an effective means of preventing and treating distant metastases continues to limit our ability to improve outcomes in

asymmetrical, poorly circumscribed, with notched, scalloped, or jagged borders and dark pigmentation with variable shades of brown. There may also be black, blue, and pink areas. The so-called 'ABCDE' (Asymmetry, Border irregularity, Color variegation, Diameter >6 mm, and Elevation) is a useful aid in clinical diagnosis (53). Bleeding and ulceration, however, are late signs of malignancy.

Distinguishing atypical nevi from early melanoma can be difficult. The use of dermatoscopy and photographic baseline records may be useful (54,55). Only lesions that have acquired the clinical features of malignant melanoma or have changed "out of step" with other pigmented lesions are considered for removal and histological assessment.

high-risk patients. Early diagnosis and adequate primary surgery are the mainstays of therapy.

Surgery

Treatment of the Primary Melanoma

Cutaneous melanomas of all sites, including the head and neck, require surgical excision but the extent of excisional margins continues to engender debate (67,68). The current recommendations, however, are based on thickness of the primary melanoma. In general a 1 cm clearance for thin melanomas (<1 mm), 2 cm for intermediate thickness (1–4 mm) and 2–3 cm for thick melanomas (>4 mm) are adequate. The evidence for these recommendations comes from the results of several randomized trials (69–74). The World Health Organization (WHO) Melanoma Group (71) compared 1 cm versus 3 cm margins in 612 patients with primary tumors less than 2 mm in thickness. Only four patients in the entire study group developed local recurrence as the first relapse, and all four of these had received a 1 cm excision margin for tumors between 1 and 2 mm thickness. The disease-free and overall survival rates at a mean follow-up of 55 months were similar in both groups at 96%. The Intergroup Melanoma Trial (69,70) compared 2 and 4 cm margins in 486 patients with intermediate thickness melanomas (1–4 mm). The local recurrence rate was the same for both groups and there was no survival difference between the two groups.

Two further European studies compared 2 cm and 5 cm excision margins. The Swedish Melanoma Study Group examined 989 patients with melanomas 0.8 to 2.0 mm in thickness (72) and the French Group for Research on Malignant Melanoma studied 326 patients with primary tumors under 2.1 mm thick (73). Neither study demonstrated a lower recurrence rate nor a better survival for the wider margin of excision.

The British Association of Plastic Surgeons collaborative study was the first to examine the efficacy of 1 cm margins for thicker depths of melanoma. They compared 1 cm versus 3 cm margins for melanomas greater than 2 mm thickness in a study of over 900 patients. The narrower excision margin was associated with a slightly higher local and regional recurrence rate, but not with a significant difference in overall survival (74).

Surgery for melanoma of the head and neck is complicated by functional and cosmetic considerations, and evidence regarding optimal margins is even less conclusive because most of the trials excluded primaries in the head and neck. About half of all head and neck melanomas occur on the face (9). Excision of these lesions requires the preservation of appearance and function, without compromising the oncologic result. In practice, a 1 cm margin usually proves to be adequate (9). Every attempt should be made to achieve primary closure using local tissues in order to avoid skin grafts on the face or neck. If primary closure is not possible or desirable, local flaps provide the best cosmetic and functional result for facial cutaneous defects without compromising survival (75). Skin grafts are both cosmetically acceptable and effective on the scalp, though aesthetically superior rotation flaps may be possible.

Desmoplastic neurotropic melanoma may be associated with a higher rate of local recurrence than other forms of the disease. A study of 280 patients accrued over a 10-year period at the SMU (32) found that the rate of local recurrence for desmoplastic neurotropic melanoma was 20%, whereas desmoplastic melanomas that did not display neurotropism were found to have a recurrence rate of only 6.8%. Wider margins are therefore justifiable for the desmoplastic variant especially if neurotropism is present. The current treatment philosophy at the SMU is to excise with at least a 1 cm margin and then follow with radiotherapy to the area. If a named nerve is involved, the radiotherapy is extended to the skull base to encompass the nerve in question. This radiotherapy has been delivered in standard daily fractions to a total of 50 to 54 Gy, but there may be a role for intensity modulated radiotherapy (IMRT) in this setting.

Management of the N0 Neck

Prior to the advent of sentinel node biopsy in the early 1990s, this issue continued to provoke controversy. Treating clinically negative lymph nodes among patients with cutaneous melanoma was thought to be appropriate because elective lymphadenectomy had the potential to remove subclinical micrometastases from the lymphatic basin at risk, and thereby prevent spread to the rest of the body. The theoretical benefit, however, did not translate into clinical reality. Elective neck dissection can improve regional control of disease and identify patients at risk of distant failure, but unfortunately no useful adjuvant therapy exists for the high-risk group.

If a decision is made to carry out an elective lymphadenectomy, a selective neck dissection based on the site of the primary melanoma is appropriate. Melanomas of the anterior scalp and face tend to drain to the parotid gland and node levels I, II and III, while those lying on the scalp through the coronal plane and those involving the ear drain to the parotid gland and levels I–V. Melanomas arising on the posterior scalp tend to drain to levels II–V including the occipital group of nodes (76). In a series of 106 patients having elective neck dissection based on these clinically predicted lymph drainage pathways, O'Brien et al (77). described a rate of geographic miss of 3%, indicating that clinical prediction of which nodes are at risk, based on the site of the primary, can be very accurate. The incidence of pathologically positive nodes in the clinically negative neck, however, was only 8%. Overall, the benefits of elective neck dissection have not been demonstrated and furthermore, length of hospital stay, cost, and morbidity can be significant. A common complication, for example, is paresis of the marginal mandibular nerve after parotidectomy combined with neck dissection (78).

A number of studies have evaluated the efficacy of elective lymphadenectomy, but the results have almost invariably been negative (79–81). A retrospective review of 534 patients with clinical stage I melanoma of the head and neck treated at the SMU and University of Alabama did reveal a significant benefit for elective lymphadenectomy in patients with intermediate tumor thickness (78). This study, however, included patients referred from outside these two institutions, creating a bias in favor of elective lymphadenectomy. In 1991 the SMU published the largest single institution experience of head and neck melanoma, and analyzed its own patient population to evaluate the benefits of elective lymph node dissection. There were 998 patients in this series; a total of 234 patients with melanomas greater than 1.5 mm thickness received prophylactic neck dissection, consistent with the philosophy of the SMU at the time. Retrospective univariate analysis of patients treated only at the SMU indicated a small survival advantage to patients with intermediate thickness melanoma treated by elective neck dissection (9). When multivariate analysis was carried out, however, no benefit could be demonstrated for elective neck dissection.

Four prospective randomized trials have been unable to demonstrate the efficacy of elective lymphadenectomy. Veronesi et al (79). carried out a study of 267 patients with extremity melanomas. Patients were randomized to receive elective lymphadenectomy or observation only, but there were no differences found in survival between the two groups or in any subset analyzed. A similar result was obtained from a subsequent WHO trial assessing melanomas arising only on the trunk (82). The Mayo Clinic in 1986 published a prospective, randomized study of 171 patients who received immediate elective lymphadenectomy, delayed elective lymphadenectomy at three months, or underwent observation only. All patients had localized (stage I) melanoma restricted to the extremities or lateral trunk. Results indicated no improvement in disease-free survival in the elective lymphadenectomy group; however, almost two-thirds of the patients in this study had thin lesions and therefore would have been at low risk for nodal metastases (80).

Many of the methodological problems of earlier studies were taken into account in the design of the Intergroup study (81). The Intergroup Melanoma Surgical Program enrolled 740 patients with stages I and II melanoma. Patients were randomized to observation of the regional lymph node basin or elective lymphadenectomy. All patients with trunk melanomas had cutaneous lymphoscintigraphy in order to identify the lymph node basins at risk and to direct lymphadenectomy. There was no difference in overall five-year survival between the observation and elective lymphadenectomy groups (86% vs. 82%; $P = 0.25$), but a subgroup of patients 60 years of age or younger with tumors 1–2 mm in thickness and no ulceration experienced an increased survival with elective lymphadenectomy (88% vs. 81%; $P = 0.04$). More than 90% of patients with regional recurrence had clinical evidence of their relapse within five years, and distant relapses were still occurring after nine years (81). The small benefit found only on subgroup analysis in this study has failed to convince surgeons of the efficacy of elective lymphadenectomy in cutaneous melanoma. In fact, this analysis has been criticized because the subgroup that appeared to benefit from elective dissection was manufactured and was not part of the original stratification process.

The four randomized trials have been subjected to a meta-analysis that, not surprisingly, found no survival advantage for patients undergoing elective lymphadenectomy. However, because of limitations of each of the studies, the authors considered the evidence insufficient to rule out a benefit for elective node dissection and found that larger randomized trials would be required (83). Such trials are unlikely to take place because of the use of sentinel node biopsy.

Sentinel Node Biopsy

The unproven benefits of elective lymphadenectomy combined with the potential cost and morbidity of the procedure have led to the development of the technique of sentinel node biopsy. This method is based on the theory that there is a "sentinel" node, or nodes, in each lymphatic basin that will be the first node to be involved with metastatic disease (84). A sentinel node is defined as a lymph node or nodes having direct and independent drainage from the primary tumor site (85). Sentinel nodes can be identified preoperatively by lymphoscintigraphy and intraoperatively by the injection of vital dye and a hand-held gamma probe.

A combination of all three methods is used at the SMU to identify the sentinel node and has been shown to improve the accuracy of sentinel node identification (86–88). Four to six injections of technetium 99 m antimony trisulfide colloid are placed intradermally in volumes of 0.05–0.1 ml around the site of the primary melanoma. This material has a small particle size of 3–12 μm that facilitates its delivery through the lymphatic network. The study must be performed prior to wide excision of the primary since wide excision, beyond simple biopsy, is likely to alter normal lymphatic drainage. Scanning is carried out immediately and in a delayed fashion 2.5 hours later (Fig. 26.6). The sentinel node or nodes are then marked with a dermal tattoo (Fig, 26.7). The surgical procedure is performed ideally within 24 hours of lymphoscintigraphy, while there is still radioactivity in the node, to take advantage of intraoperative localization with the handheld gamma probe.

At the time of surgery, the primary site is injected (Fig. 26.8) with 0.5–1 ml of patent blue-V dye (Rhone–Poulec–Rhorer, Sydney, Australia). An incision is made over the marked node and dissection is performed in order to identify the blue-stained lymphatic that is then traced to the blue-stained sentinel node (Fig. 26.9). Exploration around this may identify other blue-stained nodes. The handheld gamma probe is used to confirm the sentinel node by its high counts (Fig. 26.10) and the subsequent presence of only background radiation once the node or nodes have been removed. The sentinel node is removed and sent for histological analysis (84,89–91).

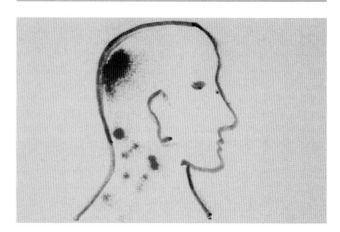

Figure 26.6 Lymphoscintigram of right posterior parietal melanoma with multiple nodes seen.

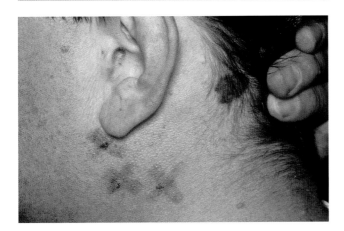

Figure 26.7 Left post-auricular melanoma with three marked sentinel nodes.

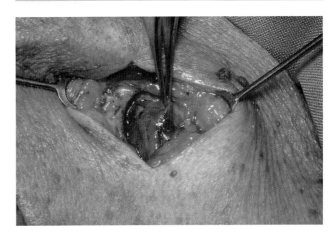

Figure 26.9 Blue-stained sentinel node, identified in the submandibular region in the patient shown in Figure 26.8.

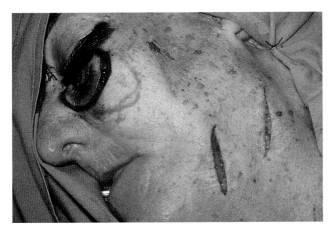

Figure 26.8 Primary infraorbital melanoma being resected following injection of blue dye. Two left neck sentinel nodes also biopsied.

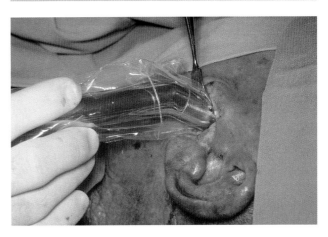

Figure 26.10 Gamma probe searching for left preauricular sentinel node.

Sentinel node biopsy in the head and neck presents special problems. It became apparent early in the experience with lymphoscintigraphy in the head and neck that there are wide variations in lymphatic drainage (92). At least one-third of primary melanomas of the head and neck will show drainage to nodal basins outside the parotid bed and neck levels usually dissected in the era of elective nodal dissections (76,93). In a study of 97 patients with head and neck melanoma, sentinel nodes were identified by lymphoscintigraphy in 95 patients. Of these patients, 50% had three or more sentinel nodes identified on lymphoscintigraphy (76). Head and neck melanoma primaries drain to more nodal basins, and to more nodes per nodal basin than primaries of the trunk or limbs (88). There may be difficulty in recognizing which of the many nodes demonstrated on lymphoscintigraphy are actually sentinel nodes (Fig. 26.11). If the primary site overlies the sentinel node, both the radiopharmaceutical injection and the blue dye injection are likely to obscure the sentinel node. In addition, the actual nodes may be small and difficult to find at the time

of surgery. Experience in the Sunbelt Melanoma Trial has shown that, even when blue dye is used, neck nodes are less likely than those in non head and neck sites to be blue-stained (94). The potential for damage to important anatomic structures, such as the spinal accessory nerve in the posterior triangle or deep in the upper neck, or the facial nerve when dissecting for parotid sentinel nodes, must also be considered. A superficial parotidectomy or selective neck dissection may be more appropriate in some circumstances. Finding these nodes during surgery is not straightforward for the reasons presented; however with increasing experience, very high rates of success in identifying sentinel nodes during surgery have been achieved. When combining the use of preoperative lymphoscintigraphy, intraoperative blue dye and gamma probe localization, success rates of 95 to 100% have been reported, with false negative results averaging 7.7% to 10% (40,76,88,95–98).

The success of the sentinel node biopsy technique has ended the need for elective lymph node dissection. Complete lymph node dissection would rarely be performed now

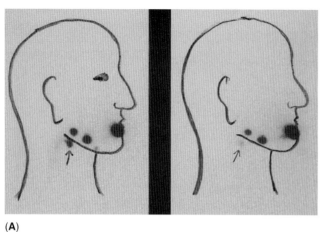 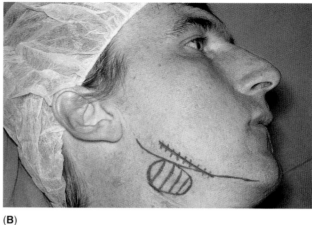

(A)   **(B)**

Figure 26.11   **(A)** These lymphoscintigrams are from a young man with melanoma of the right side of the lower lip. These are two brightly enhancing nodes seen on the initial scan (*right*) with a faint node below the line of the jaw. This latter node enhances more brightly on the delayed scan (*left*) but was thought to be a second tier node rather than a sentinel node. **(B)** Sentinel node biopsy of the two nodes seen on the initial scan was attempted through an incision marked by the blue line. The nodes were not identified. Six months later, the patient returned with an enlarged node, just below the jaw. This was shown to be the node that enhanced only faintly on the initial scan.

without first confirming the presence of metastatic disease in the relevant nodal basin. The procedure has not, however, ended the controversy about whether there is a benefit to be gained by treating subclinical nodal disease at all. Although accepted by many as being a "standard of care" (99–101), some have argued that it is inappropriate or even improper to perform sentinel node biopsy, citing potential surgical complications and lack of evidence for an overall survival benefit (102,103). Regardless of whether or not ongoing randomized trials demonstrate a survival benefit for the procedure, there are several reasons why sentinel node biopsy is a worthwhile procedure. The procedure is primarily a diagnostic staging test. It is now well-established that the status of the sentinel node is the most important predictor of survival in patients with melanoma (41). Sentinel node biopsy provides prognostic information important for guiding patients and their caregivers in decisions about potential adjuvant therapy. It facilitates early therapeutic dissection for those patients found to have nodal metastases, and potentially minimizes cost and anxiety in the follow-up of those 80% of patients without positive nodes. As outlined above, the microscopic lymph node status is incorporated into the AJCC staging system; accurate staging is important in comparing treatment outcomes, and for identifying homogeneous patient groups for entry into clinical trials of new treatments (101).

The issue of the safety and efficacy of the sentinel node biopsy technique is being studied in the first Multicenter Selective Lymphadenectomy Trial (MSLT I). This phase III study developed by Donald Morton commenced in 1994 and completed accrual of 2001 patients from 18 melanoma treatment centers in March 2002. Final results will not be available for several years, but data from the third of five planned interim analyses were published in 2006 (104). Patients with tumors 1.2 mm or greater were randomized to have wide local excision of the primary and a sentinel

node biopsy, or to have wide excision only and observation of the at-risk nodes. Complete lymph node dissection was performed immediately for a positive sentinel node, or when nodal metastases became clinically apparent in the observation arm. The report concerned the main targeted subset of patients with primaries from 1.2 to 3.5 mm in thickness. The study confirmed the prognostic significance of sentinel node biopsy, and laid to rest concerns about safety by showing no increase in local recurrence rates or in-transit metastases in the biopsy group. The five-year disease-free survival was greater in the biopsy group (78% vs. 73%), but no overall survival difference was seen between the two groups (87% vs. 86%). Among the patients who developed nodal disease, about 16% in both groups, survival was significantly greater in those undergoing dissection for microscopic disease (72.3% at five years) than those undergoing delayed dissection for macroscopic disease (52.4%) (P = 0.004). The mean number of involved nodes in the former group was 1.4 compared to 3.3 (P < 0.001) in the observation arm, implying that nodal disease progresses during observation. The validity of this comparison has been questioned (105,106), but the data do demonstrate the potential for improved outcome if early treatment is provided to those patients demonstrated to have early nodal disease, and minimal morbidity is reported in the remainder of patients (100,104).

Management of the Positive Sentinel Node

When metastatic melanoma is identified at sentinel node biopsy, current management would dictate that a therapeutic completion node dissection be performed. The practice at the SMU is now to do selective parotid and/or neck dissection guided by the drainage pattern demonstrated by the lymphoscintigraphy prior to the sentinel node biopsy. Prior experience with selective neck dissection suggests this is reasonable (42,77), but the efficacy of this approach is yet to be reported. Up to 40% of patients will have involved nodes in addition to the removed positive sentinel nodes (96,107), with the risk increasing with increasing thickness of the primary (108). In MSLT I, 20% of patients had additional positive nodes at completion node dissection, suggesting that up to four in five patients may not have benefitted from the completion node dissection. A second Multicenter Selective Lymphadenectomy Trial (MSLT II) has commenced to investigate whether immediate completion node dissection is needed in those patients who have been shown to be a higher risk of systemic disease by virtue of their positive sentinel node status. Accrual commenced in December 2004, aiming to study 1925 patients.

Management of the Clinically Positive Neck

Our current state of knowledge indicates that treatment of the clinically positive neck probably requires comprehensive neck dissection. This is because any lymph node level can be involved with disease once metastatic lymphadenopathy is present in the neck. Shah et al (56). analyzed the distribution of pathologically positive nodes in 111 radical neck dissection specimens. Levels II–IV were most commonly involved, but 23% also had level I disease and 19% had level V involvement. In addition, patients with ear, face, and anterior scalp lesions were at high risk for parotid involvement. O'Brien et al (77). evaluated 175 patients undergoing various forms of neck dissection for cutaneous melanoma. They confirmed a recurrence rate of 23% with selective neck dissection (i.e., dissection of only certain node groups), and 0% for modified radical neck dissection (a comprehensive dissection) for clinically positive neck disease. In that study, patients undergoing radical neck dissection had a 14% recurrence rate, but they were also the group that had more advanced disease. Superficial parotidectomy should be included for lesions of the face, ear, or anterior scalp that have metastasized to the neck, even in the absence of clinical parotid involvement (109).

Patients with clinical metastatic melanoma have a poor prognosis overall, however, the outlook is not hopeless. The five- and 10-year survival rates for patients treated by neck dissection at the SMU were 48% and 34%, respectively (9). Therefore, therapeutic neck dissection is a worthwhile procedure.

Radiotherapy

For much of the twentieth century, melanoma carried a reputation for resistance to radiotherapy (110,111), which has been shown to be unjustified (112). Radiotherapy has been applied successfully in a number of settings for the treatment of melanoma. In part this has been due to an improved understanding of the radiobiology of this disease. The remarkable ability of melanoma cells to repair sublethal damage has led to the development of high dose per fraction radiotherapy in an effort to overcome this phenomenon. This technique delivers the total amount of radiation in a hypofractionated course with each fraction containing a greater dose. High dose per fraction therapy aims to overcome the ability of melanoma cells to repair sublethal damage, but late radiation effects in normal tissue may be increased (113). Hypofractionated regimens have been used successfully, but a demonstrable difference in response

rates has not been shown in comparisons with standard fractionation regimens (114).

Primary Site

Radiotherapy has a limited role in the treatment of the primary site because adequate local control is usually achieved with surgery. Factors that may indicate its use as adjuvant treatment include cosmetically sensitive sites in the head and neck, close or positive margins that are not amenable to further excision, extensive lymphatic space invasion, multiple recurrences, or a desmoplastic neurotropic growth pattern (115). Desmoplastic melanoma, found predominantly in the head and neck, has relapse rates of up to 50%, which may be markedly reduced with postoperative radiotherapy (31). Foote et al. in Queensland treated 24 high-risk patients, 22 with primaries in the head and neck, with adjuvant radiotherapy, and achieved a 91% infield relapse-free survival at three years. Univariate analysis showed that the usual risk factors for local recurrence— the presence of neurotropism, close or positive surgical margins, and increasing Breslow thickness—were not predictive of recurrence, suggesting a benefit from radiotherapy. The Australian and New Zealand Melanoma Trials Group is about to commence a trial to try to confirm the benefit of adjuvant radiotherapy for desmoplastic melanoma (116).

Radiotherapy has been used as definitive treatment for primary melanomas and advanced acral lentigenous melanoma, and as a substitute for wide excision after a limited excision, with excellent control rates reported. Large lentigo maligna melanomas may be unsuitable for wide excision because of large size, proximity to facial structures, or medical comorbidities in the patients. Radiotherapy has been used with good long-term control rates and acceptable cosmetic results (115).

Regional Nodes

Most patients who die of melanoma do so with disseminated disease, while the primary site remains controlled. Consequently, the problem of regional recurrence after lymphadenectomy has received little attention. Recurrence in the parotid bed or neck, however, can cause severe morbidity and worsen prognosis (109). Therapeutic neck dissection may fail in up to 30% of cases (9). Singletary et al (117). reported even higher rates of regional recurrence with increasing number of nodes involved, noting up to 44% rates of recurrence after dissection of matted nodes. Recurrence rates after nodal dissection are found to be greater in patients with macroscopic nodes, a greater number of nodes, and the extracapsular extension of tumor (114,118), though these risk factors are likely to be interrelated. A multivariate analysis of 196 patients with positive nodes from head and neck primaries showed extracapsular extension to be the major risk factor for recurrence, with neither the number nor the size of positive nodes contributing (119). These findings indicate a potential need for adjuvant therapy after therapeutic neck dissection in order to improve locoregional control for these groups of patients.

The SMU published a non-randomized study of 152 dissected necks or parotids comparing neck dissection alone with neck dissection and adjuvant radiotherapy for pathologically positive disease. The adjuvant radiotherapy regimen used consisted of six fractions of 5.5 Gy delivered twice weekly for three weeks. The group of 45 dissected necks or parotids that received adjuvant radiotherapy demonstrated a 6.5% regional recurrence rate, whereas the group that received neck dissection only demonstrated recurrence in the neck 18.7% of the time (120). A more recent study of 160 patients treated at the M.D. Anderson Cancer Center with a similar adjuvant radiotherapy protocol produced a 94% 10-year regional control rate (121).

Although the clear benefits of high dose per fraction regimens over conventional fractionation schemes have not been definitively demonstrated for melanoma (113), the adjuvant use of radiotherapy for patients with nodal metastases does appear to improve the locoregional control of disease. Several phase I and II studies have now considered adjuvant therapy (114). Although different indications for treatment and different radiation schedules were used, recurrence rates of about 10% were uniformly reported for treatment of microscopic residual disease. Whether or not improved locoregional control improves survival is still debated. Control rates fall to about 50% when gross disease remains, stressing the importance of adequate surgery for this disease.

Resistance to the use of postoperative radiotherapy relates to presumed toxicity and the lack of evidence for a survival benefit. Irradiation to the lateral neck seems to be well-tolerated, with a self-limiting skin reaction acutely, and mild edema and subcutaneous fibrosis as a late response. A randomized intergroup trial to finally address the benefit and toxicity of adjuvant radiotherapy was commenced in 2003 by the Trans Tasman Radiation Oncology Group (TROG) and the Australian and New Zealand Melanoma Trials Group (ANZMTG), and completed accrual in early 2008. This study is comparing the outcomes of patients with completely resected nodal disease randomized to observation or adjuvant radiation (48 Gy in 20 fractions). Eligibility for head and neck patients included those with one or more parotid, or two or more neck nodes, extranodal spread, or nodes greater than 3 cm. Endpoints of the study include infield tumor control, treatment related complications, quality of life, and overall survival.

Other approaches to radiotherapy for melanoma in the neck have attempted to minimize toxicity from multimodality treatment. An early study from the M.D. Anderson Cancer Center included 76 patients who received neck irradiation after limited excision of palpable nodal disease. The control rate in the radiotherapy field was 90% at five years (122). A more recent study from the same institution assessed the role of elective irradiation for high-risk primary disease. Only 6% of the 157 patients treated reported a treatment-related complication at 10 years; the regional control rate was 89% (123). One aspect to be explored in light of these results from the M.D. Anderson Cancer Center is the future role of treatment for subclinical disease after removal of a positive sentinel node once results of the MSLT II trial are available.

Radiotherapy may also be considered for unresectable nodal disease. Standard fractionation is recommended to reduce the potential adverse effects of large fraction size on wound healing. Palliative radiation for unresectable nodal disease can be beneficial, with complete response rates of 24% and partial response rates of 25% to 48% able to be achieved (124,125).

Recurrent and Metastatic Disease

Radiotherapy has a considerable role in the palliation of advanced disease. Many patients benefit from treatment for relief of mass effect, pain, obstruction, bleeding, and fungation. Modern imaging techniques have also defined a group of patients with oligometastatic disease who could potentially benefit from recent advances in targeted stereotactic and intensity modulated radiotherapy (115).

Adjuvant Therapy in Melanoma
Immunotherapy

Chemotherapy, vaccines, and biological modifiers have been used alone and in combination as adjuvant treatment for high-risk resected melanoma, but to date high-dose interferon alpha has been the only immunotherapy agent shown reproducibly to affect disease behavior. Mature results (30 years) of studies investigating Bacillus Calmette Guérin (BCG) injections have confirmed no benefit for BCG as adjuvant treatment for Stage I to III melanoma (126). Considerable optimism about the efficacy of interferon alpha followed the publication of the initial randomized controlled trial, ECOG 1684, which showed improved relapse-free and overall survival in patients treated with high-dose interferon alpha, although this agent was employed with considerable treatment-related toxicity (127). On the basis of the trial results, the drug won approval from the U.S. Food and Drug Administration, and it remains the only agent approved for adjuvant treatment of melanoma. On subsequent follow-up, however, the improvement in overall survival was seen to lose statistical significance (128). A follow-up study (ECOG 1690) designed to compare high-dose with low-dose interferon alpha again demonstrated a modest improvement in relapse-free survival, but failed to confirm any survival benefit of interferon alpha either in high or low dosage (129). A pooled analysis of the trials (128) and systematic reviews (130,131) all confirm an improvement in median relapse-free survival of less than one year, but no improvement in overall survival. Whether these impacts on disease progression are sufficient to consider adjuvant high-dose interferon the "standard of care" continues to be debated (132–135).

Numerous trials have also investigated lower doses of interferon alpha to try to minimize toxicity. As with the high-dose trials, none have shown an improvement in overall survival, but an improvement in relapse-free survival was seen while the patients were receiving the low-dose treatment. The benefit appeared to be lost, however, when the treatment was stopped. The data suggested that better tolerated, lower doses of interferon required longer treatment regimens for patients to obtain a benefit (136). The European Organisation for Research and Treatment of Cancer (EORTC) has reported a large trial long-term administration of pegylated interferon alpha, which again showed an improved relapse-free survival in those receiving the treatment. The greatest benefit appeared to be in those patients with microscopic nodal involvement (SNB positive), who were also reported to have an improved distant-metastasis-free survival (137).

Interferon alpha, in combination with other agents, has not proven beneficial in patients with advanced (stage III and IV) disease (138). Its use in the neoadjuvant setting has been investigated, and one study showed objective clinical responses in over half the patients treated (139). The relationship between response rates and long term survival remains unclear.

A substantial number of melanoma-associated antigens have been identified, and the antibody and cellular responses to these targets characterized. Clinical trials have been, and continue to be, conducted utilizing a number of different vaccine approaches. Allogeneic and autologous whole cells, cell lysates, peptides, proteins, and glycolipid antigens have all been the subject of investigation (136,140). Several large phase III clinical trials have been performed, but none has demonstrated a significant improvement in survival of patients receiving vaccine therapy, except in some subset analyses (141–145). Phase II trials have shown enhanced survival for patients who develop a humoral and/or cellular response to a melanoma vaccine (146). On-going research seeks to determine which aspects of enhanced immunoresponsiveness improve clinical outcome. With the increasing knowledge of T cell biology over the last decade, recent approaches have searched for ways to further activate cytotoxic T cells against melanoma, trying to overcome the immune tolerance that has been observed in numerous studies.

Chemotherapy

There have been numerous studies of adjuvant chemotherapy regimens for the treatment of metastatic melanoma, but it has been argued that no trial has been sufficiently powered to show a survival benefit. None has been demonstrated to improve survival. Multi-agent regimens have proven to be no more effective than single-agent dacarbazine, which has produced response rates of no greater than 15% in recent multicenter phase III trials (136). Recent work has focused on combinations of chemotherapy, immunotherapy, and biological modifiers. The M.D. Anderson biochemotherapy regimen is the only regimen with reproducible response rates over 20%, but is associated with considerable toxicity. A current Southwest Oncology Group (SWOG) trial comparing biochemotherapy with interferon is currently being undertaken, but more effective and considerably less toxic regimens are sought.

SUMMARY

Despite advances in understanding the biology of cutaneous melanoma, an effective systemic agent for this disease remains elusive. The best chance of cure continues to be through appropriately radical surgery, and improvements in care have come through measures that minimize the morbidity of that surgery. Excision margins for primary tumors in general have become narrower, as risk factors for recurrence are better understood, and conservative margins can be used safely in the head and neck. The use of sentinel node biopsy has not entirely ended controversy about the management of lymph nodes, but the era of elective node dissection has now passed, and a more selective approach is now used. Only those demonstrated to have metastatic disease in regional nodes undergo surgery with a minimal burden of disease. In the therapeutic setting, selective and modified neck dissections have been shown to be appropriate. Aggressive surgical treatment of recurrence and systemic metastases in select patients also has a role in improving locoregional control, minimizing morbidity and offering some a potential for cure.

Ideal adjuvant treatment following surgery is also still to be defined. Current trials hope to settle many concerns about the appropriate use of adjuvant radiotherapy, and allow more selective and targeted approaches in this setting also. Although long ago noted to be an immune responsive disease, the promise of immunotherapy for treatment of melanoma has still not been realized, but there is much ongoing and promising research into the molecular pathogenesis of melanoma. While awaiting the development of effective adjuvant and systemic agents, the challenge remains to decrease the rising incidence of cutaneous melanoma by better professional and public education to ensure early diagnosis and prevention of this deadly disease.

REFERENCES

1. Wingo PA, Ries LAG, Risenberg HM et al. Cancer incidence and mortality 1973–1995—A report card for the US. Cancer 1998; 82: 1197–207.
2. Armstrong BK, Kricker A. Cutaneous Melanoma. Cancer Survey 1994; 19/20: 219–40.
3. Giles GG, Thursfield VJ, Staples MP. The bottom line: cancer mortality trends in Australia 1950–1991. Cancer Forum 1994; 18: 18–23.
4. Mackie RM, Hole D, Hunter JA et al. Cutaneous malignant melanoma in Scotland: incidence, survival, and mortality 1979–94. Br Med J 1997; 315: 1117–21.
5. Elwood JM, Gallagher RP. Body site distribution of cutaneous malignant melanoma in relationship to sun exposure. Int J Cancer 1998; 78: 276–80.
6. Jemal A, Siegel R, Ward E et al. Cancer Statistics, 2008. CA Cancer J Clin 2008; 58: 71–96.
7. Beddingfield FCr. The melanoma epidemic: *res ipsa loquitur.* Oncologist 2003; 8: 459–65.
8. Fisher S. Cutaneous malignant melanoma of the head and neck. Laryngoscope 1989; 99: 822–36.
9. O'Brien CJ, Coates AS, Petersen-Schaefer K et al. Experience with 998 cutaneous melanomas of the head and neck over 30 years. Am J Surgery 1991; 162: 310–4.
10. Ringborg U, Afzelius LE, Lagerlof B et al. Cutaneous malignant melanoma of the head and neck. Cancer 1993; 71: 751–8.
11. Andersson AP, Gottlieb J, Drzewiecki KT et al. Skin melanoma of the head and neck. Cancer 1992; 69: 1153–6.
12. Parkin DM, Muir CS, Whelan SC et al. Cancer incidence in five continents. IARC Scientific Publication No 120. 1992.
13. Armstrong BK, Kricker A. The epidemiology of UV induced skin cancer. J Photochem Photobiol B 2001; 63: 8–18.
14. Tucker MA, Goldstein AM. Melanoma etiology: where are we? Oncogene 2003; 22: 3042–52.
15. Bulliard JL, Cox B, Elwood JM. Latitude gradients in melanoma incidence and mortality in the non-Maori population of New Zealand. Cancer Causes Control 1994; 5.
16. Lee JA, Strickland D. Malignant melanoma: social status, indoor and outdoor work. Br J Cancer. 1980; 41: 757–63.
17. Cooke KE, Skegg DC, Fraser J. Socio-economic status, indoor and outdoor work, and malignant melanoma. Int J Cancer 1984; 34: 57–62.

18. Autier P, Dore J-F. Influence of sun exposure during childhood and adulthood on melanoma risk. Int J Cancer. 1998; 77: 533–7.

19. Westerdahl J, Olsson H, Ingvar C. At what age do sunburn episodes play a crucial role for the development of malignant melanoma? Eur J Cancer. 1994; 30A: 1647–54.

20. Elwood JM, Jopson J. Melanoma and sun exposure: an overview of published studies. Int J Cancer 1997; 73: 286–92.

21. Dennis LK, Beane Freeman LE, VanBeek MJ. Sunscreen use and the risk for melanoma: a quantitative review. Ann Intern Med 2003; 139: 966–78.

22. Autier P, Dore JF, Schiffers E et al. Melanoma and use of sunscreens: an EORTC case-control study in Germany, Belgium, and France. Int J Cancer 1995; 61: 749–55.

23. Balch CM, Karakosis C, Mettlin C. Management of cutaneous melanoma in the United States. Surg Gynecol Obstet 1984; 158: 311–9.

24. Bataille V, Grulich A, Saseini P et al. The association between naevi and melanoma in populations with different levels of sun exposure: a joint case-control study of melanoma in the UK and Australia. Br J Cancer 1998; 77. 505–10.

25. Kaplan EN. The risk of malignancy in large congenital nevi. Plast Reconstr Surg 1974; 53: 421–8.

26. Goldstein AM, Tucker MA. Genetic epidemiology of familial melanoma. Dermatol Clin 1995; 13: 605–12.

27. Ford D, Bliss JM, Swerdlow AJ et al. Risk of cutaneous melanoma associated with a family history of the disease. Int J Cancer 1995; 62: 377–81.

28. Goldstein AM, Tucker MA. Genetic epidemiology of cutaneous melanoma: a global perspective. Arch Dermatol 2001; 137: 1493–6.

29. Seykora J, Elder D. Dysplastic nevi and other risk factors for melanoma. Semin Oncol 1996; 23: 682–7.

30. Clark WHJ, Ainsworth AM, Bernardino EH et al. The development biology of primary human malignant melanomas. Semin Oncol 1975; 2: 83–93.

31. Carlson JA, Dickersin GR, Sober AJ et al. Desmoplastic neurotropic melanoma. A clinicopathologic analysis of 28 cases. Cancer 1995; 75: 478–94.

32. Quinn MJ, Crotty KA, Thompson JF et al. Desmoplastic and neurotropic melanoma: experience with 280 patients. Cancer 1998; 83: 1128–35.

33. Sagebiel RW. Unusual variants of melanoma: fact or fiction. Semin Oncol 1996; 23: 703–8.

34. Breslow A. Thickness, cross-sectional area and depth of invasion in the prognosis of cutaneous melanoma. Ann Surg 1970; 170: 902–8.

35. Balch CM, Soong S-J, Gershenwald JE et al. Prognostic factors analysis of 17,600 melanoma patients: Validation of the American Joint Committee on Cancer staging system. Am J Clin Oncol 2001; 16: 3622–34.

36. Azzola MF, Shaw HM, Thompson JF et al. Tumor mitotic rate is a more powerful prognostic indicator than ulceration in patients with primary cutaneous melanoma. Cancer 2003; 97: 1488–98.

37. Francken AB, Shaw HM, Thompson JF et al. The prognostic importance of tumor mitotic rate confirmed in 1317 patients with primary cutaneous melanoma and long follow-up. Ann Surg Oncol 2004; 11: 426–33.

38. Morton DL, Davtayan DG, Wanek LA et al. Multivariate analysis of the relationship between survival and microstage of primary melanoma by Clark level and Breslow thickness. Cancer 1993; 71: 3737–43.

39. Golger A, Young DS, Ghazarian D et al. Incidence and prognosis of cutaneous melanoma involving the head and neck. Arch Otolaryngol Head Neck Surg 2007; 133: 442–7.

40. Leong SPL, Accort A, Essner R et al. Impact of sentinel node status and other risk factors on the clinical outcome of head and neck melanoma patients. Arch Otolaryngol Head Neck Surg 2006; 132: 370–3.

41. Gershenwald JE, Thompson W, Mansfield PF et al. Multi-institutional melanoma lymphatic mapping experience: The prognostic value of sentinel lymph node status in 612 stage I or II melanoma patients. Am J Clin Oncol 1999; 17: 976–83.

42. O'Brien CJ, Gianoutsos MP, Morgan MJ. Neck dissection for cutaneous malignant melanoma. World J Surg 1992; 16: 222–6.

43. Martin RCW, Shannon KF, O'Brien CJ et al. The management and prognosis of cervical nodes in cutaneous melanoma. 7th International Conference on Head and Neck Cancer. San Francisco, 2008.

44. Wanebo HJ, Cooper PH, Young DV et al. Prognostic factors in head and neck melanoma: effect of lesion location. Cancer 1988; 62: 831–7.

45. Deichmann M, Benner A, Bock M et al. S100-beta, melanoma-inhibiting activity, and lactate dehydrogenase discriminate progressive from non-progressive American Joint Committee on Cancer stage IV melanoma. Am J Clin Oncol 1999; 17: 1891–6.

46. Eton O, Legha SS, Moon TE et al. Prognostic factors for survival of patients treated systemically for disseminated melanoma. Am J Clin Oncol 1998; 16: 1103–1.

47. Franzke A, Probst-Kepper M, Buer J et al. Elevated pretreatment levels of soluble vascularcell adhesion molecule I and lactate dehydrogenase as predictors of survival in cutaneous metastatic malignant melanoma. Br J Cancer 1998; 78: 40–5.

48. Sirott M, Bajorin D, Wong G et al. Prognostic factors in patients with metastatic malignant melanoma. Cancer 1993; 72: 3091–8.

49. Balch CM, Buzaid AC, Soong S-J et al. Final version of the American Joint Committee on Cancer staging system for cutaneous melanoma. Am J Clin Oncol 2001; 19: 3635–48.

50. Buzaid AC, Ross MI, Balch CM et al. Critical analysis of the current American Joint Committee on Cancer staging system for melanoma and proposal of a new staging system. Am J Clin Oncol 1997; 15: 1039–51.

51. Buzaid AC, Tinoco LA, Jendiroba D et al. Prognostic value of size of lymph node metastases in patients with cutaneous melanoma. Am J Clin Oncol 1995; 13: 2361–8.

52. Ross MI. New American Joint Commission on Cancer staging system for melanoma: Prognostic impact and future directions. Surg Oncol Clin N Am 2006; 15: 341–52.

53. Friedman RJ, Rigel DS, Kopf AW. Early detection of malignant melanoma: the role of physician examination and self-examination of the skin. CA Cancer J Clin 1985; 35: 130–51.

54. Steiner A, Pehamberger H, Wolff K. In vivo epiluminescence microscopy of pigmented lesions. II. Diagnosis of small pigmented skin lesions and early detection of melanoma. J Am Acad Dermatol 1987; 17: 584–9.

55. Menzies SW, Crotty KA, Ingvar C et al. An atlas of surface microscopy of pigmented skin lesions: dermoscopy. 2nd edn. Sydney: McGraw-Hill, 2003.

56. Shah JP, Kraus DH, Dubner S et al. Patterns of regional lymph node metastases from cutaneous melanomas of the head and neck. Am J Surg 1991; 162: 320–3.

57. Iscoe N, Kersey P, Gapski J et al. Predictive value of staging investigations in patients with clinical stage I malignant melanoma. Plast Reconstr Surg 1987; 80: 233–7.

58. Hofmann U, Szedlak M, Rittgen W et al. Primary staging and follow-up in melanoma patients—monocenter evaluation of methods, costs and patient survival. Br J Cancer 2002; 87: 151–7.

59. Damian DL, Fulham MJ, Thompson E et al. Positron emission tomography in the detection and management of metastatic melanoma. Melanoma Res 1996; 6: 325–9.

60. Rinne D, Baum RP, Hor G et al. Primary staging and follow-up of high risk patients with whole-body 18F-Fluorodeoxyglucose positron emission tomography. Cancer 1998; 82: 1664–71.

61. Holder WP, White RL, Zuger JH et al. Effectiveness of positron emission tomography for the detection of melanoma metastases. Ann Surg 1998; 227: 764–71.

62. Havenga K, Cobben DC, Oyen WJ et al. Fluorodeoxyglucose-positron emission tomography and sentinel node biopsy in staging primary cutaneous melanoma. Eur J Surg Oncol 2003; 29: 662–4.

63. Fink AM, Holle-Robatsch S, Herzog N et al. Positron emission tomography is not useful in detecting metastasis in the sentinel lymph node in patients with primary malignant melanoma stage I and II. Melanoma Res 2004; 14: 141–5.

64. Wagner JD, Schauwecker D, Davidson D et al. Inefficiency of F-18 fluorodeoxy-D-glucose-positron emission tomography scans for initial evaluation in early-stage cutaneous melanoma. Cancer 2005; 104: 570–9.

65. Brady MS, Akhurst T, Spanknebel K et al. Utility of preoperative 18F fluorodeoxyglucose-positron emission tomography scanning in high-risk melanoma patients. Ann Surg Oncol 2006; 13: 525–32.

66. Gulec SA, Faries MB, Lee CC et al. The role of fluorine-18 deoxyglucose positron emission tomography in the management of patients with metastatic melanoma: impact on surgical decision making. Clin Nucl Med 2003; 28: 961–5.

67. Handley WS. The pathology of melanotic growths in relation to their operative treatment. Lancet 1907; i: 927.

68. National Institutes of Health Consensus Development Panel on Early Melanoma. JAMA 1992; 268: 1314.

69. Balch CM, Soong S-J, Smith T et al. Long-term results of a prospective surgical trial comparing 2 cm vs. 4 cm excision margins for 740 patients with 1–4 mm melanomas. Ann Surg Oncol 2001; 8: 101–8.

70. Balch CM, Urist M, Karakousis C et al. Efficacy of 2 cm surgical margins for intermediate thickness melanomas 1–4 mm: results of a multi-institutional randomized surgical trial. Ann Sur 1993; 218: 262–7.

71. Veronesi U, Cascinelli N. Narrow excision: a safe procedure for thin cutaneous melanoma. Arch Surg 1991; 126: 438–41.

72. Cohn-Cedermark G, Rutqvist LE, Andersson R et al. Long term results of a randomized study by the Swedish Melanoma Study Group on 2-cm versus 5-cm resection margins for patients with cutaneous melanoma with a tumor thickness of 0.8–2.0 mm. Cancer 2000; 89: 1495–501.

73. Khayat D, Rixe O, Martin G et al. Surgical margins in cutaneous melanoma (2 cm versus 5 cm for lesions measuring less than 2.1-mm thick). Cancer 2003; 97: 1941–6.

74. Thomas JM, Newton-Bishop J, A'Hern R et al. Excision margins in high-risk malignant melanoma. New Engl J Med 2004; 350: 757–66.

75. Ariyan S. Plastic and reconstructive surgery in melanoma patients. In: Balch CM, ed. Surgical approaches to cutaneous melanoma. Basel: S Karger, 1985.

76. O'Brien CJ, Uren R, Thompson JF et al. Prediction of potential metastatic sites in cutaneous head and neck melanoma using lymphoscintigraphy. Am J Surg 1995; 170: 461–6.

77. O'Brien CJ, Petersen-Schaefer K, Ruark D et al. Radical, modified, and selective neck dissection for cutaneous malignant melanoma. Head Neck 1995; 17: 232–41.

78. Urist MM, Balch CM, Soong S-J et al. Head and neck melanoma in 534 clinical stage 1 patients: a prognostic factors analysis and results of surgical treatment. Ann Surg 1984; 200: 769–75.

79. Veronesi U, Adamus J, Bandiera D et al. Inefficacy of immediate node dissection in stage I melanoma of the limbs. New Engl J Med 1977; 297: 627–30.

80. Sim F, Taylor W, Pritchard D et al. Lymphadenectomy in the management of stage I malignant melanoma: a prospective randomized study. Mayo Clin Proc 1986; 61: 697–705.

81. Balch CM, Soong S-J, Bartolucci AA et al. Efficacy of an elective regional lymph node dissection of 1-4 mm thick melanomas for patients 60 years of age and younger. Ann Surg 1996; 224: 255–66.

82. Cascinelli N, Morabito A, Santinami M et al. Immediate or delayed dissection of regional nodes in patients with melanoma of the trunk: a randomised trial. Lancet 1998; 351: 793–6.

83. Lens MB, Dawes M, Goodacre T et al. Elective lymph node dissection in patients with melanoma: Systematic review and meta-analysis of randomized controlled trials. Arch Otolaryngol Head Neck Surg 2002; 137: 458–61.

84. Morton DL, Wen DRW, Wong JH et al. Technical details of intraoperative lymphatic mapping for early stage melanoma. Arch Surg 1992; 127: 392–9.

85. Uren RF, Howman-Giles R, Thompson JF et al. Lymphoscintigraphy to identify sentinel lymph nodes in patients with melanoma. Melanoma Res 1994; 4: 395–9.

86. Thompson JF, Scolyer RA, Uren RF. Surgical management of primary cutaneous melanoma: Excision margins and the role of sentinel node examination. Surg Oncol Clin N Am 2006; 15: 301–18.

87. Morton DL, Thompson JF, Essner R et al. Validation of the accuracy of intraoperative lymphatic mapping and sentinel lymphadenectomy for early-stage melanoma: a multicenter trial. Ann Surg 1999; 230: 453–63.

88. Davison SP, Clifton MS, Kauffman L et al. Sentinel node biopsy for the detection of head and neck melanoma: A review. Ann Plast Surg 2001; 47: 206–11.

89. Uren R, Howman-Giles R, Shaw H et al. Lymphoscintigraphy in high risk melanoma of the trunk: predicting draining node groups, defining lymphatic channels and locating the sentinel node. J Nucl Med 1993; 34: 1435–40.

90. Thompson J, McCarthy W, Bosch C et al. Sentinel lymph node status as an indicator of the presence of metastatic melanoma in regional lymph nodes. Melanoma Res 1995; 5: 255–60.

91. Reintgen D, Cruse W, Wells K et al. The orderly progression of melanoma nodal metastases. Ann Surg 1994; 220: 759–67.

92. Morton DL, Wen DR, Foshag LJ et al. Intraoperative lymphatic mapping and selective cervical lymphadenectomy for early-stage melanoma of the head and neck. Am J Clin Oncol 1993; 11: 1751–6.

93. de Wilt JHW, Thompson JF, Uren RF et al. Correlation between preoperative lymphoscintigraphy and metastatic nodal disease in 362 patients with cutaneous melanomas of the head and neck. Ann Surg 2004; 239: 544–52.

94. Chao C, Wong SL, Edwards MJ et al. Sentinel lymph node biopsy for head and neck melanomas. Ann Surg Oncol 2003; 10.

95. Leong SPL, Achten TA, Habib FA et al. Discordancy between clinical predictions vs. lymphoscintigraphic and intraoperative mapping of sentinel node drainage of primary melanoma. Arch Dermatol 1999; 135: 1472–6.

96. Wagner JD, Park H-M, Coleman JJI et al. Cervical sentinel node biopsy for melanomas of the head and neck and upper thorax. Arch Otolaryngol Head Neck Surg 2000; 126: 313–21.

97. Carlson GW, Murray DR, Greenlee R et al. Management of malignant melanoma of the head and neck using dynamic lymphoscintigraphy and gamma probe-guided sentinel

lymph node biopsy. Arch Otolaryngol Head Neck Surg 2000; 126: 433–7.

98. Bostick P, Essner R, Sarantou T et al. Intraoperative lymphatic mapping for early-stage melanoma of the head and neck. Am J Surg 1997; 74: 536–9.

99. WHO declares lymphatic mapping to be the standard of care for melanoma. Oncology 1999; 13: 288.

100. Balch CM, Cascinelli N. Sentinel-node biopsy in melanoma. New Engl J Med 2006; 355: 1370–1.

101. McMasters KM, Reintgen DS, Ross MI et al. Sentinel lymph node biopsy for melanoma: Controversy despite widespread agreement. Am J Clin Oncol 2001; 19: 2851–5.

102. Otley CC, Zitelli JA. Review of sentinel lymph node biopsy and systemic interferon for melanoma: Promising but investigational modalities. Dermatol Surg 2000; 26: 177–80.

103. Thomas JM, Patocskai EJ. The argument against sentinel node biopsy for malignant melanoma: its use should be confined to patients in clinical trials. Br Med J 2000; 321: 3–4.

104. Morton DL, Thompson JF, Cochran AJ et al. Sentinel-node biopsy or nodal observation in melanoma. New Engl J Med 2006; 355: 1307–17.

105. Thomas JM. Personal view of sentinel node biopsy in melanoma after the Multicenter Selective Lymphadenectomy Trial. Aust N Z J Surg 2006; 76: 98–9.

106. Kanzler MH. The current status of evaluation and treatment of high-risk cutaneous melanoma: therapeutic breakthroughs remain elusive. Arch Dermatol 2007; 143: 785–7.

107. Pu LLQ, Wells K, Cruse CW et al. Prevalence of additional positive lymph nodes in complete lymphadenectomy specimens after positive sentinel lymphadenectomy findings for early-stage melanoma of the head and neck. Plast Reconstr Surg 2003; 112: 43–9.

108. Yee VSK, Thompson JF, McKinnon JG et al. Outcome in 846 cutaneous melanoma patients from a single center after a negative sentinel node biopsy. Ann Surg Oncol 2005; 12: 1–11.

109. O'Brien CJ, Petersen-Schaefer K, Papadopoulos T et al. Evaluation of 107 therapeutic and elective parotidectomies for cutaneous melanoma. Am J Surg 1994; 168: 400–3.

110. Adair F. Treatment of melanomas. Surg Gynecol Obstet 1936; 62: 406–9.

111. Del Regato J, Spjut H. Cancer: diagnosis, treatment and diagnosis. St. Louis: CV Mosby, 1977.

112. Harwood AR, Cummings BJ. Radiotherapy for melanoma: a re-appraisal. Cancer Treat Rev 1981; 8: 271–82.

113. Sause WT, Cooper JS, Rush S et al. Fraction size in external beam radiation therapy in the treatment of melanoma. Int J Radiat Oncol Biol Phys 1991; 20: 429–32.

114. Bastiaanet E, Beukema JC, Hoekstra HJ. Radiation therapy following lymph node dissection in melanoma patients: treatment, outcome and complications. Cancer Treat Rev 2005; 31: 18–26.

115. Stevens GN, Hong A. Radiation therapy in the management of cutaneous melanoma. Surg Oncol Clin N Am 2006; 15: 353–71.

116. Foote MC, Burmeister B, Burmeister E et al. Desmoplastic melanoma: The role of radiotherapy in improving local control. Aust N Z J Surg 2008; 78: 273–6.

117. Singletary S, Byers R, Shallenberger R et al. Prognostic factors in patients with regional cervical node metastases from cutaneous malignant melanoma. Am J Surg 1986; 152: 371–6.

118. Cooper J. The evolution of the role of radiation therapy in the management of mucocutaneous melanoma. Hematol Oncol Clin North Am 1998; 12: 849–62.

119. Shen P, Wanek LA, Morton DL. Is adjuvant radiotherapy necessary after positive lymph node dissection in head and neck melanomas? Ann Surg Oncol 2000; 7: 554–9.

120. O'Brien CJ, Petersen-Schaefer K, Stevens GN et al. Adjuvant radiotherapy following neck dissection and parotidectomy for metastatic malignant melanoma. Head Neck 1997; 19: 589–94.

121. Ballo MT, Bonnen MD, Garden AS et al. Adjuvant irradiation for cervical lymph node metastases from melanoma. Cancer. 2003; 97: 1789–96.

122. Ang KK, Peters LJ, Weber RS et al. Postoperative radiotherapy for cutaneous melanoma of the head and neck region. Int J Radiat Oncol Biol Phys 1994; 30: 795–8.

123. Bonnen MD, Ballo MT, Myers JN et al. Elective radiotherapy provides regional control for patients with cutaneous melanoma of the head and neck. Cancer 2004; 100: 383–9.

124. Burmeister B, Smithers BM, Poulsen M et al. Radiation therapy for nodal disease in malignant melanoma. World J Surg 1995; 19: 369–71.

125. Corry J, Smith JG, Bishop M et al. Nodal radiation therapy for metastatic melanoma. Int J Radiat Oncol Biol Phys 1999; 44: 1065–9.

126. Agarwala SS, Neuberg D, Park Y et al. Mature results of a phase III randomized trial of Bacillus Calmette-Guerin (BCG) versus observation and BCG plus Dacarbazine versus BCG in the adjuvant therapy of American Joint Committee on Cancer stage I-III melanoma (E1673). Cancer 2004; 100: 1692–8.

127. Kirkwood JM, Strawderman MH, Ernstoff MS et al. Interferon alfa-2b adjuvant therapy of high-risk resected cutaneous melanoma: the Eastern Cooperative Oncology Group Trial EST 1684. Am J Clin Oncol 1996; 14: 7–17.

128. Kirkwood JM, Manola J, Ibrahim J et al. A pooled analysis of eastern cooperative oncology group and intergroup trials of high-dose interferon for melanoma. Clin Cancer Res 2004; 10: 1670–7.

129. Kirkwood JM, Ibrahim JG, Sondak VK et al. High- and low-dose interferon alfa-2b in high-risk melanoma: first analysis of intergroup trial E1690/S9111/C9190. Am J Clin Oncol 2000; 18: 2444–58.

130. Lens MB, Dawes M. Interferon alfa therapy for malignant melanoma: a systematic review of randomized controlled trials. Am J Clin Oncol 2002; 20: 1818–25.

131. Wheatley K, Ives N, Hancock B et al. Does adjuvant interferon-α for high-risk melanoma provide a worthwhile benefit? A meta-analysis of the randomised trials. Cancer Treat Rev 2003; 29: 241–52.

132. Kefford RE. Adjuvant therapy of cutaneous melanoma: the interferon debate. Ann Oncol 2003; 14: 358–65.

133. Sabel MS, Sondak VK. Pros and cons of adjuvant interferon in the treatment of melanoma. The Oncologist 2003; 8: 451–8.

134. Kirkwood JM, Tarhini AA, Moschos SJ et al. Adjuvant therapy with high-dose interferon α2b in patients with high-risk stage IIB/III melanoma. Nat Clin Pract Oncol 2008; 5: 2–3.

135. Bajetta E. Adjuvant use of interferon α2b is not justified in patients with stage IIB/III melanoma. Nat Clin Pract Oncol 2008; 5: 4–5.

136. Shah GD, Chapman PB. Adjuvant therapy of melanoma. The Cancer Journal 2007; 13: 217–22.

137. Eggermont AM, Suciu M, Santinami M et al. EORTC 18991:Long-term adjuvant pegylated interferon-alfa2b(PEG-INF) compared to observation in resected stage III melanoma, final results of a randomized trial. American Society of Clinical Oncology Conference. Chicago, IL, 2007; Abstract # 8504.

138. Falkson CI, Ibrahim J, Kirkwood JM et al. Phase III trial of dacarbazine versus dacarbazine with interferon alpha-2b versus dacarbazine with tamoxifen versus dacarbazine with interferon alpha-2b and tamoxifen in patients with metastatic malignant melanoma: an Eastern Cooperative Oncology Group study. Am J Clin Oncol 1998; 16: 1743–51.

139. Moschos SJ, Edington HD, Land SR et al. Neoadjuvant treatment of regional stage IIIB melanoma with high-dose interfern alfa-2b induces objective tumor regression in association with modulation of tumor infiltrating host cellular immune responses. Am J Clin Oncol 2006; 24: 3164–71.

140. Ollila DW, Kelley MC, Gammom G et al. Overview of melanoma vaccines: active specific immunotherapy for melanoma patients. Semin Surg Oncol 1998; 14: 328–36.

141. Livingston PO, Wong GYC, Adluri S et al. Improved survival in stage III melanoma patients with GM2 antibodies: a randomized trial of adjuvant vaccination with GM2 ganglioside. Am J Clin Oncol 1994; 12: 1036–44.

142. Wallack MK, Sivanandham M, Balch CM et al. Surgical adjuvant active specific immunotherapy for patients with stage III melanoma: the final analysis of data from a phase III, randomized, double-blind, multicenter, vaccinia melanoma oncolysate trial. J Am Coll Surg 1998; 187: 69–77.

143. Kirkwood JM, Ibrahim J, Sosman JA et al. High-dose interferon alfa-2b significantly prolongs relapse-free and overall survival compared with the GM2-KLH/QS-21 vaccine in patients with resected stage IIb-III melanoma: results of intergroup trial E1694/S9512/C509801. Am J Clin Oncol 2001; 19: 2370–80.

144. Hersey P, Coates AS, McCarthy WH et al. Adjuvant immunotherapy of patients with high-risk melanoma using vaccinia viral lysates of melanoma: results of a randomized trial. Am J Clin Oncol 2002; 20: 4181–90.

145. Sondak VK, Liu PY, Tuthill RJ et al. Adjuvant immunotherapy of resected, intermediate thickness, node-negative melanoma with an allogenic tumor vaccine: overall results of a randomized trial of the Southwest Oncology Group. Am J Clin Oncol 2002; 20: 2058–66.

146. Chan AD, Morton DL. Active immunotherapy with allogeneic tumour cell vaccines: present status. Semin Oncol 1998; 25: 611–22.

Complications in Head and Neck Cancer Surgery

Emma Barker, Aongus Curran, Patrick J Gullane and Jonathan C Irish

INTRODUCTION

Despite the best preoperative care, meticulous surgical technique, and attentive postoperative management, complications frequently arise in the head and neck cancer patient. Many of these individuals are elderly with concomitant medical problems and pose a constant challenge for those involved in their care. Early recognition of the symptoms and signs of complications can prevent amplification of existing problems. The purpose of this chapter is to focus on the major surgical complications and how they are best avoided or treated once they occur.

THE NECK
Vascular

Before embarking on any type of neck surgery the surgeon must have a thorough knowledge of the anatomy of the region. An understanding of vascular instruments and their use coupled with an ability to dissect and/or repair vessels will be beneficial when bleeding occurs.

Internal Jugular Vein

Bleeding. The internal jugular vein (IJV) is associated with severe hemorrhage when torn during surgery. This usually occurs at the upper or lower ends as the vein is mobilized prior to ligation and transfixion. It is best to achieve vessel control by mobilizing with blunt clamps. Use of a spreading motion perpendicular to the wall of the vein avoids trauma. A combination of sharp and blunt dissection may be used. Once the vein is mobilized circumferentially, two clamps are applied proximally and distally avoiding injury to the vagus nerve prior to vessel transfixion and ligation (both proximal and distal ends). Occasionally a tear extends from a tributary to the main vessel. Usually a jugular vein tear can be repaired with a fine vascular suture on a tapered needle.

Uncontrolled bleeding at the skull base is first controlled with tamponade. When the vein can be identified and clamped it is ligated. In situations where the vessel retracts into the temporal bone Surgicel (Ethicon Inc., Somerville, NJ), is packed into the area and may control the bleeding. At times it is necessary to skeletonize the jugular vein or sigmoid sinus to obtain control over the proximal bleeding point and rotate a local muscle flap into the area. Normally at the skull base, the vein should be divided at the level of the transverse process of the atlas taking care to identify and preserve the vagus, hypoglossal, and accessory nerves.

Some surgeons do not tie the lower aspect of the vein until most of the neck dissection is completed as back-pressure on the venous system results in troublesome intra-operative bleeding. In this situation, leaving loose silk sutures around a well-exposed vein is necessary.

Excessive bleeding from the stump of the vein as a result of a slipped ligature may be controlled by direct pressure, which prevents air embolism and controls bleeding temporarily. No blind attempts should be made to control bleeding as this may extend a tear. With good light and exposure, pressure is gradually removed and the patent vein end is identified and ligated as before. Rarely the stump retracts into the superior mediastinum necessitating a sternal split to access the internal jugular or brachiocephalic trunk.

With large venous tears, placing the patient in the Trendelenburg position is employed to reduce the risk of air embolus. In cases where the IJV is being preserved, a running 6–0 vascular suture can be used to repair a tear while holding the vessel with a DeBakey vascular forceps. Its non-crushing serrated tip prevents tissue trauma. When the vessel is to be preserved, tributaries should be ligated away from the main vessel. This avoids eddy currents and thrombosis formation of the IJV that can result in loss of a free flap when one of the venous anastomoses is into this system (1). Interestingly, IJV thrombosis is an uncommon event following radical neck surgery (2). Postoperative facial edema and raised intracranial pressure, which are typically seen following radical neck dissection, may be avoided. Increased intracranial pressure following unilateral radical neck dissection has been previously described (3). If a second side radical neck dissection is required, raised intra-cranial pressure will result. It has been shown that pressure levels of greater than 40 mm Hg can be observed in the majority of patients (4). Systemic hypertension occurs in response to elevated intracranial pressure (Cushing's reflex). Normally within 24 hours the intracranial pressure will return to normal; however, intraoperative intervention to lower intracranial pressure is generally required. Therefore, when the second IJV is sacrificed, an increase in ICP should be anticipated, monitored, and treated accordingly.

IJV rupture and subsequent hemorrhage is associated with postoperative pharyngeal fistula formation in those patients with significant tobacco history and a poor nutritional status (5). In addition, a more complete circumferential dissection of the vein low in the neck in the presence of hypopharyngeal fistula may place it at a higher risk for rupture (5).

Air embolism. This may present as a sucking noise audible over the torn vein, which is usually the IJV. This rare complication occurs when a large neck vein is inadvertently opened, causing air to be sucked into the negatively pressured venous system. A loud churning noise over the precordial area may be auscultated. Hypotension and cardiac arrest may result when a significant air embolism is not recognized and effectively managed (6). The involved vein should be immediately compressed and the patient placed in the Trendelenberg position on the operating table. Aspiration of air from the tip of a central venous pressure (CVP) catheter is often diagnostic as well as therapeutic. In the absence of a CVP catheter, nitrous oxide from the anesthetic circuit should be discontinued and airway pressures increased to raise venous pressure. A "millwheel" murmur and cardiovascular collapse are usually late clinical features. Turning the patient into the left lateral Trendelenberg position may move air from the pulmonary valve and re-establish cardiac output in the event of cardiovascular collapse. Large bubbles (up to 2.5 cm) can be observed in the IJV intra operatively in 42% of patients undergoing supine radical neck surgery (7). Their presence may potentially result in central air embolism.

Carotid Artery

Stell reported a 3% incidence of carotid artery rupture in a series of 280 patients undergoing major head and neck surgery (8). The majority died (77%) and 11% had neurological sequelae such as hemiplegia/aphasia. Factors that contribute to this complication include prior radiation, atheromatous disease, stripping of the carotid adventitia due to tumor adherence on the vessel wall and scar formation. A mortality rate of 17% and an incidence of neurological sequelae of 28% are reported after elective ligation (9), compared with a 38% mortality and 88% incidence of neurological complications following non-elective resection.

Modern CT and gadolinium-enhanced MRI provide improved detail of the tumor-artery interface that helps predict the need for resection in cases of suspected invasion. To determine the effects of carotid artery resection in the setting of tumor invasion, conventional angiography, dynamic brain scans, and balloon-occlusion techniques with somatosensory cortical evoked potentials (SCEP) are used to assess the risks of internal carotid artery (ICA) occlusion (6,10,11).

Preoperative evaluation of clinical responses and SCEPs can be performed using balloon-occlusion angiography. A non-detachable balloon is introduced on a double-lumen Swan–Ganz catheter and the patient's responses are recorded for 20 minutes post occlusion. Neurological symptoms or alterations on SCEPs indicate that complete ICA resection without prior bypass surgery would be contraindicated. In 10% of patients permanent neurological deficit will be experienced following resection of the ICA despite negative findings (11). When a tear occurs in the carotid artery during a resection a decision has to be made whether to ligate or repair the vessel. In a hemodynamically and neurologically stable patient primary repair may be feasible using a 5/0 or 6/0 nylon suture with or without shunting. When tumor invades the carotid artery a decision must be made about proceeding with surgery versus leaving gross disease. Long-term prognosis is usually very poor in patients who have carotid artery invasion despite surgical sacrifice of the carotid artery. Factors that impact on this decision include whether the patient has previously received radiation

treatment, as well as patient factors such as age, medical co-morbidity, and overall patient prognosis. If surgical resection is indicated, a graft using saphenous vein, Gore-Tex, or Dacron may be possible in a clean, non-contaminated neck and may reduce the incidence of secondary cerebrovascular events (12).

When a tear occurs close to the skull base, ligation or packing may be the only option. If ligation is impossible, reverse bleeding from the circle of Willis can be controlled by oversewing of the vessel ends. Alternatively, a balloon catheter fed up into the vessel and left in an occluded position to arrest bleeding is the approach of choice. If this fails, craniotomy and trans-temporal ligation of the internal carotid may be required.

Postoperative carotid blow-out. Risk factors include prior irradiation, necrotic cervical flaps (Fig. 27.1), or an orocutaneous fistula/pharyngocutaneous fistula. The patient may have undergone a surgical resection of a malignant mucosal lesion involving the oral cavity, pharynx, or larynx with a radical neck dissection. Prevention may be possible by excising necrotic tissue and wound toilet with antiseptic dressings; adequate packing and drainage; as well as the use of antibiotics. A sentinel bleed may precede the eventual blow-out and allow time to cover the exposed area with well-vascularized tissue. When a massive rupture occurs on the ward, direct pressure is applied to the site of bleeding, the patient is placed in the Trendelenberg position, immediate fluid replacement instituted, and the airway secured. The patient is transferred to the operating room for definitive exploration and management. The vessel stumps are exposed to healthy tissue, ligated, and transfixed. After appropriate debridement, the stumps are buried in healthy tissue and the area covered with a vascularized regional flap. Angiography with embolization offers a safe and rapid alternative method of achieving vascular control in patients

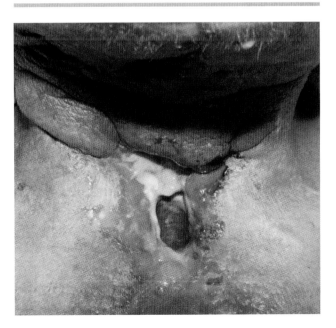

Figure 27.1 8 hours prior to a right carotid blow-out in a patient with a necrotic jejunal reconstruction.

with spontaneous rupture of the common carotid, carotid bulb, or external carotid system once the patient has been stabilized. Recent advances in imaging combined with more successful embolizing techniques have made this possible. Spontaneous late carotid-cutaneous fistulas have been reported many years after radical neck dissection (13). These are rare and associated with post-operative radiation.

Postoperative Hematoma

Hematoma is avoided by meticulous intraoperative hemostasis. Intraoperative valsalva and Trendelenburg positioning, prior to closing, may help with the identification of open, collapsed veins, at the end of the procedure. It is our practice to attach closed suction drains to a Pleuro-Vac pump or wall suction at −40 cmH$_2$O for the first 24 hours postoperatively. The source of bleeding is often from the skin edges, from small anterior cervical veins, the external jugular, or transverse cervical arterial branches. Rarely, aspiration and application of a pressure dressing is sufficient to manage this problem; however, if bleeding is brisk the source of bleeding needs to be identified and controlled. Returning the patient to the operating room, re-exploring the wound, securing the bleeding point, irrigating the wound thoroughly, and placing appropriate drains are mandatory. Clearly, a hematoma in the neck can compromise the airway due to pressure and result in a medical emergency. Therefore, management of these cases may require the neck incision to be re-opened on the ward, before the patient is returned to the operating room. In addition, a neck hematoma may significantly alter the ease of intubation, either due to mass effect, or associated edema. A senior anesthetist is essential.

Neural Complications

General Considerations

Gentle handling of soft tissues in the neck and avoiding traction on identified nerves are central to preventing injuries. Direct neural transection is often due to scar tissue or a failure to identify normal/abnormal anatomy. Scarring may also impede dissection and obscure tissue planes, thereby predisposing to injury. Careful use of cautery, suction, and ties helps prevent neural trauma. Nerve monitoring may also help to reduce neural injury.

Marginal Mandibular Nerve

This branch of the facial nerve emerges from the parotid fascia and descends between the platysma and fascia overlying the submandibular gland. Injury results in a deformity of the lower lip, which is most noticeable when smiling. Feeding may be disrupted due to loss of oral competence. Injury is less likely by (1) dividing the fascia low over the submandibular and reflecting it superiorly with the dissection; (2) ligating the posterior facial vein at the lower border of the submandibular gland and dissecting deep to this plane; (3) identifying the nerve deep to the platysma (with or without a nerve stimulator) and directly following its course. Inadvertent cutting of the nerve should be repaired with perineural 9-0 or 10-0 monofilament nylon.

Accessory Nerve (Cranial Nerve XI)

This emerges from the jugular foramen anterolateral to the IJV. The nerve supplies motor function to the sternocleidomastoid

and trapezius muscles. Sacrifice is indicated when gross metastatic disease is present in the posterior triangle, in the high jugulodigastric region, or skull base. Inadvertent injury may result in an inability to abduct the shoulder beyond 90 degrees, associated with pain and discomfort in the shoulder joint. In up to 40% of patients no symptoms are experienced after radical neck dissection despite sacrificing the nerve (14). Recent years have witnessed a trend toward a less radical approach to neck dissection with every attempt to preserve the nerve where possible. Most injuries occur during neck dissections, yet simple excision of a node within the posterior triangle, or during removal of a branchial cyst, may result in inadvertent damage to the nerve (15). Injury is less likely by (1) locating the nerve 1 cm above nerve point (16) [where the cervical roots course behind the posterior border of the sternocleidomastoid muscle (SCM)] or as it enters the trapezius (4–6 cm above the clavicle) (Fig. 27.2); (2) ensuring that the main trunk has been followed towards the jugular foramen; (3) dissecting along the anterior border of the SCM during selective neck dissection and identifying the nerve anterior to the internal jugular vein in most, but not all cases.

Once identified the accessory nerve should be cleared from surrounding muscle and handled gently, avoiding traction at all times. Complete disruption may be repaired by epineural or perineural repair with 9-0 or 10-0 monofilament suture. Shoulder function after cable grafting results in an intermediary level of function between sacrifice and preservation of the nerve (17). Intensive physiotherapy and home exercise are beneficial in relieving symptoms and avoiding a permanent "frozen shoulder." Improved shoulder function can be achieved by anastomosing the distal transected end of the spinal accessory nerve to the proximal cervical trunk at the time of neck dissection.

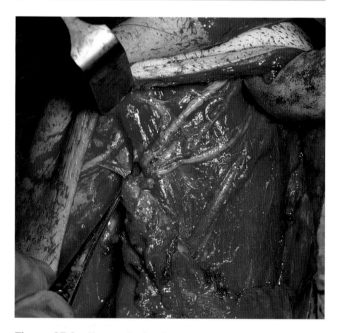

Figure 27.2 Nerve point is where the great auricular nerve (GAN) comes forward over the posterior border of the sternomastoid muscle. The accessory nerve (XI) emerges approximately 1 cm above nerve point.

If this complication is not recognized intra-operatively, pain is the most common presenting symptom, and a loss of sustained abduction the most common physical sign (18). Delayed repair has a reported variable motor improvement but importantly, should reduce pain (18).

Vagus Nerve (Cranial Nerve X)

This emerges at the mid-point of the jugular foramen and courses through the neck between the IJV and carotid artery within the carotid sheath. Ipsilateral laryngeal and pharyngeal paralysis with loss of sensation at and below the glottis occurs when the nerve is transected low in the neck. Skull-base transection results in a devastating loss of both sensory and motor nerves, including loss of sensation in the supraglottis, and paralysis of the pharyngeal musculature and the vocal cord. Both dysphagia and aspiration are likely sequelae following this type of damage. Injury is usually avoided by clearly identifying the nerve before ligating the IJV high in the neck. Vagal injuries as a result of crushing are usually temporary and will improve or recover over several months. When the nerve has been transected, nasogastric or gastrostomy tube feeding may be necessary because of dysphagia and aspiration. Improvement in speech and swallowing may be gained by immediate or delayed vocal cord injection of Teflon, glycerin, or Gelfoam (Pharmacia & Upjohn Company, New York, NY). A medialization thyroplasty (19) is a worthwhile option when no recovery of a paralyzed cord is apparent after six months. Cricopharyngeal myotomy may assist swallowing following a high vagal transection, although this is controversial. Animal model studies in the rat have demonstrated that if the recurrent laryngeal nerve has been transected, immediate suture repair and the application of basic fibroblast growth factor restored vocal fold movement (20). In addition, the phrenic nerve transfer technique, with the addition of neurotropin-3 has shown good reinnervation of the posterior cricoarytenoid muscle in the pig model (21). In addition, spontaneous reinnervation of the larynx in cats is more likely to occur if the nerve has been transected distally (the recurrent laryngeal nerve) compared to a high vagal transaction (22). The benefit gained by immediate neurorrhaphy in clinical situations where the nerve is transected is not clear but generally most surgeons would likely attempt a neurorrhaphy of the vagus nerve if intentional or iatrogenic sacrifice were to occur. When the nerve is sacrificed cardiovascular and gastrointestinal symptoms are usually not apparent.

Hypoglossal Nerve (Cranial Nerve XII)

This emerges from the hypoglossal foramen at the skull base and lies deep to the styloid muscles and posterior belly of the digastric before running deep to the mylohyoid muscle to supply the musculature of the tongue. The nerve is particularly prone to injury where it lies deep to the belly of the digastric muscle just anterosuperior to the carotid bifurcation. Attempts made to control bleeding from a complex of venae comitantes in this area may traumatize the nerve. Time spent cauterizing or ligating small vessels in this region is worthwhile as these vessels tend to retract deep to the nerve once transected. Cautery tips must be visualized at all times with no blind attempts to control bleeding.

Dysarthria and dysphagia usually compensate to an acceptable physiological level after a period of time when one hypoglossal nerve is resected. Bilateral hypoglossal nerve resection renders the patient an oral cripple. Primary neurroraphy is recommended when the nerve is inadvertently cut. Delayed repair does not result in a good clinical outcome (23).

Brachial Plexus and the Phrenic Nerve

The brachial plexus lies within the posterior triangle of the neck between the anterior and middle scalene muscles. It is protected by developing a plane between the deep cervical fascia and the overlying fat pad. Visualization of the plexus prior to clamping the posterior triangle fat pad should prevent injury. The phrenic nerve courses over the anterior scalene muscles, running from a lateral to medial direction. Injury results in an immobile elevated diaphragm, which can cause postoperative pulmonary atelectasis and pulmonary sepsis. If transection is noted intra-operatively, immediate repair is undertaken (24). This anastomosis potentially may be improved with a polyglycolic acid and collagen tube, as demonstrated in an inter-thoracic animal model (25). As dissection proceeds across the posterior triangle any cervical sensory branches should be divided high, thereby avoiding injury to the contributions to the phrenic from C3–5.

Sympathetic Plexus

Horner's syndrome (ptosis, miosis, enopthalmos, and anhydrosis) results when the sympathetic plexus is damaged. When dissecting posterior or around the carotid sheath the trunk or the superior cervical ganglion may be inadvertently injured. The middle cervical ganglion lies in close proximity to the inferior thyroid artery. The inferior ganglion lies behind the subclavian on the first thoracic vertebra.

Greater Auricular Nerve

Derived from C2, C3 and loops behind the sternocleidomastoid muscle to pass superficially on its surface and supply the pinna, parotid region, and skin over the mastoid bone, this nerve is easily divided when elevating the upper cervical flaps. Injury results in paresthesia of the pinna and on occasion the development of a painful neuroma. The nerve should be visualized on the sternocleidomastoid muscle during cervical flap elevation. A decision to preserve or sacrifice the nerve can be made once the status of the upper cervical nodes is identified.

Chyle Leaks

Chyle fistulas occur in 1–3% of neck dissections and mostly on the left side (75% of cases) (26). Chyle consists of the products of fat digestion (chylomicrons); continuous loss may result in significant electrolyte disturbance, impaired wound healing, and nutritional imbalance. A leak is recognized intraoperatively by the presence of a collection of clear/milky fluid in the lower neck or by a greasy feel to the surgical gloves (Fig. 27.3). During dissection in the level IV distribution (particularly on the left) care is taken to ligate the low neck contents between the IJV and the phrenic nerve. If the thoracic duct is identified it is carefully ligated to prevent a chyle leak.

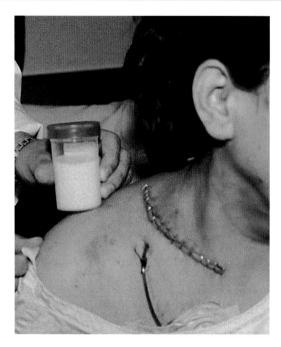

Figure 27.3 Chylous leak.

Intraoperative Management

A suspected leak should be confirmed by asking the anesthetist to apply continuous positive airway pressure (i.e., Valsalva). This increases the flow of chyle by raising the venous and lymphatic pressures. Ligation of the thinned-walled thoracic duct in isolation is not recommended and it is better to include the surrounding tissue with the duct using a non-absorbable suture. The scalene muscle can be included with this suture ligature. Ligating the cervical thoracic duct can be associated with rare complications including chylothorax or chylous ascites and very infrequently, lower-extremity lymphedema (27). Surgical glues and sclerosing agents such as tetracycline have been used with some reported success (28).

Postoperative Management

The presence of fluid with a milky appearance or continuous fluid from the neck drains once feeding begins is likely to be due to a chylous fistula. An intense inflammatory response due to chyle may cause flap compromise or loss of the overlying skin. The presence of triglycerides in this fluid confirms the diagnosis when in doubt. The goal is to optimize the patient's nutritional status and reduce the volume of chyle production. Generally two types of leak arise. The low output leak can usually be managed with aspiration, a pressure dressing, and dietary manipulation. Vivonex is a 98% fat-free solution that fulfills these requirements. Collaboration with a dietician and careful monitoring of electrolytes are necessary. Some centers also use medical agents, including octreotide, to minimize output (29). A high output leak (>500 ml/day) for three days or longer despite conservative management warrants surgical management. Persistence of this output volume necessitates neck re-exploration on the fourth or fifth postoperative day (30). Feeding the patient 100–200 ml of cream two to three hours

preoperatively will improve the chances of identifying the leak at the time of re-exploration. Placing the patient in the Trendelenburg position with the use of continuous positive pressure also helps in localization. Applying a sclerosing agent, such as tetracycline, after ligating the duct may be beneficial at this stage (28). Closed suction drainage is used and the patient is managed postoperatively with a medium chain triglyceride diet and careful electrolytic monitoring. A thoracoscopic ligation of the thoracic duct is an effective method of controlling a leak if neck re-exploration fails, particularly in situations with severe metabolic and nutritional complications, a coexisting chylothorax with respiratory compromise, or low-output fistulas (<500 cm³/day) of long duration (>14 days) (31,32).

Pharyngocutaneous Fistula

Occurring in 7–38% of patients, usually following oncologic resection of laryngeal or hypopharyngeal tumors (33), pharyngocutaneous fistula is a serious and relatively common complication associated with major head and neck surgery, especially in the irradiated patient. As saliva accumulates in the neck, flap necrosis, and carotid exposure and rupture are likely. Risk factors include poor nutritional status, prior irradiation, poor surgical technique, and any factor that impairs wound healing (34), including diabetes mellitus, preoperative hypoalbuminemia, chronic pulmonary diseases, and chronic hepatopathy. Each of these factors was shown to be an independent predictor for pharyngocutaneous fistula formation in patients undergoing total laryngectomy (35). In addition, salvage surgery, following radiation treatment, with or without induction chemotherapy, has an increased risk of fistula formation (36,37). The combined result of chemoradiation has a significant effect on the exposed soft tissues and how they will tolerate surgery, specifically relating to their healing potential and associated increased risk of fistula formation. Technical factors, such as gentle atraumatic handling of the soft tissues, achieving a watertight anastomosis, ensuring complete hemostasis, and using closed suction drains to eliminate dead space are key factors in its prevention. A pharyngocutaneous fistula initially presents with erythema and tenderness in the lower neck incision or skin flap. There may be an associated pyrexia and leukocytosis. The extent of the fistula will become apparent over a number of days and is primarily dependent on the degree of mucosal separation at the site of closure. With massive fistulas the entire neck skin may slough, exposing major neural and vascular structures. As with all surgical complications, prevention is better than cure. Free tissue transfer to reinforce the pharyngeal suture-line in failed organ-preservation patients undergoing a laryngectomy has shown variable outcomes with regard to alteration in pharyngocutaneous fistula rate. One study has shown no reduction, but fistulas that developed were small and could be managed with outpatient wound care (38). In contrast, another study showed a reduction in pharyngocutaneous fistula rates (39). Both studies agreed with a reduction in major wound complications in the free-tissue transfer group. Conflicting results have also been published regarding pharyngeal stricture requiring dilatation (38,39). Fistula management may be conservative or surgical, dictated by size and location of the fistula. Two groups are generally seen.

Group 1

With meticulous wound care, small fistulas often heal spontaneously. Wound care consists of antiseptic dressings, minimal debridement, and antibiotics. The patient is fed by nasogastric/gastrostomy tube or parenterally with careful monitoring of nutritional and biochemical status. With this form of management the majority of fistulas heal by secondary intention. Every attempt is made to divert the flow of saliva medial to the carotid artery and to minimize tracheal aspiration. Oral feeding is commenced once the integrity of the upper aerodigestive tract is ensured by contrast medium or methylene blue dye swallow. With a conservative approach, small fistulas may take up to one month or more to close.

Group 2

Massive fistulas are associated with extensive overlying skin loss and mucosal dehiscence (Fig. 27.4). Initial management consists of controlled exteriorization after surgical debridement. Residual or recurrent disease must be considered a possibility when a large fistula fails to close by secondary intention. The conservative measures described for group 1 also apply to this group of patients and once clean and fresh granulation tissue appears, the wound is usually ready for closure. The exception is the patient with major vessel exposure where urgent cover with vascularized tissue is needed to prevent carotid artery blow-out. Local, pedicled, and free flaps may initially be employed to cover exposed vascular structures in a defect based approach (40). With respect to the fistula, the goal is to ensure that mucosal continuity is maintained and adequate skin cover is established. This is typically provided by a myocutaneous pedicled flap (e.g., pectoralis major). More recently, free-tissue transfer has become the treatment of choice in some centers (41). In this situation, early tissue transfer is favored (41).

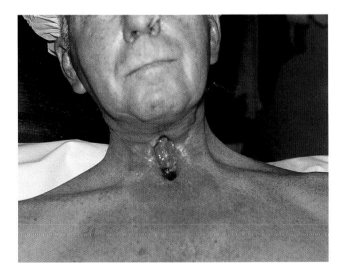

Figure 27.4 A pharyngocutanous fistula following a laryngectomy. Acknowledgements: Mr TJ O'Neill.

Tracheostomy

General Considerations

Complications may be divided into (1) intraoperative, (2) immediate postoperative, and (3) late postoperative. Anatomical factors such as an enlarged thyroid, a short fat neck, inability to extend the neck due to arthritis, or other causes may render the procedure technically difficult.

When a tracheostomy is to be performed for airway control in a head and neck cancer patient it is advisable to try to secure the airway initially with an endotracheal tube. A flexible bronchoscope will facilitate intubation in a patient with a compromised airway. Alternatively a rigid bronchoscopy can be attempted to establish an airway as complications are increased when the operation is performed on an air-hungry struggling patient. Dexamethasone may be useful in the immediate preoperative period by reducing edema.

Intraoperative Complications

Hemorrhage during tracheostomy is usually from the anterior cervical veins or thyroid gland. In an emergency, the goal is to secure the airway and control bleeding once this is established. A vertical midline incision is best in an acute airway emergency. This reduces the risk to the local vascular structures. In an elective setting damage to major vascular structures is avoided by dissecting in the midline. The suprasternal region should always be palpated to exclude a high-placed innominate artery. The thyroid isthmus is usually retracted superiorly and, if obstructing access to the trachea, is divided and oversewn. Prior to entering the airway in the elective tracheotomy, hemostasis must be complete. In the rare instance where inadvertent injury to the common carotid or innominate occurs, immediate digital pressure is necessary. The wound is opened and may require the clavicle/sternum to be split for access. Prior to repair, the injured vessel should be exposed both above and below the breach to allow vascular clamps to be applied if necessary. Unless the surgeon is skilled at vascular anastomosis, a vascular surgeon should be called for help. The vessel injury is then sutured, patched, grafted, or ligated. Other potential intraoperative complications include development of a false passage, pneumomediastinum, pneumothorax, esophageal perforation, and recurrent laryngeal nerve injury.

Early Postoperative Complications

Minor bleeding can often be controlled with light packing. If this is not successful, the patient is returned to the operating room for adequate hemostasis.

Subcutaneous emphysema. This may indicate partial tube dislodgement or simply be due to a tight wound closure. Correct tube position needs to be established by fiberoptic endoscopic evaluation of the airway or by chest X-ray. All patients should undergo a postoperative chest X-ray, to exclude a pneumothorax and pneumomediastinum.

Airway obstruction. Clots, secretions, or tube displacement may occur, especially in the first 24 hours following tracheostomy. Close monitoring of vital signs, regular suctioning, humidification, and inner cannula cleaning will reduce the possibility of this complication.

Accidental decannulation. This may result from an inappropriately sized tube or an incorrect tracheostomy incision. Securing the tracheotomy with sutures and ties will minimize the risks of dislodgement. Ties must be loose enough to allow two fingers to slip beneath them and are best secured when the patient's neck is flexed or in the neutral position. A stay suture at the level of the second tracheal ring will help to pull the trachea forward and facilitate recannulation in case of early accidental decannulation. Although our unit does not use Björk flaps, there is evidence in the literature that they are not associated with fistula formation, tracheal stenosis, or cosmetically unacceptable scarring (42).

Early tracheostomy tube change or replacement. Early tracheostomy tube change or replacement of a dislodged tube can result in pneumothorax or even death. No attempt should be made to change a tracheostomy tube without good light, suction, a range of tracheostomy tubes, and a tracheal dilator. Passing a catheter into the airway prior to removing the tracheostomy tube will serve as a guide to locating the airway in the event of tissue collapse into the wound.

Late Postoperative Complications

Innominate artery erosion or major vessel hemorrhage occurs in approximately 0.4–4.5% of cases (43). Correct tube placement between the second and third tracheal rings should prevent this complication. Visible pulsations of the tracheostomy tube may signal an impending innominate artery erosion. A sentinel bleed may precede the massive event and should prompt early evaluation of the wound, often including angiography. In the event of a massive acute hemorrhage, immediate inflation of the tube with digital pressure on the anterior tracheal wall may control the bleed while the patient is urgently taken to the operating area (44). A sternotomy is performed and the vessel repaired or ligated. In some cases the bleeding may come from the inferior thyroid artery, which should be accessible once the cervical incision is explored.

Subglottic or tracheal stenosis. This is likely in patients following prolonged endotracheal intubation, a high tracheostomy, percutaneous tracheotomy, or cricothyroidotomy (45,46). Inappropriate tube size, traumatic intubation, diabetes, and any factor that impairs wound healing are other etiological factors. In select cases, laser excision, dilatation, or stenting may be definitive forms of therapy depending on the site, degree of the stenosis, and the medical condition of the patient. Resection of the stenotic segment with a primary end-to-end anastomosis may be feasible for stenotic segments up to 4 cm in length (47) and generally has a good functional outcome (48). Risk factors for anastomotic complications include re-operation, diabetes, resection greater than 4 cm, laryngotracheal resection, age (17 years or younger), and need for tracheostomy preoperatively (49).

Tracheo-esophageal fistula. This is a rare occurrence (0.01%) and is caused by pressure necrosis from an over-inflated and often malpositioned tube (50,51). A nasogastric tube often contributes to the development of a fistula by causing post-cricoid ulceration (52). Diagnosis is confirmed with methylene blue swallow and fiberoptic examination.

Conservative management, with enteral or parenteral nutrition may be an adequate form of therapy if aspiration is minimal. The principles of surgical repair involve closing the esophagus in two layers, excising the necrotic trachea and performing an end-to-end anastomosis via a cervical incision. A local regional or free flap may be needed for tissue cover. In the pediatric population, endoscopic management of recurrent tracheoesophageal fistula has shown good results (53).

Wound Infections
General Considerations

The head and neck cancer patient is predisposed to the development of wound infection due to a number of preoperative factors such as malnutrition, prior radiation, anemia, chronic infection, advanced age, extensive tumor mass, and medical factors such as diabetes (37,54).

Careful preoperative planning is essential to try to minimize the risk of infection. Adequate nutritional support; attention to dental hygiene; and elimination of any foci of infection in the head and neck region, respiratory system, or elsewhere are important preoperative measures.

Preventative Measures

Careful skin preparation, along with draping and maintenance of sterility at all times should reduce the risk of wound infection. Incisions must be placed along relaxed skin tension lines or creases where possible. A number of surgical principles help to minimize infection, including atraumatic tissue handling, judicious use of cautery, maintaining viability of skin flaps by regular moistening with saline or water, wound irrigation, and careful placement of wound drains.

Planning incisions. Knowledge of the vascular supply of the neck is fundamental to avoiding flap ischemia or loss (55). A curvilinear incision, which can be extended by dropping a vertical limb provides excellent exposure and cosmesis. Knowledge of the dose and fields of any prior radiation therapy will facilitate a prudent choice of skin incision. It is vital to include the platysma in the skin flap because it carries the blood supply to the overlying skin. A trifurcation point should be placed well posterior to the carotid, reducing the risk of vessel exposure in the event of flap necrosis (Fig. 27.5).

Prophylactic antibiotics. Prophylactic antibiotics in adequate dosage and at the appropriate time should diminish the likelihood of sepsis. Best results are achieved when administered immediately before, during, and for 24–48 hours after surgery (56). A number of studies have demonstrated the non-efficacy of perioperative antibiotics in clean head and neck surgery. Many surgeons continue to use prophylactic antibiotics in this setting as the cost-benefit of preventing even a small number of wound infections is enormous. It is our practice to routinely use prophylactic antibiotics (a third generation cephalosporin) in clean wounds that have been previously irradiated or when dealing with malignant disease. There is a 20–30% risk of developing a wound infection when the upper aerodigestive tract is breached (clean-contaminated wound) justifying the use of antibiotics during this period (57). It is our practice to use

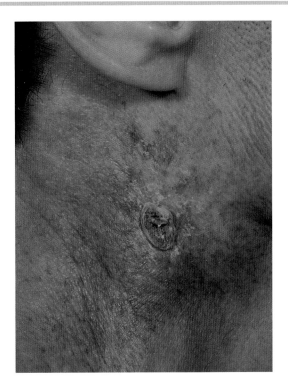

Figure 27.5 Radionecrotic breakdown of skin incision overlying the carotid artery after a radical neck dissection and post-operative radiotherapy.

a cephalosporin combined with metronidazole, which provides broad spectrum anaerobic cover in this setting.

Management

Many patients develop erythema and induration of the skin especially when previous radiation has been administered. Often this resolves over a number of days and does not progress to wound dehiscence. When the latter arises the principles of care involve regular sterile dressings, wound culture, appropriate antibiotic therapy, and attention to nutritional support. Extensive tissue loss may require a skin graft, or a myocutaneous or free flap for cover.

ORAL CAVITY

General Considerations

Cancer of the oral cavity accounts for approximately 30% of head and neck carcinomas. Surgical intervention ranges from simple excision with minimal morbidity to composite resection with its attendant complications. With large resections, speech and swallowing problems are common. This is as a result of reduced tongue mobility, intra-oral sensation and mandibular-support.

Mandibular osteotomy has become the preferred method of access for the majority of large oral cavity and oropharyngeal tumors (58,59). The improved exposure provided by this technique greatly facilitates surgical resection from these sites. Previous reports from our institution have described the complications following this procedure and outlined possible technical aspects to avoid or reduce their

incidence (60,61). Evidence regarding the most stable fixation with plating systems leans towards low-profile locking plates (62), although not all reports have shown a significant advantage over non-locking plates (63). Increased stability is associated with better healing and a lower risk of complications.

Fistula formation and wound dehiscence continue to prolong hospital stay, occasionally leading to plate exposure and subsequent surgical intervention. Postoperative sepsis related to the osteotomy site is reported to be from 13% to 21% (64,65).

Previous authors have attempted to identify factors that may predispose to mandibulotomy sepsis although no consensus has been reached as to the precise cause. Preoperative irradiation and type of fixation (wire or plate) does not appear to influence the incidence of sepsis although most studies have been retrospective in nature (66,67). Patients who undergo step osteotomy as opposed to linear cuts, and those who have a marginal mandibulectomy in combination with the resection are not at an increased risk of infection (68). Failure to achieve a watertight mucosal closure adjacent to the mandibulotomy site, even when utilizing a free flap to reconstruct the defect, is an important factor. A parasymphyseal or midline osteotomy is preferable to a more lateral osteotomy.

Orocutaneous Fistula

Management is similar to that of a pharyngocutaneous fistula: conservative, local, pedicled, or free tissue transfer. The majority of orocutaneous fistulas respond to conservative measures, except those extending over the carotid artery, or those where wound healing has failed, especially in previously irradiated wounds (Fig. 27.6). Fresh vascularized

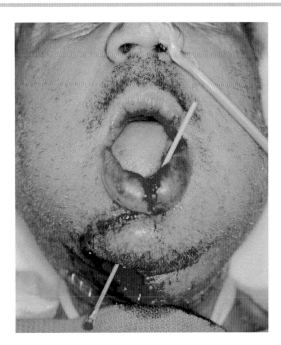

Figure 27.6 Orocutaneous fistula following composite resection and free flap repair in a previously irradiated patient.

tissue is needed in these situations. Other complications associated with mandibulotomy are dental injury, malunion, delayed union or non-union, and neural injuries.

Dental Injury

Osteotomy involving a tooth root predisposes to infection, tooth loss, and instability of the mandibulotomy site. A tooth extraction may be necessary intraoperatively when teeth are too close together. The osteotomy can be performed through the gap to prevent these complications. Care must be taken to ensure the plate is positioned below the tooth roots to avoid injury with screws. Any patient who may require radiotherapy as part of their management must have a dental assessment. Dental prophylaxis before surgery will reduce the likelihood of dental sepsis contributing to postoperative problems.

Problems with Union

Failure to accurately oppose the mandibular fragments, or inadequate immobilization, may predispose to a failure of bony union. This may lead to plate or mandible exposure. It is our practice to use a six- or eight-hole 2.4-mm titanium reconstruction plate and tension band splint with either a micro-plate or wire to ensure immobilization of the mandibular fragments following a parasymphyseal or midline mandibulotomy. A gastrostomy or nasogastric tube is used until the oral mucosa is well healed. This may take 10 days or more to prevent wound dehiscence.

Paraesthesia

Osteotomy lateral to the mental foramen is avoided as it causes anesthesia to the ipsilateral lower lip and gums. When the mandible is well realigned many patients recover sensation after three to six months.

Osteoradionecrosis

The reported incidence of osteoradionecrosis is 2–22% following radiation to the mandible or maxilla (69). Osteoradionecrosis is a serious complication of radiotherapy used to treat head and neck cancer and varies considerably in severity (Fig. 27.7). No single treatment modality has been entirely successful.

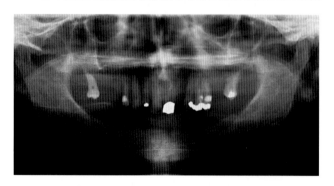

Figure 27.7   Osteoradionecrosis of the mandible.

Prevention

Patients must undergo a dental evaluation prior to therapy. Pre-radiotherapy extraction reduces the risk of osteoradionecrosis (66). Generally, teeth in the primary field of radiation that show periapical or periodontal disease and that are unlikely to be viable following radiotherapy are extracted (71). A combination of meticulous dental care and intensity-modulated radiotherapy are likely to contribute to a reduction in osteoradionecrosis (72,73).

Management

Acute infection is treated with broad spectrum antibiotics, analgesia, oral hygiene, and by avoiding irritants such as tobacco smoke and alcohol. Sequestrectomy, antibiotic treatment, and hyperbaric oxygen may benefit some patients with less extensive symptoms and/or disease state. The benefit of hyperbaric oxygen, however, is not obvious (74). Patients with intractable pain, trismus, and persistent infection, despite conservative treatment are candidates for major surgical resection. The surgical choice of reconstruction is thought to depend, at least in part, on the type of radiation that induced the osteoradionecrosis (75). Conservative management should be limited to early-onset osteoradionecrosis after brachytherapy with or without a low dose of external irradiation. Marginal mandibulectomy is appropriate for the late-onset osteoradionecrosis after brachytherapy with or without low-dose external irradiation. Segmental mandibulectomy is required for late-onset osteoradionecrosis after a high dose of external irradiation (75).

SALIVARY GLANDS
Parotidectomy
Facial Nerve Paralysis

The reported incidence of temporary paralysis is approximately 30% and permanent paralysis less than 0.5% following superficial parotidectomy (76). The risk to the nerve is increased when total parotidectomy is performed for large tumors or for malignant disease, especially with nerve involvement (77). Over 90% of temporary injuries resolve within 12 months. Apart from the severe psychological sequelae associated with total paralysis, eye function, mastication, and emotional response are also impaired.

Prevention. The anesthetist should avoid using a long-acting muscle relaxant to allow stimulation of neural tissue as the dissection proceeds. A wide surgical exposure using a modified "Blair" incision is used. Tissue landmarks for the nerve are employed to avoid inadvertent injury and include (1) the tragal pointer—the nerve is located 1 cm below and medial to this cartilaginous pointer; (2) the posterior belly of the digastric serves as a guide to the plane of the nerve; (3) the mastoid bone and tympanomastoid suture—the nerve is 6–8 mm medial to this landmark; (4) when the nerve cannot be identified by an antegrade approach, it may be possible to find a peripheral branch and trace it back to the main trunk.

Technical considerations. Once the nerve is identified it diverges laterally to the mid-gland region and the surgeon must be cognizant of this as dissection proceeds in the plane above the nerve. A nerve stimulator, initially set at 0.5 mA, is used to confirm identification. Repeated stimulation increases the likelihood of neuropraxia postoperatively. During mobilization bipolar cautery tips must be visualized at all times to avoid thermal trauma. No blind attempts are made to control bleeding and no undue pressure or traction must be placed on the nerve. Continuous facial nerve monitoring may be beneficial for large tumors, revision procedures, and malignant lesions. There is no obvious predictive benefit of intraoperative facial nerve monitoring (78). Operating loupes are used by some surgeons and may help preserve smaller peripheral branches.

Management. Unintentional division of any portion of the nerve should be followed by immediate microsurgical reanastomosis with 9-0 or 10-0 monofilament suture. Coaption must be precise and free from tension. An interposition nerve graft with sural, greater auricular, or lateral cutaneous nerve should be considered in cases where the nerve has to be sacrificed and primary reanastomosis is not an option.

All patients with facial paralysis must have appropriate eye care when the branch to the orbicularis oris has been damaged. Eye moisturizers, lubricants, and taping the eye at night will prevent corneal desiccation. An ophthalmology consultation should be obtained if any complication such as keratitis or corneal ulceration is suspected. The management of permanent facial nerve paralysis may require dynamic procedures such as interposition nerve graft, facial hypoglossal anastomosis, cross-face nerve transfer, masseter or temporalis muscle transfer to improve facial function. Adynamic procedures using gold-weighted implants for ocular rehabilitation, Gortex implants, facial slings, rhytidectomy, brow lifts, and blepharoplasty may also be helpful. The patient must be aware that it is not possible to restore complete facial function and the goal should be to improve the existing situation.

Other complications following parotidectomy include hemorrhage, infection, flap necrosis, symptomatic Frey's syndrome, and rarely salivary fistula.

Submandibular Gland
Hemorrhage
Intraoperative hemorrhage from the facial artery and veins can be troublesome unless care is taken during identification and ligation. Postoperative hematoma formation can lead to displacement of the tongue and airway compromise.

Neural Injury
Injury to the marginal mandibular branch of the facial nerve can be avoided by planning the incision 2 cm below the angle of the mandible and preserving the nerve as previously described. Lingual nerve trauma fortunately is rare, but results in loss of sensation to the anterior two-thirds of the tongue. The nerve lies deep to the mylohyoid muscle and can be identified once the muscle is retracted anteriorly. When dividing the submandibular ganglion the ligature should be placed away from the nerve to avoid injury. Hypoglossal nerve injury is rare and is best avoided by careful dissection and identification during mobilization.

SKULL BASE

Over the past two decades a multidisciplinary approach involving otolaryngologists, neurosurgeons, and plastic surgeons has evolved in the management of skull-base tumors. This has resulted in a reduction in postoperative morbidity and an increase in the number of these procedures being performed worldwide. Central to this development has been the introduction of improved, safer methods of access to the skull base coupled with an ability to reconstruct large defects with microvascular free flaps.

Complications involving these procedures may be catastrophic for the patient intraoperatively or postoperatively. The overall complication rate may be as high as 33% and may be infectious, neurovascular, or related to cranial nerve trauma. Cerebrospinal fluid (CSF) leakage and meningitis are the most common complications to arise.

Cerebrospinal Fluid Leakage
CSF leakage may arise following anterior skull-base resection, lateral skull-base resection, post-transsphenoidal hypophysectomy, or maxillectomy. The identification of the anatomical site of CSF rhinorrhoea may be difficult especially when intermittent in nature (79). Unrecognized CSF leakage can result in meningitis and possibly death (80). The overall risk of meningitis in patients with CSF rhinorrhoea was found to be 19% (81).

Diagnosis
When the leak is profuse and clear the diagnosis is obvious. Often a small and intermittent leak may be overlooked or misinterpreted when mixed throughout nasal secretions. Collection of nasal discharge for a "halo sign" on a cotton sheet or glucose content of greater than 30 mg/ml has traditionally been regarded as diagnostic of cerebrospinal fluid (82). There is a high incidence of false positive results due to contamination of fluid with lacrimal secretions and blood. Now the diagnosis is made with a beta-2 transferrin assay. This provides a highly sensitive, selective, rapid, and non-invasive test for the detection of CSF leakage (83–85). Equally important is the demonstration of an absence of beta-transferrin, which obviates the need for further investigation and/or surgical intervention.

Investigations
Intrathecal tracers, fluorescein, metrizamide, and gamma cameras with a radioisotope tracer (radioactive cisternography, RIC) have been utilized to detect the source of the leak when not obvious (86,87). Contrast CT cisternography (CCTC) has now replaced RIC yet both are invasive, time consuming, and often insensitive. Recently MRI cisternography has been used to locate the precise site of CSF fistulas (88). Compared with other techniques, MRI cisternography is fast, non-invasive, and carries no apparent risk to the patient. The demonstration of a high signal through the cribriform plate and paranasal sinuses, which is continuous and similar to that of CSF in the basal cisterns, is considered to be diagnostic of a fistula.

Prevention
Prevention of leaks may be difficult especially when dura is deliberately resected. In such circumstances the area must be carefully repaired primarily or with local or distant tissue because contamination with bacteria from the nasal cavity or sinonasal tract will result in meningitis.

Management

Conservative treatment consists of bed rest, laxatives, avoiding raising intracranial pressure by nose blowing or straining, and antibiotics. CSF-penetrating antibiotics are widely used although it is controversial whether the risk of meningitis is reduced (89). A lumbar drain may also be beneficial particularly when dealing with a vigorous leak. The patient is kept supine and CSF pressure maintained between 10 and 15 cmH$_2$O. Persistence of leakage beyond seven to ten days necessitates surgical intervention.

Leaks occurring from the pneumatized temporal bone are best managed by obliterating the mastoid space with fascia, abdominal fat, or a local temporalis muscle flap. To prevent CSF entering the eustachian tube the middle ear should be sealed from the mastoid antrum. Clivus leaks may require a free vascularized flap (e.g., rectus abdominis) to adequately seal the defect.

Anterior skull-base leaks may be repaired via an extracranial or intracranial approach. A leak accessible through the nose may be repaired transnasally either under direct vision or endoscopically (81). Fibrin glue, fat, fascia lata, and local flaps may be used to seal the defect. A successful closure in 70–80% of patients can be achieved with a transnasal repair.

Despite these excellent results it is estimated that 30–40% of all fistulas will recur after initial therapy. This failure may be due to an inadequate initial repair, a true recurrence at the original site, and/or leakage from another site on the skull base. The beta-trace protein test for postoperative screening and confirmation of dura repair success has been employed successfully and in some centers is considered the gold-standard (90).

Meningitis

Meningitis is a major cause of postoperative morbidity. Prolonged surgery, CSF leakage, and contamination with the bacterial flora of the upper aerodigestive tract are contributing factors. The use of broad spectrum antibiotics, a watertight reconstruction of the dura when feasible, and surgical precautions to minimize the potential for contaminating the operative field are vital preventative measures. Any patient with alteration in mental status, progressive headache, and persistent pyrexia not attributable to other sources should have this diagnosis suspected. Cerebrospinal fluid must be sampled by a lumbar puncture to confirm the diagnosis.

Pneumocephalus

Pneumocephalus is more commonly seen after anterior skull-base resection and becomes significant when air becomes trapped and continues to accumulate, resulting in raised intracranial pressure and displacement of intracranial contents.

Prevention

Preventative measures include complete sealing of breached dura, avoiding lumbar drains, and performing a tracheostomy to prevent air being diverted intracranially with coughing or sneezing.

Management

Needle aspiration via a frontal burr hole may suffice. Re-exploration of the wound and tacking the pericranial flap forward, and/or re-suturing the dura may be necessary if the patient continues to deteriorate.

Cranial Nerve Injury

The location of the tumor dictates which nerves are likely to be injured. Olfaction is lost when the frontal lobes are retracted during anterior skull-base approaches. Surgery in proximity to the cavernous sinus and petrous apex is likely to damage the III–IV, V, and VI cranial nerves.

The facial nerve is injured typically in lateral skull-base and posterior fossa surgery. Manipulation should be minimal when preservation of neural function is the goal. Cranial nerves IX, X, and XII are at risk during dissection of tumors near the lower clivus and foramen magnum. With benign tumors it is usually possible to dissect and preserve the nerve. Advances in intraoperative monitoring have resulted in increased neural preservation. The most devastating neuropathies occur following lateral skull-base surgery involving the lower cranial nerves IX, X, and XII.

Cerebral Edema, Infarction, and Hemorrhage

These are other potential causes of postoperative deterioration in mental status. Carotid artery vasospasm may occur especially with lateral skull-base surgery, leading to a fatal cerebrovascular accident. Significant edema and infarction are best avoided by minimal brain retraction. Epidural or subdural bleeds are evacuated unless collections are small.

Epidural Abscess Formation

This may occur in the early postoperative period or several weeks later. Acute neurological deficit is the usual presentation. Infected bone may be a contributing factor and exploration with removal is indicated. Other infectious complications include osteomyelitis and frontal sinusitis.

RECONSTRUCTIVE COMPLICATIONS
Skin Grafts

The principal complications of skin grafts are caused by hematoma formation or inadequate stabilization, which may lead to graft failure or infection. It is important to ensure adequate hemostasis and applying a graft of suitable thickness helps to prevent these complications. To minimize graft movement, adaptic gauze with saline/acriflavin-soaked cotton wool secured with a tie over the dressing was previously used; however we presently use Allevyn to maintain graft position.

Local Flaps

Errors in design or technical factors are responsible for most local flap failures. Blood supply entering the base of the flap may be altered by previous surgery or radiation (Fig. 27.8). Use of skin hooks, avoiding compression, and introducing the flap into a dry recipient bed are technical points that help maintain viability. Basing a flap inferiorly is worthwhile for facial flaps as this facilitates venous drainage. When rotation or transposition flaps require cut-backs, enough

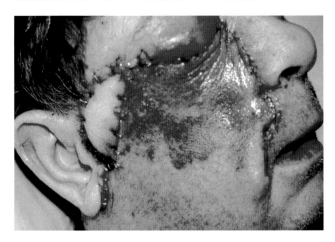

Figure 27.8 Failed transposition flap in a previously irradiated patient.

width must be preserved to avoid flap ischemia. Excessive tension on the distal aspect of the flap must also be avoided.

Postoperatively the wound should be kept moist with a topical antibiotic that helps remove nonviable tissue and uncovers healthy tissue.

Pedicled Myocutaneous Flaps

A thorough knowledge of the vascular supply of any myocutaneous flap is essential prior to elevation. Partial or complete flap necrosis may occur. Generally complete flap loss occurs in less than 10% of most series (Fig. 27.9) (91,92).

Prevention of Complications

Separating the loosely attached skin and subcutaneous tissue from the underlying muscle by shearing can avulse an already tenuous blood supply. Avoid inwardly bevelled skin incisions, which tend to compromise the skin paddle. The vascular pedicle must be identified and preserved. Kinking must be avoided, and when insetting the flap there should be no undue compression from skin flaps, tracheostomy ties, or other factors, such as the mandible or reconstruction plates.

In the postoperative period, the patient should be nursed head-up without compressive dressings. Wound drains help to prevent hematoma and flap compromise. Prompt debridement of any areas of skin necrosis prevents infection and potential loss to the underlying muscle. Bleeding, seroma, and fistulization are other potential sequelae.

Free Flaps

Over the past decade microvascular free flaps have become widely utilized in head and neck surgery. Presently, cosmetic and functional restoration is the goal following major ablative resection. Certain flaps such as the radial forearm, the anterolateral thigh, fibula, and scapula have reasonably reliable vascular pedicles and are valuable reconstructive options in head and neck surgery. Factors known to impair flap survival other than technique include prior irradiation, smoking, atherosclerosis, diabetes, advanced age, and sepsis (93).

Increasing age within a patient group has been correlated with an increased American Society of Anesthesiologists (ASA) Classification of Physical Status score, which correlated with a greater risk of postoperative medical complications (94,95). Age did not correlate, however, with postoperative surgical complications, including free-flap complications (94,95). Interestingly, it has been shown that postoperative medical complications in elderly and medically

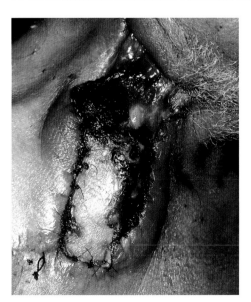

(A)

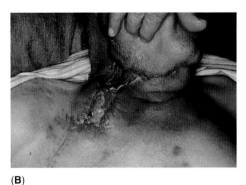

(B)

Figure 27.9 (A) Latissimus dorsi pedicled flap with partial loss of skin only. (B) Healing by granulation on a viable muscular bed.

debilitated patients, specifically with regard to both pulmonary problems and alcohol withdrawal, were significantly more important in terms of financial cost, than microsurgical costs in this group of reconstructive patients (96).

Technical Considerations

Loss of vascular perfusion or venous congestion is the main complication associated with free flaps. Donor and recipient vessels must be adequate prior to flap transfer as reanastomosis has to be speedy to prevent flap loss due to ischemia. Free jejunal flaps are particularly sensitive to ischemia (Fig. 27.1). When a vein graft is needed it should be prepared prior to dividing the vascular pedicle. Once revascularized, considerable bleeding may arise from the flap and hematoma formation must be avoided.

Checking Viability

In the postoperative period flap viability is checked visually and with Doppler. Color, bleeding to pin-prick, and capillary refill are inexpensive, simple, and reliable methods of flap monitoring. Other objective methods include measuring heat, pH, intra-flap blood pressure (BP), light absorbancy, CO_2/O_2 content and fluorescein dye inspection with a Wood's light (97,98). General flap viability can be determined by visual inspection by an experienced observer. Arterial insufficiency is recognized clinically by a flap that is cool to touch, white, and non-blanching. Venous insufficiency is more common and gives the flap a bluish appearance; it also causes swelling and dark bleeding on pin-prick testing. Vasodilators and low-molecular-weight dextrans have been used with little evidence of success in a case of impending flap compromise. Prompt re-exploration and revision is crucial because most flaps fail to recover after 10–12 hours of ischemia. Revision has a quoted success rate of 60–83% (98). Although a more realistic figure is approximately 50%. Color flow Doppler ultrasonography has been shown to be useful in postoperative monitoring of head and neck free tissue transfer (99). Buried free flaps are more problematic and can be monitored using an implantable 20-MHz ultrasonic Doppler probe. The implantable Doppler probe has been shown to be a sensitive method for postoperative monitoring of free flaps but is prone to false-positive signals. The use of color duplex sonography to confirm implantable Doppler probe findings can reduce unnecessary surgical exploration, thereby improving postoperative monitoring of free flaps (100).

Thrombosed vessels require resection on either side of the anastomosis (101). Once normal vessel wall is reached and good blood flow is re-established, a reanastomosis can be performed. Flushing the arterial or venous ends with heparinized saline helps to remove thrombus. Occasionally, an interpositional vein graft or cephalic vein mobilization is necessary to avoid excessive anastomotic tension.

Early free flap failure and other immediate postoperative complications have been correlated to the preoperative (Acute Physiology and Chronic Health Evaluation) APACHE II score (102). Late free flap failure can be defined as failure after the seventh postoperative day. In one study with 1530 patients, the late failure rate was less than 1%, occurring between day 7 and 90 (median day 21) (103). The etiology for the delayed flap failure is thought to include pressure on the pedicle, infection (abscess formation), and re-growth of residual tumor (103).

REFERENCES

1. Brown DH, Mulholland S, Yoo JH et al. Internal jugular vein thrombosis following modified neck dissection: implications for head and neck reconstruction. Head Neck 1998; 20: 169–74.
2. Harada H, Omura K, Takeuchi Y. Patency and caliber of the internal jugular vein after neck dissection. Auris Nasus Larynx 2003; 30: 269–72.
3. Tobin HA. Increased cerebrospinal fluid pressure following unilateral radical neck dissection. Laryngoscope 1972; 82: 817–20.
4. Weiss KL, Wax MK, Haydon RC III et al. Intracranial pressure changes during bilateral radical neck dissections. Head Neck 1993; 15: 546–52.
5. Cleland-Zamudio SS, Wax MK, Smith JD et al. Ruptured internal jugular vein: a postoperative complication of modified/selected neck dissection. Head Neck 2003; 25: 357–60.
6. Sekhar L, Sen C, Jho H. Saphenous vein graft bypass of the cavernous carotid artery. J Neurosurg 1990; 72: 35–41.
7. Rice JH, Gonzalez RM. Large visible gas bubbles in the internal jugular vein: a common occurrence during supine radical neck surgery? J Clin Anesth 1992; 4: 21–4.
8. Stell PK. Catastrophic haemorrhage after major neck surgery. Br J Surg 1969; 56: 525.
9. Moore OS, Baker HW. Carotid artery ligation in surgery of the head and neck. Cancer 1955; 8: 712.
10. Erba S, Horton J, Latchaw R et al. Balloon test occlusion of the internal carotid artery with stable xenon/CT cerebral flow imaging. AJNR 1989; 9: 533–8.
11. Atkinson D, Jacobs L, Weaver A. Elective carotid resection for squamous cell carcinoma of the head and neck. Am J Surg 1984; 148: 483–8.
12. Oleott C, Fee WE, Enzmenn DR et al. Planned approach to the management of malignant invasion of the carotid artery. Am J Surg 1981; 142: 123–5.
13. Rodriguez F, Carmeci C, Dalman RL et al. Spontaneous late carotid-cutaneous fistula following radical neck dissection: a case report. Vasc Surg. 2001; 35: 409–13.
14. Leipzig B, Suen JY, English JL et al. Functional evaluation of the spinal accessory nerve after neck dissection. Am J Surg 1983; 146: 526–30.
15. London J, London NJ, Kay SP. Iatrogenic accessory nerve injury. Ann R Coll Surg Engl 1996; 78: 146–50.
16. Tubbs RS, Loukas M, Salter EG et al. Wilhelm Erb and Erb's Point. Clinical Anatomy 2007; 20: 486–8.
17. Weisberger EC, Lingemen RE. Cable grafting of the spinal accessory nerve for rehabilitation of shoulder function after radical neck dissection. Laryngoscope 1987; 97: 915–18.
18. Chandawarkar RY, Cervino AL, Pennington GA. Management of iatrogenic injury to the spinal accessory nerve. Plast Reconstr Surg 2003; 111: 611–17.
19. Isshiki N, Taira T, Kojima H et al. Recent modifications in thyroplasty type I. Ann Otol Rhinol Laryngol 1989; 98: 777–9.
20. Motoyoshi K, Hyodo M, Yamagata T et al. Restoring vocal fold movement after transection and immediate suturing of the recurrent laryngeal nerve with local application of basic fibroblast growth factor: an experimental study in the rat. Laryngoscope 2004; 114: 1247–52.
21. Kingham PJ, Hughes A, Mitchard L et al. Effect of neurotrophin-3 on reinnervation of the larynx using the phrenic nerve transfer technique. Eur J Neurosci 2007; 25: 331–40.
22. Woodson GE. Spontaneous laryngeal reinnervation after recurrent laryngeal or vagus nerve injury. Ann Otol Rhinol Laryngol 2007; 116: 57–65.
23. Shahzadi S, Abouzari M, Rashidi A. Bilateral traumatic hypoglossal nerve transection in a blast injury. Surg Neurol 2007; 68: 464–5.

24. Merav AD, Attai LA, Condit DD. Successful repair of a transected phrenic nerve with restoration of diaphragmatic function. Chest 1983; 84: 642–4.
25. Yoshitani M, Fukuda S, Itoi S et al. Experimental repair of phrenic nerve using a polyglycolic acid and collagen tube. J Thorac Cardiovasc Surg 2007; 133: 726–32.
26. Conley JJ. Operative complications. In: Complications in head and neck surgery. Philadelphia: WB Saunders, 1977; 25–36.
27. Raguse JD, Pfitzmann R, Bier J et al. Lower-extremity lymphedema following neck dissection—an uncommon complication after cervical ligation of the thoracic duct. Oral Oncol 2007; 43: 835–7.
28. Kassel RN, Havas TE, Gullane PJ. The use of topical tetracycline in the management of persistent chylous fistulae. J Otolaryngol 1987; 16: 174–8.
29. Bejarano Glez-Serna D, Utrera-Glez A, Cordoncillo-Prieto JM et al. Chyle fistula. Medical management with octreotide. Cir Esp 2006; 79: 250–1.
30. Crumley RL, Smith JD. Postoperative chylous fistula prevention and management. Laryngoscope 1976; 86: 804–13.
31. Kent RB, Pinson TW. Thorascopic ligation of the thoracic duct. Surg Endosc 1993; 7: 52–5.
32. Gunnlaugsson CB, Iannettoni MD, Yu B et al. Management of chyle fistula utilizing thoracoscopic ligation of the thoracic duct. ORL J Otorhinolaryngol Relat Spec 2004; 66: 148–54.
33. Giordano AM, Adams GL. Pharyngocutaneous fistula after laryngeal surgery. Otolaryngol Head Neck Surg 1984; 92: 19–23.
34. Gullane PJ, Jabbour JN, Conley JJ et al. Correlation of pharyngeal fistulization with preoperative radiotherapy, reduced serum albumin and dietary obstruction. Otolaryngol Head Neck Surg 1979; 87: 311–17.
35. Boscolo-Rizzo P, De Cillis G, Marchiori C et al. Multivariate analysis of risk factors for pharyngocutaneous fistula after total laryngectomy. Eur Arch Otorhinolaryngol 2008; 265: 929–36.
36. Sassler AM, Esclamado RM, Wolf GT. Surgery after organ preservation therapy. Analysis of wound complications. Arch Otolaryngol Head Neck Surg 1995; 121: 162–5.
37. Ganly I, Patel S, Matsuo J et al. Postoperative complications of salvage total laryngectomy. Cancer 2005; 103: 2073–81.
38. Fung K, Teknos TN, Vandenberg CD et al. Prevention of wound complications following salvage laryngectomy using free vascularized tissue. Head Neck 2007; 29: 425–30.
39. Withrow KP, Rosenthal EL, Gourin CG et al. Free tissue transfer to manage salvage laryngectomy defects after organ preservation failure. Laryngoscope 2007; 117: 781–4.
40. Magdy EA. Surgical closure of postlaryngectomy pharyngocutaneous fistula: a defect based approach. Eur Arch Otorhinolaryngol 2008; 265: 97–104.
41. Iteld L, Yu P. Pharyngocutaneous fistula repair after radiotherapy and salvage total laryngectomy. J Reconstr Microsurg 2007; 23: 339–45.
42. Malata CM, Foo IT, Simpson KH et al. An audit of Björk flap tracheostomies in head and neck plastic surgery. Br J Oral Maxillofac Surg 1996; 34: 42–6.
43. Schlaepfer K. Fatal haemorrhage following tracheostomy for laryngeal diphtheria. JAMA 1924; 82: 1581–2.
44. Myers WO, Lawton BR, Santter RD. An operation for tracheal-innominate fistula. Arch Surg 1972; 105: 269–74.
45. Esses BA, Jakek BW. Cricothyroidotomy: a decade of experience in Denver. Ann Otol Rhinol Laryngol 1987; 96: 519–24.
46. Christenson TE, Artz GJ, Goldhammer JE et al. Tracheal stenosis after placement of percutaneous dilational tracheotomy. Laryngoscope 2008; 118: 222–7.
47. Maddaus MA, Toth JL, Gullane PJ et al. Subglottic tracheal resection and synchronous laryngeal reconstruction. J Thorac Cardiovasc Surg 1992; 104: 1443–50.
48. George M, Lang F, Pasche P et al. Surgical management of laryngotracheal stenosis in adults. Eur Arch Otorhinolaryngol 2005; 262: 609–15.
49. Wright CD, Grillo HC, Wain JC et al. Anastomotic complications after tracheal resection: prognostic factors and management. J Thorac Cardiovasc Surg 2004; 128: 731–9.
50. Thomas AN. Management of tracheoesophageal fistula caused by cuffed tracheal tubes. Am J Surg 1972; 124: 181–7.
51. Mooty RC, Rath P, Self M et al. Review of tracheo-esophageal fistula associated with endotracheal intubation. J Surg Educ 2007; 64: 237–40.
52. Freidman M, Bairn H, Shelton V et al. Laryngeal injuries secondary to nasogastric tubes. Ann Otol 1981; 90: 469–474.
53. Richter GT, Ryckman F, Brown RL et al. Endoscopic management of recurrent tracheoesophageal fistula. J Pediatr Surg 2008; 43: 238–45.
54. Hooley R, Levine H, Flores TC et al. Predicting postoperative head and neck complications using nutritional assessment: the prognostic nutritional index. Arch Otolaryngol 1983; 107: 725–9.
55. Freeland AP, Rogers JH. The vascular supply of the cervical skin with reference to incision planning. Laryngoscope 1975; 85: 714.
56. Burke JF. The effective period of preventive antibiotic action in experimental incisions and dermal lesions. Surgery 1961; 50: 161.
57. Johnson J, Myers EN, Thearle PB et al. Antimicrobial prophylaxis for contaminated head and neck surgery. Laryngoscope 1984; 94: 46–51.
58. MacGregor IA, McDonald DG. Mandibular osteotomy in the surgical approach to the oral cavity. Head Neck Surg 1983; 5: 457–562.
59. Spiro RH, Gerold FP, Shah JP et al. Mandibulotomy approach to oropharyngeal tumours. Am J Surg 1985; 150: 466–469.
60. Davidson J, Freeman J, Gullane P et al. Mandibulotomy and radical radiotherapy: compatible or not? J Otolaryngol 1988; 17: 279–81.
61. McCann K, Irish J, Gullane P et al. Complications associated with rigid fixation of mandibulotomies. J Otolaryngology 1994; 23: 210–15.
62. Engroff SL, Blanchaert RH Jr, von Fraunhofer JA. Mandibulotomy fixation: a laboratory analysis. J Oral Maxillofac Surg 2003; 61: 1297–301.
63. Chiodo TA, Ziccardi VB, Janal M et al. Failure strength of 2.0 locking versus 2.0 conventional Synthes mandibular plates: a laboratory model. J Oral Maxillofac Surg 2006; 64: 1475–9.
64. Christopoulos E, Carrau R, Segas J et al. Transmandibular approaches to the oral cavity and oropharynx. Arch Otolaryngol 1992; 118: 1164–7.
65. DeSanto LW, Whicker JH, Devine KD. Mandibular osteotomy and lingual flaps. Arch Otolaryngol 1975; 101: 652–5.
66. Bedwinek JM, Shukovsky LJ, Fletcher GH et al. Osteoradionecrosis in patients treated with definitive radiotherapy for squamous cell carcinomas of the oral cavity and naso- and oropharynx. Radiology 1976; 119: 665–7.
67. Nam W, Kim HJ, Choi EC et al. Contributing factors to mandibulotomy complications: a retrospective study. Oral Surg Oral Med Oral Pathol Oral Radiol Endod 2006; 101: e65–70.
68. Dubner S, Spiro R. Median mandibulotomy: a critical assessment. Head Neck 1991; 13: 389–93.
69. Epstein JB, Wong FLW, Stevenson-Moore P. Osteoradionecrosis: clinical experience and a proposal for classification. J Oral Maxillofac Surg 1987; 45: 104–10.
70. Bedwinek JM, Shukovsky LJ, Fletcher GH et al. Osteoradionecrosis in patients treated with definitive radiotherapy for squamous cell carcinomas of the oral cavity and naso- and oropharynx. Radiology 1976; 119: 665–7.

71. Breumer JP, Curtis TA, Firtell DN. Radiation therapy of head and neck tumours. In: Maxillofacial rehabilitation: prosthodontic and surgical considerations. St Louis: Mosby Year Book, 1979; 56–60.

72. Ben-David MA, Diamante M, Radawski JD et al. Lack of osteoradionecrosis of the mandible after intensity-modulated radiotherapy for head and neck cancer: likely contributions of both dental care and improved dose distributions. Int J Radiat Oncol Biol Phys 2007; 68: 396–402.

73. Chang DT, Sandow PR, Morris CG et al. Do pre-irradiation dental extractions reduce the risk of osteoradionecrosis of the mandible? Head Neck 2007; 29: 528–36.

74. D'Souza J, Goru J, Goru S et al. The influence of hyperbaric oxygen on the outcome of patients treated for osteoradionecrosis: 8 year study. Int J Oral Maxillofac Surg 2007; 36: 783–7.

75. Notani K, Yamazaki Y, Kitada H et al. Management of mandibular osteoradionecrosis corresponding to the severity of osteoradionecrosis and the method of radiotherapy. Head Neck 2003; 25: 181–6.

76. MeGurt M, Renahan A, Gleave EM. Clinical significance of the tumour capsule in the treatment of parotid pleomorphic adenomas. Br J Surg 1996; 83: 1747–9.

77. Huang CC, Tseng FY, Chen ZC et al. Malignant parotid tumor and facial palsy. Otolaryngol Head Neck Surg 2007; 136: 778–82.

78. Meier JD, Wenig BL, Manders EC et al. Continuous intraoperative facial nerve monitoring in predicting postoperative injury during parotidectomy. Laryngoscope 2006; 116: 1569–72.

79. Walsh MA, Curran AJ. Cerebrospinal fluid rhinorrhoea. Br J Neurosurg 1997; 11: 189–90.

80. Park J, Streizow VV, Freidman WH. Current management of cerebrospinal fluid rhinorrhoea. Laryngoscope 1983; 93: 1294–300.

81. Daudia A, Biswas D, Jones NS. Risk of meningitis with cerebrospinal fluid rhinorrhea. Ann Otol Rhinol Laryngol 2007; 116: 902–5.

82. Ornmaya AK. Spinal fluid fistulae. Clin Neurosurg 1975; 23: 363–92.

83. Meurman O, Irjala K, Juonpaa J et al. A new method of identification of cerebrospinal fluid leakage. Acta Otolaryngol 1979; 87: 366–9.

84. Ryall RG, Peacock MK, Simpson DA. Usefulness of beta-2 transferrin assay in the detection of cerebrospinal fluid leaks following head injury. J Neurosurg 1992; 77: 737–9.

85. Skedros DG, Cass SP, Hirsch BE et al. Beta-2 transferrin assay in the clinical management of cerebrospinal fluid and perilymphatic leaks. J Otolaryngol 1993; 22: 34–4.

86. Nicklaus P, Dutcher PO, Kido DK et al. New imaging techniques in the diagnosis of cerebrospinal fluid fistula. Laryngoscope 1988; 98: 1065–8.

87. Crowe HJ, Keogh C. The localization of cerebrospinal fluid fistulae. Lancet 1956; ii: 325–7.

88. Eljamel MS, Pidgeon CN, Toland J et al. MRI cisternography, localization of CSF fistulae. Br J Neurol 1994; 8: 433–7.

89. Eljamel MS. Fractures of the middle third of the face and cerebrospinal fluid rhinorrhoea. Br J Neurol 1994; 8: 289–93.

90. Meco C, Arrer E, Oberascher G. Efficacy of cerebrospinal fluid fistula repair: sensitive quality control using the beta-trace protein test. Am J Rhinol 2007; 21: 729–36.

91. Shah JP, Haribhakti V, Loree TR et al. Complications of the pectoralis major myocutaneous flap in head and neck reconstruction. Am J Surg 1990; 160: 352.

92. Biller HF, Baek SM, Lawson W. Pectoralis major myocutaneous island flap in head and neck surgery. Arch Otolaryngol 1981; 107: 23.

93. Leonard A, Brennan M, Colville J. The use of continuous temperature monitoring in the postoperative management of microvascular cases. Br J Plast Surg 1982; 35: 337–42.

94. Ozkan O, Ozgentas HE, Islamoglu K et al. Experiences with microsurgical tissue transfers in elderly patients. Microsurgery. 2005; 25: 390–5.

95. Coskunfirat OK, Chen HC, Spanio S et al. The safety of microvascular free tissue transfer in the elderly population. Plast Reconstr Surg 2005; 115: 771–5.

96. Jones NF, Jarrahy R, Song JI et al. Postoperative medical complications—not microsurgical complications—negatively influence the morbidity, mortality, and true costs after microsurgical reconstruction for head and neck cancer. Plast Reconstr Surg 2007; 119: 2053–60.

97. Dingwall JA, Lord JW. The fluorescein test in the management of tubed flaps. Bull Johns Hopkins Hosp 1943; 73: 129.

98. Goldberg J, Sepka R, Perona B. Laser Doppler flow measurements of common cutaneous donor sites for reconstructive surgery. Plast Reconstr Surg 1990; 85: 58.

99. Khalid AN, Quraishi SA, Zang WA et al. Color Doppler ultrasonography is a reliable predictor of free tissue transfer outcomes in head and neck reconstruction. Otolaryngol Head Neck Surg 2006; 134: 635–8.

100. Rosenberg JJ, Fornage BD, Chevray PM. Monitoring buried free flaps: limitations of the implantable Doppler and use of color duplex sonography as a confirmatory test. Plast Reconstr Surg 2006; 118: 109–13.

101. Tsai TM, Bennett D, Pedersen W. Complications and vascular salvage of free-tissue transfers to the extremities. Plast Reconstr Surg 1988; 82: 1022–6.

102. Grant CA, Dempsey GA, Lowe D et al. APACHE II scoring for the prediction of immediate surgical complications in head and neck cancer patients. Plast Reconstr Surg 2007; 119: 1751–8.

103. Wax MK, Rosenthal E. Etiology of late free flap failures occurring after hospital discharge. Laryngoscope 2007; 117: 1961–3.

28

Principles of Head and Neck Reconstruction

Nitin A Pagedar and Ralph W Gilbert

INTRODUCTION

The recorded history of head and neck reconstructive surgery dates back five millennia with the Edwin Smith papyrus (1), which documented Egyptian techniques for management of wounds of the head and neck. In the intervening time, reconstructive surgery has been propelled forward by the creativity of the discipline's practitioners, utilizing an ever-growing body of anatomic and physiologic information.

The modern practice of head and neck reconstructive surgery is the result of the serial advances made by surgeons the world over: Sushruta, Celsus (2), Branca, Dieffenbach (3), Gillies (4), Bakamjian (5), Taylor (6), Ariyan (7), and Yang (8) are among the many associated with new reconstructive paradigms. These innovations have created an art by which patients with increasingly complex problems can be managed more reliably with better outcomes and less morbidity. This chapter will seek to describe the current state-of-the-art of this continuously evolving field.

GENERAL PRINCIPLES OF RECONSTRUCTION
Wound Healing

The physiology of wound healing is the foundation of head and neck reconstructive surgery. After soft tissue injury, the healing response is characterized by three phases (9). The inflammatory phase is marked by neutrophil and macrophage infiltration, and lasts about four days. The proliferative phase, which lasts through the third post-injury week, is characterized by chronic inflammation, granulation, tissue formation, and fibroblast ingrowth. Finally, the months-long maturational phase results in extensive remodeling of the injured area. The cellular components of each phase are coordinated by a cascade of mediators that include growth factors and interleukins, many of which have been proposed as targets of therapeutic intervention.

As described by Ai-Aql et al. (10), the healing of bony wounds follows a similar pattern, beginning with an inflammatory phase in which mesenchymal stem cells are recruited to the wound bed. The next phase involves the initiation of both endochondral and intramembranous ossification; the latter results in formation of hard callus, while the former occurs in areas of mechanical instability and results in a cartilaginous callus. Subsequent is the phase of primary bone formation, in which cartilage becomes mineralized and replaced by bone. Finally, secondary bone formation transforms primary bone into mature bone with appropriate mechanical properties. The molecular mechanisms behind the phases of repair are the subject of active research.

The effect on wounds of radiotherapy and chemotherapy are increasingly relevant to head and neck surgeons. There are measurable changes in fibroblast function and in small-vessel endothelium after radiotherapy (11), and the resultant alterations in tissue quality are unmistakable in the vast majority of cases. Many surgical series report higher wound-related complication rates in radiated patients (12), but some series report satisfactory wound-related complication rates in radiated or chemoradiated patients (13,14).

There are many reasons why the mechanisms of wound healing are relevant to clinicians. Many wound-related and patient-related factors have been shown to affect the progression of the wound healing response (Table 28.1), and should be taken into account during the preparation of an operative plan. Mechanical instability of bone segments plays an important role in the pattern of healing, with endochondral ossification predominating and resulting in delay of mature bone formation (15). In addition, in the case of soft tissue wounds, the induction of myofibroblasts results in wound contracture, which if not anticipated by the reconstructive surgeon will have profound functional and aesthetic consequences. There are other longer-term alterations of transferred tissue that reconstructive surgeons must anticipate. Non-innervated muscle will atrophy, whereas vascularized subcutaneous fat will not. Nonvascularized bone grafts will not survive in an irradiated field or tolerate adjuvant radiotherapy.

Options for Reconstruction

The reconstructive ladder is a concept familiar to many surgeons as a means of identifying all options available for a patient after ablative surgery. Simpler options sit on the lower rungs of the ladder, and more complex procedures occupy the upper rungs. Though a useful method of recalling surgical options, the "ladder" idea leads to a sense that surgeons and patients ought not climb any higher than absolutely necessary. In clinical practice, however, what seem to be simple options can be more likely to fail and result in significantly more complex problems; ill-advised low-risk procedures can turn into high-risk situations.

Reconstructive options may be better conceptualized as a "star"; each option will have benefits and risks (Fig. 28.1). Decisions should be made after careful weighing of each option, including considerations of preservation of function, donor site morbidity, aesthetics, and the

Table 28.1   Factors Affecting Wound Healing

Patient related
    Malnutrition
    Immunodeficiency
    Diabetes mellitus
    Smoking
    Advanced age

Wound related
    Radiotherapy
    Contamination
    Infection

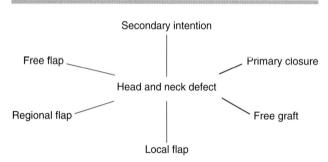

Figure 28.1   The reconstructive star demonstrates options to be considered for head and neck defects without the hierarchy introduced by the familiar "ladder."

likelihood and consequences of wound breakdown. Patient expectations may significantly impact the reconstructive calculus, especially in the setting of cutaneous facial defects. Many patients, for example, would choose soft-tissue augmentation after total parotidectomy, even if it meant a longer operation and longer hospitalization. Some patients may choose to allow an auricular helix defect to be closed primarily rather than undergoing a multistage reconstruction. Surgeons should include patient expectations in their considerations of reconstructive modalities.

Free Tissue Transfer: Special Considerations

Free tissue transfer has become increasingly popular for head and neck reconstruction in the last 20 years. It greatly expands options for patients and surgeons, and does appear to result in improved patient outcomes compared with other reconstructive techniques applied to many head and neck sites (16).

Patients undergoing free tissue transfer reconstructions should be properly selected to ensure satisfactory outcomes. Patients with peripheral vascular disease are at risk of poor results (17). Several retrospective reviews provide no convincing evidence that outcomes are worse in elderly patients, and instead indicate that comorbidities are stronger predictors of postoperative complication than age (18–20).

In addition, donor site options should be understood in the context of the patient's preoperative status, which is likely to predict postoperative functional results. For example, the authors find that elderly patients have significant difficulty mobilizing after free fibula transfer, and are thus more suited to a scapular bone flap. Young patients concerned about donor site aesthetics are more likely satisfied with the parascapular donor site compared with scapular or anterolateral thigh.

With procedures frequently lasting 12 hours, meticulous attention to the details of perioperative management is required. It is the authors' experience that patients benefit from a dedicated nursing team who ensure that none of the many precautions is missed. Patients should be positioned with sufficient padding at all pressure points, and immobilized on the operating table to allow for optimal intraoperative table positioning. Patient hypothermia is preventable and can result in poor outcomes (21); the operating room should be kept warm prior to the patient entering, as body temperature frequently falls after anesthesia induction during positioning. Core temperature should be monitored throughout the case, and a forced-air warming blanket should be present. Attention should also be paid to prevention of deep venous thrombosis, which can be accomplished with compression stockings or subcutaneous heparin. There may be increased risk of bleeding complications with the latter treatment (22), but this is justified in these patients, who are at very high risk for thrombosis.

Perioperative fluid management also may affect outcomes. Clark et al. (23), among other groups, found increased crystalloid administration during free flap procedures to be associated with medical complications. The use of certain colloid preparations may result in a hypocoagulable state, which may complicate long surgical procedures (24). In addition, multiple studies have demonstrated deleterious effects on cancer outcomes after perioperative blood transfusion (25,26). Patients are likely to benefit from the use of minimum perioperative crystalloid replacement, with colloid and blood administered only when absolutely necessary.

Thrombosis at the microvascular anastomosis remains a risk, and blood flow through the flap should be evaluated closely for several days after surgery. Several large studies have reported complication rates, most recently Bui et al. (27), who reported 1193 procedures, including 885 head and neck free flaps. Overall, 6% of flaps required re-exploration, with venous thrombosis representing the most common finding; 71% of flaps with venous thrombosis were salvaged. Interestingly, head and neck free flaps were more likely to require re-exploration and to experience late complications than other free flaps. Other recent series have confirmed the finding of overall flap failure rate less than 5% (28,29). At exploration, anastomotic failure necessitates revision, potentially with thrombectomy. Thrombosis may also be amenable to thrombolysis with streptokinase or tissue plasminogen activator delivered directly into the arterial pedicle. Finally, leeches may be used as a means of providing temporary venous outflow from a flap after irreparable venous failure. Leeches require antibiotic prophylaxis and increase transfusion requirements, but may allow salvage in difficult situations (30).

Selection of donor vessels is another factor that merits attention. Recipient arteries should be of roughly equivalent caliber to the flap pedicle vessels and should be widely accessible to the surgeon. They should also be positioned to permit a tension-free anastomosis without vessel kinking or compression by surrounding anatomy. In practice, the facial, superior thyroid, and transverse cervical arteries are used in the vast majority of cases. Jacobson et al. (31) recently described strategies for selecting vessels in necks with few available vascular options. If the internal jugular vein on the side of the defect has been sacrificed, the contralateral neck may be the best option for a recipient vein. End-to-side venous anastomoses are preferred when possible.

Many perioperative strategies are currently used successfully for free tissue transfer, and choices are largely a matter of surgeon training and preference. The authors' preference is for meticulous dissection of the vascular pedicle under loupe magnification during harvest. The surgical microscope, rather than high-powered loupes, is used for the vascular anastomosis. The Synovis™ microvascular anastomotic device provides excellent venous patency rates while decreasing operative time, and is especially valuable for small-caliber veins. The authors do not routinely use perioperative systemic anticoagulation, antiplatelet agents, or volume expanders, although many surgeons advocate their use (32). Flap monitoring is accomplished with handheld Doppler probes along with clinical observation.

The reconstructive surgeon occasionally will be faced with complications after free tissue transfer procedures. Salivary fistula, wound infection, and hematoma uncommonly occur in the postoperative period. There is little evidence to guide decision making in this setting, but there is general understanding that all of these problems increase chances of perioperative flap failure. Wound infections should be addressed early, with drainage directed as far away from the pedicle as possible; hematomas similarly require early evacuation. Fistulas similarly should be addressed early with drainage away from the pedicle; healthy transferred tissue frequently allows for secondary intention healing as long as vascularity is maintained.

COMMON FREE FLAPS
Radial Forearm
Synopsis
The radial forearm free flap is a fasciocutaneous or osteocutaneous flap based on the radial artery, its venae comitantes,

and the cephalic vein (or other superficial forearm vein). There is little anatomic variation in the harvest, and the flap usually provides a pedicle of large caliber and length. Donor site morbidity is minimal, with the exception of the risk of pathologic radius fracture with osteocutaneous harvest. The pliable skin paddle can be used to resurface internal and external defects, although color match with facial skin is not ideal. Two-team harvest is readily achieved. The radial forearm flap is the "workhorse" for head and neck soft tissue defects.

Design
The radial forearm free flap (Fig. 28.2) is based on the radial artery, and as such can include a large skin paddle from the volar surface of the forearm. The distal limit of the skin paddle is the wrist crease, although return to function is facilitated by a more proximally positioned flap. The junction of the radial and ulnar arteries represents the proximal limit of dissection. Some authors intentionally design a skin paddle that extends around the radial aspect of the forearm in order to incorporate the cephalic vein into the flap. It is generally possible, however, to keep the skin paddle on the relatively hairless volar surface while including superficial tributaries leading to the proximal cephalic vein. Subcutaneous fat proximal to the skin paddle may be included if additional bulk is desired. The flap may also include a segment of bone from the radius or the palmaris longus tendon. One useful technique for a limited defect is the "hatchet" flap (33), in which a small skin paddle is transversely oriented in the distal forearm; a proximal incision is then placed from the radial-distal forearm curving to the ulnar-proximal forearm to access the pedicle. The forearm skin can then be advanced distally to obtain a primary closure of the donor site.

Harvest
Harvest is performed under tourniquet control. Dissection is performed in the suprafascial plane except in the case of a "hatchet" flap, in which the small skin paddle

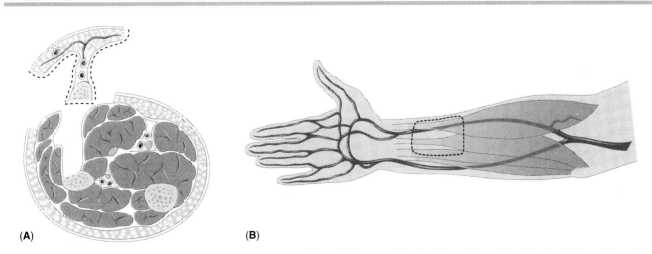

Figure 28.2 Radial forearm free flap. **(A)** The flap is comprised of the radial artery and veins, the overlying skin, and potentially a portion of the radius. **(B)** If required, the skin paddle may encompass almost the whole circumference of the forearm.

necessitates a subfascial harvest. During harvest, it is important to preserve the superficial branch of the radial nerve, which is found immediately lateral to the brachioradialis tendon. When harvesting an osteocutaneous flap, 40% or less of the circumference of the radius can be safely removed; prophylactic plating of the radius is often required to prevent postoperative fracture. The donor site requires a split thickness skin graft for closure, followed by application of a volar splint for seven days.

Inset
Fasciocutaneous flaps demonstrate excellent tolerance of ischemia, allowing most insets to be performed prior to revascularization. Anastomoses are performed with both the cephalic vein and a radial vena comitans, ideally into two independent recipient veins. The length and caliber of the vascular pedicle allows unparalleled flexibility in recipient vessel selection.

Anterolateral Thigh
Synopsis
The anterolateral thigh provides a family of free flaps based on perforators of the descending branch of the lateral circumflex femoral artery, with long and large-caliber pedicles. The flap can be harvested in cutaneous, fasciocutaneous, or myocutaneous configurations. The majority of anterolateral thigh flaps require dissection of the perforating vessels through the vastus lateralis muscle. There is usually very little donor site morbidity as long as the motor nerve to vastus lateralis is preserved, with primary closure and fast return to ambulation being the rule. The skin paddle is hair-bearing and can be thick, depending on body habitus, although it tolerates careful thinning. The fascia lata at the

deep surface of the flap may be a useful adjunct in wound closure.

Design
The descending branch of the lateral circumflex femoral artery lies between the rectus femoris and vastus lateralis muscles, and the skin paddle of the anterolateral thigh flap is based on musculocutaneous (or, less commonly, septocutaneous) perforators of the descending branch (Fig. 28.3A,B). As such, the skin paddle is designed based on the identification of the perforators by Doppler; one is usually found near the midpoint of a line connecting the anterior superior iliac spine and the superolateral aspect of the patella. A distally located perforator will result in a longer vascular pedicle; the pedicle can be traced proximally to the branch to rectus femoris, which should be left undisturbed. The medial aspect of the skin incision is made and the position of the perforator is confirmed prior to completing the incision.

Harvest
The most important initial step of the harvest is identification of the proper intermuscular septum. The rectus femoris is identifiable by its bipennate structure ("chevron pointing superiorly"), and dissection should remain lateral to it. The perforator vessel is frequently of small caliber and requires meticulous dissection. A small cuff of muscle can be left attached to musculocutaneous perforators to identify twisting during inset. During harvest, all efforts are made to preserve the motor nerve to vastus lateralis, but this is not always possible depending on the position of the perforator. Dissection is carried out in the subfascial plane. Flaps that are 8 cm in width can generally be closed

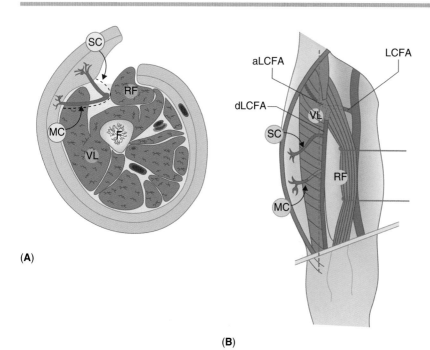

(A)

(B)

Figure 28.3 Anterolateral thigh free flap. **(A)** Skin, subcutaneous tissue, and fascia lata are supplied by perforators of the descending branch of the lateral circumflex femoral artery, which travel between rectus femoris and vastus lateralis or through the vastus lateralis. **(B)** The descending branch can be dissected superiorly to the branch to rectus femoris. *Abbreviations*: SC, Septo-cutaneous perforator; MC, Musculo-cutaneous perforator; RF, Rectus Femoris; VL, vastus lateralis; aLCFA, ascending lateral circumflex femoral artery; dLCFA, descending lateral circumflex femoral artery; LCFA, lateral circumflex femoral artery.

primarily, although some suprafascial undermining may be required. The skin is closed in two layers; to avoid compartment syndrome, no effort is made to reapproximate the fascia.

Inset

Portions of the flap may be de-epithelialized for soft tissue augmentation. Vascularized fascia lata may be useful in closure as a bed for a skin graft or to fill dead space within a wound. Fascia and the deep layers of the subcutaneous tissue can be removed for use in defects that call for thin flaps.

Fibula

Synopsis

The fibula flap is an osseous or osteocutaneous free flap based on the peroneal artery and venae comitantes. Attention should be paid to verify that the skin perforators of an osteocutaneous flap do in fact derive from the peroneal artery, as they may branch from the posterior tibial artery. Donor site morbidity is usually acceptable, especially in younger patients, although older patients may have more difficulty returning to full weight-bearing. The vascular pedicle is usually of excellent caliber and length, but is affected by atherosclerotic disease in susceptible patients. The bone flap can usually support osseointegrated implants.

Design

Prior to fibula harvest, patients should undergo arterial assessment of the lower extremities with an ultrasound-based noninvasive study or an imaging-based study; patients with clinical signs of venous insufficiency may also be unsuited to fibular harvest due to risk of donor site wound complications. The length of bone available for transfer with the fibula free flap is limited by the need to leave six centimeters of intact bone at both the knee and the ankle. In most cases, the flap pedicle is directed laterally toward recipient vessels in the ipsilateral neck; therefore, the contralateral fibula is chosen for an intraoral skin paddle. In the case of resections involving the condyle, the pedicle needs to be directed medially, so the ipsilateral fibula should be selected. The hair-bearing skin paddle is based on the perforators of the peroneal artery, and is designed as an ellipse whose long axis coincides with the posterior intermuscular septum (Fig. 28.4). Use of a more proximal skin paddle results in a shorter pedicle, but may permit a primary closure of the donor site.

Harvest

The harvest is performed under tourniquet control. The position of the vascular perforators is determined by Doppler, but the posterior incision of the skin paddle is not made until the perforators are visualized. Attention should be paid to verify that the cutaneous perforators do indeed arise from the peroneal artery, as they occasionally arise from the posterior tibial artery. The peroneal artery, which usually has two venae comitantes, can be traced proximally to its junction with the posterior tibial artery. Superficial dissection proximally should be undertaken cautiously so

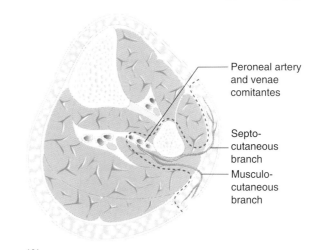

(A)

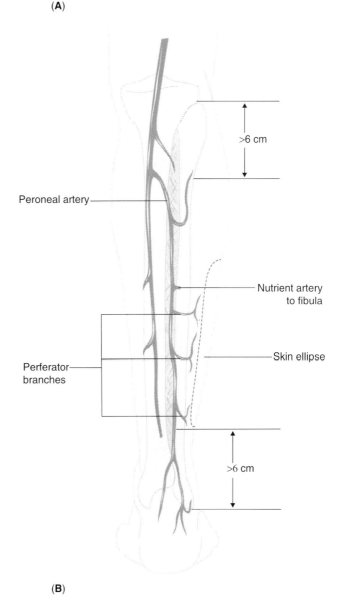

(B)

Figure 28.4 Fibula free flap. **(A)** The flap includes peroneal artery and veins, fibula, overlying skin, and potentially portions of flexor hallucis longus and soleus muscles. **(B)** Proximal dissection is limited superficially by the common peroneal nerve.

as to avoid injury to the common peroneal nerve, while the tibial nerve is in proximity at the deep aspect. The donor site may be closed primarily, or may require a split thickness skin graft, which can be elevated on the medial aspect of the ipsilateral calf. A posterior splint is applied for five days, with return to full weight-bearing at that time.

Inset

The peroneal artery maintains an intimate relationship with the fibular periosteum for a significant distance, which allows multiple osteotomies to be performed without sacrifice of vascularity. The fibula has a roughly triangular cross-section, which presents a flat surface for application of hardware (Fig. 28.5). A 2-mm reconstruction plate is contoured prior to the mandibular resection if possible, and is then used as a template for the fibular osteotomies, with monocortical drilling to prevent injury to the pedicle. For ease of access, the inset of the intraoral skin paddle is performed prior to fixation of the reconstruction plate to the native mandible.

Subscapular System

Synopsis

The subscapular artery is a branch of the axillary artery (Fig. 28.6). It travels through the axilla and divides into the thoracodorsal artery and the circumflex scapular artery. The former continues inferomedially to supply the latissimus dorsi muscle and overlying skin, while sending branches to the scapular angle and to the serratus anterior muscle. The circumflex scapular artery sends a nutrient branch into the scapula near the glenoid fossa. There are two divisions of the circumflex scapular artery: the scapular branch travels medially from the triangular space, while the parascapular branch travels inferiorly. The subscapular

artery offers a large caliber vessel for anastomosis; pedicle length depends on the components of the flap. There is usually little long-term donor site morbidity provided the muscular attachments of the scapula are restored. Color match with facial skin is usually good (34).

Design

The subscapular system of free flaps includes possibilities for three different skin paddles (scapular, parascapular, and skin based on thoracodorsal artery perforators), bulky muscle (latissimus dorsi), functioning muscle (serratus anterior),

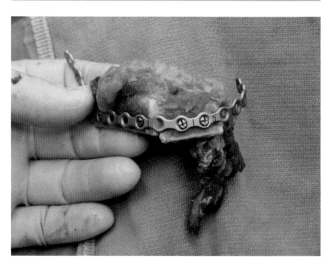

Figure 28.5 Osteotomized fibular flap affixed to reconstruction plate. *Source*: Courtesy of Richard Gilbert.

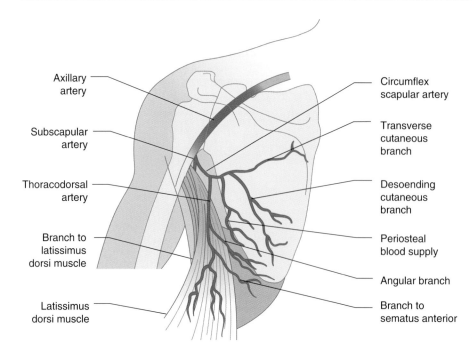

Figure 28.6 The subscapular artery and its branches. Each branch can support an independent free flap or a portion of a composite flap.

and vascularized bone (lateral border of scapula or scapular tip). Almost any combination of these components is possible, and they can be positioned in almost any orientation with respect to each other. These vessels are not commonly affected by atherosclerotic disease. Compared with the anterolateral thigh flap, the subscapular skin paddles generally display better color match with facial skin. We find that the parascapular flap leaves a scar that can be hidden or camouflaged more easily than that of the scapular flap. The skin paddle supplied by the thoracodorsal artery perforators is similar in quality but with a longer pedicle.

Harvest

Although some sources describe turning the patient onto the lateral decubitus position during scapular flap harvest, minimal technical difficulty is introduced by simply placing the patient, rotated about 30 degrees, on a beanbag cushion for both the ablative procedure and the flap harvest. Even so, two-team surgery is not possible with subscapular flaps, which results in longer operative times. The arm can be manipulated during the dissection to obtain adequate visualization of the vascular pedicle into the axilla. The vascular pedicle of any of these flaps can be lengthened by carrying the dissection proximally to the axillary artery. During dissection of the vascular pedicle in the axilla, the long thoracic and thoracodorsal nerves should be protected. Scapular bone can be vascularized by the nutrient vessel branching from the circumflex scapular artery or by the angular artery, which typically arises from either the thoracodorsal artery or the branch to the serratus anterior. The angular artery has been shown to supply the inferior 10 cm of the lateral border of the scapula. Primary closure of the defect is almost always possible. After bone harvest, it is necessary to reconstitute the detached musculature, specifically serratus anterior and teres major, via holes drilled in the residual scapula.

Inset

The bony component is osteotomized in a green-stick manner, but multiple osteotomies might result in devascularization of smaller segments. The bone is affixed to a reconstruction plate using a monocortical technique. Generally, a single vena comitans is present with the subscapular, thoracodorsal, and circumflex scapular arteries.

Rectus Abdominis
Synopsis

The rectus abdominis free flap is based on the deep inferior epigastric artery, which runs on the deep surface of the rectus abdominis muscle within the rectus sheath. It can be raised as a muscle flap or a myocutaneous flap. The pedicle is usually of intermediate caliber and length, with a single vena comitans. Incisional hernia is a risk of flap harvest, and incisional pain may limit early mobilization postoperatively.

Design

The rectus abdominis free flap is a myocutaneous or muscle flap based on the deep inferior epigastric artery. The vessels run along the deep surface of the rectus abdominis

muscle and send transmuscular perforators through the anterior rectus sheath to the overlying skin (Fig. 28.7). The myocutaneous perforators are located in proximity to the umbilicus, so the skin paddle should be designed as a paramedian ellipse. The perforating vessels are substantial in size, and allow harvest of the muscle-sparing deep inferior epigastric artery perforator (DIEP) flap, in which the skin paddle is designed around a perforator, which is dissected through the rectus abdominis to the vessel. Skin is thick and hair-bearing, and the paddle often contains a significant amount of subcutaneous fat. Color match with facial skin is usually poor.

Harvest

Harvest should begin in the superior aspect of the flap, as the posterior rectus sheath clearly delineates the deep dissection plane. Inferior to the arcuate line, there is no posterior sheath, and the vessels are dissected off the underlying transversalis fascia. It is important to obtain a primary closure of the anterior rectus sheath to prevent incisional hernia; for this reason only the periumbilical portion of the anterior sheath, through which the perforators travel, is included with the flap. The abdominal skin edges can be closed primarily. Some authors advocate use of an abdominal binder in the postoperative period for improved comfort.

Inset

The bulk and weight of the rectus abdominis flap are frequently substantial, so attention should be paid to adequate

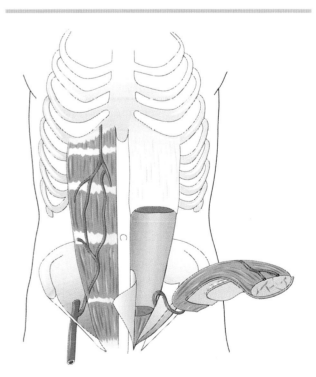

Figure 28.7 The rectus abdominis flap. The deep inferior epigastric artery runs along the deep surface of the rectus abdominis muscle. The majority of skin perforators arise near the umbilicus.

fixation during inset to prevent wound edge dehiscence. The surgeon should plan for significant atrophy of the rectus muscle in the postoperative period.

Gastro-omental
Synopsis
The gastro-omental free flap is based on the right gastro-epiploic vessels, which arise from the gastroduodenal artery. These vessels supply blood to the greater curvature of the stomach as well as the greater omentum. The greater curvature, when formed into a tube, can be used to reconstruct the pharyngeal conduit, while the attached omentum provides a second layer which seems to revascularize radiation-damaged soft tissues of the neck.

Design
The length of stomach harvested is equal to the length of the pharyngeal defect. At least 4 cm of distal stomach should be left adjacent to the pylorus to prevent postoperative gastric outlet obstruction. A segment of greater omentum should be included; this can be used to reinforce the pharyngeal anastomoses, the tracheal repair, or fill any other dead space that might accompany an extended laryngopharyngectomy.

Harvest
It is generally not possible to harvest the gastro-omental flap in a two-team manner. Through a mini-laparotomy, the greater curvature of the stomach is identified, along with the right gastroepiploic vessels. Taking care to preserve the pylorus, two gastrotomies are made along the greater curvature separated by the required length of the pharyngeal conduit. A 36 French chest tube is placed through the gastrotomies and an automated stapling device is used to simultaneously divide the flap and create a tube (Fig. 28.8). The left gastroepiploic vessels are divided, and the right gastroepiploic vessels are dissected to the gastroduodenal vessels. The abdominal wall is closed in routine fashion, with nasogastric tube decompression.

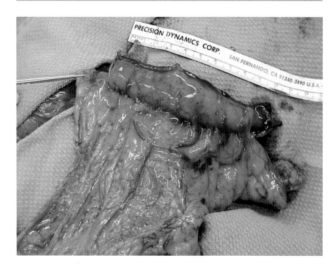

Figure 28.8   Harvested and tubed gastro-omental free flap. *Source:* Courtesy of Ralph Gilbert.

Inset
Enteric free flaps display lower tolerance for ischemia than fasciocutaneous flaps. For this reason, only the back walls of the superior and inferior suture lines should be inset prior to revascularization. After the gastric tube is inset, the attached omentum is laid on top and tacked into place.

REGIONAL MYOCUTANEOUS FLAPS
Pectoralis Major
Synopsis
The pectoralis major can be used as a pedicled myocutaneous flap or muscle flap for defects in the upper aerodigestive tract and the neck. The skin paddle can be placed internally or externally. The main blood supply to the flap is through the thoracoacromial trunk, with the lateral thoracic artery providing an independent pedicle; the skin is supplied through transmuscular perforators. Skin paddle harvest results in a cosmetic deformity that can be especially significant in women. Generally, the thickness of the subcutaneous tissue, along with donor site cosmesis, limits the applicability of this flap.

Design
The rotation point of the flap is the junction of the middle and lateral thirds of the clavicle. Based on this, a skin paddle of appropriate dimension is designed (Fig. 28.9). The inferior border of the sternum represents the inferior limit of the skin flap. Incisions are then designed to permit exposure of the entire pectoralis major muscle, either in the inframammary line or obliquely into the axilla.

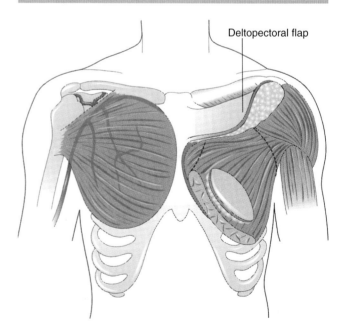

Figure 28.9   The pectoralis major flap. The muscle is mainly supplied by the pectoral branch of the thoracoacromial artery that runs along its deep surface.

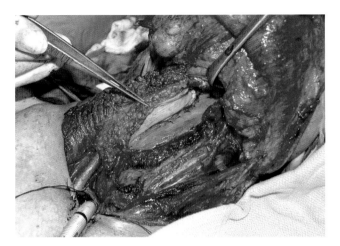

Figure 28.10 Laryngectomy with partial pharyngectomy being reconstructed with right pectoralis major myocutaneous flap. The bulk of the flap is evident. *Source:* Courtesy of Ralph Gilbert.

Harvest

During harvest, care should be taken to limit shear forces on the skin paddle, as the transmuscular perforator vessels are delicate. This is commonly accomplished by temporarily suturing the edges of the paddle to the surrounding muscle. The pedicle should be identified in its course along the deep surface of the pectoralis major. This is most easily done by identifying the space between the pectoralis major and pectoralis minor muscles in the axilla; this plane is somewhat more difficult to identify while dissecting from inferior to superior due to the multiple costal attachments of the pectoralis major. The lateral pedicle lies in the same plane; it may be preserved but often limits the arc of rotation. With the pedicle in view, the portions of muscle lying on either side can be left in situ if a narrower flap is desired.

Inset

The bulk of the muscle requires that a sizable tunnel be created over the clavicle between the chest and the neck to avoid compression of the vascular pedicle. Dissection should be carried high enough to prevent downward tension on the bulky flap (Fig. 28.10). Frequently, a split thickness skin graft is required when the neck skin cannot be closed; in this setting, a meshed graft with a very light dressing should be used.

Latissimus Dorsi
Synopsis

See the section on the subscapular system of free flaps for detailed description of general principles. This latissimus dorsi myocutaneous or muscle flap is based on the thoracodorsal vessels. In comparison to the pectoralis major flap, the latissimus dorsi flap contains a larger muscle volume and a larger skin paddle, with similar subcutaneous component. It cannot be harvested from the supine position. Vascular anatomy is similarly consistent. The pedicled flap is then passed through the axilla between the pectoralis major and minor muscles, superficial to the clavicle, and

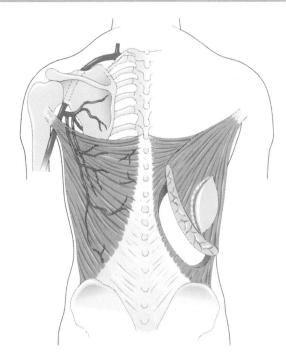

Figure 28.11 The latissimus dorsi flap. The thoracodorsal artery originates in the axilla and courses inferiorly under the anterior border of the muscle.

into the neck. Donor site cosmesis is more favorable than with the pectoralis major.

Design

The majority of the transmuscular perforators are located near the anterior free margin of the latissimus dorsi muscle. The desired paddle is designed based on this. An incision is then carried superiorly into the axilla (Fig. 28.11).

Harvest

The transmuscular perforators are larger than those of the pectoralis flap, but the edges of the skin paddle should be sutured down to the surrounding muscle to prevent shearing. After identification of the anterior border of the latissimus dorsi muscle, the thoracodorsal vessels are sought by identifying the serratus branch and tracing it superiorly. The thoracodorsal vessels are then followed into the axilla, and the thoracodorsal nerve should be divided.

Inset

A tunnel is created from the axilla over the clavicle into the neck. The tunnel must be wide enough to accommodate the bulk of the muscle, and is most commonly placed between the pectoralis major and minor muscles. Care should be taken to avoid undue tension on the muscle in the axilla to prevent brachial plexus compression (35).

SITE-SPECIFIC PRINCIPLES
Oral Cavity/Oropharynx Soft Tissue

The goals of reconstruction of oral cavity and oropharyngeal soft tissue defects are to restore swallowing and provide for speech and mastication, while separating the upper aerodigestive tract from the neck. At this anatomic site, reconstructions must find a balance between bulk and mobility: the oral tongue must be able to contact the palate and upper alveolus for proper chewing and speech; however, the posterior tongue must be substantial enough to drive boluses during deglutition.

The radial forearm free flap is an ideal choice for most oral defects. Larger defects, especially those that involve a significant portion of the tongue base, may be better suited to the bulkier anterolateral thigh flap. The decision between these two flaps is frequently determined by the patient's habitus. The anterolateral thigh flap is often not acceptable in patients with abundant subcutaneous fat. When designing cutaneous skin paddles for tongue and floor of mouth reconstruction, they should be broad enough anteriorly to maintain satisfactory distance between the tip of the tongue and the floor of mouth. Regional muscle flaps, such as pectoralis major and latissimus dorsi, are most often too large to allow satisfactory oral function. Mucosal and cutaneous regional flaps, such as the buccinator myomucosal flap (36) and the submental island flap (37), are also options for smaller defects. For small oral tongue defects, split-thickness skin grafts or secondary-intention healing may provide adequate coverage for oral defects, but cannot be applied in the setting of concurrent neck dissection. In the oropharynx, additional bulk is essential for defects involving the tongue base, even if the reconstruction extends to the lateral pharyngeal wall. Reiger et al. described their experience with radial forearm free flap reconstruction for tongue base defects, in which most patients achieved excellent swallowing and speech outcomes (38).

A free or regional flap is almost always required in patients whose tumor ablations require mandibulotomy, as well as in previously radiated patients in whom the extirpation results in continuity between oral cavity or pharynx and neck.

In the case of tumors of the posterior oral cavity and oropharynx, ablative surgery sometimes results in velopharyngeal incompetence, which can have a significant impact on speech and swallowing outcomes. There is currently no satisfactory surgical method of replicating the function of a dynamic soft palate. If a portion of innervated soft palate remains and can contact the posterior pharyngeal wall, the remainder of the velopharyngeal aperture should be statically closed. With large soft palate resections, or if the remaining palate is immobile, this closure frequently requires a superiorly-based pharyngeal flap (39).

Restoration of sensory innervation of cutaneous free flaps has been attempted in many centers. The design and transfer of sensate flaps has been shown possible, and in fact patients do achieve improved two-point discrimination in sensate flaps than non-sensate flaps (40). However, there has been no demonstration that swallowing outcomes are improved in sensate flaps (41), and they have fallen out of favor.

Mandible

Bony reconstruction after segmental mandibulectomy is required to maintain effective mastication and, for anterior defects, a competent oral sphincter. Reconstruction allows for optimal dental rehabilitation, and also permits restoration of lower facial contour. There is no consensus on optimal methods for mandibular reconstruction, and practices vary by surgeon experience. Free flaps incorporating vascularized bone have revolutionized mandibular reconstruction, with studies of free bone transfer demonstrating excellent functional outcomes (42). In contrast, there are no widely-accepted options for regional bone-containing flaps for mandible reconstruction, with some surgeons advocating a latissimus dorsi-based flap including a segment of rib. Nonvascularized bone grafts cannot be radiated or placed in a radiated bed, and in general are inadequate for mandibular reconstruction.

Another option for reconstruction is the use of a bridging mandibular reconstruction plate with intraoral soft tissue coverage. This technique may have use in patients with lateral mandibular defects that are unsuited to fibular harvest. Some series have demonstrated satisfactory outcomes (43), but others report a high rate of plate exposure requiring a revision (44). This technique is not applicable to patients with defects involving the anterior mandibular arch, as bridging plates will be inadequate to support the soft tissues of the chin, anterior floor of mouth, and anterior tongue, and will extrude through the skin. Vascularized bone flaps are the only reasonable options for these defects.

Due to the favorable donor site characteristics and quality of available bone, its workhorse of mandibular reconstruction is the fibula free flap. Even so, there are cases in which other flaps may be preferable. Patients who have large concomitant soft tissue defects may be better served with a scapular osteocutaneous free flap, whose soft tissue component is larger and more mobile relative to the bone and vascular pedicle compared to that of the fibular flap. Elderly patients may have more difficulty returning to full ambulation after fibula harvest. They may also have subclinical venous insufficiency, which can result in higher incidence of thrombosis at the venous anastomosis. Patients with peripheral vascular disease may have atherosclerosis involving the peroneal artery, which makes successful vascular anastomosis more difficult; disease of the tibial arteries may result in the peroneal artery being critical for distal perfusion of the foot. It is best to avoid the fibular donor site in such patients.

Mandibular reconstruction requires knowledge of the available hardware and instrumentation, and more importantly the principles of skeletal fixation. As restoration of functional mastication is a primary goal of reconstruction, surgeons should be familiar with techniques of mandibular osteosynthesis and intraoperative intermaxillary wire fixation (45). The authors' preference for fibular or scapular bone flaps is to use a 2.0-mm non-locking reconstruction plate; others prefer the use of locking plates (46). A heavier reconstruction plate is required in the case of reconstruction with soft-tissue only.

Mandibular osteoradionecrosis is an unfortunate consequence of head and neck irradiation that presents particular challenges to the reconstructive surgeon. Several case series have described the increased complication rates in these cases. Some authors have advocated hyperbaric oxygen in combination with nonvascularized bone grafting and regional flap soft tissue reconstruction (47). Many surgeons, however, advocate vascularized osteocutaneous free flaps as the only means of creating a stable and functional jaw (48), and limit the use of hyperbaric oxygen to patients with minimal devitalized bone (49).

Optimal reconstruction of mandibulectomy defects that involve the condyle is a subject of controversy. There is no widely accepted method of solving this difficult problem. Manufacturers of plating systems produce condylar head prostheses designed to fit into the glenoid fossa; these have a risk of becoming displaced into the middle cranial fossa over time, especially in younger patients who return to mastication. An alternative is to simply place the end of the vascularized bone graft into the glenoid fossa, secured with nonabsorbable sutures from the temporomandibular joint capsule (50). The intraarticular disc of the temporomandibular joint is left in place if possible. Patients are at risk of displacement of the neomandible from the glenoid fossa as soft tissue scar contracture occurs; they are also prone to trismus from scarring. We advocate suture fixation without condylar head protheses in most cases; patients are asked to begin range-of-motion exercises within a week of surgery.

Maxilla

Defects of the maxilla are amenable to reconstruction. Maxillectomy defects can have a profound impact on oral function and the aesthetics of the central face. Reconstructive procedures should separate the oral and nasal cavities, allow for a stable and functional dental prosthesis or placement of osseointegrated implants, support orbital soft tissues, and re-establish anterior and lateral midfacial projection. There is significantly less literature on maxillary reconstruction than on mandibular reconstruction, as prosthetic techniques historically have been found to be effective in most patients. Recent advances in osseointegrated implantation have spurred interest in reconstruction.

The choice to reconstruct palatomaxillary defects is based on the expertise of the surgical team and the desires of the patient. The idea of leaving defects open in order to monitor aggressive tumors should no more apply to the maxilla than it does to the mandible or the pharynx. Some data exist describing poorer masticatory function in prosthesis users with large defects (51). In a small study, Genden et al. (52) discovered improved functional and quality of life outcomes with bone flap reconstruction after hemimaxillectomy compared with obturation. Rogers et al. (53) discovered no difference in quality of life outcomes in another comparison of prosthesis users with reconstructed patients.

Some patients may benefit profoundly from reconstruction, and surgeons should be familiar with the options. Cordeiro et al. (54), Brown et al. (55), and Okay et al. (56) have developed classification systems for maxillary defects based on expected functional and aesthetic deficits. The latter two systems incorporate dual considerations: the proportion of remaining hard palate as well as the extent of the remaining bony support of orbital and upper midfacial soft tissues. The first determines the stability of an obturator prosthesis and therefore oral function, while the second determines deficits related to eyelid and globe position.

Although there is a bony component to all maxillary defects, bone reconstruction is necessary only for patients who would not otherwise regain functional masticatory ability. For small palate defects, including those involving the premolar and molar teeth, soft tissue reconstruction is optimal. This can be accomplished with local flaps, such as the palatal island rotation flap; or a thin soft tissue free flap, such as the radial forearm. There is no advantage to bone reconstruction in these patients, as partial dentures can provide effective dental rehabilitation.

Soft tissue flaps used for hemipalatectomy and larger defects tend to bulge persistently into the oral cavity, however, and can hinder denture use and oral function. In the case of total and subtotal palatectomy defects, there is insufficient palatal and alveolar bone to stabilize prostheses against masticatory forces, and bony reconstruction is an excellent choice. Multiple techniques have been described using iliac crest (57), fibula (58), scapular tip (59), and osteocutaneous radial forearm free flaps (60). Hemipalatectomy defects generally leave sufficient palate to be managed effectively with obturator prostheses, but bony reconstruction is an option for patients with access to osseointegrated implants.

Pharynx

After laryngopharyngectomy, reconstruction is primarily directed at restoration of an alimentary tract that permits swallowing. Reconstructions should also permit effective speech production through a tracheoesophageal puncture. Both regional and free flaps have been found to achieve satisfactory results, with no randomized studies directly comparing their respective functional outcomes. Circumferential defects are better managed with free flaps, as the regional options are problematic: the pectoralis major is frequently too bulky to maintain an adequate lumen, while the deltopectoral flap requires a controlled fistula that is closed in a second stage.

The relative benefits of jejunal and fasciocutaneous free flaps for circumferential defects have been debated for two decades. The two options are equally effective at re-establishing a conduit for swallowing. Patients are more likely to experience dysphagia after jejunal transfer (61), possibly because the jejunal graft retains peristaltic function that is not coordinated with that of the native pharynx. Fasciocutaneous flaps, in contrast, remain adynamic and passive conduits. In addition, the same study showed that, although jejunal flaps can allow for tracheoesophageal puncture speech, patients are less likely to report using their tracheoesophageal voice for routine conversation than patients who had anterolateral thigh flaps.

Circumferential pharyngeal reconstruction carries a risk of stricture; some surgeons attempt to prevent this by placing salivary bypass tubes, to stent the reconstruction while also decreasing salivary contamination of the suture lines. There is some data suggesting that fistula and stricture rates are improved with use of bypass tubes for 10–14 days (62).

The authors' preference in case of total laryngopharyngectomy is to use a tubed anterolateral thigh free flap in conjunction with a salivary bypass tube for four to six weeks (63). In patients in whom the anterolateral thigh flap is too thick, the radial forearm is the flap of choice. In the setting of salvage surgery after chemoradiotherapy or altered-fractionation radiotherapy, we also consider using a gastro-omental free flap because the presence of vascularized omentum has a salutary effect on wound healing in the neck. For noncircumferential pharyngeal defects, a radial forearm or pectoralis major myocutaneous flap is used.

Reconstruction in the setting of salvage laryngopharyngectomy after radiotherapy or chemoradiotherapy failure is particularly challenging. There is increasing evidence to support use of specialized techniques in this setting, such as routine use of regional or pedicled flaps even when primary pharyngeal closure is possible.

Parotid/Facial Nerve

The goal of reconstruction of defects involving the parotid gland is to restore normal facial contour and auricular position. Total parotidectomy results in a deep hollow between the mandibular ramus and the mastoid that is impossible to disguise. The loss of upper neck soft tissues invariably results in a deformity of the auricle, in which the lobule rotates anteriorly and medially as the wound contracts. For these reasons, soft tissue augmentation of the parotid bed is frequently desirable, with the additional goal of preventing Frey's syndrome. It generally should be performed in the primary setting, as secondary reconstruction is difficult due to the potential for facial nerve injury.

Several methods of soft tissue augmentation have been described, including use of alloplasts (64), abdominal fat grafts, local muscle flaps (65), composite free grafts of dermis and fat (66), and de-epithelialized fasciocutaneous free flaps (67). No method is uniformly accepted. Free grafts frequently undergo significant and unpredictable absorption in the postoperative period. In the case of malignant parotid disease, alloplasts such as acellular dermis may not tolerate postoperative radiotherapy. Free tissue transfer procedures require time and expertise.

Malignant parotid tumors sometimes necessitate resection of the facial nerve. There are two considerations for the reconstructive surgeon at the primary setting: facial reinnervation with a nerve graft, and static suspension to prevent morbidity related to facial paralysis. Interposition nerve grafting is an excellent option for any patient in whom proximal and distal nerve stumps are available; postoperative radiotherapy is not a contraindication (68). Older patients may have poorer outcomes from nerve grafting (69), but even a minimally functional nerve graft may add to quality of life. Many donor sites have been described; the authors find the great auricular, sural, and medial antebrachial cutaneous nerves to be useful, depending on the required branching pattern.

Static rehabilitation procedures are useful either as temporizing measures after nerve grafting or as primary treatment after nerve resection. The eyelids, eyebrow, and oral commissure are the main targets of static procedures. Gold weight implantation, lateral tarsal strip, and tarsorrhaphy are the main techniques to prevent exposure keratitis, all of which can be easily done under local anesthesia. Brow ptosis can also be corrected under local anesthesia by direct browlift or mid-forehead lift. Suspension of the oral commissure is best accomplished using autologous fascia. Fascia should be tunneled to the oral commissure and sutured to the orbicularis oris muscle both above and below the commissure using nonabsorbable suture. The fascia should be tensioned to overcorrect the position of the commissure, and then suspended from the temporalis fascia or the periosteum of the zygomatic arch.

The authors' routine is to perform soft tissue augmentation with a parascapular or anterolateral thigh free flap, de-epithelialized unless there has been resection of skin. At the same time, the oral commissure is suspended using fascia obtained from the free flap donor site or with plantaris tendon, and a tarsorrhaphy is performed. Gold weight implantation and browlift are performed as needed in the postoperative period, along with debulking of the soft tissue. Finally, patients with persistent lower lip weakness are offered lower lip suspension with a palmaris longus tendon graft, in which the tendon is passed deep to the vermilion border from the commissure to the midline so as to improve symmetry during function.

Large Composite Defects

In some circumstances, tumor resection results in large defects involving mucosal surfaces of the upper aerodigestive tract in combination with mandibular bone and external skin. Such defects require reconstructive surgeons to understand a variety of regional and free flap techniques in order to restore function.

The main principle is that the surgeon should not expect that a single reconstructive procedure will result in a perfect functional and aesthetic outcome. The primary procedure should result in a stable construct that can be modified as necessary after wound healing has taken place. In the case of malignant tumors, the primary reconstruction can be modified after adjuvant treatment has been completed.

The system of flaps based on the subscapular artery is ideal for large composite defects. Large amounts of skin, subcutaneous fat, muscle, and bone can be transferred, frequently on a single vascular pedicle. The various components of the composite flap can be contoured independently, in contrast to many other commonly-used composite flaps. There is usually very little donor-site morbidity, and the vessels are usually unaffected by peripheral vascular disease or venous insufficiency. The bone component can derive from the traditional bony nutrient artery, or for increased pedicle length from the angular branch of the thoracodorsal artery. The soft tissue component can come from the scapular or parascapular areas, or for a longer pedicle from over the latissimus dorsi, either with the muscle or as a muscle-sparing perforator flap. This flap is easily adapted to through-and-through defects requiring replacement of mucosa and external facial or neck skin. Importantly, the use of multiple simultaneous free flaps can be avoided.

REFERENCES

1. Breasted J. The Edwin Smith surgical papyrus. Chicago: The University of Chicago Press, 1930.
2. Marmelzat WL. Medicine in history. Celsus (Ad 25), plastic surgeon: on the repair of defects of the ears, lips, and nose. J Dermatol Surg Oncol 1982; 8: 1012–14.
3. Whitaker IS, Karoo RO, Spyrou G et al. The birth of plastic surgery: the story of nasal reconstruction from the Edwin Smith Papyrus to the twenty-first century. Plast Reconstr Surg 2007; 120: 327–36.
4. Sakula A. Sir Harold Gillies, FRCS (1882–1960). J Med Biogr 2004; 12: 65.
5. Bakamjian VY. Total reconstruction of pharynx with medially based deltopectoral skin flap. NY State J Med 1968; 68: 2771–8.

6. Taylor GI, Daniel RK. The free flap: composite tissue transfer by vascular anastomosis. Aust N Z J Surg 1973; 43: 1–3.

7. Ariyan S. The pectoralis major myocutaneous flap. A versatile flap for reconstruction in the head and neck. Plast Reconstr Surg 1979; 63: 73–81.

8. Yang GF. [Free grafting of a lateral brachial skin flap]. Zhonghua Wai Ke Za Zhi. 1983; 21: 272–4.

9. Shetty V, Schwartz HC. Wound healing and perioperative care. Oral Maxillofac Surg Clin North Am 2006; 18: 107–13.

10. Ai-Aql ZS, Alagl AS, Graves DT et al. Molecular mechanisms controlling bone formation during fracture healing and distraction osteogenesis. J Dent Res 2008; 87: 107–18.

11. Denham JW, Hauer-Jensen M. The radiotherapeutic injury—a complex "wound". Radiother Oncol 2002; 63: 129–45.

12. Sassler AM, Esclamado RM, Wolf GT. Surgery after organ preservation therapy. Analysis of wound complications. Arch Otolaryngol Head Neck Surg 1995; 121: 162–5.

13. Lavertu P, Bonafede JP, Adelstein DJ et al. Comparison of surgical complications after organ-preservation therapy in patients with stage III or IV squamous cell head and neck cancer. Arch Otolaryngol Head Neck Surg 1998; 124: 401–6.

14. Morgan JE, Breau RL, Suen JY et al. Surgical wound complications after intensive chemoradiotherapy for advanced squamous cell carcinoma of the head and neck. Arch Otolaryngol Head Neck Surg 2007; 133: 10–14.

15. Le AX, Miclau T, Hu D et al. Molecular aspects of healing in stabilized and non-stabilized fractures. J Orthop Res 2001; 19: 78–84.

16. Smith RB, Sniezek JC, Weed DT et al. Utilization of free tissue transfer in head and neck surgery. Otolaryngol Head Neck Surg 2007; 137: 182–91.

17. Moran SL, Illig KA, Green RM et al. Free-tissue transfer in patients with peripheral vascular disease: a 10-year experience. Plast Reconstr Surg 2002; 109: 999–1006.

18. Serletti JM, Higgins JP, Moran S et al. Factors affecting outcome in free-tissue transfer in the elderly. Plast Reconstr Surg 2000; 106: 66–70.

19. Ozkan O, Ozgentas HE, Islamoglu K et al. Experiences with microsurgical tissue transfers in elderly patients. Microsurgery 2005; 25: 390–5.

20. Shestak KC, Jones NF, Wu W et al. Effect of advanced age and medical disease on the outcome of microvascular reconstruction for head and neck defects. Head Neck 1992; 14: 14–8.

21. Kinnunen I, Laurikainen E, Schrey A et al. Effect of hypothermia on blood-flow responses in pedicled groin flaps in rats. Br J Plast Surg 2002; 55: 657–63.

22. Clagett GP, Reisch JS. Prevention of venous thromboembolism in general surgical patients. Results of meta-analysis. Ann Surg 1988; 208: 227–40.

23. Clark JR, McCluskey SA, Hall F et al. Predictors of morbidity following free flap reconstruction for cancer of the head and neck. Head Neck 2007; 29: 1090–101.

24. Stephens R, Mythen M. Optimizing intraoperative fluid therapy. Curr Opin Anaesthesiol 2003; 16: 385–92.

25. Szakmany T, Dodd M, Dempsey GA et al. The influence of allogenic blood transfusion in patients having free-flap primary surgery for oral and oropharyngeal squamous cell carcinoma. Br J Cancer 2006; 94: 647–53.

26. Taniguchi Y, Okura M. Prognostic significance of perioperative blood transfusion in oral cavity squamous cell carcinoma. Head Neck 2003; 25: 931–6.

27. Bui DT, Cordeiro PG, Hu QY et al. Free flap reexploration: indications, treatment, and outcomes in 1193 free flaps. Plast Reconstr Surg 2007; 119: 2092–100.

28. Nakatsuka T, Harii K, Asato H et al. Analytic review of 2372 free flap transfers for head and neck reconstruction following cancer resection. J Reconstr Microsurg 2003; 19: 363–8; discussion 9.

29. Panchapakesan V, Addison P, Beausang E et al. Role of thrombolysis in free-flap salvage. J Reconstr Microsurg 2003; 19: 523–30.

30. Chepeha DB, Nussenbaum B, Bradford CR et al. Leech therapy for patients with surgically unsalvageable venous obstruction after revascularized free tissue transfer. Arch Otolaryngol Head Neck Surg 2002; 128: 960–5.

31. Jacobson AS, Eloy JA, Park E et al. Vessel-depleted neck: techniques for achieving microvascular reconstruction. Head Neck 2008; 30: 201–7.

32. Spiegel JH, Polat JK. Microvascular flap reconstruction by otolaryngologists: prevalence, postoperative care, and monitoring techniques. Laryngoscope 2007; 117: 485–90.

33. Elliot D, Bardsley AF, Batchelor AG et al. Direct closure of the radial forearm flap donor defect. Br J Plast Surg 1988; 41: 358–60.

34. Ngo K, Goldstein D, Neligan P et al. Colorimetric evaluation of facial skin and free flap donor sites in various ethnic populations. J Otolaryngol 2006; 35: 249–54.

35. Siegmund CJ, Tighe JV. Sensory and motor function impairment after brachial plexus cord compression by a pedicled latissimus dorsi flap. Br J Plast Surg 2001; 54: 449–51.

36. Van Lierop AC, Fagan JJ. Buccinator myomucosal flap: clinical results and review of anatomy, surgical technique and applications. J Laryngol Otol 2008; 122: 181–7.

37. Merten SL, Jiang RP, Caminer D. The submental artery island flap for head and neck reconstruction. ANZ J Surg 2002; 72: 121–4.

38. Rieger JM, Zalmanowitz JG, Li SY et al. Functional outcomes after surgical reconstruction of the base of tongue using the radial forearm free flap in patients with oropharyngeal carcinoma. Head Neck 2007; 29: 1024–32.

39. Brown JS, Zuydam AC, Jones DC et al. Functional outcome in soft palate reconstruction using a radial forearm free flap in conjunction with a superiorly based pharyngeal flap. Head Neck 1997; 19: 524–34.

40. Kuriakose MA, Loree TR, Spies A et al. Sensate radial forearm free flaps in tongue reconstruction. Arch Otolaryngol Head Neck Surg 2001; 127: 1463–6.

41. Netscher D, Armenta AH, Meade RA et al. Sensory recovery of innervated and non-innervated radial forearm free flaps: functional implications. J Reconstr Microsurg 2000; 16: 179–85.

42. Maciejewski A, Szymczyk C. Fibula free flap for mandible reconstruction: analysis of 30 consecutive cases and quality of life evaluation. J Reconstr Microsurg 2007; 23: 1–10.

43. Head C, Alam D, Sercarz JA et al. Microvascular flap reconstruction of the mandible: a comparison of bone grafts and bridging plates for restoration of mandibular continuity. Otolaryngol Head Neck Surg 2003; 129: 48–54.

44. Wei FC, Celik N, Yang WG et al. Complications after reconstruction by plate and soft-tissue free flap in composite mandibular defects and secondary salvage reconstruction with osteocutaneous flap. Plast Reconstr Surg 2003; 112: 37–42.

45. Ellis E III, Miles BA. Fractures of the mandible: a technical perspective. Plast Reconstr Surg 2007; 120(7 Suppl 2): 76S–89S.

46. Kim Y, Smith J, Sercarz JA et al. Fixation of mandibular osteotomies: comparison of locking and nonlocking hardware. Head Neck 2007; 29: 453–7.

47. Peleg M, Lopez EA. The treatment of osteoradionecrosis of the mandible: the case for hyperbaric oxygen and bone graft reconstruction. J Oral Maxillofac Surg 2006; 64: 956–60.

48. Buchbinder D, St Hilaire H. The use of free tissue transfer in advanced osteoradionecrosis of the mandible. J Oral Maxillofac Surg: official journal of the American Association of Oral and Maxillofacial Surgeons 2006; 64: 961–4.

49. D'Souza J, Goru J, Goru S, Brown J, Vaughan ED, Rogers SN. The influence of hyperbaric oxygen on the outcome of patients

treated for osteoradionecrosis: 8 year study. Int J Oral Maxillofac Surg 2007; 36: 783–7.

50. Gonzalez-Garcia R, Naval-Gias L, Rodriguez-Campo FJ et al. Vascularized fibular flap for reconstruction of the condyle after mandibular ablation. J Oral Maxillofac Surg: official journal of the American Association of Oral and Maxillofacial Surgeons 2008 ;66: 1133–7.

51. Ono T, Kohda H, Hori K et al. Masticatory performance in postmaxillectomy patients with edentulous maxillae fitted with obturator prostheses. Int J Prosthodont 2007; 20: 145–50.

52. Genden EM, Okay D, Stepp MT et al. Comparison of functional and quality-of-life outcomes in patients with and without palatomaxillary reconstruction: a preliminary report. Arch Otolaryngol Head Neck Surg 2003; 129: 775–80.

53. Rogers SN, Lowe D, McNally D et al. Health-related quality of life after maxillectomy: a comparison between prosthetic obturation and free flap. J Oral Maxillofac Surg: official journal of the American Association of Oral and Maxillofacial Surgeons 2003; 61: 174–81.

54. Cordeiro PG, Santamaria E. A classification system and algorithm for reconstruction of maxillectomy and midfacial defects. Plast Reconstr Surg 2000; 105: 2331–2346; discussion 47–8.

55. Brown JS, Rogers SN, McNally DN et al. A modified classification for the maxillectomy defect. Head Neck 2000; 22: 17–26.

56. Okay DJ, Genden E, Buchbinder D et al. Prosthodontic guidelines for surgical reconstruction of the maxilla: a classification system of defects. J Prosthet Dent 2001; 86: 352–63.

57. Brown JS, Jones DC, Summerwill A et al. Vascularized iliac crest with internal oblique muscle for immediate reconstruction after maxillectomy. Br J Oral Maxillofac Surg 2002; 40: 183–90.

58. Peng X, Mao C, Yu GY et al. Maxillary reconstruction with the free fibula flap. Plast Reconstr Surg 2005; 115: 1562–9.

59. Clark JR, Vesely M, Gilbert R. Scapular angle osteomyogenous flap in postmaxillectomy reconstruction: defect, reconstruction, shoulder function, and harvest technique. Head Neck 2008; 30: 10–20.

60. Villaret DB, Futran NA. The indications and outcomes in the use of osteocutaneous radial forearm free flap. Head Neck 2003; 25: 475–81.

61. Lewin JS, Barringer DA, May AH et al. Functional outcomes after circumferential pharyngoesophageal reconstruction. Laryngoscope 2005; 115: 1266–71.

62. Varvares MA, Cheney ML, Gliklich RE et al. Use of the radial forearm fasciocutaneous free flap and montgomery salivary bypass tube for pharyngoesophageal reconstruction. Head Neck 2000; 22: 463–8.

63. Murray DJ, Gilbert RW, Vesely MJ et al. Functional outcomes and donor site morbidity following circumferential pharyngoesophageal reconstruction using an anterolateral thigh flap and salivary bypass tube. Head Neck 2007; 29: 147–54.

64. Govindaraj S, Cohen M, Genden EM et al. The use of acellular dermis in the prevention of Frey's syndrome. Laryngoscope 2001; 111(11 Pt 1): 1993–1998.

65. Casler JD, Conley J. Sternocleidomastoid muscle transfer and superficial musculoaponeurotic system plication in the prevention of Frey's syndrome. Laryngoscope 1991; 101(1 Pt 1): 95–100.

66. Nosan DK, Ochi JW, Davidson TM. Preservation of facial contour during parotidectomy. Otolaryngol Head Neck Surg 1991; 104: 293–8.

67. Biglioli F, Autelitano L. Reconstruction after total parotidectomy using a de-epithelialized free flap. J Craniomaxillofac Surg 2007; 35: 364–8.

68. Reddy PG, Arden RL, Mathog RH. Facial nerve rehabilitation after radical parotidectomy. Laryngoscope 1999; 109: 894–9.

69. Brown PD, Eshleman JS, Foote RL et al. An analysis of facial nerve function in irradiated and unirradiated facial nerve grafts. Int J Radiat Oncol Biol Phys 2000; 48: 737–43.

29

Reconstruction of the Oral Cavity and Oropharynx

Rajan S Patel, Patrick J Gullane, Christine B Novak and Peter C Neligan

INTRODUCTION

The oral cavity is a unique structure that serves a multitude of functions. It is the gateway to the aerodigestive tract and is vital in the production of normal speech. It houses many specific and highly specialized structures: the mandible, the teeth, the tongue, the palate, and the oropharynx. The oral cavity is lined with mucosa, which is lubricated by saliva. This mucosa covers the muscles that provide the motor functions that facilitate speech and swallowing. It is rich in nerve endings, which provide the special sense of taste as well as exquisite sensation.

When planning reconstruction of the oral cavity, there are several considerations that must be contemplated. Issues such as prognosis, the general medical condition of the patient, and the use of preoperative or postoperative radiation are important in selecting the type of repair (1–12). The extent of the resection and the tissues involved must also be considered. The fundamental question that must be answered is which tissues are being excised and consequently, which tissues need to be replaced?

RECONSTRUCTIVE TECHNIQUE

The reconstructive technique chosen can include multiple modalities, but the reconstructive ladder that applies to all defects is also applied in the oral cavity. These principles have been extensively discussed in the chapter on the principles of head and neck reconstruction. Planning of the reconstruction should consider the different reconstructive requirements of the oral cavity. These are discussed initially; thereafter, details of the various reconstructive techniques are discussed.

FLOOR OF MOUTH

Reconstruction of the floor of the mouth requires thin pliable tissue. The extent of the defect will determine which technique is most appropriate. Very small defects can be allowed to granulate and remucosalize or may be covered with a split-thickness skin graft. Local flaps may be used effectively in moderate-sized defects and include the facial artery musculomucosal flap (13), tongue flaps, palatal flaps (14), and nasolabial flaps. For larger defects, the radial forearm flap has become the workhorse within the oral cavity. It has the advantage of being thin and pliable and has the potential for reinnervation. The flap may be raised synchronously with the ablation, which reduces operative time. Access to the floor of the mouth for ablation and reconstruction is generally achieved, except for the smaller lesions, by the use of a mandibulotomy approach. A midline mandibulotomy is preferred because it provides excellent exposure and ensures maximal bone contact to the healing segments. It is important to ensure that the mandibulotomy is accurately repaired. This is achieved either with a plate or with lag screws (15–17). Accuracy is assured by applying the fixation prior to the mandibulotomy: the mandible is predrilled either at the site of plate hole placement or lag screw placement. The fixation device is then removed and the mandibulotomy is performed. At the end of the procedure the screws are merely inserted in the predrilled holes to give a perfect reduction and rigid fixation (Figs. 29.1–29.3).

When planning the reconstruction, it is important to ensure that there is adequate tissue to provide coverage of the defect and to avoid any potential tethering of the tongue, which can increase the morbidity and compromise functional rehabilitation. The defect should be carefully measured to ensure harvest of an adequately sized flap. Our flap of choice is the radial forearm flap, which is ideally suited to oral reconstruction because of its thinness, vascularity, and propensity for partial or complete spontaneous sensory reinnervation (18,19); however, objective evidence of improved sensory perception with intraoral forearm flaps reinnervated with the lateral antebrachial cutaneous nerve, has encouraged others to advocate the use of reinnervated forearm flaps because of improved functional sensation and thus an increased ability to sense food and oral secretions (20,21). The technique of raising the flap is critical and we have found it important to raise the flap in a suprafascial plane. This is well described and helps to significantly reduce donor site morbidity (20,22–25).

Xerostomia is one of the problems encountered by many oral cavity patients following radiation. To address this particular symptom, a patch of bowel can be used to reconstruct the floor of the mouth (26–29). Both colon and jejunal patches have been used for this purpose. These vascularized patches have the advantage of providing thin pliable cover as well as the potential to produce saliva. While they work well in producing mucus, the major disadvantages of these flaps relates to donor site morbidity and poor toleration of radiation.

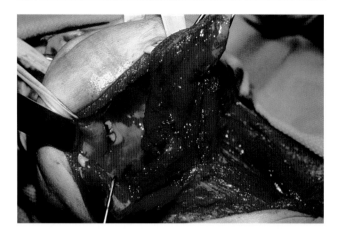

Figure 29.1 Mandibulotomy using degloving approach.

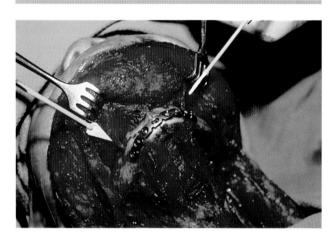

Figure 29.2 Application of fixation.

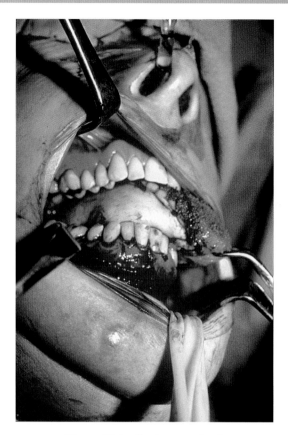

Figure 29.3 Flap inset completed.

TONGUE

The tongue is a unique muscular organ that fills the oral cavity and without which normal oral function cannot occur. The priorities for tongue reconstruction include restoration of swallowing, articulation, and airway protection (30). Normal or near-normal tongue mobility is vital for intelligible speech. The tongue also plays an important role in the initiation of swallowing by propelling the food bolus posteriorly into the pharynx. Functional reconstruction of such a vital and dynamic structure is very difficult to achieve. The result of the reconstruction as well as the most appropriate reconstructive choice depends on the size of the tongue defect. The capability to rehabilitate oral function is largely dependent on the volume of native tongue and preservation of the hypoglossal and lingual nerves. As more tongue is resected normal functional restoration becomes less likely and greater bulk is required in the reconstruction. For minor resections, a thin pliable flap such as the radial forearm flap is ideal and is the flap of choice.

It is important when insetting the flap to ensure that the remaining normal tongue is in no way tethered and is allowed to move optimally. The reconstruction can best be achieved by folding the flap along the lateral border of the tongue and insetting it in such a way that the part of the flap covering the resected surface of the tongue is functionally separate from the portion of the flap covering the adjacent floor of mouth (Figs. 29.4–29.6). Hemiglossectomy and subtotal glossectomy defects with laryngeal preservation are associated with a high incidence of significant permanent swallowing problems (Figs. 29.7–29.9). Nevertheless, with preservation of a segment of the tongue base and at least one hypoglossal nerve, rehabilitation of functional swallowing is achievable. In these cases, our preferred method of reconstruction is the anterolateral thigh flap, which provides considerably more tissue bulk than the forearm flap, and also avoids the donor site morbidity associated with the radial forearm flap. Regional flaps such as the pectoralis major provide good initial results but do not stand the test of time (31,32). Functioning muscle flaps have been advocated in order to obliterate the space between floor of mouth and palate during swallowing but the results have been disappointing (33,34).

THE LATERAL OROPHARYNX

The oropharynx is frequently involved in oral malignancies and as with areas within the oral cavity, it demands

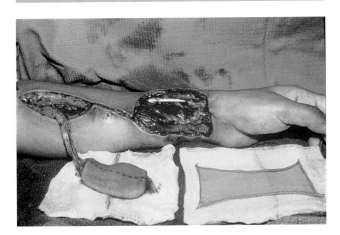

Figure 29.4   Elevated radial forearm flap.

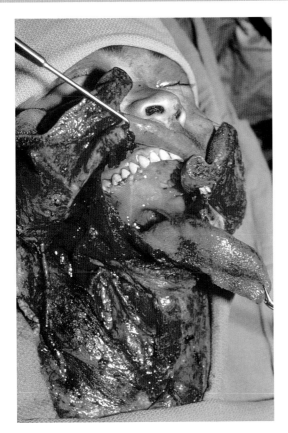

Figure 29.5   Tongue defect, mandibulotomy approach.

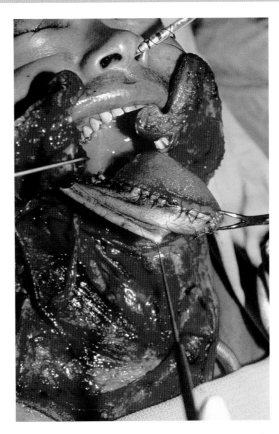

Figure 29.6   Flap folded and inset along lateral surface of tongue defect.

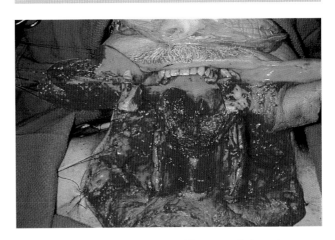

Figure 29.7   Mandibulotomy with near total glossectomy.

thin pliable cover. Again, in our practice, the radial forearm flap is the workhorse for this area. Other thin flaps, such as ulnar artery flap (35), the lateral arm (36–38), and anterolateral thigh flap have been used successfully and the selection, again, will be dictated by the size of the defect.

THE PALATE
Soft Palate

The soft palate is such a dynamic structure that reconstruction is difficult and its repair has traditionally been non-surgical, a prosthesis being frequently used to obturate the palatal defect. Fitting such a prosthesis is frequently

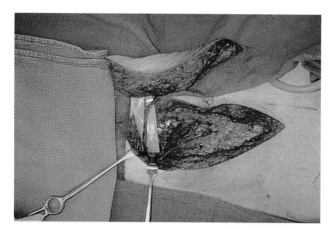

Figure 29.8 Elevation of free rectus cutaneous perforator flap on the inferior epigastric artery.

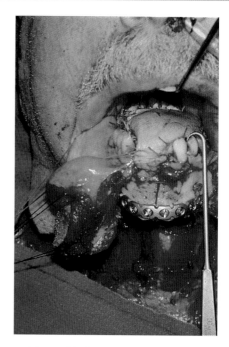

Figure 29.9 Flap inset and closure.

troublesome and the prosthesis may be difficult to wear because of mucositis. Thin sensate flaps such as the radial forearm are best suited to this area (39). Because the flap is non-dynamic, however, velopharyngeal competence cannot be achieved unless the flap touches the posterior pharyngeal wall. Urken achieves this by fashioning a pharyngoplasty incorporated within his flap (40).

Hard Palate

In the past reconstruction was frequently achieved with the use of prostheses, an obturator being attached to the dental prosthesis in order to plug the palatal hole. While this technique works extremely well in most circumstances, there are certain situations where functional rehabilitation of the patient can be enhanced with the use of vascularized free flaps incorporating bone and soft tissue, such as the scapula osteocutaneous flap. This method of reconstruction will be discussed in more detail in the chapter on principles of head and neck reconstruction.

THE MANDIBLE

Mandibular reconstruction has evolved over the past two decades from a complex and often unsuccessful venture to a very reliable but still complex technique. The main reason for this advance has been the incorporation of microsurgical techniques and the development of reliable flaps for the reconstruction (6). The concept of maintaining quality of life has become particularly important in the overall care and treatment of cancer patients (41,42). Thus, patients with even a very limited life expectancy are routinely reconstructed if it is expected that their quality of remaining life would be significantly enhanced (4). The high success rate of head and neck reconstructive procedures has allowed for significant improvement in both functional and aesthetic results and has completely changed the conceptual approach to mandibular reconstruction. Only patients who are medically unfit to tolerate a prolonged operation or have a poor prognosis are excluded as candidates for resection and immediate reconstruction.

The ideal tissue for mandibular reconstruction, which incorporates soft tissue and bone, does not exist. What we

seek is a combination of the best bone stock with the best skin paddle that produces the least morbidity at both the donor and recipient sites. Repair of a mandibular defect frequently includes bone and soft tissue, which are needed to replace intraoral lining, external skin, or both. While such flaps do exist, each reconstruction is a compromise. The price paid for reconstruction is measured in terms of donor site morbidity, functional loss, and days of life lost. This latter concept was introduced by Boyd et al. in 1995 and is a valid one (4). Given that the overall prognosis for many of these patients is limited, we must be sure that whatever intervention is performed is likely to succeed without complication. This surgery is technically demanding and the technical expertise that is required may not be universally available. It is not for the occasional reconstructive surgeon and requires a critical volume of work to maintain competence. Furthermore, these operations are resource-intensive and the postoperative care requires experienced nursing staff.

The choice of reconstruction depends on factors such as the bone and soft tissue requirements and the site of the defect (Figs. 29.10–29.17). Donor site availability and morbidity, ease of flap dissection and status of the recipient vessels in the neck, as well as the patient's overall medical condition, may also influence the final decision (6,9,43). Although microsurgery has revolutionized mandibular reconstruction, there is still also a place for more traditional techniques. Smaller defects can sometimes be repaired with reconstruction plates alone, and in certain circumstances the use of non-vascularized bone is still a reasonable approach (44). It may even be acceptable not to reconstruct the bony defect in a small subset of patients with posterolateral defects. The absolute indications for vascularized bony mandibular reconstruction are in patients who will have postoperative radiation therapy, and in those with a central

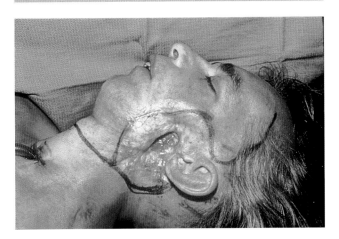

Figure 29.10 Extensive osteoradionecrosis with recurrent adenoid cystic carcinoma of the left skull base.

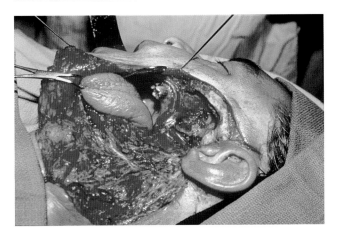

Figure 29.11 Extensive defect, bone and soft tissue.

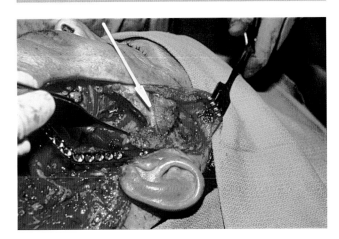

Figure 29.12 Reconstruction of hemimandible with plate. Note temporalis fascia cushion for the glenoid fossa.

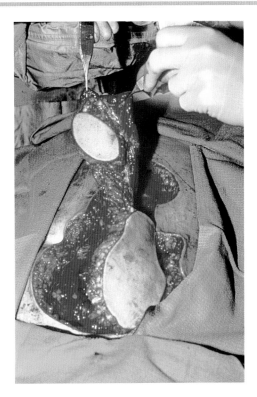

Figure 29.13 Elevation of double-paddle free myocutaneous rectus flap.

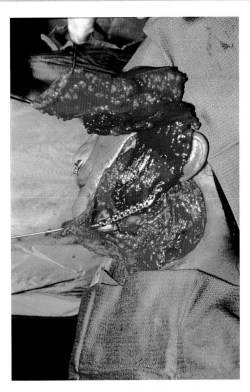

Figure 29.14 Flap inset, one paddle for lining and one for resurfacing.

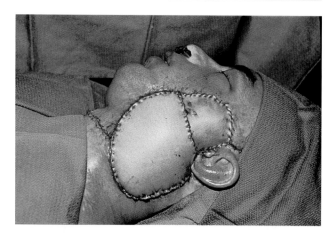

Figure 29.15 Inset and closure. Note skin graft on muscle.

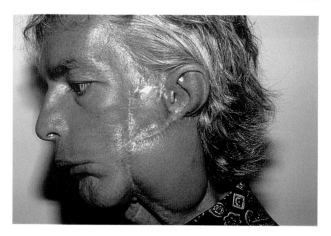

Figure 29.16 One year postoperative.

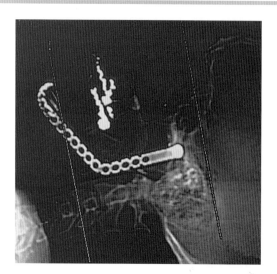

Figure 29.17 Plate at one year.

anterior mandibular defect, the C defect according to the HCL classification (45). Using alternative techniques in these cases produces unacceptable functional and cosmetic results.

Replacement of the resected mandible with a replica of what has been removed is important. There are several ways in which this can be done. The most common and simple method is to apply a mandibular reconstruction plate that will ultimately be used for fixation before resection. This ensures that when the plate is replaced, the remaining elements of the mandible will be in the same preoperative anatomical position. Thus, optimal occlusion as well as undisturbed temporomandibular joint dynamics can be assured. The plate is applied to the mandible, the holes are drilled and screws applied. The plate is then removed and used as a template for contouring the bony reconstruction.

In through and through defects of the mandible, the reconstruction plate cannot be applied to the mandible prior to resection. Some surgeons advocate the use of a template of the mandible that is designed from the preoperative CT scans. Alternatively, the mandibular elements can be stabilized with a bridging bar applied to the mandible prior to bone resection as shown in Figure 29.18. Once the mandible has been resected the reconstruction plate can be contoured appropriately.

The choice of flap is determined by the characteristics of the defect. While rib (46–48), metatarsal bone (49–51), humerus (52), and clavicle (53,54) have all been used in mandibular repair, the most widely used current donor sites include the fibula (55,56), iliac crest (57–59), scapula (60–62), and radius (63). Of these, the fibula is the workhorse flap in these situations (6,64). While iliac crest and radius have their proponents, they have for the most part been relegated to the position of secondary choice in those patients for whom the fibula, for whatever reason, is not an option. If soft tissue bulk is a requirement then the iliac crest may be a better choice and if extensive skin cover is required as, for example, in through and through defects, then the scapula may be a good option. While it has many desirable characteristics, the radial forearm flap is associated with a high rate of fracture in the residual radius, as shown in Figure 29.19.

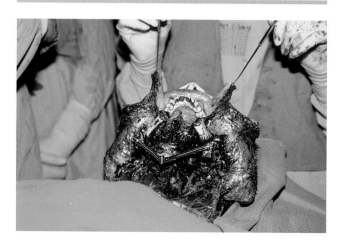

Figure 29.18 Bridging bar applied to stabilize mandibular segments prior to plate and graft repair.

FLAPS

The Radial Forearm Flap

The radial forearm flap provides excellent quality, thin, pliable skin, and has a reliable long vascular pedicle making it an ideal choice for intraoral reconstruction. Patency of the radial artery is established preoperatively with the Allen test (65). The flap is designed on the volar aspect of the forearm based on the radial artery, which is identified with its concomitant venous system running within a condensation of fascia referred to as the lateral intermuscular septum that separates the flexor carpi radialis and the brachioradialis. The flap is raised in a suprafascial plane leaving the vascular pedicle attached to this fascial condensation (Fig. 29.20). The cephalic vein is identified on the radial side of the forearm and harvested along with its tributaries that drain the skin flap. Care is taken to identify and preserve the superficial branches of the radial nerve, which provides sensation to the dorsum of the hand. Although rarely required, the radial artery may be traced all the way to the brachial artery.

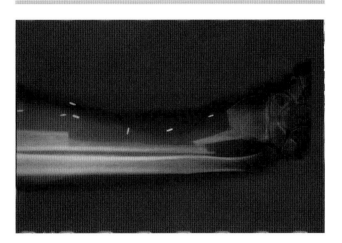

Figure 29.19 Note excess bone harvested with fracture of radius at six months.

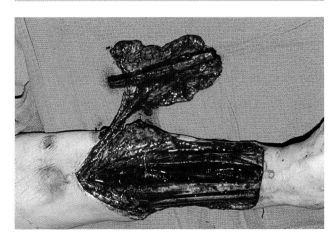

Figure 29.20 Elevation of osseocutaneous free radial forearm flap.

The Anterolateral Thigh Flap

First introduced by Song in 1984, the anterolateral thigh flap has recently been used more frequently for reconstruction of the oral cavity in those cases that require only soft tissue reconstruction (66–70). This flap can provide a large amount of soft tissue, which can include skin, muscle, and fascia if required. In many cases, the donor site can be closed primarily with no skin graft and thus minimize donor site morbidity (25,71). This flap is elevated from the lateral thigh and may extend from the greater trochanter to 3 cm proximal to the patella. The axis of the flap is based on a line between the anterior superior iliac spine and the lateral patella and the main perforator is located near the midpoint, which originates from the descending branch of the lateral circumflex femoral artery (Figs. 29.21–29.24).

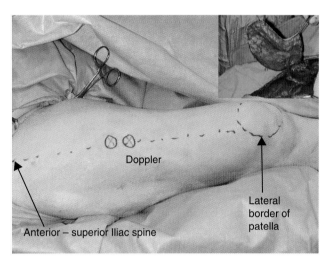

Figure 29.21 The axis of the anterolateral thigh flap is illustrated with the perforators located near the mid-point.

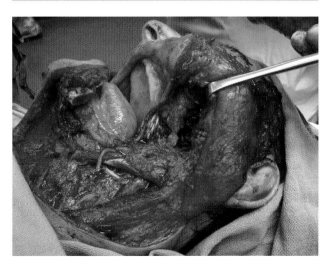

Figure 29.22 Extensive oral pharyngeal defect.

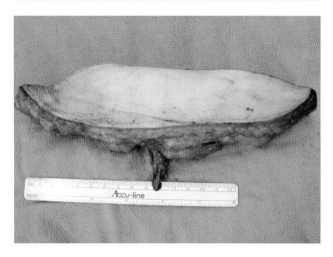

Figure 29.23 Harvested anterolateral thigh flap.

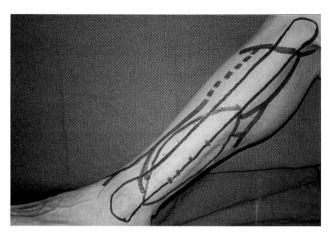

Figure 29.25 Outline of planned osseocutaneous free fibular flap. Note skin paddle designed low on the leg.

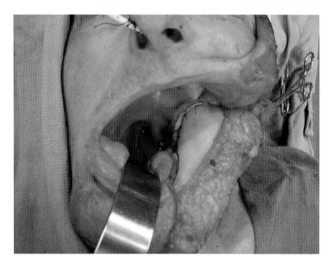

Figure 29.24 Anterolateral thigh flap inset.

The flap perforator may be either septocutaneous between the vastus lateralis and the rectus femoris muscles, or it may pierce through the vastus lateralis muscle, which will then require intramuscular dissection.

The Fibular Osseocutaneous Free Flap

The fibula can provide up to 25 cm of uniformly shaped bicortical bone and because of the profuse periosteal blood supply, it can tolerate multiple osteotomies. The bone stock is adequate to support osseointegrated implants; however, the height of the neomandible is limited relative to that of the native dentate mandible. The skin island, based on the septocutaneous blood supply is adequate in size and reliable in more than 90% of patients (72,73). The skin has the potential for innervation, but its quality is intermediate in thickness and pliability and therefore ranks behind that of

the radial forearm flap. The vascular pedicle is adequate in length and can effectively be lengthened by dissecting it off the proximal fibula. To provide soft-tissue bulk where needed, the flap can include the flexor hallucis longus muscle. Donor leg morbidity—with or without skin grafting following fibula free flap harvest—is minimal (Figs. 29.25–29.31) (74).

The Iliac Crest Osseocutaneous Flap

The ileum, based on the deep circumflex iliac artery (DCIA) and vein has a natural curvature not unlike that of the mandible. A total of 14 to 16 cm of bone can be harvested by extending the resection posteriorly to the sacroiliac joint (75). This bone can be contoured to reconstruct the anterior mandibular arch with osteotomies through the outer cortex, and is well-suited for placement of osseointegrated implants (76–78). The blood supply of the skin paddle of this osseocutaneous flap comes from an array of perforators that are located in a zone along the medial aspect of the iliac crest. It is important when insetting the skin paddle to maintain the relationship of skin to bone so as not to torque the perforators. Furthermore, the skin is bulky and not particularly pliable so that it is usually less than the optimal choice for intra-oral reconstruction. Donor site morbidity also can be substantial and because of the postoperative pain, patients are frequently slow to ambulate. Moreover, abdominal wall weakness, frank herniation and occasional gait disturbances can occur (77,79). The donor defect of the DCIA can be minimized by splitting the ileum and taking only the inner table of the bone with the flap (80). In this manner, the crest itself is left and the abdominal repair is much more secure. Holes are drilled in the remaining crest to which the three layers of abdominal musculature are attached. Furthermore, the muscles on the lateral side of the crest are undisturbed, thereby minimizing donor site morbidity. Finally, the cosmetic defect of this maneuver is significantly less than when the tradiational flap is used. The only disadvantage to this technique is that the thickness of bone harvested is generally inadequate to facilitate use of osseointegrated implants for

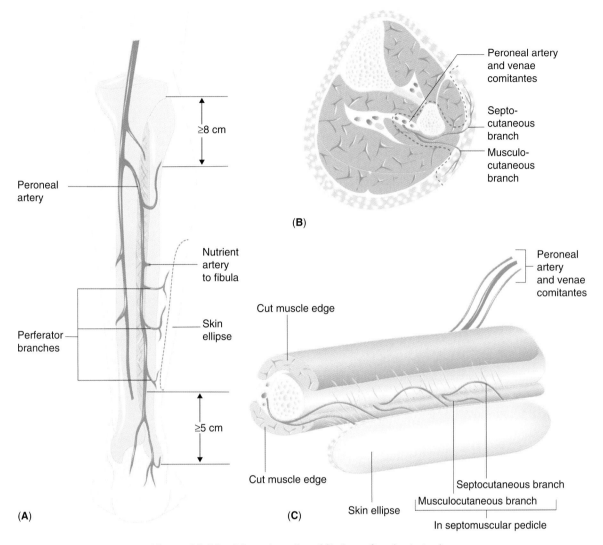

Figure 29.26 Schematic outline of fibular graft and osteotomies.

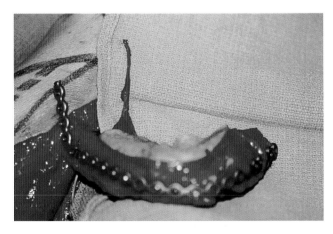

Figure 29.27 Plate contoured and then transferred to the leg, where bony osteotomies are performed; then vascular pedicle is divided and tissue transferred. This reduces ischemia time.

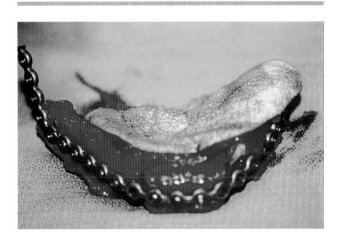

Figure 29.28 Flap transfer.

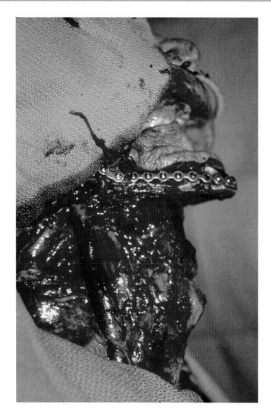

Figure 29.29   Flap inset completed.

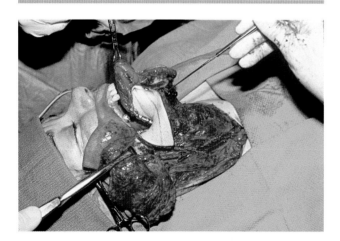

Figure 29.30   On occasion, two flaps are employed. Radial forearm for soft tissue lining, which provides thinner skin with innervation, is combined with free fibular bone flap.

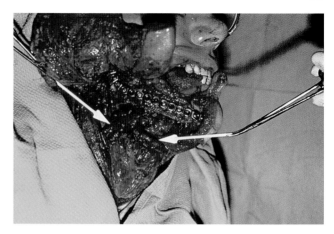

Figure 29.31   Fibula fixed with low profile titanium plate.

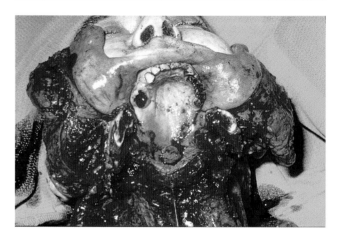

Figure 29.32   Total glossectomy and mandibulectomy.

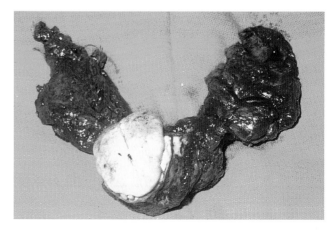

Figure 29.33   Total glossectomy and bilateral neck dissection specimen.

dental rehabilitation. The traditional criticism of this flap has been the bulk of the associated skin paddle. Using muscle instead of skin has become a popular alternative, which not only minimizes bulk but provides adequate muscle to cover most defects. This modification using the internal oblique, vascularized by the ascending branch of the DCIA, has rekindled interest in this flap for both mandibular and maxillary reconstruction (Figs. 29.32–29.39) (81–83).

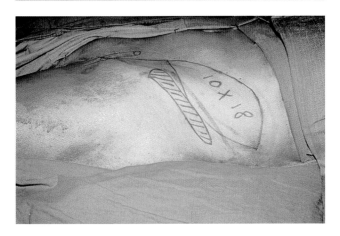

Figure 29.34 Outline of flap.

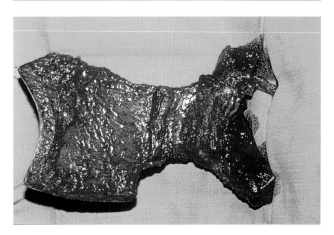

Figure 29.36 Osseocutaneous free iliac graft. Note thick skin paddle.

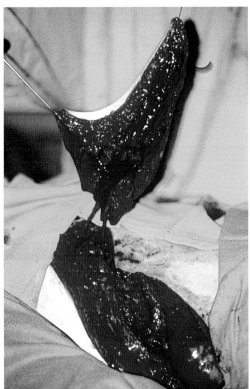

Figure 29.35 Elevation of flap.

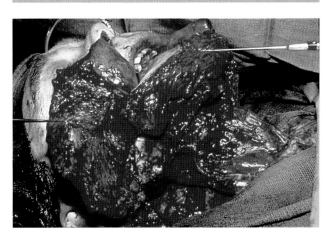

Figure 29.37 Flap inset with bone fixation using plate.

The Scapular Osseocutaneous Flap

Based on the circumflex scapular artery, this flap has the advantage of providing an extensive expanse of skin, muscle, and bone (84). Furthermore, the skin can be taken as separate skin paddles, a scapular as well as a parascapular flap based on the transverse and descending branches of the circumflex scapular artery respectively. The bony perforators, which are direct short branches from the circumflex scapular artery, supply the lateral border of the scapula and provide approximately 8 cm of good bone stock (62). The medial scapula also can be harvested with this flap (85) but harvesting lateral bone is more usual. Because of the anatomical characteristics of the vascular pedicle, the various elements of this flap (two skin paddles and bone) all can be manipulated independent of one another as there is sufficient vascular length to facilitate this. This makes the scapular osseocutaneous flap very versatile for reconstructing complex three-dimensional defects especially complex palatal defects (Figs. 29.40–29.43). It has the disadvantage, however, that the patient has to be turned in order to harvest this flap. Furthermore, while the bone stock is excellent it cannot safely be osteotomized. This limits its utility for larger bony defects greater than about 10 cm.

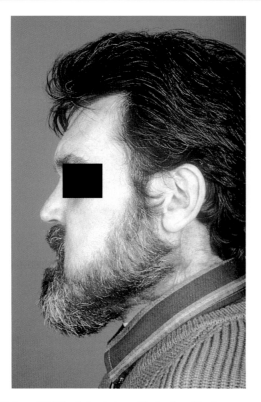

Figure 29.38   Lateral view with good profile at one year.

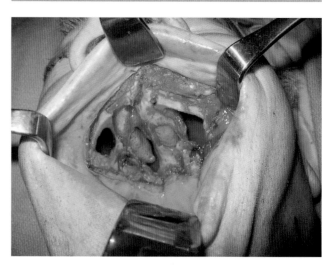

Figure 29.40   Total palatal defect.

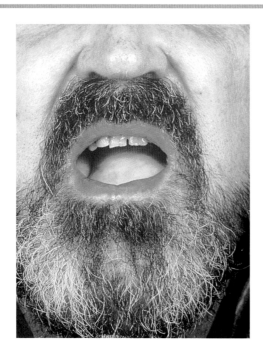

Figure 29.39   Result at one year.

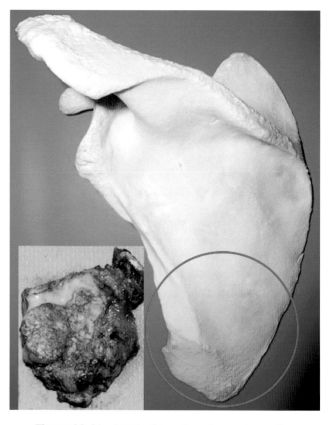

Figure 29.41   Design of scapular osteomyogenous flap.

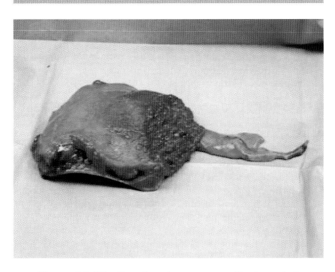

Figure 29.42 Scapular osteomyogenous flap harvested.

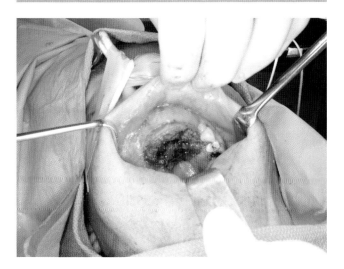

Figure 29.43 Flap inset.

SUMMARY

Reconstruction of the oral cavity is complex, which reflects the intricacies of the oral cavity itself. There is no perfect reconstruction and we have presented the current optimal choices for the various regions within the oral cavity. We are constantly seeking to improve our reconstructions in an effort to restore optimal function and quality of life to those patients who require surgical excision within the oral cavity.

REFERENCES

1. Beausang ES, Ang EE, Lipa JE et al. Microvascular free tissue transfer in elderly patients: the Toronto experience. Head Neck 2003; 25: 549–53.
2. Boyd JB. Mandibular reconstruction in the young adult using free vascularized iliac crest. Microsurgery 1988; 9: 141–9.
3. Boyd JB, Morris S, Rosen IB et al. The through-and-through oromandibular defect: rationale for aggressive reconstruction. Plast Reconstr Surg 1994; 93: 44–53.
4. Boyd JB, Mulholland RS, Davidson J et al. The free flap and plate in oromandibular reconstruction: long-term review and indications. Plast Reconstr Surg 1995; 95: 1018–28.
5. Deleyiannis FWB, Lee E, Gastman B et al. Prognosis as a determinant of free flap utilization for reconstruction of the lateral mandibular defect. Head Neck 2006; 28: 1061–8.
6. Gullane PJ, Neligan PC, Novak CB. Management of the mandible in cancer of the oral cavity. Operative Techniques in Otolaryngology 2004; 15: 256–63.
7. Neligan PC, Gullane PJ, Gilbert RW. Functional reconstruction of the oral cavity. World J Surg 2003; 27: 856–62.
8. Shpitzer T, Neligan PC, Gullane PJ et al. The free iliac crest and fibula flaps in vascularized oromandibular reconstruction: comparison and long-term evaluation. Head Neck 1999; 21: 639–47.
9. Shpitzer T, Gullane PJ, Neligan PC et al. The free vascularized flap and the flap plate options: comparative results of reconstruction of lateral mandibular defects. Laryngoscope 2000; 110: 2056–60.
10. Thoma A, Veltri K, Archibald S et al. Microsurgical reconstruction of the through-and-through defect in head and neck cancer: is it worth it? J Reconstr Microsurg 1999; 15: 401–8.
11. Thoma A, Levis C, Young JEM. Oromandibular reconstruction after cancer resection. Clin Plast Surg 2005; 32: 361–75.
12. Smith RB, Sniezek JC, Weed DT et al. Microvascular Surgery Subcommittee of the American Academy of Otolaryngology—Head and Neck Surgery. Utilization of free tissue transfer in head and neck surgery. Otolaryngol Head Neck Surg 2007; 137: 182–91.
13. Pribaz JEA. The intra-oral flap: the facial artery musculomucosal (FAMM) flap. Plast Reconstr Surg 1992; 90: 421.
14. Gullane PJ, Arena S. Palatal island flap for reconstruction of oral defects. Arch Otolaryngol 1977; 103: 598–9.
15. McCann KJ, Irish JC, Gullane PJ et al. Complications associated with rigid fixation of mandibulotomies. J Otolaryngol 1994; 23: 210–15.
16. Serletti JM, Tavin E, Coniglio JU. Transverse lag screw fixation of the midline mandibulotomy. Plast Reconstr Surg 1997; 99: 239–41.
17. Sullivan PK, Fabian R, Driscoll D. Mandibular osteotomies for tumour extirpation: the advantages of rigid fixation. Laryngoscope 1992; 102: 73–80.
18. Kerawala CJ, Newlands C, Martin I. Spontaneous sensory recovery in non-innervated radial forearm flaps used for head and neck reconstruction. Int J Oral Maxillofac Surg 2006; 35: 714–17.
19. Vriens JP, Acosta R, Soutar DS. Recovery of sensation in the radial forearm free flap in oral reconstruction. Plast Reconstr Surg 1996; 98: 649–56.
20. Boyd B, Mulholland S, Gullane P et al. Reinnervated lateral antebrachial cutaneous neurosome flaps in oral reconstruction: are we making sense? Plast Reconstr Surg 1994; 93: 1350–9.
21. Shibahara T, Mohammed AF, Katakura A et al. Long-term results of free radial forearm flap used for oral reconstruction: Functional and histological evaluation. J Oral Maxillofac Surg 2006; 64: 1255–60.
22. Chang SC-H, Miller G, Halbert CF et al. Limiting donor site morbidity by suprafascial dissection of the radial forearm flap. Microsurgery 1996; 17: 136–40.

23. Demerikan F, Wei FC, Lutz BS et al. Reliability of the venae comitantes in venous drainage of the free radial forearm flaps. Plast Reconstr Surg 1998; 102: 1544.

24. Lutz BS, Wei FC, Chang S et al. Donor site morbidity after suprafascial elevation of the radial forearm flap: a prospective study in 95 consecutive cases. Plast Reconstr Surg 1999; 103: 132–7.

25. Novak CB, Lipa JE, Noria S et al. Comparison of anterolateral thigh and radial forearm free flap donor site morbidity. Microsurgery 2007; 27: 651–4.

26. Habel G. Revascularized jejunal grafts in oral reconstruction. Ann R Aust Coll Dent Surg 1991; 11: 312–19.

27. Jones NF, Eadie PA, Myers EN. Double lumen free jejunal transfer for reconstruction of the entire floor of mouth, pharynx and cervical oesophagus. Br J Plast Surg 1991; 44: 44–8.

28. Jones TR, Lee G, Emami B et al. Free colon transfer for resurfacing large oral cavity defects. Plast Reconstr Surg 1995; 96: 1092–9.

29. Michiwaki Y, Schmelzeisen R, Hacki T et al. Articulatory function in glossectomized patients with immediate reconstruction using a free jejunum flap. J Craniomaxillofac Surg 1992; 20: 203–10.

30. Flood J, Hobar PC. Head and neck II: reconstruction. Selected Readings in Plastic Surgery 1995; 8: 17.

31. Sultan MR, Coleman JJ. Oncologic and functional considerations of total glossectomy. Am J Surg 1989; 158: 297–302.

32. Weber R, Ohlms L, Bowman J. Functional results after total or near total glossectomy with laryngeal preservation. Arch Otolaryngol Head Neck Surg 1991; 117: 512–15.

33. Haughey BH. Tongue reconstruction: concepts and practice. Laryngoscope 1993; 103: 1132–41.

34. Salabian AH, Allison GR, Rappaport I et al. Total and subtotal glossectomy: function after microvascular reconstruction. Plast Reconstr Surg 1990; 85: 513–24.

35. Lovie MJ, Duncan GM, Glasson DW. The ulnar artery forearm free flap. Br J Plast Surg 1984; 37: 486–92.

36. Katsaros J. The lateral upper arm flap: anatomy and clinical applications. Ann Plast Surg 1994; 12: 489.

37. Sullivan MEA. Lateral arm free flap in head and neck reconstruction. Arch Otolaryngol Head Neck Surg 1992; 118: 1095.

38. Yousif N, Warren R, Matloub H et al. The lateral arm fascial free flap: its anatomy and use in reconstruction. Plast Reconstr Surg 1990; 86: 1138–45.

39. Yousif NJ, Matloub HS, Sanger JR et al. Soft-tissue reconstruction of the oral cavity. Clin Plast Surg 1994; 21: 15–23.

40. Urken M. The restoration or preservation of sensation in the oral cavity following ablative surgery. Arch Otolaryngol Head Neck Surg 1995; 121: 607–12.

41. Schliephake H, Ruffert K, Schneller T. Prospective study of the quality of life of cancer patients after intraoral tumour surgery. J Oral Maxillofac Surg 1996; 54: 664–9.

42. Wilson KM, Rizk NM, Armstrong SL et al. Effects of hemimandibulectomy on quality of life. Laryngoscope 1998; 108: 1574–7.

43. Takushima A, Harii K, Asato H et al. Mandibular reconstruction using microvascular free flaps: a statistical analysis of 178 cases. Plast Reconstr Surg 2001; 108: 1555–63.

44. Gullane PJ. Primary mandibular reconstruction: analysis of 64 cases and evaluation of interface radiation dosimetry on bridging plates. Laryngoscope 1991; 101(Suppl 54): 1–24.

45. Boyd JB, Gullane PJ, Rotstein LE et al. Classification of mandibular defects. Plast Reconstr Surg 1993; 92: 1266–75.

46. Guelinckx PJ, Sinsel NK. The "Eve" procedure: the transfer of vascularized seventh rib, fascia, cartilage, and serratus muscle to reconstruct difficult defects. Plast Reconstr Surg 1996; 97: 527–35.

47. Millard DR, Dembrow V, Shocket E et al. Immediate reconstruction of the resected mandibular arch. Am J Surg 1967; 114: 605–13.

48. Netscher D, Alford EL, Wigoda P et al. Free composite myo-osseous flap with serratus anterior and rib: indications in head and neck reconstruction. Head Neck 1998; 20: 106–12.

49. Duncan MJ, Manktelow RT, Zuker RM et al. Mandibular reconstruction in the radiated patient: the role of osteocutaneous free tissue transfers. Plast Reconstr Surg 1985; 76: 829–40.

50. MacLeod AM. Vascularized metatarsal transfer in mandibular reconstruction. Microsurgery 1994; 15: 257–61.

51. Rosen IB, Bell MS, Barron PT et al. Use of microvascular flaps including free osteocutaneous flaps in reconstruction after composite resection for radiation-recurrent oral cancer. Am J Surg 1979; 138: 544–9.

52. Martin D, Breton P, Henri JF et al. Role of osteocutaneous external brachial flap in the treatment of composite loss of substance of the mandible. Ann Chir Plast Esthet 1992; 37: 252–7.

53. Seikaly H, Calhoun K, Rassekh CH et al. The clavipectoral osteomyocutaneous free flap. Otolaryngol Head Neck Surg 1997; 117: 547–54.

54. Siemssen SO, Kirkby B, O'Connor TP. Immediate reconstruction of a resected segment of the lower jaw, using a compound flap of clavicle and sternomastoid muscle. Plast Reconstr Surg 1978; 61: 724–35.

55. Hidalgo DA. Fibula free flap: a new method of mandible reconstruction. Plast Reconstr Surg 1989; 84: 71–9.

56. Hidalgo DA. Fibula free flap mandibular reconstruction. Clin Plast Surg 1994; 21: 25–35.

57. Jewer D, Boyd JB, Manktelow RT et al. Orofacial and mandibular reconstruction with the iliac crest free flap: a review of 60 cases and a new method of classification. Plast Reconstr Surg 1989; 84: 391–403.

58. Taylor GI. Reconstruction of the mandible with free composite iliac bone grafts. Ann Plast Surg 1982; 9: 361–76.

59. Taylor GI. The current status of free vascularized bone grafts. Clin Plast Surg 1983; 10: 185–209.

60. Coleman JJ III, Wooden WA. Mandibular reconstruction with composite microvascular tissue transfer. Am J Surg 1990; 160: 390–5.

61. Nakatsuka T, Harii K, Yamada A et al. Surgical treatment of mandibular osteoradionecrosis: versatility of the scapular osteocutaneous flap. Scand J Plast Reconstr Surg Hand Surg 1996; 30: 291–8.

62. Swartz WM, Banis JC, Newton ED et al. The osteocutaneous scapular flap for mandibular and maxillary reconstruction. Plast Reconstr Surg 1986; 77: 530–45.

63. Mounsey RA, Boyd JB. Mandibular reconstruction with osseointegrated implants into the free vascularized radius. Plast Reconstr Surg 1994; 94: 457–64.

64. Mehta RP, Deschler DG. Mandibular reconstruction in 2004: an analysis of different techniques. Curr Opin Otolaryngol Head Neck Surg 2004; 12: 288–93.

65. Allen EV. Thromboangiitis obliterans: methods of diagnosis of chronic occlusive arterial lesions distal to the wrist with illustrative cases. Am J Med Sci 1929; 2: 1–8.

66. Farace F, Fois VEE, Manconi A et al. Free anterolateral thigh flap versus free forearm flap: Functional results in oral reconstruction. J Plast Reconstr Aesthetic Surg 2007; 60: 583–7.

67. Celik N, Wei FC, Chih-hung L et al. Technique and strategy in anterolateral thigh perforator flap surgery, based on an analysis of 15 complete and partial failures in 439 cases. Plast Reconstr Surg 2002; 109: 2211–16.

68. Shieh S-J, Chiu H-Y, Yu J-C et al. Free anterolateral thigh flap for reconstruction of head and neck defects following cancer ablation. Plast Reconstr Surg 2000; 105: 2349–57.

69. Song YG, Chen GZ, Song YL. The free thigh flap: a new free flap concept based on the septocutaneous artery. Br J Plast Surg 1984; 37: 149–59.

70. Wei FC, Jain V, Celik N et al. Have we found an ideal soft-tissue flap? An experience with 672 anterolateral thigh flaps. Plast Reconstr Surg 2002; 109: 2219–26.

71. Lipa JE, Novak CB, Binhammer PA. Patient-reported donor site morbidity following anterolateral thigh free flaps. J Reconstr Microsurg 2005; 21: 365–70.

72. Jones NF, Monstrey S, Gambier BA. Reliability of the fibular osteocutaneous flap for mandibular reconstruction: anatomical and surgical confirmation. Plast Reconstr Surg 1996; 97: 707–16.

73. Shpitzer T, Neligan PC, Gullane PJ et al. Oromandibular reconstruction with the fibular free flap. Analysis of 50 consecutive flaps. Arch Otolaryngol Head Neck Surg 1997; 123: 939–44.

74. Shpitzer T, Neligan PC, Boyd B et al. Leg morbidity and function following fibular free flap harvest. Ann Plast Surg 1997; 38: 460–4.

75. Taylor GI, Cormack RJ, Boyd JB. The versatile deep inferior epigastric (inferior rectus abdominis) flap. Br J Plast Surg 1984; 37: 330–50.

76. Beckers A, Schenck C, Klesper B et al. Comparative densitometric study of iliac crest and scapula bone in relation to osseous integrated dental implants in microvascular mandibular reconstruction. J Craniomaxillofac Surg 1998; 26: 75–83.

77. Frodel JL Jr, Funk GF, Capper DT et al. Osseointegrated implants: a comparative study of bone thickness in four vascularized bone flaps. Plast Reconstr Surg 1993; 92: 440–55.

78. Moscoso JF, Keller J, Genden E et al. Vascularized bone flaps in oromandibular reconstruction. A comparative anatomic study of bone stock from various donor sites to assess suitability for enosseous dental implants. Arch Otolaryngol Head Neck Surg 1994; 120: 36–43.

79. Porchet F, Jaques B. Unusual complications at iliac crest bone graft donor site: experience with two cases. Neurosugery 1996; 39: 856–9.

80. Shenaq SM, Klebuc MJ. The iliac crest microsurgical free flap in mandibular reconstruction. Clin Plast Surg 1994; 21: 37–44.

81. Brown JS. Deep circumflex iliac artery free flap with internal oblique muscle as a new method of immediate reconstruction of maxillectomy defect. Head Neck 1996; 18: 412–21.

82. Moscoso JF, Urken ML. The iliac crest composite flap for oromandibular reconstruction. Otolaryngol Clin N Am 1994; 27: 1097–117.

83. Urken ML, Weinberg H, Vickery C et al. The internal oblique-iliac crest free flap in composite defects of the oral cavity involving bone, skin and mucosa. Laryngoscope 1991; 101: 257–70.

84. Clark JR, Vesely MJ, Gilbert R. Scapular angle osteomyogenous flap in postmaxillectomy reconstruction: defect, reconstruction, shoulder function and harvest technique. Head Neck 2008; 30: 10–20.

85. Thoma A, Archibald S, Payk I et al. The free medial scapular osteofasciocutaneous flap for head and neck reconstruction. Br J Plast Surg 1991; 44: 477–82.

30

Reconstruction of the Ear

David T Gault

INTRODUCTION

The aesthetic quality of the ear is extremely important. It is a mostly decorative structure of intricate twists and turns. Resection of the ear in whole or in part can cause psychological distress out of proportion to its size.

The ear components are difficult to mimic and reconstruction after major resection is a challenging task. It is worthwhile only if great attention is paid to fine detail. In addition to providing a realistic shape it is important to maintain the patency of the external auditory canal, to provide support for spectacles and, where possible, to maintain an anchor point in the lobe for earrings.

The ear is a thin sandwich of cartilage and skin. Over most of the ear, the skin tightly adheres to the cartilage and there is little excess skin available to be mobilized for cover of adjacent defects. It is more loosely attached over the helix and the lobe where a small amount of subcutaneous tissue is present. Minor defects in these zones are more readily dealt with by direct closure than elsewhere on the ear.

PATHOLOGY

Cancer of the ear is common and many tumors are induced by sun exposure. Ear cancer comprises 5–8% of all skin cancer. The decline in the wearing of hats, the adoption of shorter hair styles, the thinning of the ozone layer, and the popularity of package holidays all contribute. Even when sunscreens are applied to the face, the ear is often forgotten, allowing harmful rays unsuspected access to auricular skin. Patients on immunosuppressive therapy are especially at risk.

The majority of auricular cancer is squamous cell carcinoma (60%), followed by basal cell carcinoma (35%) and melanoma (5%). Adnexal carcinomas derived from sweat glands, hair follicles, and sebaceous glands can also occur but are less common. The ear can also be destroyed in childhood by capillary hemangioma. The current fashion for body piercing has caused massive ear keloids in some cases. Occasionally the ear structure is destroyed by infection following piercing for jewelry.

Squamous cell carcinoma arising de novo on the auricle is probably rare. Most tumors originate in areas of solar keratosis and the proper treatment of such minor lesions is therefore important. These discrete crusty lesions frequently develop on the helical rim. They are scaly and raised with thickening of both the prickle cell layer and stratum corneum. Some active lesions are infiltrated by plasma cells and lymphocytes. Squamous cell carcinoma is sometimes not aggressive on the rim of the ear but lesions of the concha and posterior surface are more worrisome and can spread to local lymph nodes.

Basal cell carcinoma of the ear is unusual in that it tends to occur in the conchal hollow and on the posterior sulcus (Fig. 30.1), areas that do not correspond to those of maximal sun exposure. Lesions of the ear often extend in a silent manner beyond the visible tumor. This, combined with the surgeon's reluctance to unnecessarily increase the postoperative deformity associated with wider margins, may explain the high recurrence rate after the excision of ear tumors.

Larger cancers (basal cell and squamous cell), above 2 cm in diameter, and recurrent tumors are especially likely to have unrecognized pockets of tumor at a distance from the visible margins. Rather than a spherical growth pattern they may have finger like projections of tumor along tissue planes. A useful guide is that the likely extension beyond visible limits is equivalent to the radius of a small primary lesion with a short history but to the diameter of a recurrent longstanding or thicker lesion.

Because there is limited subcutaneous tissue, tumors will become fixed to and invade the perichondrium at an early stage. Basal cell carcinoma in particular may spread laterally at the level of the perichondrium beyond the visual tumor limits but this deep lateral spread rarely exceeds 5–6 mm. When the perichondrium is involved the underlying cartilage must be excised.

Basal cell carcinoma presents a great diversity of appearance and can mimic a simple skin infection or a rash. Any suspicious persistent lesion near the ear should be biopsied (Fig. 30.2).

Malignant tumors of the external auditory canal are rare. Squamous cell carcinoma, basal cell carcinoma, and malignancies of the ceruminous glands may all occur.

TREATMENT

The treatment of keratosis is usually nonsurgical, using either 5-fluorouracil ointment or cryotherapy. It is important to distinguish between a keratosis and an early squamous cell carcinoma and biopsies are often necessary (Fig. 30.3). A nonhealing ulcer should be presumed to be malignant. The distinction between a basal cell carcinoma and a squamous cell carcinoma on the ear may not always be obvious.

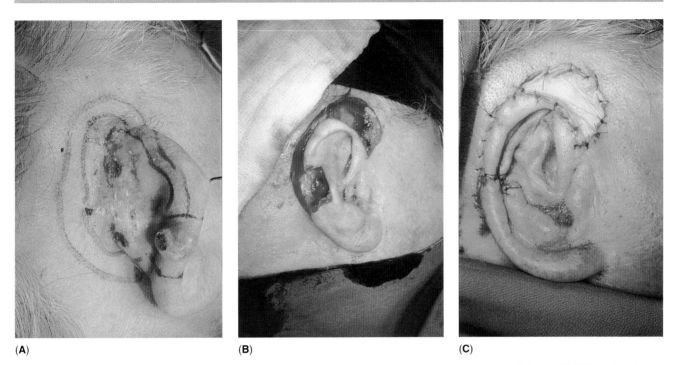

(A) **(B)** **(C)**

Figure 30.1 **(A)** An extensive basal cell carcinoma of the postauricular sulcus with a separate tumor on the rim of the ear. **(B)** Wide excision leaves an extensive defect. **(C)** The wound is closed by replacing the uninvolved external skin. A supplementary skin graft was used.

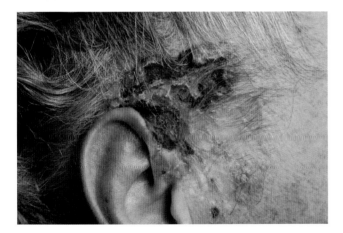

Figure 30.2 An extensive basal cell carcinoma involving the ear. This was diagnosed variously as a cold sore, psoriasis, and an atypical mycobacterial infection before a biopsy was taken.

The majority of tumors are treated with excisional biopsies and immediate reconstruction. With most lesions only a conservative margin is needed for cure. When a tumor is adherent to cartilage then wider margins of skin and cartilage should be taken because of lateral spread (Fig. 30.4). The more aggressive squamous cell tumors of the central and posterior parts of the ear should also be removed with a wider margin. The incidence of node metastasis from these sites is 6–20%. These tumors will need wide excision and regular follow-up (1–4).

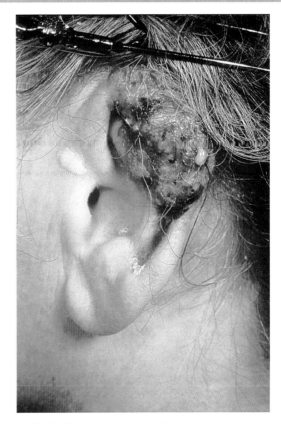

Figure 30.3 This nasty looking ear lesion was suspected to be a squamous cell cancer. Histology, however, showed this to be an irritated seborrhoeic keratosis.

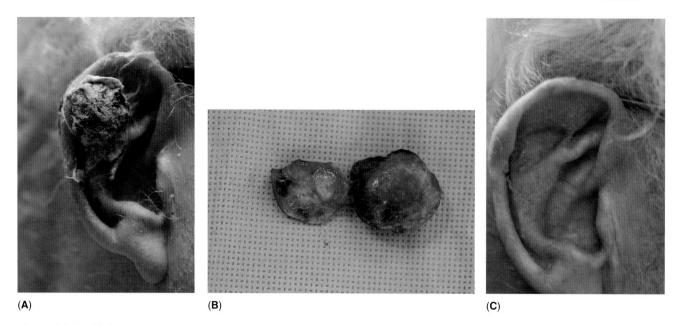

(A)   **(B)**   **(C)**

Figure 30.4 **(A)** An unusual tumor of the ear that turned out to be an atypical fibroxanthoma. **(B)** The excision biopsy and a disc of underlying cartilage. **(C)** The defect reconstructed with a skin graft.

Ablative carbon dioxide lasers can be used to excise superficial basal cell carcinoma tumors with little or no bleeding from the resulting wound bed (5). Lasers are also useful in removing keloids from the earlobe. This technique rarely cures the keloid but does appear to delay recurrence when compared to surgical excision.

Melanoma of the ear is treated first by a confirmatory excision biopsy. Subsequent treatment depends on the tumor depth. Tumors greater than 1.5 mm in thickness will require radical excision of the primary site. The old adage of 1 cm of clearance for every millimeter of tumor depth gives a useful guide.

If a melanoma or squamous cell lesion has spread to the nearby lymph nodes then a parotidectomy and neck dissection is needed. Surgery provides the mainstay of treatment. Adjuvant radiotherapy or chemotherapy is considered in special circumstances. Recurrence following radiotherapy is often considered to be chondritis, but a painful ulcer is more likely to be a recurrent tumor associated with chondritis.

Ceruminous adenocarcinoma of the external auditory canal is usually aggressive and cure rates are low. A basal cell carcinoma in the ear canal is often locally aggressive. In this hidden site the tumor may invade the petrous bone and early detection is essential for successful management. Excision of all involved tissue is a difficult surgical procedure (Fig. 30.5 and Fig. 30.6).

RECONSTRUCTIONAL ANATOMY

Reconstruction of ear defects is aided by a working knowledge of the relevant anatomy. The main nerve supply is from the great auricular nerve (C2, C3). This lies superficial to the external jugular vein and travels obliquely over the sternomastoid muscle to enter the ear through the posterior portion of the lobe. As it enters the ear it splits into several branches. Division of the nerve causes numbness of the lower two-thirds of the ear (Fig. 30.7).

The posterior surface of the ear is supplied with blood by auricular branches of the posterior auricular artery (Fig. 30.8). The lateral or external surface is supplied by the superficial temporal artery. A rich plexus of vessels around the helical rim links these systems and many reconstructive flaps are based on this ring of connecting vessels (6). Lymph drains to superficial parotid, mastoid, and superficial cervical lymph nodes.

RECONSTRUCTION AFTER TUMOR EXCISION: SIMPLE TECHNIQUES FOR SMALLER TUMORS
Direct Closure

In some patients, the skin of the helical rim is slack enough to permit direct closure when simple lesions, such as small basal cell carcinomata and chondrodermatitis nodularis helicis chronica, are removed. Incisions along the helical rim margin are particularly easy to close. When the skin is tight then skin on the posterior surface can be rotated onto the rim to assist closure. The skin on the posterior ear is less adherent and defects on the postauricular surface can often be closed directly. The scar is hidden in the groove behind the ear. Sometimes the ear is pulled a little closer to the head in the process.

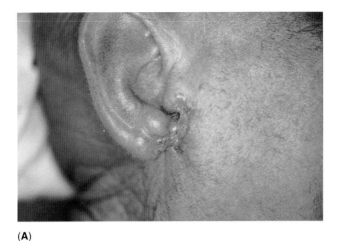

(A)

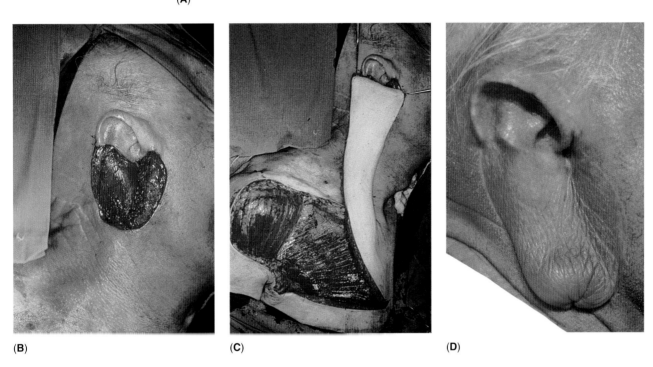

(B)   (C)   (D)

Figure 30.5 **(A)** An extensive basal cell carcinoma invading the external auditory meatus. **(B)** Wide resection was required to obtain clearance. The facial nerve was preserved. **(C)** A deltopectoral flap was used to resurface the defect. **(D)** The eventual result after return of the pedicle to the chest wall.

Skin Grafts

If the perichondrium can be preserved then a full thickness skin graft is an ideal reconstructive solution (Fig. 30.9). Both preauricular and postauricular donor sites are available. For lesions of the conchal hollow, a skin graft is a good form of reconstruction even if cartilage is excised (Fig. 30.10). The raw soft tissue behind the conchal cartilage will readily accept a skin graft. Small defects at other sites can be reconstructed with skin grafts, but it is important to preserve a round rim of cartilage and skin behind the defect. Without cartilage the helical rim margin will collapse postoperatively.

When large defects of the ear are excised, preserving the underlying perichondrium, then large split thickness skin grafts will give excellent results (Fig. 30.11).

Wedge Excisions

Defects on the helical margin can be removed as a small wedge. Some elderly patients with skin tumors have oversized ears (7–8 cm tall) and a small reduction in overall size is not readily apparent. A simple wedge should always be modified with small lateral extensions to prevent cupping of the ear when the components are joined (Fig. 30.12).

In the Antia and Buch technique (a modified wedge), the available circumference of the ear after tumor excision is enhanced by advancing (stretching) the locally available tissues along the helical rim (Fig. 30.13) (7). Large peripheral flaps of the adjacent helical margin are based on a wide postauricular skin pedicle. The earlobe varies in size, but in most patients loose tissue within the lobe can be advanced along the rim of the ear.

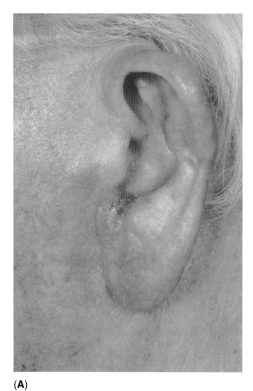

(A)

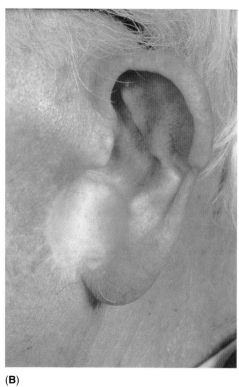

(B)

Figure 30.6   (A) A squamous cell carcinoma of the intertragal incisura. (B) The tumor was widely excised and the defect skin-grafted.

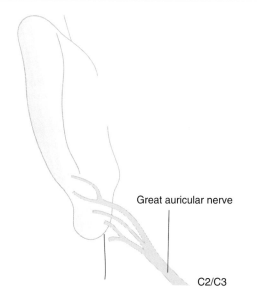

Great auricular nerve

C2/C3

Figure 30.7   Great auricular nerve entering the posterior surface of the ear lobe.

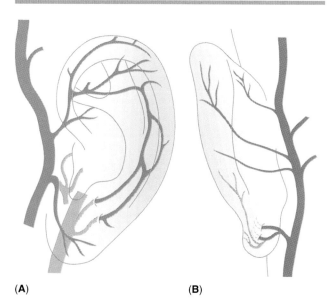

(A)   (B)

Figure 30.8   (A) The superficial temporal artery sends branches to the lateral surface of the ear. (B) The posterior auricular artery supplies the posterior surface of the ear. Both systems communicate in a ring of vessels near the helical rim.

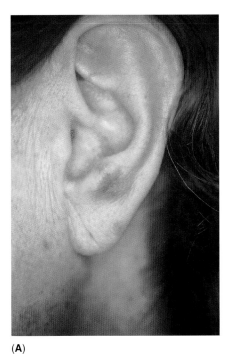

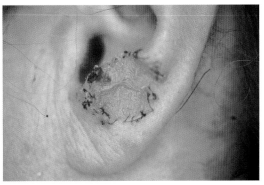

(B)

(A)

Figure 30.9 A basal cell carcinoma widely excised and reconstructed with a postauricular skin graft. **(A)** Tumor of the lower ear. **(B)** The skin graft has healed well. Some peripheral sutures have yet to be removed.

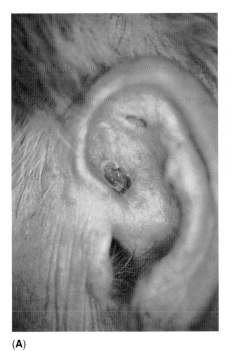

(A)

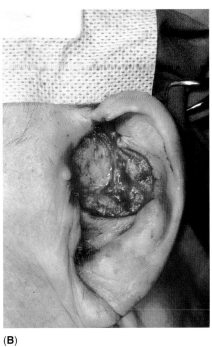

(B)

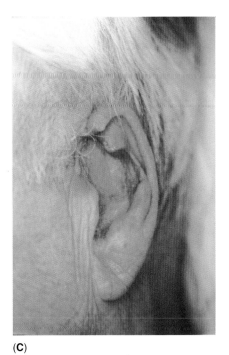

(C)

Figure 30.10 **(A)** A recurrent basal cell carcinoma of the ear after multiple attempts at cure. **(B)** Mohs micrographic surgery was used to confirm that extensions of tumor beyond the visible limits were excised. **(C)** The extensive defect has been healed with a split-thickness skin graft.

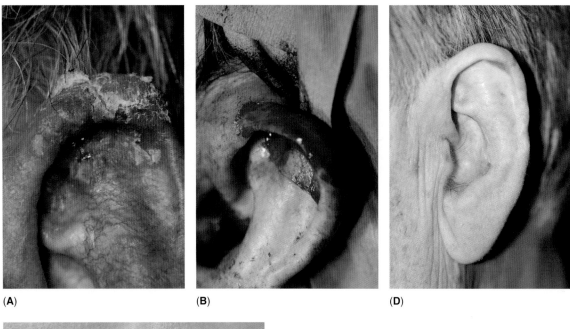

(A)   (B)   (D)

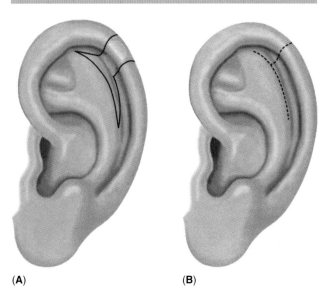

(C)

Figure 30.11   **(A)** Bowenoid actinic keratosis of the ear—a lesion that would not heal over many years complicated by erosions and infection. **(B)** The tissue was removed. **(C)** The excised lesion. **(D)** The ear resurfaced with a split thickness skin graft that was curative.

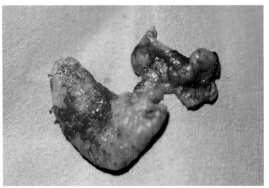

(A)   (B)

Figure 30.12   A small lesion treated by a wedge excision. The wedge is modified to prevent cupping of the ear.

This is a useful technique because the flaps are a good match for the missing helical rim. A single flap will suffice for small defects, but for larger defects the intact cephalic segment of the helical rim can be advanced into the defect as a second flap. Extension of the flap's triangular tail into the depth of the concha leaves the ear with a pleasing shape. The chondrocutaneous rim tissue is mobilized on a very wide and highly vascular pedicle and accurately apposed with fine sutures prior to skin closure.

Postauricular Pedicle Flaps

Defects on the posterior surface of the ear may be repaired by rotation flaps or transposition flaps. In the case of transposition flaps, the donor site is located in the posterior sulcus so that when this is closed, the ear is simply approximated to the side of the head. (Fig. 30.14 and Fig. 30.15)

Postauricular Pedicle Flaps to the Anterior Surface of the Ear

A large skin flap from uninvolved postauricular and adjacent mastoid skin can be used to reconstruct defects on the anterior surface of the ear. Such a flap can reach the concha

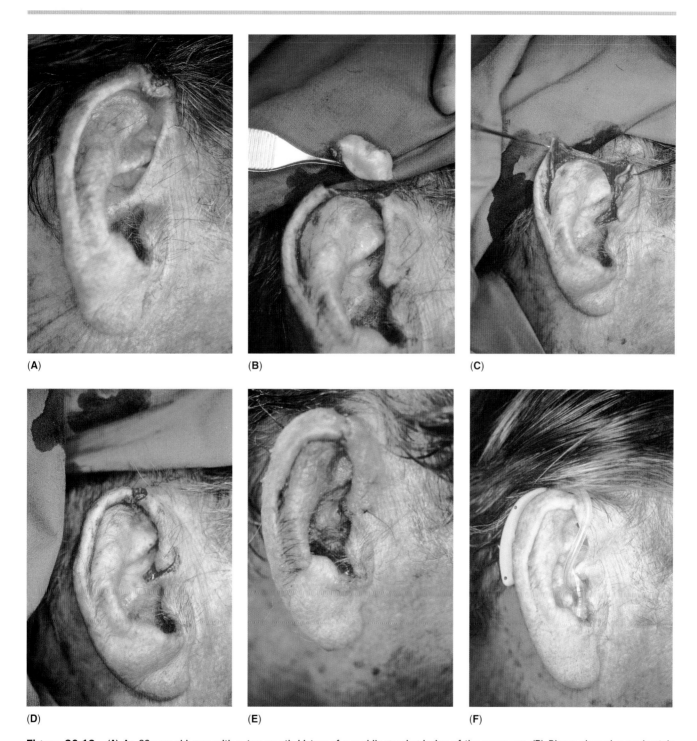

(A) (B) (C)

(D) (E) (F)

Figure 30.13 (A) An 83-year-old man with a two-month history of a rapidly growing lesion of the upper ear. (B) Biopsy showed a moderately differentiated squamous cell carcinoma with clear margins. (C) Helical rim flaps with intact postauricular skin are raised. (D) The flaps are stretched around the defect. (E) The final result. (F) The patient has been followed up regularly without recurrence. He can still wear his hearing aid.

and the scaphal hollow. It is easy to use and the skin color match is ideal. A posterior skin flap is outlined and undermined in the postauricular sulcus at a zone corresponding to the defect to be filled. A central pedicle of subcutaneous tissue is preserved. When the ear is pushed back the flap is delivered through to the external defect and secured. The donor site is closed directly.

An alternative to a subcutaneous pedicle is a de-epithelialized pedicle of dermis. Such postauricular flaps

are also flipped through the ear to the external surface and used for reconstruction of central ear defects. If both a superior and inferior dermal pedicle are preserved, then the flap is rotated into the central ear defect in the manner of a swinging door (Fig. 30.16). It is important to keep the donor defect elliptical in shape to allow easy closure. Wide undermining beneath the epidermis in the corners of the opening will allow substantial pedicles of dermis and subcutaneous tissue to nourish the flap. Small preauricular

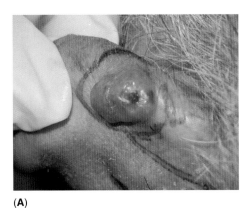

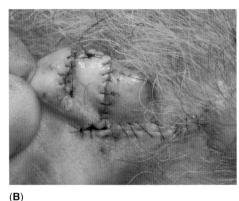

(A)   **(B)**

Figure 30.14 **(A)** A basal cell carcinoma on the posterior surface of the ear. **(B)** The defect excised and repaired with a local flap.

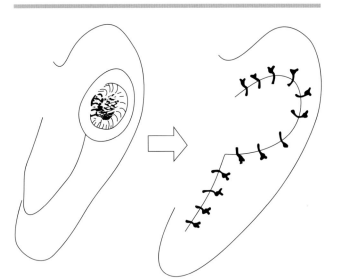

Figure 30.15   Transposition flap on posterior surface of the ear.

flaps and flaps from the concha can also be used to reach the external auditory meatus.

TECHNIQUES FOR LARGER TUMORS

When large tumors of the ear have been resected, then reconstruction will require some structural support to replace the missing cartilage. Small defects can be replaced by conchal cartilage grafts from either the same or contralateral ear. The curve of these cartilage grafts can be put to good use in mimicking a helical rim. When the missing segment is extensive, a carved costal cartilage framework is required (8). Complex shapes can be tailor-made to fit the defect after tumor excision, and this technique of reconstruction gives excellent results. In the age group that presents with auricular tumors, however, some patients are not keen on the additional discomfort of harvest of costal cartilage, and a number will opt to be fitted with a prosthesis.

AUTOGENOUS TISSUE RECONSTRUCTION
Stage 1
Preparation
Autogenous tissue reconstruction starts by mapping the shape of the normal (contralateral) ear. The shape is drawn on a see-through plastic sheet. (The section at the bottom on a chest X-ray film is ideal.) The scaphal hollow and triangular fossa parts are cut away to leave a template that can be sterilized for use throughout the operation (Fig. 30.17).

Construction of a Costal Cartilage Framework
Costal cartilage is harvested through an oblique incision overlying the costal margin anteriorly. Care is taken not to puncture the pleura. If a small hole is made, it should be closed and the final suture tied while the lungs are held fully inflated to avoid trapping air within the pleural space.

To minimize postoperative pain, a fine-bore cannula is left in the chest wound for the postoperative infusion of local anesthetic. To prevent atelectasis, it is important to consider chest physiotherapy following surgery.

The costal cartilage framework is constructed to mimic all the missing ear components. Before starting to carve the cartilage, it is essential to double-check whether a right or left ear is to be made. A cartilage segment from a floating rib is thinned to make a helical rim and blocks of cartilage from the synchondrosis are used to make a base plate and antihelical ridge. It is usually possible to carve the cartilage using scalpel blades and gauges, but in the elderly it may have calcified. If the material is excessively tough, a rotating burr may be used.

With care the cartilage segments are joined together with either 4/0 clear Prolene or fine wire sutures. Where possible, it is useful to preserve a layer of perichondrium on the external surface of the cartilage; it tends to prevent the stitches from cutting through. The cartilage edges are bevelled to abut neatly against any remaining original ear cartilage.

Insertion of Framework into Skin Pocket
The framework is next inserted into a suitable skin pocket. The siting of the incisions made to create the skin pocket requires careful planning. Wide undermining is used to

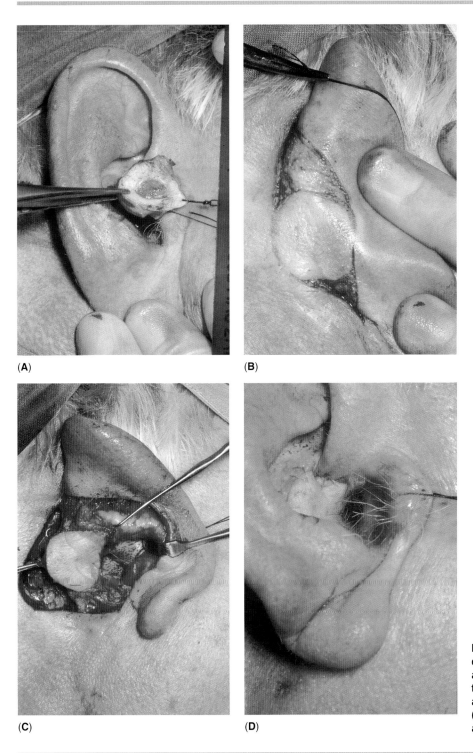

(A)

(B)

(C)

(D)

Figure 30.16 (**A**) A basal cell carcinoma of the conchal hollow of the ear treated with a postauricular flap. (**B**) An area of skin for the reconstruction is outlined. (**C**) Pedicles above and below the flap are preserved. (**D**) The flap is rotated into the conchal defect and sewn in place.

create a large pocket with broad attachments, thus preserving the skin's blood supply. Careful adjustment of the replacement framework is essential. Residual cartilage elements left behind after tumor resection are sutured to the framework, and any protruding ear remnants are blended with the reconstruction.

Skin from the posterior surface is raised and preserved as a pedicled flap. The edges are sutured together to form an airtight seal and suction drains are used to coapt the skin onto the carved cartilage framework. At the end of the operation, the ear defect has been filled by a contoured framework in the shape of an ear, albeit flat against the side of the head and without a post-auricular sulcus.

Suction is applied continuously for five days, so that the ear shape persists. Small silicone drains are used because

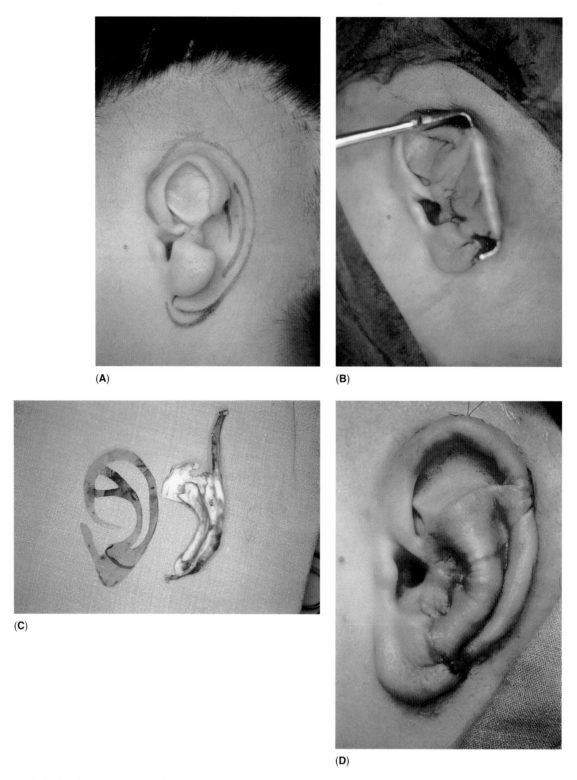

(A)

(B)

(C)

(D)

Figure 30.17   (A) A child with resection of the central portion of the ear. (B) An extensive postauricular pocket is created. This is held open with a retractor passed from the upper to the lower opening. (C) The template of the normal (contralateral) ear and the framework carved from costal cartilage. The helical rim and antehelical fold components are assembled together. (D) The skin is coapted onto the framework with suction drains to allow the detail to show through.

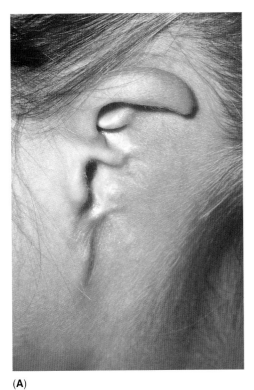
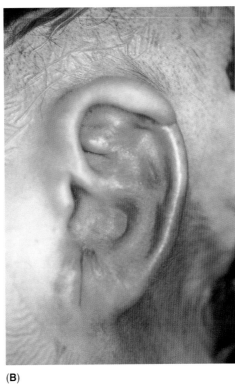

Figure 30.18 **(A)** A hemangio-pericytoma was resected in childhood. **(B)** The defect reconstructed with a costal cartilage framework.

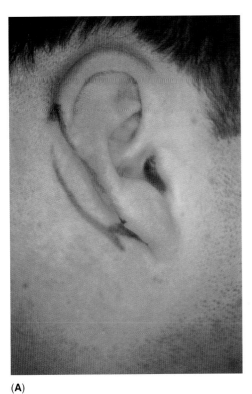
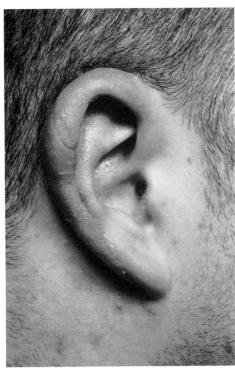

Figure 30.19 **(A)** A rim defect of the ear. **(B)** The result after reconstruction with costal cartilage.

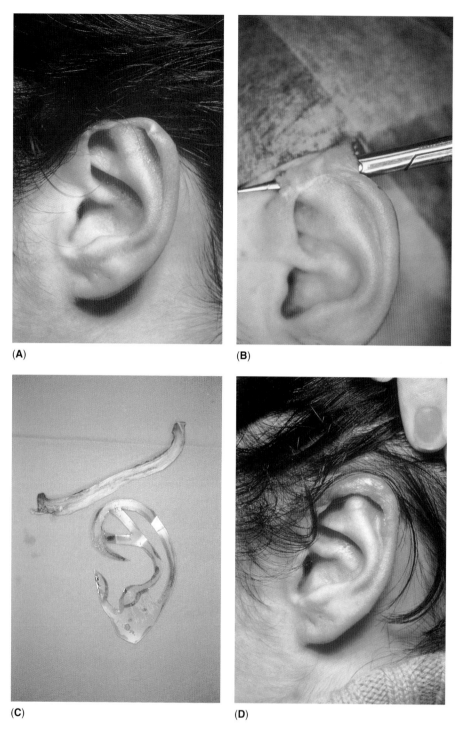

(A)   (B)

(C)   (D)

Figure 30.20   (A) An upper pole defect due to trauma. (B) The skin pocket is developed. (C) The template and the costal cartilage framework to be wound around the rim of the ear. (D) The final result.

they do not clog. The drains are connected to hollow needles that insert into Vacutainers. These containers are checked for suction (with each new tube a small splat of blood reaches the tube) and are changed regularly (when one-third full or even more often). A five-day course of antibiotic medication is recommended (Figs. 30.17–30.20).

Stage 2

Reconstruction of the postauricular sulcus is considered after a delay of 4–6 months to allow circulation to the zone of reconstruction to become established. An incision around the ear is used to elevate the whole reconstruction, taking care to preserve subcutaneous tissues over the framework to avoid framework exposure. The posterior surface of the ear is thus released from the mastoid fascia. This leaves two raw surfaces, one behind the ear and one on the side of the head. The majority of the defect on the side of the head is closed by undermining the scalp above and the neck below and closing these two flaps together. This is sometimes not easy, but the loop mattress suture can help to prevent the suture "cheese-wiring" through skin when skin edges are closed under tension (9).

The raw surface behind the ear framework is covered with a skin graft, either a thick split-thickness skin graft or full thickness graft. The graft is sutured in place with Vicryl (Ethicon, Inc, West Somerville, New Jersey, U.S.) and a Proflavine tie-over dressing is applied. Drains beneath the scalp and neck skin flaps are recommended.

An ear reconstructed using this technique is durable. Minor cuts and abrasions sustained in the future will readily heal. If a framework of artificial material is used (Silastic, Medpore), then the result is less durable, and minor skin damage causing exposure can lead to a significant infection and loss of the reconstruction.

PROSTHETIC TECHNIQUES
Glue-on Prostheses

Glue-on prostheses to replace missing ears and segments of ears are often used. It is now possible to make an auricular prosthesis that is difficult to distinguish from a normal ear. By embedding material to resemble small blood vessels, freckles, and moles, and by applying life-like coloration, excellent results are achieved by some prosthetists (Fig. 30.21).

It is important, however, that the patient feels confident that the prosthesis will remain in place regardless of his activity, and those retained by glue alone sometimes fall off. Moreover, cleaning the skin and applying glue is time consuming and messy, and some patients are, in addition, sensitive to the gluing agents.

Osseointegrated Fixation

The term osseointegration is used for a direct structural and functional connection between living bone and the surface of a load-carrying implant (10). The gold standard retention device for a prosthetic ear is currently a bone-anchored osseointegrated titanium fixture with a skin penetrating abutment (11). Auricular prostheses can be retained on this scaffold using clips or magnets.

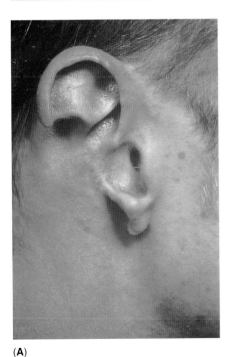
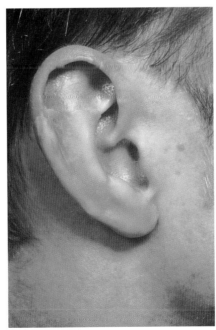
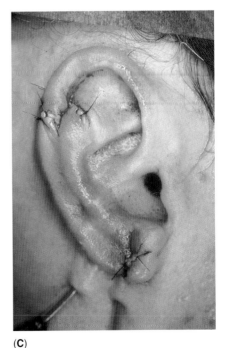

(A)   **(B)**   **(C)**

Figure 30.21 **(A)** A melanoma of the ear has been excised to leave a substantial defect. **(B)** A stick-on prosthesis replaces the missing segment. **(C)** At a later date the missing component is reconstructed with a costal cartilage framework.

Stage 1

The first stage of this process is to insert commercially pure titanium fixtures into the mastoid bone. The drill holes are sited with care so that the metal work lies beneath the antihelical fold of the prosthesis. Two fixtures are used, positioned 20–25 mm from the center of the external auditory meatus. The ideal site is at the 8 o'clock and 11 o'clock position on the right and the 4 o'clock and 1 o'clock position on the left.

A guide hole is drilled for each fixture, cooling the point of contact between drill bit and bone with normal saline throughout the process. Debris is regularly removed from the cutting surface of the drill bit to minimize heat trauma. The bottom of the hole is checked regularly to ensure that neither dura nor the sigmoid sinus is encountered. In good bone stock, a 4-mm deep hole is made. The guide drill is then replaced with a wider drill and countersink, again ensuring adequate cooling.

The final stage is to use a titanium tap at low speed (8–15 rpm). The tap is unscrewed and the fixture inserted into the threaded hole, again at low speed. A cover screw is used to protect internal threads on the outside of the fixture. Bone dust can be applied around the fixture and the periosteum carefully replaced before the incision is closed. The operation note should record the location of the fixtures. In patients who have undergone radiotherapy after tumor resection, hyperbaric oxygen treatment is advisable.

Stage 2

A second stage is undertaken some three months later when osseointegration is established. To make room for the prosthesis, auricular remnants are removed, ideally with the exception of the tragus. An incision is made 10 mm around the implant site. All subcutaneous tissue is removed as far as the pericranium, which is preserved, and the skin is thinned to approximately 1 mm thick around the implant. A hole is punched in the skin overlying the implants, the cover screws removed and the abutments screwed into place. With healing caps attached to the abutments, the thinned skin is replaced onto a thin layer of vascularized pericranium. This prevents movement at the interface between the skin and the abutments. A pressure dressing is applied.

Three or four weeks later, when the postoperative swelling has begun to settle, prosthesis manufacture is begun. An alginate copy of the defect is made. If this is done too early, it is possible to pull off the underlying skin and delay healing. Using the wound cast, an accurate silicone prosthetic ear with an acrylic base plate for fixation is manufactured. It is retained by either magnets or a clip and bar system, which attaches to the abutments (Figs. 30.22–30.24). In good conditions, a prosthesis will last two to three years. If the patient smokes or works in an oily or dirty environment, this period may be shortened. It is important to care for the abutment site, and cleaning around these pins with a soft toothbrush each day is needed.

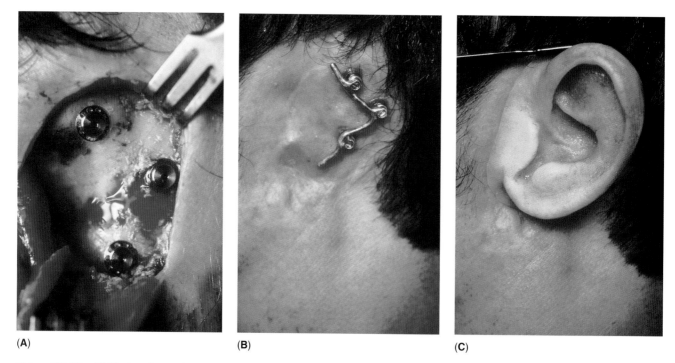

(A)   **(B)**   **(C)**

Figure 30.22   **(A)** Titanium fixtures inserted into the mastoid bone. **(B)** Abutments are screwed to the fixtures and a bar attached. **(C)** The prosthesis is securely fixed by clips to the bar mechanism.

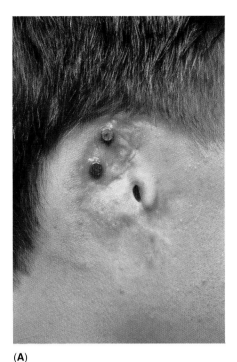

(A)

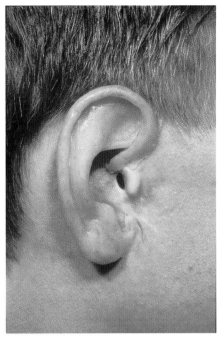

(B)

Figure 30.23 **(A)** In this patient, magnets are attached to the abutments for **(B)** prosthesis retention.

Some patients referred for reconstruction of the ear after tumor resection show no enthusiasm for either an autogenous tissue reconstruction or a prosthetic device. Where spectacle support is a problem, then a simple device can be fitted (Fig. 30.25). Other patients are grateful if enough upper pole tissue to support spectacles can be preserved (Fig. 30.27).

COMPLICATIONS AND TROUBLESHOOTING

Smoking

Smoking reduces skin blood supply and in patients undergoing surgery involving skin flaps or autogenous tissue reconstruction, this can predispose to skin loss. It is advisable to stop smoking six weeks prior to reconstruction if at all possible.

Skin Loss

Small areas of skin loss that expose autogenous cartilage will often heal in spontaneously if the area is protected by antibiotic ointment. Secondary healing may take several weeks. If the area of skin loss is greater than 1 cm in diameter, then local flap cover should be considered.

Problems with Bone-anchored Prostheses

Granulations around abutments can be removed with a carbon dioxide laser if extensive. If minor, then treatment with Aureocort ointment is helpful. Persistent soft tissue reaction around abutments may require their temporary removal. It is important to ensure that all soft tissues are removed around abutments at the initial surgery to prevent such problems. Rarely, trauma to abutments can bend them such that replacement is required. Keloid scars are also rare.

Infections

Tumors of the ear are often crusty and surrounded by keratin flakes adherent to the skin. Dermatologists have known for some time that staphylococci and streptococci can shelter there. Antiseptic solutions applied at the start of an operation may coat only the outer layers of such friable skin. Exposure of deeper tissues during tumor manipulation could increase the risk of wound infection (14).

Meticulous care with autogenous cartilage grafts is essential to avoid infection. Before reconstruction, the persisting curves and hollows of any residual ear tissue must be cleaned with a cotton bud and antiseptic skin preparation. The external auditory meatus is a particular source of potential infection. Grafts should be washed with saline prior to implantation. With precaution, infection is rare.

Hair Growth

In most cancer reconstructions that use autogenous tissues, the nonhair bearing mastoid skin is the source of local skin flaps. Unwanted hair on such flaps used to resurface the ear is best treated by excision and skin grafting. At the present time, laser treatment is able to remove unwanted

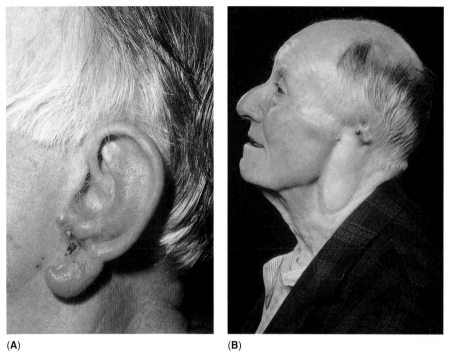

(A)

(B)

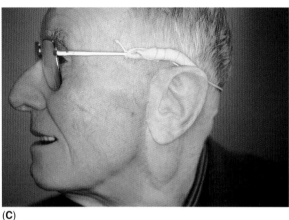

(C)

Figure 30.24 **(A)** A squamous cell carcinoma of the ear requiring wide excision. **(B)** The defect is reconstructed with a latissimus dorsi myocutaneous flap. **(C)** A bone anchored prosthesis is helpful to support his spectacles.

hair for several months but is not a permanent solution to the problem (12).

Poor Skin Quality

The presence of scars and skin grafts may render the local skin inflexible and not suitable to drape over costal cartilage when replacing resected segments of the ear. In these circumstances two devices can prove to be helpful.

Tissue Expansion

The placement of a tissue expander beneath poor quality skin requires great care. A remote incision is required for insertion. Small amounts of saline are added at weekly intervals via a remote port. The thickened capsule that surrounds the expander is removed before draping the skin created over cartilage grafts (Fig. 30.26 and Fig. 30.28) (13).

Fascial Flaps

If the superficial temporal artery is intact, then the temporoparietal fascial flap is an excellent source of thin vascularized tissue to be wrapped around a cartilage graft when no local skin is available. Skin grafts are then required to achieve healing but the results are very good. Such fascial flaps can also be used to cover areas of inadvertent cartilage exposure during a reconstruction. In patients with a low hairline these flaps are also useful (Fig. 30.29 and Fig. 30.30).

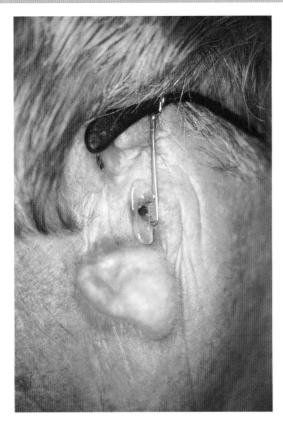

Figure 30.25   A patient with an extensive resection. He wished only to support his glasses, and a small custom-made device has been created.

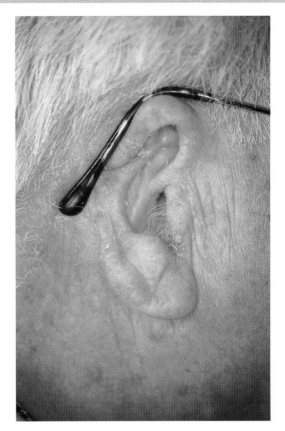

Figure 30.27   After an extensive resection of an ear tumor, enough tissue is left to support a spectacle leg.

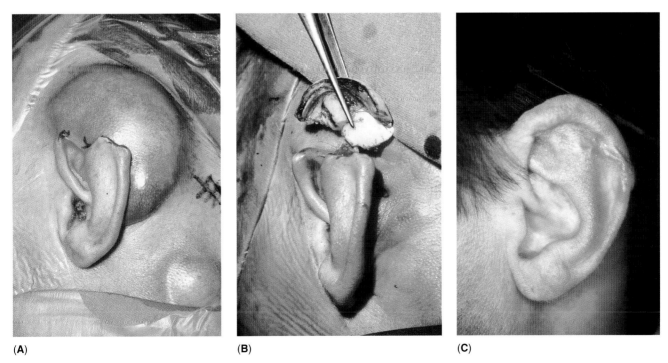

(A)   (B)   (C)

Figure 30.26   **(A)** Tissue expansion used to create extra skin for a costal cartilage reconstruction. **(B)** The cartilage framework. **(C)** The final result.

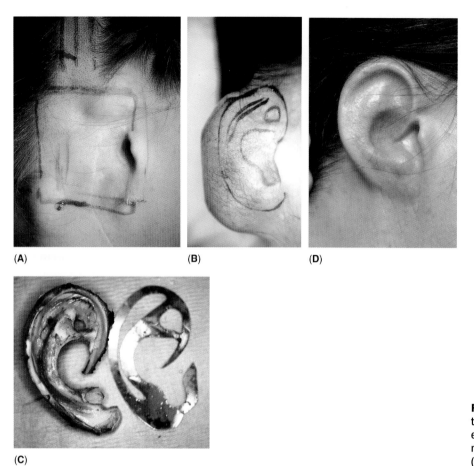

(A)   (B)   (D)

(C)

Figure 30.28 **(A)** Ear amputation to treat malignant melanoma. **(B)** A tissue expander has been used to generate extra non-hair-bearing skin. **(C)** The framework. **(D)** The reconstructed ear.

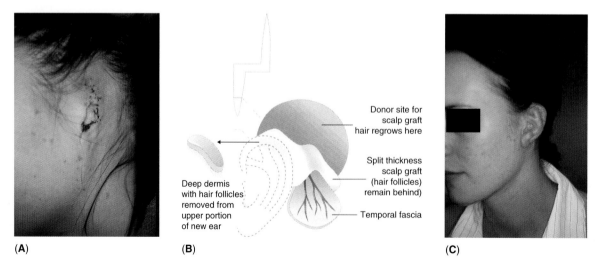

(A)   (B)   (C)

Figure 30.29 **(A)** Preoperative slide; **(B)** Diagram; **(C)** Postoperative slide. **(A)** This young girl was very distressed after her ear was removed in the treatment of a malignant melanoma. **(B)** To avoid hair appearing on the upper portion of the ear reconstruction, this zone was covered in a small facial flap and a split thickness scalp graft. **(C)** The completed reconstruction after release.

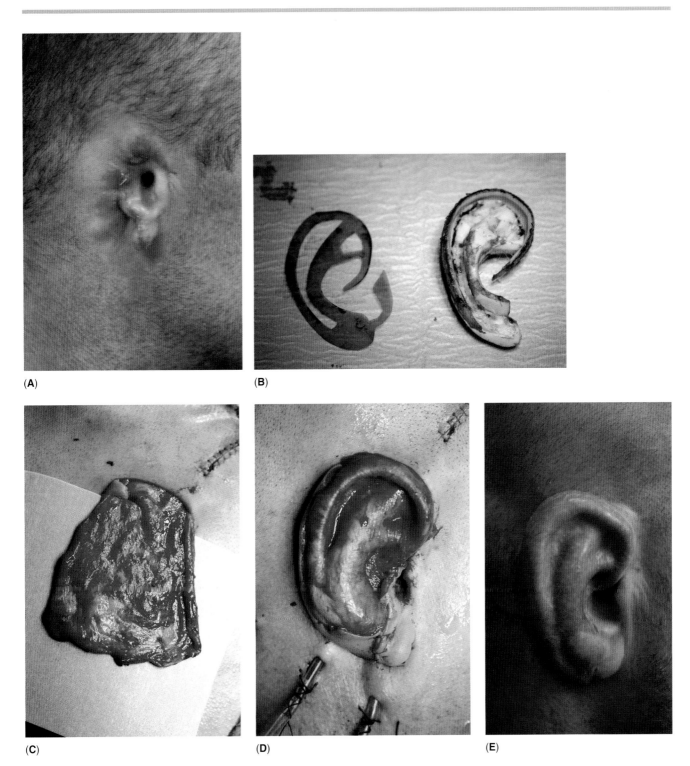

Figure 30.30 (A) An amputated ear with inadequate skin for reconstruction. (B) The costal cartilage framework. (C) The temporoparietal flap. (D) Suctions drains coapt the flap to the framework. (E) The finished result with a skin graft applied.

REFERENCES

1. Freedlander E, Chung FP. Squamous cell carcinoma of the pinna. Br J Plast Surg 1983; 36: 171.
2. Lederman M. Malignant tumours of the ear. J Laryngol 1965; 79: 85–119.
3. Lewis JS. Cancer of the ear. A report of 150 cases. Laryngoscope 1960; 70: 551–79.
4. Blake GB, Wilson JSP. Malignant tumours of the ear and their treatment. I Tumours of the auricle. Br J Plast Surg 1974; 27: 67–76.
5. Horlock N, Grobbelaar AO, Gault DT. Can the carbon dioxide laser completely ablate basal cell carcinomas? A histological study. Br J Plast Surg 2000; 53: 286–93.
6. Park C, Lineaweaver WC, Rumly TO et al. Arterial supply of the anterior ear. Plast Reconstr Surg 1992; 90: 38–44.
7. Antia NH, Buch VI. Chondrocutaneous advancement flap for marginal defects of the ear. Plast Reconstr Surg 1967; 39: 472–7.
8. Harris PA, Ladhani K, Das-Gupta R et al. Reconstruction of acquired subtotal ear defects with autologous costal cartilage. Br J Plast Surg 1999; 52: 268–75.
9. Gault DT, Brain A, Sommerlad BC, Ferguson DJP. The loop mattress suture. Br J Surg 1987; 74: 820–1.
10. Branemark PI, Hansson B, Adell R et al. Osseointegrated implants in the treatment of the edentulous jaw. Experience from a 10 year period. Scand J Plast Reconstr Surg 1977; 16: 1–132.
11. Tjellstrom A. Osseointegrated implants for replacement of absent or defective ears. Clin Plast Surg 1990; 17: 355–66.
12. Gault DT, Grobbelaar AO, Grover R et al. The removal of unwanted hair using a ruby laser. Br J Plast Surg 1999; 52: 173–7.
13. Chana JS, Grobbelaar AO, Gault DT. Tissue expansion as an adjunct to reconstruction of congenital and acquired auricular deformities. Br J Plast Surg 1977; 50: 456–62.
14. Beckett KS, Gault DT. Operating in an eczematous surgical field: don't be rash, delay surgery to avoid infective complications. J. Plast Reconstr Aesthet Surg 2006; 59: 1446–9.

31

Principles of Nasal Reconstruction

Caroline E Payne and Stefan OP Hofer

"I know of a nose that will save me from all my difficulties."
"A nose!" cried the jailer.
"A nose," said Yi Chin Ho. "A remarkable nose, if I may say so, a most remarkable nose."
A Nose For a King, Jack London 1904

INTRODUCTION

The nose has a central partnership with all the other facial units to impart conformity. It is a study of shading, curves, flow, and subtle blending with the other facial features (Fig. 31.1). The ability to master the aesthetic portrayal of the nose requires an appreciation of the light reflected off these curves and how light can significantly change the three-dimensional nasal image. The nose is a consideration and integration of angles, planes, and protrusions. The reconstruction of such a masterful piece of artwork is therefore a challenge that has emerged over the millennia.

TIMELINE OF NASAL RECONSTRUCTION

The ancient Egyptians replaced amputated ears and noses with prosthetics as the theology of Osiris, the god of the dead, stated that the body, in order to be effective during the afterlife, should be complete. The great edict of Horenheb (1319–1292 B.C.) demanded the nose to be cut off for thieving and the reality of this mutilation was punishment, humiliation as facial labeling, and an inability to attain the afterlife. During this period in ancient history and through the 2nd to 16th century A.D, nasal prostheses were fashioned from material available at the time, such as gold, silver, porcelain, leather, wood, and ivory; and for the poor, paper-maché. Ultimately, however, under the influence of a "good glass of wine" (for the patient) surgery came to the forefront in replacing what was missing.

The requirement for surgical nasal reconstruction originates in part from certain "barbaric" social customs. The symbolic significance of nose-cutting carries an underlying notion that cultural categories such as "honor" and "shame" are encoded in body morphology and affect behavior. Hence, the instigation of corporal punishment by removal of the nose for crimes such as committing adultery, abetting a thief, or stealing livestock.

The timeline for interventional nasal reconstruction follows a route mirroring the Turko-Mongol invaders as they reached India and dealt out such corporal punishment. The earliest writings in Sanskrit in the Sushruta Samhita (Vedic period around 600 B.C.), originally advances cheek skin and then develops the technique to a very sophisticated forehead flap practiced for centuries but only fully described by the Kangharia family of Kangars in the 1440s. These surgical techniques spread from India to Arabia, to Persia and Egypt, and finally Europe by trade routes, Crusades, invasions, and ultimately, printed materials.

The first European mention of nasal reconstruction is from the Branca family of Catania, Sicily. This family practiced the forehead method of reconstruction but also, imaginatively, raised the skin of the upper inner arm to rebuild the nose. It took until the middle of the 16th century to publish these methods because this surgery was carried out in the utmost secrecy to prevent knowledge of it spreading out of the family.

The University of Bologna surgeon Gaspare Tagliacozzi famously published his volume "De curtorum chirurgia per insitionem" (1597) on the aspects and undertaking of reconstructive surgeries (Fig. 31.2). At this time in history, religious belief and science were in conflict; the Pope had decreed that surgical experimentation was directly against the word of God. Even after death Tagliacozzi was exhumed from the nunnery where he had been buried and placed in unconsecrated ground for practicing these dark arts and interfering with the perfection of the Almighty.

The Indian forehead method of nasal reconstruction was finally published, centuries after its conception, in the *Madras Gazette* and conclusively in 1794 in the *Gentleman's Magazine of London* (Fig. 31.3). Mass printing and extensive distribution of this specialized current affairs periodical throughout the English-speaking world instantly sent the technique global.

In the modern era, the most common etiology of nasal defects that require reconstruction is skin cancer and to a lesser degree traumatic amputation. The quintessential characteristic of nasal surgery is the consideration that the nose is an entity that can totally disrupt a person's life. Any aesthetic and functional outcome must maximize patient satisfaction and allow patients to believe they are socially acceptable (1,2). The artist, Michelangelo di Lodovico Buonarroti Simoni (1475–1564) had his nose disfigured by Pieto Torrigiano and from then on he believed he was imperfect compared to his great contemporary at the time, Leonardo da Vinci and his "perfect face." Michelangelo would show his ruined image as minor characters in his later paintings (Fig. 31.4).

The nose performs such a pivotal role in appreciation of facial beauty that St. Aebbe the Younger (870 A.D.) cut

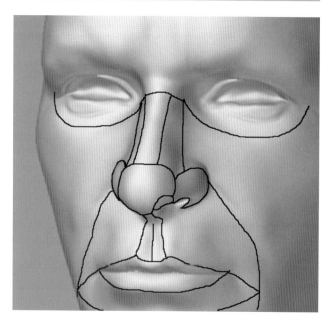

Figure 31.1. The blend of nasal and facial subunits. The importance of understanding these borders in nasal reconstruction.

off her nose ("to spite her face") so as to appear unappealing to the Viking raiders. Unfortunately, this was a Pyrrhic victory as they slaughtered her and all the other nuns as a consequence of their facial disfigurement.

THE IDEOLOGY BEHIND RECONSTRUCTION

Clinical Pearls: Goals for Nasal Reconstruction

I. Analyze defect
II. Do not fill a hole, but restore individual units
III. Nasal contours
IV. 3-D image
V. Assess subunits
VI. Resultant scars
VII. Restoration of function
VIII. Restoration of layers
  – Nasal Cover
  – Support
  – Lining

As the center of facial composition, the nose naturally attracts the eye. It is necessary to have a complete appreciation of nasal function because this acts as a guide for the reconstruction. Essentially, the reconstruction has to permit unimpeded airflow for normal breathing, speech, and smell. It may also be needed to support eyewear.

The transformation of a reconstruction into an aesthetic nasal unit requires the recognition of anatomical structural layers. The nose is divided into three main layers: the external soft tissue and skin, the osteocartilaginous framework, and the mucosal lining. The basic principle of restoration of each layer, preferably with "like for like," as in Millard's axiom, is the foundation of each reconstruction. Only by obeying the layer rule, localizing and measuring

the defect, and knowing local donor tissue availability can one establish which of the multiplicity of reconstruction techniques is the most appropriate.

The nose has its own composition of aesthetic units. Facial unity is produced when these units blend with the other facial components of lips, cheeks, orbital units, and forehead. It is imperative that they blend well because the human eye registers distortions of continuous lines, or disfigurements, causing us to stare at one another.

It is unrealistic to believe that a perfect nose can be created from surrounding tissues; the goal becomes to create acceptability, in a staring society, for the disfigured patient.

SUBUNIT PRINCIPLE

The nose is given its three-dimensional appearance by the subtleties of the convex and concave surfaces. These surface contours are the basis of the 9-aesthetic subunit principle by Burget and Menick (1985) (3) and have to be considered when recreating or adapting the defect (Fig. 31.5). When providing the external skin cover, scars are placed in the juncture of these units to make them less conspicuous. Originally defects were reconstructed in toto by means of local tissue with a disregard for the aesthetic subunits and final aesthetic outcome. The subunit principle from Millard (4,5) and expanded by Burget and Menick, takes into account the transition of skin type and the contours of the nose so that the visual topography is continued.

The other opinion outlined by Burget and Menick is to excise and replace the entire subunit if 50% or more of that subunit is deficient. The belief is that the distortion will be greatest above this percentage so it is better to replace the unit than try to repair half or more of it. This then should avoid the prominence of scars and replace correct contours so the visual line is not drawn to the reconstruction.

RECONSTRUCTION OF THE NOSE

Nasal reconstruction can vary from a minor defect to a total nasal amputation. There are local flaps in abundance for skin-only defects that may have a superior quality compared to simple skin grafts. For larger or more complex defects more specific consideration of the reconstruction of the separate layers needs to be made. The rest of the chapter will elucidate these three layers required in the provision of nasal reconstruction.

SOFT TISSUE NASAL SURFACE COVER

Nasal skin is very particular among ages, gender, and races, as it changes from thin pliable nonsebaceous skin over the rhinion, sidewalls, and dorsum to the thick, sebaceous skin interlaced with vertical septae at the tip. There are three soft tissue layers between the skin and the nasal skeleton: a superficial fatty layer, a fibromuscular level directly associated with the (superficial musculoaponeurotic system (SMAS) and then the periosteum/perichondrium. All levels play a significant role in determining skin surface reconstruction.

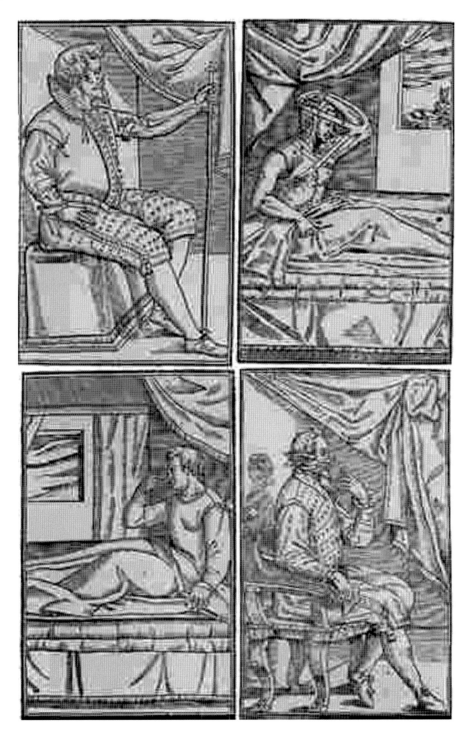

Figure 31.2 Gasparre Tagliacozzi, "De curtorum chirurgia per insitionem Libri Duo" (1597). The four levels of nasal reconstruction.

Soft tissue deficits are frequent occurrences on the nose because it is the site of several commonly found skin carcinomas, especially basal cell. There are aggressive histological subtypes, such as morphea form or infiltrating, which can easily extend to the lining and hence, have an increased incidence of recurrence. Mohs microsurgery is a complementary technique of ablative surgery that can be employed to gain clearance of these invasive cancers, but the resultant defect frequently does not conform to the subunit principle. It is a skill then to formulate a plan as to which subunits need adjustment to construct the most desired nasal restoration.

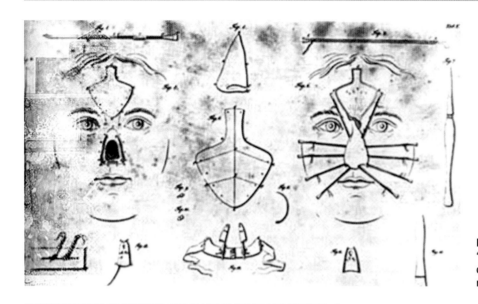

Figure 31.3 Original diagram in the "Gentleman's Magazine of London," 1794, describing the Indian method of nasal reconstruction.

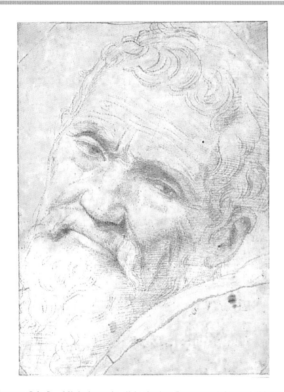

Figure 31.4 Michelangelo di Lodovico Buonarroti Simoni (March 6, 1475–February 18, 1564), Italian Renaissance painter, sculptor, architect, poet, and engineer.

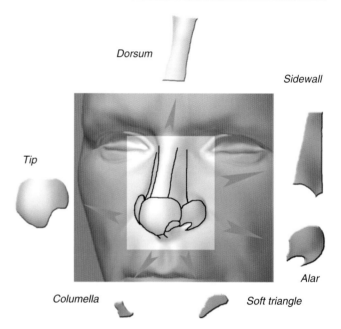

Figure 31.5 Surface topography of the nose and the nine subunits.

Grafts

When the surgical excision generates a skin-only defect, this can frequently be reconstructed with various commonly practiced plastic surgery techniques. A full-thickness graft taken from the pre- or post-auricular or neck area can provide ideal cover for defects to the nasal dorsum or sidewalls.

Small defects may comprise the alar rim subunit. This is an area of special consideration and frequently is included in cancer ablation. The alar skin alone is anatomically complex as the stratified squamous epithelium rolls over the rim to convert intranasally into hair-bearing mucosa adherent to the overlying cartilage and finally to pseudostratified columnar ciliated epithelium of the nasal mucosal lining. The tissue available that can simulate the alar architecture is found at the root of the helix, conchal bowl, or triangular fossa of the ear. The anterior auricular skin adheres tightly to the cartilage and can be harvested for use as a two-layer composite graft for lining or as a three-layer composite graft for alar rim or columella reconstruction. We believe the graft should be limited to 1 cm due to peripheral margin angiogenesis as the only source of blood supply for graft survival. Improved healing can be achieved by enlarging the subcutaneous contact surface by additional de-epithelialization when insetting the graft. This will increase the surface area for angiogenesis into the composite graft. Unfortunately, the sequence of wound contraction during the healing process usually distorts the rim with notching when these free grafts are employed. In our experience these grafts have a restricted use and often contract to some extent. The free helical root flap can be employed as an alternative and requires anastomosis to the facial vessels (6).

Skin Flaps

There are many congruous local flaps available for nasal reconstruction. The more caudal the nasal defect, the more suitable a local flap becomes as full-thickness grafts tend to demonstrate an obvious transition the farther they encroach on the zone of sebaceous skin. There are several local transposition, rotation, and advancement flaps designed to recruit the well-vascularized lax tissue found adjacent to the nose (Table. 31.1).

The most important consideration in the design of all these flaps is the donor site in the adjacent tissue and whether the flap can BLEND satisfactorily into the nasal cosmetic units without bulkiness, distortion, or pin cushioning. The tip and alar regions can easily be distorted due to flap bulk or tension and are areas of special consideration even for skin-only defects.

Bilobed Flap

The bilobed flap was described by Esser (1918) (7) and further modified by Zitelli (1989) (8) by adjusting the flap's

Table 31.1 Skin Flaps for Nasal Surface Reconstruction

Local	Bilobed
	Superiorly based NLF
	Inferiorly based NLF
	Islanded NLF
	Rhomboid
	Glabella
	Rieger
	Banner
	FAP flap
Regional	Forehead flap
	Washio
	Gullwing

Abbreviations: NLF, nasolabial flap; FAP, facial artery perforator flap.

rotational angle to a maximum of 50° each. This decreases the buckling around the pivotal point and the distal distortion that occurs with the previous bilobed design. The correct design is that the bilobed flap works best when the secondary flap is designed exactly vertically rather than obliquely and on defects no greater than 1.5 cm in diameter at the tip. Only with correct orientation and appropriate undermining of the pedicle base, as well as excision of the excess tissue at the turning point, can the flap rotate from a medial pivot point for alar defects and from a lateral point for tip, decreasing the chance of distortion and alar retraction (Fig. 31.6A, B, C)

Nasolabial Flap

The versatility of the nasolabial flap (NLF) comes from its excellent random blood supply from the multiple perforating vessels of the facial artery. It originates from the abundant mobile non–hair-bearing skin of the medial cheek, and is particularly useful in the older generation due to cheek laxity and the ability to hide the donor scar. The superiorly based flaps can be adequately thinned to the subdermal plexus to provide cover for the lower two-thirds of the nose, with cosmetic limitations to the supratip area. The pedicle to these flaps can leave a bulky distortion to the nasolabial fold that can be adjusted several weeks later to improve cosmesis. An alternative consideration initially is the islanded NLF or the facial artery perforator flap (FAP) (9). The inferiorly based NFL flap can provide nasal floor, alar, and columella reconstruction with the proviso that adjustment is needed due to bulkiness (Fig. 31.7A, B).

The Forehead Flap
Clinical Pearls: Forehead Flap

I.   Analyze all the defective layers
II. Note all subunits involved
III. Create accurate 3-D template
IV. Correct pedicle length
V.   Narrow pedicle base
VI. Three stage operation
VII. Consider lining

The forehead flap is the preferred method of cover for numerous nasal defects of differing sizes, varying from a minimal alar rim deficiency to a total nasal reconstruction. When analyzing the final defect it is important to realize that surgical ablation frequently is not restricted just to the nasal subunits. The resultant deficient area of soft tissue typically infringes on other cosmetic units, especially the cheek, and violates or effaces the nasal-facial junction. In these cases it is important to appreciate that the forehead flap needs to be combined with the cheek flap that is advanced and suspended at the nasal-facial junction. In conclusion, the focus for reconstruction must be centered on the nose and the other affected units need individual consideration and reconstruction.

The forehead flap has the history of surgery behind it, as previously described in the introduction, and over the centuries it has become a very sophisticated, robust method of reconstructing the nose. The refinements that are needed to gain the most out of this flap require patience,

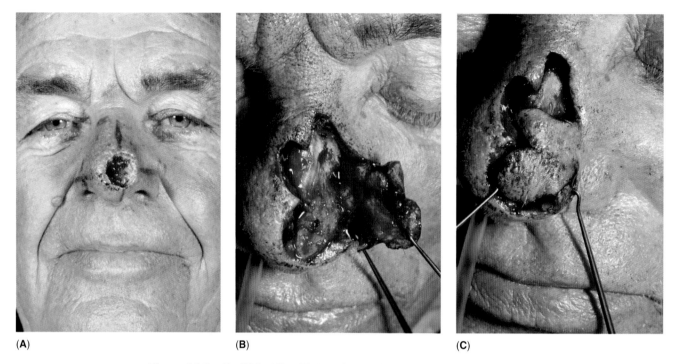

(A)   (B)   (C)

Figure 31.6.   The bilobed flap. **(A)** the defect; **(B)** flap widely undermined; **(C)** inset.

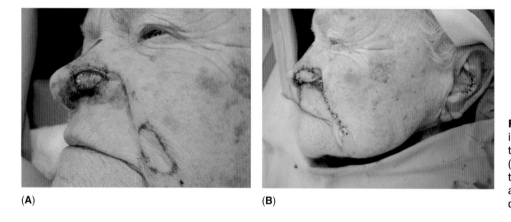

(A)   (B)

Figure 31.7 **(A)** Marking for an inferiorly based Nasolabial fold flap to reconstruct a left alar defect. **(B)** The flap after inset and closure of the donor area. Note that an anterior approach was used to harvest conchal cartilage for alar support.

dedication, and patient understanding of a prolonged, intricate process.

The forehead is the best available source of matching skin for the nose in its pliability, color, and ultimate thickness. The flap can be orientated directly in the midline of the forehead, which can result in a very cosmetically camouflaged scar; or, if preferred, the paramedian position, whereby it is based directly over the feeding vessel and can help avoid a low "widow's peak" and even lengthen the flap (Fig. 31.8). Whichever flap is decided upon, the flap's vascularity is still dependent on the unilateral median brow area. The blood supply to the area of forehead used

in flap design is complex, with contributions from the supraorbital, supratrochlear, infratrochlear, and dorsal nasal arteries that are terminal branches of the ophthalmic artery. The angular artery from the facial is also a key vessel supplying the tissue at the pedicle base where multiple collateral vessels converge and anastomose.

There is a predilection for the paramedian position because it has the additional advantage of bilateral flaps that can be raised from the forehead if unforeseen complications occur. The preoperative Doppler localization of the supratrochlear artery as the vessel enters the flaps deep surface just on the medial edge of the supraorbital rim,

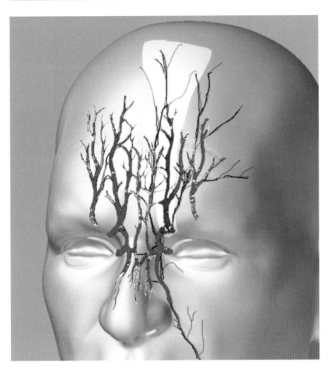

Figure 31.8 Representation of the paramedian forehead flap and blood supply from the supratrochlear, supraorbital, angular, and facial arteries.

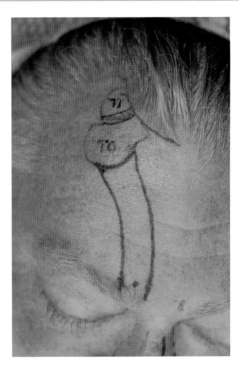

Figure 31.9 Paramedian forehead flap drawn to recreate the nasal defect over the Doppler signal for the supratrochlear vessels. This flap is planned superiorly for nasal lining.

permits a 1.2 to 1.5 cm pedicle base width to be designed with a guarantee of vessel inclusion. A narrower pedicle permits gain in vertical length when rotating the flap to the nasal defect. The course of the vessels has been well defined between the corrugator muscle deeply and the orbicularis oculi superficially. The axis is then vertical with the vascular supply of the paramedian forehead flap running superficial to the frontalis muscle inferiorly and finally subdermal at the hairline. The consequence of this is that the flap can be raised in the subdermal plane at its most cephalad point. It is exactly this piece of skin, however, that is vital to the reconstruction, usually of the alar rim, nasal tip, or columella. It is an area of surgical contention that taking it in this particular subdermal plane may venously compromise the vascularity of this skin. The preference, therefore, is to take a full-thickness flap to, or even into, the hairline, if inherent to the reconstruction. The thinning to this area is achieved at a second intermediate stage after two to three weeks when the blood supply is enhanced by the surgical delay phenomenon.

The forehead flap is templated to re-create the defective nasal subunits, but special attention to the alar base is needed to get consistently favorable results. Symmetrization of the alar bases is a difficult cosmetic component to perfect and can be accomplished by accurate three-dimensional understanding of the entire alar subunit and consideration of the alar-facial angle, which must not be compromised. This may require additional length to the flap, which is reached by either extending the flap caudally into the eyebrow, with careful dissection over the orbital rim by

up to 1.5 cm, or by extending the flap above the frontal hairline.

When managing nasal reconstruction with deficiency in more than one layer, the design of the forehead flap must take into consideration the inner lining and whether the flap will provide not just surface soft tissue cover as one layer, but also be folded to create the mucosal layer of the reconstruction (Fig. 31.9).

The forehead flap donor site is very forgiving even with the tightest closure. In lower-third nasal reconstruction the most superior area of the flap will ultimately become the TIP and must not be compromised. The three-dimensional template molded from the defect must be accurately transcribed to the forehead and into the hairline if sizeable, as erroneous transcription will give a suboptimal result. This area commonly cannot be closed directly when performing multiple subunit reconstructions, and is best left to heal by secondary intention, producing acceptable scarring that patients frequently cover with the frontal hair.

It is paramount that the forehead flap design is never compromised in order to achieve donor site closure. It is unnecessary to precede the reconstruction with tissue expansion as an immediate forehead flap of appropriate size can be taken and the donor site will always heal by secondary intention. In addition, there is some concern about subsequent contraction of the expanded forehead skin and distortion of the final nasal reconstruction.

The forehead flap is best regarded as a three-stage operation, whether used to resurface a single layer nasal

Table 31.2   Three Nasal Reconstruction Stages

Forehead flap: Three stage operation
1.   Raising, inset and lining
2.   Thinning of flap and re-inset +
     Structural support
     Week 3
3.   Division of pedicle and re-inset
     Week 6

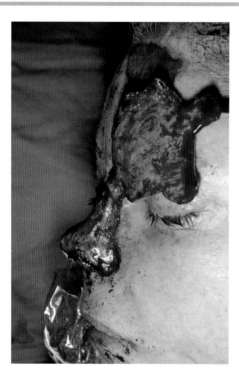

Figure 31.10   Thinning of the forehead flap at the intermediate stage.

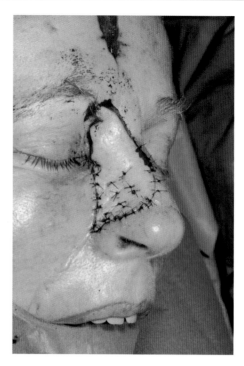

Figure 31.11   Quilting sutures placed after severe thinning of the forehead flap at stage 2.

defect or employed in a complex three-layer nasal reconstruction (Table 31.2).

The sequence of procedures allows fine-tuning of the flap and extensive thinning at week 3 when the pedicle is still intact and has a good vascular bed for inset of structural support. At this time, the flap is fully detached from the nose. Extensive thinning is tolerated by the fact that the vascularity of this "delayed" flap has improved over the first three weeks (Fig. 31.10). The flap is still very pliable and moldable at this stage. Not only is wound healing still in its early stages, but there has been no surgical trauma to the posterior surface of the dermis because the flap was initially raised in the plane underneath the frontalis muscle. It is necessary to place loose quilting sutures in the thinned area to prevent seroma and hematoma formation (Fig. 31.11). A delay of another three weeks after this second intermediate stage allows vascularization of the flap from the surrounding tissue; this permits division of the pedicle to occur six weeks from the original surgery. Further touch-up operations will now be postponed for

at least six months to let wound healing occur, swelling disappear, and the nose to soften.

Other methods are described for resurfacing the nose including the Washio flap, free radial forearm flap, free dorsalis pedis, and the construction of prelaminated flaps on the forearm for inset as the total unit of lining, support, and cover. These techniques are generally not first choice and will not be elaborated on at this point.

STRUCTURAL SUPPORT

Clinical Pearls for Nasal Structural Support

I.   Aim to achieve – Nasal length
                          Passage of air
                          Tip support/projection
II.   Graft material needs a blood supply
III. Strong support to counteract wound healing
      Contractile forces
IV.   Place graft material in previously unsupported areas
V.   Always add extra support to maintain alar opening and tip
      projection

The use of autogenous tissue to rebuild nasal support is not a modern technique. By the turn of the 19th century harvested costal cartilage was transferred to correct saddle nose deformities (10).

The surgical standards for reconstructing the nasal skeletal and cartilaginous supporting elements call for providing nasal length, tip projection, and airway patency. This must be able to maintain overall conformation and symmetry against gravity and progressive tissue contraction

Table 31.3 Nasal Structural Support

Areas:	Central nasal skeleton
	Nasal sidewalls
	Alar arches
	Lateral alar elements.
Grafts:	Nasal septum
	Auricular Cartilage
	Costal cartilage
	Split calvarial bone
	Iliac crest

due to wound healing forces. The central skeletal buttress constitute the two paired nasal bones, which have an outer surface that is concavoconvex from above downward, convex from side to side and covered by the procerus and compressor naris muscles. As these are rarely involved in ablative surgery, they conventionally provide a stable platform essential for the soft tissue cover and a solid footing for graft embedment (Table 31.3).

The rest of the nasal projection and contour is fashioned by the complex interaction between the paired upper lateral, paired lower lateral, septal, and accessory hyaline cartilage configuration. Together they subtly define the surface convexities and concavities created in the flexible lower two-thirds of the nose and buttress the soft tissue.

No one would question that when considering reconstruction there has to be an alliance between structural support and nasal airflow. Paired internal valves consisting of the caudal end of the upper lateral cartilage, the nasal septum, and the soft tissue surrounding the piriform aperture influence the natural passage of air. Unlike the external valve, the internal valve functions paradoxically: inspiration causes narrowing of this segment and nasal airflow resistance. The paired external valves are composed of the lower lateral cartilage, the columella, and the nasal floor. Active dilatation of this valve occurs with each inspiration by action of the nasalis muscles. It would be exceptional for nasal reconstruction methods to exactly recreate this distinctive anatomy. Even with accurate design patterns air turbulence can easily be created due to wound tension, nasal aperture contraction, and reconstructive bulkiness.

The lower lateral cartilages are the prime supportive elements to the sidewalls as they adhere to the septum medially, lie under the nasal bones superiorly, and extend laterally—creating the tip, soft triangles, and columella. The cartilage fans out laterally away from the alar rim so naturally there is no support in this area. In this case, one must appreciate that any defect encroaching on the free margin of the ala requires obligatory auxiliary structural support, such as an alar rim graft, in the reconstruction to keep the vestibule open and resist wound contraction forces to prevent collapse.

When reconstructing nasal support, the areas that need addressing are not only those that had actual support before—such as the central nasal skeleton, the nasal sidewalls, the alar arches—but also previously unsupported areas, such as the lateral alar elements. In all cases support needs to be stronger than before to withstand contraction and distortion from wound healing forces (Table 31.3).

Midline Support

There is no doubt a necessity for midline support, but controversy exists about which method to choose.

Cantilever Graft

A deficiency in the skeletal pyramid, which is very uncommon, can be addressed using a cantilevered split calvarial bone graft harvested from the straight region of the parietal bone. This is a reliable source of good strong bone that can be shaped and secured in position by lag screws, or plates to the remaining nasal platform.

The quality of the harvested graft prevents significant resorption and warping, and can resist wound contraction forces. This bone can be used to rebuild the lateral bony piriform aperture or premaxilla if necessary, and provide a strong foundation to build the other structures upon.

L-Strut

Midline support in the form of an L-strut as a one or two piece, longitudinal piece of bone or costal cartilage can be seated on the radix and extend along the dorsum to nasal tip, the L- then angles to be fixed to the anterior nasal spine. A block of costal cartilage can be harvested from the 7th, 8th, or 9th rib and carved into the required configuration. Cartilage grafts, especially in younger people can have a tendency for warping, so harvesting osseocartilaginous rib grafts as an alternative can help prevent this phenomenon. It is also essential to examine lateral support when placing an entire L-strut to prevent lateral instability. It is best, therefore, to view the tip support complex as a tripod structure.

Various alloplastic materials have been developed, such as Vitallium/titanium mesh and porous polyethylene implants, used alone or combined with purified acellular human dermal grafts. There is a high risk of artificial implant exposure and infection, however, and autogenous grafts are the gold standard. Tissue-engineered cartilage has received a great deal of interest over the past years. A true, easy, mainstream application of this material, however, still seems far away. In practice this would idealistically result in an autogenous implant associated with minimal donor morbidity, and be engineered into the desired three-dimensional morphology in-vitro.

Lateral Support

Central support is inadequate on its own in complex defects encompassing several subunits and requires lateral support. The upper lateral cartilages can be substituted with costal grafts or straight septal cartilage positioned on the nasal sidewall to support the middle vault against collapse (Fig. 31.12). Septal cartilage can be used as a septal hinge flap in those cases where inner lining and sidewall support are missing. This will result in a monolocular nose, which generally gives few problems.

In rebuilding lower nasal support, the conchal ear cartilage has a natural curve that can reflect the conformation of the alar cartilages and can be harvested via an anterior or posterior approach with minimal donor site morbidity (Fig. 31.13). Here it is essential to comprehend the critical introduction of non-anatomical alar rim batten grafts, preferably from the conchal bowl or septum. This will stiffen

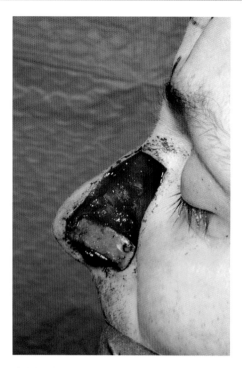

Figure 31.12   Septal cartilage alar batten graft sutured in place.

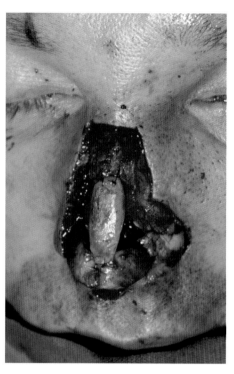

Figure 31.14   Inset of the conchal cartilage and on-lay grafts for tip and lateral support. The midline is supported by a costal cartilage graft.

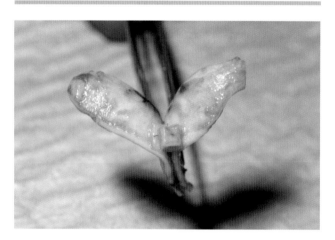

Figure 31.13   Harvested conchal graft crafted into a representation of the alar cartilages to support the lower nasal reconstruction. Two blocks of cartilage sutured in place for tip projection.

Tip Support and Enhancement of Tip Projection

The tip is the determinate of nasal refinement and gaining this demands reconstruction of the lateral projection of the left and right domes, a tip defining point, and a columella-lobular junction. This goal is achievable in aesthetic rhinoplasty when working with the original skin cover, but it is difficult to achieve this perfection when the soft tissue cover is less pliable. The tip needs individual consideration in nasal reconstruction and one can exploit to good effect aesthetic rhinoplasty techniques. These tip defining procedures include attention to the lateral cartilages, employing columella strut grafts, and securely fastening on-lay, shield, and spreader cartilage grafts to the previously positioned midline support (Fig. 31.14). Adequate tip protrusion will require over-projection of the tip framework by at least 15 mm above the septum or central midline support. In addition, every nasal tip reconstruction will require a columella strut graft to prevent loss of projection due to wound healing contraction.

Timing of Support Insertion

Originally, prevailing opinion maintained that cartilage grafts could only be introduced at the time of primary reconstruction because they demand a well-vascularized bed for survival. This was in part due to a conviction that the soft tissue had to be shaped and supported at the initial surgery, as the flap would become permanently altered by scar formation and uncorrectable at later surgery. Contrary to this belief, cartilage support can successfully be placed at the second stage of reconstruction three weeks

the rim to help prevent retraction and notching, and allow the airway to remain open on inspiration. A cartilage strip 4–6 mm wide inserted beneath the soft tissue cover and above the lining aids the vestibular opening. Alar batten grafts should be secured with a through-and-through suture placed between the graft and intranasal lining. This serves to pull the lining against the graft and obliterate the dead space, thus maximizing contact between the vascularized tissue and the cartilage graft.

later, when wound healing and contraction has not yet set in. The advantage of the intermediate stage is that the soft tissues can be radically lifted and thinned due to their improved vascularity and make an excellent bed for the graft material. Cartilage grafts, therefore, should be put in at a time when they can be well vascularized, which could be at the first stage (for primary support structures) or three weeks later at the shaping and thinning stage (for alar and tip grafts).

NASAL LINING

Clinical Pearls: Inner Lining

I. Vascularity	
II. Thinness	
III. Inner cover for cartilage support	
For:	– prevention of nostril stenosis
	– sustain grafts
	– prevention of cartilage infection
	– air passage

The nasal mucosal lining is unique and specialized for its function. There is a transition from stratified squamous epithelium intranasally to thin, well vascularized, hair-bearing mucosa in the nasal vestibule and ciliated, moist lining in the nasal vault. The lining is an essential component of functional reconstruction and maintains both the integrity of the supplemental structural support (11) and the nostril opening. Not surprisingly, it is the most difficult to reconstruct from many perspectives including poor surgical field visibility and limited surgical access.

The goal is to establish a thin, well vascularized, reliable nasal lining that will not obstruct the nasal passage and can sustain cartilage/bone grafts and prevent infection (Table 31.4). Suboptimal surgical results can frequently be traced to inadequate lining introduced at the preliminary procedure. The reconstructive surgeon is presented with a multitude of options for resurfacing the internal nose, including skin grafts, folded regional flaps, mucosal advancements, hinged nasal mucosa, and composite flaps of nasal septum. The discerning surgeon will have to decide which is the most appropriate for each separate case (Table 31.5).

Table 31.4 Lining Options

Grafts:
    Split thickness
    Full thickness
    Chondrocutaneous (auricular)
    Chondromucosal

Local flaps:
    Folded Forehead
    Nasolabial
    Nasal turn-in
    Buccal mucosal

Mucosal flaps:
    Septal door (hinge)
    Bipedicle vestibular
    Bipedicled mucosal
    Septal mucoperichondrial

Table 31.5 My Current Approach for Inner Lining

Applications:	– *full thickness defect 0.5–1.5 cm*
Advantage:	– *simple*
Limitations:	– *borderline vascularity*
	– *stiff*
	– *risk of contraction*

Grafts

Full- and split-thickness skin or mucosal grafts survive by plasma imbibition in the first two to three days until they can survive by promotion of angiogenesis from the recipient bed. The limitation of this reconstruction is the fact that they need a well vascularized bed and cannot cover exposed cartilage or bone. In the first stage of reconstruction a full-thickness graft can be proposed as lining to the forehead flap, making use of the frontalis muscle to gain an adequate blood supply. These grafts leave a dry nasal lining and are vulnerable to some distortion of the reconstruction from wound bed contraction, but are excellent for smaller (<2 cm) lining requirements. When extensive lining is required for reconstruction, flaps that have an independent blood supply should be used to minimize the risk for long-term distortion. The Gillies composite auricular skin and cartilage graft is a useful technique for some alar defects (12), but with the understanding that the graft is dependent on the recipient site vascularization. The same holds true for chondromucosal grafts. In our experience the results in reconstruction of even small defects can be unpredictable.

Regional Folded Flaps

Gillies found the laxity in the nasolabial fold provided adequate tissue to pivot inwards and line the nasal vestibule and columella (13). As expected, this tends to yield a bulky asymmetric nostril opening, which makes it very difficult to achieve an acceptable result.

The folded forehead flap, on the other hand, makes use of an extension of forehead skin that is used to replace inner lining requirements. At the first stage this yields a bulky flap as well; however, after three weeks at the intermediate thinning stage, this forehead flap extension can be cut from the forehead flap and thinned considerably. This is a consequence of the flap's incorporation into the surrounding tissues and the development of a separate blood supply. This type of lining reconstruction yields a well-vascularized thin piece of lining for small to medium-sized defects.

Hingeover Flaps

Hingeover flaps utilize the available full-thickness skin adjacent to the defect (Fig. 31.15A, B). This is a useful technique for smaller defects, mostly around the alar and soft triangle. The skin flaps can be thick, stiff, and at risk of ischemia if they are larger than 1.5 cm. If these flaps are employed for larger defects, wound healing contracture can frequently leave an inadequate internal airway (Table 31.6).

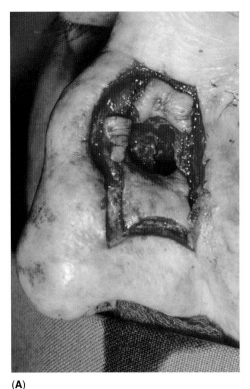
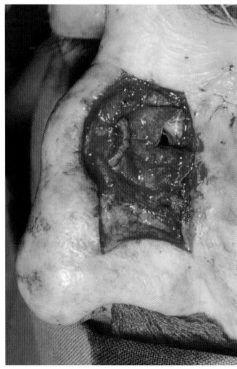

(A)   **(B)**

Figure 31.15 Hingeover flap to reconstruct a left sidewall lining deficit. **(A)** preparing the flaps; **(B)** turning the flaps in.

Table 31.6 The Hingeover Flap

Radial Forearm
   Prelaminated
   Prefabricated osseocutaneous
Dorsalis pedis
Auricular helix
First dorsal metacarpal

Mucosal Flaps

Adopting the Millard philosophy of replacing "like for like," may lead one to think that intranasal mucosal flaps are the best source of lining because the tissue is soft, thin, and well-vascularized. Unfortunately, these flaps are fragile and unforgiving to raise due to tight adherence to the underlying cartilage. The vascularity is not always what it promises to be in the most distal part of these flaps. There is also a relative paucity of available tissue, which often results in too little length to the inner lining flap.

Mucosal Advancement Flap

A very simple technique of raising a small mucosal flap and turning it down into the defect is often not sufficient, even for small defects. When lining is required to reconstruct an inadequate alar rim, a bipedicled vestibular skin advancement flap based medially on the remaining septum

and laterally on the piriform aperture can be brought inferiorly to reconstruct the deficiency (14). It is vascularized well enough to support an auricular cartilage graft.

Septal Mucoperichondrial Flap

Larger flaps are based on anatomical knowledge of the septal blood supply. The upper septum is supplied by the posterior and anterior ethmoidal artery, while the sphenopalatine artery supplies a large area of the inferoposterior septum. The important vessel is the septal branch of the superior labial artery. It enters the anteroinferior septum lateral to the nasal spine and is the basis for the septal mucoperichondrial flap, with or without cartilage. Considering the layers needed in reconstruction, two layers can be brought into the defect in one flap. The septal mucoperichondrial flap is based anterior-inferiorly or axially near to the nasal spine (Fig. 31.16A, B). It is a practical, versatile flap that can advance a large rectangle of mucosa with or without support to recreate the upper and middle nasal vault.

Septal "Trap Door" Flap

The septal chondromucosal "trap door" flap was one of the earliest flaps to re-create the nasal lining and is based on the anterior septal blood supply. The technique first requires elevation of the ipsilateral mucosal surface to access the septal cartilage. The contralateral mucosa and cartilage are incised with a wide dorsally hinged base that permits the flap to line the sidewalls of the middle and

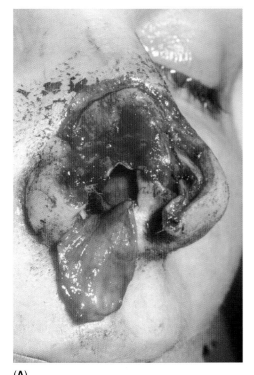

(A)

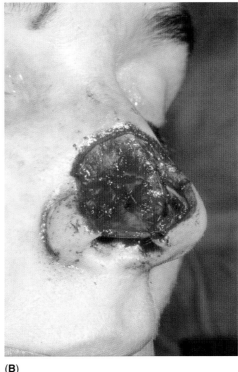

(B)

Figure 31.16 The septal mucoperichondrial flap. **(A)** The flap has been raised; **(B)** inset of flap to reconstruct the right alar lining.

upper vaults. A sufficient amount of midline dorsal septal support of at least 1 cm has to be left in place, thus limiting the flap's lateral reach. In order to be able to swing this flap, a narrow strip of septal cartilage at the anterior pivot point needs to be removed cautiously. The elevated ipsilateral mucosa can be used to reconstruct the additional lining requirement of the ala (Fig. 31.17A, B).

Large Inner Lining Reconstructions

When managing extensive defects requiring a sizable inner lining, a combination of the options described above can be used. Restoring inner lining is a creative art that will have more than one option available. We can expect, therefore, that individual cases may vary as widely as the possibilities available to reconstruct the inner lining. The ultimate single piece of inner lining that can be brought into the reconstructive play is a free flap (Table 31.7).

The traditional reconstructive surgeon's armamentarium comprises numerous regional and distant free flaps, most of which are unsuitable for inner lining reconstruction. The radial forearm flap provides a thin, pliable skin cover; however, when used for inner lining, it suddenly becomes an extremely thick flap. If used for inner lining, at initial surgery the radial forearm flap is positioned with the skin inside and the posterior surface is covered with a skin graft or folded over itself. Extensive thinning at subsequent stages is possible and can give adequate inner lining for nasal reconstruction. At that time the skin graft that had been used for cover is excised and the outer cover is then changed to a paramedian forehead flap. An alternative method of reconstruction is mapping the nasal defect on to the forearm

and prelaminating the lining on to the undersurface ready for raising and inset three weeks later. Variations to this concept are possible when cartilage grafts or bone are used at the time of prefabrication. It is very difficult to create a pleasing nose from a donor site distant from the face.

Finally, alar reconstruction can be performed with a helical root free flap. Branches from the anterior temporal artery supply the root of the helix and this area can be transferred as a composite free flap mainly to restore the alar complex (6).

CLINICAL CASES DEMONSTRATING NASAL RECONSTRUCTION

Each individual principle of nasal reconstruction described in the body of this chapter needs to be evaluated to be able to create the desired combination of reconstructive techniques for each clinical case and establish a pleasing result. For each patient there is a wide range of creativity and personal input within the boundaries of general principles. The following three cases will illustrate working within the principles of earlier described techniques for nasal reconstruction.

Case 1: Nasal Tip Reconstruction

A 42-year-old woman presented with a nasal tip deformity (Fig. 31.18). The deformity was the result of a human bite following a lovers' quarrel one year earlier that had been treated conservatively in an emergency department.

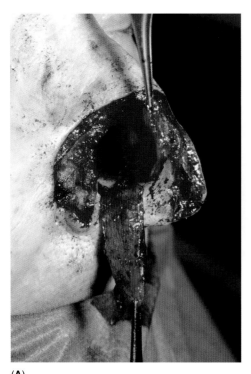

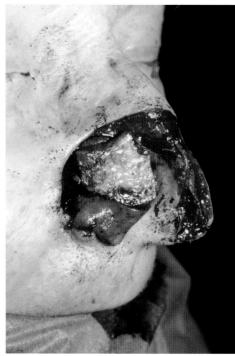

(A)   **(B)**

Figure 31.17 Septal "trapdoor" flap. **(A)** The flap has been raised, revealing the mucosal lining and the septal cartilage; **(B)** inset of the cartilage and mucosal flap.

Table 31.7 Free Flaps for Nasal Reconstruction

Defect <1.5 cm	– Hinge flap or skin graft with 3-stage forehead flap
Defect 1 cm – 3.5 cm	– 3-stage folded forehead flap or Skin graft with 3-stage forehead flap
Defect >3.5 cm	– 3-stage folded forehead flap with septal composite flap – Free flap

On close inspection it is quite hard to appreciate the full scope of her condition, as it would seem that the tip is still in decent shape with only a little ala missing (Fig. 31.19). In order to truly appreciate what has been surgically ablated in a case like this, which is very different from a fresh defect, the original defect has to be re-created. This is achieved by opening up the area through the old scars and performing a meticulous and extensive scar tissue removal. Only now is it possible to make an accurate assessment of the missing tissues (Fig. 31.20).

After re-creation of the defect, the damage is assessed as separate layers. In this case there was no shortage of inner lining after scar release and therefore no reconstruction of this layer needed.

Assessment of structural support showed that the tip defining cartilages were essentially incomplete. Therefore

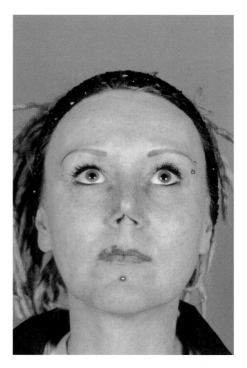

Figure 31.18 Clinical Case 1. Frontal preoperative view.

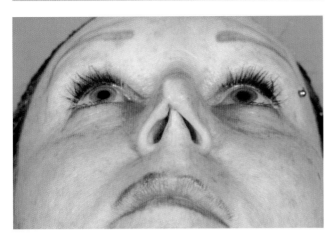

Figure 31.19 Preoperative close-up from below revealing the full extent of the tip and alar defects.

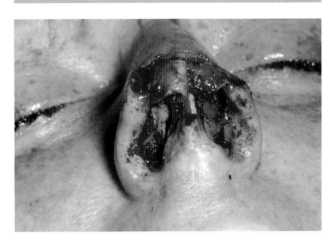

Figure 31.21 Close-up of the inserted tip grafts.

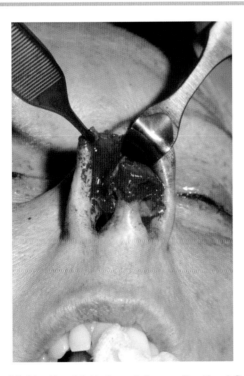

Figure 31.20 The debrided nasal tip revealing the deficient tip structures.

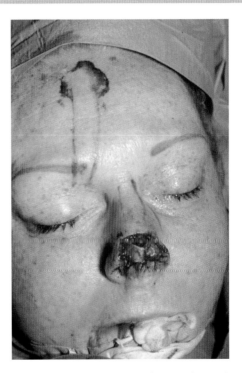

Figure 31.22 The open nasal tip with forehead flap design marked for external nasal cover.

reconstruction of the lower lateral cartilages was required. These cartilages were reconstructed with auricular conchal cartilages. To address the excessive wound healing forces that would be present after this tip reconstruction, a strut graft, harvested from the septum, was placed to protect tip projection (Fig. 31.21).

Nasal skin requirement after recreation of the defect consisted of the tip, soft triangles, and anterior-most portion of the columella. A paramedian forehead flap could easily supply this skin requirement, which was even small enough to allow primary closure of the forehead donor site (Fig. 31.22). The paramedian forehead flap was dissected in the submuscular plane in the first stage, fully lifted and thinned at the intermediate stage after three weeks, and finally divided after six weeks. A fourth operation was performed after six months to thin the cranial tip and quilt

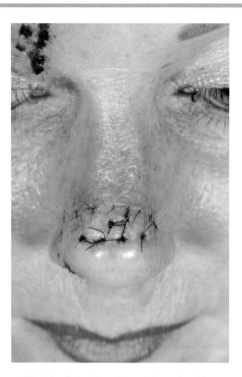

Figure 31.23 Debulking of nasal tip and quilting sutures.

the skin down to get reduction in fullness in that area (Fig. 31.23). One year after the last operation a pleasing tip shape had been achieved giving good function and appearance (Fig. 31.24A, B).

Case 2: Nasal Ala and Tip

A 75-year-old gentleman presented with a defect after Mohs resection of a basal cell skin cancer from the nose. Analysis of the defect was performed to identify the extent of damage and revealed that all three layers were involved and needed reconstruction (Fig. 31.25).

The inner lining showed a defect of approximately 1.5 × 1.0 cm. Several options are available to reconstruct this lining requirement. An important requirement in the reconstruction of this layer is to end up with a thin well-vascularized lining that would fit without excessive tension and prevent distortion. In this case a choice was made for a three-stage folded forehead flap over a skin graft or septum mucosa based flap (Fig. 31.26).

Reconstruction of structural support was required not only to replace the missing lower lateral cartilage on the left side, but also to add additional columella support to withstand wound healing contraction forces. A columella strut and an alar rim batten graft were inserted on the left side. The alar replacement and additional cartilages, which were made up of auricular conchal cartilage, could not be inserted at the first stage of the nasal reconstruction. This

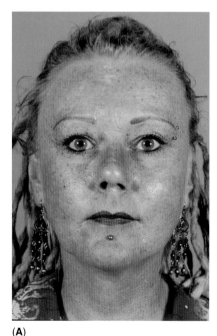

(A)

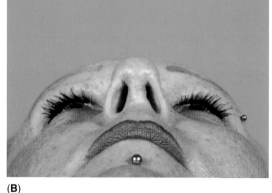

(B)

Figure 31.24.   Case 1. Postoperative view after a three-stage nasal reconstruction. **(A)** frontal; **(B)** from below.

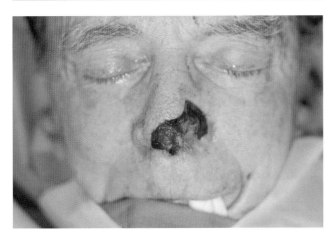

Figure 31.25 Clinical Case 2. The full extent of the tip and alar defect from the front.

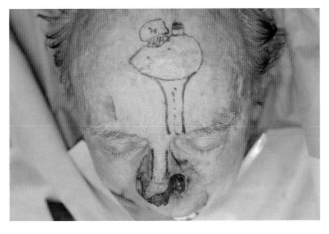

Figure 31.26 Flap designed on forehead showing the extent of the flap to include an extension for lining and based over the supratrochlear Doppler signal.

was due to the bulk of the folded forehead flap used to recreate the left ala at the first operation (Fig. 31.27A, B). All alar cartilage support was added at the intermediate thinning operation three weeks later when the forehead flap was cut at the alar rim, leaving the folded extension of the flap inside the nose for lining. This part of the flap now received its blood supply from the surrounding tissues and was not reliant on the pedicle. Aggressive thinning of this new inner lining into the subdermal plane left a well vascularized, thin piece of inner lining with sufficient blood supply to allow delayed cartilage grafts at this stage.

The nasal skin cover was reconstructed with a three-stage paramedian forehead flap. At the intermediate stage, after 3 weeks, the flap was lifted up entirely by cutting the flap distally at the level of the skin extension that had been added for inner lining. The flap was then raised completely and very thinly in a subdermal plane while it was just left attached to its original pedicle (Fig. 31.28A, B). This safe thin lifting of the flap at the intermediate stage is possible due to a delay phenomenon that occurs when cutting a forehead flap. The flap was divided six weeks after the first operation and thinned cranially while being left attached caudally (Fig. 31.29). At three months after the last operation a pleasing functional and aesthetic result had been achieved (Fig. 31.30A, B, C). Further follow-up is necessary not only for cancer purposes but also to follow whether the reconstruction was sufficiently supported to withstand all wound healing contraction forces during the first postoperative year.

Case 3 : Subtotal Nasal Reconstruction

A 43-year-old woman presented with a facial defect after Mohs resection of a sclerosing basal cell cancer of the nose (Fig. 31.31A, B). Analysis of the defect was performed to not only identify the extent of damage for each of the three layers of the nose, but also the involvement of the different adjacent aesthetic units. It was clear that there was extensive debridement of several nasal subunits and encroachment on to the upper lip and cheek units. The management of the adjacent units will not be discussed in great detail here as it lies beyond the scope of this chapter. It is important to understand, however, that all units should be reconstructed

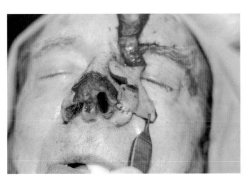

(A)

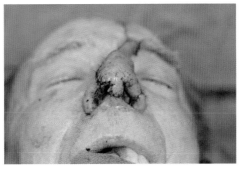

(B)

Figure 31.27 **(A)** The forehead flap has been raised. The extension is sutured to create the left alar rim and lining; **(B)** Inset of the forehead flap showing how the flap is folded to create lining.

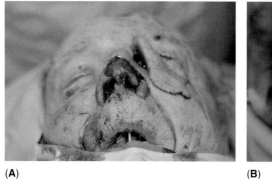   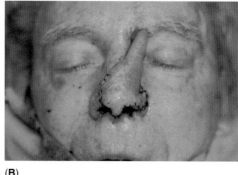

(A)   **(B)**

Figure 31.28   (A) The intermediate stage with complete raising of the forehead flap from the nose and extreme thinning; (B) inset of the thinned forehead flap.

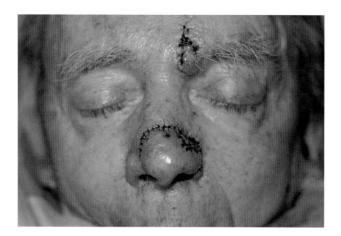

Figure 31.29   Division of the forehead flap at six weeks. The contour of the eyebrow is carefully recreated. Quilting sutures are also in place.

separately; when beginning nasal reconstruction all attention must be focused on the nose. The forehead flap cannot be used to reconstruct both the nose and cheek, or any other aesthetic unit outside of the nose. In this case the cheek was addressed with a combination of cheek and remaining upper lip units advanced to the border of the philtrum edges. At this stage the philtrum was recreated with a piece of full thickness skin graft and later reconstructed with an Abbe flap.

Returning our attention to the nose, there was a requirement in this case for a substantial inner lining reconstruction because the defect comprised most of the lining of the nasal vestibule bilaterally. We felt that the use of the septal mucosa was unreliable because there had been significant resection in the area of the septal branch of

the superior labial artery. A very large forehead flap was needed in combination with a large inner lining, so the use of a folded forehead flap seemed unpractical. The two options for inner lining we considered were either a free flap or, in light of free flap bulk, full-thickness skin grafts. Two 3.5 × 3.0 cm full-thickness skin grafts were harvested and fixed to the cranial-most extent of the remaining inner lining (Fig. 31.32). Full-thickness grafts were chosen because they tend to contract less than split-thickness grafts.

Complete reconstruction of structural support was required. Fortunately, the remaining septum provided a stable base on which to build. The inner lining was reconstructed at the first stage with full-thickness skin grafts so it was not possible to initially place the conchal cartilage grafts for alar support. The rib cartilage grafts for the columella strut and septal extension could be placed in well-vascularized areas at this time (Fig. 31.32). The remaining rib cartilage was buried in the donor site for later use. At the second stage, after three weeks, the forehead flap was lifted entirely off the neovascularized full-thickness lining. The vascular bed was now ready to receive alar cartilage grafts, which consisted of auricular conchal and rib cartilage grafts for tip reconstruction, alar rim, and sidewall support (Fig. 31.33).

The nasal skin cover was reconstructed with a three-stage paramedian forehead flap, which was cut from the forehead as required without compromising flap design for possible donor site closure considerations. The flap was cut in the submuscular plane after meticulous three-dimensional template design. The entire nasal skin was missing so a plaster cast model was constructed of the face and a proportionate neo-nose created from clay. The nasal template was made on the model and used intraoperatively. The flap was cut as designed, which resulted in a large donor site defect, which was left open (Fig. 31.34) and was only dressed with petroleum gauze. After three weeks the intermediate flap thinning stage was performed with the cartilage grafts inserted as described above. The donor site is already contracting and healing (Fig. 31.35).

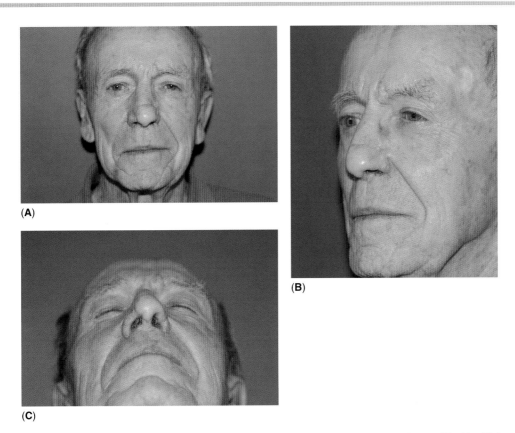

Figure 31.30 Clinical Case 2. Postoperative views after a three-stage nasal reconstruction. **(A)** frontal; **(B)** side; **(C)** from below.

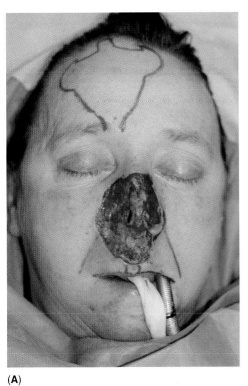

(A)

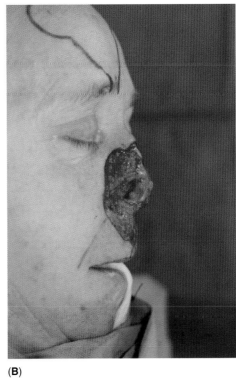

(B)

Figure 31.31 Clinical Case 3. **(A)** Frontal operative view at the first stage of reconstruction. The full extent of the nasal defect is marked out with the paramedian forehead flap. **(B)** Lateral view of same defect.

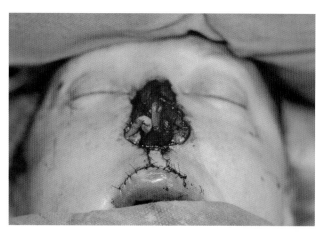

Figure 31.32   The first stage reconstruction requiring costal cartilage support and full-thickness skin graft for lining. The upper lip subunits were advanced and a full-thickness graft applied to the philtrum.

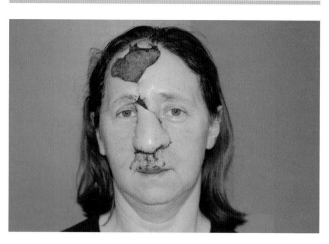

Figure 31.34   Donor site and flap at one week postoperative.

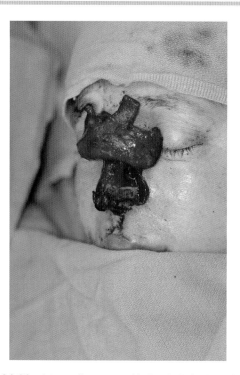

Figure 31.33   Intermediate stage with the whole forehead flap lifted for insertion of further conchal and costal cartilage support and extreme flap thinning.

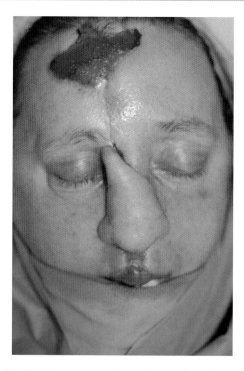

Figure 31.35   Flap and donor site at three weeks at the intermediate thinning stage.

After six weeks the original flap pedicle is divided and the flap is further thinned in the cranial region. After each stage quilting sutures are placed in the thinned areas to prevent formation of a seroma or hematoma, which would undo the thinning. Quilting sutures are applied loosely to prevent compromise of circulation. The flap pedicle is discarded, but it is important to inset the remaining flap pedicle and restore the medial eyebrow symmetrically with the contralateral side (Fig. 31.36). The patient shows a pleasing result after a three-stage nasal reconstruction and Abbe flap reconstruction of the philtrum (Fig. 31.37). Further improvements in outcome can be achieved by touch-up procedures if patients desire.

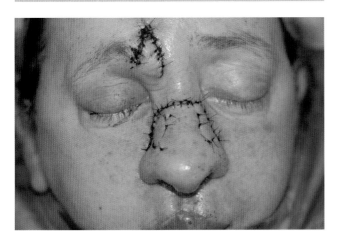

Figure 31.36 Stage 3 at six weeks, with division of the flap, adjustment to the superior edge of the flap and quilting sutures.

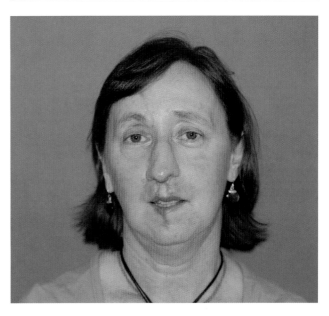

Figure 31.37 Postoperative view after an Abbe flap to reconstruct the philtrum.

REFERENCES

1. Moolenburgh SE, Mureau MA, Duivenvoorden HJ et al. Validation of a questionnaire assessing patient's aesthetic and functional outcome after nasal reconstruction: the patient NAFEQ-score. J Plast Reconstr Aesthet Surg 2008. Feb 8. [Epub ahead of print]
2. Mureau MA, Moolenburgh SE, Levendag PC et al. Aesthetic and functional outcome following nasal reconstruction. Plast Reconstr Surg 2007; 120: 1217–27; discussion 1228–30.
3. Burget GC, Menick FJ. The subunit principle in nasal reconstruction. Plast Reconstr Surg 1985; 76: 239–47.
4. Millard DR. Aesthetic reconstructive rhinoplasty. Clin Plast Surg 1981; 8: 169.
5. Millard DR. Reconstruct by units. In: Millard DR, ed. Principlization of Plastic Surgery. Boston, MA: Little Brown; 1986: 229–53.
6. Pribaz J, Falco N. Nasal reconstruction with auricular microvascular transplant. Ann Plast Surg 1993; 31: 289.
7. Esser JFS. Gestielte loakle Nasenplastik mit zweizipfligen Lappen, Deckung des sekundaren Defektes vom ersten Zipfel durch den Zweiten. Dtsch Zschr Chir 1918; 143: 385.
8. Zitelli JA. The bilobed flap for nasal reconstruction. Arch Dermatol 1989; 125: 957–9.
9. Hofer SO, Posch NA, Smit X. The facial artery perforator flap for reconstruction of perioral defects. Plast Reconstr Surg 2005; 115: 996–1003.
10. Mangoldt F yon. Reconstruction of saddle nose by cartilage overlay. Gesell Chir 1900; 29: 460. Translation published in Plast Reconstr Surg 1970; 46: 495.
11. Burget GC, Menick FJ. Nasal support and lining: the marriage of beauty and blood supply. Plast Reconstr Surg 1989; 84: 189–202.
12. Gillies H. New free graft (of skin and ear cartilage) applied to reconstruction of nostril. Br J Surg 1943; 30: 305.
13. Gillies H. The Columella. Br J Plast Surg 1950; 2: 192.
14. Kazanjian VH. Plastic repair of deformities about the lower part of the nose resulting from loss of tissue. Trans Am Acad Ophthalmol Otolaryngol 1937; 42: 338.

32

Functional Voice Restoration after Total Laryngectomy

Jan S Lewin, Peter H Rhys Evans and Eric D Blom

INTRODUCTION

Cancers of the upper aerodigestive tract, specifically the larynx, have a major impact on speech and swallowing, not only through the destructive process of the disease itself, but also through the effects of curative treatment, be it surgery, radiotherapy, or combined regimens that may or may not include chemotherapy. Functional rehabilitation of these patients has long been one of the major challenges facing head and neck surgeons, speech pathologists, and patients, but it is only in the last three decades that the emphasis on restoration of function and quality of life has become a major focus of treatment for patients with head and neck cancer. Despite significant advances in cancer therapy long-term cure rates for head and neck cancer have not changed significantly over the last 50 years. Therefore, optimal immediate rehabilitation of patients with head and neck cancer is of paramount importance and a major consideration in developing the initial treatment plan.

We are just beginning to understand the true impact of the various cancer treatments on speech and swallowing function, and the long-term consequences to quality of life for patients presenting with advanced laryngeal disease. For early-stage cancer of the larynx, definitive radiotherapy or conservation laryngeal surgery results in excellent outcomes both in terms of survival and function. For patients with advanced laryngeal carcinoma, however, the selection of the optimal treatment or treatments has become less clear and much more complicated. Data still does not tell us which patients will benefit both in survival and functional outcomes from conservative organ sparing protocols that combine radiation and chemotherapy versus those who are best treated surgically. Combined protocols that spare the larynx and preserve the voice but damage airway protection and the ability to swallow may prove less desirable than total laryngectomy. Patients who are treated with total laryngectomy and tracheoesophageal voice restoration often have better functional outcomes and quality of life than patients who are treated with organ preservation procedures that spare but cripple the larynx.

In general, treatment of patients with head and neck cancer will require precise coordination of a highly specialized multidisciplinary team, including the head and neck surgeon, radiotherapist, medical oncologist, and plastic reconstructive surgeon. Other specialists, including oncology and surgical nurses, speech pathologists, dietitians, and social workers will provide critical input to preoperative planning and counseling, nutritional support, and postoperative care. For head and neck cancer patients who undergo laryngectomy, the speech pathologist is a critical member of the multidisciplinary team because of the loss of laryngeal voice and the inability to produce audible and intelligible speech.

The several options available for voice restoration include the artificial larynx (electrolarynx), traditional methods of esophageal speech production, and surgical prosthetic alternatives [tracheoesophageal (TE) voice restoration]. This chapter will provide a brief overview of the history of alaryngeal voice restoration, including the use of the artificial larynx, and esophageal speech production, but the primary focus will be placed on the method of TE voice restoration.

HISTORICAL PERSPECTIVE

For over 100 years total laryngectomy has been used as an effective alternative for the treatment of advanced and recurrent laryngeal and laryngopharyngeal cancer. The early history associated with total laryngectomy at the end of the last century carried an operative mortality of over 90%. Despite greater cure rates, fewer complications, and improved survival associated with the advancements in the treatment for head and neck cancer, the loss of the voice, altered swallowing, and a permanent tracheostoma, continue to have profound effects on the patient's physical and psychological rehabilitation.

Watson, of Edinburgh, performed the first total laryngectomy in a patient with tuberculosis, but a few years later, in 1873, Billroth was the first to carry out the procedure for cancer. The importance of early restoration of voice was recognized and one of Billroth's associates, Carl Gussenbauer, designed a device with a vibrating reed in a bifurcated tracheal cannula (Fig. 32.1), which apparently produced satisfactory speech for several weeks before the patient eventually succumbed to recurrent disease (1).

Esophageal Speech

Not long after the relatively successful use of reed devices for production of voice some early pioneers (Table 32.1) noted that patients sometimes experienced a "vicarious" sound source in the back of the throat that they found could be developed with exercise into a useful voice. Esophageal speech occurs as a result of compression of oral air into the esophagus that is expelled past the pharyngoesophageal (PE) segment and vibrates the mucosal walls for sound production. The patient must rapidly impound air

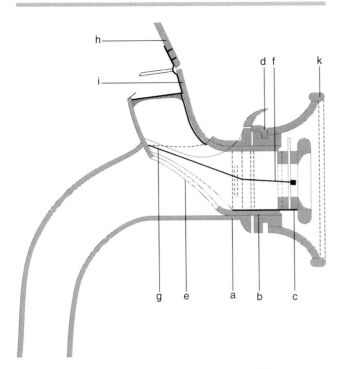

Figure 32.1 The speech device of Gussenbauer (1873).

a: trachea cannula
b: pharynx cannula
c: cannula for phonation
d: ring that can be turned for fixation of the tracheal cannula and the pharynx cannula
e: this opening enables communication with the trachea
f: window in which the metal reed is fixated
g: metal reed for sound production
h: pharyngeal flap that is held open by (i) and (k)
i: spring
k: respirator

Table 32.1 Early Pioneers of Esophageal Speech

Stoerk (Vienna)	1887
Schmid (Stettin)	1889
Solis–Cohen (Philadelphia)	1893
Gottstein (Breslau)	1900
Gutzman (Berlin)	1908

into the esophagus and then expel air into the mouth to produce fluent speech (2) (Fig. 32.2). Resonation of sound occurs in the vocal tract (pharynx, mouth, and nose) and articulation of words takes place in the mouth, similar to that produced by normal laryngeal speakers, using the lips, teeth, and tongue.

Learning esophageal speech requires determination and usually prolonged speech therapy because it does involve a complex and different technique for voice production. Many patients are not able to develop proficient skills to master the technique; less than one-third are able to speak using successful intelligible esophageal speech (3). The disadvantages of esophageal speech are that the voice is generally reduced in intensity, poorly sustained, has limited fluency interrupted by the frequent need to

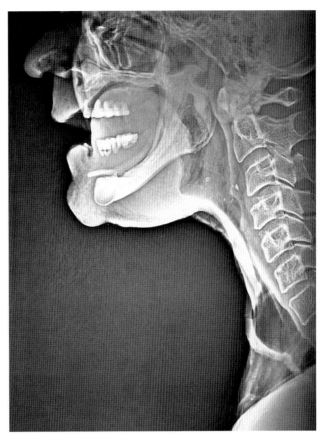

(A)

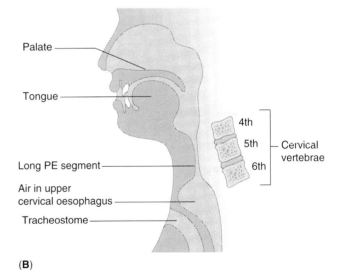

(B)

Figure 32.2 (A) Lateral xerograph of the neck in a laryngectomee phonating with good oesophageal speech showing a long tonic PE segment at C4/5/6. (B) Diagrammatic representation of (A).

inject air, and the listener is often distracted by expiratory noise from the stoma. Nevertheless, until the successful introduction of surgical voice restoration during the 1980s, this method had been the mainstay of voice rehabilitation following total laryngectomy since the early part of the century.

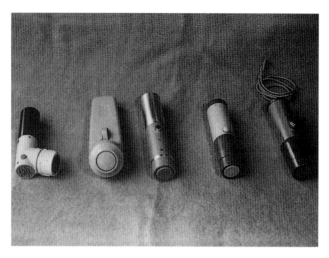

Figure 32.3 Types of artificial larynx vibrators (Bart's vibrating bell, Western Electric, Medici, Rexton, Servox – left to right).

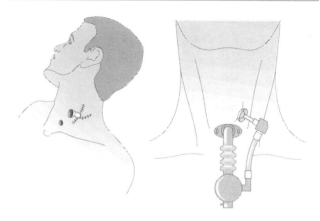

Figure 32.4 Taub's 'Voice Bak' prosthesis.

Artificial Larynx

The use of handheld electronic or pneumatic vibrating devices applied to the side of the throat or cheek or directed into the mouth via a small piece of tubing (Fig. 32.3) has provided an artificial alaryngeal voice for many patients, particularly those who are not interested in, or unable to learn or use, esophageal speech or TE speech. Voice acquisition is usually rapid and does not interfere with the subsequent acquisition of esophageal or TE speech. Early introduction of the artificial larynx often relieves the emotional frustration of not being able to speak during the immediate postoperative period. Patients often find the mechanical sound quality and the need to operate the device manually unacceptable. Despite the disadvantages, all laryngectomized patients should be encouraged to use an artifical larynx as a back-up in the event that their primary mode of alaryngeal communication fails.

Early History and Evolution of the TE Voice Prosthesis

Gussenbauer's tube (Fig. 32.1) was the prototype that combined an artificial sound source with an external shunt. The device was fitted into the tracheostoma, which conveyed air from the trachea through a reed device into the pharynx via a connecting pharyngostomy tube. The "Voice Bak" device (Fig. 32.4) introduced in 1972 by Taub and Spiro (4) was one of the more successful ones, but these methods were virtually abandoned because of problems with leakage, aspiration, and bleeding due to the close proximity of the shunt to the great vessels.

Guttmann, in 1932, is credited with the first description of an internal TE fistula in a patient who pierced his pharynx through the posterior wall of the tracheostoma with an ice-pick, establishing a shunt unintentionally. He found he was able to speak with a loud, fluent voice although the tract was prone to leakage and spontaneous closure.

Over the next 40 years a succession of techniques was proposed to create a surgical shunt to divert air from the trachea into the upper cervical esophagus or pharynx using a variety of methods including skin, mucosa, or a vein

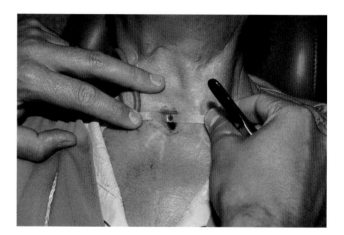

Figure 32.5 Early Blom–Singer valve in place.

graft. Consistent results proved impossible and invariably these procedures failed over time, either because the shunt stenosed or became too patulous and allowed aspiration.

Development of the Modern Voice Prosthesis

The modern era of highly successful surgical voice restoration was due to a major conceptual development in the late 1970s introduced by Blom and Singer, which transformed the expectation and quality of voice production after total laryngectomy (5). The technique involved creating a simple TE puncture between the posterior wall of the tracheostoma and the upper esophagus into which was inserted a one-way silicone valve (Fig. 32.5). This allowed air to flow from the trachea into the esophagus and the "duckbill" valve (Fig. 32.6) prevented aspiration of food and liquid. Over the next 20 years, the valve was improved and modified with introduction of the low pressure/low profile prosthesis in 1983 and an indwelling prosthesis (Fig. 32.7) in 1995 (6).

During this period of time, other investigators developed modifications of the original voice prosthesis

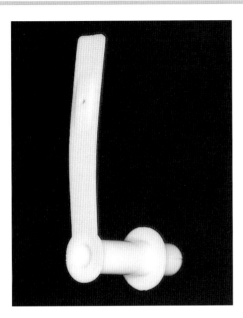

Figure 32.6 Blom–Singer 'duckbill' valve.

Table 32.2 Types of TE Voice Prostheses and Years of Introduction

Voice prosthesis	Year
Blom-singer duckbill	1979
Blom-singer low pressure	1983
Blom-singer indwelling	1995
Panje voice button	1981
Groningen voice prosthesis	1982
Provox	1988
Provox2	1997
Provox non-indwelling	2005
Bivona duckbill	1986
Bivona low-resistance	1988
Bivona ultralow	1988
Bivona colorado	1992+
Nijdam voice prosthesis	1996

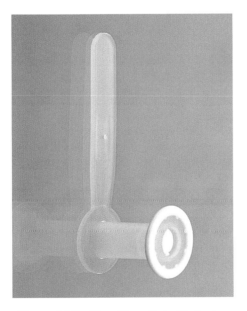

Figure 32.7 Blom–Singer 'indwelling' valve.

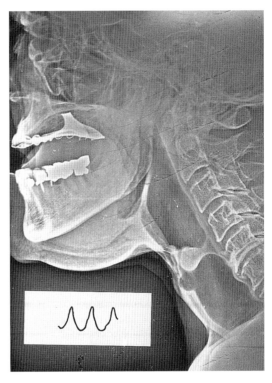

Figure 32.8 Xerograph of the neck in a laryngectomee phonating with good oesophageal speech showing a short tonic PE segment at C4/5.

introduced by Blom and Singer. These devices worked similarly by shunting air from the trachea into the esophagus for voice production while preventing aspiration of saliva and food during swallowing (Table 32.2).

THE PHYSIOLOGY OF THE PE SEGMENT
The PE Segment, Esophageal and TE Speech
The PE segment is the source of sound production for both the esophageal and TE speaker. The PE segment may vary greatly in its position, length, and muscular component. In contrast to the long circumferential segment seen in Figure 32.2, the one clearly seen in Figure 32.8 is a short, posteriorly based mucosal fold incorporating some muscle. In both cases an air reservoir is seen in the upper esophagus below the PE segment and the patients are both good esophageal speakers. A similar PE segment is shown in Figure 32.9 while the patient is phonating three days after fitting a voice prosthesis. In this case, air from the lungs is being diverted through the valve into the upper esophagus and then through the PE segment and vocal tract into the oral cavity to produce speech.

Although the vibrating PE segment, the resonating vocal tract, and the articulators are the same, the major

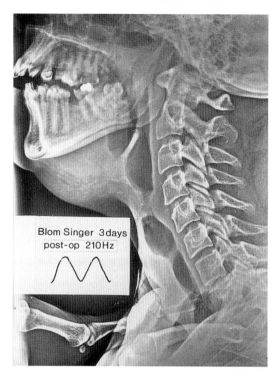

Figure 32.9 Xerograph of the neck in a laryngectomee 3 days after fitting a Blom–Singer valve showing digital occlusion of the stoma and a short tonic PE segment at C4.

Table 32.3 Comparison of Laryngeal, Esophageal and Tracheo-Esophageal Voice Production

Physical requirements	Laryngeal voice	Esophageal voice	Fistula voice
Initiator	Lungs 500 ml	Oesophageal air 40–70 ml	Lungs 500 ml
Vibrator	Vocal cords	PE segment	PE segment
Resonator	Supragl Lx orophx	Reconstructed orophx	Reconstructed orophx

Articulators: tongue, teeth, lips, soft palate.

difference between TE and esophageal speech is the volume and capacity of the air reservoirs (Table 32.3). For esophageal speech, only 40–70 ml of air can be trapped in the upper esophagus for voice production, whereas a maximum tidal capacity of 500 ml is available for TE speech. This capacity is comparable to that associated with normal lung-powered laryngeal voice. This means that TE speech is more similar to laryngeal speech in that it is much louder and more sustained than esophageal voice.

When the resection is extended beyond the larynx and includes the pharynx or the esophagus, partial or total pharyngolaryngectomy or pharyngolaryngoesophagectomy, the pharyngeal mucosa is partly or completely replaced by skin (cutaneous, myocutaneous, or free flaps) or intestinal mucosa (free jejunum or transposed stomach) rather than re-sutured pharyngeal wall. This alters the dynamics of the new PE segment and vocal tract, and may significantly influence the quality of the resulting voice.

Evaluation for Hypertonic Constrictor Spasm

The physical requirements of postlaryngectomy esophageal and TE voice are summarized in Table 32.3 where it may be seen that both rely on the PE segment to act as the vibratory source for sound production (Figs. 32.2, 32.8, and 32.9). The medial and inferior (cricopharyngeus) pharyngeal constrictor muscles need to be tonic to allow a steady stream of air through the segment to produce fluent sound. Uncoordinated disruptions in the flow of air through the PE segment, referred to as a hypertonic PE segment, will restrict or completely stop the smooth flow of air and result in what has been termed PE spasm (Fig. 32.10). PE spasm still remains one of the most common problems preventing successful TE speech production because it prevents the superior egress of air flow for sound production resulting in patient complaints of gastric filling. Several methods have been used to relieve constrictor spasm, including pharyngeal plexus neurectomy, cricopharyngeal myotomy, non-muscle closure of the pharynx, and mechanical hypopharyngeal dilation. Currently, chemical denervation with botulinum neurotoxin (Botox) injection is preferred over surgical alternatives as a noninvasive treatment for the relief of constrictor muscle spasm. It is always important to appropriately evaluate TE voice failure prior to intervention to accurately identify the etiology and select the optimal treatment approach to facilitate fluent TE voice.

Evaluation of TE Voice Failure
Videofluoroscopy

The most accurate method for assessing PE segment function after laryngectomy is with videofluoroscopy (7,8,9). This examination should be carried out routinely prior to secondary voice restoration and should be available to every laryngectomee who has voice problems or who is unable to acquire esophageal or TE speech. The results of videofluoroscopy show that approximately 60% of patients have poor or failed speech due to hypertonic or spasmodic PE segments (9). This corresponds quite well to the proportion of patients previously documented by Johnson et al. (10) who failed to achieve esophageal voice. With the help of videofluoroscopy, Lewin et al. (11) found that 91% of voice failures could eventually achieve speech if fully investigated and treated accordingly. Videofluoroscopy involves the use of a small dosage of radiation (5–10 cGy). A comprehensive videofluoroscopic examination of PE segment functioning has the following three components:

Modified Barium Swallow Study

Since TE voice production and swallowing are intimately related, any evaluation of TE voice failure should include a brief evaluation of swallowing using the modified barium swallow study. The patient is instructed to swallow barium liquid to evaluate clearance of the barium through the pharynx to differentiate spasm from stricture. The patient should be evaluated in the lateral and antero-posterior views. Any anatomical abnormality is easily visualized and evaluated as a contributory cause of either

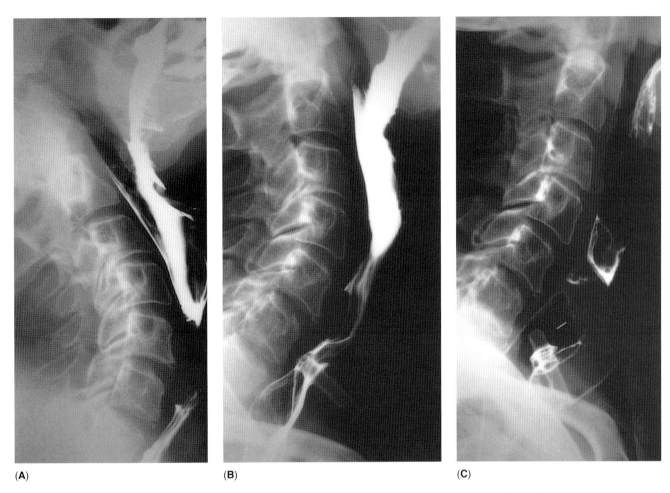

(A) (B) (C)

Figure 32.10 **(A)** Lateral X-ray of the neck during videofluoroscopy in a laryngectomee 5 years after operation with poor voice due to intense constrictor spasm (premyotomy). **(B)** Postmyotomy showing flow of barium and Blom–Singer valve. **(C)** Phonation producing strong fluent voice showing air reservoir in the oesophagus and ligaclip at lower limit of myotomy.

dysphagia or poor voice. In general, other consistencies that are routinely used for assessment of swallowing, such as purees and solid food consistencies are not needed for the evaluation of TE voice failure.

Attempted Phonation

After the mucosa of the pharynx is coated with barium, the TE speaker is asked to cover his stoma, say "ah" and count to 20, in a lateral radiographic view. Airflow either passes easily through the segment between the pharynx and esophagus or there is variable hold-up at the PE segment. Airflow through the PE segment may be restricted due to stricture, PE spasm, or both. Strictures may occur at the anastomotic site if there has been inadequate mucosal/skin reconstruction of the hypopharynx. The critical differentiation between voice failure related to spasm and voice failure related to stricture is that the liquid barium passes normally through the PE segment during swallowing in patients with constrictor spasm. In contrast, patients who have a stricture demonstrate both the stoppage of air flow and sound production during voice

attempts, as well as the stoppage of liquid barium through the PE segment during swallowing.

Esophageal Insufflation Test

Insufflation testing during videofluoroscopy is performed as a preoperative evaluation for patients considered for secondary TE puncture. A catheter is passed through the nose down into the pharynx to just below the PE segment (about 25 cm from the nasal aperture) and connected to a stomal adaptor (Fig. 32.11). The patient is asked to occlude the opening and to try to sustain phonation and count. The videofluoroscopic recording during the two voice tasks is analyzed to identify the presence of spasm or any other reason for an inability to produce sound.

Manometry

Measurement of pressures within the PE segment during TE speech production is also a useful indication of constrictor tonicity and corresponds very well with the results of videofluoroscopy (Fig. 32.12) (8). A simple pressure

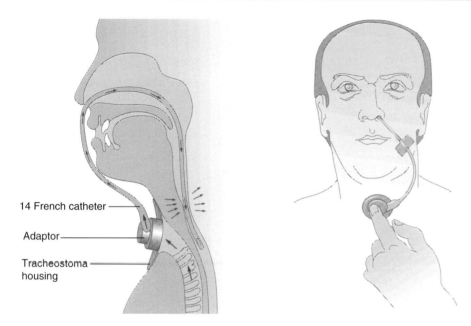

14 French catheter

Adaptor

Tracheostoma
housing

Figure 32.11   Insufflation test.

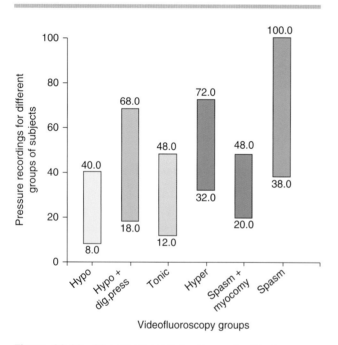

Figure 32.12   PE segment opening pressures for videofluoroscopy
groups (14).

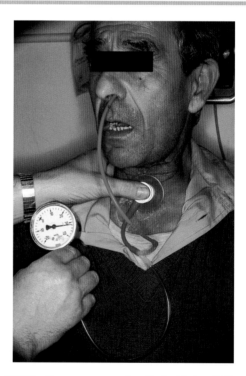

Figure 32.13   Pressure manometer attached to insufflation tubing.

manometer is attached to the tubing of the insufflation
catheter and the reading is taken during phonation of the
pressure required to open the segment and produce voice
(Fig. 32.13).

Objective intraesophageal insufflation has determined
fluent speech to be associated with intraesophageal pressure levels less than 20 mm Hg on a pressure manometer.

Three levels of TE speech fluency—fluent, nonfluent,
and nonspeaker—are associated with three ranges of
peak intraesophageal pressure measurements (11). Objective
insufflation is a useful tool to definitively identify constrictor spasm and objectively evaluate successful TE speech
outcomes after interventions, such as Botox injection, that
compromise constrictor muscle contraction (12).

TIMING OF TE VOICE RESTORATION

TE puncture may be performed at the time of laryngectomy (primary TE puncture), or may be performed as a secondary procedure several months or even years after laryngectomy. Experience has shown that patients who receive primary TE puncture are equally successful in their ability to achieve fluent TE speech as patients who receive TE puncture as a secondary procedure after healing has occurred. Furthermore, no significant differences in complication rates have been shown between the two groups. The reader is referred to the section Selection Criteria for TE Speech Restoration for further details.

Primary Voice Restoration
Surgical Considerations
There are surgical considerations that should be taken into account before making the decision to carry out a primary puncture at the time of total laryngectomy. These mainly concern the potential increased risk of developing a postoperative fistula or wound breakdown.

A large proportion of patients will have had previous high-dose radiotherapy, which has an adverse effect on healing and is associated with a higher complication rate after laryngectomy. A TE puncture is not a contraindication even in patients who have been treated with intensive radiation. As with prior irradiation, the presence of diabetes, anemia, malnutrition, and cardiovascular disease will predispose to poorer healing, but individually should not be a contraindication to primary voice restoration.

Resection of the cervical esophagus at the time of laryngectomy will open up the retrotracheal space, which increases the risk of fistula breakdown. It is therefore inadvisable to undertake a TE puncture at the time of pharyngolaryngo esophagectomy with gastric transposition or free jejunum repair. There is a similar risk if dissection between the upper trachea and esophagus has inadvertently been taken down to the level of the puncture site. This separation of the party wall is an absolute contraindication to primary puncture and must be repaired (13). If circumferential resection and reconstruction is limited to the pharynx, it may be reasonable to undertake a primary voice restoration provided that the lower anastomosis is well above the proposed puncture site.

Surgical Technique
The laryngectomy is carried out in the usual fashion conserving as much pharyngeal mucosa as possible, particularly over the postcricoid region and the piriform fossae, provided safe clearance from the tumor is obtained. For hypopharyngeal tumors the mucosa of the uninvolved piriform fossa is carefully preserved to minimize the need for flap reconstruction. Ideally a transverse mucosal width of at least 6 cm is necessary to enable adequate swallowing and effortless tracheo-esophageal speech. Augmentation of the pharynx with a flap is preferable if the residual mucosal strip is under 4 cm; otherwise stenosis, together with significant functional impairment, is likely.

Certain fundamental principles and modifications have been incorporated into the laryngectomy technique to ensure good predictable results with minimal risk of complications.

Stoma Position
A Gluck–Sorensen incision is preferred, incorporating inferolateral extensions if necessary for neck dissection. The midline horizontal portion is at the level of the planned superior border of the tracheostome, usually at the second/third tracheal ring. The curved lateral limbs extend up to the level of the hyoid bone.

Stoma Reconstruction
The central part of the lower skin flap is sutured around the curved margin of the anterior trachea to the posterior ends of the tracheal ring. Close approximation of the mucosa to the skin is necessary, covering any bare cartilage in order to avoid granulation formation. The upper flap is sutured to the margin of the trachealis muscle on the posterior wall of the trachea. This reconstruction ensures that the tracheal rings are pulled laterally to maintain an adequately sized stoma, not too large and not too small. Attention should be given to the junction of the tracheocutaneous mucosa as the shape and configuration of the stomal edge will be important in achieving successful hands-free TE speech. It is usually a good idea to put absorbable sutures between the esophageal wall and the posterior aspect of the trachealis on either side of the proposed position of the puncture in order to secure the party wall and avoid inadvertent separation.

Tracheo Esophageal Puncture
Ideally, the puncture is positioned in the midline about 10–15 mm below the mucocutaneous junction on the posterior tracheal wall. A 14-FG Foley catheter is first prepared by trimming a slither of Silastic from opposite edges near the tip to facilitate easier grasping of an otherwise awkward rounded end. The balloon is tested by inflating with 1.5 ml of saline; it is then deflated and the catheter is grasped near the tip with a small pair of curved artery forceps.

The tip of another pair of curved artery forceps is inserted through the pharyngeal defect and advanced into the upper esophagus just as far as the puncture site,

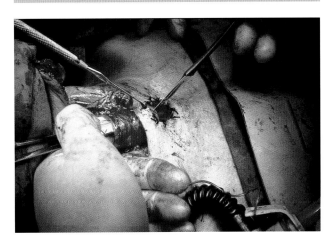

Figure 32.14 Positioning of the primary tracheo-esophageal puncture.

tenting up the mucosa (Fig. 32.14). A scalpel is used to incise horizontally through the mucosa and muscle onto the tip of the forceps, which are then advanced into the tracheal lumen and opened to grasp the tip of the Silastic catheter (Fig. 32.15). The forceps and the catheter are then withdrawn through the fistula tract and the tip of the catheter is passed distally down the esophagus to just above the cardio-esophageal junction. The catheter balloon is inflated with about 1.5 ml of saline to prevent accidental dislodgement and the catheter is anchored to the skin above the stoma. A 14 French red rubber catheter can also be used and has the advantage of no attached balloon that needs to be inflated and deflated. In addition, the red rubber catheter may also be less traumatic to the TE tract mucosa when removed.

There are several advantages of using the Foley or red rubber catheter as a feeding tube during the postoperative period. It obviates the need for a nasogastric tube, which is irritating to the nose and cosmetically unsightly. The nasogastric tube would normally pass down across the suture line of the reconstructed pharynx, through the esophagus and into the stomach, thus preventing proper closure of the cardio-esophageal sphincter. During the early postoperative period, with the patient in a recumbent position most of the time, the tube may act as a very effective syphon allowing unwanted gastric acid to reflux up the esophagus to the site of the pharyngeal reconstruction.

Cricopharyngeal Myotomy

A short posterior midline myotomy is carried out with a scalpel over a distance of 2–3 cm from the level of the TE puncture site (Fig. 32.16). This divides the circular muscle fibers in the upper esophagus and the cricopharyngeus. Effective assessment of the tone of the circular fibers is made by inserting the index finger into the lower pharynx and upper esophagus, where frequently the finger detects some resistance due to hypertonicity or spasm (14). This correlates well with manometric pressure measurements and outcome (15). The finger is kept in position and the tightness is felt to be gradually relieved as the scalpel divides the circular fibers down to the submucosal vascular plexus.

Any inadvertent cut through the mucosa should be repaired with an absorbable suture.

The myotomy carried out at the time of laryngectomy is designed to allow expansion of the upper esophagus providing an air "reservoir" below the PE segment, which is essential for good voice production (Figs. 32.2, 32.8, and 32.9). It is shorter than the myotomy carried out as a secondary procedure for voice failure due to spasm or hypertonicity, which extends from the puncture site up to the tongue base (see below).

Pharyngeal Plexus Neurectomy

A unilateral pharyngeal plexus neurectomy is an alternative method of constrictor relaxation (16) or can be carried out as well as myotomy. Usually three to five branches of the plexus entering the lateral wall of the pharynx are exposed and tested with a nerve stimulator before cautery and division.

Pharyngeal Closure

The previously widely used method of vertical closure of the pharyngeal defect is not suitable for optimum voice restoration for various reasons. It produces a long anterior scar, which contracts over a period of time producing the typical appearance on endoscopy of a pseudo-vallecula with a transverse pharyngeal mucosal bar. This also has a characteristic appearance on lateral view videofluoroscopy (Fig. 32.17). This pseudo-vallecula potentially can cause problems with speech and swallowing. In the early postoperative period it can form a small "sump" at the tongue base, which may fill with fluid and predispose to development of a fistula tract. Vertical closure produces a long narrow pharyngeal segment, which may contribute to dysphagia. On swallowing, the bolus of food may collect in the pseudo-vallecula, which enlarges, pushing the posterior wall backwards causing further narrowing of the opening into the hypopharynx. This produces a similar effect on swallowing as does the pharyngeal pouch when it obstructs the opening of the esophagus. The patient may experience difficulty in clearing food from the pharynx, taking several swallows to get the bolus into the esophagus.

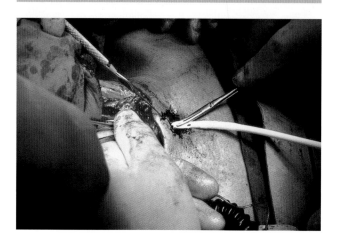

Figure 32.15   Insertion of the Foley catheter.

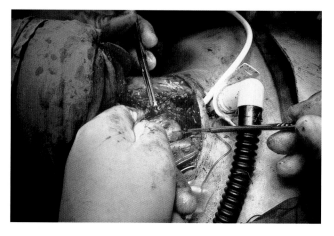

Figure 32.16   Short constrictor myotomy.

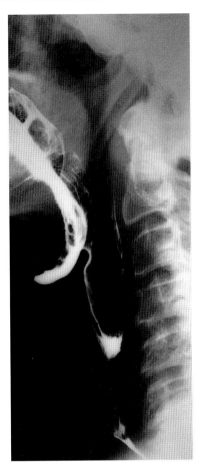

Figure 32.17 Lateral X-ray of the neck to show barium in a pseudovallecula after laryngectomy.

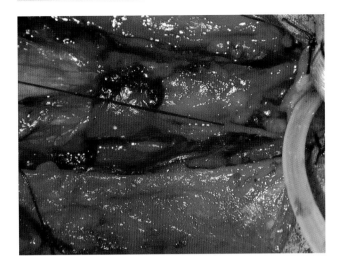

Figure 32.18 Reconstruction of the muscular PE segment and re-implantation of recurrent larngeal nerve.

Injection of air into the pharynx during esophageal speech may be affected in a similar way. TE and esophageal speakers also complain of a "gargly," wet voice that lacks intensity because of the effect of the "pouch" on mucosal vibration.

A horizontal closure of the pharyngeal defect is preferred using a continuous absorbable mucosal suture and then an interrupted muscle layer. This produces a wider pharynx above the PE segment, which has been shown to improve resonance for speech. If additional mucosa from the piriform sinus has been excised it will probably be necessary to close the pharynx in a 'T' shape in order to avoid tension. Despite the three-point junction this is still preferred to a vertical closure. Significant resection of the hypopharynx will necessitate a skin flap reconstruction (see above).

Reconstruction of the PE Segment

A 1-cm band of the thyropharyngeus constrictor muscle is brought together anteriorly with mattress sutures about 3–4 cm above the TE puncture site (Fig. 32.18). The purpose is to try to create a suitable PE segment at the optimal site in the pharynx with a good air reservoir below it and a wide resonating pharyngeal segment above. It is important, however, not to make the band too tight, otherwise it may produce a hypertonic segment.

Reinnervation of the Pharynx

The cut ends of the superior laryngeal nerves and the recurrent laryngeal nerves are reimplanted into the muscular wall of the reconstructed pharynx and upper esophagus respectively in the hope that this may restore some sensory and motor reinnervation. It is felt that this can only have a potentially beneficial effect on neuromuscular coordination of the reconstructed "neolarynx," although obviously it is difficult to measure any effect objectively (Fig. 32.18).

Primary Placement of the Voice Prosthesis

Primary placement of the voice prosthesis before closure of the pharynx at time of laryngectomy is a variation of the puncture technique that has gained some popularity primarily in Europe (13). A nasogastric tube must be inserted, however, for postoperative feeding. With the disadvantages mentioned previously, most patients find this much less acceptable than a tube passed through the puncture site. In addition, the prosthesis will require resizing and replacement within a few weeks as the postoperative edema subsides. During the acute postoperative recovery period, generally lasting 10 days postoperatively, use of the prosthesis for speech is inadvisable to ensure complete wound healing and to avoid risking fistula formation.

Closure and Postoperative Care

The wound is closed routinely with suction drainage. Feeding is continued through the Foley or red catheter and oral intake is commenced usually after seven days if no previous radiotherapy has been given, in which case it is delayed until the tenth day following a satisfactory barium swallow. Once oral feeding has commenced, the catheter is removed after two to three days and replaced with a suitable TE prosthesis (Fig. 32.19). Occasionally patients require longer recovery; however, it is inadvisable to stent the TE puncture with a catheter for an extended period of time as prolonged catheter placement may encourage enlargement

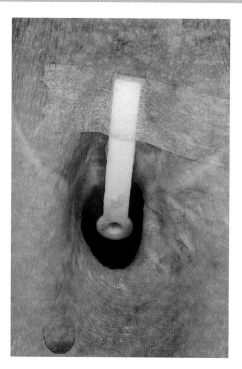

Figure 32.19   Blom-Singer prosthesis in position.

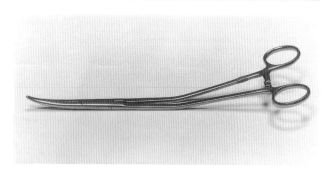

Figure 32.20   Secondary tracheo-esophageal puncture forceps.

or irregularity of the TE puncture. In these cases, it is preferable to insert a dummy prosthesis, one with a closed valve, to stent the tract during recovery.

Secondary Voice Restoration
Surgical Technique
The technique of TE puncture with prosthetic voice restoration was originally developed as a secondary procedure for those patients who had failed to achieve adequate esophageal speech (5). The method described by Singer and Blom in 1980 (5) has provided a reliable technique for restoration of good quality lung-powered speech, but significant problems associated with the rigid endoscopic technique have been described, particularly concerning access down to the stoma level (17–20). Similar problems with access using the rigid endoscope prompted the first

author to develop an alternative method (21) using a modified pair of curved Lloyd-Davies forceps (Fig. 32.20), which has been used successfully in a series of 94 secondary voice punctures since 1984, with no failed or abandoned procedures.

The forceps are inserted alongside a pharyngeal speculum into the esophageal opening under direct vision and advanced down to the level of the tracheostoma where the tip can be seen and palpated as it tents up the posterior tracheal wall in a similar way to the primary puncture technique. An incision is made through the posterior wall of the stoma in the midline on to the tips of the forceps (Fig. 32.21A), which are advanced into the trachea. The end of a 14-FG catheter is then introduced into the opened tips of the forceps (Fig. 32.21B) and withdrawn into the pharynx (Fig. 32.21C), passed caudally and released. The catheter is sutured to the skin above the tracheostoma and if a Foley catheter is used the balloon is inflated with 1.5 ml of saline to prevent dislodgement.

A normal diet is resumed after the procedure and the stenting catheter (Fig. 32.22) remains in place for a period of two to seven days depending on whether a myotomy has been carried out simultaneously. It is then removed and after measuring the length of the tract a suitable TE voice prosthesis is inserted.

Secondary TE puncture may also be performed successfully in the outpatient clinic under local anesthetic using a transnasal esophagoscope to visualize the procedure. High success rates are reported in several small retrospective series (22–25).

SELECTION CRITERIA FOR TE SPEECH RESTORATION
Patient Selection
As the medical complexity of patients who require total laryngectomy has increased, it is prudent to provide thorough assessment to determine appropriate candidacy for TE puncture. Despite the simplicity of the method of TE puncture, the complexity of managing patients with postoperative complications, involved medical histories, and those who have had salvage surgery in previously radiated fields, requires clinicians to be much more careful and prudent with their recommendations for TE puncture as well as the timing of the procedure, either primary or secondary. For a majority of patients, primary TE puncture at the time of total laryngectomy offers the optimal timing for voice restoration. This procedure has made a great difference in the management of laryngeal cancer by eliminating the major stigma of loss of voice and restoring a good quality of life. The contraindications to primary TE puncture for the standard, uncomplicated laryngectomy are few but again careful selection of patients will help to reduce disappointment and failure. It may be in the best interest of certain patients, however, to delay the TE puncture a few months to avoid postoperative problems and achieve optimal results. Successful TE voice restoration should be delayed in patients who are at high risk for postoperative complications such as fistulas, or those who require longer recovery from complex reconstructions. In these cases, management of the TE puncture causes added burden for the patient and the clinical team without the benefit of rapid voice restoration. Therefore, secondary TE

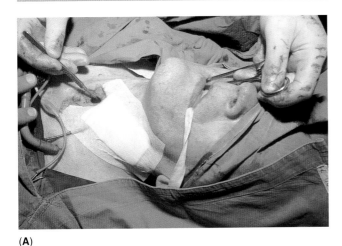

(A)

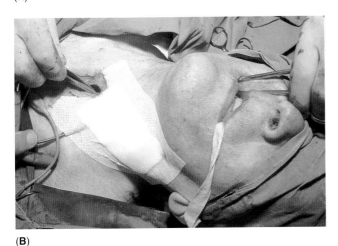

(B)

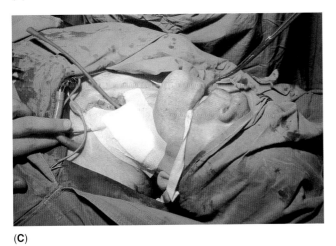

(C)

Figure 32.21 Incision being made through the posterior stomal wall.

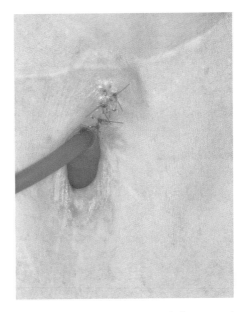

Figure 32.22 Stenting catheter before removal.

Table 32.4 Advantages and Disadvantages of Primary and Secondary TE Puncture

	Pros	Cons
1° TEP	Early voice restoration	Patient readiness
	Psychological benefit	Preoperative evaluation (especially for medically complex patients)
	May be safer (avoids further surgery, potential complications, and additional anesthesia)	Difficult in patients with complicated reconstructions
	Avoids 2nd operation	Heavily irradiated patients
	High vocal satisfaction	
	Avoids nasogastric tube	
2° TEP	Allows post-surgical healing in medically fragile patients	Delayed oral speech restoration
	Allows patient-specific prosthetic selection	Greater risk for complications
	High vocal satisfaction	Psychological sequelae

puncture may be more optimal for patients who have severe radiation sequelae or those who require extended surgery with reconstruction. Additionally, secondary TE voice restoration is often preferred for patients who do not demonstrate understanding of the method or lack a readiness for TE puncture. The relative advantages and disadvantages of primary and secondary TE puncture are described in Table 32.4 and a summary of the timing of TE voice restoration and characteristics for candidacy is described in Table 32.5.

Careful investigation and selection is even more critical for successful secondary voice restoration. With the advent of the use of Botox injection to relieve TE voice failure, there has been recent debate regarding the need for preoperative insufflation to assess TE voice potential prior to secondary TE puncture. The advantages of preoperative insufflation testing provide support for its use in all patients prior to secondary TE puncture. Insufflation testing provides a baseline measurement for objective comparison with postoperative speech results and is an excellent preoperative indicator of postoperative TE speech production for anxious

Table 32.5 Timing of the TE Puncture

Primary	Secondary	No TEP
Standard laryngectomy	Complicated medical history	Marked cognitive impairment
Patient who is motivated, compliant, and independent	Complicated surgical procedures	Severe substance abuse
Good family/significant other support	"At risk" patients	*Poor compliance** *Limited rehabilitative access**
Access to rehabilitative services	Limited readiness and independence	*No support**

*All three characteristics together are poor indicators for TE voice restoration.

patients who will benefit from hearing the potential quality of their TE voice after puncture. This is particularly true for patients whose pharynx has been reconstructed following pharyngolaryngectomy or pharyngolaryngo esophagectomy. Finally, preoperative insufflation helps to determine the functionality of the PE segment and identify patients who need further compromise of the PE musculature, surgical or pharmacological, to achieve successful TE speech (11). Videofluoroscopy should be performed in patients with suspected PE segment dysfunction, Lewin et al. (11) showed elevated intraesophageal pressures on insufflation, >20 mmHg, were associated with hypertonicity of the pharyngeal constrictors, or PE spasm.

PE Segment Function

As discussed previously, the findings from videofluoroscopy will determine the functioning of the PE segment, and whether or not compromise of the PE musculature is recommended prior to secondary TE puncture.

Manual Dexterity

The patient should ideally be able to clean, change, and maintain the prosthesis independently. If this is not possible, a relative or close live-in significant other may be able to help. Motivation is essential.

Expectations of Surgery and Rehabilitation

The expectations of surgery and rehabilitation have not been widely researched. It is important that patients and their families have realistic expectations about the limitations and advantages of TE voice restoration before the procedure is performed. This includes the quality of TE voice, the need to occlude the stoma, and the ability to appropriately manage the TE prosthesis. Although TE voice is the single alaryngeal alternative that most closely approaches "normal" laryngeal speech, it is also important that patients and their families understand that TE speech is not normal in its production, quality, loudness, or pitch. It is always beneficial to ask a fully rehabilitated TE speaker to meet with the patient and family prior to TE puncture.

Visual Acuity

Good eyesight is important for adequate management of the prosthesis. The patient should have access to a good light source and mirror. Visual acuity by itself, however, is not a sole determinant of successful TE voice production.

Alcohol or Drug Abuse

Some patients with addiction problems are unable to manage a prosthesis. Their unreliability causes unnecessary frustration and expense through repeated loss of the valve, and inability to manage the valve, which can result in persistent leakage, infection, and other problems.

Respiratory Status

Many laryngectomized patients have other smoking-related lung conditions, such as bronchitis, emphysema, and chronic obstructive pulmonary disease (COPD) of varying severity. There may be inadequate pulmonary reserve to provide the power source for TE voice. Potentially excessive bronchial secretions may hinder TE speech production by clogging the valve or preventing the use of a hands-free system. Patients with pulmonary disease or poor pulmonary function are likely better candidates for a secondary TE puncture so that intraesophageal insufflation can be performed to accurately determine candidacy.

Esophageal Speech

Patients with a well-established esophageal voice who wish to be considered for TE puncture need to be critically evaluated and the advantages and limitations of the valve clearly explained. Excellent esophageal speakers may be one of the most difficult conversions to TE speech as the entire method of esophageal speech through oral air implosion remains the antithesis of TE voice production that uses pulmonary air to power sound production. The ability to extinguish the techniques for esophageal speech production is very difficult in a well-established esophageal speaker. The patient who is unable to extinguish esophageal speech production may experience non-fluent TE voice and painful gastric distension that requires removal of the prosthesis and closure of the TE puncture.

Extent of Surgery

Satisfactory speech restoration with a TE valve is possible in the majority of patients following total pharyngolaryngectomy, as well as those with additional esophagectomy and stomach transposition (26,14,27). Depending on the type of reconstruction, the voice may be weak, liquid, cavernous, and hypotonic. Sometimes the quality and strength can be improved with digital pressure over the reconstructed segment. In most cases secondary TE voice restoration is preferred until healing has been completed to avoid additional risk of wound breakdown and to allow for preoperative air insufflation.

Tracheostoma Size and Contour

During the first few months after laryngectomy, until scar tissue has stabilized, a stoma button or tube is sometimes necessary to avoid contraction and stenosis. The stoma should ideally be adequate in size for respiration but small enough for easy occlusion. In general, a stoma 20–25 mm in diameter is ideal. If the stoma is too small it may be dilated with a laryngectomy tube or may require enlargement with stomaplasty. Often a small stoma holds an intraluminally placed button that maintains adequate stomal patency and allows for the attachment of a hands-free speaking valve. If the stoma is too large for satisfactory digital occlusion, the use of a peristomal attachment or intraluminal button may help occlude the stoma. Tracheo-stomaplasty should also be considered in these cases.

The size, shape and contour of the stoma and surrounding skin are more critical for successful "hands free" speech. Ideally the peristomal neck contour should be flat to help ensure optimal adhesion of the tracheostoma valve housing (28). In order to avoid unnecessary tracheal retraction, the trachea should not be transected too low, and the margins of the trachea can be sutured to the tendinous medial margins of the sternomastoid muscles to secure it near the skin. This may be difficult if a low transection of the trachea has been necessary, in which case a sternomastoid tendonectomy may help.

Recurrent Disease

The possibility of early recurrent disease may influence the decision to carry out voice restoration. In a strongly motivated patient, however, it may be very important to facilitate speech restoration even if it is just for a short period of time.

In summary, a patient who is otherwise in good health, strongly motivated, and determined to achieve voice after laryngectomy will usually succeed, provided that the surgeon and speech pathologist have the knowledge and expertise to manage any problems and complications that arise. Again, careful selection of patients will help ensure optimal TE speech results. New surgical techniques, along with the variety of TE prostheses now available, have widened the potential population of patients suitable for a TE prosthesis.

VOICE FAILURE AFTER LARYNGECTOMY

Historical Perspective

In their 1979 review of the literature Johnson et al. (10) estimated that the esophageal voice failure rate after laryngectomy was between 15% and 50%. Of those who achieved voice, only a small proportion were able to communicate with reasonably fluent intelligible speech. These disappointing results, often after prolonged speech therapy, were

thought to be related mainly to poor understanding or motivation of the patient.

In the same year Duguay (29) recognized that the reasons for esophageal voice failure could be categorized into four main causes: anatomical and physiological problems, psychological and social problems, teaching and learning difficulties, and a final group of "unknown" etiology. These potential causes of voice failure became more of an issue when it was recognized, after the introduction of TE puncture by Blom and Singer, that a proportion of their valve patients were not achieving good or optimal voice because of pharyngeal constrictor hypertonicity (30). Video-fluoroscopic evaluation substantiated this finding and continues to be used to evaluate the PE segment as a reason for both esophageal and TE voice failure (7,31,12). Table 32.6 describes the five categories of PE segment tonicity.

Management of Pharyngeal Constrictor Hypertonicity (Spasm)

Surgical Treatment

The recognition of pharyngeal constrictor spasm or hypertonicity as a cause of voice failure (32) by Singer and Blom in 1981 and its treatment with myotomy was a major factor in achieving good consistent results for TE speech. Experience has shown that cricopharyngeal myotomy at the time of laryngectomy is not always successful in facilitating fluent TE voice. Videofluoroscopic examinations have shown that hypertonicity may occur at any level along the pharyngeal constrictor musculature, and not just involve the cricopharyngeus (Fig. 32.23). A long myotomy from the stoma to the base of the tongue has been shown to result in more consistent TE speech outcomes (Fig. 32.10).

Surgical technique.

Identification of the pharynx An esophageal dilator (36–40 FG) is initially inserted to delineate the hypopharynx and to stretch the muscle fibers to facilitate the myotomy.

Side of approach A decision is then made on which side to approach the pharynx. Normally at laryngectomy the thyroid lobe will have been removed on the side of the tumor and it is generally more convenient to approach the pharynx from this side. The presence of a thyroid lobe does make access more difficult (Fig. 32.24) for the myotomy, particularly as it is not advisable to divide the inferior thyroid artery, which may devascularize the remaining gland if the superior thyroid artery has already been divided at the time of laryngectomy.

Incision Reopening of the Gluck–Sorensen scar from the stoma up to the level of the tongue base is preferred

Table 32.6 Videofluoroscopy Assessment of Pharyngeal Constrictor Tone

PE Segment	Ba swallow	Phonation	Assisted phonation (Taub test)
Tonic	Passes easily	Good voice	Stronger sustained voice
Hypotonic	Passes easily	Weak voice	More sustained, stronger with digital pressure
Hypertonic	Normal or slower passage	Intermittent tight voice	Intermittent tight voice Gastric distension
Spasm	Some hold-up and residue above PE segment	No voice, no air goes into esophagus	Minimal voice, explosive segment release as pressure increases Gastric distension
Stricture	Permanent hold-up	No voice	No voice

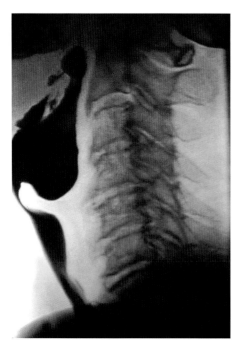

Figure 32.23 Note the collection of barium above and below the area of PE spasm.

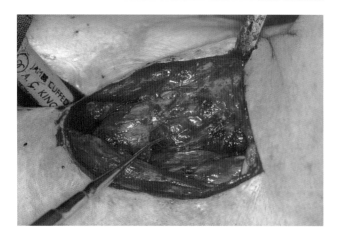

Figure 32.24 Identification of the hypertrophied pharyngeal constrictors that are partly hidden by the thyroid lobe.

to an incision between the carotid and the pharynx (32) since this gives better protection to the carotid artery. There is usually dense fibrous tissue between the carotid and the pharynx, but this is carefully divided down to the prevertebral fascia with lateral retraction of the artery.

Myotomy The pharyngeal constrictors are stretched over the dilator and incised from the level of the stoma up to the level of the tongue base (Fig. 32.25). The myotomy is taken as deep as the submucosal vessels and the muscle coat is retracted back and sutured to prevent reclosure.

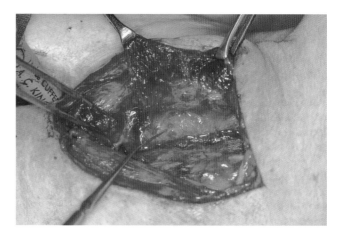

Figure 32.25 Long secondary constrictor myotomy.

Any inadvertent perforation of the mucosa is closed with absorbable suture and if this does happen the patient will have to remain tube-fed for one week, using the catheter through the trans-esophageal fistula.

The main complication following secondary myotomy is a small fistula (10–20%) (32), but most of these are recognized during surgery and sutured. If there is any doubt about the integrity of the mucosa, air can be insufflated into the pharynx to identify any leak. Cervical spine injury is not a common problem unless a rigid endoscopic puncture is carried out at the same time (17–20). Cervical osteomyelitis may occur even in the absence of a fistula (33). Satisfactory healing is verified with a barium swallow before starting an oral diet; tracheo esophageal speech is commenced with the prosthesis after one week.

Pharmacological Treatment

Botulinum toxin injection. The use of botulinum toxin (Botox) to chemically relieve constrictor hypertonicity or spasm has become the preferred method of treatment because it is a simple technique that can be performed during an office outpatient visit and does not prevent further surgical intervention if needed. Successful results that are often permanent have been achieved using a technique for EMG-guided Botox injection. Botox is reconstituted in 2cc of normal saline yielding a concentration of 50 mouse units per cc of normal saline. Usually, two to three injections are performed on one side along the neopharynx into the hypertonic segment that has been previously marked during videofluoroscopic assessment (12). Myotomy is generally reserved for circumstances in which Botox injection has been ineffective in relieving spasm.

VOICE RESTORATION FOLLOWING TOTAL PHARYNGOLARYNGECTOMY

Successful management of carcinoma of the hypopharynx or upper cervical esophagus is difficult because these tumors often present late with nodal metastases and they are generally not as radiosensitive as carcinoma of the nasopharynx or oropharynx. A large proportion of these patients will undergo pharyngolaryngectomy either primarily or for recurrence with a potential cure rate of up to 40%. This operation, however, is much more complex than total laryngectomy, particularly the reconstruction and is associated with a greater risk for complications, a higher morbidity, and potentially less successful restoration of speech and swallowing. It is therefore essential that treatment be performed by an experienced multidisciplinary team to achieve optimal results.

A variety of choices are available now for reconstruction of the hypopharynx following total pharyngolaryngectomy and the decision to select a particular method will depend on various factors. There are two main groups of reconstructive options. The first includes a variety of tubed myocutaneous flaps, the most common ones being the free radial forearm flap, the anterolateral thigh flap, the pedicled deltopectoral fasciocutaneous flap, and the pedicled pectoralis major and latissimus dorsi myocutaneous flaps. The second type of reconstruction involves transfer of alimentary tract mucosa, using either transposition of the stomach or a free jejunal graft.

Deltopectoral Flap

The modern era of reconstructive surgery for head and neck tumors dates back to 1965. Bakamjian described the deltopectoral flap for most reconstructions of the mouth and pharynx. The great advantage of this flap was that it provided a large area of skin with a good blood supply taken from outside the area of previous surgery or radiotherapy. Following total pharyngolaryngectomy the long axial pattern flap is tubed and inset into the defect leaving a controlled salivary fistula at its lower end. The pedicle of the flap is divided during a second stage operation two to three weeks later and the remaining corner of the flap is inset into the esophagus.

This technique offered significant advantages over existing methods of reconstruction, such as the Wookey flap or the distant tubed pedicle popularized by Gillies, which required many staged operations over several months. Hospitalization, however, was still prolonged and there was a considerable delay in swallowing, the development of speech production, and initiation of postoperative radiotherapy.

Results

This flap originated at a time before TE fistula techniques, but some patients were able to develop esophageal speech. It is still used now as a safe alternative in difficult situations where other flaps have failed or are not suitable. Generally, voice restoration is carried out as a secondary procedure. Vocal quality is decreased compared to the voice produced by the native pharynx.

Pectoralis Major Myocutaneous Flap

In 1979 Ariyan introduced the pectoralis major myocutaneous flap, which largely superseded the deltopectoral flap as the reconstructive workhorse of the head and neck (34). Its great advantage is that it allows one stage reconstruction of the pharynx (35) and it is also very reliable and easy to raise. For circumferential reconstruction of the hypopharynx the flap is raised and tubed before insetting into the defect. There are, however, some potential limitations. It is important to take a wide enough flap to allow for some contraction, otherwise there is potential for stenosis and swallowing problems. It is usually possible to get primary closure of the primary defect on the chest wall but sometimes a skin graft is necessary. The muscle and subcutaneous fat layers may be quite thick producing a bulky flap that may be difficult to tube and inset without tension. It is generally not suitable in women because of the additional bulk of the breast tissue and also it may result in unacceptable distortion and asymmetry of the breast. The latissimus dorsi flap is much more preferable for these patients. In men the chest flap is often hairy and may obstruct swallowing during the initial period of recovery. After a period of time the hairs atrophy.

Results

If an adequate flap has been used, swallowing and quality of speech are usually acceptable (36). Primary puncture can be done if there is sufficient length of esophagus and hypopharynx between the lower anastomosis and the stoma level. Typically with these types of cutaneous flaps, the smooth skin lining offers less resistance to the flow of air compared with jejunum and the voice is correspondingly stronger. The PE segment often becomes established at the upper anastomosis (Fig. 32.26).

Latissimus Dorsi Myocutaneous Flap

This is a versatile flap for either pedicled or free flap reconstruction in the head and neck (37). A disadvantage is that the patient needs to be turned onto one side during the procedure, but this is generally not a major problem for experienced surgeons. A large area of flap can be raised (Fig. 32.27) with good reliability and the muscle is thin and pliable and ideal for tubing. The donor site can be closed primarily. An additional advantage of this flap is that there is no hair growth.

Results

The functional outcomes for swallowing and speech are similar to the other cutaneous flaps and because of its generous size, there is less risk for stenosis.

Free Radial Forearm Flap

The advent of free microvascular tissue transfer has greatly increased the scope of reconstructive options in the head and neck. The forearm flap is thin and pliable and can be tubed for reconstruction of the hypopharynx (Fig. 32.28). Harvesting the flap can be done synchronously with the resection by the reconstructive surgeon to minimize additional operating time (38).

The area of skin available on the forearm, however, is usually not sufficient for large circumferential defects with the risk for insufficient width to allow for contracture resulting in stenosis. A flap width of 9 cm is necessary to ensure a final lumen diameter of 1 cm (36), but ideally a greater pharyngeal diameter is preferable to ensure good speech and deglutition. As with other cutaneous flaps,

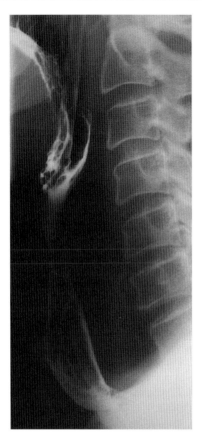

Figure 32.26   Lateral X-ray of the neck at videofluoroscopy 2 years following total pharyngolaryngectomy and reconstruction with a tubed myocutaneous flap. Long hypotonic PE segment at C4–7 with satisfactory voice (stronger with digital pressure).

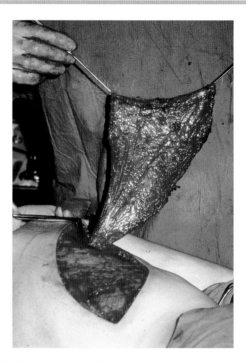

Figure 32.27   Latissimus dorsi myocutaneous flap.

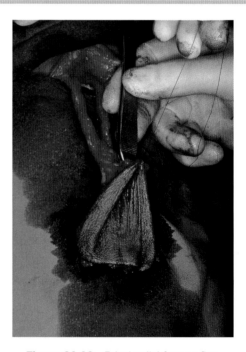

Figure 32.28   Tubed radial forearm flap.

primary puncture is usually possible and functional results are good provided that adequate width has been taken. The quality of TE voice approximates that produced by the native pharynx.

Results
The quality of TE voice approximates that produced by the native pharynx.

Anterolateral Thigh Flap
The anterolateral thigh flap (ALT) is a pliable fasciocutaneous segment that can be used to reconstruct partial or circumferential pharyngesophageal defects. For a circumferential defect, a flap width of 9.5 cm is obtained to give a diameter of 3 cm for the neopharynx after tubing the flap on itself. The distal flap-to-esophagus anastomosis is spatulated by incising the anterior esophageal end longitudinally for approximately 1.5 cm to minimize the development of stricture. Although the flap requires an additional suture line to form a tubed structure it lacks some of the disadvantages of organ transposition such as the jejunal flap. The anterolateral thigh flap provides a passive conduit

that does not secrete mucus, is less redundant, and is associated with minimal donor site morbidity. Studies have shown lower complication rates and shorter hospitalization in patients reconstructed with ALT flap compared to free jejunum transfer (27).

Results

Most patients are able to return to oral nutrition after ALT reconstruction. TE speech is more similar to the speech produced by patients after a simple laryngectomy without reconstruction. TE speech is fluent, less effortful, and has a better vocal quality.

Free Jejunal Flap

The free jejunal flap gained popularity for the repair of circumferential pharyngoesophageal defects because it is already a tubed structure lined with mucosa of similar diameter to the native pharynx and is associated with relatively low rates of fistula formation. The requirement of an additional abdominal surgery and the wet vocal quality associated with mucous secretion has lessened its popularity as the reconstructive option of choice for circumferential defects.

Although the graft also tolerates postoperative radiotherapy well (39), stenosis has been reported to occur some months or even years after the operation (40). The jejunum graft remains dependent on its own vascular pedicle because unlike other flaps the serosal surface prevents ingrowth of new vasculature from the surrounding tissue. The graft therefore remains much more vulnerable to the long-term adverse effects of postoperative radiotherapy and it is not unusual to see gradual avascular fibrosis of a graft that for some time had appeared very healthy. It is therefore important to preserve the integrity of the pedicle at any subsequent surgery, such as neck dissection, treatment of recurrence, or new primary.

Results

Tracheojejunal speech is generally characterized by a wet, cavernous, and effortful voice. Mucous secretion from the jejunum can be a problem especially during the first few months but may improve with time and after postoperative radiotherapy. The natural circular mucosal folds (Fig. 32.29) will also reduce the expiratory voice pressure by causing turbulence in the ascending flow of air. Swallowing is frequently characterized by slow transit, regurgitation, and dysmotility that can prevent a patient from resuming a complete oral diet. For these reasons, jejunal reconstruction for circumferential pharyngoesophageal defects is associated with poor patient satisfaction (41).

Surgical technique is therefore very important in achieving optimum voice quality and swallowing. It is easy to be overgenerous with the length of jejunum graft particularly when it is inset with the neck in the extended position. It should be put in under slight tension so that when the neck returns to the natural flexed position the jejunum will not be too long, otherwise it will form convolutions or redundant loops, which will further impede the flow of air and food (42).

Gastric Pull-up

Gastric transposition for reconstruction of the hypopharynx was first described in 1960 by Ong and Lee (43) and provides an effective one-stage procedure that eliminates the risk of inadequate inferior resection because it incorporates total esophagectomy as well. The incidence of fistula formation is also reduced because there is only one anastomosis

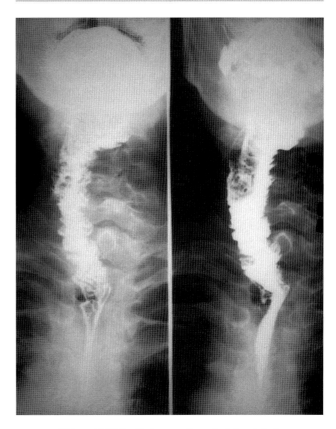

Figure 32.29 Barium swallow of a jejunal graft.

in the upper neck. The lumen itself is wide and so swallowing problems and stenosis are not seen, but tracheogastric voice is generally breathy, weak, and cavernous. Gastric filling with air is a common complaint of patients after gastric pull-up.

The operation has a high complication rate with an associated mortality of 6–12% and morbidity of up to 50% (44,45). The early postoperative problems mainly result from the complexity of the synchronous thoracic, cervical, and abdominal dissections. Later complications include the "dumping" syndrome and reflux in 23% of patients (44) and the need for small volume meals.

Results

Because of separation of the TE party wall, voice restoration is best carried out as a secondary procedure, ideally a few months after surgery, but it may be delayed by slow recovery or by postoperative radiotherapy. The quality of the voice remains poor because of the wide lumen diameter, and the presence of gastric secretions resulting in a liquid quality that many patients find unacceptable (46).

Summary

The functional results of voice restoration after pharyngolaryngectomy are generally not as predictable and are more suboptimal compared to voice restoration after simple laryngectomy. Nevertheless, for many patients it remains a viable means of communication.

Skin-lined flaps have given us the most predictable results and have the least morbidity. They are preferable provided that the length of the defect is not too long and adequate width is taken to avoid problems of stenosis. Of these, the pectoralis major flap is the easiest to harvest but it is bulky, has several limitations, and is not suitable in women. The latissimus dorsi flap is an ideal alternative and merits wider use.

The free radial forearm flap is the preferred option in several experienced institutions (36) and gives good predictable results. Its main limitation is size and also it requires a more prolonged procedure with an experienced microvascular team to achieve an acceptable complication rate. The anterolateral thigh flap is increasingly preferred (47,27) because it is associated with minimal complications and excellent functional results for both speech and swallowing.

The free jejunum flap has become a less desirable method for reconstruction because of the poor functional results for both speech and swallowing. The microvascular anastomosis and additional abdominal procedure increase the potential for operative complications and in the long term there may be problems with stenosis.

Pharyngogastric anastomosis with stomach pull-up has a high complication rate and mortality when compared with other well-established techniques. Even in experienced hands it is debatable whether it should be done as the routine method of reconstruction when safer methods are equally appropriate. It is, however, the technique of choice for cervical esophageal lesions and for reconstructions in which the resection extends close to the thoracic inlet and that may be difficult to close at the lower anastomosis of a pedicled or free flap.

TE VOICE PROSTHESIS ASSESSMENT AND FITTING

After primary voice restoration procedure the patient is fed through the tracheo esophageal catheter, usually 14-Fr, for a period of seven to ten days before fitting the TE prosthesis. If no previous radiotherapy has been given and there has been no postoperative problem with healing, an oral diet is usually commenced after seven days with discontinuation of catheter feeding. In patients who have undergone salvage laryngectomy, videofluoroscopic examination may be indicated to rule out leakage before beginning oral intake or voicing. In heavily irradiated patients, it may be safer to delay oral feeding and placement of the TE voice prosthesis for two to three more days. Following secondary puncture the prosthesis may be fitted after two to three days unless a myotomy has been carried out in which case fitting is best delayed for a week.

Assessment and Fitting of the TE Voice Prosthesis

The basic procedures for assessment, fitting, and management of the TE prosthesis are essentially the same following primary or secondary voice restoration. As a preliminary trial it is useful to try voicing with an "open tract," that is, without a prosthesis. The 14-Fr catheter, which had been placed at the time of the operation, is removed and the patient is asked not to swallow and to take a deep breath. The stoma is digitally occluded and the patient is asked to

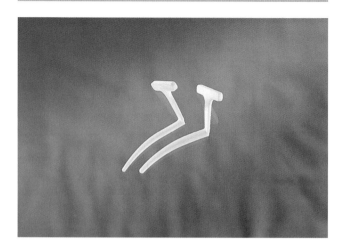

Figure 32.30   Tracheo-esophageal dilators.

exhale saying "aahhh" or to count to 10. The ability of the patient to successfully produce sound with an open tract is important. An inability to produce easy, effortless voice through an "open tract" generally suggests an anatomical or physiological problem such as acute edema or pharyngoesophageal spasm.

It is best to dilate the TE tract prior to placing the prosthesis. This may be accomplished using an 18 french silicone dilator (Fig. 32.30) or red rubber catheters (Fig. 32.31A, B) of increasing diameter. It is always best to dilate the puncture one size bigger than the size of the prosthesis to be placed. This facilitates non-traumatic insertion of the prosthesis. After dilating the TE puncture, a measuring device is inserted (Fig. 32.32). It is important to insert the measuring device fully so that the proximal end abuts the posterior tracheal wall at the inlet to the puncture. It is then gently withdrawn until resistance is felt. The size marker visible nearest the entrance to TE tract will designate the appropriate length of prosthesis to be placed. When sizing is uncertain, it is best to select the longer TE voice prosthesis to prevent underfitting that may ultimately result in closure of the TE tract.

It may be more advantageous to select a standard non-indwelling prosthesis until the postoperative edema resolves. This generally takes a period of weeks during which time the length of the tract will usually get shorter and a shorter prosthesis will be required. Once the healing process has stabilized and edema has resolved, a long-term TE prosthesis may be fitted. It is important to recognize, however, that both standard and indwelling long-term prostheses may demonstrate comparable durations of prosthetic life. In other words, standard devices may last as long as indwelling ones and vice versa. Some clinicians prefer to change prostheses every six months if the patient has not required a change sooner to prevent potential problems from occurring; other clinicians prefer to leave a prosthesis in place until it becomes a problem. Either management preference is acceptable in patients who do not present with frequent prosthetic difficulties.

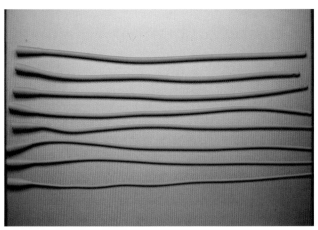

(A)

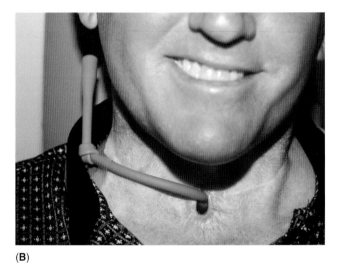

(B)

Figure 32.31 Red rubber catheters **(A)** Sizes ranging from 8 Fr to 18 Fr diameters **(B)** Red rubber catheter in situ.

Choice of Prosthesis

A variety of TE voice prostheses are available. These vary according to length, diameter, type of valve, material, retention flange, and resistance to airflow. TE voice prostheses are generally classified into one of two categories. Standard devices can be changed by the patient without medical supervision. These types of voice prostheses generally need to be replaced more frequently than do the long-term devices often referred to as indwelling type prostheses. Indwelling type prostheses require placement by the speech pathologist, physician, or other qualified clinician.

Types of TE voice prostheses

Standard "duckbill" TE prostheses. The "duckbill" valve (Fig. 32.6) incorporates a slit aperture over its tip that has a higher airway resistance than the low-pressure valve. It is available in lengths of 6–26 mm and has a diameter of 16-Fr. The duckbill valve may be easier to fit and change because of its bullet-nosed shape. It may be more resistant to the development of fungal colonies because it does not incorporate a valve and valve-seat.

Standard valved TE prostheses. The standard valved prostheses (Figs. 32.33 and 32.34) (Provox Non-Indwelling voice prothesis) are used by a majority of patients. The one-way valve allows airflow to pass easily through the shaft of the prosthesis but prevents backward propulsion of air or aspiration of food. Standard valved prostheses are associated with lower airflow resistance during voicing and are often preferred by patients because of the decreased effort associated with speaking. These prostheses are available in 16-, 17-, or 20-Fr diameters.

Indwelling type prostheses. These types of prostheses (Figs. 32.35–32.37) have more robust retention collars making them less likely to be aspirated. Indwelling type prostheses are ideal for patients who are unable or unwilling to change their TE prostheses independently. Indwelling type prostheses need to be removed and replaced by a speech pathologist, physician, or other qualified clinician.

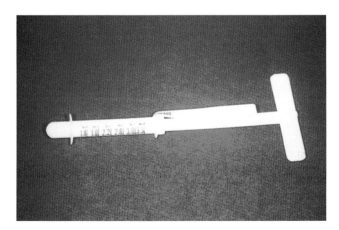

Figure 32.32   Tracheo-esophageal measurement device.

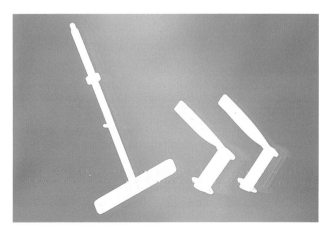

Figure 32.33   Low pressure valves with inserter.

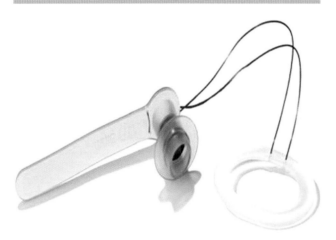

Figure 32.34   Provox Non-indwelling (NiD) voice prosthesis.

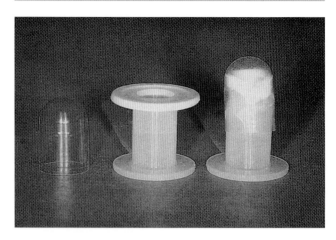

Figure 32.36   Gelcap and indwelling valve.

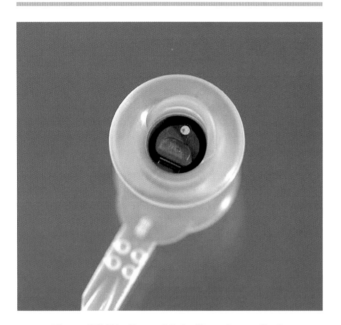

Figure 32.35   Provox 2 indwelling voice prosthesis.

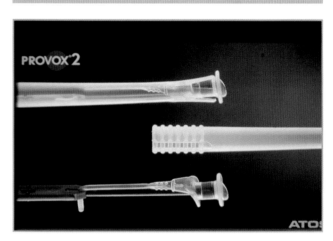

Figure 32.37   Provox tapered loading tool.

Insertion Methods

In general TE voice prostheses are placed in anterograde or retrograde procedures most often in an outpatient clinic setting. Retrograde placement of the voice prosthesis is basically similar in technique, but may be performed using a variety of devices. The duckbill and standard valved prostheses are secured on an insertion stick and are inserted directly into the TE tract after the tract has been dilated. Additionally, standard valved prostheses may be loaded into a gelcap that is fitted over the esophageal end of the valve to facilitate easy insertion. The gelcap dissolves allowing the retention collar to open within the lumen of the esophagus. Placement of indwelling type prostheses may be accomplished by gelcap insertion or the use of a

tapered loading tool to help fold and collapse the esophageal retention flange, again for easier placement (Figs. 32.36 and 32.37). Indwelling type prostheses should not be placed without a gelcap or loading tool because of the larger, more rigid flange and the potential for mucosal trauma. More recently, particularly in Europe, intraoperative placement of the TE prosthesis at the time of laryngectomy has gained popularity.

Confirming Placement

It is important to confirm accurate placement of the prosthesis after insertion. When the TE prosthesis is properly placed, the retention collar opens and seats itself within the lumen of the esophagus to hold the prosthesis in place. It should be possible to freely rotate the prosthesis to check that it is in the correct position and the patient should be able to produce a clear voice with the prosthesis. If the prosthesis is too short, the retention collar will have opened within the TE tract and will be difficult to rotate.

Videofluoroscopy or endoscopy may be used to confirm prosthetic placement if clinical assessment is unclear. Antero-posterior radiograph of the neck will show the circular radiopaque retention collar when the flange is fully opened within the esophagus. If the prosthesis is incorrectly placed antero-posterior view of the retention collar will be irregular and appear folded. Lateral videofluoroscopic assessment is used to confirm placement of the prosthesis within the lumen of the esophagus. Prostheses that are too short and do not fully stent the TE tract are easily visualized.

HANDS-FREE SPEAKING VALVES, AIRWAY FUNCTION, NASAL FUNCTION, AND HEAT AND MOISTURE EXCHANGE SYSTEMS

Hands-free Speaking Valve

As an alternative to digital occlusion, hands-free speaking valves offer patients a more normal appearing method of speaking. The hands-free speaking valve, originally developed in 1982 by Blom et al. (48) is an external valve that fits over the stoma that automatically closes on expiration to direct air through the prosthesis permitting "hands-free" TE speech (Figs. 32.38 and 32.39). Hands-free speaking valves may be attached to the stoma using peristomal adhesives and housings, or they may be attached intraluminally using specially designed buttons and tubes (Fig. 32.40) (49). Not every laryngectomy is a candidate for the use of a hands-free speaking valve. Careful selection will improve ultimate success and patient satisfaction. Generally, patients with a flat, smooth peristomal contour who generate relatively low (<35 cm H_2O) (50) intratracheal back pressure against the speaking valve are good candidates for the use of peristomaly attached speaking valves. Therefore, physicians are encouraged to release the medial heads of the sternocleidomastoid muscles during surgery to facilitate successful use of peristomally attached hands-free speaking valves.

The disadvantages associated with the need to use glues and adhesives, as well as the inability to maintain a

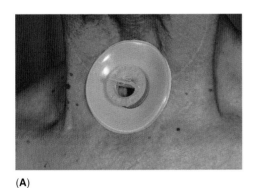

(A)

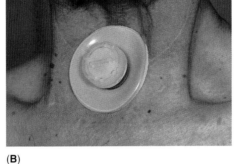

(B)

Figure 32.38 **(A)** Tracheostoma valve in the open position during quiet respiration. **(B)** Tracheostoma valve in the closed position during speech.

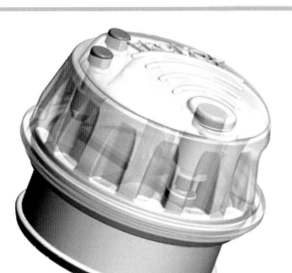

Figure 32.39 Atos Free-Hands speaking valve.

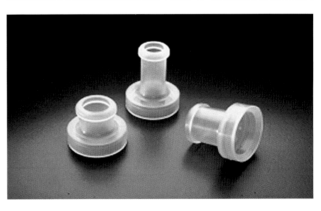

Figure 32.40 Barton-Mayo button.

long-lasting seal, have made devices that provide an intraluminal attachment for the speaking valve an attractive alternative for patients who are interested in achieving hands-free TE speech. Careful assessment of stomal configuration is critical to ensure that the patient interested in intraluminal attachment has a contiguous stomal edge or lip that will help secure the button within the tracheal lumen.

Postlaryngectomy Airway Function

Total laryngectomy has important physiological effects on the remaining airway due to separation of the nasal passage from the respiratory tract and the associated loss of all its important functions (Table 32.7). Most importantly, the loss of nasal filtration and humidification have been the subject of much recent research.

Loss of Nasal Function

Following laryngectomy, particles and micro-organisms are inhaled directly into the trachea and the patient is therefore much more susceptible to inflammation and chest infections. After laryngectomy, it is difficult to compensate for the loss of nasal function that previously filtered foreign micro-organisms and particles from entering the airway. In addition to filtration, the nasal cavity acts as an efficient "air conditioner" by regulating inhaled air temperature and humidity. This ensures that air reaching the bronchi has a temperature of 34–35°C and a humidity of 90–100%. By the time it reaches the alveoli it is 37°C and fully saturated to ensure optimal conditions for gas exchange. On expiration the heat and moisture are reabsorbed back through the nasal mucosa and only a small proportion (350 kcal of heat and 250 ml water per day) is lost to the atmosphere.

Following laryngectomy, cool and dry air is inhaled into the trachea causing significant changes to the surface mucosa. The mucus becomes thicker and more viscous; and ciliary action is impaired resulting in a much less efficient mechanism for clearing mucus. With the loss of the mechanism for normal glottic closure, coughing also becomes less effective. This can cause difficulty clearing secretions and increase the risk of lower respiratory infections by as much as 54% (51). Patients often experience an increase in excessive mucous production during the first few months after surgery. These symptoms usually stabilize after six months but are particularly disturbing in patients already suffering from chronic obstructive pulmonary disease (COPD).

Table 32.7 *Functional Alterations Following Laryngectomy*

Loss of nasal function
  Filtering
  Heat and moisture exchange
  Olfaction
  Airway resistance
Loss of glottic function
  Voice
  Airway protection
  Coughing/straining mechanism

For patients with severe COPD, TE speech production may be more difficult and the use of a hands-free speaking valve may be impossible. Therefore, it is prudent to consider secondary TE puncture for patients with severe COPD to allow for preoperative insufflation testing, thus ensuring appropriate candidacy. Patients should be counseled appropriately to provide realistic expectations as to ultimate TE speech success.

Heat and Moisture Exchangers (HMEs)

A heat and moisture exchanger (HME) is a simple and effective method for helping to restore a more normal physiological balance of the lower respiratory tract following laryngectomy. It is fitted over the tracheostoma so that all inspired and expired air passes through the device (Figs. 32.41 and 32.42) and thus it helps to restore many of the functional aspects of the nasal airway.

During inspiration the cool and dry air is filtered and gains heat and moisture as it passes through the HME significantly reducing the detrimental effect on the lower respiratory tract. It therefore helps to protect the trachea and lungs and maintains more normal mucociliary function. During expiration air passes through the heat and moisture exchanger; some of the heat is retained in the HME and water vapor condenses as the temperature drops. Airway resistance is also increased on expiration, which has been shown to improve oxygen saturation after laryngectomy (52). Airway resistance in the upper respiratory tract is particularly important during expiration as it helps to keep the lungs expanded and prevent alveolar collapse. The use of heat and moisture exchangers reduces phlegm production by 60% after one week of continuous use (53) and a prospective study in 61 patients showed a clear trend towards improvement in respiratory and psychosocial function (54).

COMPLICATIONS, PROBLEMS, AND SOLUTIONS
Leakage

Leakage at the puncture site into the trachea can occur and is usually most prominent during liquid swallows. Although leakage should trigger coughing, recent data has shown that leakage does not always induce a cough (55). It is therefore important for both the clinician and TE speaker to periodically examine the puncture site for leakage. Leakage may occur through the prosthesis or around it and the causes are quite different.

Leakage Through the Prosthesis

Leakage through the prosthesis may be due to a number of reasons. A faulty or defective valve is generally easy to recognize. Valve distortion may occur due to excessive compression of the shaft of the prosthesis, which is usually associated with a TE tract that is narrow or misaligned. This generally results in a slight gaping of the flap. Careful dilation for sufficient duration is advisable before inserting a larger diameter valve. Distortion may also occur if the valve is not inserted correctly or is inserted traumatically. Small pieces of debris or undissolved gelatin from the gelcap may hold the valve open. The prosthesis should be

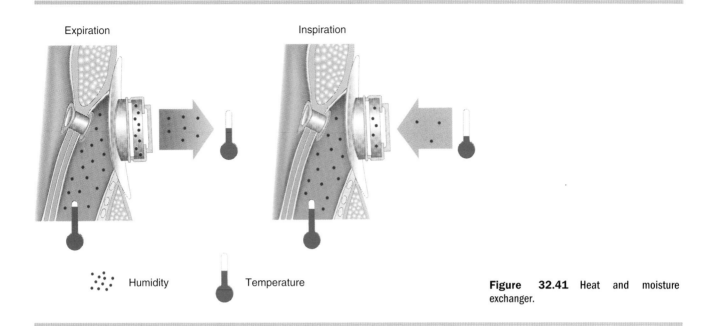

Expiration   Inspiration

:·: Humidity   Temperature

Figure 32.41 Heat and moisture exchanger.

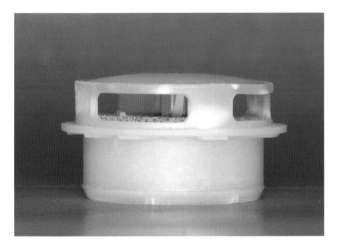

Figure 32.42 Atos heat moisture exchanger (HME).

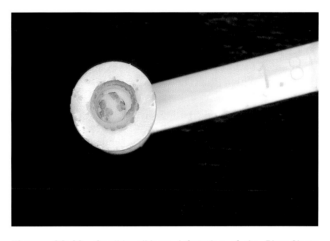

Figure 32.43 Candida albicans infestation of the Blom-Singer valve.

inspected to make sure it closes completely. Leakage through the prosthesis may be due simply to the natural lifespan of the valve that can vary from a few weeks to over a year. Careful cleaning of the delicate valve mechanism will prolong its usage. Some patients prefer to remove the prosthesis regularly; others clean it in situ. The prosthesis should be carefully cleaned before inserting it.

Microbial colonization of the prosthesis, predominantly with *Candida albicans* is the most commonly reported cause of leakage through the valve (Fig. 32.43) due to distortion of the valve mechanism. It is important, however, to consider that other microbial organisms, such as staphylococcus and streptococcus, along with gastroesophageal reflux, and potential changes in pharyngoesophageal

motility, may also contribute to leakage through a voice prosthesis. Much effort has been devoted to finding a prophylactic method of protecting the silicone prosthesis from microbial colonization.

In the absence of detectable microbial colonization, changes in pharyngoesophageal motility may make the voice prosthesis more susceptible to leakage through it. The inadvertent opening of the valve during swallowing and/or inhalation can be observed by anterograde inspection of the prosthesis in situ while the patient is swallowing or inhaling. The changes in the gradient between negative and positive pressures within the esophagus and the lumen of the prosthesis may facilitate the occurrence of leakage through the prosthesis (56).

Leakage may occur when the distal end of the prosthesis abuts the posterior esophageal wall, as is typical of duckbill prostheses that are too long. This is more frequently seen where there is osteophyte formation indenting the esophagus so that when the valve moves up and down during normal swallowing the end of the valve is distorted and may leak. This may be relieved by changing to a valved prosthesis, particularly one that does not have a protruding hood.

There are a variety of techniques that have been suggested to manage the problem of leakage through the prosthesis. The selection of prostheses with increased valve resistance, heavier weights, and different lengths has been suggested to reduce leakage. Dietary remedies include ingestion of foods and supplements high in acidophilus (57,58). There is, however, no data or consensus to define optimum use. The most common treatment still remains the use of pharmacological agents such as nystatin suspension (500,000 units twice daily swished around the mouth for four minutes) as a method to reduce colonization and increase prosthetic life span. Antireflux regimens should be adopted and adhered to after laryngectomy.

Leakage Around the TE Prosthesis

Chronic leakage around the TE voice prosthesis is one of the most difficult problems to manage and may be due to a number of reasons. A satisfactory seal around the TE prosthesis depends on the natural elasticity of the surrounding party wall tissues to provide a "snug" fit around the shaft of the prosthesis. It is also important to insert a prosthesis of appropriate length so that the prosthesis does not piston within the TE tract. This will ensure a good circumferential seal and help prevent movement or dislodgement. A prosthesis that is too long acts as a piston and dilates the tracheo esophageal tract as the prosthesis moves in and out. It is essential that the length of the tract is correctly measured and a prosthesis of appropriate length is selected, particularly during the first six months as the postoperative edema settles and the thickness of the party wall decreases.

The compromised TE wall can be associated with an increased risk for leakage. The TE wall may lose its thickness over a period of time due to radionecrosis or ischemic changes in the muscle (Figs. 32.44 and 32.45). This is often associated with loss of the muscular tone and elasticity; thus the tract loses the ability to snuggly contract around the prosthesis, usually resulting in leakage. The puncture tract may visibly appear thin with a poor surrounding seal through which leakage is inevitable. Attempts to place a larger prosthesis are ill advised and may only result in enlargement of the tract and greater leakage. Insertion of a smaller catheter to encourage contraction of the tract is rarely helpful. The use of silver nitrate or electrocautery also provides only temporary relief of leakage.

This problem may be alleviated with the use of an enlarged distal retention flange that is securely seated within the esophageal lumen. Endoscopic confirmation should be performed to ensure that the flange completely seals the dilated puncture site. It is important that the prosthesis is fitted properly so that pistoning within the TE tract is avoided. Alternatively, an injection of collagen into the party wall around the valve may help to eliminate minor

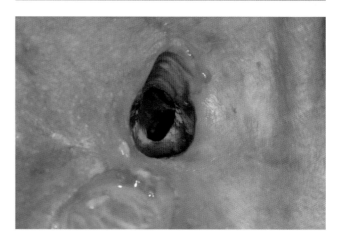

Figure 32.44 The compromised party wall: radionecrosis causing TOP leakage.

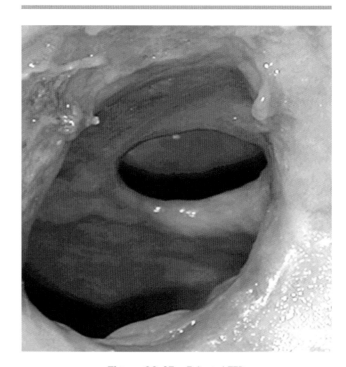

Figure 32.45 Enlarged TEP.

leakage problems, but this usually only has a temporary benefit. Studies investigating the use of other injectable materials to effectively treat this problem are ongoing.

Surgical alternatives with flap reconstruction are generally considered when conservative attempts to manage the enlarged TE puncture have failed. A thin leaking compromised party wall may be reconstructed with a decent layer of muscle, preferably non-irradiated tissue. In some cases an inferiorly based pedicled sternomastoid muscle flap can be sandwiched between the trachea and the esophagus using a three-layer closure, followed by successful repuncture of the tract about three months later. In some instances where there is significant loss of surface mucosa, a pedicled myocutaneous flap may be required to achieve satisfactory closure (Fig. 32.46).

Problems with the Fistula
Granulations

Some of the early valves had an inferiorly placed portal that frequently became blocked with granulation tissue that eventually occluded the valve lumen. This has been resolved by elimination of the inferior opening. Occasionally, granulation tissue forms around the prosthesis at the proximal or distal opening to the TE puncture as a result of trauma or irritation to the mucosa (Fig. 32.47). This may occur if the prosthesis fits too tightly within the TE tract. If the tracheal lumen is narrow, the proximal edges of the prosthesis may cut into the surrounding mucosa resulting in granular formation. Sometimes, granulation forms in response to frequent removal and replacement of the prosthesis. During the early years of TE voice restoration, patients were advised to remove the prosthesis to clean it on a daily basis. This practice is no longer recommended because of the potential formation of granulation associated with mucosal irritation.

Granulation tissue can be easily excised by a physician. A new properly sized prosthesis is then inserted.

Fibrous Ring

Similar to the formation of granulation, a fibrous ring may occur from constant prosthetic irritation to the tracheal mucosa. This is often the case when the prosthesis has been used for some period of time; it may gradually become surrounded by an increasingly thick ring of fibrous tissue that forms a "doughnut" around the tracheal end of the valve (Fig. 32.48). Like granulation, this has the effect of lengthening the tract so that the posterior end of the prosthesis is gradually drawn forward into the tract. If not recognized, the patient's voice will slowly deteriorate requiring increasing effort and eventually fail completely as the esophageal end of the fistula closes off. If the ring is not too prominent the tract can be resized and a longer valve fitted. Otherwise excision of the fibrous ring is a straightforward procedure.

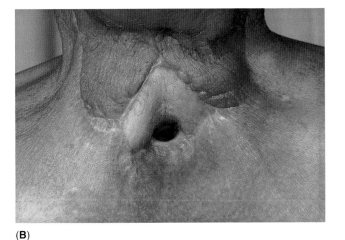

(A)

(B)

Figure 32.46 **(A)** A large radionecrotic TOP fistula. **(B)** Reconstruction with a pectoralis major myocutaneous flap.

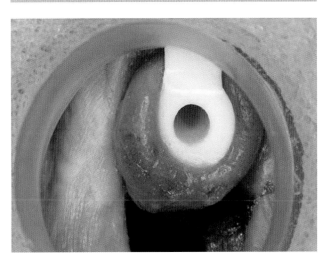

Figure 32.47 Granulation doughnut.

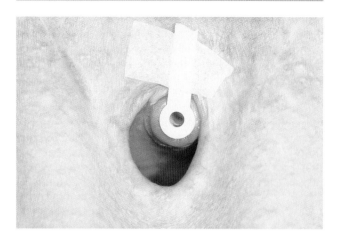

Figure 32.48 Fibrous 'doughnut' around the prosthesis.

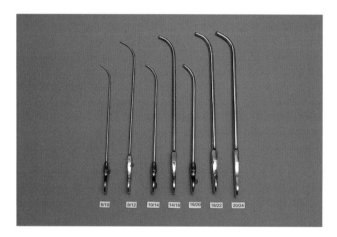

Figure 32.49 Dilating Bougies.

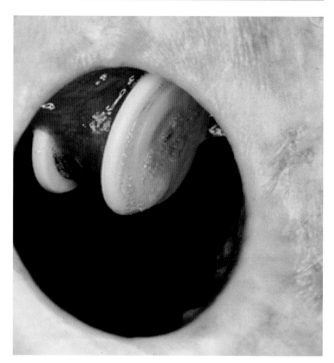

Figure 32.50 Extrusion of TE prosthesis through wall of the TE tract.

Valve Extrusion

The prosthesis may become dislodged from the TE tract during cleaning or coughing. If it is not replaced immediately, stenosis of the tract will occur, eventually resulting in complete closure of the posterior TE puncture site. A catheter or dilator may be used to stent the tract until the prosthesis can be replaced. Unless the fistula has closed down completely, it is usually possible to gradually dilate it successfully, and for this purpose a series of soft urethral catheters is useful (Fig. 32.49). Frequently, the TE voice prosthesis may extrude through the wall of the TE tract when the prosthesis is under-sized and remains in the TE tract for an extended period of time. This is usually the case with heavier indwelling-type prostheses (Fig. 32.50). Occasionally valves may need to be retrieved with bronchoscopy if inhaled.

Elective Closure of the TE Puncture

Some patients may elect to have the puncture tract closed if they cannot use the prosthesis or maintain it. Simple removal of the valve will usually allow spontaneous closure over a period of hours to days. The use of progressively smaller diameter catheters is generally recommended to facilitate closure without aspiration. In most cases, once the TE puncture has stenosed to an 8 Fr diameter, a catheter is no longer needed and the puncture will close on its own. In some patients, closure of the TE puncture may take several days to weeks. A cuffed tracheostomy tube may be useful to help prevent aspiration. Some patients may also need a nasogastric tube to prevent food and debris from interfering with closure of the TE puncture. The TE puncture may not completely close in some patients, especially in patients who have been heavily irradiated. In these cases, other interventions such as surgery or cauterization may be needed to achieve permanent closure. In rare instances, replacement with a permanently closed dummy prosthesis may be used to prevent leakage through the TE puncture in patients who are not suitable candidates for surgical intervention.

Pharyngo-esophageal Problems
Constrictor Hypertonicity/Spasm

The primary cause for TE voice failure continues to be pharyngeal constrictor hypertonicity or spasm. Despite the completion of a cricopharyngeal myotomy at the time of total laryngectomy, hypertonicity or spasm may continue to occur. This is evaluated with insufflation and videofluoroscopy as described earlier in this chapter. The treatment of choice for PE spasm is Botox injection.

Pseudo-vallecula

The pseudo-vallecula is most often related to surgical closure and seems to be typical in patients who have had a vertical closure of the pharynx at the time of laryngectomy. The anterior pouch at the tongue base, and the coronal fibrous web behind it, may cause dysphagia characterized by stasis of swallowed material within the anterior pouch that may not be cleared despite repeated swallowing. Patients may also complain of regurgitating small amounts of undigested food along with a wet, gargled TE voice. This is a problem that is quite frustrating to patients. The pseudo-vallecula appears similar to the epiglottis on video-fluoroscopic imaging (Fig. 32.17). The pseudo-vallecula may be dilated or surgically excised.

Stenosis

Stenosis, narrowing of the pharyngoesophagus, may occur if insufficient mucosa/skin has been used for reconstruction of the hypopharyngeal defect or at the anastomotic site. This problem is more common in patients who have been heavily irradiated or whose surgical closure has been tight. It may also develop slowly after jejunal transposition due to ischemic contracture if the mesenteric blood supply is compromised (42). Dilatation may be sufficient if the narrowing is not severe but in some cases surgical resection is required.

Constrictor Hypotonicity

Constrictor hypotonicity is generally associated with a flaccid pharyngoesophageal segment and results in a weak, breathy TE voice. It results from the loss or absence of muscular tone or when the pharyngoesophageal lumen is large. Voice quality may be improved by applying external pressure over the pharynx or the anterior neck. The outcomes of surgical attempts to correct this problem have been variable.

Gastric Filling

Excessive collection of air in the stomach is a disturbing and sometimes painful problem in TE voice users and may be due to several different causes. During normal respiration, negative esophageal pressures during inspiration may facilitate valve opening resulting in gastric filling. This occurs similarly in patients with a hypotonic PE segment (Fig. 32.26). In contrast, patients who have constrictor hypertonicity or spasm also complain of gastric filling because of the obstruction to the superior flow of pulmonary air into the oral cavity for speech production. Again, the use of Botox injection to eliminate PE spasm will thereby relieve gastric filling. Dilation or surgical correction is generally required for patients who complain of gastric filling related to stricture.

The use of prostheses with increased resistance to airflow may prevent gastric filling. New TE voice prostheses that are specially designed to prevent inadvertent opening of the valve are good choices for patients who complain of this problem. TE speakers who talk while eating may swallow large amounts of air and should be counseled appropriately. The esophageal speaker who also uses TE voice production may find it difficult to extinguish the exaggeration of consonants used to produce esophageal speech and will frequently complain of discomfort associated with the ingestion of air.

Stoma Problems

The tracheostoma is the anatomic site for respiratory exchange following total laryngectomy and plays a key role in restoring pulmonary function in all laryngectomized patients and in restoring speech in patients who use TE voice production. Variations in the size, shape, and location of the stoma are significant challenges to restoring pulmonary function and speech after total laryngectomy and TE puncture.

The size of the tracheostoma is important for TE speakers who will digitally occlude the stoma and for patients who will use a hands-free speaking valve. The stoma that is overly large will be difficult to seal adequately while the stoma that is very small will make prosthetic insertion next to impossible. The ideal stoma should be large enough to accommodate the TE voice prosthesis without compromising the airway yet small enough to easily occlude with a digit for speech production. A stoma that is 1.5 to 2.0 cm is usually considered large enough to accommodate a voice prosthesis without the need for a laryngectomy tube and to allow for adequate stomal hygiene.

Macrostomia

Occasionally the tracheostoma is too large for the patient to adequately occlude digitally. Sometimes the use of a silicone laryngectomy tube or a peristomal attachment may help digital occlusion or allow the patient to use a hands-free speaking valve. When the stoma is excessively large (Fig. 32.51) it becomes a greater challenge to manage than a small stoma because commercially manufactured devices that accommodate large stomas are not available. In most cases, if the stoma is overly large after normal postoperative healing it will remain so.

Custom made prosthetic devices including cotton-filled finger cots, customized washers, as well as customized

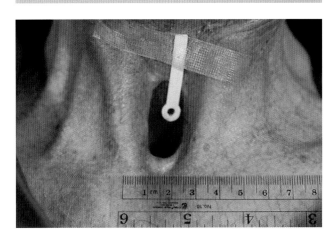

Figure 32.51 Macrostomia.

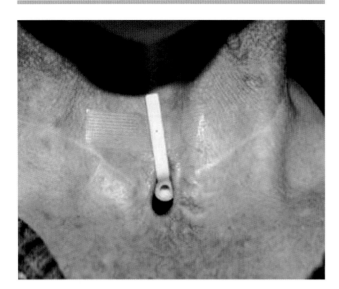

Figure 32.52 Microstomia.

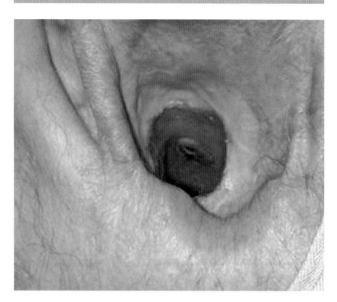

Figure 32.53 Recessed and irregular stoma.

housings are usually unacceptable to patients and ultimately ineffective. The use of fenestrated laryngectomy tubes and vents is also ineffective and frustrating to patients. The tube often rotates resulting in misalignment of the fenestrated area and TE puncture while speaking. Frequently, long-term use may cause irritation to the tracheal mucosa and result in the development of granulation tissue in the area of fenestration. Subsequent stomaplasty may be required to decrease the size of the stoma.

Microstomia

After laryngectomy, the peristomal scar tissue has a natural tendency to contract. Although many factors contribute to stomal stenosis the very small stoma (Fig. 32.52) is probably most common in patients who have had intensive radiation. When a tracheostoma is too small, the TE puncture is difficult to visualize and insertion and care of the voice prosthesis are impeded.

An overly small stoma may be progressively dilated until the circumference permits adequate visualization and easy access. In cases of a stenotic stoma, the use of specific buttons or tubes that permit attachment of hands-free speaking valves or HMEs is preferable because the button provides the same dilating benefit along with the ability to speak without using a digit to occlude the stoma. Prosthetic management of small or stenotic stomas using buttons, tubes, vents, or other devices is always the preferred intervention especially in irradiated patients who are at risk for further complications. Surgical revision of the stoma may be necessary when prosthetic management fails and stomal stenosis persists.

Stomal Shape and Position

Variations in stoma size and position also represent obstacles to TE speech production. Sometimes the trachea has to be resected low down to achieve adequate tumor clearance, but if the rim of the trachea is not sutured to the medial tendinous margins of the sternomastoid muscles it will recede into the suprasternal notch. This may cause difficulty with stoma occlusion, particularly if an outer housing and hands-free valve are used. Following standard laryngectomy the trachea should not be transected too low and should lie comfortably without tension in the same plane as the skin over the sternomastoid muscles. Vicryl sutures from the trachea to the adjacent muscle tendon may help to stabilize its position.

A recessed or irregular stoma (Fig. 32.53) will preclude an adequate stomal seal. Patients will experience air leakage during speech attempts that are often embarrassing as well as frustrating. Management techniques and outcomes are often the same as for a large stoma. Clinicians are ill advised to attempt peristomal attachment of a hands-free speaking valve in patients with irregular and deeply recessed stomas. Alternatively, the use of an intraluminal device slightly larger than the stoma has been found successful in maintaining an attachment for hands-free speech. When standardized buttons are not successful, investigations have shown that a customized device can be created to accommodate the stomal configuration and allow for successful hands-free TE speech production (48). It is generally preferable to detach the clavicular heads of the sternocleidomastoid muscles in patients with prominent muscles to achieve a flatter, less convex peristomal region, which may improve the ability to use peristomal and intraluminal devices.

Stomal Ulceration

Excessive trauma to the tracheocutaneous margins of the stoma can cause ulceration of the skin that may resemble stomal recurrence (Fig. 32.54). This is usually seen in patients with acute reactions during irradiation.

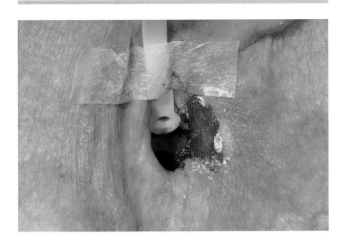

Figure 32.54 Stomal ulceration.

The peristomal skin is relatively insensate due to division of the supraclavicular nerves and therefore patients are less likely to note excessive pressure or irritation to this area. This is in contrast to the very sensitive tracheal mucosa whose inferiorly based innervation is usually unaffected by laryngectomy.

CONCLUSION

The evolution of voice rehabilitation after total laryngectomy has made an enormous difference in the treatment of laryngeal cancer and, most importantly, in the quality of life for laryngectomized patients. With the advances in design and variety of TE voice prostheses, and the ability to manage problems more simply and effectively, a greater number of patients are able to achieve a more normal conversational level of speech production after laryngectomy. Despite the potential for superior speech production after TE voice restoration, experience has shown that not every laryngectomized patient is a candidate for TE puncture nor should every TE puncture be performed or managed in the same way. Some patients are excellent candidates for primary voice restoration while other patients need time to adjust or heal before they are ready for the procedure. It is important that clinicians refrain from imposing personal preferences regarding decisions such as when to perform the TE puncture or what type of prosthesis is the best. An eclectic approach is critical to achieve the best functional outcome with the greatest patient satisfaction.

Despite the relative simplicity of the method of TE puncture, the population of head and neck cancer patients has become more challenging as the treatment paradigms for laryngeal cancer have also become increasingly more complex. The rehabilitative methods may be straightforward but more intensive treatment regimens, new surgical reconstructions, the potential for severe complications in previously treated patients, and a more informed population who demand effortless communication, are but a few of the factors that mandate the need for experienced clinicians who are expert in the management of TE speakers. TE voice restoration is certainly more than just placing a prosthesis. A strong multidisciplinary team that combines the knowledge and skills of many specialists including speech pathologists, head and neck surgeons, maxillofacial prosthodontists, anaplastologists, plastic reconstructive surgeons, radiologists, and neurologists is essential for rehabilitative success.

Given our current state of knowledge, prosthetic voice restoration has set the "gold-standard" for rehabilitation of laryngectomized patients. Despite its many advantages, TE speech production still requires daily care and management associated with increasing prosthetic and medical costs. There are still questions to be answered and problems to be solved as researchers and clinicians strive to improve the quality of life after laryngectomy.

I would like to acknowledge Mrs. Katherine A. Hutcheson, Mrs. Denise A. Barringer, and Mrs. Janet R. Hampton for their academic and editorial contributions to this chapter. Their help was invaluable.

REFERENCES

1. Gussenbauer C. Ueber cie Erste Durch Th. Billroth Am Menschen Ausgefuhrte Kehlkopf-Exstirpation Und die Anwendung Eines Kunstlichen Kehlkopfes. Archiv fur Klinische Chirurgie 1874; 17: 334–56.
2. Edels Y. Pseudo voice, its theory and practice. In: Edels Y, ed. Laryngectomy: Diagnosis to Rehabilitation. Beckenham: Croom-Helm, 1983; 117.
3. Gates GA, Hearne EM III. Predicting esophageal speech. Ann Otol Rhinol Laryngol 1982; 91: 454–7.
4. Taub S, Spiro RH. Vocal rehabilitation of laryngectomees: preliminary report of a new technique. Am J Surg 1972; 124: 87–90.
5. Singer MI, Blom ED. An endoscopic technique for restoration of voice after laryngectomy. Ann Otol Rhinol Laryngol 1980; 89: 529–33.
6. Blom ED. Evolution of tracheoesophageal voice prostheses. In: Blom ED, Singer MI, Hamaker RC, eds. Tracheoesophageal Voice Restoration Following Total Laryngectomy. San Diego: Singular Publishing Group 1998; 1–8.
7. Perry A, Edels Y. Recent advances in the assessment of failed esophageal speakers. Br J Disord Commun 1985; 20: 229–36.
8. McIvor J, Evans PF, Perry A, Cheesman AD. Radiological assessment of post-laryngectomy speech. Clin Radiol 1990; 41: 312–16.
9. Perry A. Preoperative tracheoesophageal voice restoration assessment and selection criteria. In: Blom ED, Singer MI, Hamaker RC, eds. Tracheoesophageal Voice Restoration Following Total Laryngectomy. San Diego: Singular Publishing Group 1998; 9–18.
10. Johnson JT, Casper J, Lesswing NJ. Toward the total rehabilitation of the alaryngeal patient. Laryngoscope 1979; 89: 1813–19.
11. Lewin JS, Baugh RF, Baker SR. An objective method for prediction of tracheoesophageal speech production. J Speech Hear Disord 1987; 52: 212–17.
12. Lewin JS, Bishop-Leone JK, Forman AD, Diaz EM Jr. Further experience with Botox injection for tracheoesophageal speech failure. Head Neck 2001; 23: 456–60.
13. Freeman SB, Hamaker RC. Tracheoesophageal voice restoration at time of laryngectomy. In: Blom ED, Singer MI,

Hamaker RC, eds. Tracheoesophageal Voice Restoration Following Total Laryngectomy. San Diego: Singular Publishing Group, 1998; 19–25.

14. Garth RJN, McRae A, Rhys Evans PH. Tracheo-esophageal puncture: a review of problems and complications. J Laryngol Otol 1991; 105: 750–4.

15. van Lith-Bijl JT, Zijlstra RJ, Nahieu HS et al. A manometric study of the pharyngo-esophageal segment during total laryngectomy. Proceedings of the International Voice Restoration Meeting, London.

16. Singer MI, Blom ED. Pharyngeal plexus neurectomy for alaryngeal speech rehabilitation. Laryngoscope 1986; 961: 50–3.

17. Singer MI, Blom ED, Hamaker RC. Further experience with voice restoration after total laryngectomy. Ann Otol Rhinol Laryngol 1981; 90: 498–502.

18. Sisson GA, Hurst PS, Goldman ME. Prosthetic devices in neoglottic surgery. Ear Nose Throat J 1981; 60: 55–61.

19. Silver FM, Gluckman JL, Donegan JO. Operative complications of tracheo-esophageal puncture. Laryngoscope 1985; 95: 1360–2.

20. Ward PH, Andrews JC, Mickel RA et al. Complications of medical and surgical approaches to voice restoration after total laryngectomy. Head Neck Surg 1988; 10: 124–8.

21. Rhys Evans PH. Tracheo-esophageal puncture without tears: the forceps technique. J Laryngol Otol 1991; 105: 748–9.

22. Desyatnikova S, Caro JJ, Andersen PE, Cohen JI, Wax MK. Tracheoesophageal puncture in the office setting with local anesthesia. Ann Otol Rhinol Laryngol 2001; 110: 613–16.

23. Snelling JD, Price T, Montgomery PQ, Blagnys BL. How we do it: secondary tracheoesophageal puncture under local anaesthetic, using a trans-nasal flexible laryngo-oesophagoscope (TNFLO). Logoped Phoniatr Vocol 2007; 32: 80–2.

24. Eerenstein SE, Schouwenburg PF. Secondary tracheoesophageal puncture with local anesthesia. Laryngoscope 2002; 112: 634–7.

25. Doctor VS. In-office unsedated tracheoesophageal puncture. Curr Opin Otolaryngol Head Neck Surg 2007; 15: 405–8.

26. Wilson PS, Bruce-Lockhart FJ, Johnson AP, Rhys Evans PH. Speech restoration following total laryngo-pharyngectomy with free jejunal repair. Clin Otolaryngol 1993; 19: 145–8.

27. Lewin JS, Barringer DA, May AH et al. Functional outcomes after laryngopharyngectomy with anterolateral thigh flap reconstruction. Head Neck 2006; 28: 142–9.

28. Blom ED. Tracheoesophageal valves: problems, solutions and directions for the future. Head Neck Surg; 2 (Suppl): S142–5.

29. Duguay M. Special problems of alaryngeal speakers. In: Keith RL, Darley FL, eds. Laryngectomee Rehabilitation. London: College Hill Press, 1979; 107–42.

30. Blom ED, Singer MI, Hamaker RC. An improved esophageal insufflation test. Arch Otolaryngol 1985; 111: 211–12.

31. Simpson IC, Smith JS, Gordon T. Laryngectomy: the influence of muscle reconstruction on the mechanism of esophageal voice production. J Laryngol Otol 1972; 86: 960–90.

32. Hamaker RC, Cheesman AD. Surgical management of pharyngeal constrictor muscle hypertonicity. In: Blom ED, Singer MI, Hamaker RC, eds. Tracheoesophageal Voice Restoration Following Total Laryngectomy. San Diego: Singular Publishing Group, 1998.

33. Hosni AA, Rhys Evans PH. Cervical osteomyelitis with cord compression complicating pharyngeal myotomy. J Laryngol Otol 1994; 108: 511–13.

34. Ariyan S. The pectoralis major myocutaneous flap. A versatile flap for reconstruction in the head and neck. Plast Reconstr Surg 1979; 63: 73–81.

35. Rhys Evans PH, Das Gupta AR. The use of the pectoralis major myocutaneous flap for one stage reconstruction of the base of the tongue. J Laryngol Otol 1981; 95; 809–16.

36. Huntley TC, Borrowdale RW. Tracheoesophageal voice restoration following laryngopharyngectomy and laryngopharyngoesophagectomy. In: Blom ED, Singer MI, Hamaker RC, eds. Tracheoesophageal Voice Restoration Following Total Laryngectomy. San Diego: Singular Publishing Group, 1998.

37. Davis JP, Nield DV, Garth RJN et al. The latissimus dorsi flap in head and neck surgery. Clin Otolaryngol 1992; 17: 487–90.

38. Anthony JP, Singer MI, Mathes SJ. Pharyngoesophageal reconstruction using the tubed radial forearm flap. Clin Plast Surg 1994; 21: 137–47.

39. Biel MA, Maisel RH. Postoperative radiation-associated changes in free jejunal autographs. Arch Otolaryngol Head Neck Surg 1992; 118: 1037–41.

40. Salamoun W, Swartz WM, Johnson JT et al. Free jejunal transfer for reconstruction of the laryngopharynx. Otolaryngol Head Neck Surg 1987; 96: 149–50.

41. Lewin JS, Barringer DA, May AH et al. Functional outcomes after circumferential pharyngoesophageal reconstruction. Laryngoscope 2005; 115: 1266–71.

42. Wilson PS, Bruce-Lockhart FJ, Johnson AP, Rhys Evans PH. Speech restoration following total pharyngolaryngectomy with free jejunal repair. Clin Otolaryngol 1994; 19: 145–8.

43. Ong GB, Lee TC. Pharyngogastric anastomosis after oesophagopharyngectomy for carcinoma of the hypopharynx and cervical esophagus. Br J Surg 1960; 48: 193–200.

44. Harrison DFN, Thompson AE. Pharyngolaryngoesophagectomy with pharyngogastric anastomosis for cancer of the hypopharynx: review of 101 operations. Head Neck Surgery 1986; 8: 418.

45. Wei WK, Lam KH, Choi S, Wong J. Late problems after pharyngogastric anastomosis for cancer of the larynx and hypopharynx. Am J Surg 1984; 148: 509–12.

46. de Vries EJ, Stein DW, Johnson JT et al. Hypopharyngeal reconstruction: a comparison of two alternatives. Laryngoscope 1989; 99: 614–17.

47. Yu P, Robb GL. Pharyngoesophageal reconstruction with the anterolateral thigh flap: a clinical and functional outcomes study. Plast Reconstr Surg 2005; 116: 1845–55.

48. Blom ED, Singer MI, Hamaker RC. Tracheostoma valve for post laryngectomy voice rehabilitation. Ann Otol Rhinol Laryngol 1982; 91: 576–8.

49. Lewin JS, Lemon J, Bishop-Leone JK et al. Experience with Barton button and peristomal breathing valve attachments for hands-free tracheoesophageal speech. Head Neck 2000; 22: 142–8.

50. Blom ED. Tracheoesophageal Voice Restoration Following Total Laryngectomy. San Diego: Singular Publishing Group, 1998.

51. Jay S, Ruddy J, Cullen RJ. Laryngectomy: the patient's view. J Laryngol Otol 1991; 105: 934–8.

52. McRae D, Young P, Hamilton J, Jones A. Raising airway resistance in laryngectomees increases tissue oxygen saturation. Clin Otolaryngol 1996; 21: 366–8.

53. Blom ED. Laboratory and clinical investigation of post laryngectomy airway humidification and filtration. Proceedings of the 1st EGFL Conference and 5th International Congress on Surgical and Prosthetic Voice Restoration after Total Laryngectomy, Grado, Italy.

54. Ackerstaff A, Hilgers F, Aaronson N et al. Improvements in respiratory and psychosocial functioning following total laryngectomy by use of heat and moisture exchanger. Ann Otol Rhinol Laryngol 1993; 102: 878–83.

55. Acton LM, Ross DA, Sasaki CT, Leder SB. Investigation of tracheoesophageal voice prosthesis leakage patterns: patient's

self-report versus clinician's confirmation. Head Neck 2008; 30: 618–21.

56. Hilgers FJ, Ackerstaff AH, Balm AJ et al. A new problem-solving indwelling voice prosthesis, eliminating the need for frequent Candida- and "underpressure"-related replacements: Provox ActiValve. Acta Otolaryngol 2003; 123: 972–9.

57. Free RH, van Der Mei HC, Dijk F et al. Biofilm formation on voice prostheses: influence of dairy products in vitro. Acta Otolaryngol 2000; 120: 92–9.

58. Busscher HJ, Free RH , Van Weissenbruch R et al. Preliminary observations on influence of dairy products on biofilm removal from silicone rubber voice prostheses in vitro. J Dairy Science 2000; 83: 641–7.

33

Future Developments in Head and Neck Cancer Therapy

Gideon Bachar, Patrick J Gullane and Jonathan C Irish

INTRODUCTION

Recent scientific advances have provided a platform for better understanding the biology of head and neck tumors. We now have a clearer understanding of cancer growth, response to treatment, and patterns of spread. In addition, advanced surgical techniques and the availability of various reconstructive options have improved locoregional control, with parallel improvements in aesthetics and postoperative function. Quality of life is now rightly regarded as a major consideration in the decision process. Despite these advances, the survival of head and neck cancer patients has not significantly improved. The following chapter will provide insight into the major advances achieved so far and into future directions for head and neck cancer therapy and practice.

ADVANCES IN SURGERY
Resective Techniques

Contemporary surgical strategies increasingly employ selective resections based on preoperative and highly detailed imaging. There has been a shift from radical surgery to more conservative primary and regional treatment approaches. The application of multidisciplinary therapies is made possible by collaborative treatment approaches. Multidisciplinary clinics of radiation oncologists, medical oncologists, and surgical oncologists can outline a treatment approach that maximizes survival and locoregional control while optimizing quality of life and cosmesis. Current philosophy generally advocates applying an "organ preservation approach" in the management of most head and neck malignancies while recognizing that this treatment approach must balance the results with the likelihood that the patient is going to have a functional organ at the end of treatment. The modern head and neck oncologist, therefore, is left with a menu of treatment options from which to choose. It is the responsibility of the treatment team to balance the side effects of treatment with the success of cancer ablation.

An increasingly employed modality is the utilization of endoscopic sinus techniques in both skull base surgery and endocrine surgery. After over a decade of experience of using image-guided endoscopic techniques in benign diseases of the sinuses (1), otolaryngologists—in collaboration with neurosurgeons—are now applying this technique for the removal of benign and malignant lesions of the nasal cavity, paranasal sinuses, and skull base. Many reports have described the advantages of image-guided endoscopic surgical navigation for applications in the skull base (e.g., removal of pituitary tumors, chordomas, and anterior skull base tumors). Today, surgeons can safely navigate tumor removal in difficult to access areas close to vital structures (e g ,the brain, optic nerves, and carotid arteries). The marriage of image-guidance—especially emerging real-time image guidance—with minimal access approaches will increase the confidence of tumor resection and the preservation of normal structures.

Surgery of the pituitary gland is a good example of the effect of these current advances on patient care. Resection of the pituitary gland has traditionally been performed by neurosurgeons, usually employing a trans-septal approach (submucosal dissection of the nasal septum) with removal of pituitary tumor with the assistance of the operating microscope. Due to the extensive submucosal dissection of the nasal septum, patients often require uncomfortable nasal packing for several days, and revision surgery is difficult due to significant scarring (2). With recent advances in endoscopic optical technology, transnasal endoscopic approaches to the pituitary have become the standard of care.

The last decade has yielded a rising number of publications describing endoscopic thyroidectomy and parathyroidectomy techniques. The procedures are gaining popularity due to the advantage of superior cosmetic results as compared to open procedure. The endoscopic procedure can be performed via the anterior chest approach using a neck skin-lifting technique in which the skin is lifted by a large number of hooks to create working space. This method is quite flexible and can be modified based on the size of the space needed. The fine hooks leave no scars on the anterior neck and the skin incisions are small (3). This technique and other endoscopic techniques have been shown to be feasible and safe. Preliminary results from minimally invasive procedures are almost comparable with those of conventional surgery (4), but they have additional advantages in terms of cosmetic result and postoperative pain. Endoscopic approaches might be suitable for parathyroid surgery but may have more limited application in thyroid oncologic surgery. No doubt, the endoscopic procedure will gain popularity, but aside from its cosmetic advantage, its future role is still to be determined, particularly in the treatment of thyroid neoplasia where malignancy is a real possibility.

Another developing new technology is robotic assisted surgery. The Da Vinci™ Surgical System (Intuitive Surgical, Mountain View, California) is a sophisticated "master-slave" robot that incorporates three-dimensional (3-D) visualization, scaling of movement, and wristed

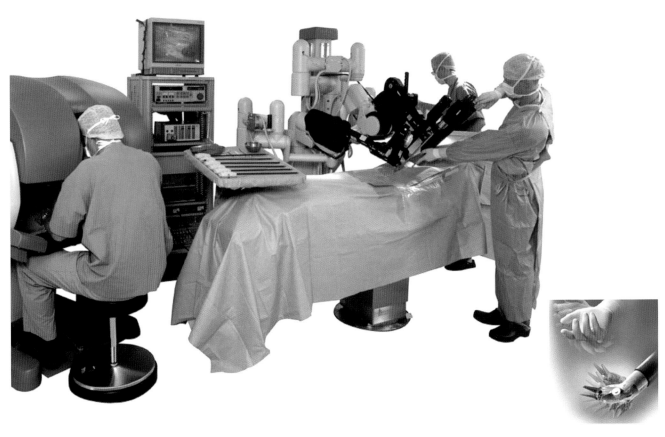

Figure 33.1 The Da Vinci™ Surgical System.

instrumentation (Fig. 33.1). The system has three multi-joint robotic arms, with one controlling a binocular endoscope and the other two controlling articulated instruments. Two lenses (0° or 30°) are used. Two finger-controlled handles, housed in a mobile console, control the two robotic arms while a foot pedal controls camera movement. Instrument movement can be scaled from 1:1, which allows exact finger movements to be transmitted to the instrument tip, to 1:3 and 1:5, which scale down the movements to allow precise and delicate dissection (Fig. 33.2). The system has been successfully applied in prostate, abdominal, ocular, sinus, and skull base surgery (5–8). It is an expensive system, however, with a capital cost of 1.2 million dollars, an annual maintenance cost of over one hundred thousand dollars, and an average instrument cost of fifteen hundred dollars per case (9). Several studies have demonstrated the efficacy of robotic assisted surgery in the head and neck. Recently, Solares and colleagues (10) reported on their experience with transoral robot-assisted CO_2 laser supraglottic laryngectomy. They concluded that the technology is feasible and has important implications on future management of supraglottic cancer. Another study describes the experience of treating three patients with trans-oral supraglottic laryngectomy. The procedure was found to be safe and offered a good surgical exposure, allowing complete surgical resection (11). Transoral robotic tongue base surgery has also been performed on cadavers, live dogs, and human

patients using the Da Vinci surgical system. The authors reported excellent three-dimensional visualization and instrument access that allowed successful surgical resections (12). In the future, more studies will describe the utilization of robots in head and neck ablative surgery. To date, the question of whether this modality provides an alternative to the conventional approach remains to be answered.

Reconstructive Techniques

Defects of the head and neck region present a challenge to the surgeon. Successful cosmetic and functional results have been achieved with both local and free tissue flaps. The flexibility of free tissue transfer, however, has dominated this area and continues to be the method of choice for reconstruction of sizable defects. The most widely used free flaps include the fibula, radial forearm, anterolateral thigh, scapula, and rectus abdominis. These free flaps reconstructions have significantly improved patient outcomes by restoring both form and function. Mandibular reconstruction with osteocutaneous free tissue transfer has allowed for single-stage surgery with full dental rehabilitation through the use of osseointegrated implants. Reconstructive surgery is at a stage where it provides restoration of almost any anatomical defect in the head and neck. Nevertheless, the next step will be to restore organ function

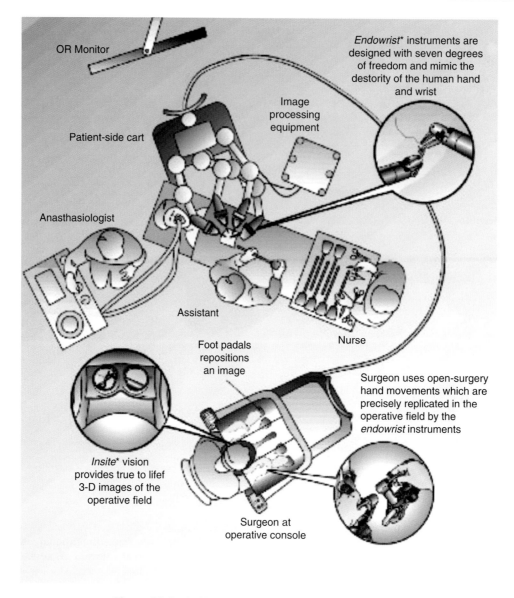

Figure 33.2   Da Vinci™ system in a general procedure setting.

such as tongue movement, swallowing, and sensation. Further refinements in flap selection and critical analysis of outcomes will also improve patient care. Application and popularization of newer flaps for the head and neck defect will continue to broaden the possibilities for reconstruction in this challenging area.

Distraction osteogenesis is a technique that involves corticotomy and subsequent distraction of the two segments. Ilizarov pioneered the technique in the former Soviet Union in the 1950s and 1960s (13), and applied it to the long bones. The apparatus is designed to hold the two sections rigidly and precisely; healing results in the formation of callus at the bone ends. Through precise separation at a rate of 1 mm per day, further callus is formed at both ends. As the segments are continuously separated, further callus is formed that gradually undergoes mineralization. As soon as separation ceases, the bone consolidates and

forms rigid mineralized bone that loses the ability for further separation.

In 1973, Snyder et al first reported the application of this technique to the mandible (14). Distraction osteogenesis has been used in the craniofacial region to treat deficiencies in mandibular growth as a result of fractures through growth centers (e.g., mandibular condyle), congenital deficiencies (e.g., Pierre Robin, Treacher Collins syndrome) and obstructive sleep apnea. It has also been used to augment bone height and width to allow for the placement of osseointegrated implants.

In so far as reconstructive treatment is concerned, there have been case reports of cyst/odontogenic tumor excisions followed by distraction osteogenesis in order to restore satisfactory mandibular length. It has yet to be determined, however, whether this could be used in the irradiated mandible. Animal experiments have shown that distraction osteogenesis applied to previously irradiated rabbit mandibles has resulted in successful osteogenesis. In addition, hyperbaric oxygen has been shown to be of additional benefit in this situation. This technique possibly could prove useful in the future for optimizing reconstructions for implant placement, particularly if radiation fields are precise and radiation dosages optimized. The most attractive feature of distraction osteogenesis is the formation of autogenous bone with no donor site morbidity. The disadvantages of this technique are the requirement for external hardware placement, as well as the fact that the technique requires time that in an oncological setting can delay the use of postoperative adjunct treatments, such as radiation therapy. The ideal mandibular rehabilitation would involve the creation of new bone identical to the missing segment without any donor site morbidity or use of external hardware.

Bone growth factors capable of inducing bone growth were first identified by Urist in the 1960s and early 1970s and named: bone morphogenetic protein (BMP) (15). BMP-1 is a regulatory protein and the remainder of the molecules in the BMP family have been identified as belonging to the transforming growth factor (TGF) superfamily of growth factors (13). The osteoinductive properties of TGF-b have been studied in both weight-bearing and non-weight-bearing bone. In a study of sheep tibial diaphyseal defects, TGF-b1 was shown to be effective in inducing new bone with structural and functional characteristics similar to normal bone (16). An increased understanding of bone growth may lead to an eventuality where segmental mandibular defects will be repaired through the production of custom-made autogenous bone segments that are subsequently implanted into the defect site.

Bone substitutes, as opposed to bone grafts, are being evaluated for use in replacing the mandibular defect. Recent developments in the field of biomaterials have seen the introduction of organic bone substitutes in the treatment of certain orthopedic injuries (17,18). These materials continue to be developed and their potential application in the craniofacial skeleton is currently being explored. In animal models, replacement of the introduced biomaterial by living bone appears to occur in a manner similar to bone remodelling (19). It is entirely possible that within the next decade, the majority of bone grafting in craniofacial reconstructive surgery may be done with biologically active synthetic bone graft substitutes rather than natural bone sources (20).

ADVANCES IN RADIOTHERAPY, CHEMOTHERAPY AND ORGAN PRESERVATION

Radiotherapy and chemotherapy have made significant progress in the last few decades demonstrating the role of nonsurgical primary or adjunctive therapies for advanced head and neck cancer. With the exception of the oral cavity, it seems that the outcome of radiotherapy with or without chemotherapy is comparable to surgery. This is not, however, without cost. Radiotherapy requires a sophisticated and costly infrastructure in order to deliver energy to the tumor while avoiding vital structures. Chemotherapy agents are expensive and not universally available. The side effects and comorbidities of nonsurgical treatments are

well documented and are not insignificant. The following section will describe the basic methods of radiotherapy and chemotherapy delivery, while focusing on the latest developments and future applications.

Radiotherapy

Several modifications have been made in radiation treatment protocols in order to improve the outcome and minimize treatment induced morbidity. Conventional fractionation generally delivers 2.0 Gy per fraction, one dose per day, for five days a week up to a total dose of 60–70 Gy, depending on the particular tumor. Altered fractionation schemes imply changing the frequency and/or the dose of the fractions in order to improve locoregional control or to reduce complications of normal tissues.

Accelerated fractionation regimens aim to improve locoregional control by reducing the treatment time as much as responding tissues can tolerate. The usual regimen for accelerated fractionation entails two or three conventional fractions of 2.0 Gy per day given up to a total dose equal to a conventional total dose. Shortening the treatment time decreases the opportunity for surviving tumor cells to repopulate during the course of treatment. The most significant limiting factor is the severe mucositis produced by accelerated fractionation requiring the reduction of the total dose to be administered (21). Techniques such as split course radiotherapy and concomitant boost have been used to try to keep the total dose as high as possible. From 1985 to 1995, a randomized controlled trial of the EORTC Cooperative Group of Radiotherapy (EORTC 22851) compared the experimental regimen of Accelerated fractionation (72 Gy/45 fractions/5 weeks) to standard fractionation and overall treatment time (70 Gy/35 fractions/7 weeks) in T2, T3 and T4 head and neck cancers (hypopharynx excluded). The end-point criteria were local and locoregional control, overall and disease-free survival, and acute and late toxicities. The authors demonstrated a higher local control rate, increased incidence of acute toxicity, as well as increased late toxicities of necrosis and fibrosis in the accelerated fractionation arm as compared to the standard protocol (22).

Hyperfractionation employs twice daily treatment, with smaller than conventional fractions, for a total dose that exceeds conventional doses. Reducing the dose per fraction is designed to decrease or minimize later complications of radiotherapy. Altered fractionation regimens are becoming increasingly routine as the results several studies are appreciated and applied. In a meta-analysis that included 15 trials with 6515 advanced head and neck cancer patients, the authors evaluated the outcome of patients treated with hyperfractionation or accelerated radiotherapy. The study demonstrated a significant increase in survival and locoregional control when compared to the conventional radiotherapy protocol (23).

Intensity-modulated radiation therapy (IMRT) delivers high doses of radiation to the tumor with very high precision, while minimizing the dose received by the surrounding normal tissues (24). IMRT is based on computer optimized treatment planning and a computer controlled treatment delivery system. The advantage as well as the limitation of IMRT is the very sharp dose fall-off gradient between the gross tumor target and surrounding normal tissue. Therefore, target volume delineation is essential. Inadequate tumor delineation will result in impaired tumor control.

High-precision delivery of radiation energy is an advantage in highly complicated anatomical areas such as the head and neck. The ability to spare the salivary glands, bony structures such as the mandible or skull base, muscles of mastication, major vascular structures and cranial nerves, results in a better functional outcome without compromising the oncological ablation. With these advances, irregularly shaped targets can be treated with highly conformal therapy; however, our knowledge of the exact extent of the tumor is still evolving. The incorporation of information obtained from computed tomography (CT), magnetic resonance imaging (MRI), and positron emission tomography (PET) into delineation of primary tumors, for highly conformal irradiation planning of head and neck cancer, is a major area of ongoing research (25). Future plans should focus on advanced functional imaging and improvement of image-guided radiation therapy. Gaining more experience with this technology will enable significant further improvements in local control, survival, and long-term toxicity profiles in the head and neck region (25).

The use of radioactively labeled antibodies to target delivery of radiation to tumor tissues is being explored as well. Isotopes capable of delivering tumoricidal doses of radiation are attached to tumor-specific antibodies. Tumors that have been treated using this approach include hepatomas, gliomas, and prostatic tumors (26). The application of this technique to head and neck cancer has been hampered by the inability to identify an antibody sufficiently sensitive and specific to be of use. Nevertheless, advances in the field of radioimmunotherapy may become more applicable to the head and neck in due course.

Chemotherapy

In the past, the role of chemotherapy in the treatment of head and neck cancer was limited to the setting of recurrent or metastatic disease. Response rates in this setting for single agent chemotherapy range from 15% to 40% with a response duration of three to six months. The single agents most frequently used are cisplatinum and methotrexate.

The use of chemotherapy with other modalities in patients undergoing curative intent therapy can be divided into adjuvant chemotherapy, concurrent chemoradiotherapy, and induction (neoadjuvant) chemotherapy. Adjuvant chemotherapy is administered as a set number of chemotherapy cycles following radiation and/or surgery. Concurrent chemoradiotherapy, which consists of a number of chemotherapy cycles administered during radiotherapy, can increase the locoregional activity of radiation by eradication of radiation-resistant cells. Two large studies (27,28) have shown that concurrent postoperative administration of cisplatinum and radiotherapy improved local and regional control. The disease-free survival was significantly longer as well. It should be noted, however, that although the effect on overall survival was significant in the European group, this was not found to be the case in the North American study. Unfortunately, chemotherapeutic toxicity increases significantly following radiotherapy.

Induction or neoadjuvant chemotherapy consists of a number of chemotherapy cycles administered prior to surgery and/or radiation. It has been extensively investigated in head and neck cancer. Induction chemotherapy

has been applied to patients with both resectable and unresectable disease. The benefit of systemic chemotherapy may lie in the reduction of systemic disease; yet, the impact on overall survival is limited (29). One philosophy in support of the use of induction chemotherapy is that it may be useful in selecting out a group of patients who respond to concurrent chemoradiation protocols while patients who do not respond may be best treated with surgical intervention.

Combined Therapy

Advanced cancers require a combined approach of either surgery with post operative radiation or chemoradiation as an organ preservation approach. The aim of organ preservation in head and neck patients is to eradicate the cancer while maintaining the basic functions of breathing, speech, and swallowing (30). Organ preservation has become an increasingly popular approach in the management of laryngeal and pharyngeal cancer due to the high morbidity associated with surgical resection.

A milestone study (29) investigated whether induction chemotherapy and definitive radiation therapy with laryngectomy reserved for salvage represented a better initial treatment approach for patients with stage 3 or 4 laryngeal cancer than total laryngectomy with postoperative radiation therapy. The study concluded that induction chemotherapy enhanced the effectiveness of definitive radiation therapy; it was also noted, however, that a direct comparison had not been made between induction chemotherapy with radiation therapy and radiation therapy alone. Another finding of the study was that local recurrence was more common and distant metastases less frequent in the chemotherapy group. It was proposed that chemotherapy may prevent or at least delay distant metastases.

The role of combined treatments in organ preservation was further investigated in the RTOG 91-11 study (31,32). Patients with advanced laryngeal cancer were randomized to one of three treatment arms. Patients in the first arm received two cycles of cisplatin and fluorouracil and were then examined. Nonresponders underwent total laryngectomy with postoperative radiotherapy. Responders underwent a third cycle of chemotherapy after which they completed radiation therapy. Patients in the second arm received concomitant chemoradiotherapy with cisplatin. Patients in the third arm were treated with conventionally fractioned radiation therapy. The rate of laryngeal preservation at a median follow-up of 3.8 years was significantly higher among patients receiving concurrent chemoradiotherapy (84%) than among those receiving induction chemotherapy (125/173) or radiotherapy alone (116/173). In fact, induction chemotherapy followed by radiotherapy when compared to radiotherapy alone, did not significantly improve the rate of laryngeal preservation. The overall two- and five-year survival estimates showed no significant difference among treatment groups with a two-year survival of 76%. Local-regional control is significantly better for patients treated with concurrent chemoradiotherapy as compared to induction chemotherapy or radiotherapy alone. Chemotherapy significantly reduces distant metastases as compared to radiotherapy alone. Laryngectomy following organ preservation treatment is associated with increased morbidity (32). Sassler et al. found that salvage surgery performed after chemoradiotherapy was associated with a 77% rate of major wound complication (33). This outcome should be taken into consideration when assessing patients for organ preservation treatment.

A significant shift is taking place with the inclusion of more aggressive chemotherapy as initial treatment prior to chemoradiotherapy. This approach is the basis of many ongoing trials. Docetaxel, cisplatin and 5-fluorouracil appear to be the most effective induction chemotherapy regimens. Patients with squamous cell carcinoma of the head and neck, who received docetaxel plus cisplatin and fluorouracil induction chemotherapy plus chemoradiotherapy, had a significantly longer survival rate than did patients who received cisplatin and fluorouracil induction chemotherapy in addition to chemoradiotherapy (34).

Does organ preservation actually preserve organ function? Side effects of organ preservation in the head and neck can result in basic organ dysfunction, including swallowing, breathing, and speech deficits. In a review article, Riegel et al. (35) criticize the functional outcomes after organ preservation approaches. They stated that most swallowing disorders after organ preservation treatment were associated with physiological changes that occurred in the movement of the tongue, pharynx, and larynx after radiotherapy. The physiological changes resulted in dysmotility of these structures and frequent episodes of aspiration, especially where the oropharyngeal musculature was involved (35). Although some function can recover with time, swallowing difficulties might be permanent, requiring long-term enteral nutrition in up to 18% of patients. Addition of chemotherapy to organ preservation regimens may result in more acute toxicity with patients requiring feeding tubes more often and losing more weight than patients treated with radiotherapy alone (35). Associated long-term swallowing issues after organ preservation for head and neck cancer include xerostomia, dysphagia, and avoidance of social eating. Xerostomia affected a large number of patients and was related to lower scores on quality-of-life measures.

Future research should evaluate the functional outcome of organ preservation treatment. Considerations in the development of organ preservation management should emphasize the understanding that comprehensive multidisciplinary management is critical. The effect on the patient's quality of life should be clarified in prospective large series. The role of salvage surgery should be investigated further, taking into account that neck management may differ from management of the primary tumor site. The relationship between the biological profile of the tumor and the host—and the effect of the treatment on both—may be of importance and predict success. It is likely, therefore, that future therapeutic prescriptions will be signed by the "molecular and biological signature" of an individual tumor rather than by the physician.

EMERGING SYSTEMIC THERAPEUTICS FOR HEAD AND NECK CANCER
Tyrosine-kinase Inhibitors and EGFR Monoclonal Antibodies

Concurrent chemoradiotherapy has been shown to improve locoregional control and survival rate as compared to radiotherapy or surgery alone. There is, however, a significant patient population who cannot benefit from the combined treatment due to the toxicity associated with chemotherapy delivery (36). In order to improve patient outcome, other strategies are now being employed, including the incorporation of novel targeted therapies into organ-preservation approaches. Several ongoing trials incorporate monoclonal antibodies or small molecules that target the epidermal growth factor receptor into combined modality regimens.

Deregulation of the epidermal growth factor receptor (EGFR) is one of the most frequently reported molecular events leading to oral carcinogenesis (37). Overexpression of EGFR is a common event in many human solid tumors, including head and neck carcinomas. The need to inhibit the tumor promoting function of the EGFR receptor has led to the development of specific tyrosine-kinase inhibitors (38) (i.e., Gefitinib, Erlotinib), which inhibit the signalling cascade, as well as monoclonal antibodies directed against the receptor molecule (i.e., Cetuximab) (39). These inhibitors are potential new anticancer drugs for a wide range of epithelial cancers. Preclinical data show the marked enhancement of antitumor activity of tyrosine-kinase inhibitors in addition to conventional chemotherapy (40). Therapies directed against the EGFR signaling pathway can also strongly influence the sensitivity and the resistance to radiation therapy (41). Cetuximab (Erbitux, ImClone Systems, New York, New York), is an IgG1 monoclonal antibody against the ligand binding domain of EGFR. It has been shown to enhance the cytotoxic effects of radiation in squamous cell carcinoma. Bonner et al. (42) have demonstrated the improvement in locoregional and survival rate in patients treated with Cetuximab and high-dose radiotherapy, compared to radiotherapy alone in patients with advanced head and neck cancer. There was no difference in toxicity between the two treatment protocols. No doubt, this regimen represents a novel and promising therapeutic option for patients with locoregionally advanced head and neck cancer and provides a potential further improvement in the outcome of cancer eradication.

Antiangiogenic Agents

Angiogenesis is the process by which new blood vessels are produced in the host. In 1972, Folkman stated that "once tumor take has occurred, every increase in tumor cell population must be preceded by an increase in new capillaries that converge upon the tumor" (43,44). The formation of new blood vessels is dependent upon migration and proliferation of endothelial cells, interactions with extracellular matrix, and soluble growth factors. Angiogenic molecules act by stimulating endothelial cell migration and division. Several angiogenic molecules have been isolated. The 14-kilodalton polypeptide angiogenin has been isolated from various solid tumors and is a potent stimulator of angiogenesis on chick embryo chorioallantoic membrane (CAM). Other factors that have been identified include acidic and basic fibroblast growth factor, transforming growth factor-alpha, tumor necrosis factor, platelet-derived endothelial cell growth factor, and angiotropin. Tumor-induced angiogenesis begins with the dissolution of the native vessel basement membrane due to production of collagenase and other metalloproteases. This is followed by migration of endothelial cells out of the vessel towards the tumor. These endothelial cells canalize into new vessels. Endothelial cell migration is a prerequisite for angiogenesis but endothelial cell division is not. Once these endothelial cells migrate and form new vessels, basement membrane is deposited and pericytes are established to support the newly formed blood vessels. Angiogenesis has been studied in several solid tumors and is also being studied in head and neck squamous cell cancer. Antiangiogenesis is being proposed as a novel treatment strategy in the setting of malignancy. Therapeutic strategies include the use of agents acting directly on tumor cells to prevent the release of angiogenic molecules, deactivating angiogenic molecules once released, or preventing the endothelial cell response to angiogenic factors (44). Antiangiogenic properties have been noted in several classes of agents including corticosteroids, interferons, and heparin substitutes. Currently, there is significant interest in the use of antiangiogenic agents in solid tumor therapy, and investigations are ongoing into the clinical applications of antiangiogenesis.

Bevacizumab (Avastin; Genentech, Inc.; South San Francisco, California) is a recombinant, humanized monoclonal antibody to vascular endothelial growth factor, a key regulator of tumor angiogenesis. Bevacizumab demonstrated potent antitumor activity in preclinical models, and also has shown biologic activity and clinical benefit in clinical studies specifically in renal cell carcinoma and colorectal cancer. Recent studies also included solid tumor of the head and neck. Recently, Fujita et al. have demonstrated for the first time the antitumor effect of Bevacizumab in head and neck squamous cell carcinoma. Although the drug did not show any advantage in vitro, the effect in vivo was significant with obvious decrease in the tumor size (45).

Retinoic Acid and Beta-carotene

At present, several trials on chemoprevention in head and neck cancer have evaluated the role of retinoids in preventing transformation of premalignant lesions and development of second primary cancers. The advantage of retinoids (synthetic analogues of vitamin A) was first observed, by chance, in cattle deprived of vitamin A. Wolbach and Howe noted that these animals had a much higher incidence of lung cancer and upper aerodigestive tract malignancies (46). Further studies using vitamin A analogs showed significant remission of premalignant lesions in the larynx and oral cavity. The primary retinoid that is being tested in cancer prevention trials is 13-cis retinoic acid (13cRA). Response rates of premalignant lesions to 13cRA have been reported to be as high as 67% in randomized studies (47). Fenretinide is a less toxic retinoid under study for oral premalignant lesions. In a randomized trial (48) at the Milan Cancer Institute, 709 subjects have been accrued in a prevention trial of basal cell carcinoma of the head and neck, and 153 patients entered a study the preliminary results showed the capability of fenretinide to prevent recurrences and new localizations of oral leukoplakia. Hong et al. (49) showed in a randomized trial that 13cRA treated patients had a significantly reduced incidence of second malignancies as compared to placebo. Unfortunately, 13cRA does have side-effects, including skin dryness, cheilitis, conjunctivitis, and hypertriglyceridemia, that limit its tolerance, especially at high doses.

Other Drugs

Docetaxel is a clinically well-established anti-mitotic chemotherapy medication mainly used so far for the treatment of breast, ovarian, and non-small cell lung cancer. Docetaxel has an approved claim for treatment of patients who have locally advanced, or metastatic, breast or non small-cell lung cancer, and have undergone anthracycline-based chemotherapy that has failed to stop cancer progression or relapse. Recently Posner et al. demonstrated that patients with squamous cell carcinoma of the head and neck who received docetaxel plus cisplatin and fluorouracil induction chemotherapy plus chemoradiotherapy had a significantly longer survival than did patients who received cisplatin and fluorouracil induction chemotherapy plus chemoradiotherapy (34).

Telomerase is a potential selective anticancer target. Telomeres are tandem repeats of DNA associated with specific proteins. These structures cap eukaryotic chromosomes and maintain the integrity of the chromosome ends. Tumors such as squamous cell carcinoma of the head and neck require telomerase to maintain telomere function; inhibition of the enzyme can lead to apoptosis. Furthermore, because most tumor cells have very short telomeres, they are more likely to succumb to telomerase inhibition than normal cells. The telomere is also involved in the repair of DNA double strand breaks, and telomere dysfunction provokes radiosensitivity. The current state of knowledge is that the telomere length, and specifically the telomerase enzyme and its cofactors, provide very attractive targets for anticancer therapeutic strategies (50).

Another class of investigational drugs aims to reduce treatment toxicity. This includes cyto-protective agents such as amifostine (51,52) for sparing of salivary gland function, or growth factors such as keratinocyte growth factor (rHuKGF, palifermin), which may have a future role in mucosal protection (53). It is too early to draw definitive conclusions on their clinical value. Prospective clinical trials of these and similar strategies are in progress.

Several cytotoxic drugs with significant activities as single agents and/or combination regimens have shown high response rates, but over the past several years, significant improvement in survival has not been achieved. New drugs, including those that target the epidermal growth factor receptor, the p53 gene, RAS protein post-translational modification, the proteosome, vascular endothelial growth factor, cyclooxygenase-2, and other molecular pathways, are promising agents in the management of head and neck cancer. Their potential is being tested in various settings, including chemoprevention, recurrent and metastatic disease, and in combination with radiation therapy and/or cytotoxic agents (54). Signal transducers and activators of transcription (STAT) proteins comprise a family of latent cytoplasmic transcription factors that become transiently activated in response to extracellular signals, leading to regulation of diverse physiological responses. There is compelling evidence that persistent activation of specific STAT molecules induces oncogenic properties in head and neck cancer. The presence of constitutively activated STAT molecules in cancer cells is mainly attributed to the dysregulation of upstream activating pathways and the aberration of negative regulatory mechanisms. The end result is induction of specific target genes that stimulate cell proliferation, prevent apoptosis, promote angiogenesis, and facilitate tumor immune evasion. The availability of multiple potential targets for interruption of aberrant STAT signaling in cancer, and the initial promising results, have generated optimism for the clinical applicability of STAT targeting in head and neck cancer (55).

IMAGING ADVANCES
Imaged-guided Surgery

The incorporation of image guidance with various methods of tumor ablation, termed "image-guided surgery" (IGS), can provide intraoperative volumetric imaging with high spatial resolution. Such technology enhances orientation and provides up-to-date intraoperative images. IGS can delineate the tumor and related structures, thereby diminishing complications and allowing preservation of adjacent vital structures, while achieving complete tumor removal. In conventional pre-captured IGS, the surgeon uses a device—be it an instrument or a pointer—to establish correspondence between intraoperative and preoperative anatomical location. Drawbacks of conventional IGS include difficulty with orientation of the image display in relation to the surgical field, and the inability to adapt to changes in normal and tumor anatomy that result from surgical manipulation. In order to overcome these potential limitations, intraoperative real-time imaging, with computed tomography (CT), magnetic resonance imaging (MRI), or ultrasound (US), has been developed (56,57). This evolving technology provides additional information about the anatomical modifications that occur during a procedure and may further increase surgical accuracy.

Image-guidance systems for planned surgical procedures should have the following attributes:

- Enable accuracy to within 2–3mm or less
- Have no loss of accuracy with body movement
- Provide the ability to use surgical instruments for image-guidance tracking
- Be easy for the surgeon and operating room personnel to operate
- Demonstrate real-time changes in anatomy
- Be cost-effective

Significant tissue distortion can take place during surgical procedures, especially in soft tissue organs. As opposed to preoperative images that do not accurately reflect the anatomical changes that occur during surgery, intraoperative CT or MR imaging do enable real-time assessment. Both these systems, however, have benefits and drawbacks that must be taken into account, particularly since studies have reported no significant differences in accuracy between preoperative and intraoperative CT scanning.

In recent decades image-guided endoscopic surgery has been used to repair cerebrospinal fluid (CSF) leaks, remove tumors of the paranasal sinuses and skull base, and explore the pterygopalatine fossa (58). Surgical navigation systems have also been instrumental in resident teaching and paranasal sinus anatomy research. Sinus and skull-base endoscopic image-guided surgery has developed rapidly in recent years. To date, it allows more thorough surgical dissections and reduces the complication rate. The next step will see the integration of

imaging with the utilization of robotics to augment the reality of the surgical field.

The development of new intraoperative imaging modalities will allow visualization of different types of images simultaneously, show structures that are normally only visible intraoperatively, and permit intraoperative navigation in areas of anatomical sensitivity. New modalities will enable preoperative surgical planning that can then be incorporated directly into the procedure. Other potential benefits of this new technology will involve smaller incisions, direct access to specific targeted areas and, as a consequence, less invasive operations (59).

One of the latest technologies being tested for clinical use is intraoperative three-dimensional (3-D) cone-beam CT scan imaging (CBCT). The technology involves the use of a flat-panel x-ray imaging detector on a surgical C-arm to achieve intraoperative "near real time" 3-D imaging. Cone-beam imaging operates on a similar principle as conventional CT, except that cone-beam imaging utilizes fluoroscopic images acquired in an 180° orbit around the patient to provide 3-D image reconstructions. In conventional CT, an x-ray source and one-dimensional (1-D) detector rotate around the patient acquiring multiple 1-D projections of the patient's anatomy. These projections are then processed to reconstruct a single slice of the patient's internal anatomy. In cone-beam imaging, a two-dimensional (2-D) fluoroscopy imaging system is used, permitting the 3-D reconstruction of multiple slices from a single rotation of source and 2-D detector. This approach vastly simplifies the acquisition geometry, allowing it to be adapted to non-ring-based geometries, such as a mobile C-arm platform (60) (Fig. 33.3).

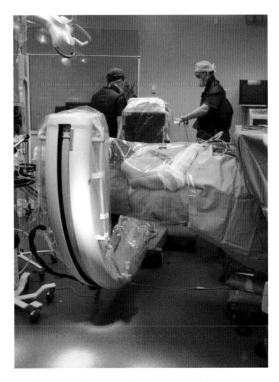

Figure 33.3 CBCT on a mobile C-arm platform in the operating room.

A broad host of applications for image-guided surgery is under consideration. All allow the surgeon to acquire high-quality, volumetric images during the procedure and overcome current limitations associated with guidance by pre-existing diagnostic image data alone. The cone beam CT application has been implemented on patients undergoing radiation therapy. Cone-beam imaging and potential applications in head and neck surgery have been investigated in the lab and are now being utilized in intraoperative patient management. Preclinical investigation conducted on 12 cadaveric specimens with and without cone-beam image guidance showed that cone-beam imaging dramatically improved surgical performance and confidence in the execution of surgical excision and landmark identification tasks. The system was found to provide volumetric images with high spatial resolution and soft-tissue visibility at imaging doses approximately one-tenth that of a diagnostic CT scan (61,62). In some cases (resection of skull base lesions), cone beam imaging afforded a two-fold increase in the sensitivity (i.e., fraction of lesion excised) of the surgical resection as compared to a traditional non-guided approach. The ability to differentiate the lesion from normal critical structures is an additional advantage of intraoperative cone-beam imaging. It permits a safer and more precise execution than existing surgical approaches, and allows for potential investigation of new, more radical surgical techniques.

The benefit from CBCT imaging is clear. Intraoperative imaging with sub-millimeter spatial resolution and soft-tissue visibility, provides quantifiable improvement in surgical performance (Fig. 33.4). This result, however, is not without cost. CBCT requires a full semicircular orbit, with gantry rotation time ranging from 5s to 60s. CBCT is computationally intense, involving 3-D reconstruction from hundreds of projections and requiring 30s for even the fastest reconstruction platforms. In addition, CBCT involves a radiation dose that, however low, is not insignificant. Tomosynthesis imaging offers a potential solution to these challenges. By acquiring projections over a limited arc of 20° to 60°, tomosynthesis can produce 3-D images at a fraction of the image acquisition time, reconstruction time, and radiation dose compared to CBCT. The trade-off is image quality, particularly in-depth resolution (Fig. 33.5).

Skull base ablation of various anatomical targets conducted on cadaver heads has demonstrated the advantage of the tomosynthesis technique. It provides the surgeon with up-to-date images of the target and related structures, overcoming limitations associated with preoperative image guidance. The images can be obtained intraoperatively in about 30 seconds, with a radiation dose delivered to the patient at about one-tenth of a CBCT. The technology provides quantifiable benefits to the surgeon: facilitating total target ablation, helping to spare surrounding vital structures, and improving the quality of surgical product.

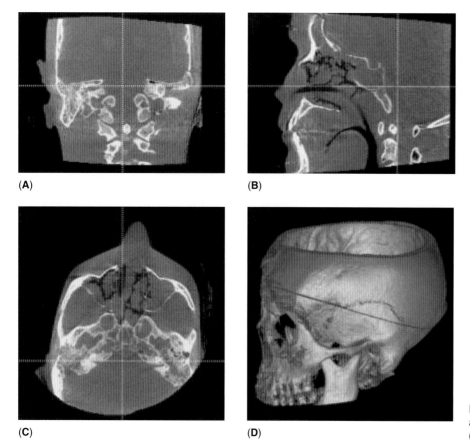

(A) (B)

(C) (D)

Figure 33.4 3D CBCT image of the head and neck. **(A)** coronal view, **(B)** sagittal view, **(C)** axial view, **(D)** volume rendering.

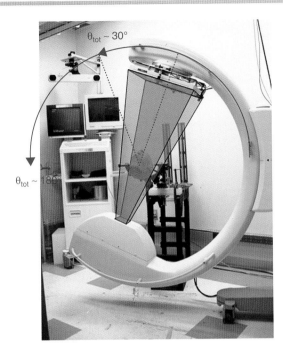

Figure 33.5 Tomosynthesis limited-angle 3D imaging acquiring projections over a limited arc.

Tomosynthesis is clearly a useful complement to CBCT. In combination it allows for high-quality images augmented by fast, repeat tomosynthesis images acquired at any point within the procedure. Growing consensus across the field of surgery is that the development of high-performance intraoperative imaging represents the next great advance in surgical intervention.

Augmented reality systems are now being developed in order to overcome intraoperative disorientation of the image display in relation to the surgical field. Augmented reality provides navigational support by direct projection of segmented structures from preoperative images onto the patient. This can be based on monocular projection in the operating microscope (63,64), head up displays, projection onto purpose built semi-translucent screens placed between the operating scene and the surgeon (64), or by projection into the binocular optics of a tracked surgical microscope. The technology's ultimate objective is to support the surgeon during the operation in the least obstructive way (65).

In conclusion, it must be stated that image-guidance systems are associated with increased operative time and expense. They are not meant for every surgeon or for every patient. There is no doubt, however, that guidance systems are useful tools for navigation of the surgical scene, but are not a substitute for sound surgical principles and a good knowledge of human anatomy.

¹⁸F-FDG PET/CT

The role of ¹⁸F-FDG PET/CT is rapidly growing in the management of head and neck cancer. Its efficacy has been extensively investigated in squamous cell carcinoma of the head and neck, as well as in thyroid and salivary gland malignancies. Physical examination and the routine use of CT and MRI imaging are the main tools used in the initial evaluation of head and neck cancer. ¹⁸F-FDG PET/CT does not provide the anatomic definition that MRI and contrast enhanced multi-slice CT can provide (66). It may have benefit in delineation of the extent of regional disease, distant metastasis, and second primary tumors. The use of ¹⁸F-FDG PET/CT may be a valuable additional tool in allowing the clinician to differentiate responders from non-responders when selecting patients for salvage surgery after radiation or chemoradiation treatment. Moreover, it offers long-term surveillance for recurrence and metastases.

¹⁸F-FDG PET/CT has a role in detecting the primary tumor in patients with unknown primary tumors. Schoder and Yeung reviewed more than 300 patients and found that the sensitivity of ¹⁸F-FDG PET/CT ranged from 10% to 60% (67). Another study revealed that the ¹⁸F-FDG PET/CT detected the primary site in 27% of patients with unknown primary that were initially negative when evaluated by physical examination and MRI. Another advantage of ¹⁸F-FDG PET/CT is its ability to identify cancer spared in unexpected locations because of its total body coverage (upper mediastinum, axilla and bone) (68,69). Quon et al. demonstrated the benefit of ¹⁸F-FDG PET/CT in detecting recurrence or persistent disease after primary treatment. They evaluated 108 patients and found that PET/CT detected local–regional persistent or recurrent head and neck squamous cell carcinoma (HNSCC) with a sensitivity of 82%, a specificity of 92%, a positive predictive value (PPV) of 64%, a negative predictive value (NPV) of 97%, and an overall accuracy of 90% (70).

In thyroid cancer PET usually does not detect normal thyroid tissue. Diffuse uptake usually suggests thyroiditis and in case of focal uptake there is a chance of up to 50% of malignancy (71). To date, there are no guidelines for the use of ¹⁸F-FDG PET/CT for HNSCC and thyroid cancer. In the future, the role of PET will be better defined and guidelines will be developed for applying PET imaging for head and neck cancer.

Autofluorescence

Autofluorescence of tissues is produced by fluorophores that occur naturally in living cells following excitation with a suitable wavelength. Collagen, elastin, keratin, and NADH are among the fluorophores included within the tissue matrix that effect tissue autofluorescence. The presence of disease changes the concentration of the fluorophores, as well as the light scattering and absorption properties of the tissue, which among other phenomena, is a result of changes in blood concentration, nuclear size distribution, collagen content, and epithelial content. Cell metabolism changes associated with malignancy, such as an increase in NADH, are also thought to be responsible for alteration of tissue fluorescence (72–74).

Autofluorescence imaging techniques involve illumination of tissue with a light source, mostly in the near-UV to green range of the spectrum (375–442 nm). Images of the fluorescence produced in the tissue and altered by absorption and scattering are recorded with a camera. Typically, normal tissue exhibits a green fluorescence. As tissues become more dysplastic, they exhibit a red and violet fluorescence (Fig. 33.6). Autofluorescence imaging, to detect

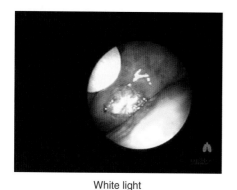

White light

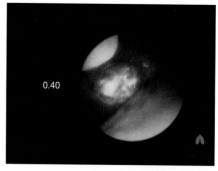

Autofluorescence

Figure 33.6 Patient with previous tonsil carcinoma treated with radiotherapy presenting with a new buccal (*right*) malignancy.

early malignancy, is being introduced in a number of clinical settings, including screening for lung, esophagus, colon, bladder, and larynx malignancies.

Subsequent research developed fluorescence spectroscopy into a fluorescence imaging technique that enables the amplification of weak fluorescence signals. Special cameras equipped with either image intensifiers or time integration facilities were included. These modifications have resulted in real-time images suitable for clinical use (72).

Investigation continues into correlating altered fluorescence profiles with changes in the underlying molecular profiles of tissues, and better understanding the clinical relevance of this new screening technique. This will not only further validate the importance of autofluorescence in early malignancy detection, but will also unravel the specific molecular events that result in altered tissue fluorescence.

TISSUE ENGINEERING

Tissue engineering utilizes techniques intended to develop biological substitutes that can restore, maintain, or improve tissue function or an entire organ. Because of the challenge that the cancer surgeon faces in reconstruction of an ablative defect there is significant interest in tissue engineering to help meet the challenge of head and neck reconstruction.

An increased effort is underway to investigate generating bone, cartilage, cornea, and vascular grafts. To date, tissue engineered bone is the only tissue type that is in routine clinical use. Bone that was engineered from BMP-2 and BMP-7 is used in orthopedics to treat lumbar fusions and long bone nonunions. Clinical application of bone tissue engineering in the head and neck is limited to case reports. There are some advances in tissue engineering with cartilage for the nose and ear in immune incompetent animal models, but there has been difficulty with generating scaffolds that do not incite an immune reaction in an immune competent model (75).

An example of tissue engineering methods for bone reconstruction in the clinical setup was reported by

Cheng et al. They described the use of a molded polymethylmethacrylate tissue chamber to explore the feasibility of using autogenous iliac morcellized bone graft in a 58-year-old patient to engineer a bone flap. The "take" and long-term durability of the engineered bone block was assessed after its transfer for mandible reconstruction and osseointegrated implant insertion. Still, it will take numerous studies before routine clinical application will be possible. More clinical research is required to develop methods to improve the quality of the engineered bone. Since the engineered bone units are presumed to be well vascularized, future studies may explore the potential feasibility of harvesting them as vascularized flaps (76).

One potential alternative to conventional skin graft reconstruction for skin defects is the development of cultured epithelial autografts. The technique is performed under local anesthesia. A 5 mm skin sample is taken from behind the ear and 50 ml of blood serum is taken. After being washed with antibiotic solution, dermis and subcutaneous tissue is removed from the skin sample under aseptic conditions. The keratinocytes are minced, isolated, and cultivated in keratinocyte growth medium under strict autologous conditions using the patient's serum. After having multiplied sufficiently, keratinocytes are seeded onto a collagen matrix (90% keratinocytes:10% fibroblasts). Next, the highly elastic collagen matrix is transferred to the wound bed, on an outpatient basis and under local anesthesia, when necessary. After transplantation, the epithelial autograft is secured with a silicone-coated wound dressing that is removed after five days. The functional as well as the cosmetic outcomes are promising (77).

PREVENTION OF HEAD AND NECK MALIGNANCY

The upper aerodigestive tract is susceptible to synchronous as well as metachronous primaries. This was partially explained under the term "field cancerization." The term was coined by Slaughter and coworkers, who described a field defect in the aerodigestive tract that allowed for independent generation of neoplastic clones at multiple sites (78). The risk of developing a second primary cancer after squamous cell cancer of the upper aerodigestive tract is 4% per year. These new cancers are about equally divided into cancers of the lungs, esophagus, and other areas of the mouth and throat. An effective intervention, to decrease the incidence of second primaries in this setting, would have a major impact on cancer control.

Smoking was found to be a significant risk factor for cancer and second primary lesions. Smoking increased considerably between 1945 and 1965. Since 1985, however, consumption has decreased in some countries. Today, there are one billion smokers worldwide. The Food and Agricultural Organization of the United Nations estimates that between the years 1986 and 2000, tobacco consumption will have decreased by 11% in developed countries but increased by 10% in developing nations. If present trends continue, the annual death rate from tobacco consumption will rise from the current 3 million to 10 million by 2025, with 7 million of these deaths in the developing nations. There are many reasons for the increase in the habit of smoking in the Third World, including an increase in population, ignorance of the health risks of smoking, and the intensive and ruthless marketing by multinational tobacco companies (79). The development of national tobacco control policies in Third World countries and education of the lower socio-economic classes is essential in order to stem the tide of increased tobacco consumption. Preventing people from taking up smoking should be a major health priority. These efforts must focus on the young because 88% of smokers start by age 18 (80). Unfortunately, current strategies such as enforcement of tobacco sales laws have not been shown to be effective, while marketing strategies of tobacco companies continue to target young people (81).

Recently, two major findings demonstrated the association between human papillomavirus (HPV) and head and neck cancer. D'Souza G et al. found that oropharyngeal cancer was significantly associated with oral HPV type 16 (HPV-16) infection. They found that DNA from HPV-16, one of the strains of HPV most commonly associated with cervical cancer, was detected in 72% of the tumor specimens. In addition, 64% of patients with cancer had antibodies for cancer-related proteins commonly found in HPV-16 (82). Other studies found that patients with HPV-positive HNSCC may have a better prognosis than patients with HPV-negative tumors. Patients with newly diagnosed, advanced HNSCC were treated with a combination of chemotherapy and radiation therapy. After a median follow-up of about 39 months, patients infected with HPV had a risk of progression that was 72% lower and a risk of death that was 79% lower than those who were uninfected. The researchers suggested that it is possible that the HPV infection causes cancers that are biologically different from other cancers (83,84). Further research will strengthen the association between presence of HPV and head and neck cancer and HPV vaccination will become an integral part of the childhood vaccination program that may affect the incidence of HPV-related malignancies.

QUALITY OF LIFE

Quality of life (QOL) is defined as the perception of one's position in life within the context of the cultural and value systems in which one lives, and in relation to their goals, expectations, standards and concerns (85). QOL is multi-dimensional with both subjective and objective aspects. Thus QOL has been measured by taking its full dimensions into account, which include the physical, mental, emotional, social, and economical aspects of the patient's health. Surgical and organ preservation treatment have a significant impact on these patients' basic functions. The main physical problems are speech difficulties, dysphagia, xerostomia, pain, and fatigue. Anxiety, depression, uncertainty, and hopelessness are the most frequently reported psychological problems. These factors all affect QOL and may influence the rehabilitation outcome (86).

Since there is no significant advance in the overall survival of head and neck cancer patients, improvement in treatment outcome can be achieved in the patient's QOL. There is a complex relationship between treatment efficacy and treatment toxicity in oncology. Therefore, careful measurement and documentation of patient functional status and QOL have become a necessary component in outcome evaluation (87).

During the past two decades an increased awareness of the importance of evaluating QOL has evolved. This is reflected in the rise of broad-based assessment tools that measure the overall impact of disease and treatment on a specific individual (87). The most common QOL questionnaires in head and neck discipline include those of the European Organization for Research into the Treatment of Cancer (EORTC), the University of Washington, and the FACT (Functional Assessment of Cancer Therapy). These tools break down the comprehensive term of QOL into multiple practical and specific domains. In years to come, the QOL evaluating tools should be developed and modified specifically for the needs of the unique head and neck cancer population. Buckley (88) has stated that the QOL tools should be quick and easy to complete, relevant, reliable, and able to reflect changes over time. QOL outcomes are likely to be strong influences on multidisciplinary team decision-making in the future management of the head and neck cancer patient.

In order to interpret the head and neck QOL literature, it is important to understand the significance and impediments of QOL assessments in the head and neck patient population. Unfortunately, the QOL literature has many limitations, including small sample size, lack of prospective data, and poor study design. Nonetheless, important insights can be obtained by reviewing the current literature (89). All of these issues should be approached in the near future. Moreover, QOL outcome should be described in terms of clinical value to the patient. It has not yet been shown whether the QOL actually has practical benefit. This has to be proven in the next few years. Specific questionnaires for the head and neck cancer population should be developed and validated in order to address the unique difficulties the head and neck patients face. There is a need for a uniform and well-accepted QOL scale that addresses the unique challenges both the patients and the clinician face during and after treatment.

THE FUTURE OF HEAD AND NECK CANCER PRACTICE

New bio-technologies, laboratory tests, imaging techniques, and clinical tools will help to shape the future practice of the head and neck surgeon. Screening, disease detection, treatment planning, and disease management in head and neck patients in the near future will likely look very different from today's practice.

Screening and detection of head and neck cancers will involve a variety of different methods, aside from basic clinical examination. In the future, patients at high risk for head and neck cancer may be screened for specific tumor antigens found in their saliva or urine, allowing for early detection of disease. Autofluorescence may also be used as a screening tool to help identify new mucosal lesions in the upper aerodigestive tract and to monitor head and neck cancer patients at risk for developing a second primary. This will result in a more limited surgical procedure with better patient outcomes.

Treatment planning for head and neck patients will be significantly altered in the future. Biopsy specimens will be used not only for histopathology diagnosis but also to characterize the unique features of a tumor, based on its genetic profile. In the near future we should expect to individualize patient treatment based on the molecular signature of the tumor. Molecular analysis of the biopsy sample will enable the clinician to predict response rates to radiation as well as to chemotherapy agents. Based on the predicted response rates, a patient may be advised to consider organ preservation, or conversely may be advised to undergo surgery. Treatment approaches will be based not only on the anatomical location and extent of disease, but also on the biological characteristics of the tumor. Oncology is expected to have the largest gains from biomarkers over the next ten years. Development of personalized medicine for cancer is closely linked to biomarkers, which may serve as the basis for diagnosis, drug discovery, and monitoring of diseases.

Treatment planning will also be influenced by the viral profile of tumors and their subtypes. HPV 16 DNA was recently detected in the majority of oropharyngeal tumor specimens and it has been suggested that HPV infection may cause head and neck cancers that are biologically different from other cancers. In the future, we might treat HPV-negative cancer patients with a more aggressive approach. In addition, the HPV vaccine will become a standard for prevention.

Surgical disease management of head and neck cancer will also look different in the near future. With image-guided endoscopic surgery, surgeons will be able to conduct procedures that are minimally invasive and highly selective. Based on further developments of anatomical, metabolic, and molecular-based imaging modalities surgeons will be able to plan ablation margins while sparing vital anatomical structures, minimizing surgical time and postoperative morbidity. This will result in better organ function and minimal surgical scaring. Augmented reality provides navigational support by direct projection of segmented structures from preoperative images onto the patient. This will provide better integration of the patient-imaging interface and will result in a higher surgical precision and better patient outcomes.

Surgical disease management may be further enhanced by the use of robotic systems. Robotic assisted surgery will continue to expand and will offer a new era where physical location is no longer a limiting factor. Complete surgical procedures that were previously performed in a relatively few specialized medical centers will be available almost anywhere. Prior to surgery, the surgeon will be able to review previous imaging electronically and communicate with the patients via a web-based conference call. During the procedure, the surgeon will operate using a remote robotic housed mobile console with a binocular endoscope. The surgeon will be able to control the robotic arms from thousands of miles away and operate on a patient without being in the actual operating room. The set-up will create borderless surgical care, making the best surgical expertise available to anyone, anywhere. Increased use of robotics will affect surgical practice and improve institutional collaboration. On the other hand, there were always be a place for radical surgical procedures in cases of salvage surgery for advanced organ preservation failure, and in patients who present with an advanced head and neck tumor that is not amenable to other treatment options.

Significant advances will also be seen in patient head and neck reconstruction. Bony as well as soft tissue defects will be planed preoperatively based on the 3-D-radiographic imaging. This will enable reconstructive surgeons to benefit from tissue-engineering techniques and use engineered products, such as tissue-engineered bone that is identical in size and shape to the tissue and bone being replaced. Once the ablation is complete, tissue-engineered bone can be transferred to the defect site. The need for a donor site and the morbidity associated with it will be avoided. In addition, in some cases surgeons will be able to avoid the use of supporting titanium plating, by instead using biological glue, other adhesive material, or absorbable plating material. Soft tissue defects such as skin defects will be reconstructed by using epithelial autografts that are harvested and cultured in advance, prior to surgery. Vascularized tissue prepared in advance may be readily available and used to provide support, protection of vital structures, and volume to fill the tissue deficit after ablation. This may partially replace the use of free flap reconstruction.

Adjuvant therapy such as chemotherapy is associated with significant tissue toxicity and is usually not advocated for elderly patients. In coming years, the introduction of EGFR monoclonal antibodies, antiangiogenic (VEGF monoclonal antibodies), and other emerging drugs will play a major role in organ preservation treatment protocols and hopefully improve the patient outcomes without increasing toxicity.

Head and neck practice may change remarkably once a vaccination against cancer is developed. The use of vaccinations will serve as a fourth treatment arm after surgery, radiation, and chemotherapy. The focus of some cancer vaccines will be on treating new cancers rather than preventing new cases. The basic principle is that the unique surface antigens that neoplastic cells present on their surface are not present on normal surrounding tissue. The cancer vaccine approach to therapy is based on the notion that the immune system could possibly mount a rejection strength response against neoplastically transformed cells. This has been demonstrated in malignant melanomas where cytotoxic T-lymphocytes can be directed against tumor-associated antigens. Therefore, as part of the molecular analysis prior to definitive treatment, the biopsy specimen will be analyzed not only for histological diagnosis and genetic analysis as previously mentioned, but also for surface antigen expression.

Immunotherapy may greatly benefit patients with advanced disease, positive post surgical margins, and only a partial response to other treatment modalities. Immunotherapy may also be applied as preventive vaccines for carcinomas. Immunotherapy will include the use of recombinant tumor necrosis factor (TNF)-related apoptosis-inducing ligand (TRAIL). It is currently being developed as a cancer therapeutic since it selectively induces apoptosis in a variety of transformed cells, but not in most normal cells. Agonistic monoclonal antibodies (mAbs) specific for human death-inducing TRAIL receptors (DR4 or DR5) are also being actively pursued. These findings suggest that antibody-based therapies that cause tumor cell apoptosis and promote T cell memory or function may be effective in fighting cancer.

It is anticipated that scientific advances over the next few years will help to greatly improve outcomes for head and neck patients. Nevertheless, it is important to remember that there is a complex relationship between treatment efficacy and toxicity in oncology. Therefore careful measurement and documentation of patient functional status and QOL will become a necessary component of outcome evaluation. QOL questionnaires specific to head and neck cancer patients will become standard of care. They will be used to assess the quality of the treatment and care provided while providing direct feedback on the patients' functional outcome. Questionnaires will be completed before and after treatment and they will become an integral part of patient care. As always, multidisciplinary teams will continue to provide comprehensive and collaborative care.

CONCLUSION

The treatment of patients with head and neck cancer continues to be both challenging, and at times frustrating, for those involved in the endeavour. New modalities for investigation and treatment of these patients will continue to improve outcomes. Each new technology must undergo rigorous testing to define its particular role in care prior to implementation. As new technology is created and implemented, it is worthwhile to remember that much head and neck cancer is preventable and that the most effective interventions may be at the level of education, prevention, and surveillance of early disease.

Once diagnosed, multiple resources are needed to allow patients to go through treatment and recovery, which can last months and often years. Those resources include nutritionists, speech and swallow therapists, social workers, psychiatrists, and dentists. It is of paramount importance that these patients have access to a multi-disciplinary clinic that can best manage the problems that will invariably arise when treatment is started.

REFERENCES

1. Anon JB. Computer aided endoscopic sinus surgery. Laryngoscope 1998; 108: 949–61.
2. Thomas RF, Monacci WT, Mair EA. Endoscopic image-guided transethmoid pituitary surgery. Otolaryngol Head Neck Surg 2002; 127: 409–16.
3. Kataoka H, Kitano H, Takeuchi E et al. Total video endoscopic thyroidectomy via the anterior chest approach using the cervical region-lifting method. Biomed Pharmacother 2002; 56(Suppl 1): 68s–71s.
4. Assalia A, Inabnet WB. Endoscopic parathyroidectomy. Otolaryngol Clin North Am 2004; 37: 871–86, xi.
5. Luke PP, Knudsen BEBE, Nguan CYCY et al. Robot-assisted laparoscopic renal artery aneurysm reconstruction. J Vasc Surg 2006; 44: 651–3.
6. Tabata MM, Cohn LHLH. Minimally invasive mitral valve repair with and without robotic technology in the elderly. Am J Geriatr Cardiol 2006; 15: 306–10.
7. Tsirbas A, Dutson E, Mango C. Robotic Ocular Surgery. Br J Ophthalmol 2006.
8. Steinhart H, Bumm K, Wurm J, Vogele M, Iro H. Surgical application of a new robotic system for paranasal sinus surgery. Ann Otol Rhinol Laryngol 2004; 113: 303–9.
9. Menon M, Shrivastava A, Tewari A. Laparoscopic radical prostatectomy: conventional and robotic. Urology 2005; 66(5 Suppl): 101–4.
10. Solares CA, Strome MM. Transoral robot-assisted CO_2 laser supraglottic laryngectomy: experimental and clinical data. The Laryngoscope 2007; 117: 817–20.
11. Weinstein GS, O'Malley BW Jr, Snyder W et al. Transoral robotic surgery: supraglottic partial laryngectomy. Ann Otol Rhinol Laryngol 2007; 116: 19–23.
12. O'Malley BW Jr, Weinstein GS, Snyder W et al. Transoral robotic surgery (TORS) for base of tongue neoplasms. Laryngoscope 2006; 116: 1465–72.
13. Woolford T, Toriumi D. Distraction osteogenesis and bone morphogenetic protein in mandibular reconstruction. In: Komisar A, ed. Mandibular reconstruction. New York: Thieme, 1997.
14. Snyder CC, Levine GA, Swanson HM et al. Mandibular lengthening by gradual distraction. Preliminary report. Plast Reconstr Surg 1973; 51: 506–8.
15. Urist M. Bone formation by osteoinduction. Science 1965; 150: 893.
16. Moxham JJP, Kibblewhite DDJ, Dvorak MM et al. TGF-beta 1 forms functionally normal bone in a segmental sheep tibial diaphyseal defect. J Otolaryngol 1996; 25: 388–92.
17. Jupiter JB, Winters S, Sigman S et al. Repair of five distal radius fractures with an investigational cancellous bone cement: a preliminary report. J Orthop Trauma 1997; 11: 110–16.
18. Kopylov P, Jonsson K, Thorngren KG et al. Injectable calcium phosphate in the treatment of distal radial fractures. J Hand Surg [Br] 1996; 21: 768–71.
19. Constantz BR, Ison IC, Fulmer MT et al. Skeletal repair by in situ formation of the mineral phase of bone. Science 1995; 267: 1796–9.
20. Costantino PD, Friedman CD. Synthetic bone graft substitutes. Otolaryngol Clin North Am 1994; 27: 1037–74.
21. Palazzi MM, Tomatis SS, Orlandi EE et al. Effects of treatment intensification on acute local toxicity during radiotherapy for head and neck cancer: prospective observational study validating CTCAE, version 3.0, scoring system. Int J Radiat Oncol Biol Phys 2008; 70: 330–7.
22. Horiot JJC, Bontemps PP, van den Bogaert WW et al. Accelerated fractionation (AF) compared to conventional fractionation (CF) improves locoregional control in the radiotherapy of advanced head and neck cancers: results of the EORTC 22851 randomized trial. Radiother Oncol 1997; 44: 111–21.
23. Bourhis J, Overgaard J, Audry H et al. Hyperfractionated or accelerated radiotherapy in head and neck cancer: a meta-analysis. Lancet 2006; 368: 843–54.
24. Lee N, Puri DR, Blanco AI et al. Intensity-modulated radiation therapy in head and neck cancers: an update. Head Neck 2007; 29: 387–400.
25. Feng M, Eisbruch A. Future issues in highly conformal radiotherapy for head and neck cancer. J Clin Oncol 2007; 25: 1009–13.

26. Slovin SF. Prostate-specific membrane antigen vaccines: naked DNA and protein approaches. Clin Prostate Cancer 2005; 4: 118–23.

27. Bernier JJ, Domenge CC, Ozsahin MM et al. Postoperative irradiation with or without concomitant chemotherapy for locally advanced head and neck cancer. N Engl J Med 2004; 350: 1945–52.

28. Cooper JS, Pajak TF, Forastiere AA et al. Postoperative concurrent radiotherapy and chemotherapy for high-risk squamous-cell carcinoma of the head and neck. N Engl J Med 2004; 350: 1937–44.

29. Induction chemotherapy plus radiation compared with surgery plus radiation in patients with advanced laryngeal cancer. The Department of Veterans Affairs Laryngeal Cancer Study Group. N Engl J Med 1991; 324: 1685–90.

30. Wolf GT, Forastiere A, Ang K et al. Workshop report: organ preservation strategies in advanced head and neck cancer—current status and future directions. Head Neck 1999; 21: 689–93.

31. Forastiere AA, Goepfert H, Maor M et al. Concurrent chemotherapy and radiotherapy for organ preservation in advanced laryngeal cancer. N Engl J Med 2003; 349: 2091–8.

32. Weber RS, Berkey BA, Forastiere A et al. Outcome of salvage total laryngectomy following organ preservation therapy: the Radiation Therapy Oncology Group trial 91-11. Arch Otolaryngol Head Neck Surg 2003; 129: 44–9.

33. Sassler AM, Esclamado RM, Wolf GT. Surgery after organ preservation therapy. Analysis of wound complications. Arch Otolaryngol Head Neck Surg 1995; 121: 162–5.

34. Posner MR, Hershock DM, Blajman CR et al. Cisplatin and fluorouracil alone or with docetaxel in head and neck cancer. N Engl J Med 2007; 357: 1705–15.

35. Rieger JM, Zalmanowitz JG, Wolfaardt JF. Functional outcomes after organ preservation treatment in head and neck cancer: a critical review of the literature. Int J Oral Maxillofac Surg 2006; 35: 581–7.

36. Garden AS, Asper JA, Morrison WH et al. Is concurrent chemoradiation the treatment of choice for all patients with Stage III or IV head and neck carcinoma? Cancer 2004; 100: 1171–8.

37. Hiraishi Y, Wada T, Nakatani K et al. Immunohistochemical expression of EGFR and p-EGFR in oral squamous cell carcinomas. Pathol Oncol Res 2006; 12: 87–91.

38. Ritter CA, Arteaga CL. The epidermal growth factor receptor-tyrosine kinase: a promising therapeutic target in solid tumors. Semin Oncol 2003; 30(1 Suppl 1): 3–11.

39. Mendelsohn J. Blockade of receptors for growth factors: an anticancer therapy—the fourth annual Joseph H Burchenal American Association of Cancer Research Clinical Research Award Lecture. Clin Cancer Res 2000; 6: 747–53.

40. Ciardiello F, Caputo R, Bianco R et al. Antitumor effect and potentiation of cytotoxic drugs activity in human cancer cells by ZD-1839 (Iressa), an epidermal growth factor receptor-selective tyrosine kinase inhibitor. Clin Cancer Res 2000; 6: 2053–63.

41. Maddineni SB, Sangar VK, Hendry JH et al. Differential radiosensitisation by ZD1839 (Iressa), a highly selective epidermal growth factor receptor tyrosine kinase inhibitor in two related bladder cancer cell lines. Br J Cancer 2005; 92: 125–30.

42. Bonner JA, Harari PM, Giralt J et al. Radiotherapy plus cetuximab for squamous-cell carcinoma of the head and neck. N Engl J Med 2006; 354: 567–78.

43. Folkman J, Merler E, Abernathy C et al. Isolation of a tumor factor responsible for angiogenesis. J Exp Med 1971; 133: 275–88.

44. Petruzzelli GJ. Tumor angiogenesis. Head Neck 1996; 18: 283–91.

45. Fujita K, Sano D, Kimura M et al. Anti-tumor effects of bevacizumab in combination with paclitaxel on head and neck squamous cell carcinoma. Oncol Rep 2007; 18: 47–51.

46. Wolbach SB, Howe PR. Nutrition Classics. The Journal of Experimental Medicine 42: 753–777, 1925. Tissue changes following deprivation of fat-soluble A vitamin. S. Burt Wolbach and Percy R. Howe. Nutr Rev 1978; 36: 16–9. http://www.ncbi.nlm.nih.gov/pubmed/342996?dopt=Citation

47. Hong WK, Endicott J, Itri LM et al. 13-cis-retinoic acid in the treatment of oral leukoplakia. N Engl J Med 1986; 315: 1501–5.

48. Costa A, Formelli F, Chiesa F et al. Prospects of chemoprevention of human cancers with the synthetic retinoid fenretinide. Cancer Res 1994; 54(7 Suppl): 2032s–7s.

49. Hong WK, Lippman SM, Itri LM et al. Prevention of second primary tumors with isotretinoin in squamous-cell carcinoma of the head and neck. N Engl J Med 1990; 323: 795–801.

50. McCaul JA, Gordon KE, Clark LJ et al. Telomerase inhibition and the future management of head-and-neck cancer. Lancet Oncol 2002; 3: 280–8.

51. Chao KS, Ozyigit G, Thorsdad WL. Toxicity profile of intensity-modulated radiation therapy for head and neck carcinoma and potential role of amifostine. Semin Oncol 2003; 30(6 Suppl 18): 101–8.

52. Bardet E, Martin L, Calais G et al. Preliminary data of the GORTEC 2000–02 phase III trial comparing intravenous and subcutaneous administration of amifostine for head and neck tumors treated by external radiotherapy. Semin Oncol 2002; 29(6 Suppl 19): 57–60.

53. Hofmeister CC, Stiff PJ. Mucosal protection by cytokines. Curr Hematol Rep 2005; 4: 446–53.

54. Rhee JC, Khuri FR, Shin DM. Emerging drugs for head and neck cancer. Expert Opin Emerg Drugs 2004; 9: 91–104.

55. Nikitakis NG, Siavash H, Sauk JJ. Targeting the STAT pathway in head and neck cancer: recent advances and future prospects. Curr Cancer Drug Targets 2004; 4: 637–51.

56. Zimmerman RRD. Is there a role for diffusion-weighted imaging in patients with brain tumors or is the "bloom off the rose"? Am J Neuroradiol 2001; 22: 1013–14.

57. Coenen VA, Krings T, Weidemann J et al. Sequential visualization of brain and fiber tract deformation during intracranial surgery with three-dimensional ultrasound: an approach to evaluate the effect of brain shift. Neurosurgery 2005; 56(1 Suppl): 133–141; discussion 133–41.

58. Wise SK, DelGaudio JM. Computer-aided surgery of the paranasal sinuses and skull base. Expert Rev Med Devices 2005; 2: 395–408.

59. Nijmeh AD, Goodger NM, Hawkes D et al. Image-guided navigation in oral and maxillofacial surgery. Br J Oral Maxillofac Surg 2005; 43: 294–302.

60. Siewerdsen JH, Moseley DJ, Burch S et al. Volume CT with a flat-panel detector on a mobile, isocentric C-arm: preclinical investigation in guidance of minimally invasive surgery. Med Phys 2005; 32: 241–54.

61. Rafferty MA, Siewerdsen JH, Chan Y et al. Intraoperative cone-beam CT for guidance of temporal bone surgery. Otolaryngol Head Neck Surg 2006; 134: 801–8.

62. Rafferty MA, Siewerdsen JH, Chan Y et al. Investigation of C-arm cone-beam CT-guided surgery of the frontal recess. Laryngoscope 2005; 115: 2138–43.

63. Roessler K, Ungersboeck K, Czech T et al. Contour-guided brain tumor surgery using a stereotactic navigating microscope. Stereotact Funct Neurosurg 1997; 68: 33–8.

64. Roessler K, Ungersboeck K, Aichholzer M et al. Frameless stereotactic lesion contour-guided surgery using a computer-navigated microscope. Surg Neurol. 1998; 49: 282–8. PMID: 9508116.

65. Wagner A, Ploder O, Enislidis G et al. Virtual image guided navigation in tumor surgery—technical innovation. J Craniomaxillofac Surg 1995; 23: 217–13.

66. Quon A, Fischbein NJ, McDougall IR et al. Clinical role of ^{18}F-FDG PET/CT in the management of squamous cell carcinoma of the head and neck and thyroid carcinoma. J Nucl Med 2007; 48(Suppl 1): 58S–67S.

67. Schoder H, Yeung HW. Positron emission imaging of head and neck cancer, including thyroid carcinoma. Semin Nucl Med 2004; 34: 180–97.

68. Goerres GW, Schmid DT, Gratz KW et al. Impact of whole body positron emission tomography on initial staging and therapy in patients with squamous cell carcinoma of the oral cavity. Oral Oncol 2003; 39: 547–51.

69. Schmid DT, Stoeckli SJ, Bandhauer F et al. Impact of positron emission tomography on the initial staging and therapy in locoregional advanced squamous cell carcinoma of the head and neck. Laryngoscope 2003; 113: 888–91.

70. Ryan WR, Fee WE Jr, Le QT et al. Positron-emission tomography for surveillance of head and neck cancer. Laryngoscope 2005; 115: 645–50.

71. Choi JY, Lee KS, Kim HJ et al. Focal thyroid lesions incidentally identified by integrated ^{18}F-FDG PET/CT: clinical significance and improved characterization. J Nucl Med 2006; 47: 609–15.

72. Tsai T, Chen HM, Wang CY et al. In vivo autofluorescence spectroscopy of oral premalignant and malignant lesions: distortion of fluorescence intensity by submucous fibrosis. Lasers Surg Med 2003; 33: 40–7.

73. Kulapaditharom B, Boonkitticharoen V. Laser-induced fluorescence imaging in localization of head and neck cancers. Ann Otol Rhinol Laryngol 1998; 107: 241–6.

74. Gillenwater A, Jacob R, Ganeshappa R et al. Noninvasive diagnosis of oral neoplasia based on fluorescence spectroscopy and native tissue autofluorescence. Arch Otolaryngol Head Neck Surg 1998; 124: 1251–8.

75. Nussenbaum B, Teknos TN, Chepeha DB. Tissue engineering: the current status of this futuristic modality in head neck reconstruction. Curr Opin Otolaryngol Head Neck Surg 2004; 12: 311–15.

76. Cheng MH, Brey EM, Ulusal BG et al. Mandible augmentation for osseointegrated implants using tissue engineering strategies. Plast Reconstr Surg 2006; 118: 1e–4e.

77. Kim DM, Schwerdtner O, Schmidt-Westhausen AM et al. Cultured epithelial autografts in the treatment of facial skin defects: clinical outcome. J Oral Maxillofac Surg 2007; 65: 439–43.

78. Slaughter DP, Southwick HW, Smejkal W. Field cancerization in oral stratified squamous epithelium; clinical implications of multicentric origin. Cancer 1953; 6: 963–8.

79. Mackay JJ, Crofton JJ. Tobacco and the developing world. Br Med Bull 1996; 52: 206–21.

80. Tobacco use and usual source of cigarettes among high school students--United States, 1995. Office on Smoking and Health. J Sch Health 1996; 66: 222–4.

81. Rigotti NA, DiFranza JR, Chang Y et al. The effect of enforcing tobacco-sales laws on adolescents' access to tobacco and smoking behavior. N Engl J Med 1997; 337: 1044–51.

82. D'Souza G, Kreimer AR, Viscidi R et al. Case-control study of human papillomavirus and oropharyngeal cancer. N Engl J Med 2007; 356: 1944–56.

83. Fakhry C, Westra WH, Li S et al. Improved survival of patients with human papillomavirus-positive head and neck squamous cell carcinoma in a prospective clinical trial. J Natl Cancer Inst 2008; 100: 261–9.

84. Fakhry C, Westra WH, Sigui Li et al. Prognostic significance of human papillomavirus (HPV) tumor status for patients with head and neck squamous cell carcinoma (HNSCC) in a prospective, multicenter phase II clinical trial. J Clin Oncol 2007; 25: 18s.

85. Study protocol for the World Health Organization project to develop a Quality of Life assessment instrument (WHOQOL). Qual Life Res 1993; 2: 153–9.

86. Ledeboer QC, Velden LA, Boer MF et al. Physical and psychosocial correlates of head and neck cancer: an update of the literature and challenges for the future (1996–2003). Clin Otolaryngol 2005; 30: 303–9.

87. Cella DF, Tulsky DS, Gray G et al. The Functional Assessment of Cancer Therapy scale: development and validation of the general measure. J Clin Oncol 1993; 11: 570–9.

88. Buckley JJG. The future of head and neck surgery. J Laryngol Otol 2000; 114: 327–30.

89. Murphy BA, Ridner S, Wells N et al. Quality of life research in head and neck cancer: a review of the current state of the science. Crit Rev Oncol Hematol 2007; 62: 251–67.

Index

Note: Page numbers in *italics* indicate figures or tables.